Smith and Aitkenhead's Textbook of Anaesthesia

Content Strategist: *Laurence Hunter*
Content Development Specialist: *Fiona Conn/Veronika Watkins*
Content Coordinator: *Susan Jansons*
Project Manager: *Janish Ashwin Paul*
Design: *Patrick Ferguson*
Illustration Manager: *Paula Catalano*
Marketing Manager: *Deborah Watkins*

Smith and Aitkenhead's Textbook of Anaesthesia

Seventh Edition

Edited by

Jonathan Thompson
Honorary Professor and Consultant in Anaesthesia & Critical Care
University of Leicester and University Hospitals of Leicester NHS Trust
Leicester, UK

Iain Moppett
Professor of Anaesthesia & Perioperative Medicine | Honorary Consultant Anaesthetist
Anaesthesia and Critical Care Section, Division of Clinical Neuroscience,
University of Nottingham
Nottingham, UK

Matthew Wiles
Consultant
Department of Anaesthesia, Sheffield Teaching Hospitals NHS Foundation Trust,
Sheffield, UK

For additional online content visit ExpertConsult.com

ELSEVIER   Edinburgh   London   New York   Oxford   Philadelphia   St Louis   Sydney   2019

First edition 1985
Second edition 1990
Third edition 1996
Fourth edition 2001
Fifth edition 2007
Sixth edition 2013
Seventh edition 2019

Notices

Practitioners and researchers must always rely on their own experience and knowledge in evaluating and using any information, methods, compounds or experiments described herein. Because of rapid advances in the medical sciences, in particular, independent verification of diagnoses and drug dosages should be made. To the fullest extent of the law, no responsibility is assumed by Elsevier, authors, editors or contributors for any injury and/or damage to persons or property as a matter of products liability, negligence or otherwise, or from any use or operation of any methods, products, instructions, or ideas contained in the material herein.

ISBN: 978-0-7020-7500-1
International ISBN: 978-0-7020-7499-8

Printed in Poland

Last digit is the print number: 9   8   7   6   5   4   3   2

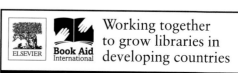

Working together
to grow libraries in
developing countries

www.elsevier.com • www.bookaid.org

Contents

v

Contents

vi

List of Contributors

The editors would like to acknowledge and offer grateful thanks to the authors, without whom this new edition would not have been possible.

John C Andrzejowski, FRCA, FFICM
Consultant Anaesthetist, Sheffield Teaching Hospitals NHS Foundation Trust, Sheffield, UK

Joseph E Arrowsmith, FRCP, FRCA, FFICM
Consultant in Cardiothoracic Anaesthesia, Papworth Hospital, Cambridge, UK

Mark Barley, MRCP, FRCA
Consultant Anaesthetist, Nottingham University Hospitals NHS Trust, Nottingham, UK

Jonathan Barratt, PhD, FRCP
Professor, Department of Infection, Immunity & Inflammation, University of Leicester, Honorary Consultant, Nephrologist, University Hospitals of Leicester NHS Trust, Leicester, UK

Nigel M Bedforth, FRCA
Consultant Anaesthetist and Honorary Associate Professor, Nottingham University Hospitals NHS Trust and University of Nottingham, UK

Martin Beed, FRCA, FFICM, DM
Consultant in Intensive Care Medicine & Anaesthesia, Nottingham University Hospitals, Hucknall Road, Nottingham; and Honorary Assistant Professor, Nottingham University Hospitals NHS Trust and University of Nottingham, UK

Ricky Bell, MRCP, FFICM
Consultant in Intensive Care Medicine, University Hospitals of Leicester NHS Trust, Leicester, UK

David Bogod, LLM
Consultant, Department of Anaesthetics, Nottingham University Hospitals NHS Trust, Nottingham, UK

Emily Bonner, FRCA
Consultant Anaesthetist, Freeman Hospital, Newcastle upon Tyne, UK

Christopher Bouch, MB, ChB, FRCA, EDICM, FFICM
Consultant in Anaesthesia & Critical Care Medicine, University Hospitals of Leicester NHS Trust, UK

Matthew Charlton, MBChB, FRCA, FFICM
Honorary Clinical Lecturer in Anaesthesia and Intensive Care Medicine, University of Leicester and University Hospitals of Leicester NHS Trust, Leicester, UK

Nicholas J Chesshire
Consultant Anaesthetist, Royal Derby Hospital, Derby, UK

Alfred Chua, FANZCA
Senior VMO Anaesthetist, Royal Prince Alfred Hospital, Sydney, Australia

Lesley Colvin, PhD, FRCA, FFPRMCA, FRCP(Edin)
Professor of Pain Medicine/Honorary Consultant in Anaesthesia & Pain Medicine, University of Dundee and Ninewells Hospital, Dundee, UK

Tim Cook, BA (Cantab.), FRCA, FFICM
Consultant in Anaesthesia and Intensive Care Medicine, Royal United Hospitals Bath NHS Foundation Trust, Bath, UK

Jugdeep Kaur Dhesi, PhD, FRCP
Ageing and Health, Guy's and St Thomas' NHS Trust, London, UK

Damian Doyle, FRCA
Consultant Anaesthetist, Sheffield Teaching Hospitals Trust, Sheffield, UK

Jake Drinkwater
Sheffield Teaching Hospital NHS Foundation Trust, Sheffield, UK

Satya Francis
Consultant Anaesthetist and Honorary Senior Lecturer, University Hospitals of Leicester NHS Trust, Leicester, UK

Sally Hancock, MB, ChB, FRCA
Department of Anaesthesia, Nottingham University Hospitals NHS Trust, Nottingham, UK

Jonathan G Hardman, BMedSci (Hons), BM, BS, EWC, FRCA, FANZCA, DM
Professor and Consultant Anaesthetist, Anaesthesia and Critical Care, Division of Clinical Neuroscience, School of Medicine, University of Nottingham, Nottingham, UK

List of Contributors

Lorraine Harrington, MBChB, Bsc (Immunology), MRCP, FRCA, FFPMRCA
Consultant in Anaesthesia and Pain Medicine, Department of Anaesthetics and Pain Medicine, St John's Hospital, Livingston, UK

Daniel John Roberton Harvey, BMBS, BMedSci, MRCP, FRCA, DICM, FFICM
Critical Care, Nottingham University Hospitals NHS Trust, Nottingham; Honorary Assistant Professor of Intensive Care, Department of Anaesthesia and Intensive Care, University of Nottingham, Nottingham, UK

Christopher Hebbes, MBChB, BSc, MMedSci, FRCA, FFICM
Clinical Lecturer and Specialist Registrar, Department of Cardiovascular Sciences, University of Leicester, Leicester, UK

David W Hewson, BSc (Hons), PGCert, FHEA, MBBS, FRCA
Specialty Registrar and Clinical Assistant Professor, Anaesthesia and Critical Care, Division of Clinical Neuroscience, School of Medicine, University of Nottingham, Nottingham, UK

Anil Hormis, MBChB, FCARCSI, AFICM
Consultant in Anaesthesia and Critical Care Medicine, The Rotherham NHS Foundation Trust, Rotherham, UK

Simon Howell, MA(Cantab), MB BS, MRCP(UK), FRCA, MSc, MD
Leeds Institute of Biomedical and Clinical Sciences, University of Leeds, Leeds, UK

Jennifer M Hunter, MBE, MB, ChB, PhD, FRCA, FCARCSI (Hon)
Emeritus Professor of Anaesthesia, University of Liverpool, UK

James Ip, BSc, MBBS, MA, FRCA
Fellow in Anaesthesia, Anaesthetics, Great Ormond Street Hospital, London, UK

David Kirkbride, BMedSci (Hons), BMBS, FRCA
Consultant Anaesthetist, Department of Anaesthesia, Leicester Royal Infirmary, Leicester, UK

Andrew A Klein, MBBS, FRCA, FFICM
Consultant in Cardiothoracic Anaesthesia, Papworth Hospital, Cambridge, UK

Chandra M Kumar, MBBS, DA, FFARCSI, FRCA, EDRA
Senior Consultant in Anaesthesia and Professor, Newcastle University, Department of Anaesthesia, Khoo Teck Puat Hospital, Yishun, Singapore

Paramesh Kumara, MBCHB, FRCA
Anaesthetic Department, Leeds Teaching Hospital NHS Trust, Leeds, UK

Dave Lambert, BSc (Hons), PhD, SFHEA, FRCA
Professor of Anaesthetic Pharmacology, Department of Cardiovascular Sciences, University of Leicester, Leicester, UK

Andrew Lumb, MB, BS, FRCA
Consultant Anaesthetist, Department of Anaesthesia, St James's University Hospital, Leeds, UK

Patrick Magee, PhD, FRCA
Consultant Anaesthetist, Circle Hospital, Peasedown-St-John, Bath, UK

Alexa Mannings, BMedSci, BMBS, MMedSci(Clin Ed), FRCA
Consultant Anaesthetist, Sheffield Teaching Hospitals NHS Foundation Trust, Sheffield, UK

Kate McCombe, MBBS, MRCP, FRCA, MA
Anaesthesia, Mediclinic City Hospital, Dubai, UAE

Iain Moppett, MB, BChir MA, MRCP, FRCA, DM
Professor of Anaesthesia & Perioperative Medicine, Honorary Consultant Anaesthetist, Anaesthesia and Critical Care Section, Division of Clinical Neuroscience, University of Nottingham, Nottingham, UK

David Mulvey, BSc, MBBS, MD, FRCA
Consultant Anaesthetist, Department of Anaesthesia and Critical Care, Royal Derby Hospital, Derby, UK

Mary C Mushambi, MBChB, FRCA, LLM
Consultant Anaesthetist and Honorary Senior Lecturer, Department of Anaesthetics, University Hospitals of Leicester, Leicester, UK

Michael Nathanson, MB, BS, MRCP, FRCA
Consultant Neuroanaesthetist, Nottingham University Hospitals NHS Trust, Queens Medical Centre, Nottingham, UK

Alexander Ng, MB ChB, MD, FRCA, FFICM
Consultant Anaesthetist, Royal Wolverhampton Hospital NHS Trust, Wolverhampton, UK

Jerry P Nolan, FRCA, FFICM, FRCP, FRCEM
Honorary Professor of Resuscitation Medicine, School of Health Sciences, University of Bristol, Bristol, UK

Mary O'Regan MBBS, DA, FRCA
Consultant Anaesthetist, Department of Anaesthesia & Critical Care, Hywel Dda University Health Board, Haverfordwest, West Wales, UK

Arani Pillai, MBBS, Bsc (Hons), MRCP, FRCA
Consultant Anaesthetist, Nottingham University Hospitals NHS Trust, Nottingham, UK

Catherine L Riley, MBBS, MA, MRCP, FRCA
Specialty Registrar in Anaesthesia, Sheffield Teaching Hospitals NHS Foundation Trust, Sheffield, UK

Simon W M Scott, MA, BM, BCh, FRCA, FFICM
Consultant in Anaesthesia and Critical Care, Department of Anaesthesia and Critical Care, University Hospitals of Leicester NHS Trust, Leicester, UK

Ian Shaw, MB, ChB, FRCA
Consultant Anaesthetist, The
Department of Anaesthetics, Sheffield
Teaching Hospital NHS Foundation Trust,
Sheffield, UK

Martin Shields, MD, FCAI, FRCA
Department of Anaesthetics, Royal
Victoria Hospital, Belfast, UK

Chris Snowden, FRCA,
BMedSCi (Hons), MD
Consultant Anaesthetist and Hon. Senior
Lecturer, Freeman Hospital, Newcastle
Hospitals NHS Trust and University of
Newcastle upon Tyne, Newcastle upon
Tyne, UK

Nguk Hoon Tan, MB BS,
FRCA, FFICM
Consultant in Cardiothoracic
Anaesthesia, University College of Wales
School of Medicine, Cardiff, UK

Emma Temple, MD
Fellow in Neuroanaesthesia, Department
of Anaesthesia, Sheffield Teaching
Hospitals NHS Foundation Trust,
Sheffield, UK

Mark Thomas, BSc, MBBChir, FRCA
Consultant Paediatric Anaesthetist,
Anaesthesia, Great Ormond St Hospital,
London, UK

Jonathan Thompson, MB, ChB,
BSc (Hons), MD, FRCA, FFICM
Professor of Anaesthesia & Critical Care,
University of Leicester and University
Hospitals of Leicester NHS Trust,
Leicester, UK

Rachel Tibble, MB, ChB, FRCA
Anaesthetics Department, Royal Derby
Hospital, Derby, UK

Pamela Wake, BMedSci, BM,
BS, FRCA
Consultant Anaesthetist, Nottingham
University Hospitals, Nottingham, UK

Isabeau Walker, BSc, MB
BChir, FRCA
Consultant Anaesthetist, Anaesthetics,
Great Ormond Street Hospital, London;
Honorary Senior Lecturer, UCL Great
Ormond Street Institute of Child Health,
London, UK

Cameron Weir, BSc (Hons), MBChB,
FRCA, PhD
Consultant Anaesthetist & Honorary
Senior Lecturer, Institute of Academic
Anaesthesia, Ninewells Hospital &
Medical School, Dundee, UK

Zoe Whitman, MB, ChB,
FRCA, FFICM
Specialty Registrar, University Hospitals
of Leicester NHS Trust, Leicester, UK

Matthew Wiles, MMedSci(Clin Ed),
MRCP, FRCA, FFICM
Consultant, Department of Anaesthesia,
Sheffield Teaching Hospitals NHS
Foundation Trust, Sheffield, UK

Gareth Williams, MB BS,
FRCA, FFICM
Adult Intensive Care Unit, Leicester
Royal Infirmary, Leicester, UK

Jonathan Wilson, BSc, MB, ChB,
FRCA
Dept of Anaesthetics, York Teaching
Hospitals NHS Foundation Trust,
York, UK

Hakeem Yusuff, MBBS, MRCP,
FRCA, FFICM
Consultant in Cardiothoracic
Anaesthesia, Intensive Care Medicine
and ECMO, Glenfield Hospital,
Leicester, UK

Acknowledgements

We are extremely grateful to our chapter authors for their commitment and goodwill; they have given their time and energies to the seventh edition in addition to their full-time clinical and academic roles.

We would also like to thank the authors from the sixth and earlier editions whose work has provided the basis for some of the revised chapters: Martin Beed, Andrew Bodenham, Margaret Bone, Beverly Collett, David Coventry, Melanie Davies, Charles Deakin, John Deloughry, Eric de Melo, David Duthie, Lorna Eyre, David Fell, Simon Flood, Richard Griffiths, Tim Hales, Jeremy Langton, Ravi Mahajan, Graeme Mcleod, Susan Nimmo, Graeme Nimmo, Nick Reynolds, Justiaan Swanevelder, Elaine Tighe, and Sean Williamson.

We would also like to thank Veronika Watkins and all those at Elsevier who have made the seventh edition of *Smith and Aitkenhead's Textbook of Anaesthesia* possible. Finally, we are indebted to Graham Smith and Alan Aitkenhead for their professional guidance and support over many years.

Jonathan Thompson, Leicester
Iain Moppett, Nottingham
Matthew Wiles, Sheffield
2019

Preface

First published as the *Textbook of Anaesthesia* in 1985 as a core text for novice and practice anaesthetists, *Smith and Aitkenhead's Textbook of Anaesthesia* is now in its seventh edition. Previous editions have enjoyed an excellent reputation worldwide because of their inclusion of the sciences underpinning practice in anaesthesia, critical care and pain management together with details of clinical anaesthesia and perioperative care. In combining these aspects, anaesthetists new to the specialty have found the textbook useful particularly during the first few years of their training as well as when preparing for professional examinations. It has also been a very useful day-to-day reference for allied professionals such as operating department practitioners and physician assistants who need an understanding of clinical practice in anaesthesia and related specialties.

Our aim in producing the seventh edition has remained to equip the reader with the basic knowledge and practical considerations required to administer anaesthesia and perioperative care for a whole range of surgical conditions in patients with all common medical comorbidities. Reflecting the expanding role of anaesthesia beyond the operating theatre, we have also included essential material related to safety and quality assurance, consent, resuscitation, intensive care medicine, prehospital care and chronic pain management.

The sixth edition involved a major revision, including seven new chapters and almost half of the chapter authors were new. In preparing this seventh edition we have included 30 new contributors, replacing those authors who have retired from clinical practice, to provide a new perspective or to contribute new chapters. The text has been thoroughly revised, updated and reorganised. Four new chapters have been added, both to reflect the UK postgraduate anaesthetic examination syllabus and changes in clinical practice. For clarity we have made extensive use of new line drawings and diagrams and, for the first time, many of these are available in colour. We have also restructured the book into sections: Basic Sciences; Physics and Apparatus; Fundamentals of Anaesthesia and Perioperative Medicine; and Clinical Anaesthesia. The newly included chapters are: Anaesthesia in the older patient; Anaesthesia in resource-poor areas; Management of critical incidents; and Data, statistics and clinical trials. Previous chapters restricted to cardiovascular and respiratory pharmacology, as well as those on analgesics and drugs acting on the kidney, have been completely revised to incorporate the relevant physiology. Airway equipment and management are now included in a single chapter. The chapter on critical incidents is deliberately different in style and is intended to be a useful *aide-memoire* for the emergency situation in clinical practice. Chapters have been extensively cross-referenced to aid the reader and avoid repetition so we have been able to include substantially more information without increasing the overall size of the book.

At the outset we decided to map the content of each chapter to much of the syllabus of the primary FRCA examination with reference links in the electronic version of the book. We have also provided specimen questions and answers with each chapter, available in the electronic version, and linked to the relevant part of each chapter. These are new features to aid candidates or their teachers involved in preparing for the examinations.

A review of the sixth edition stated that *'Smith and Aitkenhead's Textbook of Anaesthesia has become the book of choice for the trainee anaesthetist and is essential reading for candidates for the Fellowship of the Royal College of Anaesthetists and similar examinations. It is also a highly trusted, practical guide for all anaesthetists and other healthcare professionals involved in the perioperative period.'* We hope that the seventh edition will be equally useful.

Jonathan Thompson, Leicester
Iain Moppett, Nottingham
Matthew Wiles, Sheffield
2019

Section | 1 |

Basic sciences

Chapter | 1 |

General principles of pharmacology

Dave Lambert, Christopher Hebbes

Basic principles

A drug is a molecule or particle that produces a therapeutic effect by modifying how a biological system responds to a physical or chemical stimulus. This effect can occur locally at the site of administration or after absorption and delivery to a more distant site of action through carriers or mass transit. Most drugs undergo passive or active transport across membranes as part of this process. Drugs may be organic or inorganic and of peptide or non-peptide origin. Organic molecules have a carbon skeleton, with functional classification dependent on the associated functional groups (giving rise to compounds such as esters and amines). Inorganic molecules arise from non–carbon-based structures. Examples of inorganic substances used as drugs include salts of lithium and magnesium. Chemical structure and other characteristics influence the effects of drugs on the body (pharmacodynamics) and the handling of the drug by the body (pharmacokinetics).

The activity of a drug is determined by its ability to interact with its target; these interactions may be selective or non-selective. The former describes interaction with a single type of receptor (e.g. atenolol is cardioselective as it has greater effects on the β_1 myocardial adrenoceptors than the β_2 bronchial adrenoceptors). Selective drug interactions with receptors and enzymes occur because a specific region on the ligand fits a complementary region on the effector molecule. This lock and key mechanism is critical to the functioning of some drugs. Some interactions occur without the recognition of a molecular structure or motif. These non-specific interactions are known as physicochemical effects and include neutralisation of stomach acid by antacids, or molecular adsorption onto activated charcoal.

The interaction and transportation of drugs within the body is determined by factors specific to both the drug and the patient. Drug-related factors include the nature of the drug itself, chemical structure, size, lipid and water solubility, ionisation and charge. Patient-related factors influencing drug uptake and subsequent effects include regional blood flow, barriers to uptake such as membranes, the presence of specific transport or acceptor molecules and the presence of other modifying drugs or hormones.

Chemical structure

Organic molecules consist of functional groups organised around a carbon skeleton. These structures may adopt different conformations allowing specific and non-specific interactions with receptors and binding with proteins and other molecules within the body. The physical organisation of the drug's molecules, functional groups and charge determines further interactions between groups on the same or other molecules. The exposure of charges and hydrophobic or hydrophilic groups may influence a drug's ability to cross membranes, reach a site of action or be excreted.

Isomerism

Isomers are molecules sharing the same chemical formula but with a differing physical arrangement of atoms. Different forms (enantiomers) may interact with other molecules in a variable way and this, therefore affects function. There are several different classes of isomer (Fig. 1.1).

Structural isomerism describes the organisation of functional groups within an organic molecule, where either the carbon skeleton, functional group or position of functional groups along a chain differs. Isoflurane and enflurane share the formula $C_3H_2ClF_5O$ but have differences in solubility, metabolism, potency (as defined by the minimum alveolar concentration, or MAC) and other characteristics. The different positions of the highlighted F and Cl atoms in

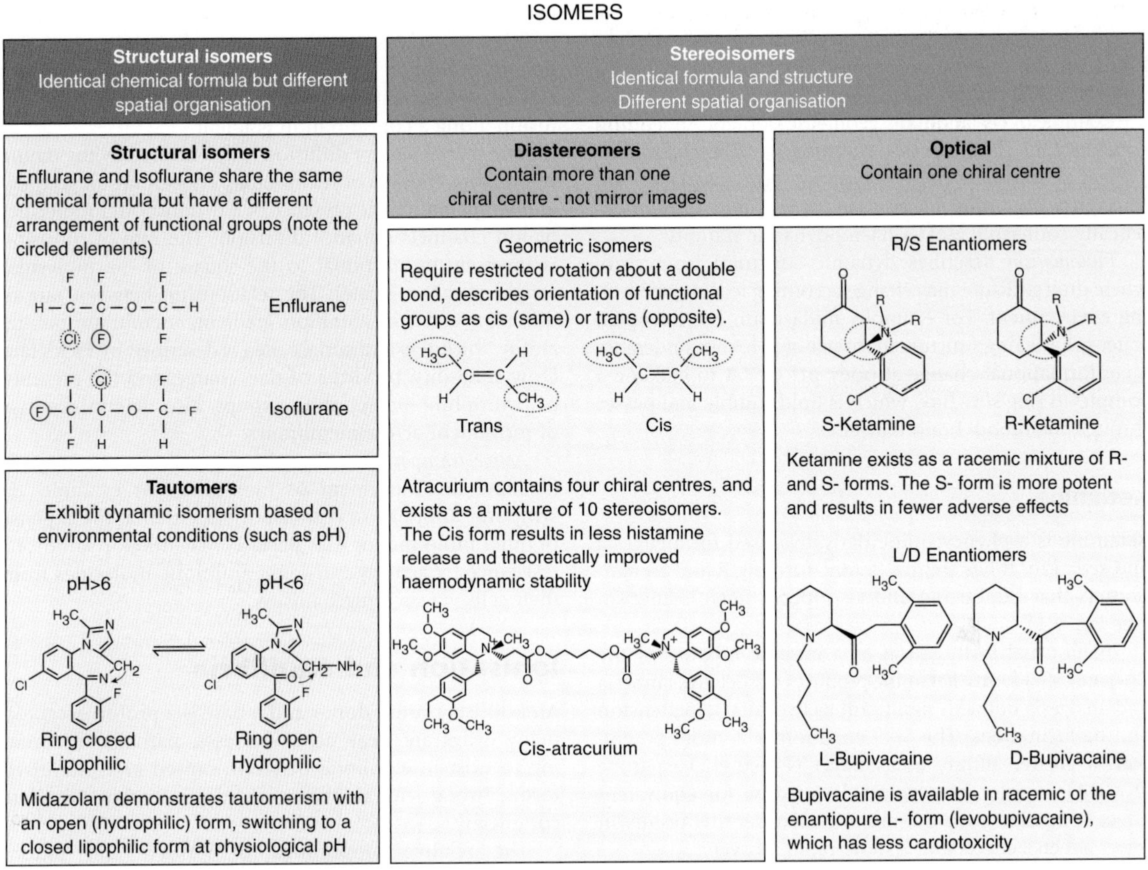

ISOMERS

Fig. 1.1 Classification of isomers with examples from anaesthetic practice.

Fig. 1.1 distinguish these different isomers. Because of the molecular size, spatial conformation and charges contained within these functional groups, the different configurations can affect end function and particularly interaction with receptors and target molecules.

Stereoisomerism refers to molecules with identical chemical and molecular structures but a different spatial organisation of groups around a chiral atom (usually carbon). Chiral atoms are present in all stereoisomers and have bonds entirely occupied by dissimilar functional groups. Stereoisomers are subclassified by the direction in which they rotate plane polarised light (optical isomerism) and/or by the spatial arrangement of atomic groups around the chiral centre. When polarised light is travelling towards the viewer, it can be rotated clockwise (termed dextrorotatory (*d*) or +) or anticlockwise (laevorotatory (*l*) or −). The *dextro* (+) and *laevo* (−) enantiomers of a compound are non-superimposable geometric mirror images of each other. The alternative R/S classification organises compounds according to the atomic number of groups of atoms attached directly to the chiral centre. When viewed with the lowest priority (lowest atomic number) facing away, the priority of the other groups can decrease clockwise (R form) or anticlockwise (S form). These correspond to 'right-handed' (rectus) or 'left-handed' (sinister) forms. Note that the *laevo/dextro* (or +/−) and R/S properties of a drug are independent.

The different configurations are known as enantiomers. Naturally occurring compounds (including some drugs) contain R and S forms in equal proportions – a *racemic mixture*. However, as enantiomers may have different properties (including receptor binding, activity and effects) it may be advantageous to use an enantiopure drug formulation that contains a single enantiomer. Examples include S(+) ketamine and levobupivacaine, as discussed later.

3

Molecules containing more than one chiral centre are described as *diastereomers*, which may form geometric isomers, based on the orientation of functional groups around a non-rotational carbon-carbon double bond. Fig. 1.1 shows the example of cis- and trans-geometric isomers. Atracurium contains four chiral centres, resulting in 10 stereoisomers present in solution. The enantiopure form, cisatracurium, causes less histamine release than the non-pure form, theoretically conferring greater haemodynamic stability.

Tautomerism describes dynamic structural isomerism, where drug structure may change according to the surrounding environment. For example, midazolam has an open, water-soluble ring structure in storage at pH 3 but undergoes a conformational change at body pH of 7.4 to become a completed ring structure, which is lipid soluble and passes through the blood–brain barrier.

Ketamine

Ketamine is a phencyclidine derivative used for analgesia and sedation. It has a chiral centre, forming R and S enantiomers that exhibit (+) and (−) optical stereoisomerism (see Fig. 1.1).

In its usual formulation as a racemic mixture of the R(−) and S(+) forms, ketamine produces dissociative amnesia and analgesia but with significant tachycardia, hypertension and hallucinations. The S(+) enantiomer is more potent, with a greater affinity at its target N-methyl-D-aspartate (NMDA) receptor, requiring a lower dose for equivalent effect compared with the racemic mixture; this results in fewer adverse effects and a more rapid recovery.

Bupivacaine

Bupivacaine is a local anaesthetic containing a chiral centre and adopts *dextro* and *laevo* forms. The enantiopure *l* form is less cardio- and neurotoxic and has an equivalent potency to the racemic mixture; therefore levobupivacaine is often preferred to reduce the potential for toxicity.

Stereoselectivity describes the differences in response at a given receptor for the different enantiomers (such as the response discussed for S(+) ketamine). The opioid and NMDA receptors also exhibit stereoselectivity.

Transport of drugs

Most drugs must pass from their site of administration to their site of action (effect site) before metabolism and elimination, usually via the kidneys or liver. This occurs by local diffusion across plasma membranes, and subsequently mass transport in the blood through dissolution or carriage by transport proteins.

Transmembrane movement is either active or passive. The former is undertaken by transporter proteins with the hydrolysis of adenosine triphosphate (ATP) or movement of other molecules, and the latter occurs by diffusion with no net utilisation of energy. Facilitated diffusion utilises carrier proteins within the cell membranes to increase diffusion along a concentration gradient.

The rate of passive diffusion is determined by the nature of the drug, barriers or membranes, concentration gradient and temperature. The presence of any transporter molecules or ion channels enhance diffusion. The rate of diffusion is inversely proportional to the square of the molecular weight (Graham's law). The relationship between rate of diffusion and concentration gradient, membrane permeability, thickness and surface area is described by Fick's law. Drug solubility, by virtue of size, charge, and the presence of hydrophilic or lipophilic groups, also determines ease of movement across membranes.

Active transport describes the expenditure of energy to facilitate the movement of molecules, for example via symports, antiports or cotransporters, either at the expense of other molecules or ATP. Bacteria may develop antibiotic resistance by actively extruding antibiotic molecules from their cells via such mechanisms.

Ionisation and equilibria

An acid is a proton donor and a base is a proton acceptor; many drugs are weak acids or bases, partially dissociating to exist in equilibria between ionised and unionised forms. Strong acids and bases are substances that dissociate completely.

The relative proportions of ionised and unionised forms for a given drug may be derived from the Henderson–Hasselbalch equation (Eq. 1.1) and depend on the environmental pH and the pKa, the pH at which a given drug exists as equal proportions of its ionised and unionised forms. The pKa is determined by the chemical nature of a drug and is independent of whether it is acidic or basic.

Only the unionised forms of a drug or molecule are highly lipid soluble and can cross cell membranes easily, so the environmental pH determines the action of many drugs.

The Henderson–Hasselbalch equation (see Eq. 1.1) can be rearranged to derive the relative proportion of ionised and unionised forms of a drug, given a known pKa and pH.

$$pH = pKa + \log_{10}\left(\frac{[proton\ acceptor]}{[proton\ donor]}\right) \quad \text{(Eq. 1.1)}$$

For a weakly acidic drug dissociating to H^+ and A^-, substituting these into Eq. 1.1 (Eq. 1.2) and rearranging gives the relative proportions of the ionised, A^-, and unionised form, HA (Eq. 1.2C). Similarly for a base, accepting a proton to form BH^+, the same principles apply.

$$pH = pKa + \log_{10}\left(\frac{[proton\ acceptor]}{[proton\ donor]}\right)$$

For an acidic substance

$$HA \rightleftharpoons H^+ + A^- \quad \text{(Eq. 1.2A)}$$

$$\downarrow$$

$$pH = pKa + \log_{10}\left(\frac{[A^-]}{[HA]}\right) \quad \text{(Eq. 1.2B)}$$

$$\downarrow$$

$$10^{pH-pKa} = \frac{[A^-]}{[HA]} \quad \text{(Eq. 1.2C)}$$

For a basic substance

$$B + H^+ \rightleftharpoons BH^+ \quad \text{(Eq. 1.2A)}$$

$$\downarrow$$

$$pH = pKa + \log_{10}\left(\frac{[B]}{[BH^+]}\right) \quad \text{(Eq. 1.2B)}$$

$$\downarrow$$

$$10^{pH-pKa} = \frac{[B]}{[BH^+]} \quad \text{(Eq. 1.2C)}$$

(Eq. 1.2)

The equilibria given are dynamic and follow the law of mass action depending on the prevailing [H$^+$]. The pKa is the negative logarithm to the base 10 of the dissociation constant. It is an intrinsic property of a drug or molecule and is also the pH at which half of all molecules are ionised. The ionised (BH$^+$) form of a weak base predominates at a pH lower than its pKa, whereas the converse is true for weak acids. The principles of this are shown in Fig. 1.2.

Local anaesthetics are weak bases (i.e. proton acceptors) with pKa values of approximately 8. Therefore at physiological pH (7.4) the environment is relatively acidic compared with the drug, and this renders local anaesthetics ionised. The addition of alkali favours the unionised form (by mass effect) and aids passage of local anaesthetic molecules across the neuronal membrane. Once inside the neuronal tissue, the molecule then becomes charged inside the nerve and is trapped, facilitating interaction with its target, the sodium channel. Acidic environments (in infected tissue) promote the ionised form, preventing entry into nerve tissues, rendering local anaesthetics less effective.

Weak acids, such as thiopental, have the opposite relationship, with the proportion of unionised molecules decreasing with increasing pH (see Fig. 1.2A).

Urinary alkalinisation traps the ionised form of acidic compounds in the renal tubules, preventing reabsorption, and is hence sometimes used in the management of poisoning (e.g. by salicylic acid).

How do drugs act?

Drugs may act at one or more specific molecules, such as a receptor, enzyme or carrier, or at non-specific sites, for example acid neutralisation by sodium citrate.

Fig. 1.3 and Table 1.1 summarise these intra- and extracellular mechanisms of drug action.

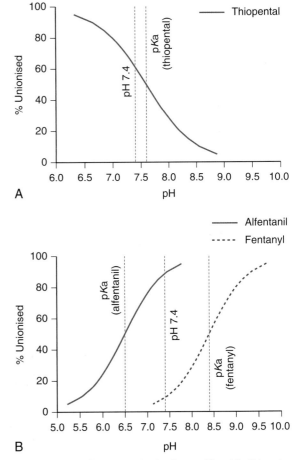

Fig. 1.2 Effect of pH on ionisation for weakly acidic (A) and basic (B) substances.

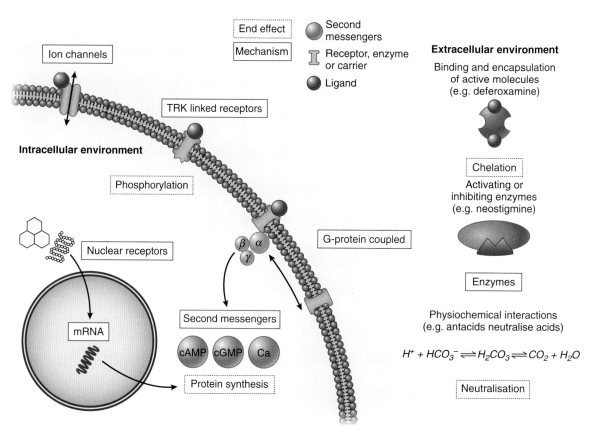

Fig. 1.3 Major targets *(solid boxes)* and mechanisms *(dashed boxes)* of drug action, intra- or extracellular and resulting biochemical changes and second messenger cascades. Targets include channels, carriers and receptors. *mRNA,* Messenger RNA; *TRK,* tyrosine kinase–linked receptors.

The extracellular environment may be affected by chelation, enzymatic breakdown of components or the neutralisation of substances. Receptors are a mechanism for transducing extracellular signals to produce an intracellular response, either via molecules on the cell surface or in the nucleus.

Receptor-mediated effects

Most drugs act at specific receptors. A receptor is a protein that produces an intracellular response when a ligand (which may be a drug or an endogenous molecule) binds to it. In the unbound state, receptors are functionally silent. Increasing knowledge of the molecular structure of the binding regions of receptors and the complementary region on drug molecules

facilitates the design of specific, targeted drugs and opens the possibility of reverse pharmacology – the discovery of new ligands for a given receptor structure.

Receptors enable cells to adapt to environmental conditions outside (in the case of membrane-bound receptors) or inside (in the case of nuclear receptors). Receptors may initiate responses locally (such as the opening or closure of ligand-gated ion channels) or via secondary messenger systems. Through activating second messengers, events on the cell surface may be amplified and cause intracellular changes.

The structure of the receptor is fundamental to its function and production of a specific response to ligand binding. The binding regions are unique to each receptor, but there are some common motifs between classes (Table 1.2).

Table 1.1 Mechanisms of drug action with clinical examples

Enzymes

Target	Inhibitor	Clinical effect and uses
Acetylcholinesterase	Neostigmine Pyridostigmine Organophosphates *Edrophonium*	Increase acetylcholine concentration at neuromuscular junction; reverse non-depolarising neuromuscular blockade. *Edrophonium*, rapidly reversible inhibitor of acetylcholinesterase, increases acetylcholine concentrations used to aid diagnosis of myasthenia gravis (improves symptoms) and cholinergic crisis (worsens symptoms). *Pyridostigmine* and *neostigmine* cause formation of a carbamylated enzyme complex with slow rate of acetylcholine hydrolysis and a long duration of action. *Organophosphates* cause irreversible inhibition of the enzyme, causing a cholinergic crisis.

Cyclo-oxygenase (COX)	Non-specific
	  Aspirin
	  Ibuprofen
	  Diclofenac
	COX 2-specific
	  Meloxicam
	  Celecoxib
		Anti-inflammatory; reduce production of prostacyclin, and leukotrienes.
		Salicylates (e.g. *aspirin*), propionic acids (e.g. *ibuprofen*), acetic acid derivatives (e.g. *diclofenac*) inhibit both COX-1 (constitutive) and COX-2 (inducible), reducing inflammation, but subject to renal injury and gastric erosions because of reduced constitutive production of protective prostaglandins.
		Oxicams (e.g. *meloxicam*) and pyrazoles (e.g. *celecoxib*) are COX-2 preferential, reducing the proinflammatory effects but without causing renal and gastric damage (although not in use because of increased cardiovascular risk).

Carbonic anhydrase	Acetazolamide	Reduced formation of carbonic acid; therefore causes urinary alkalinisation. Used as a diuretic, to correct alkalosis and in treatment of glaucoma.

Voltage-gated ion channel

Target	Activator	Inhibitor	Clinical effect and uses
Voltage-gated calcium channel		Verapamil Amlodipine Dipyridamole	Reduce nodal conduction and smooth muscle contraction; reduce chronotropy and vasodilation. Used to treat angina and tachyarrhythmias by blocking L-type calcium channels. Phenylalkylamines (e.g. *verapamil*) have preferential nodal action and are used to reduce heart rate. Dihydropyridines (e.g. *amlodipine*) and benzothiazepines (e.g. *diltiazem*) bind to calcium channels on smooth muscle, reducing vasoconstriction, lowering blood pressure.
Voltage-gated sodium channel		Lignocaine Bupivacaine Cocaine	Inhibit sodium channels, reducing depolarisation of nerves (and myocardium); used for local anaesthetic nerve blocks, topically for chronic pain. Occasionally used for antiarrhythmic effect. May be classified as amide (e.g. *lignocaine*) or ester (e.g. *cocaine*).
Voltage-gated potassium channel	Nicorandil		Potentiate opening of K^+ channels, hyperpolarising myocardial tissue and reducing myocardial work; also increases cGMP in smooth muscle, promoting relaxation.

Continued

Table 1.1 Mechanisms of drug action with clinical examples—cont'd

Ligand-gated ion channel

Target	Agonist	Antagonist	Clinical effect and uses
GABA$_A$ receptor	Benzodiazepines		The GABA$_A$ receptor is a chloride channel found in diffuse areas of the brain. Benzodiazepines (e.g. *midazolam*) bind to an allosteric site, potentiating the response to native GABA, an inhibitory neurotransmitter, causing anxiolysis, hypnosis and amnesia.
Nicotinic AChR	suxamethonium	Rocuronium Atracurium	Nicotinic acetylcholine receptors are found at nerve synapses and on neuromuscular junctions. Depolarising neuromuscular blocking agents (NMBs) (e.g. *suxamethonium*) bind to and activate the channel, producing neuromuscular stimulation, rendering the muscle relaxed and refractory after initial stimulation. Non-depolarising NMBs may be aminosteroid (e.g. *rocuronium*) or benzylisoquinolone (e.g. *atracurium*). Both are nicotinic receptor antagonists preventing acetylcholine from binding and opening the channel.
Serotonin (5-HT$_3$)		Ondansetron	Found throughout the central nervous system, ligand-gated ion channel permeable to Na$^+$, K$^+$ and Ca^{2+}. Antagonism causes antiemesis.

Nuclear receptors

Target	Agonist	Antagonist	Clinical effect and uses
Steroid receptors	Hydrocortisone Prednisolone		Reduce transcription of proinflammatory cytokines. All contain steroid nuclei, which are lipophilic, permitting intracellular passage and interaction with nuclear receptors and reduction of downstream transcription and protein synthesis.

G protein–coupled receptors

Target	Activator	Antagonist	Clinical effect and uses
Opioid receptors (G$_{i/o}$)	Morphine	Naloxone	Opioid receptors cause reduction in cAMP, opening of potassium channels and reduction of intracellular calcium. This causes neuronal hyperpolarisation, analgesia, drowsiness, respiratory depression and constipation, the effects of opioid agonists such as *morphine*. *Naloxone* is an opioid antagonist, binding to the receptor but having no effect.
α_1-Adrenoceptors (G$_q$)	Phenylephrine	Doxazosin	Located on blood vessels and smooth muscle, cause vasoconstriction. *Phenylephrine* is a synthetic amine, a pure α_1 agonist, causing vasoconstriction. *Doxazosin* produces selective antagonism at α_1, reducing vasoconstriction, and is used in the treatment of hypertension.

Table 1.1 Mechanisms of drug action with clinical examples—cont'd

Target	Activator	Antagonist	Clinical effect and uses
α_2-Adrenoceptors (G_i)	Clonidine Dexmedetomidine	Yohimbine	Located presynaptically, reduces endogenous noradrenaline release and therefore sympathetic tone by reducing cAMP and opening potassium channels. *Clonidine* is used to treat hypertension, and the widespread distribution of α_1 adrenoceptors produces other effects such as analgesia, anxiolysis and sedation. *Yohimbine* reversibly antagonises the effects of α_2 agonists.
β_1-Adrenoceptors (G_s)	Isoprenaline	Atenolol	β_1 adrenoceptors are located in the myocardium and conducting system and predominately increase inotropy, chronotropy and dronotropy through increasing cAMP formation via G_s and adenylate cyclase. *Isoprenaline* is a synthetic catecholamine and a non-selective agonist at the β_1 adrenoceptor used in the treatment of bradycardias. *Atenolol* is a β_1 selective antagonist used in the treatment of hypertension and tachyarrhythmias.
β_2-Adrenoceptors (G_s)	Salbutamol		β_2 stimulation predominately causes bronchodilation. Salbutamol is a typical β_2 agonist, causing bronchodilation, and is used in the treatment of asthma. This may promote tachyarrhythmias and lactic acidosis through non-selective β_1 effects. There are no clinically useful β_2 antagonists.
Muscarinic receptors M_1 (postsynaptic) – G_q M_2 (cardiac) – G_i M_3 (smooth muscle) – G_q	Pilocarpine	Atropine Glycopyrronium bromide	Muscarinic receptors cause increases in salivation (M_1), bradycardias (M_2) and bronchoconstriction (M_3). *Pilocarpine* is used in the treatment of glaucoma to cause pupillary constriction and permit drainage of aqueous humour, reducing intraocular pressure. *Atropine* and *glycopyrronium bromide* are tertiary amines used in the treatment of bradycardias through antagonism at the muscarinic receptors.

Drugs acting via physicochemical mechanisms

Target	Mechanism	Drug	Clinical effect and uses
Acids	Neutralisation	Sodium citrate	Sodium citrate is used before general anaesthesia in obstetric practice to neutralise stomach acid.
Rocuronium	Chelation	Sugammadex	*Sugammadex*, a cyclodextrin, acts to engulf and chelate rocuronium, reversing its effect at the acetylcholine receptor
Multiple	Adsorption	Activated charcoal	Activated charcoal adsorbs various chemicals on to its surface preventing toxicity from their systemic absorption.

AChR, Acetylcholine receptor; *cAMP*, cyclic adenosine monophosphate; *cGMP*, cyclic guanosine monophosphate.

Table 1.2 Structural features found in major receptor classes

Type	Structural features	Examples of drugs
Nuclear receptors	Zinc fingers	Steroids
Tyrosine kinase receptors	Dimers	Insulin
Ligand-gated ion channels	Multiple subunits, have a pore and ligand binding sites	Local anaesthetics
G protein–coupled receptors	7-transmembrane domains	Adrenaline

G protein–coupled receptors

The largest superfamily of receptors contains 7-transmembrane domains and couple to G-proteins. G protein–coupled receptors act as adapters between extracellular signalling and intracellular downstream second messenger systems, the endpoint of receptor activation (Fig. 1.4). Upon activation, the receptor undergoes a conformational change, causing the α subunit of the G protein to exchange bound guanosine diphosphate (GDP) for guanosine triphosphate (GTP) (see Fig. 1.4A), which then causes it to dissociate from the G protein–coupled receptor and move to an effector molecule (see Fig. 1.4B). Whilst influencing the effector the bound GTP is hydrolysed to GDP by the GTPase of the α subunit (see Fig. 1.4C), which then returns to the intracellular

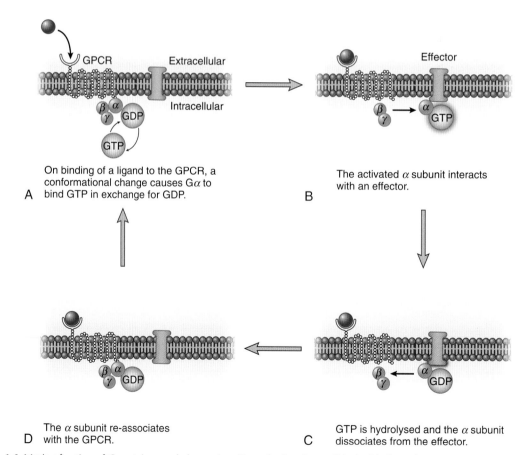

A — On binding of a ligand to the GPCR, a conformational change causes Gα to bind GTP in exchange for GDP.

B — The activated α subunit interacts with an effector.

C — GTP is hydrolysed and the α subunit dissociates from the effector.

D — The α subunit re-associates with the GPCR.

Fig. 1.4 Mode of action of G protein–coupled receptors. From the basal state (A), the binding of an agonist causes conformational change, and the G protein dissociates after exchanging guanosine triphosphate (GTP) for bound guanosine diphosphate (GDP). The α subunit interacts with an effector molecule (B), subsequently hydrolyses the bound GTP (C), and returns to the basal state (D).

Table 1.3 G-proteins and second messenger systems

G protein	Second messenger	Effect	Receptor and example of agonist drug
G_s	Adenylate cyclase	↑ cAMP	*Isoprenaline* (β-adrenoceptor)
G_i	Adenylate cyclase	↓cAMP	α_2 adrenoceptor *clonidine*
G_q	Phospholipase C	↑Ca^{2+}	α_1 adrenoceptor *phenylephrine*
cAMP, Cyclic adenosine monophosphate.			

terminus of the receptor and reassociates with the βγ subunits (see Fig. 1.4D).

There are three major types of G protein (Table 1.3) capable of interacting with the second messengers adenylate cyclase ($G_{i/o}$ and G_s) and phospholipase C (G_q). A single receptor may activate many G proteins, and this amplifies the initial signal. Drugs can target different parts of this receptor cascade by interacting with the receptor (e.g. opioids), the G protein (e.g. botulinum toxin) or further downstream (e.g. Ca^{2+}).

Second messenger systems

Second messenger systems are the endpoint of a number of different inputs. They are a further level of amplification, enabling a small extracellular signal to effect a large and significant change to the intracellular environment.

Second messengers can enable other functions, such as protein phosphorylation. The result of protein phosphorylation can influenceion transport (e.g. acetylcholine, glutamate, γ-aminobutyric acid (GABA) receptors), and receptor activation state.

What influences the response of a receptor?

Ligands bind to receptors and are classified according to their effect, either to increase (agonist) or to have no effect (antagonist) on receptor response. Ligand-receptor kinetics, biological reactions and enzyme kinetics are all subject to the law of mass action, which states that the rate of reaction is proportional to the concentration of biologically active species present at a given time.

The classic rectangular hyperbolic dose–response relationship of an agonist is shown in Fig. 1.5A. As the number of agonist molecules increases, the receptor response increases until all binding sites are fully occupied and response is maximal (see Fig. 1.5A). This rectangular hyperbolic shaped

curve is conventionally transformed to a semilogarithmic scale to produce a sigmoid-shaped curve that is approximately linear between 20% and 80% of maximum effect, allowing comparison of the effects of different agonists (see Fig. 1.5B). Agonists are described by the size of the effect they can produce (efficacy) and the dose required to elicit a given effect (potency).

The pEC_{50} is a log-transformed measure of the ligand concentration required to elicit a half-maximal response for the drug, a measure of potency. A rightward shift on the logarithmic scale indicates that the drug has lower potency; therefore an increased dose is required to achieve the same effect. Efficacy is the size of the response produced by ligand-receptor interaction. E_{MAX} is the maximal response. Therapeutic ligand-receptor interactions may produce unwanted adverse effects (such as the respiratory depression caused by agonism at the μ opioid receptor).

Full agonists can elicit a maximal effect, whereas partial agonists can never achieve maximum effect irrespective of dose and so have lower efficacy. Fig. 1.5B shows the effects of agonists A, B and C. B is less potent than A, but both are full agonists. B and C have the same potency, but C is a partial agonist as it is not able to elicit a full response, irrespective of concentration.

Antagonists bind to the receptor but produce no intrinsic effect. Competitive antagonists bind to the receptor, and displace endogenous ligands or other drugs therefore reducing receptor response. Non-competitive antagonists do not compete with endogenous ligands for the same binding site. They chemically or structurally modify the receptor, reducing the response induced by ligands occupying the binding site. Unlike competitive antagonists they cannot be overcome by increasing agonist concentration.

In the presence of a competitive antagonist, the log[dose]–response curve of an agonist is shifted to the right but the maximum effect remains unaltered (curves A and B in Fig. 1.5C). The effects of these antagonists can be overcome with an increasing agonist concentration. Examples of this

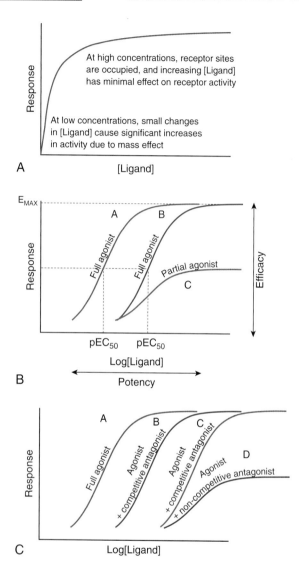

Fig. 1.5 Receptor response increases with ligand concentration for an agonist (A); the potency of different agonists may be compared by examining the pEC$_{50}$ values after semilogarithmic transformation (B). The combination of agonists and antagonists causes a rightward shift of the curve (C, *curves A, B* and *C*). Irreversible non-competitive antagonists reduce the maximal response by reducing the available receptor pool (C, *curve D*).

effect include the displacement of morphine by naloxone and endogenous catecholamines by β-blockers.

A non-competitive (irreversible) antagonist also shifts the dose–response curve to the right but, with increasing concentrations, reduces the maximum effect (curve D in Fig. 1.5C) as the receptor pool is effectively limited. Examples

of irreversible antagonism include the platelet inhibitors clopidogrel and aspirin. Organophosphates cause irreversible modification of acetylcholinesterase, causing increased cholinergic effects.

Drug actions on enzymes

An enzyme is a protein to which other molecules (substrate) may bind and undergo chemical modification in some way, such as breakdown or synthesis of other products. Drugs may act by binding reversibly or irreversibly to the active site of the enzyme and acting as substrates or to block binding of endogenous substrate. Some drugs bind to an alternative (allosteric) site to modify the activity of the enzyme.

Enzyme kinetics

The relationship between an enzyme, substrate and rate of reaction is described in Fig. 1.6A.

When an enzyme joins with appropriate substrate at the active site, the complex undergoes chemical modification to yield products. This equation (Eq. 1.3) is governed by the law of mass action, and therefore, where substrate concentrations are high, the equilibrium shifts to the right, favouring the generation of products.

$$Enzyme + Substrate \rightleftharpoons Complex \rightleftharpoons Enzyme + Products$$

(Eq. 1.3)

Where the substrate is at low concentration, its availability is rate limiting, whereas where substrate exceeds the enzyme's capacity, then enzymatic activity is the limiting factor.

Fig. 1.6A and B shows how, at low substrate concentrations, a small increase in substrate produces a significant increase in enzymatic activity, whereas at high substrate concentrations, the activity remains maximal and independent of substrate concentration. The effects of different enzymes are compared and modelled using the V$_{MAX}$ (the maximal enzyme reaction rate) and k$_M$ (substrate concentration at which half V$_{MAX}$ is achieved).

Knowledge of enzyme kinetics is useful for predicting drug metabolism and pharmacokinetics. Drugs processed by first-order kinetics are metabolised by a large pool of enzymes and therefore overall enzyme activity is increased at high drug concentration; this increases the rate of metabolism and also reduces the chance of toxicity (Fig. 1.6C). However, where the enzymatic pool is small or the dose so high that the available enzymes become saturated, the rate of breakdown becomes fixed irrespective of drug concentration (Fig. 1.6D). This is known as zero order, or saturation kinetics, and is an important consideration in the metabolism of phenytoin, paracetamol and alcohol, sometimes requiring the monitoring of plasma drug concentrations.

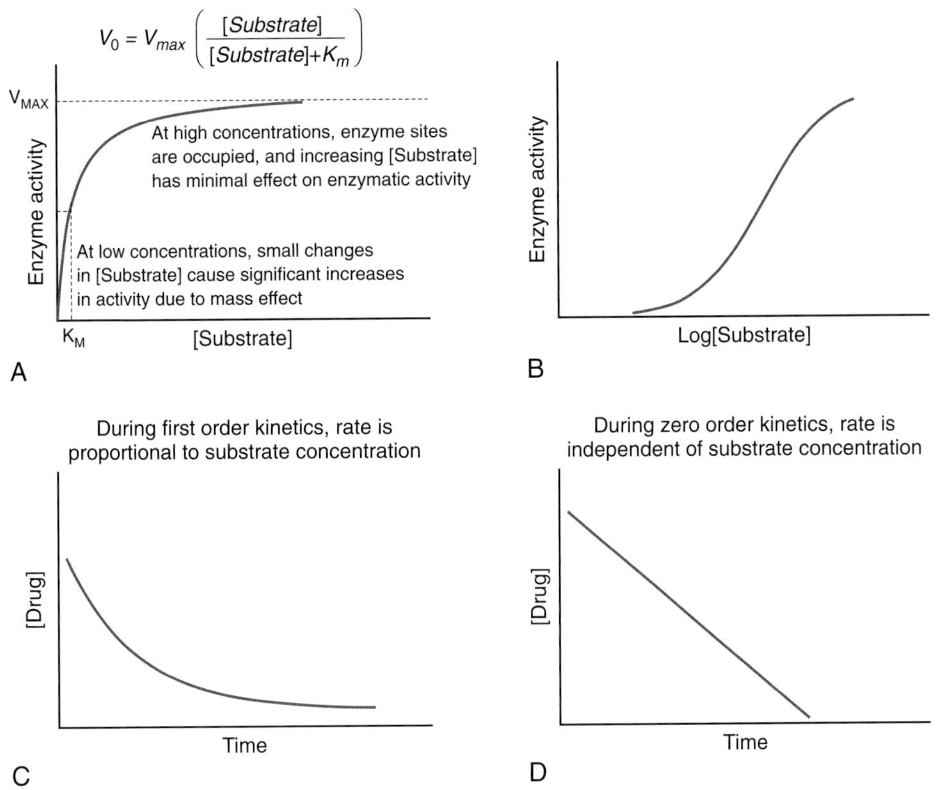

$V_0 = V_{max}\left(\frac{[Substrate]}{[Substrate]+K_m}\right)$
V_{MAX}
Enzyme activity
At high concentrations, enzyme sites are occupied, and increasing [Substrate] has minimal effect on enzymatic activity
At low concentrations, small changes in [Substrate] cause significant increases in activity due to mass effect
K_M
[Substrate]
A
Enzyme activity
Log[Substrate]
B
During first order kinetics, rate is proportional to substrate concentration
[Drug]
Time
C
During zero order kinetics, rate is independent of substrate concentration
[Drug]
Time
D

Fig. 1.6 Increasing concentrations of substrate cause increased enzyme activity (A and B) in a saturable manner. Initially, response is first order, proportional to the substrate concentration (C), but becomes zero order, independent of substrate concentration, when the number of substrate molecules exceeds the available binding sites (D).

Drugs may modulate enzymes by increasing or decreasing intrinsic activity or by competing with endogenous substrate molecules at the active site. As with receptor kinetics, reversible inhibition is caused by competition for the active site and may be overcome by an increase in the endogenous substrate. Examples include the reversible antagonism of acetylcholinesterase (by neostigmine), phosphodiesterase (by aminophylline), and angiotensin converting enzyme (by lisinopril). Irreversible enzyme inhibition occurs when a stable chemical bond is formed between drug and enzyme, resulting in prolonged or permanent inactivation. Examples include the irreversible inhibition of gastric hydrogen-potassium-ATPase (by omprazole), cyclo-oxygenase (by aspirin) and acetylcholinesterase (by organophosphates). *Allosteric modulation* refers to binding to a site other than the active site to influence enzyme activity – for example, the antiretroviral reverse transcriptase inhibitor efavirenz.

Physicochemical properties

The physicochemical properties of drugs produce other effects outside receptor, enzyme or secondary messenger pathways. These non-specific mechanisms often rely on physical properties such as pH, charge or physical interactions with other molecules (via chelation or adsorption).

pH-based interactions include the neutralisation of acid with alkali. Sodium citrate, aluminium and magnesium hydroxide neutralise gastric acid via this mechanism.

Chelating agents combine chemically with compounds, reducing their toxicity and enhancing elimination of the inactive complex. Such drugs include sugammadex (chelates rocuronium), deferoxamine (chelates iron and aluminium), dicobalt edetate (cyanide toxicity), sodium calcium edetate (lead) and penicillamine (copper and lead).

Molecular adsorption describes the interaction and binding of a molecule to the surface of another, reducing the free fraction available for absorption from the gastrointestinal tract. This mechanism may be useful in the treatment of drug toxicity to prevent an oral overdose from being absorbed (activated charcoal) or in the management of hyperkalaemia (calcium resonium reduces the GI absorption of potassium).

How does the body process drugs (pharmacokinetics)?

Absorption

Absorption describes the process by which a drug is taken up from the initial site of administration into the blood. The rate and amount of absorption affects the final plasma concentration and therefore drug concentration at the effect site. For drugs requiring multiple doses, these principles will also affect peak plasma concentration and time to maximal concentration.

Absorption is influenced by factors specific to both drug and patient, as discussed earlier. The pathway from site of administration to final effect site includes passage across membranes and blood transport (see Transport of drugs and Routes of administration). Drugs may have specific formulations which affect the rate of drug release or facilitate delivery to the target site. These are covered in more detail in Pharmacokinetic principles.

Distribution

Protein binding

Many drugs are bound to proteins in the plasma; this permits transport around the body but reduces the active unbound, ionised drug fraction. Changes in protein binding may therefore have significant effects on the active unbound concentration of a drug and thus its actions.

Albumin is the most important and abundant protein contributing to drug binding and is responsible mainly for the binding of acidic and neutral drugs. Globulins, especially α_1-acid glycoprotein, bind mainly basic drugs. If a drug is highly protein bound (>80%), any change in plasma protein concentration or displacement of the drug by another with similar binding properties may have clinically significant effects. For example, most NSAIDs displace warfarin, phenytoin and lithium from plasma binding sites, leading to potential toxicity.

Plasma albumin concentration is often decreased in the elderly, in neonates and in the presence of malnutrition, liver, renal or cardiac failure and malignancy. α_1-acid glycoprotein concentration is decreased during pregnancy and in the neonate but may be increased in the postoperative period, in infection, trauma, burns and malignancy.

Metabolism

Most drugs are lipid soluble, and the majority are metabolised in the liver. Metabolites are mostly pharmacologically inactive, ionised (water soluble) compounds which are then excreted in bile or by the kidneys. However, some metabolites may be active and cause prolonged clinical effect after the parent compound has been broken down or removed from the circulation. Some drugs are metabolised outside the liver (by kidneys, lungs, plasma and tissues).

Medications that are absorbed enterally undergo first-pass metabolism before passing from the portal circulation into the systemic circulation.

First-pass metabolism may increase or decrease drug effect to a variable extent. A substance is termed a *prodrug* if it is inactive in the form administered and its pharmacological effects depend on the formation of active metabolites. Codeine is a prodrug, undergoing metabolism via gluconuridation (50%–70%), *N*-demethylation (10%–15%) and *O*-demethylation (0%–15%). Morphine, resulting from *O*-demethylation of codeine by CYP2D6, is the most active metabolite and has greater activity at the opioid receptor. CYP2D6 exists as slow, rapid and ultra-rapid phenotypes, which affect the therapeutic response to codeine. Those with inactive CYP2D6 may derive no analgesia from codeine, whereas ultra-rapid metabolisers may have significant drowsiness, respiratory depression and features of opiate toxicity.

Drugs undergo two types of reactions during metabolism: phase I and phase II. Phase I reactions include reduction, oxidation and hydrolysis. Drug oxidation occurs in the smooth endoplasmic reticulum, primarily by the cytochrome P450 enzyme system. This system and other enzymes also perform reduction reactions. Hydrolysis is a common phase I reaction in the metabolism of drugs with ester or amide groups (e.g. meperidine). Amide drugs often undergo hydrolysis and oxidative *N*-dealkylation (e.g. lidocaine, bupivacaine).

Phase II reactions involve conjugation of a metabolite or the drug itself with an endogenous substrate. Conjugation with glucuronic acid is a major metabolic pathway, but others include acetylation, methylation and conjugation with sulphate or glycine.

Extra-hepatic or extra-renal metabolism is independent of liver or renal function. Typically this leads to a rapid offset of drug action because of the abundance of enzyme sites for metabolism. Drugs metabolised via these routes can be useful in those with hepatic or renal failure. For example, suxamethonium and mivacurium are metabolised by plasma cholinesterase, esmolol by erythrocyte esterases, remifentanil by tissue esterases and, in part, dopamine by the kidney and prilocaine by the lungs. Occasionally drugs will undergo spontaneous degradation to generate active or inactive metabolites. These processes are also independent of hepatic or renal pathways – such as the spontaneous breakdown of atracurium by Hofmann degradation.

Elimination

Ionised compounds with a low molecular weight (MW) are excreted mainly by the kidneys. Most drugs and metabolites diffuse passively into the proximal renal tubules by the process of glomerular filtration, but some are secreted actively (e.g. penicillins, aspirin, many diuretics, morphine, lidocaine and glucuronides). Ionisation is a significant barrier to reabsorption at the distal tubule. Consequently, basic drugs or metabolites are excreted more efficiently in acidic urine and acidic compounds in alkaline urine. Urinary alkalinisation is sometimes used in the treatment of aspirin and tricyclic antidepressant overdose.

Some drugs and metabolites, particularly larger molecules (MW >400 D), are excreted in the bile (e.g. glycopyrronium bromide, vecuronium, pancuronium and the metabolites of morphine and buprenorphine). Ventilation is responsible for excretion of volatile anaesthetic agents.

Pharmacokinetic principles

Pharmacokinetics describes the processing of a drug by the body. This allows modelling of the likely behaviour and actions of a drug in the body and enables predictions of plasma concentration and clinical effect at a given time. Important variables are volume of distribution (V_D), clearance (Cl) and half-life ($t_{1/2}$). Whilst pharmacokinetic predictions and models have generic value, the effects in an individual depend on existing physiology, age, disease, drug interactions and other factors.

Compartment models

For simplicity, drug pharmacokinetics are usually described using one-, two- or three-compartment models (Fig. 1.7). Drugs are added to and eliminated from a central plasma compartment and equilibrate with peripheral tissues and the effect site (see Fig. 1.7 A, B, and C respectively). The rate of equilibration depends on the drug (pKa, degree of ionisation, lipid solubility, formulation), route of administration, regional blood flow and compartment sizes.

When a drug is administered and reaches the central compartment, the plasma concentration initially increases rapidly and then falls as the drug passes into the other compartments and later is eliminated completely. The changes in measured plasma drug concentration during the time for absorption, redistribution and elimination are represented as an exponential decay (Fig. 1.8). The simplest model, a single compartment, represents plasma concentration decline only as a result of metabolism or clearance, whereas two- and three-compartment models include concentration changes caused by redistribution into other tissues, a more physiological approximation.

The rate at which drug distribution and subsequent elimination occurs is described in terms of equilibria between the various compartments (see Fig. 1.7). These are additive and result in concentration–time curves with two or three phases of decay attributable to redistribution (rapid and slow in the three-compartment model) and elimination.

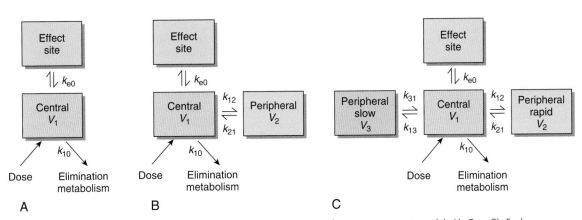

Fig. 1.7 Pharmacological compartments are described as one-, two-, or three-compartment models (A, B or C). Each compartment consists of a central region from which drug is added or removed, the effect site, and other areas within which drugs may be sequestered. The different models have peripheral compartments of varying vascularity to simulate equilibria and model pharmacokinetic drug characteristics.

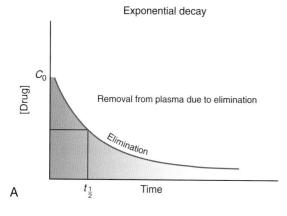

Exponential decay

[Drug] axis, C_0

Removal from plasma due to elimination

Elimination

A $t_{\frac{1}{2}}$ Time

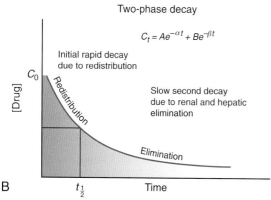

Two-phase decay

$$C_t = Ae^{-\alpha t} + Be^{-\beta t}$$

Initial rapid decay
due to redistribution

Redistribution

C_0

Slow second decay
due to renal and hepatic
elimination

Elimination

B $t_{\frac{1}{2}}$ Time

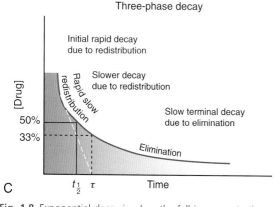

Three-phase decay

Initial rapid decay
due to redistribution

Rapid slow
redistribution

Slower decay
due to redistribution

50%

33%

Slow terminal decay
due to elimination

Elimination

C $t_{\frac{1}{2}}$ τ Time

Fig. 1.8 Exponential decay is when the fall in concentration depends on the amount of substance present at a given time. Therefore constant proportion of substance disappears per unit time. The phases relate to the number of compartments for redistribution and the terminal elimination.

The equilibria, k_{12} and k_{13}, both influence drug concentration at the final effect site (k_{e0}) and for elimination (k_{10}). The resultant concentration–time curve is a one-, two- or three-phase exponential decay (see Fig. 1.8).

In the two-compartment model, one compartment represents the plasma and the other represents the remainder of the body. In this model, after intravenous injection of a drug, the plasma concentration (C_P) decreases because of removal by elimination and redistribution into peripheral tissues. Fig. 1.8C shows the relationship between the *half-life* ($t_{1/2}$, time for the starting concentration to decay by 50%) and *time constant* (τ, the time to completion if the initial rate of change continued, or the time to decay to 33% of the initial concentration).

If the natural logs of the concentrations are plotted against time (semi-logarithmic plot), a straight line is produced in one, two or three phases depending on the compartment model used (Fig. 1.9A and B and C).

Consider a single-compartment model (see Fig. 1.8A and Fig. 1.9A). The concentration–time plot indicates $t_{1/2}$. After semilogarithmic transformation (see Fig. 1.9A), the gradient of this line (k) and the initial concentration (C_0) can be extrapolated. The gradient is the elimination rate constant k, which is related to $t_{1/2}$ in the following equation (Eq. 1.4):

$$k = \frac{ln2}{t_{1/2}} \qquad \text{(Eq. 1.4)}$$

Using the concentration–time plots and their semilogarithmic transformations, the concentration at any time can be described in terms of an exponential decay (Eq. 1.5)

$$C_P = C_0 e^{-kt} \qquad \text{(Eq. 1.5)}$$

where t is the time after administration, k is the elimination rate constant, C_0 is the initial concentration and C_P is the plasma concentration at time t.

In the two- and three-compartment model, (Fig. 1.9B and C) the plasma concentration at a given time t represents the sum of the decay processes. The two lines α and β represent decline by redistribution and elimination, respectively, each of which have their own k values (α and β), starting concentrations (A and B) and half-lives ($t_{1/2\alpha}$, $t_{1/2\beta}$).

These biexponential decays are modelled using standard exponential equations (see Eq. 1.5), and therefore C_P at any time in a two-compartment model after bolus intravenous administration is the sum of the elimination and redistribution phases (Eq. 1.6).

$$C_P = Ae^{-\alpha t} + Be^{-\beta t} \qquad \text{(Eq. 1.6)}$$

where α and β are the redistribution and elimination rate constants, respectively, and A and B are the extrapolated

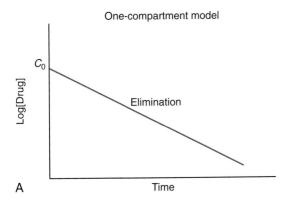

One-compartment model

C_0

Elimination

A   Time

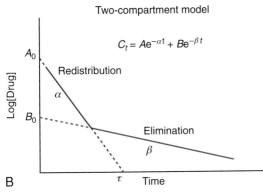

Two-compartment model

$C_t = Ae^{-\alpha t} + Be^{-\beta t}$

A_0

Redistribution

α

B_0

Elimination

β

B τ Time

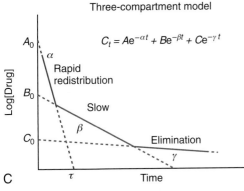

Three-compartment model

$C_t = Ae^{-\alpha t} + Be^{-\beta t} + Ce^{-\gamma t}$

A_0

α

Rapid redistribution

B_0

Slow

β

C_0

Elimination

γ

C τ Time

Fig. 1.9 Semilogarithmic transformation of concentration–time curves demonstrates a single-phase, biphasic and triphasic exponential decay. This transformation generates linear relationships for each of the phases of redistribution and elimination, allowing the calculation of initial concentration C_0, concentration at a given time, and therefore bolus or infusion requirements to achieve steady state.

starting points (see Fig. 1.9). In the three-compartment model, drug redistribution is initially rapid to well-perfused tissues and then slow into poorly perfused areas before terminal elimination, a triexponential model.

After drug administration, the clinical effect depends on the drug reaching the site of action from the central compartment. Half of this equilibration occurs in $t_{1/2}\,k_{e0}$. Therefore the $t_{1/2}\,k_{e0}$ reflects time to peak concentration at the effect site and thus time to peak clinical effect. Equilibration at the effect site during an i.v. drug infusion occurs in four to five half-lives ($t_{1/2}\,k_{e0}$), which is the time to change in effect after a change of infusion rate.

Volume of distribution

Volume of distribution is the theoretical volume into which a drug distributes immediately to give the plasma concentration observed at that time. As the concentration cannot be measured instantaneously, semilogarithmic plots (see Fig. 1.9) allow the initial concentration to be derived by extrapolation. Where the dose given and initial plasma concentration are known (C_0), the volume of distribution (V_D) may be calculated by rearranging Eq. 1.7 to form Eq. 1.8.

$$C_0 = \frac{dose}{V} \qquad \text{(Eq. 1.7)}$$

where C_0 is the initial concentration. Therefore:

$$V_D = \frac{dose}{C_0} \qquad \text{(Eq. 1.8)}$$

A more accurate measurement of V_D is possible during constant-rate infusion when the distribution of the drug in the tissues has time to equilibrate; this is termed volume of distribution at steady state (V_{Dss}).

Large, water-soluble, polar drugs that remain in the plasma and do not pass easily to other tissues have a small V_D and therefore a large C_0. Other factors such as plasma protein binding also reduce diffusion out of the plasma. Drugs with a large V_D are often lipid soluble and therefore accumulate in tissues outside the plasma (e.g. intravenous anaesthetic agents).

Some drugs accumulate outside the plasma, making values for V_D greater than total body water volume. Large V_D values are often observed for drugs highly bound to proteins outside plasma (e.g. local anaesthetics, digoxin).

Several factors may affect V_D and therefore C_0 after bolus injection of a drug. Patients who are dehydrated or have lost blood have a significantly greater plasma C_0 after a normal dose of intravenous anaesthetic agent, increasing the likelihood of concentration-dependent adverse effects. In the case of intravenous anaesthetics, this often manifests as haemodynamic instability caused by cardiac depression and reduced vascular tone. Neonates have a proportionally greater volume of extracellular fluid compared with adults, and water-soluble drugs (e.g. neuromuscular blockers) tend to have a proportionally greater V_D. Factors affecting plasma protein binding (see earlier) may also affect V_D.

Finally, V_D can give some indication of the half-life. A large V_D is often associated with a relatively slow decline in plasma concentration; this relationship is expressed in a useful pharmacokinetic equation (Eq. 1.9–1.10).

Elimination

Elimination describes the removal of active drug from the body, which may include renal excretion, metabolism to other forms or elimination via bile, sweat or exhalation.

Drug half-life can be derived from the plasma concentration–time graph (see Fig. 1.8) but is also related to clearance and to metabolism (Eq. 1.9).

$$t_{1/2} \propto \frac{V_D}{Cl} \qquad \text{(Eq. 1. 9)}$$

or

$$t_{1/2} = constant \times \frac{V_D}{Cl}$$

The constant in this equation (elimination rate constant) is the natural logarithm of 2 (ln 2) – that is, 0.693. Therefore:

$$t_{1/2} = 0.693 \times \frac{V_D}{Cl} \qquad \text{(Eq. 1.10)}$$

For simple receptor–ligand equilibria, half-life reflects duration of drug action, although where binding or action is irreversible or active metabolites are produced, the clinical effect will be prolonged relative to the plasma $t_{1/2}$.

Clearance

Clearance is defined as the volume of blood or plasma from which the drug is removed completely per unit time. Drugs may be eliminated from the blood by the liver, kidney or occasionally other routes (see earlier). The relative proportion of hepatic and renal clearance of a drug is important. Most drugs used in anaesthetic practice are cleared predominantly by the liver, but some rely on renal or non–organ-dependent clearance. Excessive accumulation of a renally cleared drug may occur in patients in renal failure. For example, morphine is metabolised primarily in the liver, and this is not affected significantly in renal impairment. However, the active metabolite morphine-6-glucuronide is excreted predominantly by the kidney.

As with volume of distribution, clearance may predict the likely properties of a drug. For example, if clearance is greater than hepatic blood flow, factors other than hepatic metabolism must account for its total clearance. Apparent clearance greater than cardiac output may indicate metabolism in the plasma (e.g. suxamethonium) or other tissues (e.g. remifentanil). Clearance is an important (but not the only) factor affecting $t_{1/2}$ and steady-state plasma concentrations achieved during constant-rate infusions (see later).

Clearance may be derived also by calculation of the area under the concentration–time curve (see Fig. 1.8) extrapolated to infinity (AUC_∞) and substituted into Eq. 1.11.

$$Cl = \frac{dose}{AUC_\infty} \qquad \text{(Eq. 1.11)}$$

Metabolism

Enzyme induction and inhibition
Some drugs may enhance the activity of enzymes responsible for hepatic metabolism, particularly the family of cytochrome P450 enzymes and glucuronyl transferase. Drugs enhancing enzyme activity include phenytoin, carbamazepine, barbiturates, ethanol, steroids and some inhalational anaesthetic agents (halothane and enflurane). Cigarette smoking also induces cytochrome P450 enzymes.

Drugs with a non-enzymatic primary mechanism may also have secondary interactions with enzyme systems. For example, etomidate inhibits the synthesis of cortisol and aldosterone – an effect which may explain the increased mortality observed when it was used as a sedative agent in the critically ill. Cimetidine is a potent enzyme inhibitor and may prolong the elimination of drugs such as diazepam, propranolol, oral anticoagulants, phenytoin and lidocaine. Troublesome interactions with enzyme systems can be unpredictable and are not always clear until the early stages of testing in phase 2 or 3 studies.

Routes of administration
Oral

The oral route of drug administration is often the most convenient when it is available. However starvation for anaesthesia or the pathophysiological effects of disease sometimes preclude enteral administration. Absorption from the gut is affected by drug- and patient-based physiological and pathological processes.

Drug and physiological factors relating to the passage of drugs across membranes have been considered previously. Drug formulation is an important consideration; tablets or capsules are more poorly absorbed than liquids, and some drugs may be given as slow release or enteric-coated modified release preparations. The combination of naloxone and oxycodone found in the drug targinact is an example of the local delivery of (non-absorbable) naloxone to the gastrointestinal tract to counteract the constipation caused by the (absorbed) oxycodone acting on local μ opioid receptors in the bowel.

The rate of absorption, and therefore effect of the drug, may be influenced significantly by its molecular size, lipid solubility and formulation. Most preparations dissolve in gastric acid, and the drug is absorbed in the small bowel after passing through the stomach; therefore formulations suitable for oral administration must not be subject to breakdown by stomach acid or peptidases.

Enterally administered drugs are subject to first-pass metabolism, and this can affect the dose required to achieve a given plasma concentration.

Gastric emptying

Most drugs are absorbed only when they have left the stomach. The effects of surgery can delay gastric emptying and promote ileus. This can affect absorption and can lead to drug accumulation in the stomach, risking unpredictable effects on plasma concentrations and clinical action.

Any factor increasing upper intestinal motility (such as drugs, surgery or the effects of autonomic dysfunction) reduces the time available for absorption and may decrease the total amount of drug absorbed.

Bioavailability

Oral bioavailability is the percentage of an enterally administered drug dose which is absorbed into the systemic circulation. This is derived from a graph of plasma concentration against time for both oral and intravenous administration of the same dose of drug in a given individual on separate occasions (Fig. 1.10). Bioavailability is calculated as the ratio of the areas under the concentration–time curves for oral, and i.v. administration. A high bioavailability indicates that a high proportion of the orally administered dose reaches the effect site, and indicates suitability oral administration (e.g. codeine >90%), whereas the opposite is true for low bioavailability, requiring administration via a non-enteral route (e.g. glyceryl trinitrate <1%).

Lingual, buccal and nasal

The oral mucosa has a rich blood supply, and therefore lipid-soluble drugs are absorbable via this route. The avoidance of first-pass metabolism and rapid absorption make this an ideal route for some drugs, such as fentanyl, buprenorphine and glyceryl trinitrate.

The nasal mucosa has a rich blood supply, is readily accessible and avoids first-pass metabolism. The rapid absorption afforded by this route allows use where intravenous access is not practical, such as for paediatric sedation or analgesia

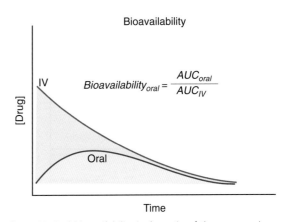

Fig. 1.10 Oral bioavailability is the ratio of the areas under the plasma concentration–time curves for enteral and parenteral routes of administration.

$$Bioavailability_{oral} = \frac{AUC_{oral}}{AUC_{IV}}$$

using midazolam or diamorphine. Topical drugs are used to facilitate nasal surgery, although the rich blood supply risks systemic toxicity and is often offset with the addition of a vasoconstrictor such as phenylephrine or adrenaline (e.g. coadministration of lignocaine and phenylephrine in nasal surgery for analgesia and to reduce bleeding).

Intramuscular and subcutaneous

Both intramuscular and subcutaneous routes avoid the need for intravenous access, the effects of first-pass metabolism and the rapid increases in plasma drug concentration seen with i.v. boluses. However, differences in regional blood flow to the skin and to muscles affects absorption unpredictably. Intramuscular administration can be particularly painful.

Variations in absorption may be clinically relevant. For example, peak plasma concentrations of morphine may occur at any time from 5 to 60 minutes after intramuscular administration, resulting in unreliable analgesia.

Intravenous

The intravenous characteristics of drugs vary depending on whether they are given as a bolus or as fixed, variable rate or target controlled infusions. Using the intravenous induction agent propofol as an example, the effects of these modes are described in Fig. 1.11 and in the following sections.

Bolus

The majority of drugs used in anaesthetic practice are given by intravenous bolus. This is a convenient and rapid method of drug delivery. However, it requires intravenous access. Plasma concentrations of propofol rise rapidly after intravenous bolus administration. This results in a fast onset of clinical effect because the propofol crosses the blood–brain

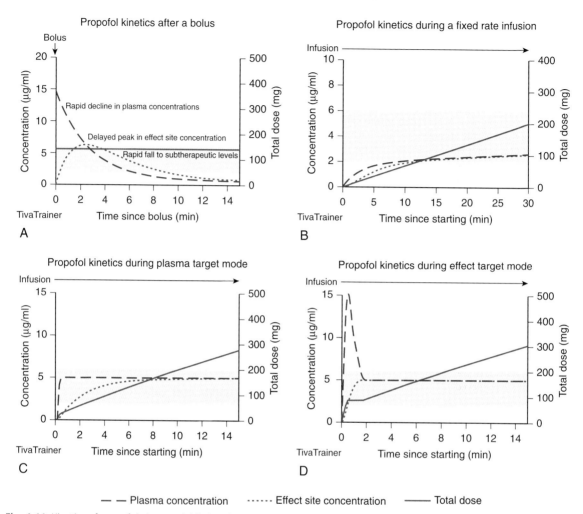

Fig. 1.11 Kinetics of propofol given as (A) bolus, (B) fixed rate infusion, (C) target controlled Schnider plasma concentration or (D) target controlled Schnider effect site. All data are for a 70-kg man, targeted at 5 mcg ml⁻¹. Therapeutic range shaded. (Data derived from Tivatrainer Simulation Software, Gutta BV, Aerdenhout, the Netherlands.)

barrier rapidly with its concentration gradient to reach its effect site. Plasma concentration falls quickly with offset of clinical effect as the drug redistributes (see Fig. 1.11A). As propofol is highly lipid soluble, offset is rapid and occurs because of redistribution from the effect site. Overshoot is a concern following bolus administration of drugs with a narrow therapeutic index. Therefore it is an important general rule that drugs administered intravenously should be given slowly and titrated to effect, except where there is a clinical need such as in rapid sequence induction.

Plasma concentration after an intravenous bolus dose is determined by the dose, speed of injection and cardiac output. Therefore an elderly, sick or hypovolaemic patient

undergoing intravenous induction of anaesthesia is likely to suffer significant side effects if the drug is given at the same dose or rate as would be used in a normal, healthy young adult.

Infusions

Fixed-rate infusions

Drugs may be given by constant-rate infusion, a method often used for propofol, neuromuscular blocking agents, opioids and many other drugs. Plasma concentrations achieved during fixed rate infusions may be described by a wash-in exponential curve (see Fig. 1.11B).

When starting or adjusting an infusion rate, a steady state plasma concentration is achieved within four to five plasma half-lives for the individual drug. As $t_{1/2}$ is the main factor influencing time to achieve steady state, use of fixed rate infusion for drugs with a short half life can avoid significant accumulation and achieve steady state rapidly. During and after infusion, drugs equilibrate between central and peripheral compartments through redistribution. To maintain a steady state plasma concentration, therefore, the rate of drug infusion must be equal to the rate of removal through redistribution and elimination. However, the clinical effect is determined by $t_{1/2}\ k_{e0}$, which relates to effect site concentration rather than plasma concentration.

The rate of a fixed infusion required to achieve a given steady state plasma concentration is dependent on drug clearance (Eq. 1.12).

$$Rate\ of\ Infusion = Cl \times C_{SS} \qquad \text{(Eq. 1.12)}$$

Eq. 1.12 shows the relationship between clearance and steady-state concentration for drugs delivered via infusions at a given rate, where C_{ss} is the steady state plasma concentration.

Many pathological conditions reduce drug clearance and may therefore result in unexpectedly high plasma concentrations during infusions. Half-life does not influence C_{ss}, only how quickly it is achieved.

Total intravenous anaesthesia and target controlled infusions

Total intravenous anaesthesia (TIVA) refers to the practice of administering anaesthesia via a continuous intravenous infusion, commonly either as fixed rate or via a computer-controlled pump. TIVA algorithms are designed to achieve and maintain a steady-state plasma or effect site concentration, by administering an initial bolus followed by an infusion (see Fig. 1.11B–D). Target controlled infusions deliver the drug according to pharmacokinetic models to give a predicted plasma or effect site concentration based on assumptions about compartment size, clearance and the effects of redistribution based on equations 1.13–1.16 below.

$$\frac{Dose}{Volume} = Concentration \qquad \text{(Eq. 1.13)}$$

$$Dose = Volume \times Concentration \qquad \text{(Eq. 1.14)}$$

$$Loading\ dose = V_{DSS} \times Plasma\ concentration \qquad \text{(Eq. 1.15)}$$

$$Infusion\ rate = Cl \times Plasma\ concentration \qquad \text{(Eq. 1.16)}$$

Pharmacokinetic models are drug specific and tailored to adults or children. Models in common use include include Marsh, Schnider and Paedfusor (propofol), and Minto (remifentanil). Models exist for adult and for paediatric

practice to take into account the differences in compartment size and physiology. These allow targeting to effect site (C_e) or plasma (C_p) concentration.

The Schnider model is used for propofol infusions and uses a fixed central compartment volume of 4.7 l. Volumes of the other compartments, the rate constants and elimination rate constant are determined by age, weight and lean body mass as calculated by the pump's algorithm. When running in C_P mode (see Fig. 1.11C), a small initial bolus is given, followed by an infusion, whereas in C_e mode (see Fig. 1.11D), the bolus is larger to account for equilibration with the effect site. In both modes there is a lag between the increase in plasma concentration and effect site concentration because of the time taken for equilibration. The time to peak effect is related to the half-life.

Context-sensitive half-time

Following administration by an infusion, the drug will have redistributed into more peripheral compartments to a variable extent, depending on its V_D, clearance and the duration of the infusion. When the infusion is stopped, the drug redistributes along concentration gradients, back into the plasma and effect sites. Hence the offset of clinical effect can be unpredictable, as it depends on the dose, duration of infusion, intrinsic properties of the drug and factors such as metabolism and organ function. Predictably, a drug with high V_D and high intrinsic clearance should have a similar half-life to a drug with low V_D and clearance – however, this is not the case. Therefore the context-sensitive half-time (CSHT) gives a realistic model for drug behaviour after prolonged infusion.

Context-sensitive half-time is defined as the time taken for the plasma concentration to decrease by half after stopping an infusion designed to maintain a steady-state concentration; CSHT allows some prediction of how long drug effects persist after an infusion is stopped.

Comparing the opioids fentanyl, remifentanil, alfentanil and morphine (Fig. 1.12) illustrates some aspects of their clinical pharmacology in practice. The CSHTs for fentanyl and morphine increase steadily with infusion duration, whereas the increase for alfentanil is shallower and plateaus. Remifentanil has a fixed, flat CSHT irrespective of infusion duration.

Remifentanil is rapidly broken down by non-specific esterases, resulting in a short CSHT independent of infusion duration. Fentanyl is highly lipid soluble and has high intrinsic clearance. However, the very large V_D at steady state results in significant accumulation after infusion or repeated boluses. Therefore, prolonged infusion of fentanyl can result in delayed offset. The pKa and relative insolubility of alfentanil result in a smaller V_D and a lower CSHT, although there is some accumulation and delayed offset after an infusion because intrinsic clearance of the drug is low. Morphine accumulates, and offset is further delayed

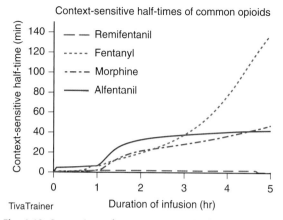

Context-sensitive half-times of common opioids

— — Remifentanil
----- Fentanyl
-·-·- Morphine
——— Alfentanil

TivaTrainer

Fig. 1.12 Comparison of context-sensitive half-times for remifentanil, fentanyl, morphine and alfentanil. All data are for a 70-kg man. (Data derived from Tivatrainer Simulation Software, Gutta BV, Aerdenhout, the Netherlands.)

after a sustained infusion because of a large V_D, which is not overcome by a relatively high clearance.

Rectal

The rectal route negates first-pass metabolism and may be used where the enteral route is unavailable. It is used in children and adults (e.g. for delivery of paracetamol, diclofenac or ibuprofen) for postoperative analgesia. The proportion of drug absorbed via this route is highly variable.

Transdermal

Drugs with a high lipid solubility and potency may be given transdermally. Drug effects locally or systemically depend on the drug crossing the dermis in sufficient quantities. The drug is either embedded in a patch with a reservoir and membrane to control delivery or in a matrix that promotes slow continuous release.

The most commonly used transdermal medications in anaesthetic practice are the local anaesthetic creams (e.g. lidocaine/prilocaine (EMLA), tetracaine (Ametop)). Here the intent is to allow sufficient transdermal penetration to achieve local anaesthesia, but without causing excessive plasma concentrations. Local absorption is encouraged by use of high concentrations and occlusive dressings.

Glyceryl trinitrate is sometimes administered transdermally for the relief of local vascular insufficiency or for the systemic treatment of ischaemic heart disease. Glyceryl trinitrate is ideal for this indication as it is potent, highly lipid soluble and has a short half-life. Transdermal administration avoids first-pass metabolism and may be used

where the enteral route is unavailable. The stable plasma concentrations afforded by the slow, continuous release of transdermal preparations avoid significant peaks and troughs in plasma concentrations. The favourable pharmacokinetic profile and steady-state kinetics of transdermal administration are useful for opioid analgesics, such as fentanyl, avoiding the nausea and drowsiness associated with a high plasma concentration but maintaining a steady state plasma concentration.

It may take some time before a steady-state plasma concentration is achieved through transdermal administration, and many delivery devices incorporate large amounts of drug in the adhesive layer to provide a loading dose, which reduces this period. At steady state, transdermal delivery has several similarities to intravenous infusion. In contrast to intravenous delivery, on removing the adhesive patch, plasma concentrations may decline relatively slowly because of a depot of drug in the surrounding skin.

Iontophoresis is a technique using the application of an electric current to a transdermal patch to allow charged drug molecules to diffuse through the skin. This allows controlled drug administration (as in a fentanyl patch PCA) and improves the delivery of drugs with poor transdermal absorption.

Inhalation

Drugs are delivered via the inhalational route for their local effects on the lungs, and their systemic effects because of rapid absorption into the bronchial circulation. Drugs acting locally on the bronchial tree are commonly given via this route for bronchodilation or the treatment of inflammatory conditions. Whilst systemic toxicity is reduced, the rich vascular supply to the respiratory tree inevitably leads to systemic absorption.

Inhaled volatile agents are given for systemic effect and are discussed elsewhere. Opioids such as fentanyl and diamorphine may be given as nebulised solutions, but this technique is not routine.

Epidural

Epidural delivery is a common route of administration in anaesthetic practice for central neuraxial effect. The epidural space is highly vascular, and significant amounts of drug may be absorbed systemically, even if inadvertent intravenous administration is avoided. Opioids diffuse across the dura to act on spinal opioid receptors, but much of their action when given via the epidural route is the result of systemic absorption. Complications of this route include epidural haematoma and abscess, inadvertent dural puncture with consequent headache or accidental spinal administration of the drug.

Spinal/Intrathecal (subarachnoid)

When given intrathecally, drugs have free access to the neural tissue of the spinal cord. Small drug doses have profound, rapid effects, an advantage and also a disadvantage of the technique. Protein binding is not a significant factor as CSF protein concentration is relatively low.

Pharmacological variability

Individual responses to medications vary for numerous reasons which require adjustment of drug doses or the use of medications directed at different targets. Causes for individual variable responses may be physiological, pathological or iatrogenic and heritable or acquired.

The changes in drug response with age and in pregnancy are good examples of this. Similarly, the use of concurrent drugs or medications may affect the response to new drugs.

Pathological causes for variability may be acquired (such as obesity) or inherited (such as the variable metabolism seen in mutations of the Cytochrome P450 genes).

The effect of age on pharmacokinetics

There are significant changes in physiology throughout aging, which affects the pharmacokinetics of many medications. Changes in body composition during aging affect the distribution of many drugs, with subsequent, predictable effects on plasma and effect site concentrations, accumulation and onset and offset of action.

The normal ageing process causes a decline in the function of many organs, particularly the kidneys, and therefore drugs dependent on renal clearance may have significantly prolonged effects in the elderly.

The cumulative effects of acquired pathology throughout life can affect the response to various medications.

In the neonatal period, increased total body water and a relatively low proportion of body fat results in high volumes of distribution. Lower concentrations of plasma proteins increase the fraction of unbound, active drug in the plasma. Overall, this results in an increased per-weight dose requirement for most drugs, although those that are highly protein bound may need to be adjusted to account for the increased free drug fraction.

Metabolic pathways and renal elimination are immature in neonates; therefore drugs that are activated by cytochrome P450 are rendered ineffective, and drugs that undergo hepatic clearance, such as midazolam, risk accumulation.

With increasing age there is a general decline in lean body mass and total body water. The proportion of body fat increases in middle age and declines in the elderly. This results in a reduced volume of distribution, thereby increasing plasma concentrations.

Additionally, the age-related decline in renal function results in reduced clearance. The combination of these effects can result in increased plasma concentrations of drugs, requiring dose adjustment.

The combination of increased plasma concentrations with a frailty phenotype and coexistent multisystem decline and development of pathological conditions can result in enhanced response to many medications, necessitating cautious titration, particularly for anaesthetic agents.

The effects of obesity on pharmacokinetics

With increasing total body weight, there is an increase in both lean and fatty mass, although in the obese the majority of the additional weight is due to adipose tissues. This results in an increased volume of distribution for fat-soluble drugs and presents a significant risk of drug accumulation and delayed offset.

Clearance increases linearly with increases in lean body mass, although the excess adiposity of obesity does not reflect any further increase in clearance. Therefore using total body weight for drug dosing may be associated with drug toxicity, and for the majority of drugs, lean body weight is used. The major exceptions to this are suxamethonium and atracurium (dosed by total body weight).

Pharmacogenetics

Pharmacogenetics refers to genetic differences in metabolic pathways which can affect individual responses to drugs, both in terms of therapeutic effect and adverse effects.

Codeine is an example of the importance of pharmacogenetics. As a prodrug, codeine is metabolised to morphine by the cytochrome P450 system (CYP2D6). There are several common genetic variants of this, resulting in inactivation, slow, rapid or ultra-rapid metaboliser phenotypes. Where administered to an individual with an ultra-rapid phenotype, the plasma concentration of morphine and active metabolites after a dose of codeine can result in opioid toxicity. As the cytochrome P450 oxidases are heavily involved in drug metabolism, these variations can result in altered responses to a large number of drugs processed by this system.

The depolarising muscle relaxant suxamethonium is metabolised by butyrylcholinesterase. Genetic variants of this enzyme may show reduced activity; when an individual is homologous for an inhibited enzyme, the duration of action of suxamethonium is significantly prolonged.

Drug interactions and adverse drug effects

There are three basic types of drug interaction, pharmaceutical, pharmacokinetic and pharmacodynamic.

Pharmaceutical

In pharmaceutical interactions, drugs mixed in the same syringe or infusion bag react chemically, with adverse results which may include neutralisation, hydrolysis, precipitation. For example, mixing suxamethonium with thiopental (pH 10–11) hydrolyses the former, rendering it inactive. Before mixing drugs, data should be sought on their compatibility to avoid this form of interaction.

Pharmacokinetic

Pharmacokinetic interactions occur where coadministration of drugs affects the processes of absorption, distribution, metabolism or elimination. Absorption of a drug, particularly if given orally, may be affected by other drugs because of their action on gastric emptying (see earlier). Interference with protein binding (see earlier) is a common cause of drug interaction. Drug metabolism is discussed in some detail and there are many potential sites in this process where interactions can occur (e.g. competition for enzyme systems, enzyme inhibition or induction).

Pharmacodynamic

Pharmacodynamic interactions are the competing or additive observed effects of coadministered drugs, and are the most common type of interaction in anaesthetic practice. A typical anaesthetic is a series of pharmacodynamic interactions. These may be adverse (e.g. increased respiratory depression with opioids and volatile agents) or advantageous (e.g. reversal of muscle relaxation with neostigmine). An understanding of the many subtle pharmacodynamic interactions in modern anaesthesia accounts for much of the difference in the quality of anaesthesia and recovery associated with the experienced compared with the novice anaesthetist.

Adverse drug reactions

Adverse drug reactions are described as A or B, representing augmented or idiosyncratic reactions, respectively. Type A reactions are related to an increase in the expected pharmacological effect of a drug, which may either relate to the desired effect (e.g. prolonged muscle relaxation) or undesirable effects (e.g. nausea and vomiting from opioids). These are often dose related and are common. Sometimes individual drug variability may result in an increase in the expected drug effect – such as an enhanced codeine effect for fast-metabolising individuals expressing rapid or ultra-rapid CYP450 mutations.

Type B reactions are idiosyncratic and unrelated to the expected properties of a drug. These include immune and idiopathic reactions. Examples include anaphylactoid reactions seen with morphine and atracurium and malignant hyperthermia in susceptible individuals exposed to volatile anaesthetic agents or suxamethonium.

Chapter | 2 |

Data, statistics and clinical trials

Iain Moppett

S tatistics is the science of learning from data – from collection and organisation through to analysis, presentation and dissemination. Like all sciences, it has its own vocabulary and can sometimes appear somewhat impenetrable to the uninitiated. This chapter gives an overview of statistical processes and methods, but readers are advised to consult more detailed texts on medical statistics for further information.

Whenever data are collected, in a more or less systematic fashion, statistics can be produced: How many things? What size? How old? The science of statistics is concerned with turning this information into something useful. Generally, this is either to *describe* the things we are measuring or to make some *inference* or *prediction* from them. Often within medicine there is a question attached – commonly of the form, 'Is one group somehow different from another group?'

Types of data

The type of data collected makes a big difference to what can be done with them using statistics.

At the most basic level, it is fairly straightforward to count things. How many patients died? How many were sick after surgery? How many of the patients who were sick were women? Sometimes these are simple categories with no order or value. Apples and oranges are not usually described as better or larger than the other. They are just *categories* or *names* of fruit. Male/female; blood groups A/B/O – these are all simple *categorical* or *nominal* data. The categories may be somewhat arbitrarily defined, with the possibility of overlap. Clear **rules** are therefore needed to define what goes in which category.

Sometimes the categories may have an *order* – mild/moderate/severe pain has a natural order as does easy/

difficult/impossible mask ventilation. These are called *ordinal* data. Some of these data lend themselves to having numbers attached, but these numbers are no more than labels for ordinal data. The Glasgow Outcome Scale has five categories, from 1 (dead) through to 5 (good recovery). Clearly, 1 is a worse outcome than 5, but there is no suggestion that the intervals between the numbers are the same. However, because the data have an order, the median value has some meaning. The special cases of rating scales (such as pain and anxiety scales) are discussed later.

Data that correspond to measurements of physical constructs are usually amenable to the use of *interval* and *ratio* scales. An interval scale is an ordered sequence of numbers in which there is a constant interval between each point in the scale. For instance, the difference in temperature between $1\,°C$ and $2\,°C$ is the same as between $101\,°C$ and $102\,°C$. However, the zero point is arbitrary, so ratios are not appropriate – $100\,°C$ is not twice as hot as $50\,°C$. A ratio scale is a type of interval scale where there is a true zero – negative numbers cannot exist. For example, there is no temperature below 0 Kelvin, and there is no such thing as a negative length. This does allow ratios to be used; 100 Kelvin is twice as hot as 50 Kelvin, and someone who is 2 m tall is twice the height of someone who is 1 m tall. Interval and ratio data can be described using the mean, although this may not always be appropriate.

Summarising data

When describing data, it is often helpful to have some idea of a representative value – the *average*, in common parlance. In statistical terms, this is a value that describes the central tendency of a set of data. In general there are three types of average: mean, median and mode. Within this chapter the term *average* is used commonly and deliberately to encompass any of these.

- *Mode* is simply the commonest value. It is used for categorical data.
- *Median* is the middle value (or halfway between the two middle values if there is an even number of data points). It is used for ordinal data.
- *Mean* is the representative value used for interval data. The arithmetic mean is most commonly used, but it is only one of three Pythagorean means, the other two being the geometric and harmonic means.

Arithmetic mean (AM) is the sum of all the values divided by the number (n) of values ($x_1 \ldots x_n$). In algebraic notation:

$$AM = \frac{1}{n} \sum_{i=1}^{n} x_i = \frac{x_1 + x_2 + \cdots + x_n}{n}$$

The *geometric mean* (GM) is found by multiplying all the numbers together and then taking the nth root.

$$GM = \sqrt[n]{\prod_{i=1}^{n} x_i} = \sqrt[n]{x_1 x_2 \cdots x_n}$$

The geometric mean is used when factors have a multiplicative effect and we want to find the average effect of these. It is most commonly used in finance (average interest rates) but is used in medicine when the mean of logarithmically transformed values is used.

The *harmonic mean* (HM) is the rather wordy reciprocal of the arithmetic mean of the reciprocals of the values.

$$HM = \frac{1}{\frac{1}{n} \sum_{i=1}^{n} \frac{1}{x_i}} = \frac{n}{\frac{1}{x} + \frac{1}{x_2} + \cdots \frac{1}{x_n}}$$

It is the most appropriate mean for comparing rates (such as speeds) or ratios. It is also used when calculating the effect of parallel resistances.

There are some other special means, of which the root mean square (RMS) or *quadratic mean* (QM) is perhaps the most widely quoted.

$$QM = \sqrt{\frac{1}{n}(x_1^2 + x_2^2 + \cdots + x_i^2)}$$

This is used to describe the average value of a varying quantity such as sine waves. Most notably it is the method used to describe the average voltage of an AC current.

The means give some idea of the typical value, but it is usually helpful to have some idea of the *spread* of the values. At the simplest level, the range, or maximum and minimum, give an idea of the spread. Similarly, the interquartile range (25th and 75th centiles) describes the middle 50% of the dataset. The standard deviation (SD)

is a useful description of the variation around the mean because it can be manipulated in statistical tests. It is defined as the square root of the variance. If we have data from the whole population (which is relatively uncommon), then the population SD is:

$$\sigma = \sqrt{\frac{1}{N} \sum_{i=1}^{N} (x_i - \mu)^2}$$

where N is the number of items in the population, and μ is the population mean.

If we only have a sample, then the sample SD is given by:

$$s = \sqrt{\frac{1}{N-1} \sum_{i=1}^{N} (x_i - \bar{x})^2}$$

where $\bar{x}$ is the sample mean.

The use of $N-1$ rather than N is known as Bessel's correction and is needed to account for the fact that the sample SD is less accurate than that of the whole population. Clearly, as the sample becomes larger, the effect of $N-1$ becomes smaller.

Sampling

It is relatively unusual to measure the whole population of interest because it is usually impractical, expensive and unnecessary. In most situations a sample is taken from the population and the items of interest recorded. Generally it is hoped that the sample represents the total population as closely as possible. If the sample is a truly random selection from the population, then quite robust inferences about the whole population can be made. The randomness of the selection is very important; if the sample is not truly random, then the statistical models used generally do not work well.

Probability

If an event or measurement is variable, then whenever we measure it, it could have one of a range of values. Probability is simply the proportion of times that the value (or range of values) occurs. Probability is the chance of something occurring and always lies between 1 (always occurs) and 0 (never occurs). If one out of every hundred people is allergic to penicillin, then the probability of meeting someone allergic to penicillin is 1 in 100, or 0.01.

The probabilities of exclusive events are additive, and the sum of all mutually exclusive probabilities must always equal 1. In other words, if the probability of the patients on the emergency theatre list being from gynaecology wards is 0.3 and the probability of them being from general surgical wards is 0.5, then the probability of them being from neither specialty is 0.2 (*1 – (0.3 + 0.5)*). If probabilities are independent (i.e. the probability of one event is not affected by the outcome of another), then they can be multiplied. For instance, the probability of a general surgical patient being female might be 0.6, in which case the probability of meeting a female general surgical patient on the list would be 0.5 × 0.6 = 0.3. Sometimes we are interested in relative probabilities; what is the chance of something occurring in one group compared with the chance of something occurring in another group? There are various methods used to describe this, which are discussed later in this chapter.

Data distributions

Often, there is apparently random variation in events or processes. If we toss a coin, it falls randomly either heads or tails; similarly, a dice will land on any number between one and six at random. If we measure the weights of children attending for surgery, they will vary at random around some central value. The probability of any one value, or range of values, is described by the *probability distribution*. Although medicine often refers to the *normal*, or *Gaussian*, distribution, this is only one of many possible probability distributions.

Uniform distributions

The mean value from a six-sided dice throw is 3.5; if you throw the dice many times and add up the total score and divide by the number of throws, it will be close to 3.5. However, the probability of throwing numbers close to the mean (3 or 4) is the same as the probability of throwing numbers at the extremes (1 or 6). In fact, the probability of any number is the same (1 in 6) – a *uniform distribution*. Uniform distributions are used to generate random numbers – the chance of any particular value is the same. In theory the probability of being on call on a particular day is also a uniform distribution, provided there are no special rules.

Non-uniform distributions

Most biological data come from non-uniform distributions. Often, these are centred on the average, and the probability of a particular value is greater if it is closer to the average. Extreme values are possible but less likely. The most well-known of these non-uniform distributions is the *normal distribution* – so called because most normal events or processes approximate to it (or can be transformed in some

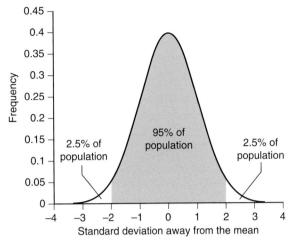

Fig. 2.1 A normal distribution curve, with a mean of zero and standard deviation of one. The unshaded areas which are greater than 1.96 standard deviations above and below the mean each encompass 2.5% of the population. The shaded area (mean ± 1.96 standard deviations) therefore covers 95% of the population.

way to approximate it). It is also known as the Gaussian distribution after the polymath Carl Friedrich Gauss (also of Gauss lines in MRI). This distribution is defined mathematically based on two values (parameters) – the mean and standard deviations. The probability frequency distribution is a bell-shaped curve. The mode, median and mean are identical, and the degree of spread is governed by the ratio of the SD to the mean. It is important to understand that the normal distribution is only one of an infinite number of bell-shaped curves. A bell-shaped probability distribution is not necessarily normal.

The normal distribution has some useful properties, not least that it is possible to calculate the probability of finding a range of values based solely on the SD (Fig. 2.1). The 97.5th centile of the normal distribution is 1.96 SD away from the mean. Therefore the probability of finding a value more extreme than this (there are two sides to the distribution) is 5%. Conversely, 95% of values, if selected at random, would be expected to be found within ±1.96 SD of the mean. Similarly, 68.3% of values would be expected to be within 1 SD on either side of the mean.

Sometimes, distributions are skewed – the mean, median and mode are not identical. If the long tail is to the right, this is termed a right-skew (or positive skew), and pulled to the left is a left-skew (negative skew). In general, for a left-skew distribution, the mean is less than the median and both are less than the mode. The converse holds for right-skewed distributions (Fig. 2.2).

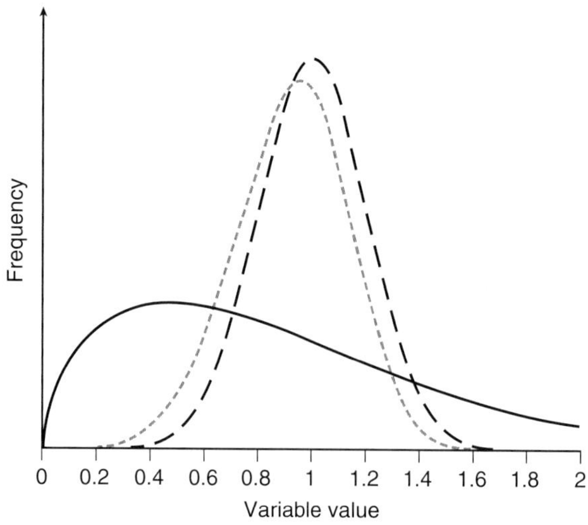

Fig. 2.2 Different types of frequency distribution curve.
——— right/positive skew distribution.
------- Weibull distribution. Note that, although it is bell shaped, it is not a normal distribution.
— — — Normal distribution.

Skew distributions are not so easy to handle with statistical tests, but often the data can be transformed to create a normal distribution. Commonly, taking the logarithm of the data will transform mildly skewed data into a normal distribution.

Chi-squared distribution

The chi-squared distribution (χ^2) is most commonly seen when used as the basis for comparing proportions of observed versus expected events. However, it is also fundamental to the t-test and analysis of variance (ANOVA). It is defined by only a single number; k is the number of degrees of freedom in the data.

Inferring information from a sample

If we were to measure some aspect of a complete population (e.g. the weight of every member of the anaesthetics department), we would be able to state with absolute confidence what the average and spread of that value were. If we measured everyone but one, we would be very confident, but there would be some error in our estimate of the average. If we measured only a few (selected at random), then we would still have an estimate of the average, but we would be less certain still about exactly what it was. Using various statistical tests (see later) we can quantify the degree of confidence that we have in our estimate of the population average.

Bias

All of the previously stated assumptions about sampling from a population assume that the sample is taken at random and is therefore representative of the whole population. However, there are many sources of bias which can invalidate this assumption. Some may be caused by the design of the experiment, some by the behaviour (conscious or unconscious) of the investigator or the subject of the investigation (e.g. a patient or volunteer). No study has ever been conducted without bias somewhere. The role of investigators, regulators, research community, funders and end users of research is to minimise this bias and account for it as far as possible.

Selection bias

Topic selection

The questions asked by researchers are a complex function of their interests and skills, the resources available and their ability to attract sufficient funding. It is widely recognised that there is a distortion of research funding. Pharmaceutical companies have a legitimate interest in research in their product areas, but these may not be the most beneficial for patients overall; charities target their resources, and government funders may sometimes follow political rather than healthcare imperatives.

Population selection

Some patient groups are easier to study than others, but the findings in one patient population may not be applicable to others. Within anaesthesia, this is perhaps most evident in the relative lack of pharmacological studies in the very young and the very old. Similarly, most clinical studies are run from large teaching hospitals, whereas most patients are treated in smaller hospitals. Outcomes are not necessarily the same for these groups – although not always better in the larger hospitals.

Inclusion/exclusion bias

Even if the appropriate population is studied, there is always a risk that the sample itself will be unrepresentative of the population. Some individuals or groups of patients may be more likely to be approached for involvement in a research study, and some may be more likely to consent or refuse.

Methodological bias

Head-to-head comparisons may be deliberately or accidentally set up to favour one group over another. A study of an adequate dose of a new oral opioid compared with a small dose of paracetamol (acetaminophen) is likely to demonstrate better analgesia with the opioid. Other more subtle biases are common in many anaesthesia and pain research studies.

Outcome bias

Detection bias

If an investigator (or patient) has an opinion about the relationship between group membership and outcome, then an outcome may be sought, or reported, more readily in one group than another. This may be conscious or unconscious. Most anaesthetists believe that difficult intubation is more common in pregnant women. A simple survey of difficult intubation is likely to reinforce this finding because this is the group in which cases are most likely to be sought. Similarly, because of preconceptions about the relative effectiveness of regional anaesthesia, a patient who has received regional anaesthesia may be more likely to report good analgesia than one allocated to receive oral analgesics.

Missing outcomes

It is not possible to measure every outcome in a study, so the investigator has to make a decision about which ones to choose. If an important variable is not measured, this may lead to a biased perception of the effects of a treatment.

Reporting bias

Research with positive results is more likely to be published in high-quality journals, and negative studies are less likely to be published at all. Some of this is bias from the journals, and some of it is bias by researchers who choose not to submit negative findings. Occasionally, commercial organisations restrict publication of studies which do not portray a favourable view of their product. The effect of this is that there is a bias in the literature in favour of positive studies. To use a coin tossing example, if researchers only ever published data when they got six or more heads in a row, the literature would soon be awash with data suggesting that the coins were biased. Subtler is the non-reporting of measured outcomes. A study which finds a positive effect in a relatively minor outcome may fail to report a neutral or negative effect on a major outcome. This is extremely hard to detect because it relies on transparency from investigators about what they measured. Outright fraud is still thought to be relatively rare, but there are several high-profile cases of researchers fabricating or manipulating data to fit their beliefs and even publishing studies that never took place.

Testing

Within medicine and anaesthesia, professionals strive to achieve the best outcomes possible for patients. It is therefore very common to ask a question of the form 'Is the outcome in group A better than in group B?' We already know that if we take a sample from a population (e.g. the total population of group A) we will be able to estimate the true population average. If we do the same for group B, this will provide an estimate for population B. Because of simple random variation, the average value for A and B will always be different, provided we measure them with sufficient precision. What we really want to know is how confident we are that any differences that we see are not just due to chance. As shown in Fig. 2.3, if the degree of separation of the two groups is small or the spread of either is relatively large, then there is a reasonable chance that the average estimated for group B could have come from population A. Conversely, if the separation is larger or the spread is smaller, the chance of the estimated average for B being found in population A is small (but never zero).

This is the fundamental principle behind most statistical testing: What is the probability that the result found has occurred simply by chance? Note that this does not mean that the result could definitely *not* have occurred by chance, just that it is sufficiently unlikely to support the hypothesis that the groups really are different. By way of a simple example, the probability of tossing six heads in a row with an unbiased coin is 0.5^6 (0.0156), or 1 in 64. This is by definition unlikely, so you would be suspicious of the coin being biased towards heads. However, it is clearly not impossible and does occur (1 in 64 times, on average).

An important principle with statistical testing is the concept of **paired tests**. There is inherent variability between things being measured – people, times, objects. This variability between things increases the spread of values we might measure, making it harder to demonstrate a difference between groups. However, if we measure the difference within an individual, then the difference may be easier to find. To take a trivial example, if we want to see whether fuel consumption is better with one fuel compared to another, we might take 20 cars with one fuel and compare them with 20 cars with another – an *unpaired* test. However, the 40 cars will all have other factors influencing fuel consumption, and this variability will hinder our ability to detect a difference. If we take 20 cars and test them with both fuels (choosing at random which fuel to test first), then we have a much better chance of demonstrating a difference. A paired test is one in which the results of some intervention are tested within the individuals in the group, not between groups. Within anaesthesia, *paired* tests are relatively unusual

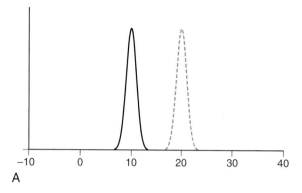

A

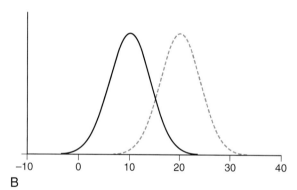

B

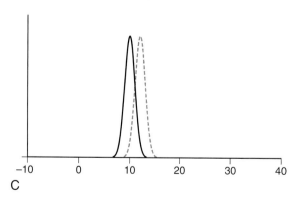

C

Fig. 2.3 The effect of changing mean and standard deviation on overlap of frequency distributions. (A) *Solid line* – mean 10, standard deviation 1; *dotted line* – mean 20, standard deviation 1. (B) *Solid line* – mean 10, standard deviation 4; *dotted line* – mean 20, standard deviation 4. (C) *Solid line* – mean 10, standard deviation 1; *dotted line* – mean 12, standard deviation 1.

because we do not normally have situations in which we can test more than one thing on one individual. There are some examples, such as physiological experiments studying the effects of drugs during anaesthesia.

When data (or their transforms) can be legitimately modelled as coming from a defined probability distribution, they are described as being from a *parametric* distribution. Most commonly, this is the normal distribution, but binomial, Poisson, and Weibull are all defined distributions. Data from undefined probability distributions are *non-parametric*. In general, parametric statistical tests are more powerful than non-parametric tests and so should be used *if appropriate*. Non-parametric tests rely on far fewer assumptions and are considered more robust. They can also be used on parametric data.

Before performing any statistical tests, there are a few simple rules and questions which reduce the likelihood of applying the wrong test or misinterpreting the results.

- What question do you want to answer?
- What type of data do you have? Categorical data require a different approach to ordinal or interval data. Survival analysis, comparison of measurement techniques, and others will require different approaches.
- Plot the data using scatter plots and frequency histograms. Summary statistics may completely hide a skewed distribution or bimodal data.
- Are there any obvious erroneous data? Transcription errors are fairly common, so always check that the data are accurate.
- Are the data paired or unpaired?
- Can a parametric test be used? If not, can the data be transformed so that a parametric test can be used?
- Is there an element of multiple testing?

A flow chart suggesting rules to guide selection of tests is shown in Fig. 2.4. A brief summary of the tests described is given in the next section. The flow chart is not an exhaustive list; there are many other tests and situations not covered, but researchers should always explain if they feel the need to use more obscure approaches.

Chi-squared test

The χ^2 test compares the expected number of events with the actual numbers. Data are tabulated in a *contingency table*; 2×2 tables are the simplest, but larger tables can be used. In general, the number of *degrees of freedom* is the number of columns in the table minus 1 multiplied by the number of rows minus 1 (i.e. for a 2×2 table, the degrees of freedom would be $(2 - 1) \times (2 - 1) = 1$).

$$x^2 = \sum_{i=1}^{n} \frac{(O_i - E_i)^2}{E_i}$$

If the expected frequencies are not known (e.g. 50/50 for male/female), the expected value for each cell (E_i) is

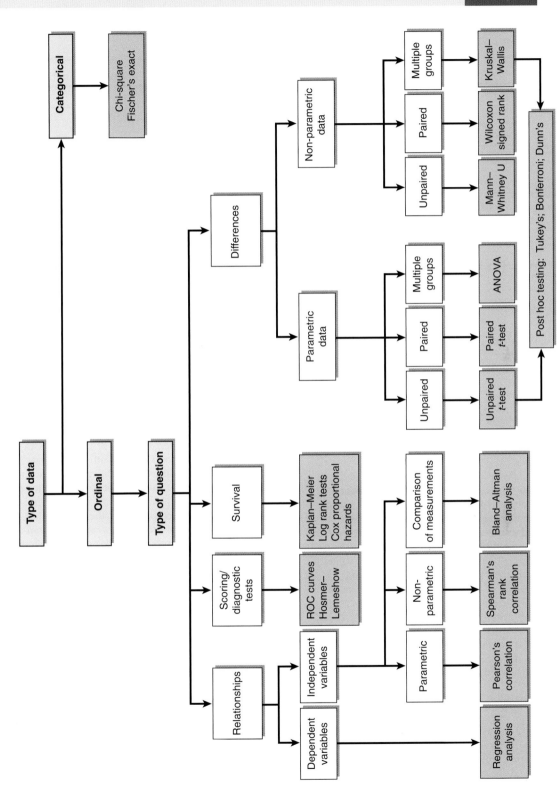

Fig. 2.4 Flow chart suggesting rules to guide selection of statistical tests. *ANOVA*, Analysis of variance; *ROC*, receiver operative characteristic.

Table 2.1 Example of a contingency table for calculation of χ^2

	With treatment	Without treatment	Row marginals
Good outcome	A	B	E = A + B
Bad outcome	C	D	F = C + D
Column marginals	G = A + C	H = B + D	N (total) = A + B + C + D

Table 2.2 A worked example of a contingency table for calculation of χ^2

	WONDER DRUG		PLACEBO		Row marginals
	Observed	Expected	Observed	Expected	
Lived	15	10.9 (21 × 55)/106	6	10.1 (21 × 51)/106	21
Died	40	44.1 (85 × 55)/106	45	40.9 (85 × 51)/106	85
Column marginals	55		51		106

determined by the number of observed events in that cell's row multiplied by the number of events in that cell's column, divided by the total number of events. An example is shown in Table 2.1. The *expected* frequency for cell A is (A + B) × (A + C)/N.

The calculated χ^2 statistic is then compared with a table of probability values for χ^2 for each degree of freedom. This gives a probability that the observed frequencies came from the same population as the expected frequencies.

A worked example is shown in Table 2.2. The *expected* columns are inserted to show the calculations. The basic table is 2 × 2. χ^2 is the sum of the $(O - E)^2/E$ values for each cell:

$$\{(15-10.9)^2/10.9\} + \{(40-44.1)^2/44.1\} +$$
$$\{(6-10.1)^2/10.1\} + \{(45-40.9)^2/40.9\} = 4.0$$

The critical value from the χ^2 tables for $P = .05$ and one degree of freedom is 3.84. The χ^2 is greater than this, making it unlikely that the distribution of data comes from a single population.

There are some standard assumptions with χ^2 tests. There should be sufficient samples; the expected cell counts should all be >5 in 2 × 2 tables or >5 in at least 80% of cells in larger tables. If these conditions are not satisfied, then alternative approaches are used, such as Yates' continuity correction or Fisher's exact test.

Rank tests

If data are ranked in order, then if two groups are sufficiently different, we would expect the sum of these ranks to be much smaller for one group than the other. The bigger the groups, the smaller the difference in the sum of these ranks which we would accept. This concept is the basis for the Wilcoxon signed rank and Mann–Whitney U tests. Essentially the sum of the ranks, corrected for the sample sizes, is compared with a table of probabilities calculated from the *U distribution*. The Wilcoxon signed rank and Mann–Whitney U (or Wilcoxon rank sum) tests are non-parametric tests used for paired or independent (unpaired) samples, respectively. Because these rank tests do not perform any statistical tests on the values themselves, they are robust to the presence of outliers. It does not matter how extreme a particular value is; only its rank is important.

t-Tests

Provided that the data approximate closely enough to a normal distribution, t-tests provide a powerful method for assessing differences between two groups. Unlike the rank tests, the t distribution uses the data values themselves – the calculation uses the mean, standard deviations and sample sizes of the two groups. Again, although it can be done by hand, it is more robust to use one of the myriad statistical software packages available.

Rating scales are extremely popular in anaesthetics research – pain, nausea, satisfaction and anxiety are all commonly measured using verbal, numerical or visual analogue scales. The safest way to analyse these is using non-parametric statistical tests because these avoid any assumptions about the interval between points. However, in practice, many researchers assume the data behave as though normally distributed and analyse them using t-tests.

Multiple testing

Sometimes we may want to look for differences between multiple groups or at multiple times within groups. In this case the obvious answer might be to perform several tests. However, this leads to a problem about probability. If we had three groups (A, B, C), there would be three comparisons: A–B, A–C and B–C. The chance of obtaining a positive finding purely by chance is now rather greater. As the number of comparisons increases, the number of chance findings will inevitably increase. If we perform 20 experiments, we would expect one of these to be positive with $P < .05$ purely by chance.

There are numerous approaches to this problem. One is simply to correct the overall P value, so that it remains correct, by adjusting the P values for the individual tests. This is the principle of the *Bonferroni correction*. This is simple to calculate (the P value for each comparison is approximated by the overall P value divided by the number of comparisons), but it may be too conservative in some situations. An alternative approach, which is widely used (and abused), is to employ the family of statistical tests known as *ANOVA* (ANalysis Of VAriance). When properly constructed, ANOVA can provide information about the likelihood of significant variation between or within groups. ANOVA requires various assumptions about the distribution of the data, including normality. The non-parametric equivalent is the *Kruskal–Wallis* test. When applied to two groups, ANOVA is a t-test and Kruskal–Wallis a Mann–Whitney U. If these tests suggest a significant difference, there are various *post hoc* tests used to identify where the difference lies without falling foul of the multiple testing issues described earlier. Tukey's honestly significant difference is commonly used in medical research.

Relationship testing

Sometimes, rather than asking the question of whether groups are different, we want to know how certain factors relate to each other. When there are several variables, tests from the family of regression techniques are used, of which *logistic regression* is the best known. Essentially, the strength of association between a set of variables (e.g. age, sex, presence of active malignancy) and an outcome (e.g. length of stay in intensive care) is tested. It is important to note that association does not imply causation, and if important variables are left out, then erroneous conclusions can be drawn. For example, yellow staining of the fingers is associated with the diagnosis of lung cancer but is not the cause.

Sometimes a more straightforward relationship is sought. How does weight vary with age in children? Correlation statistics give an idea of the strength of such an association; in other words, how much scatter around the expected value we might expect. To take the example of children's weight and height, there is a reasonable correlation – hence the various formulae for estimation of children's weight. However, there is considerable scatter from other factors – nutrition, genetic predisposition, sex – so the correlation is not perfect.

The most commonly used correlation analysis is *Pearson's* or *least squares correlation*. This gives an estimated equation predicting one variable (y) from another (x) (of the form $y = mx + c$) and a correlation coefficient (R^2) – a summary statistic of how close the variables lie to this predicted line. Truly random association would have a correlation coefficient of 0 and perfect association, 1.

This approach is insensitive to changes in scale of either variable. This is to be expected – the correlation between height and weight should be the same regardless of whether metric or imperial units are used. However, this does mean that correlation can tell us nothing about whether the prediction of one value from another is accurate – only that as one increases, the other increases by a similar relative amount. Second, the statistical interpretation of R^2 is determined by the sample size. A large sample may have low (near zero) R^2 but still have a statistically significant association between the two variables. The shape of the relationship is important – always look at the data. As seen in Fig. 2.5, curvilinear relationships may have apparently reasonable correlations. A similar approach can be taken to correlations between non-parametric data using *Spearman's rank correlation*.

Comparison of techniques

It is relatively common for anaesthetists to wish to find out whether measurements taken with one device are interchangeable with those from another. For instance, is cardiac output measured by pulse contour analysis equivalent to that obtained by thermodilution? Correlation describes the relationship between two set of measurements – does one increase as the other increases? – but does not adequately describe the accuracy of the technique. This is more appropriately done using the Bland–Altman technique (Fig. 2.6).

Paired measurements of the variable of interest are taken, such as cardiac output with bolus thermodilution (A) and a new monitor (B). The mean of these values ($(A + B)/2$) is plotted against the difference (A – B). The mean difference between the measurements is the *bias*. The *limits of agreement* are usually defined as the bias ± 1.96 SD of the differences.

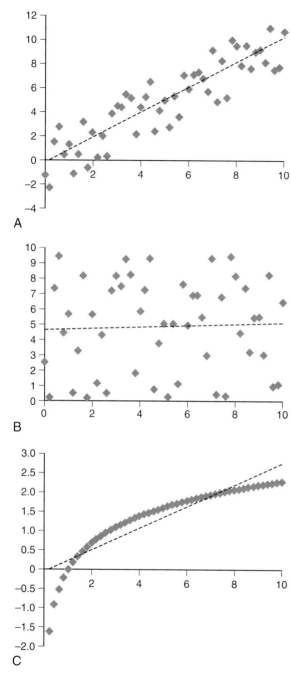

Fig. 2.5 Linear regression. Scatter plots of two possibly related variables. The lines show the calculated regression lines. (A) Reasonably well correlated data. $R^2 = 0.8$. (B) Data with no correlation at all. $R^2 \approx 0$. (C) Data which shows reasonable correlation ($R^2 = 0.83$) though in fact are better fitted by a non-linear relationship (logarithmic in this case).

It should be noted that these *limits of agreement* are purely descriptive. They do not define what is clinically acceptable – that is a matter for the investigator to justify. Often these limits of agreement are described as percentages of the overall mean value.

Within medicine, there is usually not a true gold standard against which to compare a new device. There is inaccuracy even in the best devices compared with the true value (e.g. real cardiac output). This has important implications for evaluating new devices. A perfect new device would inevitably have some degree of variation compared with current devices. Two devices of equivalent accuracy, when compared with each other, would be expected to have wider limits of agreement than each alone. An example of this is the comparison of thermodilution and other methods of estimating cardiac output. The error for thermodilution against true cardiac output is around 20%. If a new technique has similar accuracy, then the limits of agreement for the two devices compared would be expected to be around 30%. The Bland–Altman approach was originally designed for single pairs of measurements from multiple subjects. Corrections are required if the approach is used with multiple measurements from the same subject.

Predictive testing and scoring systems

In clinical practice, anaesthetists often use some form of test to predict the presence or absence of a certain condition, such as difficult tracheal intubation, malignant hyperthermia or postoperative mortality. In an ideal world the tests available would be completely accurate, cheap, quick and easy to apply in normal practice. Unfortunately, none of the tests we use meets these criteria. The degree to which the available tests match these criteria dictate how we should use them.

Test accuracy

There are several interrelated characteristics of a diagnostic test. *Sensitivity* is calculated as the proportion of those with a condition *(true positives)* who are correctly identified by the test. Therefore a *sensitive* test identifies all individuals with the condition, and if a highly sensitive test is negative, it is unlikely that an individual will have the condition. This is usually at the expense of incorrectly identifying individuals who do not actually have the condition *(false positives)*. Conversely, *specificity* is calculated as the proportion of those without a condition *(true negatives)* who are correctly identified by the test. Hence a highly *specific* test identifies only those individuals who definitely have the condition of interest – the false positive rate is low; the trade-off is

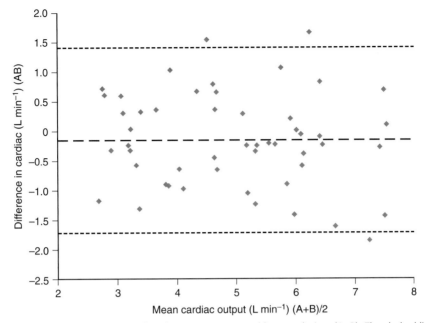

Fig. 2.6 Bland–Altman plot. Hypothetical data of cardiac output measured by two devices (A, B). The *dashed line* represents the bias (mean difference), the *dotted lines* represent the upper and lower 95% limits of agreement between the two devices. Note that in this example both devices were given a 20% error. The combined limits of agreement are approximately 30%.

that individuals with the condition may be missed *(false negatives).*

A well-used memory rule for these is *Spin and Snout* – a positive *SPecific* test rules an individual *IN (they have the condition)*; a negative *SeNsitive* test rules them *OUT (they don't have the condition).* However, this should be used with caution, as the usefulness of a test depends on both sensitivity and specificity.

The *positive predictive value* (PPV) of a test is the probability that an individual with a positive test result actually has the condition of interest. The *negative predictive value* is the probability that an individual with a negative test is truly free of the condition. It is extremely important to realise that the positive and negative predictive values of tests depend upon the prevalence of the condition in the population as well as the accuracy of the test technique itself. To take an extreme example, over-the-counter pregnancy tests have very high positive and negative predictive values for detecting pregnancy in women of childbearing age. The negative predictive value is actually higher in men (there are no false negatives), but the positive predictive value is zero (positive tests will occur, but there are no pregnant men). The sensitivity and specificity of the test itself are unchanged. Examples are given in Tables 2.3–2.5.

Often diagnostic tests are not truly dichotomous (yes *vs.* no). Rather, some threshold value is used. As this threshold varies, so the sensitivity and specificity of the test varies. To take the pregnancy test example again, the higher the concentration of β–human chorionic gonadotropin (hCG) required for a positive test, the greater the specificity, but at the loss of sensitivity.

This trade-off was investigated systematically in the development of aircraft radar systems, which were monitored by receiver-operators. At one end of the scale, all objects will be identified (aeroplanes and birds), a highly sensitive threshold, but at the cost of a lack of specificity, resulting in a lot of false positives. At the other end of the scale, a positive signal will almost certainly be an aeroplane – very specific, but at the cost of missing quite a few planes. This can be assessed statistically using the so-called receiver operating characteristic curves – usually shortened to ROC curves (Fig. 2.7).

These plot the false positive rate (1 – specificity) against the true positive rate (sensitivity). A near ideal test would form a right angle. A test which was no better than tossing a coin would lie on the line of identity. Most tests, of course, lie somewhere in between. Various summary statistics can be derived from ROC curves. The most common is the area under the curve (AUC). A perfect discriminant curve has an AUC of 1; a non-discriminatory test AUC is 0.5. There is no consensus for acceptable AUC, but 0.9–1.0 is considered excellent, 0.8–0.9 good and <0.6 poor. The point on the curve closest to the top left corner (false positive rate 0, true positive rate 1) is sometimes viewed as the best trade-off

Table 2.3 Sensitivity, specificity, positive (PPV) and negative (NPV) predictive values

		Disease positive						
		Yes	No	Totals				
Test positive	Yes	A	B	A + B	Sensitivity	A/(A + C)	PPV	A/(A + B)
	No	C	D	C + D	Specificity	B/(B + D)	NPV	D/(C + D)
	Totals	A + C	B + D	A + B + C + D	Prevalence	(A + C)/(A + B + C + D)		
Test positive	Yes	True positive	False positive (type I error)		Sensitivity	True positives/ all disease positive	PPV	True positive/ all test positives
	No	False negative (type II error)	True negative		Specificity	True negatives/ all disease negative	NPV	True negative/ all test negatives

Table 2.4 Effect of changing prevalence on results

		True cholinesterase deficiency						
A: General population		Yes	No	Total				
Cholinesterase activity test	Yes	9	50	59	Sensitivity	0.33	PPV	0.15
	No	18	2000	2018	Specificity	0.98	NPV	0.99
	Totals	27	2050	2077	Prevalence	1.3%		
B: Family history of cholinesterase deficiency								
		Yes	No					
Cholinesterase activity test	Yes	9	5	14	Sensitivity	0.33	PPV	0.64
	No	18	200	218	Specificity	0.98	NPV	0.92
	Totals	27	205	232	Prevalence	12%		

In the two groups (A, a general population; B, a group with a known family history of cholinesterase deficiency), the prevalences of cholinesterase deficiency are 1.3% and 12%. The tests' sensitivity and specificity are unchanged, but the positive and negative predictive values are different.
NPV, Negative predictive value; *PPV,* positive predictive value.

between sensitivity and specificity, but in practice the thresholds used for diagnostic tests are influenced by wider costs (of the test, of subsequent intervention or further testing and of false negatives).

Risk scoring

In peri-operative medicine, we are often interested in estimating the risk of an event occurring. This is slightly different from diagnostic testing. The question is not whether a person has a certain condition, but what is the risk (probability) of an event (such as death, postoperative nausea and vomiting (PONV), morbidity) occurring. Such systems are useful for discussions with patients and relatives, helping to plan treatments (e.g. critical care, PONV prophylaxis), benchmarking outcomes against self or others and designing research studies.

There are various approaches to creation of such scoring systems. First, predictor variables are chosen based on some combination of investigator opinion, clinical experience and previous or ongoing research. The strength of association between the variables and the outcome of interest is assessed, often using logistic regression, in a development cohort. This may then allow creation of a score whereby relative

Table 2.5 Effect of changing tests on sensitivity and specificity

		Difficult Intubation						
		Yes	No	Totals				
Previous difficult intubation	Yes	7	2	9	Sensitivity	0.14 (7/50)	PPV	0.78 (7/9)
	No	43	1148	1191	Specificity	0.998 (1148/1150)	NPV	0.96 (1148/1191)
	Totals	50	1150	1200				
Mallampati 3–4	Yes	39	168	207	Sensitivity	78	PPV	0.19
	No	11	982	993	Specificity	85	NPV	0.99
	Totals	50	1150	1200				

These data show that, within the same population, some tests are more specific and less sensitive (previous history of difficult intubation), whereas others may be more sensitive (higher Mallampati score).
NPV, Negative predictive value; *PPV*, positive predictive value.
(Data from Arné, J., Descoins, P., Fusciardi, J., Ingrand, P., Ferrier, B., Boudigues, D., Ariès, J. (1998) Preoperative assessment for difficult intubation in general and ENT surgery: Predictive value of a clinical multivariate risk index. *British Journal of Anaesthesia*. 80 (2), 140–146.)

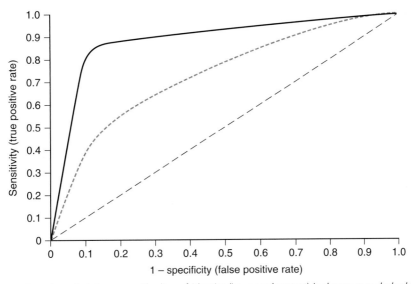

Fig. 2.7 Receiver operating characteristic curves. The line of identity (i.e. a useless test) is shown as a *dashed line*. The *dotted line* shows a moderately discriminatory test (AUC = 0.73), whereas the *solid line* is rather better (AUC = 0.88). *AUC*, Area under the curve.

values (points) are ascribed to each of the variables and summed to create an overall score. The ability of the score to identify risk correctly should then be tested against a separate validation cohort and, ideally, against a cohort from outside the original research population. The most common method of assessing the *calibration* of scoring systems is to use the *Hosmer–Lemeshow* test. This is an application of the χ^2 test using the observed and predicted outcomes in the population.

Survival analysis

Rather than looking at events at a specific time interval, we sometimes wish to investigate the effects over time (e.g.

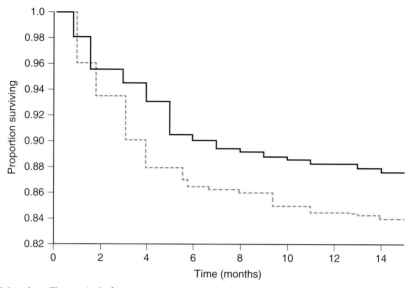

Fig. 2.8 Kaplan–Meier plots. The survival of two groups over time is shown. Each vertical step represents an event. Early on, random variation means that it is not possible to discern the difference in survival between the two groups.

disease-free survival after different types of cancer surgery or death after different modes of anaesthesia). These are usually analysed using *Kaplan–Meier* plots (Fig. 2.8) and differences between groups assessed using *log rank* or *Cox proportional hazards* tests. The number of survivors (as a proportion of the at-risk population) is plotted against time. Note that the at-risk population becomes smaller as the time horizon becomes longer because fewer individuals are available for follow-up. *Log rank tests* assess the overall difference between survival curves when there are discrete groups (e.g. regional anaesthesia *vs.* general anaesthesia). *Cox proportional hazards* are used for estimating the effect of continuous variables (such as gene expression) on risk.

Types of error

Most statistical questions can be framed with a so-called *null hypothesis*. This is a statement of the form 'There is no difference between A and B'. Experiments are designed to test this hypothesis. If the set of observations obtained are sufficiently unlikely to have occurred were the null hypothesis true, then the null hypothesis is *rejected*. Conversely, if there is insufficient evidence to reject the null hypothesis, then the experiment has *failed to reject* it. The null hypothesis is never proven. There are two important consequences of this approach. First, the results are degrees

of uncertainty; a finding that is unlikely is not impossible. Second, statistically significant results do not imply clinically significant results. Clinical research is awash with small but statistically significant differences that are of no clinical relevance.

The whole of this chapter has been predicated on the idea that statistics give some idea of the probability of an event occurring by chance. This has led statisticians to describe two classical types of statistical error, although more have been proposed.

Type I error or α *error* is the probability of a false positive result, falsely rejecting the null hypothesis. It is the probability (*P*) value used to describe the results and is the type of error most familiar to anaesthetists. For mainly pragmatic reasons within medicine, an accepted type I error rate is .05, or 1 in 20. There is no fundamental truth to this value: a study with a reported *P* value of .051 is not really any different to one with a *P* value of .049.

Type II error or β *error* occurs when the null hypothesis is false but fails to be rejected. It is directly related to the power of a study (power = 1 – β). Conventionally, studies have been designed with 80% power – that is, an 80% chance of rejecting the null hypothesis if it truly should be rejected. More recently, there has been a move towards increasing the power of studies. The power of a study is related to the number of participants, the variability in the measurement, the size of difference being sought and the acceptable α error (Fig. 2.9). There are several formulae for

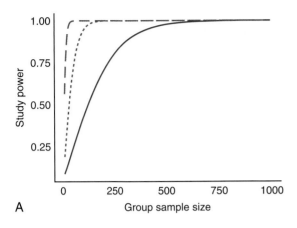

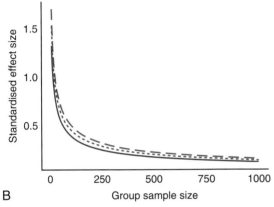

Fig. 2.9 Sample size and power. (A) As the group size increases, the study power increases. The three lines show the impact of the standardised effect size (difference between groups/standard deviation): *red/plain:* 0.25; *green/dotted:* 0.5; *blue/dashed:* 1.0. (B) As group size increases, the standardised effect size that can be detected decreases. The three lines show the impact of the varying study power: *red/plain:* 0.8; *green/dotted:* 0.9; *blue/dashed:* 0.95.

estimating the number of participants required for a given power; a simple one is shown here:

$$n = \frac{2\sigma^2 \left(Z_\beta + Z_{\alpha/2} \right)^2}{\Delta^2}$$

n: sample size for each group

σ: standard deviation of outcome variable

Z_β: standardised value based on the desired power (0.84 for 0.8 power)

Z_α: standardised value based on the desired significance (1.96 for two-sided, α = 0.05)

Δ: clinically significant difference between means

From this, it is straightforward to see that the number of participants needed for a study increases with:
- increasing variability (σ);
- increasing power (Z_β increases as β decreases);
- decreasing type I error (Z_α increases as α decreases);
- smaller clinically significant differences.

Other categories of error

Although not part of the traditional categorisation of type I and II errors, there are other types of conceptual error, all of which occur within medical research:
- *Type III:* correctly rejecting the null hypothesis but for the wrong reason.
- *Type IV:* giving the correct answer to the wrong question.
- *Type V:* solving the right problem in the right way, but too late.

Confidence intervals

Confidence intervals are often misunderstood. The probability attached to a confidence interval (e.g. 95%) refers to the confidence interval itself. So, for a given test or trial, if it were repeated and the 95% confidence interval was computed each time, 95% of the confidence intervals would contain the population mean. This is not the same as saying that the true mean is 95% likely to be within a given confidence interval, even though that is how it is often interpreted. In practical terms, confidence intervals tell us two things:
1. how confident are we with our estimate of some parameter (proportion, mean, sensitivity, correlation, etc.);
2. that if confidence intervals of different groups overlap or cross a value indicating no difference (such as a difference of zero or a ratio of 1), then it is possible that the observed differences have occurred purely by chance.

Bayesian statistics

The preceding paragraphs have largely described so-called frequentist statistical methods. There is a complementary approach that is being seen more often and that probably allies more closely to clinical reasoning. The Bayesian approach (named after Thomas Bayes' work in 1763) is about inferring our current state of uncertainty (beliefs) pertaining to some parameter (such as a proportion or a mean) on the basis of both previous knowledge and new data. The important terms are *prior* – the current knowledge about our beliefs; *likelihood* – what the (new) data tell us about our estimate; and *posterior* – our new beliefs about our parameter, based on the combination of prior and new knowledge.

In simple terms, if a new piece of information (e.g. a trial or diagnostic test) is very discordant with current understanding, then the overall result is that the new understanding (the posterior) is shifted towards, but not all the way to, the new data. Conversely, if our current beliefs are very uncertain, then our new beliefs (the posterior) will be much more strongly influenced by new data. How much our understanding moves is dependent on the degree of uncertainty of both the prior and the likelihood (Fig. 2.10).

This approach is helpful not only for interpreting the results of clinical trials but also clinical tests. If we have a high degree of confidence in a diagnosis already, then clinical tests, particularly if of low certainty, are unlikely to change our belief, regardless of their outcome.

Clinical trials

'A clinical trial is a carefully and ethically designed experiment with the aim of answering some precisely framed question.' This definition by Sir Austin Bradford Hill, a pioneer of clinical trials, is worth remembering because it encapsulates the fundamentals of good clinical trials: They must be careful, ethical and have a clear question.

In broad terms, clinical studies can be divided into purely observational studies and interventional studies. Both of these *must* fulfil the requirements listed earlier.

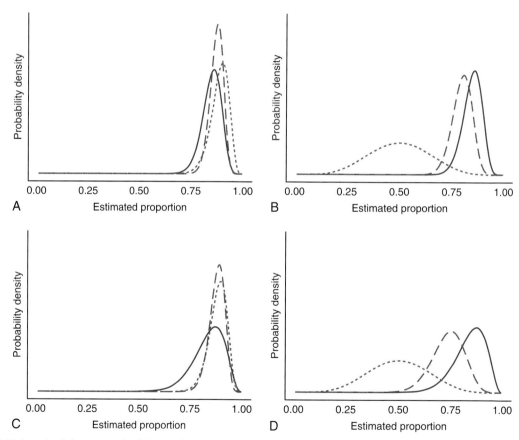

Fig. 2.10 Bayesian inference. Each of the graphs shows the prior (what is currently known; *green, dotted*); the likelihood (new data; *red, plain*); and the posterior (the new inference based on all the data; *blue, dashed*). The impact of relative certainty or uncertainty in the prior or likelihood on the posterior is shown. Although the graphs are estimating proportions, the principle is the same for any parameter (e.g. the mean). (A) Prior and likelihood relatively certain (narrow) and similar to each other. Posterior is similar to prior and likelihood. (B) Low certainty prior (wide) much lower than higher certainty likelihood. Posterior closer to likelihood. (C) More uncertainty in likelihood than prior but estimate is similar. Little change in posterior. (D) Low certainty prior, somewhat lower estimate than moderate certainty likelihood. Moderate certainty posterior.

Observational studies

Observational studies generally answer questions such as:
- Is there an association between factor *x* and outcome *y*?
- What is the natural history of a particular condition?

There are three main types of observational study: cohort, case control and cross-sectional studies.

Cohort studies

Cohort studies may be prospective or retrospective. A cohort is a group of people who share a common experience (e.g. all having cancer surgery, first-time labouring women, children aged <3 y). Exposures of interest are recorded by the investigators. This cohort is then followed up for sufficient time for the outcome of interest to occur: cancer recurrence; long-term backache; psychological testing at school entry. The relative risk of developing the outcome of interest with and without exposure is then calculated. As with all observational studies, association can be shown but not causality. Confounding factors are a particular issue. To take the three earlier examples:
- Regional anaesthesia may be associated with a lower cancer recurrence rate than general anaesthesia, but this may be due to patient selection or surgical technique.
- Backache may be associated with epidural analgesia, but women requesting epidural analgesia may be those with other reasons to develop postpartum back pain.
- Intellectual ability may be associated with general anaesthetic exposure in childhood, but anaesthesia is always administered in conjunction with surgery or investigations.

Prospective studies take a long time to complete and suffer from loss to follow-up. They have the advantage that the investigators have control over the nature and timing of data collection. They can give information about the *incidence* and *prevalence* of a disease or condition.

Incidence is the **rate** of occurrence of a condition. It is usually expressed relative to the population at risk. For example, the UK incidence of stroke in 2010 was 1.15/1000 person-years: in other words, just more than 1 stroke for every 1000 people in 1 year.

Prevalence is the **proportion** of people with the condition. For example, for the same period, the prevalence of people who have had a stroke was around 2% of the UK population.

Retrospective studies are sometimes easier to perform but can suffer from poor-quality data collection, bias in data recording and incomplete cohorts.

Case control studies

For rare diseases it may be impractical to identify and follow up a sufficiently large cohort. Instead, cases are identified and matched with controls – individuals without the condition. The odds ratio of exposure for case and controls is then used to estimate risk. The classic example of a case control study is the work of Sir Richard Doll demonstrating the link between tobacco smoking and lung cancer. Within anaesthesia, case control studies have been used to investigate relatively unusual events such as postoperative mortality and failed tracheal intubation. By definition, case control studies are retrospective because they rely on already identified cases.

Cross-sectional studies

Cross-sectional studies involve data collected from a defined population at a single period. This is unlike cohort and case control studies, which involve some collection of data over time. Cross-sectional studies can therefore be used to determine the *prevalence* of conditions. One of the best known cross-sectional studies in peri-operative medicine was the EPIC study, which recorded the prevalence of intensive treatment unit infections in more than 1400 units across Europe on a single day.

Interventional studies

These studies intervene in some way, such as:
- using a new or different drug;
- delivering care in a different way; or
- using a different technique.

The gold standard for interventional studies is the multicentre, randomised, controlled, multiply blinded trial. However, there are many situations in which this cannot occur for ethical, practical and financial reasons, and modifications of the design may be used.

Before undertaking any interventional trial, it is important to consider patient and public involvement (PPI) in the study design. There is increasing recognition that PPI enhances the research process and results in better designed trials, improved trial efficiency and studies that are more relevant to patients. Good PPI engages with non-researchers early and throughout the research process – from planning through to analysis and dissemination. In the UK the National Institute for Health Research funds INVOLVE (http://www.invo.org.uk) to support active public involvement in NHS research. Most hospitals and universities now have active PPI groups to help researchers.

Before starting any study, an investigator needs to have a clear concept of why the research is needed and how it is to be carried out. There are many structures used to assist in this, but a common device is the *EPICOT* framework. This stands for *Evidence, Population, Intervention, Comparison, Outcome* and *Timeliness*. The framework applies to observational studies, interventional studies and systematic reviews.

Evidence

What is the existing research and clinical evidence within the field? Have distinct gaps in knowledge been identified?

This requires thorough and systematic searching and appraisal of the literature. Systematic reviews and meta-analyses may already have been done or, if not, may be required.

Population

Many research studies fail to identify clearly the appropriate research population. This needs to be relevant, plausible and accessible to the researcher. For instance, the author's main research interest is fragility hip fracture. However, there are many studies purporting to be of hip fracture which include sizeable numbers of young patients or patients undergoing elective hip arthroplasty. In the same group, undisplaced intracapsular fractures almost never need blood transfusion, so there is little to be gained from undertaking transfusion-related studies in this group. Inclusion and exclusion criteria need to be clearly defined and justified for any study. If these are too restrictive, the generalisability of the study may be questioned. Conversely, overly lax criteria reduce the power of the study. This issue is of particular concern when trial evidence is used to drive practice. Recent investigations suggest that study generalisability is poor, especially in older people and the very young.

Intervention

Even apparently straightforward drug trials need care in defining the intervention. Consider a hypothetical antiemetic study. What dose should be used? When should it be given? By which route? There is not usually a single perfect answer to these questions, so it is up to the researchers to justify their choices.

Comparison

If the intervention can be hard to pin down, the comparison can be even trickier. Head-to-head drug trials (e.g. cyclizine *vs.* a new antiemetic) usually define two intervention groups, but often the comparator is normal or standard care. If standard care is too loosely defined and practice varies greatly within the comparator groups, then it becomes difficult to define exactly what the intervention is being compared with. Conversely, a rigidly defined normal care group may lack relevance to real life. This problem is confounded by the changing practice of standard care. The inevitable delay between starting a study and final publication of results may mean that standard care is now quite different to at the start of the trial.

Outcome

Most clinicians want to know whether something is better than something else. Unfortunately, better is very much in the eye of the beholder. Researchers therefore need to be absolutely clear about the outcome they wish to assess. There is usually a trade-off between practicality of a study and the outcomes of real interest to patients and clinicians. There are myriad studies of intubating devices such as videolaryngoscopes. The outcome of interest in these studies is often well defined (e.g. time to successful insertion of tracheal tube) but may not be particularly relevant to patients. Conversely, studies to demonstrate differences in airway-associated mortality would require vast, probably impractical, numbers of participants. As the research develops from an idea into a full proposal, this section should expand into a fully worked through data collection and statistical analysis plan.

There is a move towards (a) standardising endpoints so that trials report the same outcomes, and (b) designing trials around endpoints that really matter to patients. In addition, researchers are moving towards the concept of minimal clinically important difference (MCID), the smallest change in an outcome that a patient would identify as important.

Timeliness

Funders need to know that there is some pressing reason for research to be undertaken now. This may be because practice has changed, new drugs are available or the population has changed.

Regulatory approvals

All research requires some regulatory approval. There are various legal and ethical requirements set out in guidance and national statutes such as the EU Good Clinical Practice Directive, the Medicines for Human Use (Clinical Trials) Regulations 2004 (and similar legislation internationally) and the Declaration of Helsinki.

Ethical review

A properly constituted ethical review committee must consider the proposed study and whether the research is ethical and scientifically sound. The role of the ethical review committee is to safeguard the rights, safety, dignity and well-being of people participating in research.

Sponsorship

All research requires a sponsor. This is an organisation (or occasionally an individual) that takes responsibility for:
- implementing and maintaining quality assurance and quality control systems;
- securing written agreements with all involved parties to ensure direct access to:
  - all trial-related sites and
  - source data and documents;

- reports for the purpose of monitoring and auditing by the sponsor and inspection by regulatory agencies; and
- applying quality control measures to each stage of data handling to ensure that all data are reliable and have been processed correctly.

These responsibilities are usually taken on by pharmaceutical companies, universities or hospitals. To meet these responsibilities, the sponsor will have standard operating procedures covering all stages of the research process and regular systematic audit of the research it sponsors.

Local approvals

The site where the research is to occur needs to approve the research before it can start. This is to ensure that there are adequate facilities and resources to undertake the study in a safe and timely fashion and that there are no undue conflicts with other ongoing studies.

National approvals

There may be other regulatory bodies which need to be involved, depending on the country and type of research. For instance, in the UK, drug-related studies require approval from the Medicines and Healthcare Products Regulatory Agency (MHRA), and gamete and embryo research requires approval from the Human Fertilisation and Embryology Authority (HFEA).

Trial registration

In an attempt to reduce the risks of selective reporting, it is now an international standard for publication in a medical journal that clinical trials are registered in a publicly accessible trials registry such as ClinicalTrials.gov or the International Standard Randomised Controlled Trial Number (ISRCTN) register. The intended consequence of these approval processes is that investigators comply with a strict framework that should protect the rights and well-being of participants, as well as ensure the quality of research. The ethical review should ensure that research studies are presented to potential participants in an open, understandable and unbiased fashion. The research governance frameworks of the sponsor facilitate the design of high-quality and efficient research. The downside is an increase in bureaucracy and costs.

Specific aspects of trial conduct

Informed consent

Involvement in clinical research is a voluntary activity, for which individuals are free to give or withhold their consent. There are strict rules about the amount and type of information which individuals should be given as part of the research process. Investigators must be extremely careful to ensure that potential participants understand the purpose of the research and what it will involve for them and that they have adequate time to consider the study and discuss it with other people if they wish.

For some areas of research, particularly in perioperative and critical care, it may not be possible to give participants a prolonged period to consider inclusion in a study. Wherever possible, investigators should confirm continued consent to study participation at a later date. There may be occasions on which participants cannot consent for themselves, such as patients who have temporarily lost capacity (such as those who are unconscious after trauma or in an ICU) or who have longstanding conditions (such as dementia) meaning they are incapable of understanding the information given to them. In these situations the ethical review committee will consider carefully the balance of risks and benefits to potential participants before granting approval for studies.

Randomisation

As discussed earlier in the chapter, a truly random allocation of study participants to treatment groups is very important. Although in theory tossing a coin should be adequate, in practice this is a fallible approach, and more and more sophisticated systems have been introduced. Most studies now use some form of computerised system. A good randomisation system should ensure several aspects of good trial conduct.

- *A truly random allocation.* Usually the allocations are made with reference to computer-generated random number tables. The investigator has no influence at all on the allocation.
- *An audit trail of randomisations.* It is possible for the sponsor to verify who has been randomised and when.
- *Entry validation.* Screening questions can be included in the randomisation process which ensure that only eligible participants are randomised.
- *Concealment of allocation.* For placebo-controlled studies, the allocation is usually to a pack number, made up elsewhere, to reduce the risk of the investigator knowing the treatment allocation. This also means that the randomisation must be sufficiently robust that investigators cannot make educated guesses about current, future or past allocations.

Blinding/concealment

To reduce investigator and participant bias, ideally all parties would be completely unaware of treatment allocation. The use of the terms *single-blind* or *double-blind* are probably best avoided because they do not clearly define who is blinded to what. Such complete blinding is only really possible for drug trials with a placebo or active comparator which has an identical formulation and no easily discerned physiological effects (e.g. bradycardia with β-blockers).

Even though this gold standard is not often achievable, investigators should design their studies in ways to reduce the risk of bias to a minimum. Individuals responsible for data collection should be unaware of treatment allocation, data should be analysed before code breaking as far as possible and clear definitions of outcomes of interest should be provided before data collection starts.

Completeness of follow-up

It is extremely important that, as far as possible, data are recorded for all participants in a study. This is to ensure that results are not biased by disproportionate loss of follow-up between groups. Excessive loss to follow-up may raise questions about either the tolerability of the protocol or the adequacy of the research team.

Stages of drug trials

Anaesthetists have a professional interest in new drugs. To be available for general human use, new drugs have to go through a rigorous process of testing. There are various phases of research, outlined in Table 2.7. Many drugs fail at the phase 2 stage, often because of unexpected toxicity. Early trials generally demonstrate *efficacy* (the treatment works in ideal conditions). Postmarketing surveillance (phases 4 and 5) evaluates *effectiveness* (the treatment does more good than harm in real clinical practice) and is an important part of drug development.

Publication

All research should be disseminated to a wider audience in some way. Traditionally this has been through the media of scientific conferences and printed publication in peer-reviewed journals. Increasingly the internet is changing the way research results are disseminated. In addition, funders are keen to see their research reach relevant parties such as patients; non-research clinicians; industry and policymaking groups such as charities, medical colleges and associations; and government bodies. The presentation of material for each of these audiences is different – one style does not suit all. Researchers often find it difficult to explain their findings in ways that are meaningful to non-experts, and even the most experienced researcher is likely to benefit from lay advice. Peer-reviewed journals all have their own style, which should be adhered to. However, they all have common core standards. These include the following:
- *Transparency and probity*. Sufficient detail should be given of the research so that others can understand what has been done. There should be no suspicion of hidden data.

- *Intelligible writing*. Published research is wasted if no one can understand what is being presented.
- *Relevance*. Most journals have a target audience and will not publish material which is unlikely to be of interest to their subscribers.
- *Single publication*. With some exceptions, journals will not tolerate duplicate publication (i.e. publication of a paper that has been previously published elsewhere in whole or in part). This is partly an issue of honesty, but duplicate publication also distorts the scientific record by exaggerating the results of research.

Publication checklists

In the same way that the research governance framework should ensure that research is performed well, there are international consensus statements and checklists which journals encourage or require authors to use when submitting.
- CONSORT (Consolidated Standards of Reporting Trials) is a 25-item checklist and flow diagram. It aims to guide authors in reporting all stages of trial design, participant flow, analysis and interpretation (http://www.consort-statement.org).
- PRISMA (Preferred Reporting Items for Systematic Reviews and Meta-Analyses) is a similar approach for systematic reviews (http://www.prisma-statement.org)
- STROBE (STrengthening the Reporting of OBservational studies in Epidemiology) is a similar approach for observational studies (http://www.strobe-statement.org/).

Presentation of results

Journals have their own styles for presentation of summary data and probability values, and these should be followed. One area of considerable confusion is presentation of the magnitude of effect of a treatment or exposure. Although most of the terms are mathematically interchangeable, the interpretation of each by clinicians, patients and managers may be very different.
- *Absolute risk (AR)*. This is simply the probability of an event occurring without reference to anything else. For instance, the absolute risk of PONV is usually quoted as around 30%. It gives no information about which factors might influence the risk.
- *Relative risk (RR)*. This is the ratio of risk between those with and without exposure. For instance, smokers are about 10 times more likely to get lung cancer than non-smokers, so their relative risk is 10. Importantly, the relative risk gives no information about the absolute risk. A doubling of risk for a very rare event still makes the event very rare.
- *Absolute risk reduction (ARR)*. Absolute risk reduction is the difference in absolute risk between two groups. For instance, in designing the BAG-RECALL study (to compare

the incidence of accidental anaesthetic awareness when bispectral index (BIS) or end-tidal gas monitoring was used to regulate depth of anaesthesia), the investigators estimated that the absolute risk of awareness in their two groups would be 0.5% (5 in 1000) in the end-tidal agent monitoring group and 0.1% (1 in 1000) in the BIS group. The estimated absolute risk reduction was therefore 0.4% (4 in 1000).

- *Relative risk reduction (RRR)*. Relative risk reduction is the proportional difference in risk. Taking the BAG-RECALL example earlier, the estimated RRR was 0.4%/0.5% = 80%.
- *Number needed to treat (NNT)*. The number needed to treat is the number of individuals who would need to be treated with the new treatment rather than the old one for one to benefit. It is the reciprocal of the absolute risk reduction. Again, using the BAG-RECALL example, the estimated NNT was 250 (1/0.04).
- *Number needed to harm (NNH)*. Given that all drugs have adverse effects, the equivalent to the NNT can also be calculated. For instance, a meta-analysis of opioids added to single-shot intrathecal anaesthesia found an NNH for fentanyl-induced pruritus of 3.3. In other words, the absolute risk increase was 30% (1/3.3).
- *Odds ratio*. In some situations, odds ratios are the appropriate statistical measure, particularly for logistic regression–based techniques. Unfortunately, they are slightly counterintuitive. The odds of an event occurring are the number of events divided by the number of non-events. The odds ratio is simply the ratio of two groups. The odds ratio overestimates relative risk. This effect becomes smaller as the absolute risk decreases, so for uncommon events the odds ratio *approximates* relative risk. For example, data from a meta-analysis of type of anaesthesia and thrombotic events after major orthopaedic surgery is shown in Table 2.6.

Evidence-based medicine

Evidence-based medicine (EBM) is an approach that promotes deliberate, explicit and judicious use of appropriate evidence to support clinical decision-making in partnership with patient values and clinical experience. It originated from a realisation that many aspects of medical treatment were based on opinion, anecdote and historical practice. Much of the discussion about EBM focusses on the use of systematic review and meta-analysis to underpin guidelines and recommendations. However, unthinking of application of guidelines and recommendations without consideration of patient, context and clinical experience has never been appropriate.

Table 2.6 Calculation of odds ratio, absolute risk and relative risk for complications caused by venous thromboembolism (VTE)

	GA	Neuraxial
Major VTE and VTE-related mortality	73	101
No major VTE and VTE-related mortality	1658	3204
Total	1731	3305
Odds	0.044 (73/1658)	0.032 (101/3204)
Odds ratio	1.4 (0.044/0.032)	
Absolute risk	0.042 (73/1731)	0.031 (101/3305)
Relative risk	1.35 (0.042/0.031)	

Evidence-based medicine places evidence in a hierarchy (Table 2.8), and recommendations can then be made on the basis of assessment of all the evidence (Table 2.9).

There are many critics of this approach, particularly the dominant role of the randomised controlled trial. These criticisms relate mainly to the lack of generalisability of a specific trial result to an individual patient, the lack of evidence relating to all the decisions to be made, poor quality of research in general, bias in published literature and a discounting of clinical experience.

Systematic review and meta-analysis

Systematic review and meta-analysis are undertaken in an attempt to provide unbiased descriptions of the current state of knowledge. In broad principle a systematic review is a reproducible method of collating relevant results. As with primary research, a good systematic review requires careful planning.

There are several stages to a systematic review: defining the question, searching for relevant data, extracting the data, assessing the quality of the data and analysing and/or combining the data (if appropriate). Each of these stages involves decisions by the reviewers, and different decisions may lead to quite different conclusions. The data included in a systematic review are only ever as good as the original studies; an appropriate conclusion from a systematic review may be that there is no good evidence. An important risk to systematic reviews is bias (see earlier). All the biases discussed tend to exaggerate positive effects and diminish negative effects and adverse events.

Table 2.7 Phases of drug development

Phase	Outcomes	Doses used	Participants (typical numbers)	Comments
Preclinical	Mode of action, toxicity, pharmacokinetics, interactions	Wide range	*In vitro* *In vivo* animals Different species and ages	How does the drug work? Is it likely to be safe to use in humans?
Phase 0	Human pharmacodynamics and pharmacokinetics	Very low – subtherapeutic	Healthy volunteers (10)	Often combined with phase 1 No information about efficacy or safety Used to rank candidate drugs to take forward to phase 1
Phase 1	Dose ranging, safety	Very low and increasing doses Maximum doses are below toxic doses in animals	Healthy volunteers (20–80)	Is the drug safe to use in phase 2 studies? Single and multiple dosing studies
Phase 2	Efficacy and more safety data	Range of therapeutic doses	Patients with relevant conditions (100–300)	Does the drug actually work? (2a) What dose should be used? (2b)
Phase 3	Efficacy in trials	Range of therapeutic doses	Patients in clinical trials with relevant conditions (1000–3000)	Does the drug work in patients? Randomised clinical trials and open-label studies
Phase 4	Postmarketing surveillance	Therapeutic doses	Clinical use (thousands)	Rare side effects Use in wider populations
Phase 5	Effectiveness research	Therapeutic dose	Clinical use (thousands)	Clinical effectiveness Cost–benefit

Meta-analysis is a statistical technique for combining study results. In theory the use of a wider source of evidence increases confidence in the conclusions drawn. The analysis presupposes that the combined studies are similar enough (in population, intervention and outcome) to be reasonably combined. This is a contentious issue – examples from anaesthesia and critical care include combining (or not) studies of the very old and the very young or critical care and elective anaesthesia. Although various approaches have been refined to assist reviewers in deciding whether studies should be included or not, there is no perfect system. Where possible, meta-analyses conduct sensitivity analyses. These are repeated analyses investigating the effect of including or excluding particular studies (e.g. older studies, smaller studies, studies with small sample sizes). If the results are robust to these changes, reviewers tend to have more confidence in the results. Conversely, large changes in results raise questions.

The main tools in the meta-analysis toolbox are the forest plot and the funnel plot. The forest plot (Fig. 2.11) is a graphical representation of the individual study results and their uncertainty, along with a summary estimate of the overall effect and its uncertainty. This is a weighted summary (i.e. not all studies contribute equally to the estimate). An estimate of the between-study heterogeneity is usually given. This is not a precise science, but large degrees of heterogeneity will raise questions about the appropriateness of combining studies. The funnel plot is a graphical approach to assessing publication bias in included studies. Study results are expected to vary randomly around the central value, and more variation is expected in smaller studies. Therefore studies should be approximately evenly distributed within a funnel around the overall summary effect. A preponderance of positive studies may suggest a publication bias with missing negative studies.

Table 2.8 Levels of evidence

Level of evidence	Descriptor
1a	Systematic reviews (with homogeneity) of randomised controlled trials
1b	Individual randomised controlled trials (with narrow confidence interval)
1c	All or none randomised controlled trials (met when all patients died before the treatment became available, but some now survive on it; or when some patients died before the treatment became available, but none now die on it)
2a	Systematic reviews (with homogeneity) of cohort studies
2b	Individual cohort study or low-quality randomised controlled trials (e.g. <80% follow-up)
2c	"Outcomes" research; ecological studies
3a	Systematic review (with homogeneity) of case control studies
3b	Individual case control study
4	Case series (and poor-quality cohort and case control studies)
5	Expert opinion without explicit critical appraisal or based on physiology, bench research or 'first principles'

Similar categorisations can be used for prognostic, diagnostic and economic analysis studies.
(Adapted from Centre for Evidence-Based Medicine. (2009) *Levels of evidence.* Available from: http://www.cebm.net/oxford-centre-evidence-based-medicine-levels-evidence-march-2009/)

Table 2.9 Grading of recommendations

A	Consistent level 1 studies
B	Consistent level 2 or 3 studies *or* extrapolations from level 1 studies
C	Level 4 studies *or* extrapolations from level 2 or 3 studies
D	Level 5 evidence *or* troublingly inconsistent or inconclusive studies of any level

Audit, research and service evaluation

There are numerous definitions of research, but most have some concept of finding out generalisable new knowledge. Audit, on the other hand, is generally concerned with finding whether something is being done a standard, and service evaluation is finding out what standard a service achieves.

The distinctions are sometimes unclear, but research requires (in the UK) a different set of legal and ethical approvals for audit and evaluation. A commonly used decision tree asks questions about the following:

- *Intent.* Is the aim of the study to derive generalisable new knowledge?
- *Allocation.* Are participants allocated at random to different treatments?
- *Standard of care.* Are participants being given non-standard care with relatively little supporting evidence?

If the answer to any of these questions is yes, then the study is categorised as research.

In part because of the regulatory hurdles of declaring a study as research, individuals and departments may be tempted to label a project as audit or service evaluation. This carries two important risks. First, the governance of research is primarily in place to protect the rights and well-being of participants. Bypassing this may put patients at unnecessary risk. Second, the strictures of research governance support well-constructed studies. Good audit and evaluation requires the same rigour as good research. The use of audit and service evaluation to support quality improvement is discussed more fully in Chapter 18.

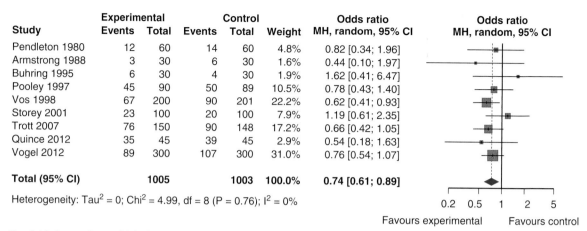

Study	Experimental Events	Total	Control Events	Total	Weight	Odds ratio MH, random, 95% CI
Pendleton 1980	12	60	14	60	4.8%	0.82 [0.34; 1.96]
Armstrong 1988	3	30	6	30	1.6%	0.44 [0.10; 1.97]
Buhring 1995	6	30	4	30	1.9%	1.62 [0.41; 6.47]
Pooley 1997	45	90	50	89	10.5%	0.78 [0.43; 1.40]
Vos 1998	67	200	90	201	22.2%	0.62 [0.41; 0.93]
Storey 2001	23	100	20	100	7.9%	1.19 [0.61; 2.35]
Trott 2007	76	150	90	148	17.2%	0.66 [0.42; 1.05]
Quince 2012	35	45	39	45	2.9%	0.54 [0.18; 1.63]
Vogel 2012	89	300	107	300	31.0%	0.76 [0.54; 1.07]
Total (95% CI)		**1005**		**1003**	**100.0%**	**0.74 [0.61; 0.89]**

Heterogeneity: $Tau^2 = 0$; $Chi^2 = 4.99$, df = 8 (P = 0.76); $I^2 = 0\%$

Fig. 2.11 Forest plot. Individual studies' results are tabulated and plotted (as odds ratios in this case). Conventions vary, but in this case the weight of the study is proportional to the area of the study box. A summary estimate of the average effect size and its uncertainty is provided (diamond). If the summary estimate crosses the point of no difference (odds ratio = 1), then an overall effect is unlikely. Note that in this example, only one of the included studies demonstrated a significant effect, whereas the overall summary estimate is in favour of the experimental treatment.

References/Further reading

Altman, D.G., 2005. Practical statistics for medical research, second ed. Taylor & Francis, London.

Browner, W.S., 1994. A simple recipe for doing it well. Anesthesiology, 80, 923.

Cruikshank, S., 1998. Mathematics and statistics in anaesthesia. Oxford University Press, Oxford.

Greenhalgh, T., 2014. How to read a paper – the basis of evidence-based medicine, fifth ed. Wiley Blackwell, London.

Hill, A.B., 1955. Introduction to medical statistics, 5th ed. Lancet Monograph.

Masic, I., Miokovic, M., Muhamedagic, B., 2008. Evidence based medicine – new approaches and challenges.

Acta Informatica Medica, 16 (4), 219–225.

Rowntree, D., 1991. Statistics without tears. Penguin, London.

Statistically speaking article series: Anaesthesia 2016 onwards.

Yentis, S.M., 2016. Research not research. Anaesthesia, 71 (8), 871–874.

Chapter 3

Inhalational anaesthetic agents and medical gases

Emma Temple, Matthew Wiles

Inhalational and volatile anaesthetic agents are used widely for the induction and maintenance of general anaesthesia throughout the world. Since the famous demonstration of an ether anaesthetic by William Morton in 1846, the development of volatile anaesthetic agents paved the way for the introduction of modern surgical practices, procedures and techniques. Early agents such as diethyl ether, chloroform, ethyl chloride, cyclopropane and trichloroethylene, although effective, were either highly flammable or toxic. Halothane, discovered in 1955, had a much improved safety profile and heralded the modern era of fluorinated compounds.

Inhalational agents in current use include the fluorinated ethers (isoflurane, sevoflurane and desflurane), halogenated hydrocarbon (halothane) and nitrous oxide (N_2O). Xenon is an inert noble gas found in the Earth's atmosphere in trace amounts and has demonstrated impressive anaesthetic properties. It is not currently in widespread use, largely because of significant production costs.

The volatile anaesthetic agents are delivered to the patient via a 'carrier gas' mixture. This is most commonly an air/oxygen or oxygen/nitrous oxide combination.

Kinetics of inhaled anaesthetic agents

Inhalational anaesthetic agents exert their effect on the CNS to produce loss of consciousness and loss of response to noxious stimuli. The magnitude of the response is proportional to the partial pressure of the anaesthetic at its effect site. This is not easily measurable, and, therefore, alveolar (end-tidal) anaesthetic partial pressure is used as a surrogate for effect-site concentration. At steady state, the partial pressure of inhaled anaesthetic agent within the alveoli is in equilibrium with that in arterial blood and subsequently the partial pressure in the CNS (the effect site). Steady state, however, is rarely achieved within clinical practice.

Mechanism of action

Despite being widely used in clinical practice for more than 170 years, the exact mechanism by which agents cause a reversible loss of conscious awareness and loss of response to noxious stimuli (antinociceptive effect) is still largely unknown. The inhalation agents are a diverse group and belong to no recognisable or unifying chemical class. This has led to the belief that there is no single distinctive CNS 'receptor' upon which these agents exert their effect. The two main theories for their action focus on direct interaction with two components of the cell membrane.

Lipid theory (Meyer–Overton relationship)

In the early 1900s, Meyer and Overton showed a close relationship between the lipid solubility of the inhalational agent and its potency of anaesthetic activity. They noticed that there was a straight line relationship between log minimum alveolar concentration (MAC; i.e. potency) and the lipid solubility; the more lipid soluble the agent (represented by a higher log oil/gas partition coefficient), the greater the potency. This led to the theory that anaesthetic agents could penetrate the cell membrane lipid bilayer and alter the molecular arrangement of the phospholipids and cause disruption of the usual function of membrane-spanning ionic channels. This theory has, however, been largely dismissed in favour of the more popular protein theory.

Protein site of action theory

Throughout the CNS, there are many excitatory and inhibitory ligand-gated ion channels. There is increasing evidence that anaesthetic agents act by inhibiting excitatory (serotonergic, neuronal nicotinic and N-methyl-D-aspartate (NMDA)) channels and activating inhibitory channels (γ-aminobutyric acid A (GABA$_A$) and glycine). The relationship between lipid solubility and potency can be explained by the lipophilic nature of the specific binding sites.

GABA$_A$ is a pentameric ligand-gated ion channel receptor. It comprises two α, two β and one γ subunit which together span the phospholipid bilayer of the cell membrane and surround a chloride ionophore. When activated, the channel permits passage of chloride ions into the cell, resulting in hyperpolarisation and therefore inhibiting postsynaptic neuronal excitability. Volatile anaesthetics are thought to cause activation by binding to the α subunits.

More recently, other similar ion channels have been discovered as potential sites of action of the volatile anaesthetic agents. These include pre- and postsynaptic two-pore domain potassium channels that are responsible for setting the resting membrane potential of a cell. Volatile anaesthetic agents have been found experimentally to enhance the activity of the channels, leading to hyperpolarisation.

Minimum alveolar concentration

The MAC is a measure of the potency of an inhalational anaesthetic agent. It is analogous to the ED50 of a drug; that is, the median effective dose that produces an effect in 50% of the population that receives it. As such, MAC is a misnomer, as *median alveolar concentration* would be a more accurate term.

One MAC is defined as 'the minimum concentration (in volumes percent) of inhalational anaesthetic agent in the alveoli, at equilibrium, at one atmosphere pressure, in 100% oxygen, which produces immobility in 50% of unpremedicated adult subjects when exposed to a standard noxious stimulus.'

In clinical practice, MAC correlates with end-tidal anaesthetic agent concentration and is used as a guide to the depth of anaesthesia. Because of the differing potencies between the volatile agents, the end-tidal anaesthetic agent concentration required to achieve 1 MAC varies. For example, in an oxygen–air mixture, sevoflurane has a MAC of 1.8%, whereas desflurane requires an end-tidal concentration of 6.6% to achieve a MAC of 1. Although 1 MAC of sevoflurane is equal in potency to 1 MAC of desflurane, it does not follow that the agents are equipotent at 2 MAC. However, in general terms, 0.5 MAC of one agent, in combination with 0.5 MAC of another, approximates to 1 MAC in total. The MAC values for anaesthetic agents in common use are shown in Table 3.1. The standard deviation for MAC values is around 10%; this means that MAC plus two standard deviations (i.e. 1.2 MAC) will produce immobility in approximately 95% of patients.

Other MAC concepts have also been described:
- MAC awake or MAC$_{aw}$: the alveolar concentration halfway between that allowing a response to verbal command and that preventing it. This is thought to be approximately 0.33 MAC for desflurane, isoflurane and sevoflurane.
- MAC blocks adrenergic response or MAC$_{bar}$: the brain concentration sufficient to prevent adrenergic response (i.e. increase in heart rate and/or arterial pressure) to skin incision. This has been found to be 1.3 MAC for isoflurane and desflurane and may be 2.0–3.0 MAC for sevoflurane. However, these values are decreased with the coadministration of opioids (e.g. MAC$_{bar}$ for isoflurane

Table 3.1 Comparison of modern volatile anaesthetic agents

	Isoflurane	Sevoflurane	Desflurane	Halothane
Molecular mass; Da	184.5	200	168	197
Boiling point; °C	49	58.5	23.5	50
Blood/gas partition coefficient	1.4	0.68	0.42	2.5
Oil/gas partition coefficient	98	47	18.7	224
MAC (40-year-old patient); %	1.17	1.8	6.6	0.75
Preservative	None	None	None	Thymol
Stability in carbon dioxide absorbers	Stable	Unstable	Stable	Unstable?[a]

[a]Halothane may be decomposed by soda lime but is still safe to use.
MAC, Minimum alveolar concentration.

Box 3.1 **Factors affecting the minimum alveolar concentration (MAC) of inhalational anaesthetic agents**

Factors leading to an increase in MAC

Decreasing age (peak at 6 months of age)
Hyperthermia
Hypernatraemia
Thyrotoxicosis
Elevated CNS catecholamine release: anxiety states, iatrogenic (e.g. hypercapnia), drugs (e.g. ephedrine, acute amphetamine/cocaine use, MAOIs)
Chronic alcohol or opioid use

Factors leading to a decrease in MAC

Acute intake of sedative or analgesic drugs (e.g. opiates, benzodiazepines, nitrous oxide)
Increasing age
Pregnancy
Hypothermia
Hypotension
Hypothyroidism
Hyponatraemia
Acute alcohol ingestion
Drugs that reduce CNS catecholamine release (e.g. reserpine, methyl dopa, clonidine, dexmedetomidine, chronic amphetamine/cocaine use).

MAOIs, Monoamine oxidase inhibitors.

and desflurane falls to 0.40–0.60 MAC when administered with i.v. fentanyl 1.5 μg kg^{-1}).
There are many pharmacological and physiological factors that can affect (increase or decrease) MAC (Box 3.1).

Pharmacokinetics of inhaled anaesthetic agents

There are many factors affecting the CNS (effect site) concentration of an anaesthetic agent and therefore speed of onset of volatile anaesthesia.
1. *Inspired agent concentration.* Put simply, the higher the concentration of the inhaled anaesthetic agent, the faster the onset. A high concentration of anaesthetic agent in the alveolus leads to a large concentration gradient between the alveolus and blood, favouring rapid diffusion across the alveolar membrane and therefore faster delivery to, and onset at, the effect site.
2. *Alveolar ventilation.* Increased alveolar ventilation results in a more rapid onset of anaesthesia. Alveolar volatile agent taken up by the pulmonary blood flow is rapidly

replaced, thereby maintaining the concentration gradient. Volatile anaesthetic agents such as desflurane and isoflurane which interfere with alveolar ventilation (e.g. because of breath holding or coughing) are therefore unsuitable for gaseous induction of anaesthesia.
3. *Functional residual capacity (FRC).* Patients with a larger FRC will experience a slower onset of anaesthesia, as this will dilute the inspired concentration of gas, thereby reducing the alveolar partial pressure of the volatile agent.
4. *Cardiac output and pulmonary blood flow.* A higher cardiac output results in more rapid alveolar uptake into blood and slower build-up of alveolar concentration; thus equilibration and anaesthesia will occur slowly. A lower cardiac output state will favour faster equilibration between agent in the alveolus and pulmonary blood; in addition, a greater proportion of cardiac output is directed to the cerebral circulation, further increasing the clinical effects. These effects are more pronounced in agents with greater solubility (see next).
5. *Blood/gas partition coefficient (solubility).* The blood/gas partition coefficient is defined as the ratio of the amount of an anaesthetic agent in blood and gas when the two phases are of equal volume and pressure and in equilibrium at 37°C. Thus the higher the blood/gas coefficient, the more soluble an agent is in blood and the longer it takes for the partial pressure of the agent in blood to rise. As previously alluded to, anaesthesia occurs when the partial pressure, not total amount, of an anaesthetic agent at the effect site reaches a certain value. Consequently, the higher an agent's blood/gas coefficient, the slower its anaesthetic effect (Fig. 3.1). Similarly, the rapidity of recovery from anaesthesia is inversely proportional to the solubility of the anaesthetic (Fig. 3.2).
6. *Second gas effect.* This describes the faster onset of anaesthesia that occurs when a volatile agent is coadministered with nitrous oxide and is a direct result of the concentration effect. The second gas effect is used in clinical practice to reduce anaesthetic induction time, particularly in gaseous inductions (see below).

The second gas effect

Nitrous oxide is rapidly absorbed across the alveolar membrane into the pulmonary capillaries. Nitrous oxide is around 20 times more soluble in blood than oxygen or nitrogen. At high concentrations of nitrous oxide, a significantly greater volume of nitrous oxide is entering pulmonary blood than oxygen or nitrogen is entering the alveolus. This results in two phenomena, which together increase the speed of onset of anaesthesia:
- *Concentration of the gases in the alveolus – the concentration effect.* As nitrous oxide is rapidly absorbed, the alveolar volume decreases, leading to a fractional concentration of the remaining gases in the alveolus. This results in an

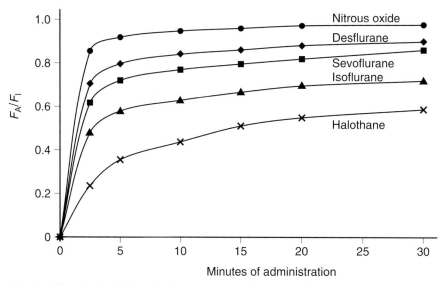

Fig. 3.1 Ratio of alveolar (F_A) to inspired (F_I) fractional concentration of nitrous oxide, desflurane, sevoflurane, isoflurane and halothane in the first 30 min of anaesthesia. The plot of F_A/F_I expresses the rapidity with which alveolar concentration equilibrates with inspired concentration. It is most rapid for agents with a low blood/gas partition coefficient.

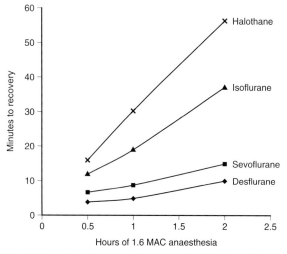

Fig. 3.2 Rapidity of recovery from anaesthesia is inversely proportional to the solubility of the anaesthetic: the most rapid recovery is with the least soluble anaesthetic (desflurane). The difference is amplified by duration of anaesthesia. Note that the difference in time of recovery between the least (desflurane) and most soluble anaesthetic (halothane) is greater after 2 h of anaesthesia than after 0.5 h of anaesthesia.

increased concentration gradient between the alveolus and pulmonary blood, favouring alveolus to blood transfer of anaesthetic agent.

• *Augmentation of alveolar ventilation.* As nitrous oxide is rapidly absorbed, the volume and pressure in the alveolus falls, creating a pressure/volume gradient between the conducting airways and the alveolus. This augments alveolar ventilation by drawing more gas down its pressure gradient into the alveolus, thus increasing speed of onset of anaesthesia. Similarly, use of nitrous oxide will accelerate the offset of anaesthesia. During emergence from anaesthesia, nitrous oxide administration is ceased and an oxygen or oxygen/air mixture is delivered. Nitrous oxide rapidly diffuses from the bloodstream across the alveolar membrane into the alveolus. This dilutes the volatile agent in the alveolus (and therefore the partial pressure), resulting in a faster offset of anaesthesia. This also causes diffusion hypoxia, which is discussed in detail later in the chapter.

The combination of the concentration effect and the augmentation of alveolar ventilation is employed to reduce induction time with the volatile anaesthetics and thus describes the second gas effect (Fig. 3.3).

Individual anaesthetic agents

There is no inhalational anaesthetic agent that fulfils the criteria of the ideal inhalational anaesthetic agent (Box 3.2). Although there are many inhaled anaesthetic agents available, only three are in regular use in economically advantaged countries: isoflurane; sevoflurane; and desflurane. Halothane is still in use in resource-poor environments (see Chapter 45); however, its popularity has declined because of its less

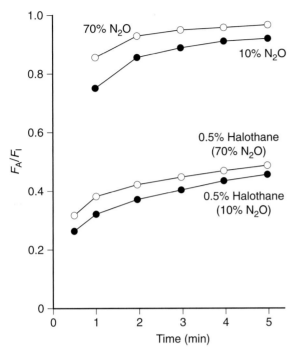

Fig. 3.3 The concentration and second gas effects. High concentrations of nitrous oxide increase the alveolar (F_A) to inspired (F_I) ratio for nitrous oxide (the concentration effect) and for a volatile agent administered with nitrous oxide (the second gas effect).

favourable kinetics and higher incidence of adverse effects. The chemical structures of the volatile agents are shown in Fig. 3.4.

Isoflurane

Uses

1. Maintenance of general anaesthesia.
2. Treatment of severe asthma in patients requiring mechanical ventilation in ICU.

Physical properties

Isoflurane is a halogenated ethyl methyl ether (1-chloro-2,2,2-trifluoroethyl difluoromethyl ether) and is a geometric isomer of enflurane. Isoflurane is a clear, colourless, volatile liquid with a pungent odour. It is presented in amber-coloured bottles and requires no preservatives for storage. It is stable, does not react with metal or other substances and is non-flammable in clinical concentrations.

Systemic effects

RS:
- Dose-dependent depression of ventilation with depression of the ventilatory response to carbon dioxide.
- Decrease in tidal volume but an increase in ventilatory rate in the absence of opioid drugs.

Box 3.2 **Properties of the ideal anaesthetic agent**

Physical

Stable compound (unaffected by light or heat)
Non-flammable/does not support combustion
SVP high enough to allow easy vaporisation and production of a clinically relevant concentration
Inert when in contact with regularly used equipment e.g. rubber, plastic, glass, soda lime
Cheap to manufacture
Environmentally friendly
Easy to administer
Long shelf life without need for preservatives
Non-irritant and non-pungent (to allow gaseous induction)

Pharmacological

Low blood/gas coefficient (to allow rapid onset/recovery)
High oil/gas coefficient (low MAC, high potency; allows delivery with a high FIO_2)
Minimal metabolism with pulmonary excretion (i.e. unaffected by renal/hepatic impairment)

Non-toxic/non-allergenic, with no trigger for malignant hyperthermia
No interactions with other drugs
Not teratogenic or carcinogenic
CVS:
　No cardiovascular depression
　No decrease in coronary blood flow
　No sensitisation of myocardial tissue to catecholamines
RS:
　No respiratory depression
　Bronchodilation
CNS:
　Analgesic properties
　Non-epileptogenic
　No increase in CBF or ICP
　No effect on cerebral autoregulation
　Muscle relaxation
GI/GU:
　Antiemetic properties
　No effect on uterine tone

CBF, Cerebral blood flow; *FIO₂*, fraction of inspired oxygen; *ICP*, intracranial pressure; *MAC*, minimum alveolar concentration; *SVP*, saturated vapour pressure.

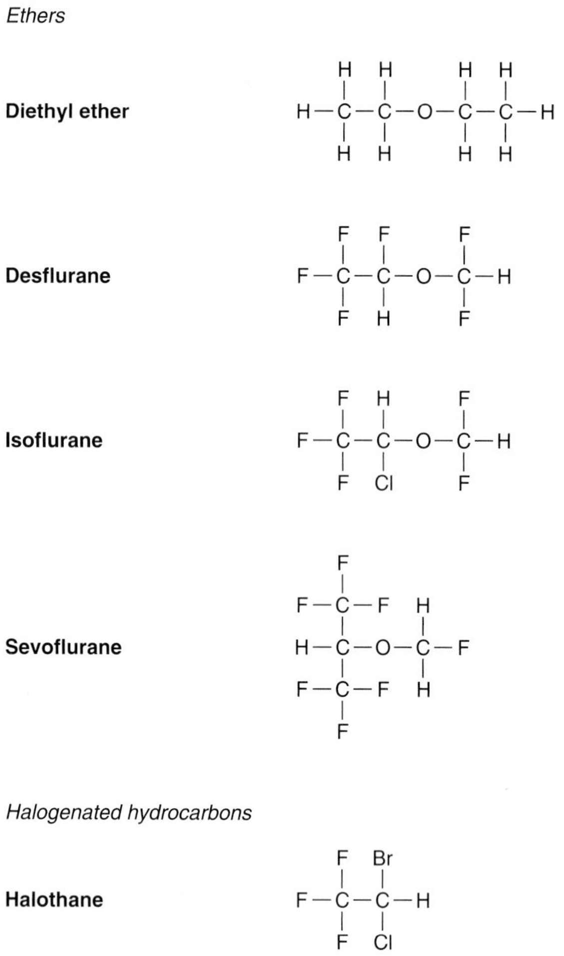

Ethers

Diethyl ether

Desflurane

Isoflurane

Sevoflurane

Halogenated hydrocarbons

Halothane

Fig. 3.4 Structural formulae of inhalational anaesthetic agents.

- Respiratory tract irritation and laryngospasm, making inhalational induction unfavourable.
- Inhibition of hypoxic pulmonary vasoconstriction (thereby increasing shunt fraction).
- Bronchial smooth muscle relaxing properties, particularly in the context of bronchoconstriction caused by histamine and acetylcholine.

CVS:
- Dose-related reduction in MAP, primarily by reduction in systemic vascular resistance (SVR), although isoflurane also has a negatively inotropic effect.
- Reflex tachycardia.
- Arrhythmias are uncommon, and there is little sensitisation of the myocardium to catecholamines.
- Coronary vasodilatation with the possibility of 'coronary steal'. Dilatation in normal coronary arteries offers a low

resistance to flow and may reduce perfusion through stenosed neighbouring vessels, causing distal ischaemia. However, although this remains a theoretical concern, it does not appear to be of any clinical significance.

CNS:
- Causes general anaesthesia and reduction in cerebral metabolic rate.
- At concentrations >1 MAC causes cerebral vasodilatation and increases cerebral blood flow (CBF), leading to raised ICP.
- Does not cause seizure activity on the EEG.
- Induces dose-dependent muscle relaxation and depression of neuromuscular transmission with potentiation of non-depolarising neuromuscular blocking agents (NMBAs).

GI/GU:
- Reduction in renal blood flow, although this is not thought to affect renal function in clinical use.
- Uterine relaxation.
- No effect on hepatic function or blood flow.
- Increased risk of postoperative nausea and vomiting (PONV).

Other:
- Trigger for malignant hyperthermia (MH).

Pharmacology

Uptake:
- With its relatively low blood/gas partition coefficient, alveolar and blood partial pressures equilibrate rapidly compared with older agents such as halothane but more slowly than desflurane and sevoflurane.
- Rate of recovery is slower than that associated with desflurane or sevoflurane because of its greater solubility (higher blood/gas partition coefficient).

Metabolism:
- Less than 0.2% metabolised by liver (defluorination via cytochrome P450 (CYP2E1) producing hexafluoroiso-propanol (HFIP)).

Excretion:
- Majority of the delivered drug is excreted unchanged through the lungs.
- Less than 0.2% renal excretion; HFIP is excreted in urine after conjugation with glucuronic acid.

Desflurane

Uses

1. Maintenance of general anaesthesia.

Desflurane is the most recent volatile agent to enter mainstream anaesthetic practice. It has been welcomed for surgical techniques where a fast onset and rapid recovery from anaesthesia are particularly desirable, such as major head and neck surgery. In addition, its low solubility (blood/gas coefficient) and subsequent smaller volume of distribution are beneficial to patients undergoing lengthy surgery or bariatric patients, in whom the volume of distribution of lipid-soluble drugs is greater.

Physical properties

Desflurane is a colourless agent which is stored in amber-coloured bottles without preservative. It is non-flammable at commercial concentrations. Desflurane is stable in the presence of soda lime but should be protected from light. Desflurane has an ethereal and pungent odour.

Desflurane has a boiling point close to room temperature (23.5°C) and a vapour pressure of 88.5 kPa at 20°C. A standard vaporiser cannot be used to deliver desflurane as small temperature and/or pressure fluctuations would result in a variable output. A special vaporiser (TEC 6) has been developed which heats the desflurane to 39°C and pressurises it to 2 atmospheres (see Chapter 16). The TEC 6 vaporiser therefore requires a source of electricity.

Systemic effects

RS:
- Dose-dependent respiratory depression, with depression of the ventilatory response to $PaCO_2$. This exceeds the effect of other volatile agents at concentrations >1 MAC.
- Irritant to the upper respiratory tract, particularly at concentrations > 6%.
- Stimulation of coughing, breath holding and laryngospasm precludes its use as an induction agent.

CVS:
- Dose-related reduction in SVR, myocardial contractility and MAP.
- Heart rate unchanged at lower steady-state concentrations but increases with higher concentrations.
- Cardiac output tends to be maintained as per isoflurane.
- In concentrations >1 MAC, an increase in sympathetic activity, leading to increased HR and MAP.
- No detectable coronary steal.
- Does not sensitise the myocardium to catecholamines.

CNS:
- Causes general anaesthesia and reduction in cerebral metabolic rate.
- Dose-dependent EEG depression.
- Does not induce seizure activity at any depth of anaesthesia.
- Dose-dependent alteration in cerebral autoregulation (vasodilatation) at concentrations > 1 MAC, which can result in an increase in ICP.
- Dose-dependent muscle relaxation.
- Potentiation of effects of NMBAs.

GI/GU:
- Uterine relaxation.
- Increased risk of PONV.

Other:
- Malignant hyperthermia trigger.

Pharmacology

Uptake:
- With a blood/gas partition coefficient of 0.42, equilibration of alveolar with inspired concentrations of desflurane is rapid compared with other available volatile agents. This leads to a rapid onset and recovery from anaesthesia.

Metabolism:
- Approximately 0.02% of inhaled desflurane is metabolised in the body.

Excretion:
- Approximately 99.98% is excreted unchanged from the lungs.

Sevoflurane
Uses

1. Induction and maintenance of general anaesthesia.
2. Sedation on ITU.
3. Treatment of severe asthma in patients whose lungs are mechanically ventilated.

Sevoflurane is a polyfluorinated isopropyl methyl ether (fluoromethyl-2,2,2-trifluoro-1-ethyl ether). Unlike the other volatile agents, sevoflurane is achiral.

Physical properties

Sevoflurane is non-flammable and has a pleasant smell. It has a low blood/gas partition coefficient close to those of desflurane and nitrous oxide. During storage, where the concentration of added water is less than 100 ppm, it is susceptible to attack by Lewis acids (defined as any substance that can accept an electron pair) resulting in the release of hydrofluoric acid, which is highly toxic. This can be compounded if sevoflurane is stored in glass bottles as the hydrofluoric acid can corrode glass, formulating further Lewis acids. Consequently, sevoflurane is formulated with 300 ppm water and stored in polyethylene naphtholate or epoxy phenolic resin–lined aluminium bottles to ensure stability.

Systemic effects

RS:
- Non-irritant to the upper respiratory tract; suitable for gaseous induction.
- Dose-dependent depression in tidal volume.
- Reduced respiratory drive in response to hypoxaemia.

55

- Reduced respiratory drive in response to raised $PaCO_2$ to a similar degree to other volatile agents.
- Increased respiratory rate.
- Inhibits hypoxic pulmonary vasoconstriction.
- Bronchial smooth muscle relaxation.

CVS:
- Increased HR (less than that of isoflurane).
- Not associated with coronary steal.
- Dose-related reduction in SVR, myocardial contractility and MAP.
- Does not sensitise the myocardium to exogenous catecholamines.

CNS:
- Causes general anaesthesia.
- Dose-dependent reduction in cerebral vascular resistance and cerebral metabolic rate.
- Preferred volatile agent for neuroanaesthesia. Although ICP is increased at high inspired concentrations (> 1.5 MAC) this effect is minimal over the 0.5–1.0 MAC range. This is thought to be due to preserved cerebral autoregulation of CBF.
- No excitatory effects on EEG.
- Potentiation of NMBAs.
- Dose-dependent muscle relaxation.

GI/GU:
- No demonstrable renal toxicity clinically despite concerns of fluoride ion exposure.
- Preservation of renal blood flow.
- Uterine relaxation.
- Increased risk of PONV.

Other:
- Trigger for MH.
- Production of potentially toxic compounds when in prolonged contact with soda lime (see next section).

Sevoflurane and carbon dioxide absorbers

Sevoflurane is absorbed and degraded by both soda lime and baralyme. When mixed with soda lime in artificial situations, five breakdown products are identified. These are termed compounds A, B, C, D and E and are thought to be toxic in rats, primarily causing renal, hepatic and cerebral injury.

In clinical situations, it is predominantly compound A and, to a lesser extent, compound B, that are produced. Evidence suggests that the concentration of compound A produced is well below the level that is toxic to animals. The use of baralyme is associated with production of higher concentrations of compound A, and this may be related to the higher temperature attained when baralyme is used. The presence of moisture reduces compound A formation. The concentration of compound A is highest during low-flow anaesthesia (<2 L min^{-1}) and is reduced by increasing fresh gas flow rate. The toxicity of sevoflurane in combination with carbon dioxide absorbers is probably more a theoretical than clinical concern.

Pharmacology

Uptake:
- Rapid onset/offset because of a low blood/gas partition coefficient.

Metabolism:
- Approximately 2%–3% of the absorbed dose is metabolised (by defluorination) in the liver (CYP450 2E1) to HFIP, carbon dioxide and inorganic fluoride. Inorganic fluoride concentrations peak within 2 h of the end of anaesthesia and have a half-life of 15–23 h. There have been no reports of fluoride toxicity in clinical studies investigating sevoflurane.

Excretion:
- Approximately 98% is excreted unchanged from the lungs. Hexafluoroisopropanol is conjugated with glucuronic acid as excreted as urinary metabolite.

Halothane

Uses

1. Induction and maintenance of general anaesthesia.

The halogenated hydrocarbon, halothane (2-bromo-2-chloro-1,1,1-trifluoroethane), was the first of the 'modern' volatile agents to be synthesised and remains the standard to which new volatiles are compared. It is seldom used in Western practice now.

Physical properties

Halothane is a colourless liquid with a relatively pleasant, characteristic smell. It is presented in amber-coloured bottles with of 0.01% thymol for stability as it undergoes decomposition in the presence of light. It should be stored in a closed container away from light and heat. Although decomposed by soda lime, it may be used safely with this mixture. In the presence of moisture, it corrodes aluminium, tin, lead, magnesium and alloys. It is known to corrode metals in vaporisers and breathing systems.

Systemic effects

RS:
- Non-irritant and pleasant to breathe during induction of anaesthesia.
- Rapid loss of pharyngeal and laryngeal reflexes.
- Inhibition of salivary and bronchial secretions.
- Dose-dependent increase in ventilatory rate.
- Dose-dependent reduction in tidal volume.
- $PaCO_2$ increases as the depth of halothane anaesthesia increases.
- Dose-dependent decrease in mucociliary function.
- Relaxation of bronchial smooth muscle.

CVS:
- Dose-dependent decrease in myocardial contractility and coronary blood flow.
- Dose-dependent reduction in CO and SVR.
- Bradycardia, thought to be caused by halothane-induced vagal stimulation.
- Marked sensitisation of myocardium to catecholamines, and can cause arrhythmias. This is increased in the presence of hypercapnia, hypoxaemia or increased circulating catecholamines (endogenous or exogenous).

CNS:
- Causes general anaesthesia.
- Increases CBF/ICP.
- Does not cause seizure activity on EEG.
- Induces skeletal muscle relaxation and potentiates NMBAs.
- Postoperative shivering is common; this increases oxygen requirements and results in hypoxaemia unless supplemental oxygen is administered.

GI/GU:
- Inhibits gastrointestinal motility.
- Increases risk of PONV, but this is seldom severe.
- Induces uterine muscle relaxation.
- Can cause significant hepatic dysfunction (see later).

Other:
- Trigger for MH.

Pharmacology

Uptake:
- Halothane has a high blood/gas solubility coefficient, which renders it very soluble, and therefore onset and recovery from anaesthesia are the slowest of the modern volatile agents.
- It is non-irritant to the airway and therefore inhalational induction with halothane is relatively rapid; however, it may take at least 30 min for the alveolar inspired concentration to reach 50% of the inspired concentration.

Metabolism:
- Approximately 20% of halothane is metabolised in the liver. This is greatest of the volatile anaesthetic agents in current use.

Excretion:
- The end products are excreted in the urine. The major metabolites are bromine, chlorine, trifluoroacetic acid and trifluoroacetylethanol amide.

Halothane-associated hepatic dysfunction

Halothane hepatitis is the most serious adverse effect from halothane anaesthesia. Two types of liver dysfunction may occur after halothane anaesthesia:

1. *Halothane-associated hepatic dysfunction.* This is mild and is associated with transient derangement of liver function tests which generally resolves within a few days. Similar changes in liver function tests have also been reported after enflurane and, to a lesser extent, isoflurane anaesthesia. This subclinical type of hepatic dysfunction, evidenced by an increase in glutathione-S-transferase concentrations, probably occurs as a result of halothane metabolism in the liver, where it reacts with hepatic macromolecules, resulting in tissue necrosis. This necrosis is worsened by hypoxaemia.

2. *Halothane hepatitis.* This is extremely uncommon and takes the form of severe jaundice, progressing to fulminating hepatic necrosis. The risk of developing halothane hepatitis increases with repeated exposure, and the mortality varies between 30% and 70%. The mechanism of hepatotoxicity is thought to be secondary to an immune response to certain fluoroacetylated liver enzymes which are formed in the process of halothane metabolism. As a result of the concerns regarding halothane hepatitis, the UK Committee on Safety of Medicines made the following recommendations in respect of halothane anaesthesia:
   - A careful anaesthetic history should be taken to determine previous exposure and any previous reaction to halothane.
   - Repeated exposure to halothane within a period of 3 months should be avoided unless there are overriding clinical circumstances.
   - A history of unexplained jaundice or pyrexia after previous exposure to halothane is an absolute contraindication to its future use in that patient.

The incidence of halothane hepatotoxicity in paediatric practice is extremely low, although there have been case reports in children.

Comparison of isoflurane, desflurane, sevoflurane and halothane (Table 3.2)

Systemic effects

RS:
- All inhalational agents cause dose-related respiratory depression, resulting in reduced tidal volume, increased respiratory rate and reduced minute ventilation (desflurane > isoflurane, halothane or sevoflurane) (Fig. 3.5).
- Nitrous oxide does not cause hypercapnia. Thus the reduction in inspired volatile anaesthetic concentration permitted by addition of nitrous oxide is associated with less overall ventilatory depression.
- With all volatile agents, depression of ventilation is associated with depression of whole-body oxygen consumption and carbon dioxide production.
- Halothane and, to a lesser extent sevoflurane and isoflurane, cause bronchodilation.

Table 3.2 Advantages and disadvantages of the modern volatile anaesthetic agents

	Isoflurane	Sevoflurane	Desflurane
Advantages	• Low cost; approximately 70% cheaper than sevoflurane • Bronchodilator • No significant toxic metabolites • Non-arrhythmogenic	• Good for inhalational induction • Non-irritant to airways • Faster onset/offset than isoflurane • Non-arrhythmogenic	• Fast onset/recovery from anaesthesia • Minimal, non-toxic metabolites
Disadvantages	• Concerns about coronary steal syndrome • Irritant to airways	• Expensive • Metabolised to toxic metabolites (not thought to be of clinical concern) • Formation of potentially toxic compounds on interaction with soda lime/baralyme (not thought to be of clinical concern)	• Expensive • Irritant to airways • Causes tachycardia at higher concentrations • Heated/pressurised vaporiser required for delivery

All volatile agents:
- may trigger malignant hyperpyrexia in susceptible individuals;
- have a higher incidence of PONV compared with total intravenous anaesthesia;
- have a possible association with postoperative cognitive dysfunction (see Chapter 31);
- are environmental greenhouse gases; and
- cause dose-dependent CVS/RS depression.

PONV, Postoperative nausea and vomiting.

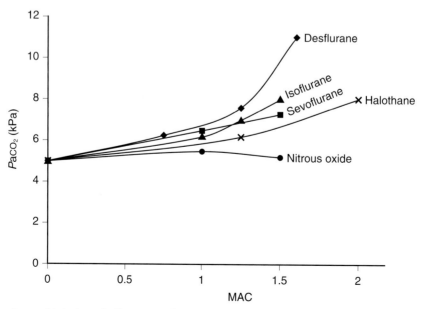

Fig. 3.5 Effects on $PaCO_2$ of halothane, isoflurane, sevoflurane, desflurane and nitrous oxide at equivalent MAC during spontaneous ventilation by healthy volunteers (nitrous oxide administered in a hyperbaric chamber).

CVS:

- All agents reduce MAP because of reduced SVR and myocardial depression (Figs 3.6 and 3.7).
- Desflurane and isoflurane maintain CO, decreasing MAP mainly by decreasing SVR (Fig. 3.8).
- Halothane reduces MAP principally by decreasing CO, with little effect on SVR.
- Isoflurane and desflurane increase HR as a result of sympathetic stimulation, whereas halothane and sevoflurane cause a reduction in heart rate.
- Some of the cardiovascular effects of volatile agents are antagonised by the addition of nitrous oxide.

- During spontaneous ventilation, the modest hypercapnia which occurs with all agents also offsets some of the changes. With isoflurane, for example, CO may be increased compared with pre-anaesthesia concentrations, although there is little effect on MAP.
- Desflurane, isoflurane and sevoflurane do not sensitise the myocardium to endogenous or exogenous catecholamines, but halothane predisposes to arrhythmias (Fig. 3.9).
- Isoflurane causes coronary vasodilatation and experimentally was found to cause coronary steal syndrome. This is now known to be of little or no clinical significance. Sevoflurane causes some coronary vasodilatation but does not appear

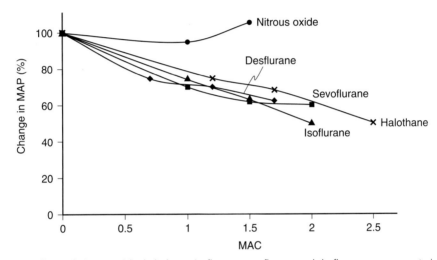

Fig. 3.6 Comparative effects of nitrous oxide, halothane, isoflurane, sevoflurane and desflurane on mean arterial pressure (MAP) in healthy volunteers.

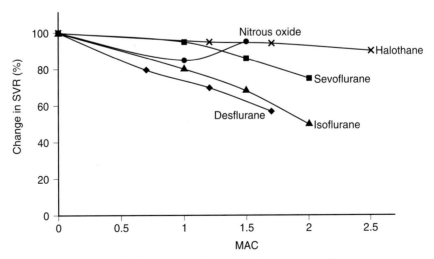

Fig. 3.7 Comparative effects of nitrous oxide, halothane, isoflurane, sevoflurane and desflurane on systemic vascular resistance (SVR) in healthy volunteers.

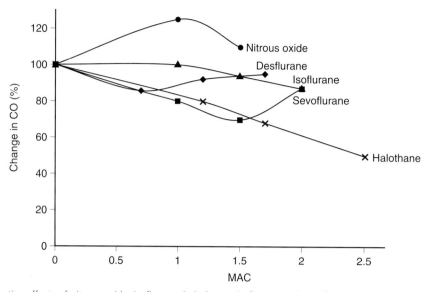

Fig. 3.8 Comparative effects of nitrous oxide, isoflurane, halothane, desflurane and sevoflurane on cardiac output in healthy volunteers.

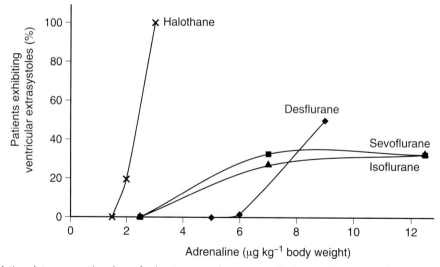

Fig. 3.9 Cumulative plots representing dose of subcutaneous adrenaline required to produce ventricular extrasystoles in normocapnic patients receiving 1.25 MAC of halothane, isoflurane, sevoflurane or desflurane.

to cause coronary steal syndrome. Halothane and desflurane do not cause any coronary vasodilatation.

CNS:

- All agents cause dose-related depression of cerebral activity.
- All agents uncouple cerebral autoregulation (desflurane > isoflurane > sevoflurane).
- All the agents decrease cerebrovascular resistance and increase ICP in a dose-related manner.
- All agents produce muscle relaxation sufficient to perform lower abdominal surgery in slim, spontaneously breathing patients.
- All agents potentiate NMBAs. In this respect, isoflurane, sevoflurane and desflurane are similar and cause

markedly greater potentiation than that produced by halothane.

GI/GU:

- Halothane and isoflurane relax uterine muscle in a dose-related manner. There is limited experience with desflurane and sevoflurane in the obstetric population. Sevoflurane appears to have similar uterine effects to isoflurane.
- Halothane is associated with life-threatening liver toxicity.

Pharmacology

Distribution:

- Uptake/offset of desflurane is faster than that of any of the other volatile agents and similar to that of nitrous oxide (see Figs 3.1 and 3.2).
- Potency is related to the lower oil/water solubility. Sevoflurane and desflurane are less potent than the older agents, as reflected by higher MAC values.

Metabolism:

- Desflurane (0.02%) < isoflurane (0.2%) < sevoflurane (2%–3%) < halothane (20%).
- Halothane and sevoflurane are both metabolised to potentially toxic metabolites, although the metabolites of sevoflurane are not thought to be clinically significant.

Carbon dioxide absorbers:

- Sevoflurane and halothane react with soda lime; desflurane and isoflurane do not.

Nitrous oxide

Nitrous oxide is an inorganic gas first synthesised by Joseph Priestley in 1772. Despite early knowledge of its analgesic and anaesthetic properties, however, it was not introduced into mainstream medical/dental practice until the late 1800s.

Uses

1. Adjuvant to the induction and maintenance of general anaesthesia.
2. Analgesic agent, especially as Entonox (see later).
3. A refrigerant in cryosurgery.

Presentation and storage

Nitrous oxide is presented as a liquid in French-blue cylinders at a pressure of 44 bar. The gauge pressure, however, bears no correlation with the cylinder content until all the nitrous oxide is in the gaseous phase. The volume of liquid nitrous oxide in a cylinder is determined by the 'filling ratio' (see Chapter 15). This is the ratio of the mass of nitrous oxide in the cylinder to the mass of water that the cylinder could hold if it were full. In temperate regions (such as the UK) the filling ratio is 0.75; in warmer climates it is reduced to

0.67 to avoid cylinder explosions. Cylinders should be kept upright and undergo regular testing, the details of which should be recorded on the plastic disc between the cylinder valve and neck and engraved onto the cylinder body. It is also presented as piped medical gas and vacuum (PMGV) at 4 bar.

Manufacture

Nitrous oxide is prepared commercially by heating ammonium nitrate to a temperature of 245–270°C. Various impurities are produced in this process: ammonia; nitric acid; nitrogen; nitric oxide; and nitrogen dioxide.

After cooling, ammonia and nitric acid are reconstituted to ammonium nitrate, which is returned to the beginning of the process. The remaining gases then pass through a series of scrubbers. The purified gases are compressed and dried in an aluminium dryer. The resultant gases are expanded in a liquefier, with the nitrogen escaping as gas. Nitrous oxide is then evaporated, compressed and passed through another aluminium dryer before being stored in cylinders.

The higher oxides of nitrogen dissolve in water to form nitrous and nitric acids. These substances are toxic and produce methaemoglobinaemia and pulmonary oedema if inhaled. There have been several reports of death occurring during anaesthesia as a result of the inhalation of nitrous oxide contaminated with higher oxides of nitrogen.

Physical properties

Nitrous oxide is a sweet-smelling, non-irritating, colourless gas with the following properties:

- Molecular weight 44 Da
- Boiling point −88°C
- Critical temperature (the temperature above which a gas cannot be liquefied however much pressure is applied) 36.5°C
- Critical pressure (the minimum pressure that causes liquefaction of a gas at its critical temperature) 72.6 bar

Nitrous oxide is not flammable but it supports combustion of fuels in the absence of oxygen.

Mechanism of action

Nitrous oxide appears to exert its activity at different types of receptors. It has an inhibitory action on NMDA glutamate receptors and stimulatory activity at dopamine, α_1- and α_2-adrenergic and opioid receptors. The analgesic action of nitrous oxide is probably mediated by activation of opioid receptors in the periaqueductal area of the midbrain (see Chapter 6). This leads to modulation of nociceptive pathways through the release of noradrenaline and activation of the α_2-adrenoreceptors in the dorsal horn of the spinal cord. Because of its analgesic properties, nitrous oxide is used in combination with volatile agents as part of a general anaesthetic, which reduces the MAC of volatile anaesthetic agent required.

Systemic effects

RS:
- Decreases tidal volume but increases respiratory rate and hence maintains minute ventilation.
- Reduces the ventilatory response to hypoxaemia and hypercapnia.
- Depresses tracheal mucociliary flow and neutrophil chemotaxis and may increase the incidence of postoperative respiratory complications.
- Non-irritant and does not cause bronchospasm.
- Can cause diffusion hypoxia (see next section).

Diffusion hypoxia

Diffusion hypoxia is the reverse of the second gas effect. The rate of transfer of nitrous oxide from pulmonary blood back into the alveolus exceeds that of nitrogen and oxygen; this effectively dilutes alveolar air and oxygen, thereby reducing the P_{AO_2}, producing hypoxia. For this reason, the delivery of oxygen-enriched air is recommended for emergence from a nitrous oxide–based anaesthetic (as per standard care in PACU; see Chapter 29).

CVS:
- Direct myocardial depression.
- Indirectly mediated, sympathoadrenal stimulation and increased SVR; this outweighs the myocardial depressant effects, and healthy patients exhibit little change in MAP.
- Increase in pulmonary vascular resistance.

CNS:
- Increases CBF, cerebral metabolism and ICP.
- Changes are more marked in patients with abnormal cerebral autoregulation and may result in reduced cerebral perfusion.
- Prolonged exposure can cause neuropathy (see later).
- Does not appear to potentiate the action of NMBAs.

GI/GU:
- Increases risk of PONV.

Other:
- Causes increase in pressure/volume in enclosed gas-filled spaces (see later).
- Long exposure can cause megaloblastic anaemia (see later).
- Potentially teratogenic and should be avoided in first trimester of pregnancy.

Pharmacokinetics

Nitrous oxide is often said to be a good analgesic but a weak anaesthetic. The latter refers to the fact that its MAC value is 105%. This value was calculated theoretically from its low oil/water solubility coefficient of 3.2 and has been confirmed experimentally in volunteers anaesthetised in a pressure chamber compressed to 2 atmospheres. As it is essential to administer a minimum F_{IO_2} 0.3 during anaesthesia, nitrous oxide alone is insufficient to produce an adequate depth of anaesthesia. Therefore nitrous oxide is usually administered in combination with a volatile agent.

Nitrous oxide has a low blood/gas solubility coefficient (0.47 at 37°C). Therefore the rate of equilibration of alveolar with inspired concentrations is very fast (see Fig. 3.1).

Metabolism/excretion:
- Does not undergo metabolism in the body and is excreted unchanged.

Effects on closed gas spaces

When blood containing nitrous oxide equilibrates with closed air-containing spaces inside the body, the volume of nitrous oxide that diffuses into the cavity exceeds the volume of nitrogen diffusing out. In compliant spaces, such as the bowel lumen or the pleural or peritoneal cavities, there is an increase in volume of the space. However, if the space cannot expand (e.g. sinuses, middle ear) there is an increase in pressure. When nitrous oxide is administered in a concentration of 75%, the volume of a cavity may increase to as much as three to four times the original volume within 30 min. This can result in significant injury such as pneumothoraces, bowel perforation, tympanic membrane perforation and an increase in the size of air emboli in blood and tissues.

A similar problem arises during prolonged procedures where nitrous oxide diffuses into the cuff of the tracheal tube and may increase the pressure exerted on the tracheal mucosa. Either avoiding the use of nitrous oxide or inflating the cuff with saline or nitrous oxide may prevent this.

A complication of the effect of nitrous oxide on closed gas spaces that has been described is the loss of vision caused by expansion of intraocular perfluoropropane gas used in vitreoretinal surgery. The visual loss is caused possibly by central retinal artery occlusion as a result of expansion of the gas by nitrous oxide, resulting in increased intraocular pressure.

The use of nitrous oxide in at-risk patients should be avoided.

Effects on blood and the nervous system

Nitrous oxide oxidises the cobalt ion present in vitamin B12, which is required as a cofactor for methionine synthetase. This results in reduced DNA synthesis in both leucocytes and erythrocytes. Exposure of patients to nitrous oxide for ≥ 6 h may result in megaloblastic anaemia. Agranulocytosis may occur after longer exposure (days). Occupational exposure to nitrous oxide may result in myeloneuropathy. This condition is similar to subacute combined degeneration of the spinal cord and has been reported in dentists and individuals addicted to inhalation of nitrous oxide.

Environment

Nitrous oxide is a greenhouse gas; it is 200–300 times more effective in trapping heat than carbon dioxide and therefore may contribute to global warming. However, the contribution to the greenhouse effect is very small as anaesthesia only accounts for <1% of global nitrous oxide emission.

Other agents

Xenon

Xenon is a dense, colourless gas found in the Earth's atmosphere in trace amounts. Cullen and Gross first reported the anaesthetic properties of xenon in humans in 1951.

Xenon offers many advantages over nitrous oxide, for which it could theoretically become a suitable replacement. Unfortunately it is difficult to manufacture, which makes it extremely expensive, precluding its use in mainstream anaesthesia. However, anaesthetic machines with the ability to deliver xenon are likely to become available thanks to a mechanism by which xenon can be recovered and recycled, making it far more economical.

Xenon, in common with nitrous oxide and ketamine, acts by non-competitive inhibition of NMDA receptors in the CNS.

Physical properties

Xenon has a blood/gas partition coefficient of 0.14–0.2, which is lower than that of nitrous oxide (0.47) and therefore provides rapid induction of and recovery from anaesthesia. Xenon is more potent than nitrous oxide, with a MAC of 70%. It does not undergo biotransformation, and it is harmless to the ozone layer.

Systemic effects

Studies so far have found no cardiorespiratory adverse effects or reduction in local organ perfusion; in fact, to date it has demonstrated both cardio- and neuroprotective properties through a variety of mechanisms.

It is not irritating to the respiratory tract. Xenon is a competitive inhibitor of the 5-HT$_3$ receptor and is therefore thought to reduce the incidence of PONV.

Enflurane

The halogenated methyl ethyl ether enflurane is a geometric isomer of isoflurane and boasts similar properties. It is no longer in use in modern clinical practice largely because of some unfavourable adverse effects. Enflurane has been associated with: tonic–clonic muscle activity; epileptiform EEG changes; sensitisation of the myocardium to catecholamines causing dysrhythmias; and hepatotoxicity as a result of its significant liver metabolism.

Diethyl ether

Ether is no longer used in modern anaesthetic practice, although it is still useful in resource-poor environments. It is discussed in detail in Chapter 45.

Medical gases

Oxygen

Oxygen comprises 21% of the Earth's atmosphere and is the third most abundant element in the universe by mass after hydrogen and helium. It is a highly reactive non-metal with the atomic number 8 and chemical symbol O.

Uses

1. Management of cellular hypoxia (either caused by hypoxaemia or low cardiac output states).
2. Treatment of carbon monoxide poisoning.
3. Treatment of anaerobic infections.
4. Treatment of decompression sickness.

Presentation and storage

Oxygen is a colourless, tasteless and odourless gas at room temperature and pressure. It supports combustion and, in the correct circumstances, is explosive. It has a specific gravity of 1.105 and a molecular mass 32. At atmospheric pressure, it liquefies at −183°C.

There are two common means of oxygen storage for hospital use:
1. *Cylinders.* Traditionally cylinders containing oxygen have a black body with white shoulders, although there are now lightweight, fibreglass cylinders in use that are fully white in colour. Both types of cylinders store oxygen at a pressure of 137 bar (13,700 kPa) at 15°C when full.
2. *Vacuum insulated evaporator (VIE).* The VIE is a large vessel that stores liquid oxygen at approximately −160°C and 7 bar and is used in medical or industrial facilities where oxygen demand is high (usually in excess of 150,000 l week^{-1}). Oxygen is delivered to the hospital from either the VIE or a cylinder manifold through PMGV and is regulated to 4 bar (see Chapter 16 and Fig. 16.1).

Manufacture

Oxygen can be manufactured from air in two main ways:

1. *Fractional distillation of air.* Oxygen is manufactured commercially by fractional distillation of liquid air. Before liquefaction of air, carbon dioxide is removed and liquid oxygen and nitrogen separated by means of their different boiling points (oxygen $-183\,°C$; nitrogen $-195\,°C$).

2. *Oxygen concentrators.* Oxygen concentrators produce oxygen from ambient air by absorption of nitrogen onto types of alumina silicates. Oxygen concentrators are useful both in hospitals and in long-term domestic use in remote areas such as in developing countries (see Chapter 45) and in military surgery. The gas formed by oxygen concentrators contains small quantities of inert gases (e.g. argon); these are harmless but reduce the maximal concentration of oxygen that can be produced.

Adverse pulmonary effects

Oxygen is one of the most commonly prescribed drugs in hospital; when given for the correct reasons and in the correct dose it is lifesaving. However, it is becoming increasingly recognised that inappropriate supplemental oxygen can have significant deleterious effects (see Chapter 10).

Hyperoxia can result in the formation of reactive oxygen intermediates, depleting antioxidant stores and causing widespread cellular damage through direct and proinflammatory effects. The respiratory tract is exposed to the highest concentration of oxygen and therefore is at greatest risk of adverse effects and oxygen toxicity. Pulmonary effects include the following:

1. *Absorption atelectasis.* In high-inspired concentrations, oxygen washes out the nitrogen from alveoli and, because of its rapid absorption across the alveolar membrane, causes alveolar collapse (atelectasis). This will increase the shunt fraction and can cause atelectrauma during re-expansion. Although this is likely to be minor in young, healthy individuals, it can contribute to worsening hypoxia and lung injury in susceptible patients.

2. *Accentuation of hypercapnoea.* High inspired concentrations of oxygen can paradoxically increase $PaCO_2$ via a number of mechanisms:

   - Although mild respiratory depression is seen in healthy individuals delivered high inspired oxygen concentrations, this is likely to be clinically insignificant. In contrast, patients with chronic hypercarbia are often dependent on mild hypoxia to maintain respiratory drive. In these individuals, administration of high inspired concentrations may abolish this drive and render them apnoeic.
   - Increasing dead space ventilation by reversal of physiological hypoxic pulmonary vasoconstriction.
   - The Haldane effect – increasing blood oxygen tension favours offloading of carbon dioxide from haemoglobin.

3. *Airway and parenchymal injury.* The reactive oxygen intermediates can cause direct airway and parenchymal injury, tracheobronchitis, airway oedema, worsening of airspace disease in acute respiratory distress syndrome (ARDS) and diffuse alveolar damage. Bronchopulmonary dysplasia (seen in neonates after neonatal respiratory distress syndrome) has been partially attributed to the effect of oxygen on the immature lung.

Adverse systemic effects

Cardiovascular depression

An increase in PaO_2 leads to direct vasoconstriction in peripheral, cerebral, coronary, hepatic and renal vasculature. Hyperbaric pressures of oxygen also cause direct myocardial depression. In patients with severe cardiovascular disease, elevation of PaO_2 from the normal physiological range to 80 kPa may produce clinically evident cardiovascular depression.

Central nervous system oxygen toxicity

Convulsions, similar to those of grand mal epilepsy, occur during exposure to hyperbaric pressures of oxygen. The administration of 100% oxygen can also result in cerebral vasoconstriction and a subsequent decrease in CBF.

Retrolental fibroplasia

Retrolental fibroplasia (RLF) is the result of oxygen-induced retinal vasoconstriction, with obliteration of the most immature retinal vessels. There is subsequent new vessel formation at the site of damage, resulting in a proliferative retinopathy. Leakage of intravascular fluid leads to vitreo-retinal adhesions and even retinal detachment. Retrolental fibroplasia occurs in infants exposed to hyperoxia in the paediatric intensive care unit and is related not to the FIO_2 *per se* but to an elevated retinal artery PO_2. It is not known what the threshold of PaO_2 is for the development of retinal damage, but an umbilical arterial PO_2 of 8–12 kPa is associated with a very low incidence of RLF and no signs of systemic hypoxia. It should be stressed, however, that there are many factors involved in the development of RLF in addition to arterial hyperoxia.

Depressed haemopoiesis

Long-term exposure to elevated FIO_2 leads to depression of haemopoiesis and anaemia.

Medical air

Uses

1. Driving gas for mechanical ventilators.
2. To operate power tools (e.g. orthopaedic drills).
3. As a carrier agent for inhalational anaesthetic agents.

Nitrous oxide is still commonly used in combination with a volatile agent to maintain anaesthesia. However, there is growing concern regarding its toxic effects and cost. Consequently, medical air in combination with oxygen is now being used increasingly during anaesthesia.

Medical air is obtained from the atmosphere near to the site of compression. Great care is taken to position the air intake to avoid contamination with pollutants such as carbon monoxide from car exhausts. Air is compressed to 137 bar and then passed through columns of activated alumina to remove water.

Air for medical purposes is supplied in cylinders (grey body and black and white shoulders in the UK) or as a piped system. A pressure of 4 bar is available for attachment to anaesthetic machines and 7 bar for orthopaedic tools. Its composition varies slightly depending on location of compression and moisture content.

Entonox

Uses

1. Inhalational anaesthetic agent (in conjunction with a volatile agent).
2. Inhalational analgesic agent.
   a. During labour.
   b. For breakthrough pain when regional anaesthesia is used (e.g. tourniquet pain (see Chapter 25) and caesarean section (see Chapter 43)).
   c. During painful short procedures, such as change of burns dressings, manipulations of fractures/ dislocations and cleaning of wounds in paediatric patients.

Entonox is a 50:50 mixture of oxygen and nitrous oxide. It is produced by bubbling oxygen through liquid nitrous oxide. The two gases dissolve into each other, creating a gas mixture that does not behave in a way that could be predicted from their individual properties – the Poynting effect.

Entonox is presented as a gas in French-blue cylinders with white and blue checked shoulders at a pressure of 137 bar when full. Below temperatures of $-7°C$ (pseudocritical temperature), Entonox can separate into its constituent parts because of liquefaction of nitrous oxide. This can potentially result in the delivery of a hypoxic mixture as the cylinder empties.

Helium

Uses

1. In medical devices, such as an intra-aortic balloon pump.
2. Improves flow dynamics in patients with airway obstruction.
3. Measurement of FRC (helium dilution technique).

Presentation and storage

Helium is a light inert gas, present in air and natural gas. It is the second most abundant element after hydrogen. It is presented as either Heliox (79% helium and 21% oxygen) in white cylinders with white and brown quartered shoulders or as 100% helium in brown cylinders at 137 bar.

Properties

Helium has a lower density than air, nitrogen and oxygen. The low density of gas results in a lowering of the Reynolds' number and thus a return from turbulent to laminar flow in some situations (see Chapter 15). By increasing laminar flow, the efficiency of breathing is increased. This physical characteristic is used to treat patients with upper airway obstruction to reduce the work of breathing and improve oxygenation.

As a result of its lower density, patients receiving helium have a typical squeaky voice because higher frequency vocal sounds are transmitted. Helium is used in the measurement of lung volumes because of its very low solubility.

Chapter | **4** |

Intravenous anaesthetic agents and sedatives

David Mulvey

A wide variety of therapeutic and non-therapeutic substances will obtund cerebral function and produce a continuum of cognitive states from almost fully awake to unexpected death (Table 4.1). The clinically useful part of this spectrum is characterised by the American Society of Anaesthesiologists as levels of sedation and general anaesthesia (Table 4.2). Any centrally acting depressant agent may produce sedation or general anaesthesia depending on the dose, route and rate of administration, mechanism of action and physicochemical properties. Anaesthetic drugs used at reduced dosage produce sedation, and agents used primarily as sedatives can provide a form of general anaesthesia. However, the dose required for some 'sedative' agents to achieve surgical anaesthesia is so high that recovery is significantly delayed, hence they are unsuitable for this purpose. Consequently only a few drugs are used routinely to induce anaesthesia by i.v. injection (see Table 4.1). When these agents are to produce sedation, seamless progression from a level of sedation with anxiolysis (with retention of verbal contact and protective airway reflexes) to general anaesthesia may occur unexpectedly. The level of sedation also depends on the intensity of surgical stimulation and can alter rapidly without alteration in drug dosage. Healthcare professionals providing sedation must possess the necessary skills and equipment to manage an unexpected progression to general anaesthesia and a detailed guide been produced by the Academy of Medical Royal Colleges. As a precaution, patients requiring deep levels of sedation should be assessed and prepared (including fasting) as though listed for planned general anaesthesia. The 5th National Audit Project report on accidental awareness during general anaesthesia (NAP5) recommended that patients are informed that awareness or recall is possible despite sedation. Clinicians must explain that the intention is to improve procedural comfort and reduce anxiety and that sedation is not equivalent to general anaesthesia.

Intravenous anaesthetic drugs

Intravenous induction of anaesthesia is smooth and rapid compared with inhalational induction with most volatile anaesthetics. Combinations of i.v. drugs (e.g. propofol, midazolam, opioids) are often used together for coinduction of anaesthesia because their actions are synergistic, allowing reduced dosages for a given clinical end-point and potentially fewer adverse effects. Intravenous agents may also be used for maintenance of anaesthesia if administered as repeated boluses or by continuous i.v. infusion (either as a sole agent or in combination with opioids and/or nitrous oxide). Other uses include sedation during endoscopic procedures, regional anaesthesia, for patients in ICU and in the treatment of status epilepticus. The compounds used as i.v. anaesthetics (with the exception of propofol) are chiral molecules (see Chapter 1). Thiopental and ketamine are administered as racemic mixtures, etomidate as a pure R-enantiomer (Fig. 4.5), dexmedetomidine as a pure S-enantiomer (Fig. 4.13) and a formulation of S-ketamine (Fig.4.4) is available in Europe. Therapeutic activity resides mainly in one of the enantiomers, whilst the other can have undesirable properties, different therapeutic activities, be pharmacologically inert or have a different rate of metabolism.

Mechanism of action

Intravenous anaesthetics exert their action at γ-aminobutyric acid A (GABA$_A$) or *N*-methyl-D-aspartic acid (NMDA)

Table 4.1 Substances used to depress cognitive function

	Chemical group	Example
Agents used primarily for induction of anaesthesia	Alkyl phenol Phencyclidine Imidazole Barbiturate Inhalational agent	Propofol Ketamine Etomidate Thiopental Sevoflurane $\pm$ N_2O
Agents used primarily for sedation	α_2 Adrenergic agonist Benzodiazepine Z-drug Butyrophenone Atypical antipsychotic Opioid Inhalational agent Other	Dexmedetomidine, clonidine Midazolam, temazepam, lorazepam, diazepam Zopiclone, zolpidem and zaleplon Haloperidol, droperidol, Olanzapine Fentanyl, alfentanil, remifentanil, morphine, sufentanil Isoflurane, sevoflurane, methoxyflurane, N_2O Melatonin
Non-therapeutic agents		Ethanol γ-Hydroxybutyrate (GHB) Hydrocarbon solvents Petroleum products

Table 4.2 Continuum of depth of sedation (American Society of Anesthesiologists 2014 revision)

	Minimal sedation ("anxiolysis")	Moderate sedation/ analgesia ("conscious sedation")	Deep sedation/analgesia	General anaesthesia
Responsiveness	Normal response to verbal stimulation	Purposeful[a] response to verbal or tactile stimulation	Purposeful[a] response following repeated or painful stimulation	Unarousable even with painful stimulus
Airway	Unaffected	No intervention required	Intervention may be required	Intervention often required
Spontaneous ventilation	Unaffected	Adequate	May be inadequate	Often inadequate
Cardiovascular function	Unaffected	Usually maintained	Usually maintained	May be impaired

[a]Reflex withdrawal from a painful stimulus is *not* considered a purposeful response.

receptors, which are both ligand-gated ion channels. The $GABA_A$ receptor is a large pentameric protein with separate allosteric binding sites for propofol, benzodiazepines, barbiturates and ethanol (Fig. 4.1). Binding of an agonist enhances the affinity of the $GABA_A$ receptor for its endogenous ligand, which increases the frequency of channel opening and intracellular chloride ion conductance. Hyperpolarisation of the postsynaptic membrane results, and this inhibits synaptic transmission. The $GABA_A$ receptors with specific β subunits appear to mediate sedative ($\beta2$) and anaesthetic ($\beta3$) activity.

Benzodiazepines bind to the $GABA_A$ receptor at the α/γ subunit interface. The binding of other compounds to the benzodiazepine site explains their synergistic activity and the development of cross-tolerance. Propofol and barbiturates also potentiate the effects of glycine at glycine receptors (chloride influx and inhibition of synaptic transmission) both in the brain and spinal cord. Propofol has further inhibitory actions on voltage-gated sodium channels and activity at $5HT_3$ receptors; the latter may explain its antiemetic effects.

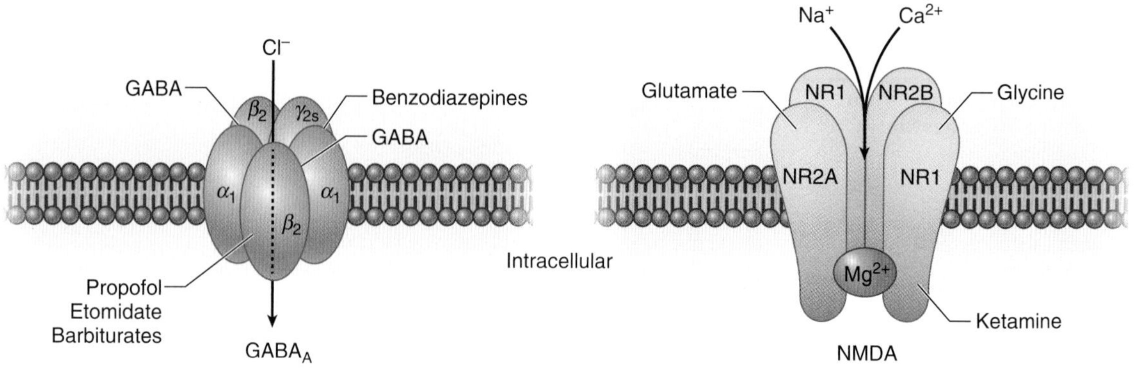

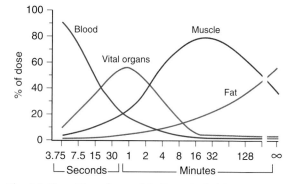

Fig. 4.1 Representation of the principle receptors mediating the action of i.v. anaesthetic drugs. Binding of agents to the GABA$_A$ receptor increases inward conductance of Cl$^-$ ions and membrane hyperpolarisation. The pentameric structure consists of different sub-types of α, β, and γ units. Agonist binding to the NMDA receptor inhibits inward conductance of Ca^{2+} and Na$^+$ ions and outward conductance of K$^+$ ions, which impairs synaptic transmission. NMDA NR1 units bind the co-agonist glycine and NR2 units bind the neurotransmitter glutamate. Genetic variations in sub-unit structure imparts variable activity to both of these receptors types. (With permission from Garcia, B., Whalin, M. K., & Sebel, P. S. (2013) Intravenous anaesthetics. In: Hemmings, H. & Egan, T. (eds.) *Pharmacology and Physiology for Anesthesia*. Philadelphia, Saunders Elsevier.)

Ketamine (in common with nitrous oxide and xenon) acts predominantly at tetrameric excitatory NMDA receptors that usually bind glycine and glutamate (see Fig. 4.1). Binding of ketamine to the NMDA receptor is non-competitive and reduces synaptic transmission by inhibiting conductance of positively charged ions. Ketamine appears to have no effect at GABA$_A$ or glycine receptors but may partially exert clinical action via cholinergic receptors and at voltage-gated ion channels for sodium, potassium and calcium.

Pharmacokinetics

Bolus administration of an i.v. anaesthetic causes a rapid increase in plasma concentration followed by an exponential decline (Fig. 4.2) (see Chapter 1). Hypnosis results from diffusion of drug along a concentration gradient between arterial blood and the brain. The initial rate of transfer into the brain and onset of effect are regulated by factors outlined next. In general, factors increasing the plasma concentration of free drug also increase the intensity of adverse effects.

Speed of injection

Rapid i.v. injection results in high initial plasma concentration of drug, which enhances diffusion into the brain and increases speed of induction. However cardiovascular and respiratory adverse effects are also more pronounced as the

Fig. 4.2 Disposition of propofol after a single intravenous bolus dose. The diagram assumes non-physiological instantaneous mixing in the entire blood volume. A high drug concentration is achieved rapidly in the brain and other vital organs with high blood flow, but this diminishes with time as the drug re-distributes to the tissue compartments with medium (muscle) or slow (fat) blood flows. (With permission from Nagelhout, J. J., Elisha, S. & Plaus, K. L. (2013) *Nurse Anesthesia*, 5th edn. Philadelphia, Saunders Elsevier.)

peak drug concentration in both brain and peripheral tissues also increases.

Blood flow to the brain

Reduced cerebral blood flow (CBF) results in slower delivery of drug to the brain. However, if CBF is reduced because of low cardiac output, initial blood concentrations are higher, and despite a slower onset, the effects will be enhanced.

Protein binding

Only unbound drug is free to cross the blood–brain barrier. Protein binding may be reduced by low plasma protein concentrations or by binding of other drugs, resulting in higher plasma concentration of free drug and an exaggerated hypnotic effect. Protein binding is also affected by changes in blood pH and is decreased by hyperventilation.

Extracellular pH and pKa of the drug

Only the unionised fraction of unbound drug in the plasma can penetrate the blood–brain barrier. Consequently the speed of induction depends on pKa because this determines the degree of ionisation at the pH of extracellular fluids.

The relative solubility of the drug in lipid and water

High relative lipid solubility enhances transfer into the brain and increases potency.

Offset of hypnotic effect

The clinical action of the i.v. anaesthetics (see Table 4.1) is terminated by redistribution away from the brain. The plasma concentration decreases exponentially and causes diffusion away from the brain along a reversed concentration gradient. Fig. 4.2 shows how the percentage of an injected propofol bolus changes with time in four groups of body tissues. Well-perfused vital organs (e.g. brain, heart, liver and kidneys) receive a high percentage of the dose initially. Uptake into muscle is slower because of lower lipid content but becomes quantitatively important because of the relatively large tissue mass and good blood supply. Despite high lipid solubility, i.v. anaesthetics distribute more slowly into fatty tissue because of lower blood flows. Fat contributes little to the termination of action of a single bolus of agent, but fat depots ultimately contain a large proportion of the injected drug (see Fig. 4.2). Drug is released back to the plasma slowly over time but fails to achieve an anaesthetic brain concentration because of high clearance from the plasma by the liver. This dynamic alters when these agents are used to maintain anaesthesia for some hours by continuous infusion. In this situation the drug concentration in organs with high or medium blood flow is in equilibrium with the plasma. When the infusion stops, distribution to fatty tissue and hepatic clearance of drug from the plasma become more important in reducing brain concentration. As a consequence, plasma concentration declines more slowly than after a single bolus (context-sensitive half-time (CSHT)) and time to consciousness increases. Complete elimination of drug from the body may be delayed in the obese because of retention in the high fat mass. Metabolism of i.v. anaesthetics occurs predominantly in the liver and may contribute to the recovery of consciousness if the process is rapid. However, elimination of a typical i.v. agent takes many hours or days because they have a high volume of distribution. A small proportion of drug may be excreted unchanged in the urine depending on the drug's degree of ionisation and the pH of urine.

Precautions when using i.v. anaesthetics

Special care is required in some circumstances as the drug may be contraindicated or the injected dose and rate of administration may need modification (Table 4.3).

Pharmacology of individual intravenous anaesthetic drugs

Propofol

Propofol, an alkylphenol, became available commercially in 1986.

Chemical structure

The chemical structure of propofol is 2,6-di-isopropylphenol (Fig. 4.3).

Physical properties and presentation

Propofol is extremely lipid soluble but almost insoluble in water, so the drug is presented as a white aqueous emulsion

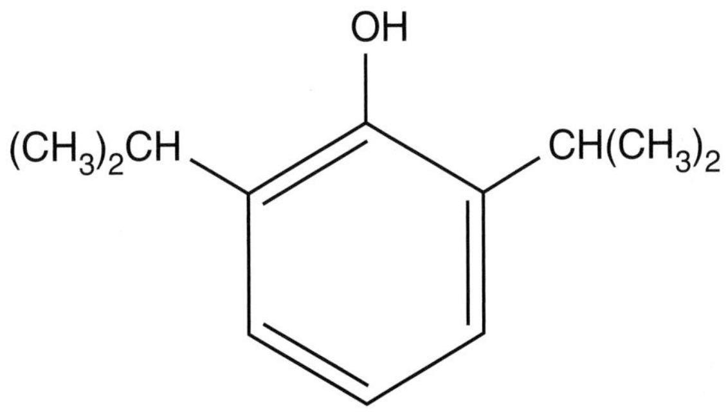

Fig. 4.3 Chemical structure of propofol.

Table 4.3 Precautions when using an i.v. anaesthetic agent

Consideration	Comment
Known hypersensitivity to the chosen drug	This is an absolute contraindication.
Airway obstruction	This may be considered a contraindication to i.v. induction of anaesthesia because it is possible to precipitate failure of oxygenation (see Chapter 23).
Cardiovascular disease	Patients with hypovolaemia, myocardial disease, cardiac valve stenosis or constrictive pericarditis are particularly likely to develop reduced stroke volume and cardiac output.
Cardioactive drugs	Medications such as β-blockers, calcium channel antagonists, angiotensin converting enzyme inhibitors and angiotensin receptor antagonists will enhance hypotension from i.v. induction.
Respiratory depression	This is exaggerated in patients with pre-existing impairment of ventilatory drive or neuromuscular disease.
Elderly patients and those with significant comorbidities	Such patients show an enhanced hypotensive response to a typical mg kg^{-1} adult dose.
Severe hepatic disease	Reduced protein binding results in higher plasma concentration of free drug, and metabolism may be impaired. Usually little effect on early recovery after a single bolus.
Renal disease	Protein binding is reduced and urinary excretion of metabolites may be delayed.
Obesity	Dose should be adjusted according to ideal body weight (see Chapters 1 & 32) to avoid overdosage.
Pregnancy, obstetric practice and breastfeeding	A lack of formal toxicity studies leads manufacturers to recommend that i.v. anaesthetics be avoided in these circumstances. However, propofol and thiopental are used for Caesarean section requiring general anaesthesia (see Chapter 43; also see NAP5 report).
Adrenocortical insufficiency	Propofol, thiopental and etomidate reduce cortisol synthesis in tissue and animal preparations. Only etomidate causes significant enzyme inhibition in humans after routine induction of anaesthesia and sedation in ICU.
Bacterial infections	Propofol preparations support the growth of micro-organisms and must be drawn up aseptically; any unused solution should be discarded if not administered promptly.

containing soya bean oil and purified egg phosphatide. The triglyceride component varies between manufacturers and may be long chain (12–20 carbon atoms) or medium chain (6–10 carbon atoms), which is claimed to reduce pain on injection. The lipid load of the latter formulation is more readily tolerated and metabolised in humans. Propofol is available in concentrations from 20 to 0.5 mg ml^{-1} (2%–0.5%), and the lower concentration is preferred for paediatric practice. Prefilled 50 ml syringes are available for use in target-controlled infusion (TCI) techniques (see later). Dosing schemes are shown in Table 4.4.

Pharmacology

Central nervous system
Diffusion from the blood is relatively slow compared with agents such as thiopental. Loss of verbal contact is a useful marker of anaesthetic onset, and loss of response to vigorous jaw thrusting indicates sufficient depth for insertion of a supraglottic airway device (SAD). The EEG frequency decreases and amplitude increases with a dominant slow wave α/δ pattern; this is accompanied by reductions in cerebral metabolic requirement for oxygen (CMRo$_2$), CBF and intracranial pressure. Non-epileptic myotonia may be evidenced by irregular muscular activity. Propofol reduces the duration of seizures induced by electroconvulsive therapy (ECT) in humans, but there are reports of convulsions after its use. Propofol has been used successfully in the management of status epilepticus, and epilepsy is not a contraindication. Recovery of consciousness is rapid, and there is a minimal hangover effect even in the immediate postanaesthetic period. Propofol is the preferred agent for volunteer studies on the neurophysiological mechanisms that underlie sedation and general anaesthesia.

Table 4.4 Dosing schemes and principal indications for i.v. anaesthetic agents

Drug	Use	Dose range		Onset of effect after bolus (s)	Time to peak effect after bolus (s)	Duration of effect after bolus (min)	Principal indications
Propofol	Bolus i.v. dose	Adult Frail adult 1–12 years 16 years	1.5–2.5 mg kg^{-1} Reduce by 50% 3–3.5 mg kg^{-1} Use adult doses	30–60	90–120	5–10	Induction of anaesthesia Maintenance of anaesthesia using TCI/TIVA Procedural sedation
	Sedation Maintenance	Use TCI With analgesics	0.5–1.5 µg ml^{-1} 2–4 µg ml^{-1}				
	TCI target Antiemesis	No analgesics	4–8 µg ml^{-1} 10–20 mg bolus, then 1–2 mg kg^{-1} h^{-1} PRN				
Ketamine	Bolus i.v. Bolus i.m. Oral sedation Analgesia	Children	2 mg kg^{-1} 8–10 mg kg^{-1} 6–10 mg kg^{-1} 0.1–0.5 mg kg^{-1} bolus, then 0.1–0.2 mg kg^{-1} hr^{-1} PRN, max 15 mg hr^{-1}	15–45	60	10–20	Induction of anaesthesia in emergency patient Paediatric sedation Analgesia
Etomidate	Bolus Infusion		0.2–0.3 mg kg^{-1} 0.04–0.05 mg kg^{-1} hr^{-1}	15–45	Unknown	3–12	Induction of anaesthesia ICU sedation (very rarely)
Thiopental	Bolus Infusion		3–6 mg kg^{-1} 1–15 mg kg^{-1} hr^{-1}	<30	40–60	5–10	Induction of anaesthesia Sedation in neurocritical care or status epilepticus

TCI, Target-controlled infusion.

Cardiovascular system

Arterial pressure decreases to a greater degree than with thiopental. This results principally from the vasodilatation caused by reduced sympathetic neural activity, but there is also a dose-dependent negative inotropic effect. Decreases greater than 40% may occur in elderly and frail patients. Hypotension is mitigated partially by slower administration (more than 30–60 s) and by allowing sufficient time for diffusion into the brain before additional bolus dosing. The pressor response to tracheal intubation is attenuated to a greater degree by propofol than thiopental. Heart rate may increase slightly after induction of anaesthesia, but there have been occasional reports of severe bradycardia or

asystole after administration of propofol. Caution is needed in patients with a pre-existing bradycardia or if propofol is given with other vagomimetic drugs (e.g. remifentanil), and a vagolytic agent (e.g. glycopyrronium bromide or atropine) may be required.

Respiratory system

Apnoea occurs more commonly and for longer than with thiopental. During an infusion of propofol, tidal volume is lower and respiratory rate higher compared with the conscious state, with a depressed ventilatory response to carbon dioxide. These effects are more marked if opioid coinduction is used. Propofol has no effect on bronchial muscle tone, and laryngospasm is particularly uncommon. Laryngeal reflexes are suppressed to a greater extent than by thiopental, and there is a lower incidence of coughing or laryngospasm on insertion of a SAD provided that an adequate depth of anaesthesia is achieved.

Skeletal muscle
Tone is reduced, but movements may occur in response to surgical stimulation as the spinal cord action of propofol is limited compared with volatile agents. Coadministration of an opioid, nitrous oxide or a neuromuscular blocking agent is necessary to prevent such responses.

Gastrointestinal system
Propofol has no effect on gastrointestinal motility in animals and reduces the incidence of postoperative nausea and vomiting. The lipid load imposed by a continuous propofol infusion has been cited as a rare cause of pancreatitis in critically ill patients.

Uterus and placenta
Propofol has been used extensively in patients undergoing gynaecological surgery and does not appear to have any clinically significant effect on uterine tone. Propofol crosses the placenta, but its safety in the neonate has not been formally established.

Hepatic/renal
There is a transient decrease in renal and hepatic perfusion secondary to reductions in arterial pressure and cardiac output. Liver function tests are not deranged after infusion of propofol for 24 h.

Endocrine
Plasma concentrations of cortisol are decreased after administration of propofol, but a normal response occurs to the administration of adrenocorticotrophic hormone (Synacthen test).

Pharmacokinetics

The distribution of propofol after a single i.v. bolus is rapid (see Fig. 4.2). Clearance of drug from the plasma is greater than expected if it were metabolised only in the liver, and extrahepatic sites (e.g. lungs) are proposed. The kidneys excrete the metabolites of propofol (mainly glucuronides), and only 0.3% of the administered dose is excreted unchanged. The terminal elimination half-life of propofol is 3–4.8 h, although the duration of clinical effects is much shorter because of redistribution to other tissues (see Chapter 1). The distribution and clearance of propofol are altered by concomitant administration of drugs that alter cardiac output. Constant infusions lasting many hours do increase CSHT but less so than with other agents. This causes little

effect on the offset of effect after termination of an infusion, and propofol is particularly suited to maintenance of intravenous anaesthesia.

Adverse effects

Pain on injection
Pain on injection occurs in 40% of patients and is caused by free propofol in the aqueous phase of the preparation. The incidence is greatly reduced if a large vein is cannulated, propofol is injected into a running fluid infusion, a small dose (10 mg) of lidocaine is injected shortly before induction, or lidocaine is mixed into the propofol syringe (10–20 mg per 200 mg). Preparations containing medium-chain triglycerides cause a lower incidence of pain, which is less severe. Accidental extravasation or intra-arterial injection does not cause adverse effects.

Sedation in ICU
Propofol infusion is used for adult patients in ICU. The lipid load administered must be incorporated into calculations of nutritional requirement and may interfere with functioning of blood gas analysers. Propofol-related infusion syndrome (PRIS) is a rare consequence of prolonged high-dose administration and is often fatal. It is characterised by bradycardia, metabolic acidosis, hyperlipidaemia, rhabdomyolysis and/or heart failure and is associated with head injury or the use of vasopressors. The syndrome is more common in children and adolescents, and propofol is not indicated for long-term sedation of critically ill patients younger than 16 years, but is used safely by intravenous infusion including TCI techniques, in the operating theatre.

Awareness during induction of anaesthesia
Propofol is now the drug of choice for i.v. induction of general anaesthesia in most cases. Rapid redistribution and clearance of propofol from the plasma may increase the risk of awareness during difficult tracheal intubation or if there is a delay in administering an adequate concentration of inhaled anaesthesia, especially during neuromuscular blockade (see NAP5 report). This is also true for the other i.v. anaesthetic agents (see Table 4.1).

Other adverse effects
Other adverse effects are listed in Table 4.5.

Precautions

The general precautions for i.v. agents listed in Table 4.3 apply to propofol.

Ketamine hydrochloride

Ketamine hydrochloride is a phencyclidine derivative and was introduced in 1965. It produces dissociative anaesthesia

Table 4.5 Pharmacological properties of i.v. anaesthetic agents

	Propofol	Ketamine	Etomidate	Thiopental
Properties				
Water soluble	–	+	+[a]	+
Stable in solution	+	+	+	–
pH of solution	7–8	3.5–5.5	6.5–8 (lipid formulation)	10.8
pKa	11	7.5	4.7 (lipid formulation)	7.6
Protein binding	98%	12%–50%	76%	80%
Long shelf-life	+	+	+	–
Pain on i.v. injection	++[b]	–	++[b]	–
Non-irritant on subcutaneous injection	Yes	No	No	No
Sequelae from intra-arterial injection	No	+++	Not in animal studies	+++
Low incidence of venous thrombosis	Yes	Yes	No	Yes
Accumulation	–	–	–	++
Features at induction				
Excitatory effects	+	+	+++	–
Respiratory complications	+	–	–	–
Cardiovascular depression	++	–	+	+
Other features				
Analgesia	–	++	–	–
Allergic reactions	Rare; history of soya or egg allergy does not contraindicate propofol administration	Rarely reported	Very rare reports with lipid formulation	Estimated 1 : 30,000
Interaction with relaxants	–	–	–	–
Salivation	–	++ Anticholinergic necessary	–	–
Postoperative vomiting	–	++	+	–
Emergence delirium, nightmares & hallucinations	–	++	–	+
Safe in porphyria	Yes	Yes	No	No

[a]Aqueous solution not commercially available.
[b]Pain may be reduced by using emulsion formulation with medium-chain triglycerides.

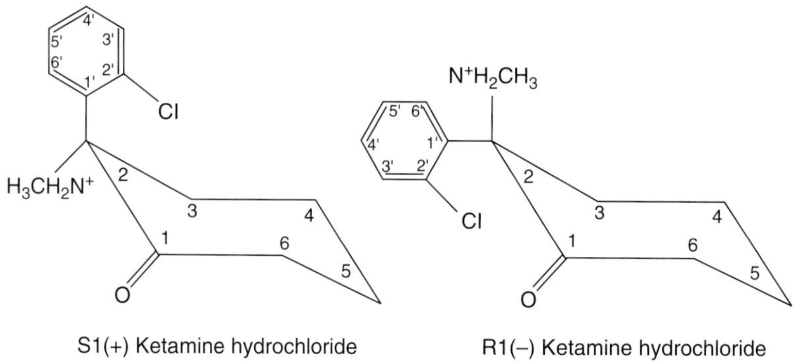

Fig. 4.4 Enantiomers of ketamine – currently a racemic mixture is used in the UK. (With permission from Vuyk, J., Sitsen, E., & Reekers, M. Intravenous anesthetics. In: Miller, R., Eriksson, L., Fleisher, L., Wiener-Kronish, J., Cohen, N., & Young, W. (eds) *Miller's Anesthesia*, 8th edn. Philadelphia, Saunders Elsevier.)

(via non-competitive antagonism at the NMDA receptor) rather than classical generalised depression of the CNS and is a useful adjunctive analgesic. Ketamine has no action at $GABA_A$ receptors.

Chemical structure

The chemical structure of ketamine is 2-(*o*-chlorophenyl)-2-(methylamino)-cyclohexanone hydrochloride (Fig. 4.4).

Physical characteristics and presentation

Ketamine has a single chiral centre and is usually presented as a racemic mixture of its R(−) and S(+) stereoisomers in water solutions at concentrations of 10, 50 and 100 mg ml^{-1}. The S(+) enantiomer has more potent analgesic effects (approximately fourfold), allowing lower doses to be used, with fewer adverse effects and a more rapid clinical recovery than the racemic mixture, but its pharmacokinetics are identical. The enantiopure formulation of S(+) ketamine is not currently available in the UK. Dosing schemes are shown in Table 4.4.

Pharmacology

Central nervous system

Ketamine is extremely lipid soluble. Amnesia often persists for up to 1 h after recovery of consciousness. It is a potent somatic analgesic at lower doses. Induction of anaesthesia is smooth, but emergence delirium may occur with restlessness, disorientation and agitation. Vivid and unpleasant nightmares or hallucinations may occur during recovery and for up to 24 h. The incidences of emergence phenomena are reduced by avoidance of verbal and tactile stimulation during recovery and by concomitant administration of benzodiazepines and/or opioids. Unpleasant dreams may

persist but are reported less commonly by children and elderly patients. The EEG changes caused by ketamine are dissimilar to those seen with other i.v. anaesthetics, and consist of loss of α rhythm and predominant θ activity, which causes processed EEG (pEEG) depth of hypnosis devices to give paradoxical indications of arousal. Traditionally, head injury and neuroanaesthesia were considered contraindications to ketamine because it was thought to increase $CMRO_2$, CBF and intracranial pressure. However, recent studies have found that ketamine has minimal cerebrovascular effects when used in patients who are normocapnic and receiving a hypnotic agent with $GABA_A$ activity. Clinical data indicate that ketamine can contribute usefully to the sedation/analgesia required by neurocritical care patients and reduces inotropic requirements for normal cerebral perfusion. NMDA receptor blockade by ketamine may provide additional neuroprotection by preventing unbalanced activation of these receptors by toxic extracellular concentrations of glutamate. These occur after brain injury and increase Ca^{2+} flux and cellular injury.

Cardiovascular system

Arterial pressure increases by up to 25% and heart rate by approximately 20%. Cardiac output and myocardial oxygen consumption may increase, and there is increased myocardial sensitivity to adrenaline. The positive inotropic effect may be related to increased Ca^{2+} influx, mediated by cyclic adenosine monophosphate (cAMP). Sympathetic stimulation of the peripheral circulation is decreased, resulting in vasodilatation in tissues innervated predominantly by α-adrenergic receptors and vasoconstriction in those with β-receptors.

Respiratory system

Transient apnoea may occur after i.v. injection, but ventilation is well maintained thereafter and may increase slightly unless high doses are given. Pharyngeal and laryngeal reflexes and a patent airway are adequately maintained in comparison with other i.v. agents. However, airway patency cannot be guaranteed and normal precautions must be taken to protect the airway and prevent aspiration. Bronchial muscle is dilated and ketamine infusion is a useful adjunct in the ICU management of status asthmaticus.

Skeletal muscle

Muscle tone is usually increased. Spontaneous movements may occur, but reflex movement in response to surgery is uncommon.

Gastrointestinal system

Salivation is increased.

Uterus and placenta

Ketamine crosses the placenta readily. Fetal concentrations are approximately equal to those in the mother.

Eye

Intraocular pressure increases, although this is often transient. Nystagmus, pupillary dilatation and lachrymation occur. Eye movements often persist during surgical anaesthesia.

Pharmacokinetics

Protein binding is lower than other i.v. agents (see Table 4.5). Redistribution after i.v. injection occurs more slowly than with other i.v. anaesthetic agents, and the elimination half-life is approximately 2.5 h. Ketamine undergoes extensive hepatic metabolism by demethylation and hydroxylation of the cyclohexanone ring. Metabolites include norketamine, which is pharmacologically active (20%–30% of the activity of ketamine). Approximately 80% of the injected dose is excreted via the kidneys as glucuronides; only 2.5% is excreted unchanged. After i.m. injection, peak concentrations are achieved after approximately 20 min.

Adverse effects

See Table 4.5.

Specific indications

The high-risk patient

Ketamine is considered useful in the patient with shock because of maintenance of cardiovascular function, but arterial pressure decreases in the presence of hypovolaemia. High-risk patients often receive postoperative sedation in ICU which minimises the risk of emergence phenomena.

Paediatric anaesthesia

Children undergoing minor surgery, invasive investigations (e.g. cardiac catheterisation), ophthalmic examinations or radiotherapy may be managed successfully with ketamine administered orally or by i.m. or i.v. injection.

Difficult locations and developing countries

Ketamine has been used successfully on scene in trauma, for analgesia and anaesthesia in casualties of war and in resource-poor locations where there is limited equipment for inhalational anaesthesia and trained staff are in short supply.

Analgesia and sedation

Ketamine may be used in lower doses for its analgesic effects – such as for changing wound or burn dressings or positioning patients in pain before regional anaesthesia (e.g. fractured neck of femur).

Absolute contraindication

Conditions in which a rapid and uncontrolled increase in blood pressure would be hazardous (e.g. cerebral aneurysm or intracranial bleeding) are absolute contraindications.

Precautions

The general precautions for i.v. agents listed in Table 4.3 apply.

Etomidate

Etomidate, a carboxylated imidazole compound, was introduced in 1972.

Chemical structure

The chemical structure of etomidate is D-ethyl-1-(α-methylbenzyl)-imidazole-5-carboxylate (Fig. 4.5).

Physical characteristics and presentation

Etomidate is soluble but unstable in water. It is typically presented as the active R(+) enantiomer dissolved in

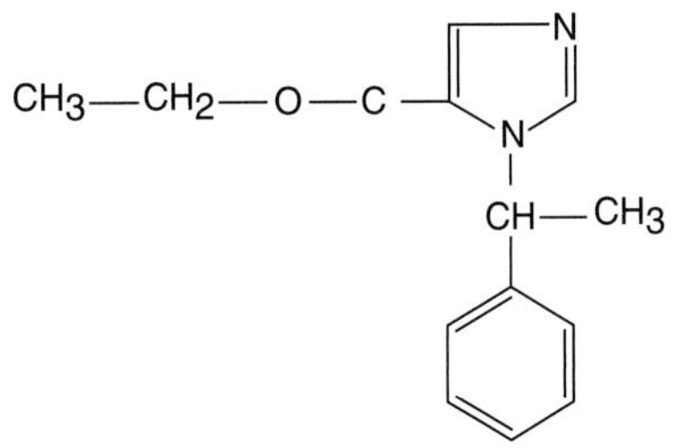

Fig. 4.5 Chemical structure of etomidate. (With permission from Vuyk, J., Sitsen, E., & Reekers, M. Intravenous anesthetics. In: Miller, R., Eriksson, L., Fleisher, L., Wiener-Kronish, J., Cohen, N., & Young, W. (eds) *Miller's Anesthesia*, 8th edn. Philadelphia, Saunders Elsevier.)

propylene glycol or as a lipid emulsion containing medium-chain triglycerides. Ampoules contain 2 mg ml^{-1} etomidate in 10 ml. Dosing schemes are shown in Table 4.4.

Pharmacology

Etomidate is a rapidly-acting general anaesthetic agent with a short duration of action. It produces less cardiovascular depression than propofol in healthy patients, but this benefit is limited if the cardiovascular system is compromised (e.g. by severe hypovolaemia). Large doses may produce tachycardia. Respiratory depression is less than with other agents.

Pharmacokinetics

Etomidate redistributes rapidly in the body, and rapid elimination also occurs. It is metabolised in the plasma and liver, mainly by ester hydrolysis, and the metabolites are excreted in the urine; 2% is excreted unchanged. The terminal elimination half-life is 2.4–5 h. There is little accumulation when repeated doses are given. The distribution and clearance of etomidate may be altered by concomitant administration of synthetic opioids. Metabolism is inhibited by fentanyl.

Adverse effects

Adverse effects include the following:

- *Suppression of adrenal enzymes.* Etomidate impairs adrenal cortisol synthesis by inhibition of the enzyme 11β-hydroxylase and response to adrenocorticotrophic hormone (ACTH). This effect occurs after a single bolus and lasts for several hours. At much higher doses, other enzymes such as 18β-hydroxylase are inhibited, reducing aldosterone and other steroid hormone synthesis. Long-term infusions of the drug in intensive care are associated with increased infection and mortality, probably related to impaired immunological competence.
- *Venous thrombosis.* This is more common than with other agents if the glycol preparation (*Hypnomidate*) is used.
- *Other.* See Table 4.5.

Specific indications

Outpatient anaesthesia

Etomidate may be suitable in this situation, but the incidence of excitatory phenomena is unacceptably high unless combined with a benzodiazepine/opioid. Use of the lipid-based formulation does not prevent the adverse effects listed in Table 4.5.

Compromised cardiovascular status

Depression is minimal with etomidate compared with other agents. However, etomidate should be avoided in patients who are expected to require level 3 intensive care postoperatively (e.g. after surgery for sepsis) because it causes adrenal suppression.

Precautions

The general precautions for i.v. agents listed in Table 4.3 apply to etomidate.

Thiopental sodium

Barbiturate compounds for i.v. anaesthesia were introduced in the 1920s, but their unpredictable action and prolonged recovery proved significant limitations. Manipulation of the barbituric acid ring (Fig. 4.6) provided anaesthetic compounds with shorter durations of action (Table 4.6) and thiopental is the most widely used worldwide. Controversies over the use of this agent in legally sanctioned executions led to its withdrawal from US practice in 2011.

Chemical structure

The chemical structure of thiopental is sodium 5-ethyl-5-(1-methylbutyl)-2-thiobarbiturate.

Physical characteristics and presentation

Thiopental sodium is a highly lipid-soluble sulphur barbiturate compound. It is presented as 500 mg of yellowish powder in single-dose ampoules for dissolution in 20 ml of sterile water to produce a 25 mg ml^{-1} (2.5%) alkaline solution (pH 10.8). Thiopental is 99% ionised in this solution

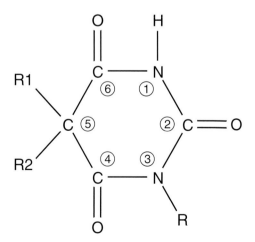

Fig. 4.6 Chemical structure of parent barbiturate ring – clinical activity is determined by the attachments to the molecule at positions 2, 3, and 5.

Table 4.6 Chemical structure of three barbiturates used as i.v. induction agents

Agent	Group	Position 2	Position 3R	Position 5R$_1$	Position 5R$_2$
Thiopental	Thiobarbiturate	S	H	C_2H_5	$CH(CH_3)C_3H_7$
Methohexital	Oxybarbiturate	O	CH_3	$CH_2CH=CH_2$	$CH(CH_3)C\equiv CC_2H_5$
Thiamylal	Thiobarbiturate	S	H	$CH_2CH=CH_2$	$CH(CH_3)C_3H_7$

Methohexital and thiamylal are no longer available for human administration in the UK. The high number of carbon atoms in the side chains at position 5 enhances the potency of these agents. Direct substitution with a phenyl group at position 5 confers anticonvulsant activity (e.g. phenobarbital).

but becomes predominantly unionised at body pH. Nitrogen gas in the unopened ampoule prevents reaction with atmospheric carbon dioxide, and sodium carbonate is added to increase solubility in water. Freshly prepared solution may be stored for 24 h.

Pharmacology

Central nervous system

Thiopental produces anaesthesia within 30–45 s because of its high lipid solubility and 61% is unionised at plasma pH; consciousness is usually regained in 5–10 min. There is progressive depression of the CNS (including spinal cord reflexes), but it has poor analgesic effect, and surgical anaesthesia is difficult to achieve unless large doses are used. The CMRO$_2$ is reduced, and there are secondary decreases in CBF, cerebral blood volume and intracranial pressure. Thiopental is a very potent anticonvulsant. It depresses sympathetic more than parasympathetic nervous system activity, and bradycardia may occur. However, tachycardia is more common after induction of anaesthesia because of baroreceptor inhibition and loss of vagal tone in young healthy adults.

Cardiovascular system

Myocardial contractility is depressed and peripheral vasodilatation occurs when large doses are administered rapidly. Arterial pressure decreases, and profound hypotension may occur in the patient with hypovolaemia or cardiac disease. Heart rate may decrease, but there is often a reflex tachycardia.

Respiratory system

Ventilatory drive is decreased by thiopental, and a short period of apnoea commonly follows a few deep breaths. When spontaneous ventilation is resumed, ventilatory rate and tidal volume are usually reduced, but they increase in response to surgical stimulation. Bronchial muscle tone increases, although frank bronchospasm is uncommon. Laryngeal spasm may be precipitated by insertion of a SAD

or when secretions or blood are present in the pharynx or larynx.

Skeletal muscle

Skeletal muscle tone is reduced at high blood concentrations, but there is poor muscle relaxation and no significant direct effect on the neuromuscular junction.

Uterus and placenta

There is little effect on resting uterine tone, but uterine contractions are suppressed at high doses. Thiopental crosses the placenta readily, although fetal blood concentrations do not reach maternal concentrations.

Eye

Intraocular pressure is reduced by approximately 40%. The pupil dilates then constricts, but the light reflex remains present until surgical anaesthesia is attained. The corneal, conjunctival, eyelash and eyelid reflexes are abolished.

Hepatic/renal function

The functions of the liver and kidney are impaired transiently after administration of thiopental. Hepatic microsomal enzymes are induced, and this may increase the metabolism and elimination of other drugs.

Pharmacokinetics

Thiopental is highly bound to albumin, and free drug availability is increased in hypoproteinaemia. Protein binding is decreased by alkalaemia, hyperventilation and some drugs that occupy the same albumin binding sites, thereby increasing unbound thiopental concentrations. Metabolism occurs predominantly in the liver, and the metabolites are excreted by the kidneys. Only a small proportion is excreted unchanged in the urine. The terminal elimination half-life is approximately 11.5 h (longer in the elderly). Elimination after an infusion is a zero-order process with 10%–15% of the remaining drug metabolised each hour. Up to 30% of the original dose may remain in the body at 24 h, and a hangover effect is common. Accumulation may result if further doses of thiopental are administered within 1–2 days.

Adverse effects

Adverse effects include the following:
- *Tissue necrosis.* Local necrosis may follow subcutaneous injection. If such injection occurs, the cannula should be left in place and hyaluronidase injected.
- *Intra-arterial injection.* This may result from placement of an i.v. cannula into the brachial artery in the antecubital fossa. The patient usually complains of intense burning pain, and injection should be stopped immediately. The forearm and hand may become blanched, and blisters may appear distally. Intra-arterial thiopental causes profound arterial constriction, local release of norepinephrine and crystal formation in arterioles. Thrombosis is caused by endarteritis, adenosine triphosphate (ATP) release from damaged red cells and aggregation of platelets and may cause distal ischaemia or gangrene. The cannula should remain *in situ* and used to administer a vasodilator (e.g. papaverine 20 mg). Stellate ganglion or brachial plexus block may reduce arterial spasm. Heparin should be given i.v., and oral anticoagulants should be prescribed after operation.
- *Laryngeal spasm.* The causes are discussed earlier.
- *Bronchospasm.* This is unusual but may be precipitated in asthmatic patients.
- *Other.* More adverse effects are listed in Table 4.5.

Indications

Indications include the following:
- *Maintenance of anaesthesia.* Thiopental is suitable for short procedures only, because accumulation occurs with repeated doses, and infusions are reserved for status epilepticus.
- *Reduction of intracranial pressure.* This can be utilised in neurocritical care (see Chapter 40).

Absolute contraindication

Porphyria is an absolute contraindication because barbiturates may precipitate lower motor neurone paralysis or severe cardiovascular collapse in patients with porphyria.

Precautions

The general precautions for i.v. agents listed in Table 4.3 apply to the use of thiopental.

Obstetrics
Thiopental is used for induction of anaesthesia for Caesarean section, and the NAP5 report highlighted issues with accidental awareness in this circumstance. Propofol is increasingly deployed for such procedures (see Chapter 43 and NAP5 report).

Maintenance of anaesthesia using i.v. agents

Maintenance of anaesthesia using i.v. drugs is technically more demanding compared with using volatile agents, and patients are more likely to have idiosyncratic or variable responses. This may deter the clinician, but there are situations where volatile anaesthesia is contraindicated (e.g. malignant hyperthermia risk) or inappropriate because of a lack of equipment for vapour delivery (e.g. during transfer of an unconscious patient). Consequently it is recommended that all anaesthetists should be competent with infusion anaesthesia to prevent unintended patient awareness. Three techniques using i.v. hypnotics are outlined here; each must incorporate the bolus elimination and transfer (BET) principle to achieve and maintain a brain concentration of drug which prevents awareness.
- *Bolus.* This creates the concentration gradient between the plasma and brain, which drives drug diffusion and rapidly achieves an appropriate depth of hypnosis.
- *Elimination.* Additional drug must be given to sustain the equilibrium between plasma/brain concentrations despite losses from the plasma to excretion and metabolism.
- *Transfer.* Further drug is administered simultaneously to replace losses from the plasma to other viscera.

Any of the i.v. anaesthetic agents detailed earlier may be used by repeated boluses or continuous infusion to maintain anaesthesia. The pharmacokinetic principles underlying i.v. drug infusions are described in Chapter 1. Etomidate has the most suitable pharmacokinetic profile because prolonged administration has limited effect on CSHT, but it also has the worst adverse effect profile and is very rarely used. Thiopental has a marked increase in CSHT following continuous infusion and causes an unacceptable delay in recovery. CSHT is more prolonged for propofol and ketamine compared with etomidate, but this has an insignificant effect on duration of their clinical action; propofol is preferred as its adverse effects are minimal and acceptable. Propofol provides no analgesia and very limited immobility through spinal cord suppression compared with volatile agents (see Chapter 3). Consequently a continuous propofol infusion requires supplementation with analgesics (e.g. opioid and/or inhaled nitrous oxide) to prevent response to noxious stimuli. Coadministration of analgesic supplements, midazolam or a volatile agent allows the hypnotic concentration of propofol in the plasma/brain to be reduced. Total i.v. anaesthesia (TIVA) describes the use of propofol as the sole hypnotic

Box 4.1 Indications for TIVA

- Malignant hyperthermia risk
- Long QT syndrome (QTc ≥500 ms)
- History of severe PONV
- 'Tubeless' ENT and thoracic surgery
- Patients with anticipated difficult intubation/extubation
- Neurosurgery to limit intracranial volume
- Surgery requiring neurophysiological monitoring
- Neuromuscular disorders (e.g. myasthenia gravis) and situations where NMBAs are of disadvantage
- Anaesthesia in non-theatre locations
- Transfer of an anaesthetised patient between locations
- Daycase surgery
- Trainee teaching
- Patient choice

ENT, Ear, nose, and throat; *NMBA*, neuromuscular blocking agent; *PONV*, postoperative nausea and vomiting.

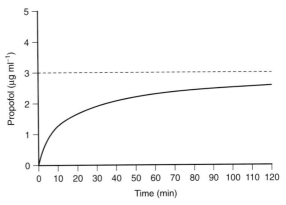

Fig. 4.7 Plasma concentration of propofol achieved by MCI technique using a continuous infusion at 6 mg kg^{-1} hr^{-1} but without an initial bolus. Note that a clinically useful concentration of 3 µg ml^{-1} is not attained after 2 h of infusion.

for general anaesthesia, or its exclusive combination with other i.v. drugs. Some indications for TIVA are given in Box 4.1.

Practical techniques for i.v. maintenance of anaesthesia

Intermittent injection

An initial bolus dose induces anaesthesia, and further smaller boluses are repeated at regular intervals for the duration of surgery. The size and timing of subsequent boluses are usually determined by clinical experience, as there is no accurate way of controlling plasma/brain concentration. Some clinicians are skilled in maintenance of anaesthesia using this method, but more typically the hypnotic effect fluctuates widely. Intermittent injection is acceptable for short procedures in unparalysed patients who can move if an inadequate effect is achieved.

Manually controlled infusion

Manually controlled infusion (MCI) of propofol is associated with a high incidence of unintended awareness. A fixed rate infusion fails to obey the BET principle, and consequently the plasma and effect site (brain) propofol concentrations increase very slowly. For example, a propofol MCI started at 6 mg kg^{-1} h^{-1} without an initial bolus requires 2 h to achieve a clinically useful effect site concentration of 3 µg ml^{-1} (Fig. 4.7). Adding an initial bolus does not necessarily correct this if redistribution of propofol away from

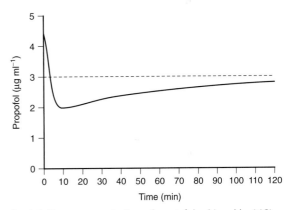

Fig. 4.8 Plasma concentration of propofol achieved by MCI technique using an initial bolus dose followed by a fixed-rate infusion at 6 mg kg^{-1} h^{-1}. Note that a clinically useful concentration of 3 µg ml^{-1} is exceeded by the bolus dose, but this infusion scheme fails to sustain this plasma concentration during a 2 h infusion.

the plasma is unaccounted for in the infusion scheme (Fig. 4.8). There is a significant risk of awareness with both these schemes if noxious stimuli are applied when the effect site concentration is subhypnotic. A variable-rate infusion obeying the BET principle is needed to achieve adequate brain concentrations within an appropriate time frame. The Bristol technique is a validated MCI regimen that utilises an initial bolus of 1 mg kg^{-1}, followed by infusion at 10 mg kg^{-1} h^{-1} for 10 min, 8 mg kg^{-1} h^{-1} for the next 10 min, and a maintenance rate of 6 mg kg^{-1} h^{-1} thereafter. This regimen typically achieves a 3 µg ml^{-1} brain concentration after 12 min and

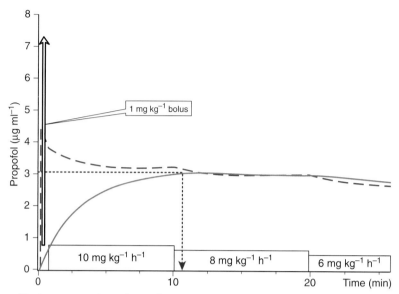

Fig. 4.9 The plasma and brain concentrations of propofol achieved by the Bristol variable-rate MCI as predicted by Tivatrainer 9 software (www.eurosiva.eu) using Marsh plasma targeting model. Dashed line = plasma concentration, solid line = brain concentration, dotted line shows time to achieve brain concentration of 3 μg ml^{-1}. It is important to note that this methodology is a plasma targeting protocol and 3 μg ml^{-1} is not achieved until 12 mins after the bolus dose. There is risk of accidental awareness if noxious stimuli or NMB are applied in the absence of analgesics before this time point; a simultaneous fentanyl bolus of 3 μg ml^{-1} and 66% inhaled nitrous oxide are required to ensure adequate surgical anesthesia. Note that the plasma and brain concentrations decline below 3 μg ml^{-1} after 25 mins.

provides adequate hypnosis in unparalysed patients who simultaneously receive fentanyl and nitrous oxide (Fig. 4.9). However, this technique is not guaranteed to prevent awareness without additional analgesics. Higher effect site concentrations can be achieved by increasing the bolus dose and infusion rates, but this increases the incidence of cardiovascular instability. The Bristol variable-rate MCI is only a guide, and administration must be adjusted by clinical signs and data from a pEEG device (see Chapter 17). The disadvantage of any MCI is dose titration when an infusion is already running; it is very difficult to account for the drug already present when calculating additional bolus doses or infusion rates. Consequently both under- and overdosing are much more likely with an MCI.

Target-controlled infusion

Target-controlled infusion (TCI) devices are syringe drivers programmed with three-compartment pharmacokinetic models (see Chapter 1) that describe the ongoing transfer of i.v. drugs into the brain and other tissues. Complex mathematics enables precise estimation of drug concentration in each compartment, and a given plasma *or* brain concentration target can be achieved rapidly and maintained indefinitely. The anaesthetist enters the desired target concentration and

changes it in response to clinical signs and pEEG data. Calculations are typically checked every 10 s and the infusion rate adjusted accordingly. The initial bolus is administered at 1200–2400 ml h^{-1} (depending on device manufacturer), and the infusion slows progressively as tissue concentrations approaches equilibrium with the plasma/brain target. When the plasma and tissue concentrations reach steady state (after 23–24 h for propofol), the infusion rate matches excretion and metabolism only. If the target concentration is increased, the algorithms take account of drug already administered and calculate an appropriate additional bolus and higher infusion rate to achieve the new target. When the target is decreased, the syringe driver stops infusing temporarily until the new concentration has been achieved and then restarts at a lower rate (Fig. 4.10). The advantages of TCI are simplicity and avoidance of potentially dangerous calculation errors. It should be noted that the actual concentration achieved by a TCI device may be ±20%–30% of the target set. This variability is not a disadvantage if the anaesthetist appreciates that a specific numeric target does not necessarily represent a particular clinical end-point; patients receiving any form of anaesthesia must be monitored for evidence of inadequate or excessive effect. Elderly and frail patients have an exaggerated response to any given target, and a lower concentration should be chosen initially. In the UK, propofol

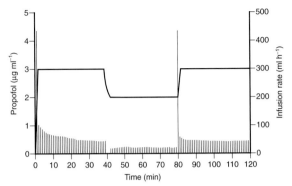

Fig. 4.10 Plasma concentration of propofol generated by a TCI device in plasma targeting mode. The narrow vertical lines are the rate of infusion required to achieve and maintain the target. A concentration of 3 µg ml⁻¹ is set initially and reduced to 2 µg ml⁻¹ after 40 min. The infusion stops at this point to allow plasma concentration to reach the lower target before re-starting at an appropriately slower rate. The target is increased to 3 µg ml⁻¹ at 80 min, and the TCI device uses a very fast infusion rate to acquire the new target, followed by an appropriately higher infusion rate. Note that the infusion rate beyond this point reflects that propofol is already present in the plasma and has been re-distributed to viscera; consequently these rates are slower than those used to sustain the 3 µg ml⁻¹ target at the start of the infusion.

and remifentanil are the i.v. agents used most often by TCI (although pharmacokinetic models exist for many other compounds). Coadministration of these agents by separate TCIs is an ideal method of TIVA, delivering a rapid and controllable effect followed by rapid awakening. Synergy between these agents allows a range of targets to be blended, and use of a low-propofol/high-remifentanil combination is usually favoured. It must be remembered that remifentanil has poor hypnotic action even at extremely high doses. Propofol targets of <3 µg ml⁻¹ should not be used in the absence of pEEG data, particularly when neuromuscular blockers are used. The detailed guide to TIVA produced by the Association of Anaesthetists and UK Society for Intravenous Anaesthesia provides details of the methodology and fundamental principles.

Closed-loop systems

Target-controlled infusion pumps can be used in conjunction with a pEEG device as a closed-loop system to control the depth of hypnosis. Feedback on effect from the cerebral monitor is relayed to the infusion pump, which increases or decreases the hypnotic and/or opioid infusion rates according to predictive algorithms. At present this is a research tool.

Box 4.2 Properties of the ideal intravenous hypnotic

- Rapid onset – agent is largely unionised at blood pH and is highly lipid soluble
- Low volume of distribution
- Rapid recovery – agent is metabolised by blood and tissue enzymes
- Duration of action independent of hepatic clearance
- No active metabolites
- High therapeutic index with steep dose–response curve
- Minimal cardiovascular and respiratory depression at hypnotic concentrations
- Water-soluble formulation
- No pain on injection
- Antiemetic action
- Analgesic at subanaesthetic concentrations
- No excitatory phenomena on induction (e.g. coughing, hiccup, involuntary movement)
- No emergence phenomena (e.g. nightmares)
- No interaction with neuromuscular blocking agents
- No sequelae from venous administration
- Safe if injected inadvertently into an artery
- Anticancer activity
- Minimal effect on the fetus/lacks teratogenicity
- No toxic effects on major organs or endocrine/exocrine axes
- No release of histamine or hypersensitivity reactions
- Long shelf life at room temperature
- Safe in porphyria

Future developments in i.v. anaesthetic drugs

None of the currently available i.v. anaesthetic agents is ideal (Box 4.2), and researchers worldwide are investigating potentially improved new drugs. Remimazolam (Fig. 4.11) is a benzodiazepine with high affinity for the GABA_A receptor. It contains a carboxylic ester moiety allowing rapid metabolism by plasma and tissue esterases. Early studies indicate a more rapid onset, greater sedation, and more rapid recovery than midazolam but with similar safety and adverse effect profiles.

Sedative and anxiolytic drugs

In addition to i.v. anaesthetics, several other drugs are used to depress consciousness or cognitive function. Inhalational anaesthetics (see Chapter 3) can be used as sedatives (e.g. nitrous oxide 50%–70% in children, sevoflurane 0.3%–0.5%

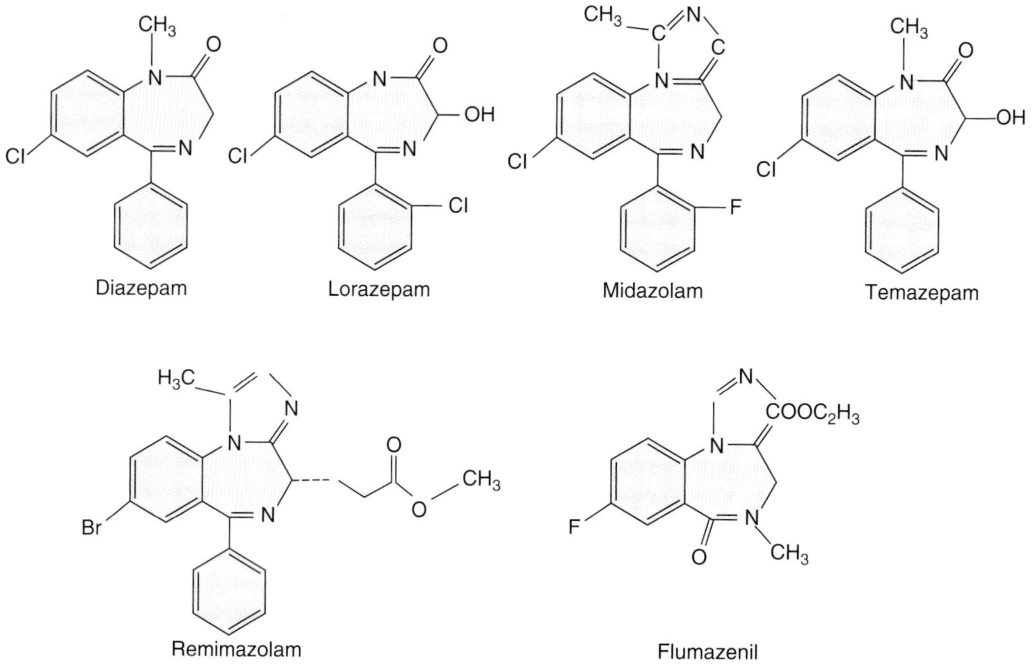

Fig. 4.11 Structure of five benzodiazepines which are relevant to anaesthetic and critical care practice; remimazolam is a new agent degraded by plasma and tissue esterases. (With permission from Vuyk, J., Sitsen, E., & Reekers, M. Intravenous anesthetics. In: Miller, R., Eriksson, L., Fleisher, L., Wiener-Kronish, J., Cohen, N., & Young, W. (eds) *Miller's Anesthesia*, 8th edn. Philadelphia, Saunders Elsevier.)

Box 4.3 Relative contraindications to the use of sedation without airway control

- Patients at significant risk of aspiration
- Marked respiratory or cardiac failure
- Depressed level of consciousness
- Significant muscle weakness from neurological/myopathic disease
- CPAP-dependent sleep apnoea

---

or isoflurane 0.5%–1% in patients in ICU) and analgesics (e.g. nitrous oxide 50%, methoxyflurane 6 ml inhaled from Penthrox inhaler). Administration of sedation for procedures requires skill and vigilance because unanticipated progression to general anaesthesia may occur. There are several relative contraindications (Box 4.3). Sedation is typically achieved using intermittent i.v. boluses of hypnotic and opioid drugs in combination, titrated to effect. The use of TCI propofol is increasingly popular.

Indications for the use of sedative drugs

Indications of the use of sedative drugs include the following:

- *Premedication.* Sedative drugs may be given for preoperative anxiolysis, particularly in young children and patients with learning difficulties. Premedication augments the action of subsequent i.v. and volatile anaesthetic agents. Parenteral administration is rarely indicated; the oral route is preferred. Benzodiazepines are used most commonly, but fentanyl (as a lozenge or lollipop), oral clonidine and ketamine are useful in children.
- *Procedural sedation.* This is defined as a minimal or moderate level of sedation (see Table 4.2) to allow tolerance of unpleasant or prolonged procedures and usually, but not always, provide amnesia. Sedatives typically have no analgesic action and are ineffective for painful procedures unless opioids are also given. However, such combinations increase significantly the incidence of airway obstruction and hypoxaemia; naloxone should be readily available.

- *Supplementation of general or regional anaesthesia.* Coinduction of general anaesthesia using an anaesthetic/benzodiazepine/opioid combination was considered earlier. Patients having surgery with regional anaesthesia may also request sedation. Propofol by TCI is used increasingly for this purpose.
- *Awake fibreoptic intubation.* Sedatives are often used to supplement topical anaesthesia in a patient with a difficult airway. Care must be taken not to depress consciousness or respiratory drive as airway obstruction may be precipitated. Remifentanil infusion (either MCI or TCI) is often used as an antitussive agent, but it has no amnesic action and may not reduce anxiety.
- *Critical care.* Critically ill patients usually require sedation to tolerate mechanical ventilation and therapeutic interventions; particular considerations apply (see Chapter 48).

Drugs used as sedatives

Drugs used therapeutically for their sedative action may be categorised as:
- benzodiazepines and related non-benzodiazepine hypnotics (Z-drugs);
- α_2 adrenoceptor agonists;
- high-dose opioids;
- antipsychotics and related agents; and
- miscellaneous.

Benzodiazepines

Benzodiazepines were developed in the 1960s as a safer alternative to oral barbiturates. They have anxiolytic and anaesthetic properties. Thirty-five compounds are used in human medicine worldwide but only a few are used as i.v. sedatives (Fig. 4.11, Table 4.7). Oral chlordiazepoxide is sometimes used for acute drug and alcohol withdrawal. The term *benzodiazepine* derives from the parent molecule's structure, which is a fusion of benzene and diazepine rings. Modification of this parent provides agents with variable durations of action and potency, which determines their therapeutic use.

Pharmacology

Benzodiazepines exert their effect by binding non-selectively to the BZ$_1$ and BZ$_2$ subtypes of the GABA$_A$ receptor (see Fig. 4.1) to increase Cl$^-$ conductance when GABA is already bound and reduce synaptic transmission. Sedation and amnesia are mediated through the α_1 subunit of the BZ (GABA$_A$) receptor, whereas action at the α_2 and α_3 subunits

appears to be involved in sleep regulation and anxiolysis. Flumazenil occupies the benzodiazepine binding sites but has minimal intrinsic activity, and it is used to antagonise the action of benzodiazepines. Ethanol also binds to the same site, and benzodiazepines (e.g. chlordiazepoxide, lorazepam) can be used to prevent or manage acute withdrawal from alcohol. Benzodiazepine binding sites are found throughout the brain and spinal cord, with the highest density in the cerebral cortex, cerebellum and hippocampus and a lower density in the medulla. The absence of GABA$_A$ receptors outside the CNS explains the cardiovascular safety profile of benzodiazepines. Binding of other compounds to the GABA$_A$ benzodiazepine site explains the synergy between benzodiazepines and other drugs and the potential for dangerous CNS depression by drug combinations. Dependency is common with continued use of oral preparations, and a potentially fatal benzodiazepine withdrawal syndrome (characterised by confusion, toxic psychosis, delirium tremens and convulsions) may be precipitated by abrupt discontinuation. Elderly patients are particularly sensitive to their effects, so benzodiazepines should be avoided if possible and dosage reduced. A form of 'pseudodementia' can develop with repeated use.

Physical properties of benzodiazepines

Most benzodiazepines are relatively hydrophobic but highly lipid-soluble molecules. Parenteral preparations of diazepam and lorazepam are dissolved in solvents (e.g. glycols) or lipid emulsions, whereas midazolam is water soluble.

Systemic effects

CNS effects

Benzodiazepines cause anxiolysis, sedation, anterograde amnesia and antiepileptic activity. The degree to which a particular agent produces these features is variable and may be related to its affinity for particular subtypes of the GABA$_A$ receptor. Anxiolysis occurs at low dosage and is useful in premedication. Higher doses produce moderate sedation, as receptor occupancy is low, but progresses to general anaesthesia as occupancy increases with repeated dosing. Benzodiazepines have a high therapeutic index because the medulla has a lower receptor density than the cortex and is less sensitive to depression. However, airway patency can be lost before profound sedation occurs in overdose and may cause death. Anterograde amnesia follows i.v. administration of benzodiazepines and is useful for patients undergoing unpleasant or repeated procedures. Prevention of the subcortical spread of seizure activity produces anticonvulsant effects, and i.v. lorazepam and diazepam are used to terminate seizures, whereas clonazepam is a useful adjunct in chronic antiepileptic therapy. Benzodiazepines increase the threshold to seizure activity in local anaesthetic toxicity but may also mask the early signs. Benzodiazepines decrease $CMRO_2$ and CBF in a dose-dependent fashion; cerebrovascular response to carbon dioxide is preserved, but depression of ventilation can result in increased $PaCO_2$. They are suitable for sedation of patients with intracranial pathological conditions, but benzodiazepines do not prevent the increases in ICP caused by laryngoscopy, tracheal intubation and hypoventilation. Unwanted CNS side effects include drowsiness and impaired psychomotor performance. Even when residual sedative effects are minimal, cognitive function and motor coordination may be impaired, which should be considered when assessing fitness for discharge after ambulatory surgery.

Table 4.7 Properties of benzodiazepine and related agents

Drug group	Routes of administration	Dose range	Onset of action	Offset of clinical effect	Principal indications	Precautions
Benzodiazepines						ALL – synergy with opioids, ethanol and CNS depressants
Midazolam	Bolus i.v.	0.025–0.05 mg kg^{-1}	90 s 90 s	2 h	Procedural sedation and anxiolysis Status epilepticus and febrile convulsions	Active metabolite hydroxymidazolam accumulates with infusions in patients with renal impairment Significant increase in CSHT with continuous infusion
	Infusion i.v.	0.03–0.1 mg kg^{-1} bolus, then 0.03–0.1 mg kg^{-1} hr^{-1}				
	Buccal	0.3 mg kg^{-1} (max 10 mg) repeated at 10 min PRN	10 min			
	Nasal	0.2 mg kg^{-1} (max 10 mg) Half to either nostril	2–5 min			
Temazepam	Oral	10–30 mg	1–2 h	2–10 h	Preoperative anxiolysis Night sedation	May cause residual drowsiness, dizziness and a hangover effect
Lorazepam	Oral Sublingual i.v.	2-5 mg 2–4 mg 1–4 mg	1–3 h 1–2 h 1–5 min	8–12 h	Preoperative anxiolysis Night sedation Withdrawal phenomena Status epilepticus	As per temazepam but more likely to occur Prolonged amnesia possible
Diazepam	Oral i.v. i.m. Rectal	5–20 mg 5–10 mg 10–20 mg 1–10 mg	30–90 min 1-5 min 15–30 min 5-10 min	24–36 h	Preoperative anxiolysis Night sedation Withdrawal phenomena Status epilepticus	As per lorazepam Should not be used to manage psychosis
Related non-benzodiazepines (Z-drugs)						ALL – synergy with opioids, ethanol and CNS depressants
Zopiclone	Oral	3.75–7.5 mg	1.5–2 h	8–12 h	Night sedation	
Zolpidem	Oral	5–10 mg	1–2 h	5–10 h	Night sedation	Visual hallucinations and amnesia occur
Zaleplon	Oral	5–10 mg	0.7–1.4 h	3–6 h	Night sedation	

Table 4.7 Properties of benzodiazepine and related agents—cont'd

Drug group	Routes of administration	Dose range	Onset of action	Offset of clinical effect	Principal indications	Precautions
Benzodiazepine receptor antagonist						
Flumazenil	Bolus i.v.	100 µg bolus repeated at 1-min intervals to effect (1 mg max, 2 mg in ICU)	60–120 s	20 min–2 h	Reversal of iatrogenic overdose or self-harm attempt	Risk of seizures if a benzodiazepine forms part of antiepileptic therapy Withdrawal symptoms may be precipitated in benzodiazepine dependence Anxiety reactions after rapid reversal of heavy sedation Sudden increase in ICP possible in patients with severe head injury
	Infusion	100–400 µg hr^{-1} after effective bolus				

CSHT, Context-sensitive half-time.

Muscle relaxation

Benzodiazepines produce a mild reduction in muscle tone, which may be advantageous during mechanical ventilation in ICU, when reducing articular dislocations or during endoscopic procedures. However, muscle relaxation is partly responsible for the airway obstruction that may occur with i.v. use. Muscle relaxation is unrelated to any effect at the neuromuscular junction but results from suppression of the internuncial neurons of the spinal cord and depression of polysynaptic transmission in the brain.

Respiratory effects

Benzodiazepines produce dose-related central ventilatory depression and diminish the responses to hypercarbia and hypoxia. Patients with hypoventilation syndromes or hypercapnic respiratory failure are particularly sensitive. Synergy occurs if opioids and benzodiazepines are coadministered, when a 75% reduction in the benzodiazepine dose should be used.

Cardiovascular effects

Benzodiazepines produce modest cardiovascular effects and have a wider margin of safety than i.v. anaesthetic agents. A decrease in systemic vascular resistance causes a small decrease in arterial pressure, but significant hypotension may occur in the presence of hypovolaemia.

Pharmacokinetics

Benzodiazepines are well absorbed orally and pass rapidly into the CNS, though midazolam undergoes significant first-pass hepatic metabolism with oral bioavailability of 36%–50%. Volume of distribution is large, as would be expected for highly lipid-soluble compounds. All benzodiazepines are extensively protein bound (>96%). After intravenous bolus administration, termination of action occurs largely by redistribution and hepatic metabolism (as described before for i.v. anaesthetics). Benzodiazepines take longer to equilibrate with the brain compared with propofol, and adequate time must be allowed for the clinical effect to develop before further incremental doses are given. Elimination is by hepatic metabolism followed by renal excretion of the metabolites. There are two main pathways of metabolism involving either microsomal oxidation or conjugation with glucuronide; oxidation is much more likely to be affected by age, hepatic disease, drug interactions and other factors which alter the concentration of cytochrome P450. Some benzodiazepines such as diazepam and chlordiazepoxide have active metabolites which greatly prolong their clinical effects. Renal dysfunction results in the accumulation of metabolites and is an important factor in delayed recovery after prolonged use in intensive care. Benzodiazepines do not induce hepatic enzymes.

Midazolam

Midazolam is the most commonly used parenteral sedative in anaesthetic practice. The structure of midazolam is altered by local changes in pH (*tautomerism*), and the two different forms confer either water or lipid solubility to the drug (Fig. 4.12) (see Chapter 1). At pH <4 the benzodiazepine nucleus opens because of an ionisable amine group in the molecule's structure, and this increases water solubility. At plasma pH the amine group is incorporated back into the unionised ring form of the molecule, which is highly lipid soluble and diffuses rapidly into the brain. A concentrated preparation (5 mg ml^{-1}) is available for i.m. injection and absorption is rapid compared with diazepam. Midazolam undergoes hepatic oxidative metabolism and has an elimination half-life of 2–4 h. The major metabolite is 1-hydroxymidazolam, which is biologically active. Midazolam has been used as a sole hypnotic for TIVA and produces superior procedural amnesia compared with propofol, but CSHT increases significantly when used by continuous infusion, and this delays recovery. Clinical studies demonstrate the inferiority of midazolam in terms of time to onset of desired sedation score, slower recovery, less clear-headedness, and significantly longer period of postoperative amnesia compared with propofol.

Flumazenil

Flumazenil is a competitive antagonist at the $GABA_A$ benzodiazepine binding site for all other ligands. It rapidly reverses the CNS and dangerous physiological effects of benzodiazepines following iatrogenic overdose or deliberate self-harm. It has no effect on benzodiazepine metabolism. Flumazenil is rapidly cleared from plasma and metabolised by the liver and has a very short elimination half-life (<1 h). Its duration of action depends on the dose administered and the duration of action of the drug to be antagonised; repeated administration or infusions may be necessary.

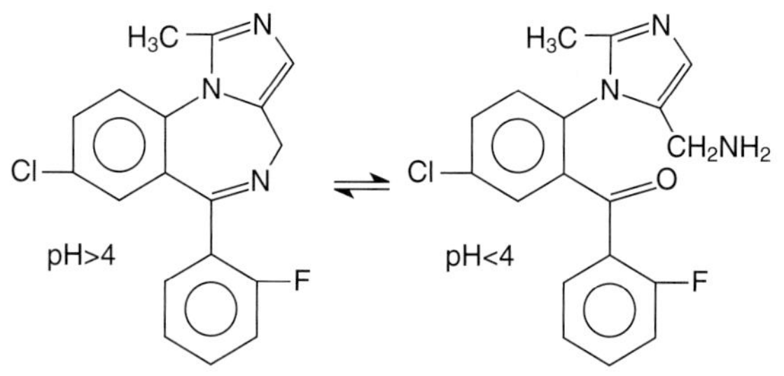

Fig. 4.12 Tautomerism exhibited by midazolam with pH change. The open form of the molecule is water soluble, and the closed form is lipid soluble.

Non-benzodiazepine hypnotics (Z-drugs)

Anaesthetists are most likely to encounter Z-drugs (see Table 4.7) when taking a preoperative history. Zopiclone, zolpidem and zaleplon have dissimilar chemical structures to benzodiazepines but exert similar clinical effects by binding to BZ_1 and BZ_2 subtypes of the $GABA_A$ receptor. Z-drugs were introduced in the late 1980s to have minimal residual sedation and to improve on the disruption of sleep architecture caused by benzodiazepines when used for insomnia. They are rapidly absorbed after ingestion and are potentially useful for preoperative anxiolysis but are licensed for 1- to 6-month courses in the management of insomnia.

α_2-Adrenoceptor agonists

Pharmacology

α_2-Adrenoceptor agonists (α_2 agonists) treat a variety of disorders, including hypertension, attention-deficit/hyperactivity disorder, panic states, and withdrawal symptoms after alcohol, opioid, benzodiazepine, and tobacco cessation. Uses in anaesthetic practice include sedation, analgesia and as an adjunct to general anaesthesia. α_2-Adrenoceptors are G-protein coupled (see Chapter 1), and three types have been identified in various anatomical locations (including platelets). In human neural tissue, these receptors are found pre-, post- and extrasynaptically in both peripheral and central locations. Activation of presynaptic receptors decreases the release of norepinephrine as a neurotransmitter at these sites and causes neuronal hyperpolarisation. Central α_2 agonists produce sedation, anxiolysis and analgesia, and an important site of action is the locus coeruleus. This is a small neuronal nucleus in the upper brainstem which contains the major noradrenergic cell group in the CNS and is an important modulator of wakefulness. This locus has connections to the cortex, thalamus and vasomotor centre, and descending fibres from this area decrease nociceptive central transmission at a spinal level. α_2-Adrenoceptor-agonists also occur in primary sensory neurons and in the dorsal horn of the spinal cord; activity at these sites may contribute to the analgesia provided by these agents. Drugs used clinically as α_2-agonists are imidazole compounds that also have activity at imidazoline receptors in the brain. Imidazoline I_1 receptors in the medulla are involved with regulation of arterial pressure, which may explain the hypotension and bradycardia seen with α_2 agonists; activity at imidazoline I_2 receptors may contribute to the analgesic action through their interaction with opioid receptors. α_2 Receptors in non-neural tissue mediate a variety of somatic effects, including decreased salivation, decreased secretion and motility in the gastrointestinal tract, contraction of vascular smooth muscle, inhibition of renin release, increased glomerular filtration rate and excretion of sodium and water via the kidney, decreased intraocular pressure and decreased insulin release.

Dexmedetomidine

Dexmedetomidine is the S-enantiomer of the veterinary anaesthetic medetomidine (Fig. 4.13). It has highly selective activity at α_2 adrenoceptors ($1600:1$ $\alpha_2:\alpha_1$) and eight times more affinity than clonidine for this site. Dexmedetomidine is licenced in the UK for i.v. sedation of adult patients in intensive care, although there is off-licence use, such as for procedural sedation during an awake craniotomy.

CNS effects

Dexmedetomidine has sedative, analgesic and anxiolytic properties and a minimum alveolar concentration (MAC)–sparing effect of up to 90%. Patients given dexmedetomidine require little or no additional medication to achieve a desired sedative end-point. A unique feature is the ease with which patients can be aroused from an effective level of sedation.

CVS effects

Adverse effects are predominantly cardiovascular (and contributed to by activity at imidazoline receptors as described earlier). Decreases in heart rate, myocardial contractility and systemic vascular resistance reduce myocardial oxygen requirements. This may be advantageous for patients with cardiac risk factors, but undesirable cardiovascular depression may limit use of this agent. Care is

required in patients with pre-existing bradycardia or conduction delay because there is a reduction in sympathetic tone and an increase in parasympathetic tone.

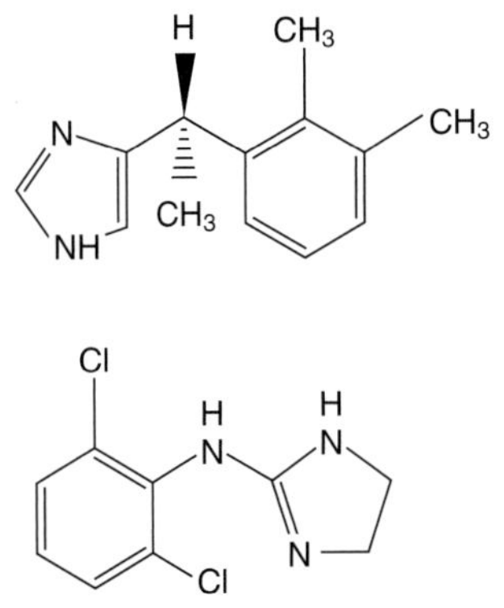

Respiratory

There is very little respiratory depression if used as a sole agent.

Endocrine

At therapeutic doses, dexmedetomidine has no significant effect on ACTH secretion, but response to ACTH may be reduced after prolonged use or at high doses.

Metabolism

Dexmedetomidine is metabolised via hepatic glucuronidation, and clearance is reduced in patients with liver impairment. Very little unchanged drug reaches the urine, but 95% of degradation products are excreted this way (4% in faeces). There is a theoretical possibility of accumulation of metabolites in patients with renal failure, but toxicity has not been described because active metabolites of dexmedetomidine have not been identified at present.

Pharmacokinetics

Dexmedetomidine is freely soluble in water and has a pKa of 7.1. The pharmaceutical formulation is a clear, colourless preservative-free solution with a pH of 4.5–8. Protein binding of dexmedetomidine is 94%, with negligible displacement by drugs commonly used in anaesthetic and ICU practice. The elimination half-life is approximately 2 h and the steady-state volume of distribution is 118 l. There are no significant differences in the pharmacokinetic profile in the elderly, but an enhanced clinical response is seen.

Dosage

Dosage of dexmedetomidine is as follows:
- ICU sedation: infusion at an average of 0.7 μg kg^{-1} h^{-1} (normal range 0.2–1.4 μg kg^{-1} h^{-1}).
- Procedural sedation: 1 μg kg^{-1} over 10 min, then infusion at an average of 0.6 μg kg^{-1} hr^{-1} (normal range 0.2–1.0 μg kg^{-1} hr^{-1}).

Fig. 4.13 Chemical structure of dexmedetomidine (above) and clonidine (below). (With permission from Vuyk, J., Sitsen, E., & Reekers, M. Intravenous anesthetics. In: Miller, R., Eriksson, L., Fleisher, L., Wiener-Kronish, J., Cohen, N., & Young, W. (eds) *Miller's Anesthesia,* 8th edn. Philadelphia, Saunders Elsevier.)

Clonidine

Clonidine is a highly selective α_2-agonist ($\alpha_2:\alpha_1 = 200:1$). It was introduced as a centrally acting antihypertensive, but abrupt discontinuation of therapy results in potentially dangerous rebound hypertension and it has fallen out of favour.

CNS effects

Clonidine produces sedation, anxiolysis and analgesia. It also has a MAC-sparing effect, but there is a ceiling to the reduction because of the potential for activity at α_1 receptors when used at higher doses.

CVS effects

The cardiovascular effects of clonidine probably involve α_1 receptors and imidazoline receptors as with dexmedetomidine. Clonidine lowers the set point around which arterial pressure is regulated.

Respiratory effects

Clonidine has minor respiratory effects, causing only a small reduction in minute ventilation.

Pharmacokinetics

Clonidine is lipid soluble and rapidly absorbed after oral administration, with a peak plasma concentration occurring in 60–90 min. Oral, intravenous and intramuscular routes may be used for sedation or analgesia. In addition, epidural and intrathecal clonidine is used to augment regional anaesthesia, but perineural administration is of limited or no effect. The elimination half-life is 9–13 h and is prolonged in renal failure. Fifty percent of an administered dose is excreted unchanged by the kidneys, and 50% is metabolised in the liver to inactive metabolites.

Dosage

Dosage for clonidine is as follows:
- Premedication: 150–300 µg orally given 1–2 h preoperatively.
- Critical care: 0–4 µg kg^{-1} hr^{-1} i.v. as a sedative, especially for agitation in drug-dependent individuals.

Opioids

Opioid analgesics have some hypnotic and amnesic action but do not provide anaesthesia even at very high doses. Infusions of opioids such as morphine, alfentanil, fentanyl and remifentanil (at rates that cause apnoea) are often used for their analgesic and sedative effects either as sole agents or combined with other sedatives in ICU. Significant prolongation of CSHT of alfentanil and fentanyl occurs with such infusions. Clinicians may use the term *remifentanil sedation* when referring to its use as an antitussive agent (e.g. during fibreoptic airway procedures). The use of remifentanil as a component of a conscious sedation technique has a high incidence of bradycardia, apnoea and hypoxaemia at subanalgesic levels. Morphine by continuous infusion is used for sedation in critical care, but it has an active metabolite (morphine-6-glucuronide) which is largely responsible for its analgesic action. Morphine-6-glucuronide is likely to accumulate in patients in ICU because of altered pharmacokinetics and impaired renal function and will prolong recovery when the infusion is discontinued.

Antipsychotics

The antipsychotic drugs used in psychiatry (also called neuroleptics) have potentially useful sedative action. *Neurolepsis* describes an altered state of awareness with suppression of spontaneous movement and a placid, compliant affect without loss of consciousness and with intact spinal and central reflexes. Since the advent of i.v. benzodiazepines, neuroleptics are rarely used for sedation of behaviourally normal patients. They provide no procedural amnesia, and patients may subsequently report unpleasant mental agitation despite a calm outward demeanour. The concept of neuroleptanalgesia was introduced in the late 1950s as a method for allowing light general anaesthesia without an inhaled volatile agent. The combination of a neuroleptic (usually droperidol), a synthetic opioid (typically fentanyl) and nitrous oxide was used to cause unconsciousness. It was a popular technique for ophthalmic surgery, cardiac surgery, and neurosurgery and for high-risk patients but has been superseded by modern hypnotics and regional anaesthesia.

Pharmacology

The drugs used in anaesthetic practice are structurally similar with a high therapeutic index and flat dose–response curve; hence the incidence of respiratory depression in overdose is low. Antipsychotics act principally by central antagonism of dopaminergic pathways, but few are clean agents as they exert activity at multiple CNS receptor types. An antiadrenergic effect may cause hypotension and syncope in the elderly. The agents described later in this section have the potential for causing long QT syndrome and fatal cardiac arrhythmia and must be used cautiously when combined with other drugs which have adverse effects on QT interval (such as ondansetron). Dopamine receptor blockade potentially causes extrapyramidal side effects, including tardive dyskinesia (involuntary movements of tongue, face and jaw), Parkinsonian symptoms, akathisia (restlessness) and dystonia (abnormal face and body movements). Neuroleptic malignant syndrome, a rare but potentially fatal adverse reaction, is characterised by hyperthermia, muscle hypertonicity, autonomic instability and fluctuating levels of consciousness. It has features in common with malignant hyperthermia and is treated with dopamine agonists (e.g. bromocriptine) in addition to dantrolene and supportive measures.

Haloperidol

Haloperidol is a butyrophenone with a long duration of action. It has little α-adrenoceptor blocking activity and minimal effect on the cardiovascular system. It is an effective antiemetic but has a high incidence of extrapyramidal adverse effects. Haloperidol may be used in the short-term management of the acutely agitated patient (when sinister causes of confusion such as hypoxaemia and sepsis have been excluded) and in the management of delirium in ICU (see Chapter 48). The duration of action of haloperidol is approximately 24–48 h.

Dosage

Dosage for haloperidol is as follows:
- Sedation: 2–10 mg i.v. or i.m. (max. 18 mg per 24 h).
- Antiemesis: 1.25 mg i.v. for prevention of postoperative nausea and vomiting (PONV).

Droperidol

Droperidol is a butyrophenone that has potent antidopaminergic (D$_2$) activity and mild α$_2$-blocking actions. It produces sedation and anxiolysis and is an effective antiemetic (see Chapter 7). Adverse effects include vasodilatation and hypotension, and at higher doses, dystonic reactions can occur. Droperidol was used for premedication and in neuroleptanaesthesia until reports of death from long QT syndrome led to its withdrawal in 2001. It has recently been reintroduced and licenced at lower doses for prevention of postoperative nausea and vomiting. Droperidol has an onset of 3–10 min after i.v. injection and duration of action of 6–12 h. It undergoes hepatic metabolism, but

approximately 10% of the drug is excreted unchanged in the urine.

Dosage

As prophylaxis for PONV, the dosage of droperidol is 0.625–1.25 mg i.v. 20–30 min before the end of surgery.

Olanzapine

Olanzapine is classed as an atypical antipsychotic and is considered a first-line agent in the management of newly diagnosed psychosis. It has a similar mechanism of action to classical antipsychotics but with a lower incidence of adverse events. Olanzapine rarely produces hypotension and has less potential for QT prolongation. It is used in the management of delirium in ICU (see Chapter 48).

Dosage

Dosage for olanzapine is as follows:
- Sedation: 5–10 mg orally (maximum 20 mg daily).
- Urgent control of mania: 10 mg i.m. (5 mg in the elderly).

Miscellaneous

Melatonin

Melatonin is a pineal gland hormone that modulates circadian rhythms. It is used primarily in the treatment of sleep disorders but has also been used as a sedative in adults and children. Its mechanism of action at CNS melatonin receptors is not fully elucidated, but it may be via enhancement of GABA activity.

Dosage

Melatonin dosage is 2–10 mg orally, starting at 2 mg per day.

References/Further reading

Academy of Medical Royal Colleges. Safe Sedation Practice for Healthcare Procedures: Standards and Guidance. https://www.rcoa.ac.uk/document-store/safe-sedation-practice-healthcare-procedures-standards-and-guidance.

Nimmo, A.F., Absalom, A.R., Bagshaw, O., et al., 2018. Guidelines for the safe practice of total intravenous anaesthesia (TIVA). doi:10.1111/anae.14428.

Pandit, J.J., Cook, T.M. (Eds.), the NAP5 Steering Panel, 2014. NAP5. Accidental Awareness During General Anaesthesia. https://www.nationalauditprojects.org.uk/NAP5home#pt.

Roberts, F.L., Dixon, J., Lewis, G.T., Tackley, R.M., Prys-Roberts, C., 1988. Induction and maintenance of propofol anaesthesia: a manual infusion shceme. Anaesthesia 43, 14–17.

Whitehouse, T., Snelson, C., Grounds, M., 2014. Intensive Care Society Review of Best Practice for Analgesia and Sedation in Critical Care. London. http://www.ics.ac.uk/ICS/guidelines-and-standards.aspx.

Chapter 5

Local anaesthetic agents

Zoe Whitman and Jonathan Thompson

Local anaesthetics are analgesic drugs that suppress action potentials by blocking voltage-activated sodium ion (Na^+) channels (VASCs) in excitable tissues. Examples include the amides (e.g. lidocaine, bupivacaine, levobupivacaine, ropivacaine) and esters (e.g. cocaine and procaine) (Table 5.1). Other drugs that can inhibit VASCs, such as diphenhydramine (a first-generation histamine H_1 receptor antagonist) and amitriptyline (a tricyclic antidepressant), also have local anaesthetic properties. The blockade of VASCs accounts for both their analgesic effects, mediated through inhibition of action potentials in nociceptive neurons, and their systemic effects. The inhibition of action potentials in the heart contributes to local anaesthetic toxicity and also accounts for the antiarrhythmic actions of intravenous lidocaine (see Chapter 9). Unlike general anaesthetics (see Chapters 3 and 4), local anaesthetics do not diminish consciousness when administered correctly.

Local anaesthetics block sensation at the site of administration by inhibiting action potentials in all sensory nerve fibres. Therefore, unlike other analgesic drugs such as the anti-inflammatory agents and opioids, the effects of local anaesthetic are similar for all peripheral causes of pain. Opioid analgesics (morphine, fentanyl, codeine etc.) and other central analgesic drugs such as the α_2-adrenergic agonists (clonidine, dexmedetomidine) activate metabotropic, G protein–coupled receptors within the membranes of specific neurons located within the pain pathway, but their main actions are centrally mediated (described in Chapter 6).

Mechanism of action of local anaesthetics

The VASC is one of many membrane proteins in the phospholipid bilayers that encapsulate neurons (Fig. 5.1). Voltage-activated Na^+ channels provide selective permeability to Na^+ when the cell becomes depolarised from the resting potential (approximately −70 mV), which is maintained in quiescent neurons by the tonic activity of potassium ion (K^+) channels.

Pain transmission begins as a depolarisation in the nerve ending of the primary afferent neuron initiated by the activation of cation channels. When the depolarisation reaches the threshold for activation of VASCs (approximately −45 mV), an action potential is generated, resulting in rapid depolarisation to approximately +20 mV (Fig. 5.2). Each action potential is brief (approximately 2 ms) because VASCs rapidly inactivate, leading to closure of their inactivation gates and halting of Na^+ influx, while at the same time VASCs activate, leading to an increase in the permeability of the cell membrane to K^+. As a result, the membrane potential travels rapidly back towards the K^+ equilibrium potential, and this period is known as the afterhyperpolarisation; this phenomenon contributes to the refractory period during which generation of another action potential is unlikely (see Fig. 5.2).

Mechanism of local anaesthetic inhibition of the voltage-activated Na^+ channel

Local anaesthetics inhibit action potentials in primary afferent nociceptive neurons: the pain-sensing neurons that transmit to the dorsal horn of the spinal cord (see Chapter 6). Their mechanism of action is that they access the open VASC from the inside of the cell and bind to specific amino acids lining the channel lumen to inhibit VASC activity (see Fig. 5.1). They bind preferentially to the open channel and are therefore said to be use-dependent (or open channel) blockers. First the local anaesthetic must cross the cell membrane, which requires it to be lipid soluble. The molecule must then diffuse into the aqueous environment within the

Table 5.1 The features of individual local anaesthetic drugs

Local anaesthetic	Ester or amide link	pKa	% Protein bound	Octanol partition coefficient	Relative potency[a]	Half-life (h)	Relative duration of action[a]	Toxicity	Main use
Lidocaine	Amide	7.9	64	43	1	1.6	1	Medium	Infiltration, nerve block, topical, epidural
Mepivacaine	Amide	7.7	77	21	1	2–3	1	Medium	Dental infiltration
Prilocaine	Amide	7.9	55	25	1	1.6	1.5	Low	Infiltration, nerve block, IVRA, topical (as EMLA)
Bupivacaine	Amide	8.1	95	346	4	3.5	2–4	Medium	Epidural, spinal, nerve block
Levobupivacaine	Amide	8.1	>97	346	4	2.6	2–4	Medium	Epidural, spinal, nerve block
Ropivacaine	Amide	8.1	94	115	3	1.9	2–4	Medium	Epidural, nerve block
Articaine	Amide	7.8	76	257	0.5	0.3	2	Medium	Dental infiltration
Cocaine	Ester	8.7	95	n/a	1	1.5	0.5	Very high	Topical
Benzocaine	Ester	3.5		n/a	n/a	n/a	2	Low	Topical
Tetracaine/amethocaine	Ester	8.4	76	n/a	4	n/a	2	High	Topical
Chloroprocaine	Ester	9.1		9	1	0.11	0.75	Low	Spinal

[a]Dosing equivalent to lidocaine = 1. NB: Published figures vary.
n/a, Not available or not applicable (not used in solution); *IVRA*, intravenous regional anaesthesia.
Strichartz, G. R., Sanchez, V., Arthur, G. R., Chafetz, R., & Martin, D. (1990) Fundamental properties of local anesthetics. II. Measured octanol:buffer partition coefficients and pKa values of clinically used drugs. *Anesthesia and Analgesia*. 71, 158–170.

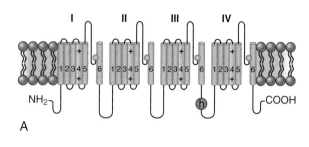

A

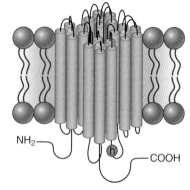

B

Fig. 5.1 Topology of the voltage-activated sodium ion channel (VASC) α subunit. (A) The subunit has 24 membrane-spanning segments arranged in four domains with positively charged amino acid residues in the fourth segment of each domain providing voltage sensitivity. Pore loops between segments five and six line the channel and have negatively charged amino acids which attract Na⁺ into the channel's outer vestibule. The intracellular loop between domains three and four contains the inactivation gate (or h gate). (B) The four domains come together to form a channel. The ancillary β subunits, which modulate channel function, are not shown.

ion channel. Amide and ester local anaesthetics possess both lipophilic and hydrophilic properties and are described as amphipathic (Fig. 5.3). They exist in basic (uncharged) and cationic (charged) forms, and the relative proportion of each (determined using the Henderson–Hasselbalch equation) depends on the pH of the solution and the pKa of the local anaesthetic (see also Chapter 1):

$$pKa = pH + \log \frac{[\text{Cationic LA}]}{[\text{Uncharged LA}]}$$

$$\log \frac{[\text{Cationic LA}]}{[\text{Uncharged LA}]} = pK_a - pH$$

Local anaesthetics are weak bases, and most have a pKa between 7.7 and 8.5 (see Table 5.1). Therefore they exist predominantly in the charged form of the molecule compared with the uncharged molecule at physiological pH:

$$\log \frac{[\text{Cationic LA}]}{[\text{Uncharged LA}]} = 1$$

$$\frac{[\text{Cationic LA}]}{[\text{Uncharged LA}]} = 10$$

An alkaline solution speeds the onset of analgesia by increasing the proportion of uncharged local anaesthetic on the outside of the nerve, resulting in more rapid passage through the cell membrane to the inside of the cell. Once inside, the balance of isoforms is re-established by the intracellular pH. In contrast, infected and inflamed tissue has a relatively low (acidic) pH, leading to a further increase in the proportion of the charged cationic local anaesthetic component, and higher doses are needed to achieve analgesia.

The voltage-activated Na⁺ channel

Local anaesthetics gain access to their binding site within the inner lumen of the VASC when the activation gate opens in response to depolarisation. The VASC is formed by a large protein (the α subunit) consisting of 24 membrane-spanning segments arranged in four repetitive motifs (see Fig. 5.1). The fourth segment of each motif is a voltage sensor: a series of positively charged amino acids (arginine and lysine residues) lying within the membrane. Depolarisation causes electrostatic repulsion of the voltage sensors, providing the energy required to open the activation gate (see Fig. 5.2). Na⁺ ions, selected by the filter formed by the four pore loops (between the fifth and sixth segments) lining the outer vestibule of the channel, are then free to pass down their concentration gradient into the cell, generating a depolarising electrical current. However, Na⁺ current is inhibited by local anaesthetic bound within the inner vestibule of the channel. The inactivation gate, formed by intracellular components of the channel, closes rapidly after depolarisation (see Fig. 5.2) and local anaesthetics stabilise the inactivated state.

There are multiple subtypes of VASCs, named after the identity of their α subunit (Na$_V$1.1–Na$_V$1.9) encoded by one of nine different genes (SCN1A–SCN5A, SCN8A–SCN11A) which are differentially expressed in tissues throughout the body and have differing pharmacological and biophysical properties. This heterogeneity provides the potential (to date unmet) for selectively targeting VASCs in pain-sensing neurons. Nociceptive neurons predominantly express Na$_V$1.7, Na$_V$1.8 and/or Na$_V$1.9 α subunits. Mutations in the *SCN9A* gene, which encodes Na$_V$1.7, are associated with several pathological pain conditions. Aspects of systemic toxicity relate to the ability of local anaesthetics to block VASCs outside the pain pathway. Cardiac VASCs are of the Na$_V$1.5 subtype, and local anaesthetics such as ropivacaine

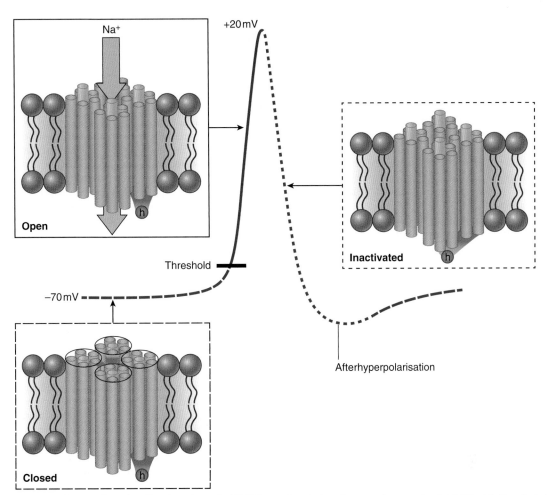

Fig. 5.2 Most voltage-activated sodium ion channels (VASCs) are closed at resting membrane potential (−70 mV). Depolarisation activates VASCs once the threshold potential is reached. Open VASCs enable greater depolarisation until channels become inactivated and no longer support Na⁺ influx because of closure of the h gate. Voltage-activated K⁺ channels (not shown) enable K⁺ efflux, leading to hyperpolarisation.

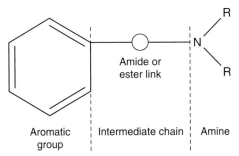

Fig. 5.3 General formula for local anaesthetic drugs.

and levobupivacaine are thought to have less systemic toxicity because of their lower affinity for cardiac channels. Additional VASC heterogeneity is conferred by four genes that encode ancillary β subunits.

Pain fibres

Different peripheral nerve fibres have differing sensitivities to blockade by local anaesthetics and are classified as A, B and C according to their conduction velocities, A being the fastest conductors and C the slowest. Aδ and C fibres both conduct pain (see Chapter 6). Other subtypes of A fibre supply skeletal muscles (α and γ) and conduct tactile sensation (β), whereas type B are preganglionic autonomic fibres. Aδ fibres are heavily myelinated and rapidly conduct acute stabbing pain. Myelination enables a remarkably high velocity of transmission (approximately 20 m s^{-1}) through a mechanism known as saltatory conduction. VASCs are segregated within the neuronal membrane of Aδ fibres at gaps in the myelin sheaths (nodes of Ranvier), enabling action potentials effectively to 'jump' from one node to the next. Aδ fibres are of small diameter and therefore have little ability to conduct changes in membrane potential once VASC activity has been inhibited. This makes them particularly sensitive to local anaesthetic block. Unlike Aδ fibres, C fibres are unmyelinated and their velocity of conduction from the skin to the spinal cord is relatively slow (approximately 1 m s^{-1}). Local anaesthetics block the transmission of dull, aching pain, mediated by C fibres very effectively. The fibre diameter is very small (approximately 1 μm) and therefore there is little passive conduction, making transmission reliant on the activity of VASCs. C fibres are activated by inflammatory mediators, and therefore the pain resulting from their stimulation can also be treated by anti-inflammatory agents.

Local anaesthetic structure

Local anaesthetics of the amide and ester classes share three structural moieties: an aromatic portion, an intermediate chain and an amine group (see Fig. 5.3). The aromatic portion is lipophilic, and lipid solubility is further enhanced in local anaesthetics that have longer intermediate chains. The amine group is a proton acceptor, providing the potential for both charged and uncharged isoforms. This means that local anaesthetics are amphipathic – that is, the molecule contains both polar (water soluble) and non-polar (water insoluble) parts. Amide and ester anaesthetics are so named because of their distinctive bonds within the intermediate chain. A convenient mnemonic is that the names of esters contain one letter *i* whereas those of amides contain two letter *i*s. The presence of either an amide or an ester bond determines its metabolic pathway. This has important implications regarding allergy potential and pharmacokinetic profile. For example, replacement of the tertiary amine by a piperidine ring increases lipid solubility and duration of action; addition of an ethyl group to lidocaine on the α carbon of the amide link created etidocaine; and addition of a propyl or butyl group to the amine end of mepivacaine results in [p]ropivacaine and bupivacaine, respectively. Halogenation of the aromatic ring of procaine produces chloroprocaine, an ester with faster hydrolysis and shorter duration of action.

Pharmacological properties of local anaesthetics

Several factors influence the pharmacological properties of local anaesthetic drugs (see Table 5.1), in particular pKa, lipid solubility, protein binding and vasodilator activity. Speed of onset is related to the concentration of unionised (lipid soluble) drug at the site of action, which relates mainly to the pKa, but also the lipid solubility, initial dose and the pH of the tissues. Potency is closely related to lipid solubility; duration of action is proportional to the degree of protein binding. Both potency and duration of action may also be affected by the addition of vasoconstrictors.

- pKa is the pH at which the ionised and unionised forms of a compound are present in equal amounts and is an important determinant of the speed of onset of a drug. For basic drugs such as local anaesthetics, the greater the pKa, the greater the ionised fraction. As diffusion across the nerve sheath and nerve membrane requires unionised drug, a local anaesthetic with a low pKa has a fast onset of action, whereas one with a high pKa has a slow onset of action. For example, lidocaine (pKa 7.9) has a fast onset compared with bupivacaine (pKa 8.1), because, at pH 7.4, 25% of lidocaine exists in the unionised base form compared with only 15% of bupivacaine.
- *Lipid solubility* is the ratio of aqueous and lipid concentrations when a local anaesthetic is introduced into a mixture of oil- and water-based solvents; it is commonly expressed as the octanol/water partition coefficient. Drugs with a higher lipid solubility are more potent but also have greater toxicity.
- *Molecular weight* influences the rate of transfer of drug across nerve membranes, including into the CNS. In theory, drugs with a lower molecular weight should transfer more quickly. However, drug mass increases with the length of side chains, which tend to be more lipid soluble.
- *Protein binding*, including local anaesthetic attachment to protein components of the nerve membrane, increases the duration of action of a local anaesthetic. In plasma, amide anaesthetics bind predominantly to α-acid glycoprotein (AAG), a high-affinity limited capacity protein, and albumin, a low-affinity large capacity protein. The bioavailability of anaesthetic is determined by the availability of plasma proteins; high plasma AAG concentrations permit greater binding of anaesthetic, and so plasma concentrations of free drug are lower. After surgery, trauma or malignancy, AAG concentrations increase significantly and serve to decrease the potential for toxicity in patients receiving local anaesthetic epidural or perineural infusions.

- *Vasodilator activity* influences potency and duration of action. Most local anaesthetics cause vasoconstriction at lower doses and vasodilatation at higher doses. Intrinsic vasodilator properties are in the order lidocaine > bupivacaine > levobupivacaine > ropivacaine. Vasodilatation reduces the amount of drug at the site of injection, increasing systemic absorption and potential toxicity. In practice, a vasoconstrictor may be added to prolong the duration of effect and reduce systemic effects (e.g. adrenaline 1:80,000 to 1:200,000 with lidocaine, bupivacaine or mepivacaine). This is more relevant for infiltration or nerve/plexus blocks than for neuraxial blockade. Felypressin, an octapeptide derivative of vasopressin, is a potent vasoconstrictor and is added to a formulation of prilocaine for dental use.

Differential sensory and motor blockade

Local anaesthetics provide differential sensory and motor block, dependent on fibre size. Smaller pain fibres are more sensitive to the effects of local anaesthetics; this is most apparent with lower drug concentrations. For example, epidural administration of 0.5% bupivacaine provides excellent sensory and motor block for Caesarean section, yet administration of 0.1% bupivacaine, often combined with fentanyl 2 µg ml^{-1}, can provide analgesia during labour but with full lower limb movement.

Pharmacokinetics

Absorption

Absorption from the injection site depends on the site itself, dose and rate of injection, pharmacological properties, and use of a vasoconstrictor. The rank order of plasma concentration after injection at various sites is intrapleural > intercostal > lumbar epidural > brachial plexus > sciatic > femoral, which reflects the relative vascularity of these tissues. First-pass pulmonary metabolism limits the concentration of local anaesthetic reaching the systemic circulation. Maximum recommended doses are shown in Table 5.2.

The local absorption (and effectiveness) of topical local anaesthetics (e.g. tetracaine, eutectic mixture of local anaesthetics (EMLA)) is considerably enhanced by using occlusive dressings.

Distribution

Tissue distribution is proportional to lipid solubility and local perfusion. Local anaesthetic drugs are distributed rapidly to brain, heart, liver and lungs but more slowly to muscle and fat, which have less blood supply. Tissue blood flow also depends on the patient's age, cardiovascular status and hepatic function.

Metabolism

Amide metabolism depends on hepatic blood flow. Toxicity is more likely in the elderly and with infusions or repeated

Table 5.2 Maximum doses of local anaesthetics administered as a bolus

	Plain (mg)	Plain per kg (mg kg^{-1})	With adrenaline (mg)	With adrenaline (mg kg^{-1})	Over 24 h (mg)
Chloroprocaine	800	11	1000 mg	13	
Prilocaine	400	6	600 mg	8	
Lidocaine	200	3	500 mg	7	
Mepivacaine	400	6	500 mg[a]	8[a]	
Bupivacaine	150	2	225 mg	3	400
Levobupivacaine	150	2	n/a	n/a	400
Ropivacaine	250	3	n/a	n/a	800

[a]With felypressin.
n/a, Not available.
Adapted from McLeod, G. A., Butterworth, J. F., & Wildsmith, J. A. W. (2008) Local anesthetic systemic toxicity. In: Cousins, M. J., Bridenbaugh, P. O., Horlecker, T. T., & Carr, D. B. (eds.) *Cousins & Bridenbaugh's Neural Blockade* (4th edn). Philadelphia, Lippincott, Williams & Wilkins, pp. 114–132.

doses, though the increase in AAG after surgery attenuates the rise in plasma concentrations. Esters are hydrolysed rapidly in plasma by pseudocholinesterase to the metabolite para-aminobenzoic acid (PABA), which can generate an allergic reaction. Amides are not metabolised to PABA and so allergic reactions to the local anaesthetic itself are very rare. Allergy to excipients can still occur.

Clearance

Clearance of amides depends on hepatic metabolism, and metabolites may accumulate in renal failure.

Placental transfer

Protein binding determines the rate and degree of diffusion of local anaesthetics, including placental transfer. The relative concentration of bupivacaine between umbilical vein and maternal circulation is 0.3, but foetal toxicity depends primarily on the free fraction of local anaesthetic, which is the same in mother and foetus.

Clinical preparation of local anaesthetics

Local anaesthetics are presented clinically as hydrochloride salts with pH 5–6 because they are unstable in solution at alkaline pH. Alteration of pH influences the rate of onset. For example, the addition of bicarbonate to lidocaine before administration increases the amount of unionised drug and so onset of action is quicker. Conversely the onset and efficacy of local anaesthetics are reduced in an acidic tissue environment (see earlier).

Enantiomer pharmacology

Bupivacaine is a chiral molecule comprising two structurally similar, non-superimposable, mirror images called enantiomers (Table 5.3). The nomenclature of enantiomers is based on the Cahn–Ingold–Prelog priority rules whereby the smallest atom is placed to the rear of the central atom about which the molecule rotates, and the sequence of the remaining three atoms is determined. For example, an increase in atomic mass in a clockwise direction is indicative of an S (sinistra) or *laevo* enantiomer, whereas an increase in atomic mass in an anticlockwise direction is indicative of an R (rectus) or *dextro* enantiomer. The + and – refer to the rotation of polarised light and are not equivalent to the S/R nomenclature. Levobupivacaine is the *laevo* (S–) enantiomer of bupivacaine; ropivacaine is the (S–) enantiomer from the

Table 5.3 Chiral terminology

Chirality	Spatial arrangement of atoms, non-superimposable on each other
Isomer	Molecule with the same atomic composition but different stereochemical formulae and hence different physical or chemical properties
Stereoisomers	Identical isomers which differ in the arrangement of their atoms in space
Enantiomer	One of a pair of molecules which are mirror images of each other and non-superimposable
Racemate	An equimolar mixture of a pair of enantiomers

propyl derivative of bupivacaine. Enantiomers are discussed further in Chapter 1.

Pharmacology of individual local anaesthetics

Lidocaine

Lidocaine is the most widely used local anaesthetic. It has a rapid onset and short duration of action. Lidocaine is rapidly and extensively metabolised in the liver and is safe at recommended doses. Efficacy is enhanced markedly and duration of action prolonged by addition of adrenaline. Lidocaine is less toxic than bupivacaine; a testament to this relative safety is that lidocaine is used intravenously as a class 1b antiarrhythmic and as an i.v. infusion to treat refractory chronic pain. Lidocaine solutions for injection are available in concentrations of 1% and 2%, with or without adrenaline. It is also available as a spray (4% or 10%), cream (2% or 4%), ointment or medicated plaster (both 5%) for topical application.

Bupivacaine

Bupivacaine is a chiral compound used clinically for 50 years, with a slower onset, greater potency and longer duration of action than lidocaine. Initial benefits of bupivacaine were sensory–motor separation and minimal tachyphylaxis, unlike repeated doses of lidocaine. However, it has greater potential for cardiac toxicity, related to its avid binding to and slow dissociation from cardiac Na^+ channels. Inadvertent intravenous administration may result in systemic toxicity (see later), and it is contraindicated for intravenous regional anaesthesia (see Chapter 25). Bupivacaine is commonly used for epidural administration in obstetrics and postoperative pain management. A hyperbaric preparation containing 80 mg ml^{-1} glucose is available for spinal anaesthesia.

Levobupivacaine

This is the *laevo* (S−) enantiomer of bupivacaine, with similar properties to the racemic mixture, though it has slightly higher protein binding and clearance and hence a lower potential for cardiac and CNS toxicity. In practice, several other factors contribute to local anaesthetic toxicity (see later), and the recommended maximum doses remain the same. Its formulation is expressed as percentage weight per unit volume of free base; racemic bupivacaine is expressed as percentage weight per unit volume of hydrochloride salt. Levobupivacaine therefore contains 13% more active molecules for a given dose.

Ropivacaine

This is a single (S−) enantiomer, similar in structure to bupivacaine. Substitution of a propyl for the butyl side chain of bupivacaine reduces lipid solubility; this leads to reduced potential for toxicity and also greater separation between sensory and motor blockade. Efficacy is similar, but motor block is reduced compared with equianalgesic doses of racemic bupivacaine.

Prilocaine

Prilocaine is less toxic than lidocaine, with a high clearance, attributable to metabolism in the lungs, kidneys and liver. It is associated with methaemoglobinaemia at doses >600 mg. It is sometimes used at a concentration of 0.5% for the provision of intravenous regional anaesthesia (see Chapter 25), and a combination of prilocaine 3% with felypressin is available for low-volume local infiltration anaesthesia in dental surgery. A 2% formulation is also available for spinal anaesthesia. Prilocaine is also formulated in a eutectic mixture with lidocaine (EMLA) for topical anaesthesia (see later).

Other local anaesthetic drugs

Mepivacaine has similar properties to lidocaine but a slower onset of action. It is used in dentistry for nerve block or infiltration at concentrations of 3% plain solution or 2% with adrenaline.

Articaine is an amide that also contains an ester linkage, which is hydrolysed rapidly so that the duration of action is short. It is available as a 4% solution with adrenaline for infiltration anaesthesia in dentistry.

Tetracaine, also known as **amethocaine,** is the most potent and lipid-soluble ester local anaesthetic and has significant potential for toxicity if used systemically. It is commonly used as a 4% gel for topical application to decrease the pain from venous puncture or cannulation.

Chloroprocaine is an ester that is metabolised rapidly by ester hydrolysis, so its duration of action is short and potential for cardiac toxicity relatively low. It can be used as a preservative-free solution for spinal anaesthesia for surgical procedures up to 40 min in duration.

Cocaine is derived from the leaves of the *erythroxylum coca* plant and was first used as an anaesthetic by Karl Koller in 1884. It is a potent vasoconstrictor, blocking reuptake of noradrenaline, but has significant potential for systemic toxicity. Cocaine has been used in nasal surgery as a paste or 4% solution for its properties of topical anaesthesia and vasoconstriction.

Benzocaine is an atypical ester that remains unionised at body pH and is therefore insoluble in water but useful for topical application. When used as oral lozenges or topical anaesthesia, it has a rapid onset (<1 min) and offset (5–10 min) of action, but it is limited by its potential to cause methaemoglobinaemia, especially with repeated doses.

Eutectic mixture of local anaesthetics (EMLA) is a eutectic mixture of 2.5% lidocaine and 2.5% prilocaine formulated as an oil/water emulsion for topical anaesthesia. A eutectic mixture is a combination of two compounds in a ratio that inhibits the crystallisation of each so that the melting point of the mixture is as low as possible, and lower than either compound alone. In EMLA, both drugs are in the unionised state in the preparation and only become ionised after absorption into the skin. EMLA is used for topical anaesthesia but should be avoided in infants aged <12 months because of the potential for methaemoglobinaemia. It should not be applied to mucous membranes.

Local anaesthetic toxicity

Toxicity is mainly caused by the intrinsic effects of local anaesthetics in blocking conduction in all excitable tissues, particularly the CNS and heart. They are also directly toxic to nerve and muscle tissues. The CNS is more sensitive than the heart to the toxic effects of local anaesthetics, and CNS symptoms and signs usually present first. These include circumoral paraesthesia, tongue numbness, tinnitus and blurred vision, proceeding to agitation, muscle twitching, drowsiness, respiratory depression and convulsions. Local anaesthetics decrease the rate of depolarisation, action potential duration and refractory period in cardiac conducting tissues. In toxicity, the ECG may show prolongation of the PR interval and QRS duration, progressing to ventricular arrhythmias and cardiac arrest; these are more likely in the presence of acidosis or hypoxia. Direct intravascular injection (especially arterial injection in the head and neck) can lead to blindness, aphasia, hemiparesis, convulsions, respiratory depression, coma or cardiac arrest. Systemic toxicity is also related to lipid solubility and potency; for example, bupivacaine is more toxic than lidocaine.

Systemic toxicity depends on the drug and mass injected, site of injection and use of vasoconstrictors. Type 1 hypersensitivity reactions may occur with ester local anaesthetics. Prilocaine, and less commonly benzocaine or lidocaine, may cause methaemoglobinaemia.

Mechanisms of systemic toxicity

Cardiovascular effects are caused by blockade of cardiac VASCs and K^+ channels. Levobupivacaine and ropivacaine are thought to be less likely to interact with cardiac VASCs. Convulsions may be caused by the blockade of γ-aminobutyric acid A ($GABA_A$) receptors in the CNS and respond to positive modulators of $GABA_A$ receptor function (barbiturates, propofol and benzodiazepines).

Systemic toxicity

Despite the introduction of agents such as levobupivacaine and ropivacaine, systemic toxicity remains a problem in clinical practice. Risk factors include:

- proximal injection site (e.g. intercostal, head and neck or upper limb blocks);
- surgical use of high drug volumes for procedures such as tissue infiltration and tumescent anaesthesia;
- use of high-concentration compound local anaesthetic mixtures;
- inappropriate use of medical devices; and
- administration at greater than the recommended dose.

For example, the incidence of convulsions has been estimated at 1 in 130 after supraclavicular and interscalene block, 1 in 827 after axillary block and 1 in 8435 after epidural anaesthesia. Tumescent anaesthesia for liposuction using doses of lidocaine > 50 mg kg^{-1} has been associated with a mortality rate between 1 in 5000 and 1 in 10,000. Deaths have also been reported after application of 6%–10% lidocaine and tetracaine compound local anaesthetic cream with cellophane wrapping to the legs before laser hair removal. Inadvertent, fatal intravascular injection of local anaesthetics (e.g. unintentional connection of epidural infusions to intravenous lines) has also been reported.

Prevention of severe local anaesthetic toxicity

Regional blocks should always be performed in an area equipped to deal with cardiorespiratory collapse, such as an anaesthetic room or block room within the theatre suite.

Doses should be adjusted according to the patient's age, weight and physical condition.

Syringes of local anaesthetics and perineural and epidural infusions should be labelled clearly. Use of premixed sterile solutions is encouraged.

Gentle aspiration of the syringe should precede every injection, but anaesthetists should be aware that negative aspiration for blood does not guarantee extravascular positioning of the needle tip.

Verbal contact with the patient must be maintained both during and after drug administration.

An appropriate test dose should be given depending on the situation. For example, a test dose of 3 ml epidural bupivacaine 0.5% (15 mg) injected accidentally into the intrathecal space will provide a definitive outcome – spinal anaesthesia. Injection of 0.5–1 ml during an ultrasound-guided perineural block is usually sufficient to differentiate between intraneural and extraneural injection.

Examples of alternative epidural test doses are 3–5 ml lidocaine 2% or adrenaline 15–25 mcg, but neither test is specific or sensitive for non-epidural injection.

Ultrasound allows visualisation of the position of the needle or catheter, their relationship to other structures – both nerves and large blood vessels – and the spread of local anaesthetic solution.

Management of severe local anaesthetic toxicity

Treatment of severe systemic toxicity from local anaesthetics is detailed in Chapter 27.

Chapter | 6 |

Physiology and pharmacology of pain

Lesley Colvin

The International Association for the Study of Pain (IASP) defines pain as 'an unpleasant sensory and emotional experience associated with actual or potential tissue damage or described in terms of such damage'. It is clear from this definition that the degree of tissue damage and perception of pain are not necessarily correlated.

Pain perception is a complex phenomenon, involving sensory, emotional and cognitive processes. Thus, although analgesic drugs can be effective in relieving both acute and chronic pain, other factors may also need to be addressed. Modulating patient expectation can have a major effect on perceived pain, reflecting the importance of communication and explanation for both acute and chronic pain management.

Mechanisms of pain

To manage pain effectively, it is important to have a good understanding of the underlying pain pathways and how these may be modulated at different concentrations by analgesic agents. Melzack and Wall, in their gate control theory of pain, introduced the concept in the 1960s that there was the potential for modulation of pain and nociception on many levels. This moved away from the Descartian philosophy that pain was a sensation transmitted from the periphery to central areas in the brain. High threshold nociceptors (non-specialised bare nerve endings) are activated by a noxious stimulus, with subsequent generation of action potentials. These are transmitted along nerve fibres (primary afferent neurons), predominantly unmyelinated C fibres and small myelinated Aδ fibres (Table 6.1 and Fig. 6.1). The nerve cell bodies are located in the dorsal root ganglia (sympathetic neuronal cell bodies are also found here), where the sensory nerve fibres enter the dorsal aspect of the spinal cord. The first central synapses of sensory neurons

are found in Rexed's laminae (I–X), with their exact location being dependent on nerve fibre type. The substantia gelatinosa (comprising mainly laminae II) and lamina V are where nociceptive inputs are normally processed. The majority of second-order projection neurons cross to form the lateral spinothalamic tract, with a smaller number of fibres ascending on the side of origin. The neurobiology of the pain pathway (Fig. 6.2) changes in response to tissue injury and also in response to treatment. For example, if an individual is taking opioids long term, his or her responses to pain and analgesics will be modified. This is at least partly because of alterations in pain pathway neurobiology: the neurotransmitters released and their target receptors may both change (Table 6.2). Furthermore, the surrounding milieu is important, particularly the peripheral and central immune responses to inflammation (see below).

Central sensitisation may occur; this is amplification of peripheral input caused by glutamate activating the N-methyl-D-aspartate (NMDA) receptor (a non-selective cation channel that is normally blocked by a Mg^{2+} ion) in a voltage-dependent manner (Fig. 6.3). With increased and repeated noxious stimulation, more glutamate is released from primary sensory neurons. This results in increases in postsynaptic effects, including unblocking of the NMDA receptor (see Chapter 4). This can occur rapidly and is seen in many different pain states. Activation of the NMDA receptor triggers a number of downstream events within the postsynaptic neuron. There is the potential for developing novel analgesics that target specific parts of this pathway (see Table 6.2).

Inflammation

The classical combination of *rubor* (redness), *calor* (heat), *tumor* (swelling) and *dolor* (pain) may occur in response to tissue injury or as part of a more general inflammatory process (e.g. inflammatory arthropathies such as rheumatoid

Table 6.1 Classification of nerve fibres

Fibre type	Conduction velocity (ms⁻¹)	Diameter (μm)	Function
Large, myelinated			
Aα	70–120	12–20	Proprioception, motor
Aβ	30–70	5–12	Light touch, pressure
Aγ	15–30	3–6	Motor to muscle spindles
Small, myelinated			
Aδ	12–30	2–5	Pain ('first' pain, e.g. pin prick), cold, touch
B	3–15	<3	Preganglionic autonomic
Unmyelinated			
C	0.5–2	0.4–1.3	Pain: 'second' pain (e.g. slow, burning), temperature, postganglionic sympathetic fibres

Data from Erlanger J & Gasser HS. Electrical Signs of Nervous Activity. Philadelphia, 1937; From Colvin L.A., and Fallon M.T., Pain physiology in anaesthetic practice, In Hardman J.G., et al. Oxford Textbook of Anaesthesia, 2017.

arthritis). Peripheral changes occur with the release of a host of proinflammatory mediators including cytokines and chemokines, leading to peripheral sensitisation, where there is a decrease in nociceptor activation threshold and increased primary afferent drive. Fig. 6.4 outlines some of the peripheral processes involved in inflammatory pain. More recently, the importance of CNS changes has been emerging, with central inflammatory processes modulating pain neurobiology. Alterations in number, size and function of both astrocytes and microglial cells have been found, which may contribute to the development and maintenance of chronic pain syndromes.

Neuropathic pain

If nerve injury occurs, neuropathic pain may result, with characteristic changes in neurotransmitters and receptors, alterations in electrical activity and a shift to a hyperexcitable state. These include the following:

- Changes in Na⁺ channel subtypes in the peripheral nervous system, with spontaneous generation of action potentials in the absence of noxious stimulation. This may be the mechanism of the spontaneous pain often found in neuropathic pain syndromes.
- Alterations in the balance between the descending inhibitory pathways and pronociceptive pathways, with amplification of pain signals from the spinal cord.
- Alterations in the balance of neurotransmitters – for example, downregulation of substance P and calcitonin gene–related peptide (CRGP) and increases in dynorphin.

Visceral pain

Whereas somatic pain usually follows a fairly precise somatotopic map, visceral pain is much more diffuse. Visceral hyperalgesia can develop in chronic pain states such as chronic pancreatitis and irritable bowel syndrome. As with somatic pain, there are many points along the pain pathway between periphery and the brain where changes can occur in sensory processing alongside modulation from inflammatory mediators, particularly in the gut mucosa and immune system. Neuroimaging studies in patients with chronic visceral pain from irritable bowel syndrome have shown increased activity in brain areas involved in affective and cognitive processing, such as the dorsolateral and ventrolateral prefrontal cortices.

Pharmacology of analgesic drugs

The ideal analgesic drug should relieve pain with minimal adverse effects. However, patients continue to suffer pain despite the wide range of analgesics available. When devising a management plan for both acute and chronic settings, it may be helpful to use *balanced* or *multimodal analgesia*. These terms refer to the use of combinations of drugs acting by different mechanisms or at different sites within the pain pathway. Analgesic combinations may have additive or synergistic actions. This allows reductions in dose and adverse effects. Effective and repeated assessment is essential in determining optimal analgesic management (Table 6.3).

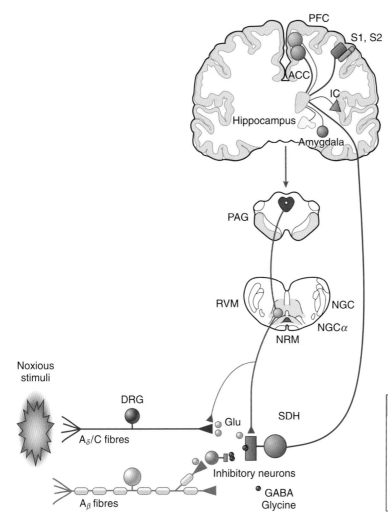

Cortical process of pain

ACC, IC: two major cortical regions responding to physiological pain, critical for pain perception and unpleasantness
S1, S2: important for pain transmission, information about pain modality, location
PFC: is also activated by pain

Other related structures

Hippocampus: pain-related spatial memory and mood disorders
Amygdala: pain-related fear, anxiety and pain modulation

Endogenous biphasic modulation

PAG: midbrain analgesic neurons
RVM: exert biphasic descending modulation of spinal pain transmission. It contains NGC, NGCα, NRM and other raphe nuclei

Spinal dorsal horn

First central pain synapse in the CNS
Local gating control of pain and descending biphasic modulation; biphasic modulation is mediated by multiple transmitters
Descending modulation may act by presynaptic and postsynaptic mechanisms

Fig. 6.1 An outline of peripheral to central pain pathways. *ACC,* Anterior cingulate gyrus; *DRG,* dorsal root ganglion; *GABA,* gamma-aminobutyric acid; *IC,* insular cortex; *NGC,* nucleus gigantocellularis; *NRM,* nucleus raphe magnus; *PAG,* periaqueductal grey matter; *PFC,* prefrontal cortex; *RVM,* rostral ventromedial medulla; *S1,* primary somatosensory cortex; *S2,* secondary somatosensory cortex; *SDH,* spinal dorsal horn. (From Zhuo, M. (2008) Cortical excitation and chronic pain. *Trends in Neurosciences.* 31 (4), 199–207.)

Opioids

Opioids are the most commonly used analgesics for the treatment of moderate to severe pain. Despite this, there are still major gaps in our knowledge of their clinical pharmacology; the choice of drug and dose is largely empirical. Although they may be highly effective, control of dynamic (pain on movement) or incident (breakthrough) pain may be poor and side effects a significant problem. The term *opioid* refers

to all drugs, both synthetic and natural, that act on opioid receptors. Opiates are naturally occurring opioids derived from the opium poppy *papaver somniferum.* A variety of different opioids are available, but morphine is the most widely used. Incomplete cross-tolerance occurs between opioids, so an alternative should be tried if morphine is poorly tolerated. There is increasing evidence that individual analgesic response and adverse effect profile are both partly related to genetic make-up. Differences in single nucleotide polymorphisms (SNPs) almost certainly contribute to this variability in response between different opioids, with

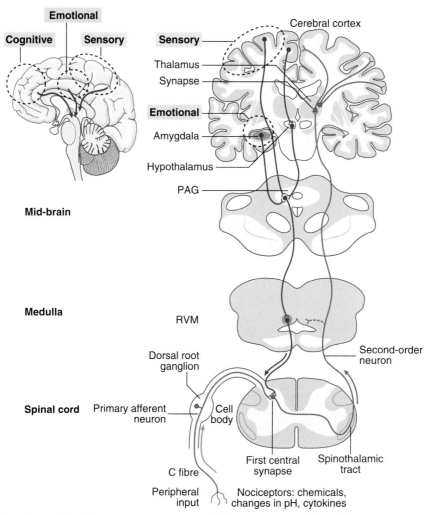

Fig. 6.2 Basic pain pathway. *PAG*, Periaqueductal grey matter; *RVM*, rostroventral medulla. (With permission from Ralston, S., Penman, I., Strachan, M., & Hobson, R. (eds.) (2018) *Davidson's Principles and Practice of Medicine.* 23rd ed. London, Elsevier.)

potential candidate genes including *ABCB1* (encoding p-glycoprotein, a membrane transporter), *STAT6* (signal transducer and activator of transcription 6) and β-arrestin (intracellular protein involved in receptor internalisation).

Dose conversion between different opioids is an inexact science; suggested equianalgesic doses (Table 6.4) are based on relative potencies, often derived from studies not designed for dose equivalence calculations.

Mechanism of action

Opioid receptors belong to the G protein–coupled family of receptors that have seven transmembrane domains, an extracellular N-terminal and an intracellular C-terminal.

Activation results in changes in enzyme activity such as adenylate cyclase or alterations in calcium and potassium ion channel permeability (see also Chapter 1).

Opioid receptors were originally classified by pharmacological activity in animal preparations and later by molecular sequence. The three main receptors were classified as μ (mu), or OP3; κ (kappa), or OP1; and δ (delta), or OP2. More recently, an opioid-like receptor, the NOP (or nociceptin/orphanin FQ) receptor, has been identified. Receptor nomenclature has changed several times in the last few years; the current International Union of Pharmacology (IUPHAR) classifications are MOP (μ), KOP (κ), DOP (δ) and NOP (nociceptin/orphanin FQ peptide) receptors (Table 6.5).

Table 6.2 Some of the neurotransmitters and receptors important in nociceptive processing, with changes in particular pain states

Neurotransmitter/agonist	Receptor	Comments
Amino acids		
Glutamate	AMPA	Excitatory; fast synaptic transmission; permeable to cations such as Ca^{2+} and Na^+.
	NMDA	Excitatory; normally blocked at resting membrane potential by Mg^{2+}. Activated by repeated high-intensity stimulation; involved in central sensitisation and wind-up; permeable to cations such as Ca^{2+} and Na^+.
	Metabotropic	Depending on site, may be excitatory or inhibitory. Linked to G proteins; at least three different groups (mGLuRI–III) may decrease glutamate release.
Glycine		Inhibitory.
GABA		Inhibitory.
Neuropeptides		
Substance P	Neurokinin	One of the first neuropeptides shown to be involved in nociceptive processing; NK antagonists had limited analgesic effect in clinical trials; some antiemetic activity; G protein–coupled receptor; increases in inflammatory conditions; decreases in nerve injury.
CGRP		Inhibits SP breakdown and thus prolongs its duration of action; increases in inflammatory conditions; decreases in nerve injury.
CCK	CCKRs1–8	Excitatory; clinical trials of antagonists.
Thermal sensation and pain		
Heat >42°C, capsaicin	TRPV1	Activated by noxious heat; topical capsaicin (low-dose cream or high-dose patch) used in chronic pain (cream: osteoarthritis; patch: neuropathic pain); selectively desensitises subset of C fibres expressing TRPV1 receptor.
Cool (8°C–28°C), menthol (in low concentrations)	TRPM8	Activated by non-noxious cold (cooling); increased expression of receptor in chronic pain; analgesic effect by receptor activation.

AMPA, α-Amino-3-hydroxy-5-methylisoxazole-4-propionic acid; *CCK*, cholecystokinin; *CGRP*, calcitonin gene–related peptide; *GABA*, γ-aminobutyric acid; *M*, melastatin; *NK*, neurokinin; *NMDA*, N-methyl-D-aspartate; *SP*, substance P; *TRP*, transient receptor potential; *V*, vanilloid.

Opioid receptors are distributed widely in both central and peripheral nervous systems, and this explains their widespread effects, both therapeutic and adverse. Complex interactions at various receptors underlie the different effects of currently available opioids. Several endogenous neuropeptide ligands are active at opioid receptors (see Table 6.5); they function as neurotransmitters, neuromodulators and neurohormones. The endogenous tetrapeptides endomorphins 1 and 2 are potent agonists acting specifically at the MOP receptor; they play a role in modulating inflammatory pain.

The analgesic action of morphine and most other opioids is related mainly to agonist activity at the MOP receptor. Unfortunately, many of the unwanted effects of opioids are also related to MOP agonism. At a cellular level, MOP receptor activation has an overall inhibitory effect via (1) inhibition of adenylate cyclase; (2) increased opening of potassium channels (hyperpolarisation of postsynaptic neurons, reduced synaptic transmission); and (3) inhibition of calcium channels (decreases presynaptic neurotransmitter release).

Some opioids or their metabolites also have activity at other receptors; for example, methadone acts at the NMDA

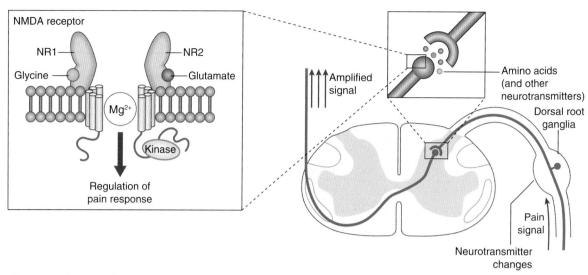

Fig. 6.3 Mechanisms of central sensitisation. *NMDA, N*-methyl-D-aspartate; *NR,* NMDA receptor (subunits). (With permission from Ralston, S., Penman, I., Strachan, M., & Hobson, R. (eds.) (2018) *Davidson's Principles and Practice of Medicine.* 23rd ed. London, Elsevier.)

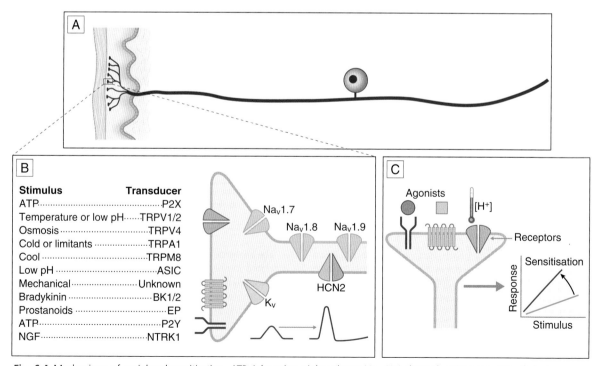

Fig. 6.4 Mechanisms of peripheral sensitisation. *ATP,* Adenosine triphosphate; *Na$_v$,* Na$^+$ channel; *NGF,* nerve growth factor. (With permission from Ralston, S., Penman, I., Strachan, M., & Hobson, R. (eds.) (2018) *Davidson's Principles and Practice of Medicine.* 23rd ed. London, Elsevier.)

Table 6.3 Approach to multimodal analgesia

Analgesic	Mode of action	Use in acute pain	Use in chronic pain	Comments
Paracetamol	Poorly understood; COX inhibition?	Yes – oral, rectal or intravenous.	Yes – reduce dose in frail elderly.	May be synergistic with some other analgesics (e.g. codeine); antipyretic.
NSAIDs	Reduce inflammatory response.	Yes.	Caution with long-term use, particularly for adverse cardiovascular side effects.	COX-2 selective drugs may have better GI profile; all can impact on renal function, especially if fluid depleted.
Opioids	Main analgesic action is via μ-opioid receptor, with inhibitory effects at spinal and supraspinal levels.	Yes – often by parenteral route if oral not available.	Very limited evidence of long-term efficacy, with increasing concerns about harms.	Harms from long-term use include addiction, tolerance, misuse, endocrine dysfunction, increased fracture risk. Major increase in prescribing for chronic pain over last 10–20 years.
Local anaesthetics	Interrupt neuronal transmission via Na^+ channel block.	Yes – very useful for perioperative pain control, with opioid-sparing effect; some evidence for intravenous use, although potential safety issues from toxicity.	Specific interventions, to allow peripheral and regional nerve blocks.	Via neuraxial route; can be useful in the management of cancer pain (especially movement-related pain).
Adjuvants/ antineuropathic agents	Depends on agent (e.g. TCAs): likely to increase descending inhibition; gabapentinoids reduce excitatory synaptic activity, probably via reduced release of glutamate.	Gabapentinoids – variable evidence from systematic reviews of efficacy as an opioid-sparing technique.	Yes – for neuropathic pain.	CNS effects often additive with opioids. Need dose titration to effect, with onset of analgesia consequently taking a number of weeks.

receptor. These particular actions are discussed for individual agents later in this chapter. The more general effects of opioids are described in this section.

Analgesic action

MOP, and to a lesser extent KOP, receptor agonists produce analgesic effects, as does activation of spinal DOP receptors in certain situations. Opioids should be titrated against pain; if higher than necessary doses are given, respiratory depression and excessive sedation may result. If the pain is incompletely opioid responsive, as may occur with neuropathic pain, care must be taken with dose titration, and a detailed reassessment of analgesic response is essential. Opioids exert their analgesic effect by:

- supraspinal effects in the brainstem, thalamus and cortex, in addition to modulating descending systems in the midbrain periaqueductal grey matter, nucleus raphe magnus and the rostral ventral medulla;
- inhibitory effects within the dorsal horn of the spinal cord both pre- and postsynaptically; and
- a peripheral action in inflammatory states: MOP receptors modulate immune function, and nociceptors are important in regulating peripheral sensitisation.

Central nervous system

Opioids have much wider ranging effects than simply analgesia. These include effects on the CNS, cardiovascular, GI, endocrine and immune systems (Table 6.6).

Opioid structure

The structures of opioid analgesics are diverse (Figs 6.5 and 6.6), although for most opioids the active compound is usually the laevorotatory *(laevo)* stereoisomer. Agents in current use include phenanthrenes (e.g. morphine), phenylpiperidines (e.g. meperidine [pethidine], fentanyl) and diphenylpropylamines (e.g. methadone). Structural modification affects agonist activity and alters physicochemical properties such as lipid solubility. A tertiary nitrogen is necessary for activity, separated from a quaternary carbon by an ethylene chain. Chemical modifications that produce a quaternary nitrogen significantly reduce potency as a result of decreased CNS penetration. If the methyl group on the nitrogen is changed, antagonism of analgesia may be produced.

Other important positions for activity and metabolism include the C-3 phenol group (the distance of this from the nitrogen affects activity) and the C-6 alcohol group. With regard to morphine, potency may be increased by hydroxylation of the C-3 phenol; oxidation of C-6 (e.g. hydromorphone); double acetylation at C-3 and C-6 (e.g. diamorphine); hydroxylation of C-14 and reducing the double bond at C-7/8. Further additions at the C-3 OH group reduce activity. A short-chain alkyl substitution is found in mixed agonist-antagonists, and hydroxylation or bromination of C-14 produces full antagonists, and removal or substitution of the methyl group reduces agonist activity.

Pharmacokinetics and physicochemical properties

Knowledge of the specific physicochemical properties and pharmacokinetics of individual agents is important in determining the optimal route of drug delivery. This is needed to achieve an effective receptor site concentration for an appropriate duration of action. All opioids are weak bases. The relative proportion of free and ionised fractions depends on plasma pH and the pKa of the particular opioid. The amount of opioid diffusing to the site of action (diffusible fraction) is dependent on lipid solubility, concentration gradient and degree of binding (see Chapter 1). Plasma concentrations of albumin and α_1-acid glycoprotein as well as tissue binding determine the availability of the unbound, unionised fraction. This diffusible fraction moves into tissue sites in the brain and elsewhere; the amount reaching

Table 6.4 Suggested equi-analgesic doses for opioids

| Opioid | ~ EQUI-ANALGESIC DOSE | |
	Parenteral	Oral
Morphine	10 mg	30 mg
Meperidine (pethidine)	100 mg	300 mg
Oxycodone	15 mg	20 mg
Fentanyl	100 μg	NA
Hydromorphone	1.5 mg	7.5 mg
Methadone	1–10 mg	10 mg (use with caution)
Codeine	N/A	200 mg

This is a guide only, and careful assessment of individual factors must be considered when transferring between opioids, particularly at higher doses. Methadone may be particularly problematic, because of its long half-life and inter-individual variability. *N/A*, Not applicable.

Table 6.5 Classification of opioid receptors as defined by the International Union of Pharmacology

Receptor	Previous classifications	Endogenous ligand	Site
MOP	Mu (μ); OP3	Endomorphin 1 and 2; met-enkephalin	Pre- and postsynaptic neurons in spinal cord, periaqueduct grey matter, limbic system, caudate putamen, thalamus, cerebral cortex; peripheral inflammation.
KOP	Kappa (κ); OP2	Dynorphin A and B; β-endorphin	Cerebral cortex, nucleus accumbens, nucleus raphe magnus (midbrain), hypothalamus, spinal cord.
DOP	Delta (δ); OP1	Leu- and met-enkephalins; β-endorphin	Olfactory centres, cerebral cortex, nucleus accumbens, caudate putamen, spinal cord, some limited distribution in areas involved in nociception.
NOP	Nociceptin/orphanin FQ; ORL-1	Nociceptin/orphanin FQ (nociceptin)	Nucleus raphe magnus, spinal cord, afferent neurons, peripheral immune cells.

Table 6.6 Non-analgesic effects of opioids

Effect	Comment
Sedation	Additive with other CNS depressant drugs. There is a dose-related reduction in minimum alveolar concentration (MAC) for volatile anaesthetics, though there is a floor to this effect. Opioids alone do not act as reliable anaesthetic agents.
Sleep	Interfere with rapid-eye-movement sleep with EEG changes (includes progressive decrease in EEG frequency; production of δ waves; burst suppression is *not* seen, even with large doses).
Mood	Significant euphoria is uncommon when used to treat pain. Dysphoria (possibly via a KOP receptor action) and hallucinations (often visual) can occur.
Miosis	KOP receptor effect on the Edinger–Westphal nucleus of the oculomotor nerve.
Tolerance (increasing doses to achieve the same effect)	Can occur acutely or chronically. At a cellular level, there is a progressive loss of active receptor sites combined with uncoupling of the receptor from the guanosine triphosphate (GTP)–binding subunit. NMDA receptor and intracellular second messenger systems are also involved, with a rationale for use of ketamine in acute tolerance.
Physical dependence	NOT addiction; physical symptoms occur with opioids cessation or in the case of precipitated withdrawal by administering an opioid antagonist. Includes anxiety, myalgia, hydrosis, GI upset.
Addiction	Craving for continued use, despite evidence of harm. Complex mechanisms, possibly involving the reward systems.
Opioid-induced hyperalgesia	This is a paradoxical response where an increase in opioid dose results in hyperalgesia. It may be part of the spectrum of opioid toxicity or can occur in isolation. It has been found to occur after systemic administration of potent short-acting opioids such as remifentanil but can occur with any opioid.
Respiratory depression	Particularly occurs in the elderly, neonates and when given without titrating effect to analgesic response; less problematic in chronic use (tolerance). Increased risk if nociceptive input is reduced or removed, such as after a nerve block. Sensitivity to CO_2 is reduced (MOP effect) via depression of neuronal sensitivity (ventral medulla).
Airway/cough reflex	Suppress stress response to laryngoscopy and airway manipulation; suppress cough activity and mucociliary function. This may cause inadequate clearing of secretions and hypostatic pneumonia.
Gastrointestinal	Nausea and vomiting (may be mediated both centrally and peripherally: direct effect on the chemoreceptor trigger zone; delay in gastric emptying). Increased gastrointestinal muscle tone and decreased motility. Constipation common (direct action on opioid receptors in gut smooth muscle); increase in biliary pressure with gallbladder contraction.
Cardiovascular	Some opioids are associated with bradycardia. If normovolaemic, no significant cardiovascular depressant effect, unless histamine release occurs. There is no direct effect on cerebral autoregulation, although an increase in $PaCO_2$ from respiratory depression may increase cerebral blood flow. Opioids decrease central sympathetic outflow, which can manifest as haemodynamic compromise, especially with rapid intravenous bolus. QTc prolongation with some opioids (e.g. methadone). Increased risk of myocardial infarction with long-term use.
Fracture	Increased risk with long-term use, especially in elderly patients taking high doses.
Endocrine	Central action via hypothalamic pituitary axis; adrenal insufficiency; sexual dysfunction, infertility can all occur with long-term use.
Immune system	Exact effects are unclear, but may impair immune response with long-term use; limited evidence for effects on cancer cells.

Continued

Table 6.6 Non-analgesic effects of opioids—cont'd

Effect	Comment
Other	Myoclonic jerks can occur, especially with opioid toxicity. Urinary retention is possible. Pruritus is common after neuraxial administration; low-dose MOP antagonist may help. Muscle rigidity, especially after intravenous bolus administration of potent phenylpiperidines, may cause significant problems with ventilation because of chest wall rigidity and decreased respiratory compliance. May be minimised by coadministration of opioids with intravenous anaesthetic agents and benzodiazepines, reversed by naloxone or prevented by neuromuscular blocking agents. Thermoregulation impaired, similar to volatile agents.

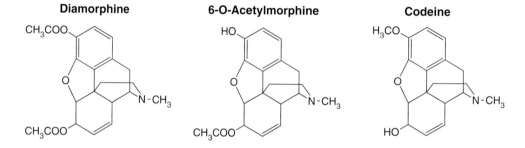

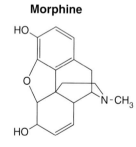

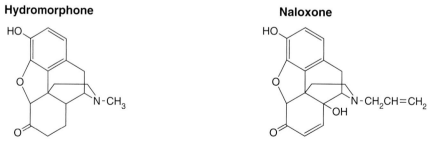

Fig. 6.5 The structures of morphine and the phenanthrenes.

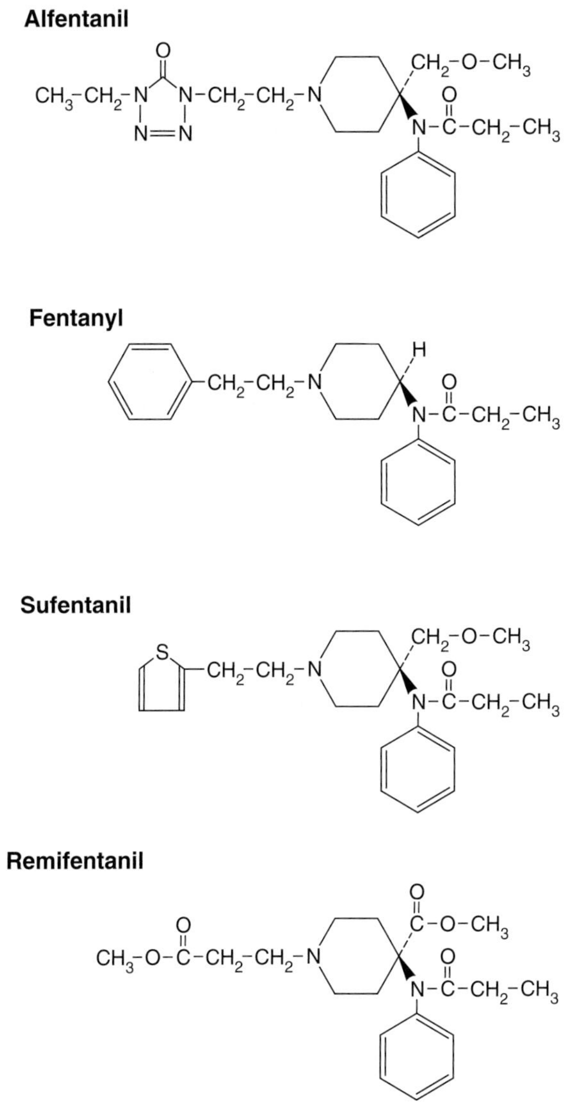

Alfentanil

Fentanyl

Sufentanil

Remifentanil

Fig. 6.6 The structures of phenylpiperidine opioids.

receptors is dependent not only on lipophilicity but also on the amount of non-specific tissue binding, such as CNS lipids.

The ionised, protonated form is active at the receptor site. This has important implications for speed and duration of activity. For example, morphine is relatively hydrophilic and penetrates the blood–brain barrier slowly. However, a large mass of any given dose eventually reaches the receptor site because of low concentrations of non-specific tissue binding. The offset time may be prolonged, resulting in a longer duration of action than would be expected from the plasma half-life.

Most opioids have a very steep dose–response curve. Therefore if the dose is near the minimum effective analgesic concentration (MEAC), very small fluctuations in plasma or effect-site concentrations may lead to large changes in analgesia.

Opioids tend to have a large volume of distribution (V_D) because of their high lipid solubility. A consequence of this can be that redistribution, particularly after a bolus dose or short infusion, can have significant effects on plasma concentrations. In addition, first-pass effects in the lungs may remove significant amounts of drug from the circulation, reducing the initial peak plasma concentration. However, the drug re-enters the plasma several minutes later. Plasma concentrations of opioids such as fentanyl, sufentanil and meperidine are affected by this; the effect is negligible for remifentanil. Other lipophilic amines such as lidocaine and propranolol are affected similarly and may reduce pulmonary uptake of coadministered opioids.

After prolonged infusion, significant sequestration in fat stores and other body tissues occurs for highly lipid-soluble opioids. Context-sensitive half-life (see Chapter 1) is increased after prolonged infusion for most opioids apart from remifentanil. For example, the elimination $t_{1/2}$ for fentanyl after bolus administration is 3–5 h but increases markedly after repeated boluses or prolonged infusion.

Most opioid metabolism occurs in the liver (phase 1 and 2 reactions) with the hydrophilic metabolites predominantly excreted via the kidneys, although a small amount may be excreted in the bile or unchanged in the urine. As a result, hepatic blood flow is one of the major determinants of plasma clearance. Enterohepatic recirculation may occur when water-soluble metabolites excreted in the gut may be metabolised by gut flora to the parent opioid and then reabsorbed. Lipid-soluble opioids may diffuse into the stomach, become ionised because of the low pH and then be reabsorbed in the small intestine; this results in a secondary peak in plasma concentration.

Details of the pharmacological properties of some opioids are shown in Tables 6.7 and 6.8. Metabolism (including production of active metabolites), distribution between tissues and elimination can all differ between individuals (see Chapter 1) to produce clinically important variations in effect.

Factors affecting pharmacokinetics of opioids include the following:

- *Age.* Dose is often calculated on body weight, although there is little evidence to support this in adult clinical practice. Age is often more important because of both pharmacokinetic and pharmacodynamic factors. Metabolism and volume of distribution are reduced in the elderly, leading to increased free drug concentrations in the plasma. Hepatic blood flow may have declined by 40%–50% by age 75 years, with reduced clearance of opioids. Increased CNS sensitivity to opioid effects also occurs in the elderly.

109

Table 6.7 Metabolism and excretion of some opioids

Drug	Metabolism	Excretion
Naturally occurring opioids		
Morphine	Liver: glucuronidation, sulphation N-dealkylation; also microsomal UDP glucuronyl transferases (UDPGT) in liver, kidney and intestine; some active metabolites	Mainly urine; 90% in 24 h (10% morphine; 70% glucuronides; 10% 3-sulphate; 1% normorphine; 3% normorphine glucuronide)
Codeine	Liver: O-demethylation, glucuronidation; some active metabolites	Mainly urine; 86% in 24 h (5%–10% codeine; 60% codeine glucuronide; 5%–15% morphine (mainly conjugated); trace normorphine)
Semisynthetic		
Diamorphine	Liver: O-deacetylation, glucuronidation; some active metabolites	Mainly urine; 80% in 24 h (5%–7% morphine; 90% morphine glucuronides; 1% 6-acetylmorphine; 0.1% diamorphine)
Oxycodone	Liver; CYP3A4, CYP2D6 (phase 1 metabolism); glucuronidation	Mainly urine; noroxycodone is weaker metabolite
Hydromorphone	Liver: no phase 1 metabolism; glucuronidation; active metabolite: hydromorphone-3-glucoronide	Some active metabolites excreted in urine (HM-3-glucuronide), dose adjustment recommended in renal impairment
Buprenorphine	Liver: glucuronidation, N-dealkylation	70% mainly unchanged in faeces; 2%–13% in 7 days; mainly N-dealkylbuprenorphine (and glucuronide); buprenorphine-3-glucuronide
Synthetic opioids		
Meperidine (pethidine)	Liver: N-demethylation, hydrolysis	70% in 24 h (10% meperidine; 10% normeperidine; 20% meperidinic acid; 16% meperidinic acid glucuronide; 8% normeperidinic acid; 10% normeperidinic acid glucuronide; plus small amounts of other metabolites)
Fentanyl	Liver: N-dealkylation, hydroxylation; no phase 2 metabolism	9% excreted in faeces; rest in urine: 70% in 4 days (5%–25% fentanyl; 50% 4-N-(N-propionylanilino-piperidine) plus other metabolites); very little excreted unchanged in urine
Alfentanil	Mainly hepatic metabolism (phase 1: CYP3A4), inactive metabolites	Very little excreted unchanged in urine
Sufentanil	Mainly hepatic metabolism phase 1 (including CYP3A4), some active metabolites	Very little excreted unchanged in urine
Remifentanil	Plasma: rapid hydrolysis – plasma and tissue non-specific esterases; non-saturable, clearance greater than hepatic blood flow; *not* affected by plasma cholinesterase deficiency or hepatic or renal dysfunction	Remifentanil acid – main metabolite, excreted in urine, no clinically significant activity
Methadone	Liver: N-dealkylation, no active metabolites	30% excreted in faeces; 60% in 24 h (33% methadone; 43% EDDP; 10% EMDP plus small amounts of other metabolites)

Table 6.7 Metabolism and excretion of some opioids—cont'd

Drug	Metabolism	Excretion
Tapentadol	Liver: via glucuronidation (main route)	1% unchanged in faeces; majority excreted in urine (3% unchanged, remainder conjugates and other metabolites)
Tramadol	Liver: phase 1(CYP3A4, CYP2D6) to active drug, O-desmethyltramadol, plus inactive metabolite, nortramadol; no phase 2 metabolism	~30% of dose excreted unchanged in urine; metabolites excreted in urine, dose adjustment in renal impairment

EDDP, 2-ethylidene-1,5-dimethyl-3,3-diphenylpyrrolidine; *EMDP*, 2-ethyl-5-methyl-3,3-diphenylpyrroline.

Table 6.8 Pharmacokinetics and physicochemical properties of some opioids

Opioid	pKa	Protein binding (%)	Octanol:water partition coefficient	Terminal half-life (h)	Clearance (ml kg^{-1} min^{-1})	Volume of distribution (L kg^{-1})	Duration of action (h)
Morphine	7.9	30	6	1.7–3.0	15–20	3–5	3–5
Oxycodone	8.5	45		3–4	13	2–3	2–4
Codeine	8.2	20	0.6	2–4		2.5–3.5	
Meperidine (pethidine)	8.5	70	39	3–5	8–18	3–5	2–4
Fentanyl	8.4	90	813	2–4	10–20	3–5	1–1.5
Alfentanil	6.5	91	128	1–2	4–9	0.4–1	0.25–0.4
Remifentanil	7.3	70	18	0.1–0.2	40–60	0.3–0.4	2–5 min
Sufentanil	8.0	93	1778	2–3.5	10–15	2.5–3	0.8–1.3
Methadone	8.3	90	26–57	15–20	2	5	4–8

- *Hepatic disease* has unpredictable effects, although there may be little clinical difference unless there is coexisting encephalopathy. Reductions in plasma protein concentrations increase the plasma concentrations of free unbound drug.
- *Renal failure* may have significant effects for opioids with active metabolites excreted by the kidney, such as morphine, diamorphine and meperidine.
- *Obesity* results in a larger V_D and prolonged elimination $t_{1/2}$. This may be a particular problem if infusions are used.
- *Hypothermia, hypotension and hypovolaemia* may also result in variable absorption, altered distribution and metabolism.

Routes of administration

Peak plasma concentrations may be affected by site of administration and haemodynamic status. Opioids may be given by many routes; variations between specific agents are discussed later. It is unclear how much cross-tolerance exists for different routes of administration, such as intravenous versus epidural.

The choice of route depends on the clinical situation, and several factors should be considered:

- If GI transit time is delayed, the biological half-life of agents administered orally may be prolonged. Similarly, if GI transit time is rapid or area for absorption reduced, then drug absorption may decrease, particularly with long-acting agents.
- Intrathecal administration is associated with fewer supraspinal effects, although both urinary retention and pruritus may be more common. Highly lipid-soluble opioids (e.g. fentanyl) do not spread readily in CSF. It is claimed that they are less likely than water-soluble opioids (e.g. morphine) to cause late respiratory depression because of rostral spread.
- Dural penetration from epidural administration is dependent on molecular size and lipophilicity For example, only 3%–5% of morphine crosses into the CSF,

with a peak concentration after 60–240 min; fentanyl peaks at approximately 20 min.

MOP agonists

Morphine is the standard opioid against which other agents are compared. Other MOP agonists have a similar pharmacodynamic profile but differ in relative potency, pharmacokinetics and biotransformation to other active metabolites.

Phenylpiperidine opioids (see Fig. 6.6) are potent MOP receptor agonists with moderate (alfentanil) to high (sufentanil) lipid solubility and good diffusion through membranes. Both potency and time to reach the effect site vary considerably. In contrast to morphine, these agents do not cause histamine release. All except remifentanil may cause postoperative respiratory depression as a result of secondary peaks in plasma concentrations. This may be caused by release from body stores if large doses have been infused intraoperatively.

Morphine

Morphine is a relatively hydrophilic phenanthrene derivative. It may be given orally (immediate or modified release), rectally, topically, parenterally and via the neuraxial route. The standard parenteral dose for adults is 10 mg, although many factors affect this and the dose should be titrated to effect. Its oral bioavailability is dependent on first-pass hepatic metabolism and may be unpredictable (35%–75%). Single-dose studies of morphine bioavailability indicate that the relative potency of oral to intramuscular morphine is 1:6, although with repeated regular administration, this ratio becomes approximately 1:3. The dose of short-acting morphine for breakthrough pain should be approximately one-sixth of the total daily dose. Morphine has a plasma half-life of approximately 3 h and duration of analgesia of 4–6 h.

Morphine is metabolised, at least in part, by microsomal UDP glucuronyl transferases (UDPGT) in the liver, kidney and intestines. Several of these metabolites may have clinically significant effects (see later). Although morphine conjugation occurs in the liver, extrahepatic sites may also be important, such as the kidney and GI tract. The site of conjugation on the molecule also varies, leading to a variety of metabolites (see Table 6.7). After glucuronidation, metabolites are excreted in urine or bile, dependent on molecular weight and polarity; more than 90% of morphine metabolites are excreted in the urine. The main metabolite in humans is morphine-3-glucuronide (60%–80%), and this may have an excitatory effect via CNS actions not related to opioid receptor activation. Morphine-6-glucuronide (M-6-G) is active at the MOP receptor, producing analgesia and other MOP-related effects. It is significantly more potent than morphine. Therefore M-6-G produces significant clinical effects despite only 10% of morphine being metabolised in this way. As it is excreted via the kidneys, it may accumulate in patients with impaired renal function, causing respiratory depression. Accumulation of morphine metabolites, especially M-6-G, may become significant when creatinine clearance declines to 50 ml min^{-1} or less.

Codeine

Codeine is a constituent of opium. Up to 10% of a dose of codeine is metabolised by the hepatic microsomal enzyme CYP2D6 to morphine, which contributes significantly to its analgesic effect. The rest is metabolised in the liver to norcodeine and then conjugated to produce glucuronide conjugates of codeine, norcodeine and morphine. Codeine is considerably less potent than morphine. Around 8% of Western Europeans are deficient in the CYP2D6 enzyme and may not experience adequate analgesia with codeine. Similarly, with super-metabolisers, there may be problems with opioid toxicity; particular care is needed in the breast-feeding mother as morphine is transferred in milk. Codeine can cause significant histamine release, and intravenous administration should be avoided. It has marked antitussive effects and also causes significant constipation. It is often combined with paracetamol.

Diamorphine

Diamorphine is available for parenteral and oral use. It is more lipid soluble than morphine, affecting distribution and tissue penetration. One advantage over morphine is in settings where high concentrations are required in relatively low volumes, such as palliative care. Furthermore, when lipid solubility is important in regulating site of action (e.g. epidural, intrathecal use), some practitioners believe that diamorphine has specific advantages over morphine.

Diamorphine is a prodrug. It is inactive at opioid receptors but is converted rapidly to the active metabolites 6-monoacetylmorphine (6 MAM), morphine and M-6-G. Presence of 6-MAM in urine or salvia can be used to differentiate between morphine and heroin (diamorphine) consumption. Further metabolism is similar to that of morphine (see Table 6.7); similar problems may arise in renal impairment.

Oxycodone

Oxycodone is a potent semisynthetic opioid that has been in use for many years. In addition to actions at the MOP receptor, it may also have analgesic effects mediated via the KOP receptor, resulting in incomplete cross-tolerance with morphine. It has a good oral bioavailability, and its plasma concentrations are more predictable than those of morphine after oral administration. It is available in both long- and short-acting oral preparations and, more recently, in a parenteral formulation. Oral oxycodone is roughly 1.5 times more potent than oral morphine.

Hydromorphone

Hydromorphone, a potent opioid, is used mainly in the palliative care setting or in patients who are not opioid naive. It can be useful if considering opioid rotation. Hydromorphone 1.3 mg is approximately equianalgesic to morphine 10 mg. Both immediate- and sustained-release preparations are available.

Meperidine (pethidine)

Meperidine (pethidine) is available as parenteral and oral preparations. There is no evidence that this opioid provides any advantage over morphine, such as treatment of colicky-type pain. Its analgesic action is fairly short, but the metabolite normeperidine can accumulate ($t_{1/2} \sim 15$ h) if repeated doses are given and especially if there is renal dysfunction. Normeperidine is a CNS stimulant and can cause seizures. Its clearance is significantly reduced in hepatic disease. Chronic use may result in enzyme induction and an increase in normeperidine plasma concentrations. Its metabolism is decreased by the oral contraceptive pill.

Meperidine has other significant effects related to activity at non-opioid receptors. For example, its atropine-like action may cause a tachycardia, in addition to direct myocardial depression at high doses. It was used originally as a bronchodilator. It can also reduce shivering related to hypothermia or epidural anaesthesia, although the mechanism for this is not fully understood. Meperidine also has a local anaesthetic-like membrane stabilising action.

Fentanyl

Fentanyl is available in a variety of preparations for parenteral, transdermal and transmucosal (including buccal) administration. Because of high first-pass metabolism (~70%) it is not given orally. It is approximately 80–100 times more potent than morphine in the acute setting, although it is approximately 30–40 times as potent when given chronically (e.g. slow-release transdermal patches). With transdermal administration, the patch and underlying dermis act as a reservoir, and plasma concentration does not reach steady state until approximately 15 h after initial application. Plasma concentration also declines slowly after removal ($t_{1/2}$ ~15–20 h).

Fentanyl is very lipophilic, with a relatively short duration of action. There are several new buccal/transmucosal preparations developed for rapid-onset breakthrough pain. These aim to have a very rapid onset in approximately 10 min, although this may not be the case in clinical practice. Fentanyl has a large V_D with rapid peripheral tissue uptake, limiting initial hepatic metabolism. This may result in significant variability in plasma concentrations and secondary plasma peaks. It binds to α_1-acid glycoprotein and albumin; 40% of the protein-bound fraction is taken up by erythrocytes. The lungs may be important in exerting a first-pass effect on fentanyl (up to 75% of the dose), thus buffering the plasma from high peak drug concentrations.

Alfentanil

The low pKa of alfentanil (6.9) results in it being largely unionised at plasma pH, allowing rapid diffusion to the effect site ($t_{1/2}k_{eo}$ ~1 min) and rapid onset of action despite it being less lipid soluble than other opioids. It does not bind strongly to opioid receptors, and the effect-site concentration also decreases rapidly as plasma concentrations decrease. Alfentanil is metabolised by the hepatic cytochrome P450 isoform CYP3A4. Genetic variability in the activity of this enzyme may result in two- to threefold variations in pharmacokinetic values when given by infusion. Low, medium or high metabolisers have been identified; this has implications for duration of action when prolonged use is contemplated.

Sufentanil

Sufentanil is one of the most potent opioids; it has a rapid onset of action after i.v. administration, and peak analgesic effect is at approximately 8 min. It is 625 times more potent than morphine and 12 times more potent than fentanyl. However, diffusion to tissues is slower than alfentanil because, although sufentanil is highly lipid soluble, it is also highly protein bound, resulting in low unbound plasma fractions at body pH. It has very low concentration of non-specific binding that may increase potential effect-site concentrations. The speed of onset of a large dose is caused by saturation of receptors and non-specific sites, with potential for overdose. One of its metabolites (desmethylsufentanil) is active at the MOP receptor (10% of sufentanil's potency).

Remifentanil

Remifentanil is a MOP agonist with a similar potency to fentanyl and approximately 20 times more than alfentanil. It has a rapid blood–brain equilibration time of just over 1 min, with a short context-sensitive half-life of 3–5 min, which is unaffected by duration of infusion. This makes it ideally suited for infusion during anaesthesia and in critical care. It may be titrated rapidly to achieve the desired effect. Remifentanil is available as a lyophilised white crystalline powder containing glycine; it should not be administered via the epidural or intrathecal routes. There may be increased opioid sensitivity in hepatic disease, resulting in a lower dosage requirement. Other situations requiring a reduction in dose include haemorrhage and shock and when administering in elderly patients. The high clearance and low V_D imply that the offset of effect is caused by metabolism rather than redistribution. Hypothermia, such as may occur in cardiac surgery, may reduce clearance by up to 20%.

There is some evidence to suggest that acute opioid tolerance and hyperalgesia may occur, particularly after remifentanil infusions. If high doses are used without neuromuscular blockade, muscle rigidity may be a problem, though this is less likely if using a concentration of 100 μg ml^{-1} or less and an infusion rate of 0.2–0.5 μg kg^{-1} min^{-1}. Bradycardia has also been reported.

Methadone

Methadone is a diphenylpropylamine. It has very good oral bioavailability (~85%) with an oral to parenteral ratio of 1:2. Its plasma half-life can be highly variable (3–50 h, average 24 h) but its duration of action is relatively short. With repeated dosing, problems with accumulation can occur because of this discrepancy between half-life and analgesic effect. Careful monitoring is therefore required when converting patients to long-term methadone. Also, there is incomplete cross-tolerance with morphine. The racemic mixture in common use has agonist actions at the MOP receptor (mainly the *laevo* isomer) as well as antagonist activity at the NMDA receptor (*dextro* isomer). Given the importance of this receptor in central sensitisation in a variety of pain states, there may be cases where methadone offers particular advantages over and above other opioids (e.g. neuropathic pain).

Plasma concentrations of methadone can be reduced by carbamazepine, and its metabolism is accelerated by phenytoin.

Dihydrocodeine

Dihydrocodeine is a synthetic opioid developed in the early 1900s. Its structure and pharmacokinetics are similar to codeine, and it is used for the treatment of postoperative and chronic pain. Both immediate- and sustained-release preparations are available. Despite its common use, there are very few clinical trials demonstrating efficacy. It has significant abuse potential.

Tramadol

Tramadol is thought to produce analgesia by two distinct actions. First, it has agonist activity at the MOP and KOP receptors. Tramadol itself is a prodrug, with most of its analgesia mediated by a metabolite – O-desmethyltramadol – that has a 200-fold higher affinity for the MOP receptor. It is metabolised by cytochrome P450 (CYP2D6 and CYP3A4), and its potency is therefore affected by a patient's CYP genetics, with rapid and poor metabolisers. Second, it

enhances the descending inhibitory systems in the spinal cord by inhibiting noradrenaline reuptake and releasing serotonin from nerve endings. It is available in immediate- and sustained-release oral preparations and for parenteral administration. Its use is contraindicated in patients receiving monoamine oxidase inhibitors (MAOIs). Caution must also be exercised in hepatic impairment as its clearance is reduced to a much greater extent than morphine and related agents.

Tapentadol

Tapentadol, a relatively new opioid, also has distinct mechanisms of analgesic action. It is a MOP receptor agonist more potent than tramadol. It also acts by selectively inhibiting reuptake of noradrenaline, and therefore there may be a rationale for using it in patients with pain with neuropathic features.

Mixed agonist–antagonist opioids

Mixed agonist–antagonist opioids have a ceiling effect for analgesia and possibly respiratory depression. They have agonist effects at the KOP receptor and weak antagonist effects at the MOP receptor. Dysphoria and hallucinations are relatively common, and withdrawal effects may occur if given to patients taking MOP agonists. Pentazocine may be given orally or parenterally but is now rarely used. It may increase pulmonary and aortic blood pressure and myocardial oxygen demand. Hallucinations and dysphoria occur less commonly with nalbuphine.

Partial agonists

Partial agonists have high affinity for the MOP receptor but limited efficacy (see Chapter 1). A ceiling effect is seen in the dose–response curve at less than the maximal analgesic effect of full MOP agonists. If given with a full MOP agonist, there may be a reduction in the maximal analgesic effect.

Buprenorphine

Buprenorphine is the only partial agonist in common use. It binds to the MOP receptor and dissociates from it very slowly. Consequently, although significant respiratory depression is less likely compared with morphine, it may be more difficult to reverse. It has poor oral bioavailability, and parenteral, sublingual or transdermal formulations are used. In addition to partial agonism at the MOP receptor, it is also a partial agonist at the NOP receptor and an antagonist at the KOP receptor. This may contribute to some of its analgesic effects. Increasingly it is also used instead of methadone for the management of opioid abuse (usually in relatively large doses up to 24 mg day^{-1}).

Opioid antagonists

Naloxone is a short-acting opioid antagonist that is relatively selective for the MOP receptor. It is structurally similar to morphine, with some modifications resulting in antagonist activity, including an OH group at C-14. It can reverse opioid-induced respiratory depression, but repeated administration may be required because of its short duration of action; it can be given by continuous infusion. However, sudden and complete reversal of the analgesic effects of opioids may be accompanied by major cardiovascular and sympathetic responses. Naloxone has a very low oral bio-availability (~3%), allowing its use in combination with oxycodone (see later) to reduce GI effects.

Naltrexone is a long-acting opioid antagonist used in the management of opioid dependence. It is available only in oral formulation.

New developments in opioid pharmacology

There is considerable interest in developing opioid analgesics with an improved side effect profile, and there are some promising recent developments in this area. It has been recognised that by using agents which act on more than one type of opioid receptor there may be beneficial effects (Fig. 6.7). Some recently developed agents include the following:

- *Oxycodone/naloxone (Targinact)* uses a fixed ratio of oxycodone and naloxone (2:1). The oral naloxone has a greater affinity for opioid receptors in the gut than oxycodone and therefore preferentially binds to these receptors. As a result, GI side effects may be reduced without any change in the central analgesic effect of oxycodone.
- *MoxDuo* is a novel opioid combination of morphine and oxycodone in a 3:2 ratio, with promising evidence of at least 50% decrease in clinically significant side effects such as nausea, vomiting and dizziness compared with either opioid alone. This seems to be achieved by the

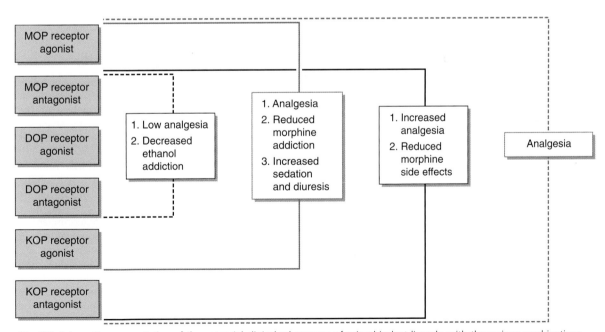

Fig. 6.7 Schematic representation of the potential clinical advantages of using bivalent ligands, with the various combinations of pharmacophores (antagonists and agonists). *DOP*, δ Opioid; *KOP*, κ opioid; *MOP*, μ opioid. (Adapted from Dietis, N., Guerrini R., Calo, G., et al. (2009) Simultaneous targeting of multiple opioid receptors: a strategy to improve side-effect profile. *British Journal of Anaesthesia.* 103, 38–49.)

need to use lower doses of both morphine and oxycodone to reach an equivalent analgesic effect.

Paracetamol

Paracetamol (acetaminophen) was first used in 1893 and is the only remaining *p*-aminophenol available in clinical practice. It is the active metabolite of the earlier, more toxic drugs acetanilide and phenacetin. Its structure is shown in Fig. 6.8. Paracetamol is an effective analgesic and antipyretic but has no anti-inflammatory activity. In recommended doses, it is safe and has remarkably few adverse effects.

Mechanism of action

The mechanism of action of paracetamol is not well understood, but it may act in a similar fashion to NSAIDs, with inhibition of cyclo-oxygenase enzymes COX-1 and COX-2 (see later) to reduce the phenoxyl radical formation required for COX-1 and 2 activity and prostaglandin synthesis. It has selectivity for inhibition of prostaglandin synthesis with low concentrations of peroxidases and arachidonic acid, but limited effect at higher concentrations and, therefore, has limited anti-inflammatory effects. Unlike opioids, paracetamol has no well-defined endogenous binding sites. In some circumstances, it may exhibit a preferential effect on COX-2 inhibition. There is growing evidence of a central antinociceptive effect of paracetamol. It has also been found to prevent prostaglandin production at the cellular transcriptional concentration, independent of COX activity.

Pharmacokinetics

Paracetamol is absorbed rapidly from the small intestine after oral administration; peak plasma concentrations are reached after 30–60 min. It may also be given rectally and intravenously (either as paracetamol or the prodrug

propacetamol). It has good oral bioavailability (70%–90%); rectal absorption is more variable (bioavailability ∼50%–80%) with a longer time to reach peak plasma concentration. The plasma half-life is approximately 2–3 h.

Paracetamol is metabolised by hepatic microsomal enzymes mainly to the glucuronide, sulphate and cysteine conjugates. None of these metabolites is pharmacologically active. A minimal amount of the metabolite *N*-acetyl-*p*-amino-benzoquinone imine is normally produced by cytochrome P450–mediated hydroxylation. This reactive toxic metabolite is rendered harmless by conjugation with liver glutathione, then excreted renally as mercapturic derivatives. With larger doses of paracetamol, the rate of formation of the reactive metabolite exceeds that of glutathione conjugation, and the reactive metabolite combines with hepatocellular macromolecules, resulting in cell death and potentially fatal hepatic failure. The formation of this metabolite is increased by drugs inducing cytochrome P450 enzymes, such as barbiturates or carbamazepine.

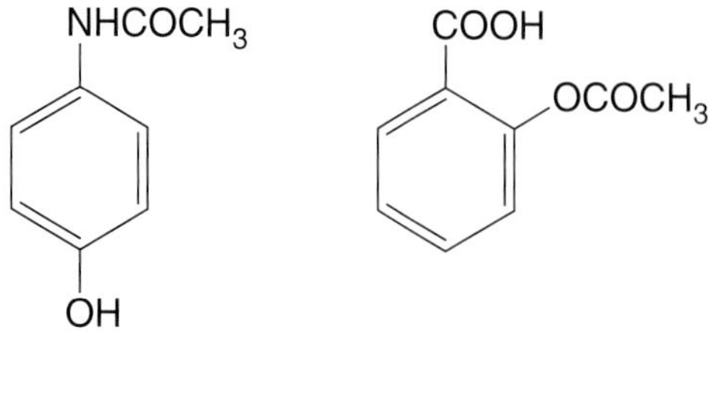

Pharmacodynamics

Paracetamol is effective in both acute and chronic pain and is available for oral or intravenous use. It is an effective postoperative analgesic but probably less effective than NSAIDs in many situations. It may reduce postoperative opioid requirements by up to 30%. The combination of paracetamol with an NSAID also improves efficacy. Paracetamol is also a very effective antipyretic, a centrally mediated effect.

Overdose and hepatic toxicity

In overdose there is the potential for the toxic metabolite described earlier to cause centrilobular hepatocellular necrosis, occasionally with acute renal tubular necrosis. The threshold dose in adults is approximately 10–15 g. Accidental overdosage can occur if combined preparations such as co-codamol are used together with paracetamol. Doses of more than 150 mg kg^{-1} taken within 24 h may result in severe liver damage, hypoglycaemia and acute tubular necrosis. Individuals taking enzyme-inducing agents are more likely to develop hepatotoxicity. More recently there has been debate about lowering the standard recommended dose of 4 g daily (or 1 g qds) for safety reasons, particularly in frail or elderly patients.

Early signs include nausea and vomiting, followed by right subcostal pain and tenderness. Hepatic damage is maximal 3–4 days after ingestion and may lead to liver failure and death. Treatment consists of gastric emptying and the specific antidotes methionine and acetylcysteine. The former offers effective protection up to 10–12 h after ingestion. Acetylcysteine is effective within 24 h and perhaps beyond. The plasma paracetamol concentration related to time from ingestion indicates the risk of liver damage. N-acetylcysteine

NHCOCH₃ structure (Paracetamol) with OH; COOH and OCOCH₃ structure (Aspirin)

Paracetamol   **Aspirin**

Fig. 6.8 The structures of paracetamol and aspirin.

is given if the plasma paracetamol concentration is more than 200 mg L^{-1} at 4 h and 6.25 mg L^{-1} at 24 h after ingestion.

Non-steroidal anti-inflammatory drugs (NSAIDs)

The analgesic, anti-inflammatory and antipyretic effects of salicylates, derived from the bark of the willow tree, were described as early as 1763. Acetylsalicylic acid (aspirin) was first produced in 1853. More recently, many other NSAIDs have been developed with actions similar to aspirin (Fig. 6.9 and Table 6.9). Perioperative analgesia using NSAIDs is free from many of the adverse effects of opioids, such as respiratory depression, sedation, nausea and vomiting and GI stasis. NSAIDs are effective analgesics in acute and chronic conditions, although significant contraindications and adverse effects limit their use.

Mechanism of action

All NSAIDs have the same basic mechanism of action – inhibition of cyclo-oxygenase (COX) enzymes. The mechanism of action of aspirin was discovered in the 1970s. It was found to irreversibly inhibit the production of prostanoids from arachidonic acid released from phospholipids in cell membranes (see Fig. 6.9). The basal rate of prostaglandin production is low and regulated by tissue stimuli or trauma that activate phospholipases to release arachidonic acid. Prostaglandins are then produced by the enzyme prostaglandin endoperoxide synthase, which has both cyclo-oxygenase and hydroperoxidase sites. At least two subtypes of cyclo-oxygenase enzyme have been identified in humans: COX-1 and COX-2. COX-1 is constitutively expressed in many tissues, with a wide variety of homeostatic functions, but can also be induced, for example, during angiogenesis. The prostanoids produced by COX-1 are functionally active in many areas, including the GI tract, kidney, lungs and cardiovascular systems. COX-1 is the only isoenzyme expressed in platelets. By contrast, the functional COX-2 enzyme is normally found less widely, e.g. brain, spinal cord, renal cortex, tracheal epithelium and vascular endothelium, with very low basal levels of activity. However, COX-2 messenger RNA (mRNA) is widely distributed, and in response to specific stimuli, especially those associated with inflammation, the expression of COX-2 isoenzyme is induced or upregulated, leading to increased local production of prostaglandins. A range of specific prostanoid receptors (e.g. EP1-4) are involved in peripheral sensitisation associated with inflammation.

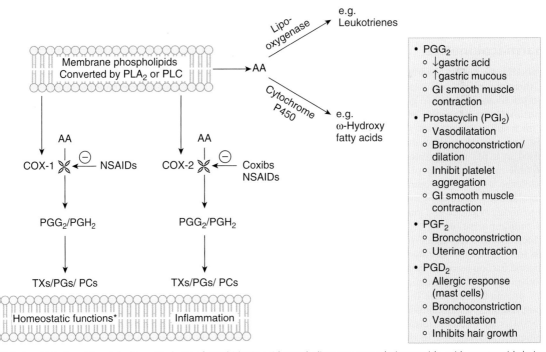

Fig. 6.9 Arachidonic acid metabolism. Products of arachidonic acid metabolism are termed eicosanoids, with prostanoids being a subgroup of these, consisting of prostacyclins, thromboxanes and prostaglandins, produced through the cyclo-oxygenase pathways. *AA*, Arachidonic acid; *COX*, cyclo-oxygenase; *PG*, prostaglandin; *PL*, phospholipase; *TXs*, thromboxanes.

Table 6.9 Classification of NSAIDs on the basis of chemical structure and selectivity for inhibition of COX-1 and COX-2 isoenzymes

Classification: chemical structure	Drugs	Classification: COX-1/COX-2 selectivity	Drugs
Salicylic acid and derivatives	Aspirin; sulfasalazine	Group 1 (poorly selective, strong inhibition)	Aspirin, naproxen, diclofenac, ibuprofen, piroxicam
Indol and related compounds	Indomethacin, sulindac, etodolac	Group 2 (preferential strong COX-2 inhibition)	Meloxicam, celecoxib, etodolac
Aryl-propionic acids	Ibuprofen, naproxen, ketoprofen, flurbiprofen, aceclofenac	Group 3 (weak inhibition of both COX-1 and COX-2)	Nabumetone
Anthranilic acids	Mefenamic acid		
Alkanones	Nabumetone		
Enolic acids	Meloxicam, piroxicam, tenoxicam		
Hetero-aryl acetic acids	Diclofenac, ketorolac		
Diarylheterocyles	COX-2 selective agents: celecoxib, etoricoxib, parecoxib		

NSAIDs also have central effects as cyclo-oxygenases are widely distributed in both the peripheral and central nervous systems. NSAIDs may also have other mechanisms of action independent of any effect on prostaglandins, including effects on basic cellular and neuronal processes. NSAIDs are non-selective; they inhibit both COX-1 and COX-2.

Pharmacokinetics

All NSAIDs are rapidly absorbed. They are weak acids and are therefore mainly unionised in the stomach, where absorption can occur. When given orally, most absorption occurs in the small intestine because the absorptive area of the microvilli of the small intestine is much more extensive. Most have pKa values lower than 5 and are therefore 99% ionised at a pH value greater than 7. Most are almost insoluble in water at body pH, although the sodium salt (diclofenac sodium, naproxen sodium) is more soluble. Ketorolac trometamol is the most soluble and can be given intravenously as a bolus and intramuscularly with less chance of significant irritation.

Most NSAIDs are highly protein bound (90%–99%), with low volumes of distribution ($\sim$0.1–0.2 l kg^{-1}). The unbound fraction is active. NSAIDs may potentiate the effects of other highly protein-bound drugs by displacing them from protein-binding sites (e.g. oral anticoagulants, oral hypoglycaemics, sulphonamides, anticonvulsants).

NSAIDs are mostly oxidised or hydroxylated and then conjugated and excreted in the urine. A few have active metabolites. For example, nabumetone is metabolised to 6-methoxy-2-naphthyl acetic acid, which is more active than the parent drug.

The interaction between NSAID and cyclo-oxygenase enzyme is often complex, and plasma half-life may not reflect pharmacodynamic half-life. Diclofenac has a terminal half-life of 1–2 h. It is conjugated to glucuronides and sulphates, with 65% being excreted in the urine and 35% in the bile. The metabolites are less active than the parent compound. Ketorolac trometamol has a terminal half-life of 5 h, and more than 90% is excreted renally. Naproxen has a terminal half-life of 12–15 h and is excreted almost entirely through the kidney as the conjugate. Tenoxicam is cleared mainly through the urine as the inactive hydroxypyridyl metabolite, although approximately 30% is via biliary excretion as the glucuronide.

Pharmacodynamics

NSAIDs are very effective analgesics, although their use is limited by adverse effects because of their general effect on prostanoid synthesis and the ubiquitous nature of prostanoids. Generally, the risk and severity of NSAID-associated adverse effects are increased in the elderly population and those with other significant comorbidity.

Analgesia

NSAIDs have well-demonstrated efficacy both as postoperative analgesics and in chronic conditions such as rheumatoid arthritis and osteoarthritis. They can have significant opioid-sparing effects. NSAIDs are insufficient alone for severe pain after major surgery but are valuable as part of a multimodal analgesic regimen.

Gastrointestinal system

The gastric and duodenal epithelia have various protective mechanisms against acid and enzyme attack, and many of these involve prostaglandin production via a COX-1 pathway. Acute and particularly chronic NSAID administration can result in gastroduodenal ulceration and bleeding; the latter is exacerbated by the antiplatelet effect.

Cardiovascular

The potential adverse effects of inhibition of the COX pathways on cardiovascular risks (including acute myocardial infarction and stroke) were first highlighted in studies of COX-2 selective agents. Subsequent large-scale studies indicate that this increased risk is probably related to all NSAIDs, not just COX-2 selective agents. There are recommendations to use with care, or not at all, in high-risk patients with ischaemic heart or cerebrovascular disease. Their use in others should be guided by individual risk assessments for each patient. Some drugs have been withdrawn.

Platelet function

Platelet COX-1 is essential for the production of the cyclic endoperoxides and thromboxane A_2 that mediate the primary haemostatic response to vessel injury by producing vasoconstriction and platelet aggregation. Aspirin acetylates COX-1 irreversibly, whereas other NSAIDs do so in a reversible fashion. This can result in prolonged bleeding times, and increased perioperative blood loss has been reported in some studies. The presence of a bleeding diathesis or coadministration of anticoagulants may increase the risk of significant surgical blood loss or bleeding related to regional techniques.

Renal function

Renal prostaglandins have many physiological roles, including the maintenance of renal blood flow and glomerular filtration rate in the presence of circulating vasoconstrictors, regulation of tubular electrolyte handling and modulation of the actions of renal hormones. NSAIDs can adversely affect renal function. High circulating concentrations of the vasoconstrictors renin, angiotensin, noradrenaline (norepinephrine) and vasopressin increase production of intrarenal vasodilators, including prostacyclin, and renal function may be particularly sensitive to NSAIDs in these situations. Coadministration of other potential nephrotoxins, such as gentamicin, may increase the likelihood of renal toxicity.

Aspirin-induced asthma

Aspirin-induced asthma may affect up to 20% of persons with asthma; it may be severe, and there is often cross-sensitivity with other NSAIDs. Patients with coexisting chronic rhinitis and nasal polyps appear to be at most risk. A history of aspirin-induced asthma is a contraindication to NSAID use after surgery. There is no reason to avoid NSAIDs in other patients with asthma if previous exposure has not been associated with bronchospasm. However, patients should be warned of potential problems and advised to stop taking them if their asthma worsens. The mechanism of this problem is unclear; it may be that cyclo-oxygenase inhibition increases arachidonic acid availability for production of inflammatory leukotrienes by lipo-oxygenase pathways.

Contraindications

Specific contraindications to NSAID administration include a history of a bleeding diathesis, peptic ulceration, significant renal impairment or aspirin-induced asthma. Care should be taken in high-risk groups, such as the elderly, those with cardiovascular disease and the dehydrated.

COX-2–specific inhibitors

COX-2–specific inhibitors are anti-inflammatory analgesics that reduce prostaglandin synthesis by specifically inhibiting COX-2, with little or no effect on COX-1 (relative specificity varies between drugs). They were developed as an alternative to traditional NSAIDs with the aim of avoiding COX-1–mediated side effects, primarily gastric ulceration and platelet effects.

Mechanism of action

The mechanism of action is similar to that of traditional NSAIDs (see Fig. 6.7). Both COX-1 and COX-2 enzymes have very similar active sites and catalytic properties, although COX-2 has a larger potential binding site because of a secondary internal pocket. This has allowed the design of drugs to target predominantly COX-2. COX-2 is induced at sites of inflammation and trauma, producing prostaglandins, and these drugs inhibit this process. However, COX-2 is an important constitutive enzyme in the CNS, including the spinal cord, and inhibition at this site is thought to be an important mechanism also.

Pharmacodynamics
Analgesia

Systematic reviews and meta-analyses indicate similar efficacy to non-selective NSAIDs in both acute postoperative pain and for chronic conditions such as osteoarthritis. Agents are available orally (e.g. celecoxib, etoricoxib) and parenterally (parecoxib).

119

Gastrointestinal

One of the commonest side effects of NSAIDs is GI toxicity. Approximately 1 in 1200 patients receiving chronic NSAID treatment (>2 months) die from related gastroduodenal complications. COX-1 isoenzyme is the predominant cyclo-oxygenase found in the gastric mucosa. The prostanoids produced here help to protect the gastric mucosa by reducing acid secretion, stimulating mucus secretion, increasing production of mucosal phospholipids and bicarbonate and regulating mucosal blood flow. Specific COX-2 inhibitors have less of an effect on these processes.

Short- to medium-term treatment with specific COX-2 inhibitors (up to 3 months) is associated with a significant reduction in the incidence of gastroduodenal ulceration. However, this effect is reduced during prolonged treatment and in patients taking low-dose aspirin. It is likely that the degree of COX-2 specificity is related to the efficacy of gastric protection.

Haematological

COX-2–specific agents have very little adverse effect on platelet function. This is potentially advantageous compared with non-specific NSAIDs with respect to perioperative or GI bleeding.

Renal

COX-2 is normally found in the renal cortex and is therefore inhibited both by conventional NSAIDs and COX-2 inhibitors. There is the potential both for peripheral oedema and hypertension, as well as direct effects on renal excretory function with oliguria and decreased creatinine clearance.

Conclusion

The neurobiology of pain is complex. It is important to have an understanding of the underlying mechanisms and how these are modified by different classes of analgesics. Multimodal analgesia may be an effective way to manage pain, particularly in the perioperative period. Key to good pain control is proper assessment of pain and regular reassessment of response to any intervention. Effective and targeted use of currently available analgesics should provide good pain control in the majority of individuals.

References/Further reading

Erlanger, J., Gasser, H.S., 1937. Electrical signs of nervous activity. University Pennsylvania Press, Philadelphia.

Honore, P., Rogers, S.D., Schwei, M.J., et al., 2000. Murine models of inflammatory, neuropathic and cancer pain each generates a unique set of neurochemical changes in the spinal cord and sensory neurons. Neuroscience 98, 585–598.

Julius, D., Basbaum, A.I., 2001. Molecular mechanisms of nociception. Nature 413, 203–210.

Melzack, R., Wall, P.D., 1965. Pain mechanisms: a new theory. Science 150, 971–979.

Chapter | 7 |

Postoperative nausea and vomiting

Cameron Weir

It is estimated that up to 80% of patients experience postoperative nausea and vomiting (PONV) within the first 24 h after surgery. If risk factors are identified and acted upon, PONV can be easily managed, but for a small, high-risk cohort of patients, symptoms can be extremely distressing and disabling. Fortunately, the aetiology of PONV is multifactorial; therefore a variety of different treatments and interventions can be used to minimise the risk of developing PONV. Prevention, along with prompt and effective treatment, decreases adverse effects, limits the length of inpatient stay and reduces hospital costs. Importantly, successful prevention of PONV greatly improves patient satisfaction.

Definitions

Nausea is derived from the Greek word *naus*, meaning 'ship' and was used originally to describe the feeling of seasickness. Nausea is an unpleasant sensation caused by afferent signals emanating from the upper gastrointestinal (GI) tract and pharynx. It is associated with dizziness and the urge to vomit. Assessment of nausea is extremely difficult because symptoms are subjective, entirely patient dependent and often difficult to quantify. For this reason, the incidence of postoperative nausea is often underestimated. *Retching* is the involuntary process of unproductive vomiting. It is characterised by the synchronous contraction of diaphragmatic and abdominal muscles against a closed mouth and glottis. Retching is extremely distressing and is usually accompanied by feelings of intense nausea. *Vomiting* represents the final common pathway of a highly coordinated sequence of events involving GI, abdominal, respiratory and pharyngeal muscles, which results in the active and rapid expulsion of contents from the stomach and upper intestine. In contrast to the rather subjective assessment of nausea, vomiting is easily identifiable and measurable!

Mechanisms of nausea and vomiting

Vomiting centre

The vomiting reflex probably developed as an evolutionary protective mechanism against ingestion of harmful substances or toxins. However, nausea and vomiting also occur in response to a wide range of pathological and environmental triggers including sight, smell, motion and GI disturbances. Other important triggers include pregnancy, migraine, head injury, vestibular problems and severe pain. Afferent signals mediated by the vagus, vestibular and higher cortical nerves are carried to discrete areas within the brainstem collectively known as the 'vomiting centre' (Fig. 7.1). Traditionally the vomiting centre was thought to be a single anatomical entity, but there is increasing evidence that it is made up of a disparate group of interconnected cells and nuclei located in the lateral reticular formation of the medulla and the nucleus tractus solitarius (NTS). All information entering the vomiting centre is processed and coordinated via autonomic, sensory and motor nerves into a highly complex series of neuronal signals known as the 'vomiting reflex'.

Chemoreceptor trigger zone

The chemoreceptor trigger zone (CTZ) consists of several nuclei found within the area postrema at the caudal end of

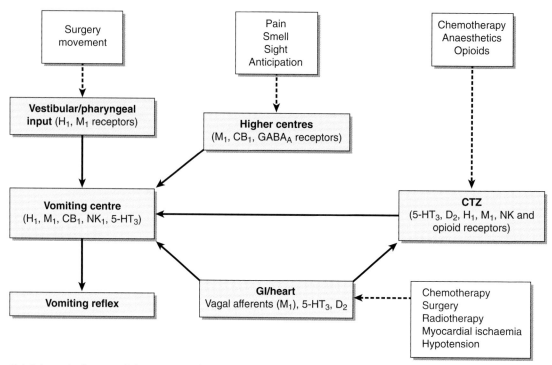

Fig. 7.1 Schematic diagram of the vomiting reflex. See text for details. *CB,* Cannabinoid; *CTZ,* chemoreceptor trigger zone; *D_2,* dopaminergic 2; receptors; *$GABA_A$,* γ-aminobutyric acid A; *H1,* histaminergic 1; *5-HT_3,* 5-hydroxytryptamine 3; *M_1,* muscarinic-1; *NK_1,* neurokinin 1.

the fourth ventricle. Although the CTZ is anatomically located within the central nervous system, its unusual pattern of endothelial fenestrations and generous blood supply allows it to 'sense' chemicals not only within cerebrospinal fluid but also within peripheral blood. In other words, the highly vascularised CTZ uses its defective blood–brain barrier to detect potentially harmful substances present within the circulation. The CTZ contains an abundance of cholinergic (muscarinic M_1), dopaminergic (D_2), histaminergic (H_1), serotonergic (5-HT_3) and opioid (mainly μ) and neurokinin (NK_1) receptors which send afferent projections to the vomiting centre. Stimulation of the CTZ contributes significantly to the nausea and vomiting experienced by surgical patients; therefore pharmacological manipulation within the CTZ forms an important strategy in the prevention and treatment of PONV.

Stimulation of the vomiting centre

Fig. 7.1 outlines the various triggers and neural connections involved in the initiation of the vomiting reflex. The vomiting centre acts as the final processor for all sensory information received from central and peripheral receptors; therefore

blocking afferent or efferent signalling in this area will potentially have an antiemetic effect. Alternatives include direct stimulation of cannabinoid (CB_1) receptors within the vomiting centre using synthetic cannabinoid derivatives (e.g. nabilone), or NK_1 receptor antagonists (e.g. aprepitant), which antagonise substance P at NK_1 receptors. These agents decrease chemotherapy-induced vomiting (CIV), although their use in the perioperative period is currently under review. Other important causes of emesis are described later.

Gastrointestinal tract

The normal functioning of the GI tract is dependent on fully integrated neural feedback mechanisms. As part of this dynamic process, numerous mechano- and chemoreceptors send information to the central nervous system via vagal nerve afferents. Any threat to the integrity of the GI system, such as gastric distension, irritation, damage, drugs or toxins, triggers an increase in ascending vagal activity which relays directly or indirectly to the vomiting centre. For example, delayed gastric emptying and reduced lower oesophageal sphincter tone induced by hormonal changes, compounded by increased intra-abdominal pressure, significantly increase the risk of nausea and vomiting during pregnancy. Cholinergic M_1, serotoninergic 5-HT_3 and dopaminergic D_2 receptors are the principal mediators of signal transduction within the gut mucosa. Stimulation of one or all of these receptors initiates a key step in the vomiting reflex; therefore pharmacological antagonism at these sites is a logical approach to managing symptoms.

Vestibular system

Motion sickness is an unpleasant consequence of aberrant vestibular or visual activity. Susceptible individuals develop motion sickness in childhood, with the incidence peaking during early adolescence. Fortunately, symptoms diminish with advancing age. Numerous studies report that females are more prone to motion sickness than males. The neurophysiological mechanisms responsible for motion sickness are largely unknown, but it is likely that an imbalance in the vestibular–cerebellar–visual axis together with stimulation of higher autonomic nerves triggers activation of the vomiting reflex. Therefore female patients with a history of motion sickness have two independent predictors of PONV (see later).

Cardiovascular system

Anaesthetists should recognise that nausea may represent an important sign of underlying hypotension, particularly in patients undergoing regional anaesthesia. Myocardial ischaemia and infarction are also associated with nausea and vomiting. It is likely that retrograde autonomic signalling to the brainstem is responsible for these early warning signs of cardiovascular compromise. Similarly, autonomic disturbances may contribute to the nausea and emesis in patients presenting with severe pain.

Cortical inputs

Higher cortical centres and the limbic system are intimately involved with initiation and modification of the vomiting reflex. For example, unpleasant sights, sounds or smells, fear or emotional stress can induce nausea. In this context, cholinergic M_1 antagonists (e.g. hyoscine) or γ-aminobutyric acid A ($GABA_A$) receptor potentiators (e.g. benzodiazepines) may be useful, with or without behaviour-modifying techniques.

Gag reflex

The gag reflex reduces the risk of ingestion of noxious material and airway obstruction. The glossopharyngeal nerve (cranial nerve IX) mediates the afferent limb of this reflex, synapsing directly within the nucleus solitarius in the brainstem. The efferent limb is coordinated by the vagus nerve (cranial nerve X). This primitive reflex is one of the strongest triggers of emesis and is particularly active after oral insertion of airway adjuncts in semiconscious patients.

Neural and muscular coordination during nausea and vomiting

Nausea usually precedes vomiting and consists of several symptoms, including pallor, salivation, shivering and the urge to vomit. The synchronised neuromuscular events mediating the vomiting reflex are divided into two distinct phases: retching and expulsion. Retching is associated with rhythmic contraction of the abdominal, intercostal and diaphragmatic muscles, whereas expulsion occurs when abdominal muscle contraction causes intragastric pressure to exceed lower and upper oesophageal pressure. Complex neuromuscular coordination using motor, sensory and autonomic nerves ensures the glottis is closed during the ejection phase to prevent aspiration of gastric contents into the trachea and lungs.

Adverse effects of PONV

Some clinicians dismiss PONV as an inevitable consequence of anaesthesia and surgery, but from the patient's perspective, PONV is almost always associated with distress and dissatisfaction. Importantly, if nausea or vomiting persist, there is a risk of potentially serious perioperative morbidity (Box 7.1). Intact laryngeal reflexes ensure glottic closure during vomiting, but in the immediate postoperative phase, laryngeal reflexes may be obtunded because of residual effects of general anaesthesia and centrally acting analgesics, resulting in aspiration of gastric contents if the upper airway is not protected. The physical act of vomiting may lead to pain, wound dehiscence, haemorrhage, haematoma or possibly oesophageal rupture (Boerhaave's syndrome). If PONV

Box 7.1 **Adverse effects of PONV**

Patient distress and dissatisfaction
Pulmonary aspiration
Postoperative pain
Wound dehiscence/haemorrhage
Dehydration, electrolyte disturbance and/or requirement for intravenous fluids
Delayed oral intake of fluids, nutrition and drugs
Delayed mobilisation
Delayed discharge

persists, dehydration, reduced oral intake, electrolyte imbalance and delayed mobilisation can result in significant morbidity and increased healthcare costs associated with delayed discharge and unplanned admissions.

Identifying patients at risk

Many different approaches have been used to stratify patients according to their individual risk of PONV. Risk stratification allows clinicians to optimise prevention and treatment for patients at moderate or high risk of PONV whilst minimising indiscriminate prescribing and adverse drug reactions in patients at lower risk.

Patient factors

Although it is impossible to identify every patient at risk of PONV, several factors contribute (Box 7.2). Numerous studies report that non-smoking habits, female sex and a history of PONV or motion sickness are all strong independent predictors for PONV. Anxiety and obesity may increase the risk; however, the evidence for these associations is weaker. Children older than 3 years and young adults are also at high risk, but the incidence decreases in later life. Vomiting, rather than nausea, is often used as an outcome measure

---

> ### Box 7.2 Risk factors for PONV
>
> **Patient**
>
> Female sex
> Non-smoker
> History of PONV or motion sickness
> Children (age >3 years) and young adults
>
> **Anaesthetic**
>
> Volatile anaesthetics
> Opioids
> Nitrous oxide
> Postoperative pain
> Hypotension
> Neostigmine at doses >2.5 mg
> Bag-mask ventilation and airway irritation
>
> **Surgical**
>
> Long duration (>30 min)
> Type
>   Gynaecological
>   Squint
>   Middle ear surgery
>   Abdominal

---

in paediatric studies because of the difficulties in assessing and quantifying nausea in young children.

Anaesthetic factors

Gastric insufflation as a result of 'enthusiastic' bag-mask ventilation or postextubation airway irritation can increase the risk of nausea and vomiting. Identification of specific pharmacological triggers is difficult because several drugs are used as part of a standard general anaesthetic technique. However, there is incontrovertible evidence that opioids and some volatile agents induce PONV. Opioid administration by whatever route (oral, intramuscular, intravenous, epidural or spinal) is associated with a high incidence of PONV. Activation of peripheral and central opioid receptors by exogenous opioids leads to stimulation of the CTZ, direct activation of the vomiting centre and reduced gastric emptying. Increased sensitivity of the vestibular nerve (possibly as a result of activation of histaminergic H_1 and muscarinic M_1 receptors) may also play a role in the genesis of PONV. This is particularly prevalent during movement in the immediate postoperative phase. Preoperative opioids contribute to a higher prevalence of PONV, and opioid-based premedication has largely been superseded by the use of non-opioid anxiolytic agents (e.g. benzodiazepines). Ineffective postoperative analgesia and pain can induce significant nausea and vomiting in susceptible individuals. In this situation, a non–opioid-based analgesic approach is justified (e.g. simple analgesics and nerve blocks). Alternatively, careful titration of opioids may be appropriate.

Most intravenous anaesthetic induction agents induce PONV, but at subhypnotic concentrations, propofol exhibits significant antiemetic activity. It is thought that this beneficial pharmacodynamic action is caused by antagonism of dopaminergic D_2 and 5-HT_3 receptors. The increasing popularity of TIVA techniques exploits the intrinsic antiemetic activity of propofol while avoiding the strong emetogenic stimuli from the volatile agents (see Chapter 4).

Though often blamed, the evidence for nitrous oxide causing PONV is less compelling. If used as part of a gas and oxygen mixture (e.g. Entonox), nitrous oxide does induce nausea and vomiting. However, studies using a combination of nitrous oxide with volatile agents do not report a consistently increased incidence, particularly in patients at high risk of PONV.

The non-depolarising neuromuscular reversal agent neostigmine has been implicated as a possible trigger for PONV. Anticholinesterases increase GI motility and retrograde vagal nerve activity by activation of M_1 receptors in the gut. However, these effects are normally antagonised by the coadministration of antimuscarinic agents (e.g. glycopyrronium bromide). It is only when higher doses of neostigmine are required (>2.5 mg) that PONV becomes problematic.

Surgical factors

Some types of surgery are associated with an increased risk of PONV. For example, stimulation of vestibular or pharyngeal nerves after surgery on the middle ear, larynx or pharynx is associated with an increased prevalence of emesis. Similarly, squint correction surgery (usually in children) has a disproportionately high incidence of PONV. Patients undergoing gynaecological procedures are often recruited into antiemetic studies because they are perceived as being at high risk for PONV, but this may be a consequence of female sex rather than the surgery per se. The cumulative doses of volatile agents and opioids are greater after lengthy surgical procedures; therefore it is unsurprising that PONV is more common particularly in procedures associated with delayed gastric emptying (e.g. abdominal surgery).

Postdischarge nausea and vomiting

Increasing numbers of surgical procedures are now carried out on a day-case basis. Despite meeting strict discharge criteria, many patients experience postdischarge nausea and vomiting (PDNV) after leaving hospital. Of those, up to 35% do not have any symptoms before discharge. This discrepancy may relate to the relatively short durations of action of current antiemetic agents. One strategy to minimise the incidence of PDNV involves the use of different classes of drug, routes of administration and dosing schedules during the perioperative period. For example, administration of i.v. dexamethasone at induction of anaesthesia and i.v. ondansetron at the end of surgery followed by oral ondansetron before hospital discharge significantly reduces PDNV compared with single-dose regimens. It should be remembered that most patients have limited or no access to antiemetic treatment after leaving hospital, However, postoperative antiemetic prophylaxis for every patient is neither beneficial nor cost effective. Prophylaxis is best targeted towards patients at moderate to high risk of PONV, who should be offered oral antiemetics as part of their take-home medication.

Pharmacology

The numerous afferent and efferent components of the vomiting reflex lend themselves to pharmacological manipulation at multiple peripheral and central receptor sites. Antagonism of one or more of the four key neurotransmitters involved in the vomiting reflex (dopamine, histamine, acetylcholine and 5-HT$_3$) forms the basis of established treatment regimens for PONV (Table 7.1). Not all the drugs listed in Table 7.1 are suitable or have been licensed for the treatment of PONV in the UK. The table indicates current or potential drug development strategies.

Dopamine (D$_2$) receptor antagonists

Peripheral and central dopaminergic D$_2$ receptors are located within the GI tract and the CTZ, respectively. D$_2$ receptors mediate GI activity and dopaminergic neurotransmission within the CTZ. The antiemetic efficacy of D$_2$ receptor antagonists relates to a combination of increased gut motility and raising the emetogenic threshold within the CTZ. Butyrophenones, phenothiazines and benzamides act primarily as D$_2$ receptor antagonists, although most dopaminergic antagonists also act on other receptor systems (Table 7.2).

Butyrophenones

Droperidol was withdrawn from clinical practice in 2001 because of concerns over QTc prolongation associated with chronic treatment. After successful campaigning (mainly by anaesthetists), droperidol was reintroduced specifically for the acute management of PONV. It acts mainly as a D$_2$ receptor antagonist, but it also has weak α_1-adrenergic blocking activity. Intravenous droperidol (0.625–1.25 mg) administered 30 min before the end of surgery is economical and generally effective at reducing PONV. It can also be co-administered with opioids using PCA pumps. Adverse effects such as sedation, extrapyramidal effects and GI upset may limit treatment. Droperidol is contraindicated in patients with long QT syndrome. Oral domperidone is generally well tolerated and causes less central effect compared with the phenothiazines, but its use has diminished after a Medicines Healthcare and Products Regulatory Agency (MHRA) report warning of serious cardiac arrhythmias.

Phenothiazines

Phenothiazines were introduced originally to treat psychotic states, including mania and schizophrenia. Subsequently, many were found to have useful antiemetic properties and are now used routinely during cancer chemoradiotherapy. The main mechanism of action of the phenothiazines is antagonism of D$_2$ receptors, but some of their clinical effects may arise from blockade of other relevant neurotransmitters (see Table 7.2). Prochlorperazine is used routinely in the treatment of PONV and labyrinthine disorders. It can be administered via intramuscular, oral or buccal routes. Adverse effects include sedation, hypotension and extrapyramidal features.

Perphenazine is not licensed for treatment of PONV in the UK but has proved to be useful as an oral antiemetic preparation.

Benzamides

Metoclopramide has been used extensively in the treatment of nausea and vomiting secondary to GI disease and

Table 7.1 Drugs used in management of PONV

Drug	Dose	Elimination $t_{1/2}$ (h)	Timing	Comments	Common adverse effects
5-HT₃ receptor antagonists					
Ondansetron	4–8 mg i.v. / i.m. / p.o.	3.5–5.5	End of surgery	Max 16 mg/24 h	Abnormal liver function, headache, dizziness Caution: QT prolongation (less common with granisetron)
Granisetron	1 mg i.v. / p.o.	6	Before induction	Max 9 mg/24 h	
Palonosetron	0.075–0.250 mg i.v. / p.o.	40		Not licensed for PONV in the UK	
Tropisetron	2 mg i.v.	5–6		Not available in the UK	
Dopamine (D₂) receptor antagonists					
Benzamides					
Metoclopramide	10 mg i.v. / i.m. / p.o.	4–6	At induction	Not recommended for children and young adults	Acute dystonic reactions involving facial and skeletal muscle spasms and oculogyric crises
Butyrophenones					
Droperidol	0.625–1.25 mg i.v.	2–3	End of surgery		Sedation, EPE, agitation Contraindicated with concomitant use of drugs prolonging QT interval MHRA alert issued in 2014 for domperidone because of risk of cardiac adverse effects
Domperidone	10 mg p.o.	7–8	End of surgery	Max 30 mg/day	
Phenothiazines					
Prochlorperazine	12.5 mg i.m. 5–10 mg p.o. 3 mg buccal	6–7	Recovery room	Not licensed for use in children	Sedation, EPE, hypotension
Perphenazine	8 mg p.o.	8–10	—	Not licensed for PONV in the UK	
Anticholinergics (M₁ receptor antagonists)					
Hyoscine (scopolamine)	1.5 mg transdermal patch	9–10	Night before surgery	Antispasmodic and useful for motion sickness Not licensed for PONV in the UK	Antimuscarinic effects; blurred vision; dry mouth; gastrointestinal disturbances; hallucinations; headache; psychomotor impairment; tachycardia: twitching; urinary retention

Table 7.1 Drugs used in management of PONV—cont'd

Drug	Dose	Elimination $t_{1/2}$ (h)	Timing	Comments	Common adverse effects
Antihistamines (H₁ receptor antagonists)					
Cyclizine	50 mg i.v. / i.m. / p.o.	14–16	At induction (i.v. / i.m.)	Max 150 mg/ 24 h Avoid in acute porphyria	Antimuscarinic effects; blurred vision; dry mouth; gastrointestinal disturbances; hallucinations; headache; psychomotor impairment; tachycardia; twitching; urinary retention
Promethazine	20 mg p.o.	5–14	—	Useful for motion sickness – not licensed for PONV in the UK	
Glucocorticoids					
Dexamethasone	3.3–6.6 mg i.v. Note: A 3.3-mg ampoule expressed as the dexamethasone base is equivalent to a 4-mg ampoule expressed as its phosphate salt	3-4	At induction	All dosage recommendations for i.v. use are now given in units of dexamethasone base (i.e. 3.3 mg c.f. 4 mg)	Perineal discomfort after rapid i.v. injection
NK₁ antagonists					
Aprepitant	40–80 mg p.o.	9–13	1–3 h before induction	Not licensed for PONV in the UK	Headaches, dizziness, hiccups
Fosaprepitant (prodrug of aprepitant)	80–150 mg i.v.	10–12	At induction	Not licensed for PONV in the UK	
Cannabinoids					
Nabilone	1–2 mg p.o.	2–35 (includes metabolites)	—	Not licensed for PONV in the UK	Mood changes, dry mouth, ataxia

EPE, Extrapyramidal effects; *MHRA,* Medicines and Healthcare Products Regulatory Agency; *PONV,* postoperative nausea and vomiting.

chemoradiotherapy. Surprisingly, there is little evidence for its efficacy in PONV. At standard doses, it blocks D_2 receptors in the gut and CTZ, but at higher doses, it also acts as a 5-HT$_3$ receptor antagonist. Current preparations are available for intravenous, oral and intramuscular administration. Adverse effects include extrapyramidal symptoms, hypotension and sedation. Extrapyramidal symptoms are dose related and occur most often in children and young adults. It is recommended that intravenous administration take place over 1–2 min to reduce the risk of adverse effects.

Histamine (H₁) receptor antagonists

Histamine (H_1) receptors are located in the CTZ, vomiting centre and possibly within the vestibular apparatus. Most antihistamines display dual activity at histaminergic (H_1) and cholinergic (M_1) receptors and, at higher doses, cause D_2 receptor blockade. Combined activity at H_1 and M_1 receptors make antihistamines particularly useful in the treatment of motion sickness. Cyclizine is used for PONV because it has less of a central sedative effect compared with

Table 7.2 Relative receptor specificities

Drug	Serotonin 5-HT$_3$	Dopamine D$_2$	Acetylcholine M$_1$	Histamine H$_1$
5-HT$_3$ antagonists (e.g. ondansetron)	++++	–	–	–
Benzamides (e.g. metoclopramide)	++	+++	+	–
Butyrophenones (e.g. droperidol)	+	++++	–	+
Phenothiazines (e.g. prochlorperazine)	–	++++	+	+
Anticholinergics (e.g. hyoscine)	–	+	++++	+
Antihistamines (e.g. cyclizine)	–	++	++	+++

other drugs in its class. It can be administered via the oral, intramuscular and intravenous routes. Adverse effects include dry mouth, sedation and blurred vision, all of which are related to inherent anticholinergic activity. Rapid intravenous injection of cyclizine induces tachycardia. It should be used with caution in patients with heart failure.

Cholinergic (M$_1$) receptor antagonists

Hyoscine (scopolamine) is not specifically indicated for the management of PONV. It is used mainly as an antispasmodic, antisialagogue premedicant and in the prevention of motion sickness. Various preparations are available for administration using intramuscular, intravenous, subcutaneous, oral or transdermal routes. Some reports suggest a reduction in PONV with perioperative use of a transdermal hyoscine patch. In susceptible individuals, hyoscine causes significant sedation, dry mouth, visual disturbance and, rarely, central anticholinergic syndrome.

Serotonin (5-HT$_3$) receptor antagonists

Serotoninergic 5-HT$_3$ receptor antagonists are indicated for use in the management of PONV and in the management of nausea and vomiting induced by chemoradiotherapy. 5-HT$_3$ receptors are located in the CTZ, vomiting centre and GI tract. 5-HT$_3$ plays an important role in detecting and transmitting emetogenic signals from the CTZ to the vomiting centre, whereas peripheral serotonergic receptors stimulate vagal afferents in response to damaging stimuli within the gut mucosa. In addition, 5-HT is also released in the area postrema in response to increased vagal activity. Therefore it is likely that the efficacy of 5-HT$_3$ antagonists results from a combination of central and peripheral effects.

Ondansetron and granisetron are both licensed for treatment of PONV in the UK. Ondansetron has a shorter half-life than granisetron and can be administered via oral, intramuscular, intravenous or rectal routes. Other 5-HT$_3$ receptor antagonists (including tropisetron and dolasetron) are not currently available in the UK. Ondansetron and granisetron are free from sedative and extrapyramidal adverse effects, but in susceptible individuals, they may induce QTc prolongation and impair liver function.

Corticosteroids

Dexamethasone is a corticosteroid with high glucocorticoid activity and virtually no mineralocorticoid activity. Its mechanism of action as an antiemetic is unknown, but it is possible that either direct genomic or indirect non-genomic effects on 5-HT$_3$ and GABA$_A$ receptors contribute to its antiemetic activity. Many of the original studies were carried out using 8–10 mg of dexamethasone phosphate, but smaller doses (2.5–4 mg) provide equal antiemetic efficacy with minimal risk of adverse effects. Concerns relating to adrenal suppression and other steroid-induced adverse effects (including increased risk of bleeding) after a single dose of dexamethasone remain largely unfounded. One of the most unpleasant adverse effects of dexamethasone involves intense perineal stimulation after rapid i.v. injection.

Substance P (NK$_1$) antagonists

Substance P, neurokinin A (NKA) and neurokinin B (NKB) are genetically related neuropeptides (tachykinins) that activate G protein-coupled NK$_1$, NK$_2$ and NK$_3$ receptors within peripheral and central compartments. Substance P is thought to play a key role in emesis by binding to

NK_1 receptors in the gut and also centrally within the NTS and area postrema. In theory, blocking substance P activity should be highly effective in the treatment of PONV, but NK_1 antagonists are no better (i.e. non-inferior) at reducing postoperative *nausea* than standard ondansetron therapy. In contrast, they can significantly reduce the incidence of postoperative *vomiting*. Further investigation of NK_1 antagonists is needed to determine whether they have a place in the management of PONV. Two NK_1 antagonists (aprepitant and its i.v. formulation, fosaprepitant) are licensed for use in the UK, but both are currently restricted to treatment of chemotherapy-induced nausea and vomiting (CINV).

Cannabinoids

Nabilone is a synthetic cannabinoid that targets endogenous CB_1 and CB_2 cannabinoid receptors. Nabilone's UK licence is currently restricted to the treatment of CINV because the results for prevention and treatment of PONV have so far been disappointing. Moreover, the potential for serious adverse effects (including psychosis, behavioural changes and ataxia) has led to the recommendation that all patients be closely monitored during cannabinoid administration.

Alternative pharmacological approaches

The α_2 agonists, including clonidine and dexmedetomidine, have shown some promise in the prevention and treatment of PONV. The mechanisms responsible for their antiemetic activity are unknown, but an opioid-sparing effect or direct α_2 receptor agonism is likely. Preoperative oral gabapentin has been found to be as equally efficacious as i.v. dexamethasone for certain types of urological surgery, with the combination of both drugs providing a superior antiemetic effect. Interestingly, low-dose i.v. midazolam (2 mg) at the end of surgery is as effective as i.v. ondansetron but superior to metoclopramide for select groups of surgical patients. These findings highlight the difficulties in extrapolating results from small, controlled studies into meaningful conclusions about PONV risk reduction within the general population.

Management

Prevention

Prevention is the key to effective management of PONV; therefore it is important to identify all patients at risk. In simple terms, patients can be stratified into three groups: low-, moderate- or high-risk. One of the most widely adopted scoring systems was developed by Apfel and colleagues (1998)

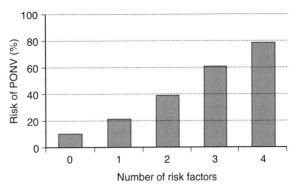

Fig. 7.2 Relationship between the number of risk factors and the incidence of postoperative nausea and vomiting *(PONV)*. (From Fero et al. (2011).)

and colleagues and uses four independent predictors (see Box 7.2) to determine the likelihood of PONV. These are:
- female sex;
- non-smokers;
- history of PONV or motion sickness; and
- use of opioids.

Each positive predictor is assigned a score of 1. Using this system, a score of 0, 1, 2, 3 or 4 predicts the chance of developing PONV as approximately 10%, 20%, 40%, 60% or 80% (Fig. 7.2). Other scoring systems include the duration and type of anaesthesia, but these have not been found to have any additional predictive value beyond that of Apfel's simplified version. Patients at low risk do not usually require pharmacological intervention, and some advocate adopting a wait and see policy. Simply reducing baseline risk by avoiding key triggers, such as opioids and volatile agents, or using loco-regional techniques may be sufficient. For those at moderate risk, the combination of two agents (e.g. 5-HT_3 receptor antagonist, butyrophenone or antihistamine) along with dexamethasone has been found to be more effective than a single agent. For patients at highest risk, avoiding key triggers combined with a multimodal antiemetic regimen usually works best.

Treatment

Despite careful planning and risk reduction, some patients still experience troublesome PONV. In these cases, it is vital that all possible causes of PONV are ruled out to avoid missing important signs of a serious underlying pathology. The most common causes of PONV are highlighted in Box 7.3. Each patient should be thoroughly assessed to exclude treatable triggers of PONV and, when these have been excluded, an appropriate antiemetic strategy devised. If prophylaxis has already been given, repeat dosing may

129

Box 7.3 **Other causes of PONV**

Hypotension
Hypoxaemia
Drugs
Opioids
Antibiotics
Intra-abdominal pathological conditions
Psychological factors (e.g. fear, emotional stress)
Early mobilisation
Dehydration
Pain

can be supplemented using one or more of the available D_2, M_1, H_1 or 5-HT_3 receptor antagonists.

Other techniques

Baseline risk reduction plays a key role in preventing PONV – for example, avoiding general anaesthesia and/or using locoregional techniques instead. If general anaesthesia is required, TIVA will exploit the antiemetic properties of propofol whilst avoiding the emetogenic effects of inhalational anaesthetic agents. Minimising opioid use and maintaining adequate hydration are other important aspects of baseline risk reduction. Non-pharmacological methods include acupuncture or acupressure targeted at the P6 (Neiguan) point between the flexor carpi radialis and the palmaris longus. In some studies, stimulation of the P6 point was as effective as a single dose of ondansetron or droperidol. Symptomatic relief was achieved for up to 6 h and could be extended if treatment was repeated. A variety of options (including transcutaneous nerve stimulation and oral ginger) have been assessed for the prevention and treatment of PONV, but the evidence base for these interventions is currently lacking.

be required, depending on the pharmacokinetic profile of the initial agent, bearing in mind that a second dose may be ineffective and might simply increase the risk of adverse effects. The next stage involves the use of drugs acting at different receptors. This multimodal approach maximises antiemetic efficacy whilst minimising the risk of adverse drug events. For example, PONV prophylaxis using a glucocorticoid

References/Further reading

Apfel, C.C., Greim, C.A., Haubitz, I., et al., 1998. A risk score to predict the probability of postoperative vomiting in adults. Acta Anaesthesiol. Scand. 42 (5), 495–501.

Diemunsch, P., Joshi, G.P., Brichant, J.F., 2009. Neurokinin-1 receptor antagonists in the prevention of postoperative nausea and vomiting. Br. J. Anaesth. 103, 7–13.

Fero, K.E., Jalota, L., Hornuss, C., Apfel, C.C., 2011. Pharmacologic management of postoperative nausea and vomiting. Expert Opin. Pharmacother. 12, 2283–2296.

Gan, T.J., Diemunsch, P., Habib, A.S., et al., 2014. Consensus guidelines for the management of postoperative nausea and vomiting. Anesth. Analg. 118 (1), 85–113.

Guidelines on the Prevention of Postoperative Vomiting in Children. https://www.apagbi.org.uk/sites/default/files/inline-files/2016%20APA%20POV%20Guideline-2.pdf (Accessed October 2018).

Watcha, M.F., White, P.F., 1992. Postoperative nausea and vomiting. Its etiology, treatment and prevention. Anesthesiology 77, 162–184.

Chapter | 8 |

Muscle function and neuromuscular blockade

Jennifer Hunter, Martin Shields

In the last 70 years, neuromuscular blocking drugs have become an established part of anaesthetic practice. They were first administered during abdominal surgery in 1942, when Griffith and Johnson in Montreal used Intocostrin, a biologically standardised mixture of the alkaloids of the Indian rubber plant *chondrodendron tomentosum* to facilitate muscle relaxation during cyclopropane anaesthesia. Previously, only inhalational agents had been used during general anaesthesia, making surgical access for some procedures difficult. To achieve significant muscle relaxation, it was necessary to deepen anaesthesia, which often had adverse cardiac and respiratory effects.

At first, neuromuscular blocking agents were used only occasionally, in small doses, as an adjunct to aid in the management of a difficult case. A tracheal tube was not always used, the lungs were not ventilated artificially and residual block was not routinely reversed; all these approaches caused significant morbidity and mortality, as demonstrated in the retrospective study by Beecher and Todd (1954). By 1946, however, it was appreciated that using drugs such as curare in larger doses allowed the depth of anaesthesia to be lightened, and it was suggested that incremental doses should also be used during prolonged surgery, rather than deepening anaesthesia – an entirely new concept at that time. The use of routine tracheal intubation and artificial ventilation then evolved.

In 1946, Gray and Halton in Liverpool reported their experience of using the pure alkaloid tubocurarine in more than 1000 patients receiving various anaesthetic agents. Over the following 6 years, they developed a concise description of the necessary ingredients of any anaesthetic technique; narcosis, analgesia and muscle relaxation were essential – the *triad* of balanced anaesthesia. A fourth ingredient, controlled apnoea, was added at a later stage to emphasise the need for fully controlled ventilation, reducing the amount of NMBA required.

This concept is the basis of the use of neuromuscular blocking agents in modern anaesthetic practice. In particular, it has allowed seriously ill patients undergoing complex surgery to be anaesthetised safely and to be cared for postoperatively in the intensive therapy unit.

Physiology of neuromuscular transmission

Acetylcholine, the neurotransmitter at the neuromuscular junction, is released from presynaptic nerve endings on passage of a nerve impulse (an action potential) down the axon to the nerve terminal. The neurotransmitter is synthesised from choline and acetylcoenzyme A by the enzyme *choline acetyltransferase* and stored in vesicles in the nerve terminal. The action potential depolarises the nerve terminal to release the neurotransmitter; entry of Ca^{2+} ions into the nerve terminal is a necessary part of this process, promoting further acetylcholine release. On the arrival of an action potential, the storage vesicles are transferred to the active zones on the edge of the axonal membrane, where they fuse with the terminal wall to release the acetylcholine (Fig. 8.1). Three proteins, synaptobrevin, syntaxin and synaptosome-associated protein SNAP-25, are involved in this process. These proteins along with vesicle membrane-associated synaptotagmins cause the docking, fusion and release (exocytosis) of acetylcholine from the vesicles. There are about 1000 active sites at each nerve ending, and any one nerve action potential leads to the release of 200–300 vesicles. In addition, small *quanta* of acetylcholine, equivalent to the contents of one vesicle, are released at the neuromuscular junction spontaneously, causing miniature end-plate potentials (MEPPs) on the postsynaptic membrane, but these are insufficient to generate a muscle action potential.

The active sites of release are aligned directly opposite the acetylcholine receptors on the junctional folds of the

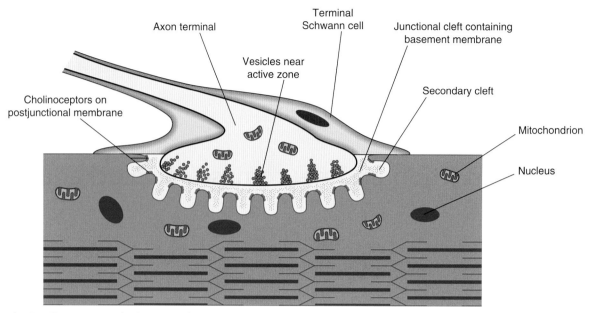

Fig. 8.1 The neuromuscular junction with an axon terminal, containing vesicles of acetylcholine. The neurotransmitter is released on arrival of an action potential and crosses the junctional cleft to stimulate the postjunctional receptors on the shoulders of the secondary clefts. (Reproduced with the kind permission of Professor W.C. Bowman.)

Table 8.1 Subtypes of nicotinic receptors involved in neuromuscular blockade

Name	Location	Type	Role in neuromuscular transmission
$\alpha_3\beta_2$	Presynaptic	Neuronal	Involved in regulation of acetylcholine release, especially during higher rates of stimulation. Inhibition by non-depolarising NMBAs results in fade of the TOF response. Very low affinity for suxamethonium.
$\alpha_2\beta\delta\epsilon$	Postsynaptic	Muscle	Main site of action for NMBAs.
$\alpha_2\beta\delta\gamma$	Postsynaptic	Muscle	Present in denervation states and other neuromuscular disorders. Slower onset of neuromuscular blockade and increased duration of paralysis with NMBAs.
α_7	Postsynaptic	Neuronal	Expressed mainly in denervation states and other neuromuscular disorders. Possible role in inflammation regulation.

NMBAs, Neuromuscular blocking agents; *TOF,* train of four.

postsynaptic membrane, lying on the muscle surface. The junctional cleft, the gap between the nerve terminal and the muscle membrane, has a width of only 60 nm. It contains the enzyme *acetylcholinesterase,* which is responsible for the ultimate breakdown of acetylcholine. This enzyme is also present in higher concentrations in the junctional folds in the postsynaptic membrane (see Fig. 8.1). The choline produced by the breakdown of acetylcholine is taken up across the nerve membrane to be reused in the synthesis of the transmitter.

Several differing nicotinic acetylcholine receptors are located at the neuromuscular junction. These are classified initially as either muscle-type or neuronal acetylcholine receptors, with further subclassification on the basis of the subunits that form each receptor (Table 8.1). The muscle-type nicotinic acetylcholine receptors on the postsynaptic membrane are organised in discrete clusters on the shoulders of the junctional folds (see Fig. 8.1). Each cluster is about 100 nm in diameter and contains a few hundred receptors. Each receptor consists of five subunits, two of which, the α (molecular weight (MW) = 40,000 Da), are identical. The other three slightly larger subunits are the β, δ and ε. In fetal muscle, the ε is replaced by a γ subunit. Each subunit of the receptor is a glycosated protein coded by a different gene. The receptors are arranged as a cylinder which spans the membrane, with a central, normally closed, channel – the ionophore (Fig. 8.2). Each of the α subunits carries a single acetylcholine binding region on its extracellular surface. They also bind neuromuscular blocking drugs.

Activation of the receptor requires both α sites to be occupied, producing a structural change in the receptor complex that opens the central channel running between the receptors for a very short period, about 1 ms (see Fig. 8.2). This allows movement of cations such as Na^+, K^+, Ca^{2+} and Mg^{2+} along their concentration gradients. The main change is influx of Na^+ ions, the *end-plate current*, followed by efflux of K^+ ions. The summation of this current through a large number of receptor channels lowers the transmembrane potential of the end-plate region sufficiently to depolarise it and generate a muscle action potential sufficient to allow muscle contraction.

At rest, the transmembrane potential is about −90 mV (inside negative). Under normal physiological conditions, a depolarisation of about 40 mV occurs, lowering the potential from −90 to −50 mV. When the *end-plate potential* reaches this critical threshold, it triggers an *all-or-nothing* action potential that passes around the sarcolemma to activate muscle contraction.

Each acetylcholine molecule is involved in opening one ion channel only before it is broken down rapidly by acetylcholinesterase; it does not interact with any of the other receptors. There is a large safety factor in the transmission process in respect of both the amount of acetylcholine released and the number of postsynaptic receptors. Much more acetylcholine is released than is necessary to trigger the action potential. The end-plate region is depolarised for

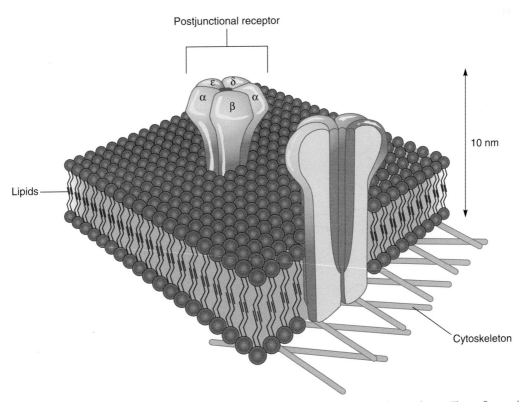

Fig. 8.2 Two postjunctional receptors, embedded in the lipid layer of the postsynaptic muscle membrane. The α, β, ε and δ subunits are demonstrated on the surface of one receptor, and the ionophore is seen in cross-section on the other receptor. On stimulation of the two α subunits by two molecules of acetylcholine, the ionophore opens to allow the passage of the end-plate current. (Reproduced with the kind permission of Professor W.C. Bowman.)

only a very short period (a few milliseconds) before it rapidly repolarises and is ready to transmit another impulse.

Acetylcholine receptors are also present on the presynaptic area of the nerve terminal. These are of a slightly different structure to the postsynaptic nicotinic receptors ($\alpha_3\beta_2$; see Table 8.1). It is thought that a positive feedback mechanism exists for the further release of acetylcholine such that some of the released molecules of acetylcholine stimulate these presynaptic receptors, producing further mobilisation of the neurotransmitter to the readily releasable sites, ready for the arrival of the next nerve stimulus (Fig. 8.3). Acetylcholine activates sodium channels on the prejunctional nerve membrane, which in turn activate voltage-dependent calcium channels (P-type fast channels) on the motor neuron, causing an influx of Ca^{2+} into the nerve cytoplasm to promote further acetylcholine release.

The wave of depolarisation spreads from the postsynaptic membrane along the plasma membrane of the muscle fibres. Deep clefts in the membrane, called T-tubules, allow this wave to penetrate into close proximity with L-type calcium channel receptors, which in turn interact with ryanodine receptors in the sarcoplasmic reticulum to cause the release of Ca^{2+} into the myoplasm. The Ca^{2+} ions interact with troponin C to counter the inhibitory effect of troponin I and tropomyosin on the sarcomere complex, thus allowing thin actin myofilaments to slide over the thicker myosin microfilaments to generate muscle tension. As Ca^{2+} is reabsorbed into the sarcoplasmic reticulum, the actin and myosin become less tightly bound and muscle tension reduces.

In health, postsynaptic acetylcholine receptors are restricted to the neuromuscular junction by a mechanism involving the presence of an active nerve terminal. In many disease states affecting the neuromuscular junction, this control is lost, and acetylcholine receptors of the fetal and α_7 types develop on the adjacent muscle surface. The excessive release of K^+ ions from diseased or swollen muscle on administration of suxamethonium is probably the result of stimulation of these *extrajunctional receptors*. They develop in many conditions, including polyneuropathies, severe burns and muscle disorders.

Pharmacology of neuromuscular transmission

Neuromuscular blocking agents (NMBAs) used regularly by anaesthetists are classified into *depolarising* (or *non-competitive*) and *non-depolarising* (or *competitive*) agents. The individual neuromuscular blocking agents differ in the following aspects:

- Potency (effective dose for tracheal intubation in 95% of patients: ED_{95})
- Onset time
- Duration of action
- Metabolism
- Mode of elimination

Those with a lower potency, such as rocuronium and suxamethonium, tend to have shorter onset times. The intubating dose recommended for routine use typically equates to twice the ED_{95} for each NMBA. Increasing this dose to three or four times the ED_{95} shortens the onset further, forming the basis for drug choice during rapid-sequence induction. At these doses the duration of action is markedly increased for the non-depolarising agents, and the therapeutic index also narrows, increasing the likelihood of adverse effects, especially those related to histamine release. Suxamethonium and rocuronium are the drugs of choice for rapid-sequence induction.

The duration of action of suxamethonium is mainly determined by its rapid metabolism in the plasma. In contrast, the elimination half-life of non-depolarising agents far exceeds their duration of clinical effects. Redistribution of these drugs away from the muscle accounts for most of the offset of action. The concept of the *ideal neuromuscular blocking agent* has been described based on its putative pharmacokinetic and pharmacodynamic properties; some such properties are presented in Box 8.1.

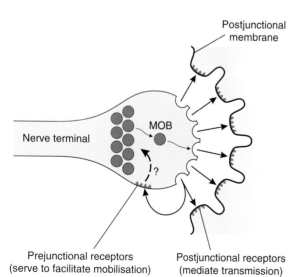

Fig. 8.3 Acetylcholine receptors are present on the shoulders of the axon terminal as well as on the postjunctional membrane. Stimulation of the prejunctional receptors mobilises *(MOB)* the vesicles of acetylcholine to move into the active zone, ready for release on arrival of another nerve impulse. The mechanism requires Ca^{2+} ions. (Reproduced with the kind permission of Professor W.C. Bowman.)

Box 8.1 **Properties of an ideal neuromuscular blocking agent**

- Non-depolarising
- Ultra-short onset of action (<1 min)
- Short duration of action and suitable for infusion
- Metabolised, independent of renal or hepatic function, to inactive compounds
- Complete recovery from block in predictable and short time (with or without reversal agents)
- Absence of antimuscarinic or other adverse effects
- Does not cross blood–brain barrier or placenta
- Stable compound at room temperature; supplied as a solution
- Similar effect in all individuals
- Inexpensive

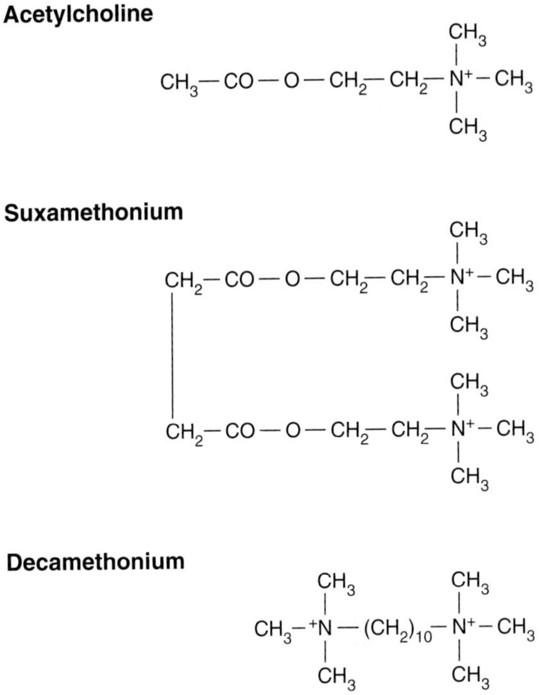

Depolarising neuromuscular blocking agents

The only depolarising NMBA now available in clinical practice is suxamethonium. Decamethonium was used clinically in the UK for many years, but it is now available only for research purposes.

Suxamethonium (succinylcholine chloride)

This quaternary ammonium compound is comparable to two molecules of acetylcholine linked together (Fig. 8.4). The two quaternary ammonium radicals, $N^+(CH_3)_3$, have the capacity to cling to each of the α units of the postsynaptic acetylcholine receptor, altering its structural conformation and opening the ion channel, but for a longer period than does a molecule of acetylcholine. Administration of suxamethonium therefore results in an initial depolarisation and muscle contraction, termed *fasciculation*. As this effect persists, however, further action potentials cannot pass down the ion channels, and the muscle becomes flaccid; repolarisation does not occur.

The dose of suxamethonium necessary for tracheal intubation in adults is 1.0–1.5 mg kg^{-1}. This dose has the most rapid and reliable onset of action of any of the NMBAs presently available, producing profound block within 1 min. Suxamethonium is therefore of particular benefit when it is essential to achieve tracheal intubation rapidly, such as in a patient with a full stomach or an obstetric patient.

The drug is metabolised predominantly in the plasma by the enzyme *plasma cholinesterase,* at one time termed

Acetylcholine

Suxamethonium

Decamethonium

Fig. 8.4 The chemical structures of acetylcholine and suxamethonium. The similarity between the structure of suxamethonium and two molecules of acetylcholine can be seen. The structure of decamethonium is also shown. The quaternary ammonium radicals $N^+(CH_3)_3$ cling to the α subunits of the postsynaptic receptor.

pseudocholinesterase, at a very rapid rate. Recovery from neuromuscular block may start to occur within 3 min and is complete within 12–15 min. The use of an anticholinesterase such as neostigmine, which would inhibit such enzyme activity, is contraindicated (see later). About 10% of the drug is excreted in the urine; there is very little metabolism in the liver, although some breakdown by non-specific esterases occurs in the plasma.

If plasma cholinesterase is structurally abnormal because of inherited factors, or if its concentration is reduced by acquired factors, then the duration of action of the drug may be altered significantly.

Inherited factors

The exact structure of plasma cholinesterase is determined genetically by autosomal genes, and this has been completely defined. Several abnormalities in the amino acid sequence of the normal enzyme, usually designated E_1^u, are recognised. The most common is produced by the atypical gene, E_1^a, which occurs in about 4% of the Caucasian population. Thus a patient who is a *heterozygote* for the atypical gene (E_1^u, E_1^a) demonstrates a longer effect from a standard dose of suxamethonium (about 30 min). If the individual is a *homozygote* for the atypical gene (E_1^a, E_1^a), the duration of action of suxamethonium may exceed 2 h. Other, rarer, abnormalities in the structure of plasma cholinesterase are also recognised, such as the fluoride (E_1^f) and silent (E_1^s) genes. The latter has very little capacity to metabolise suxamethonium, and thus neuromuscular block in the homozygous state (E_1^s, E_1^s) lasts for at least 3 h. In such patients, non-specific esterases gradually clear the drug from plasma.

It has been suggested that a source of cholinesterase such as fresh frozen plasma should be administered in such cases, or an anticholinesterase such as neostigmine be used to reverse what has usually developed into a *dual block* (see later). However, it is wiser to:

- keep the patient anaesthetised and the lungs ventilated artificially, and
- monitor neuromuscular transmission accurately until full recovery from residual neuromuscular block.

This condition is not life-threatening, but the risk of awareness is considerable, especially after the end of surgery, when the anaesthetist, who may not yet have made the diagnosis, is attempting to waken the patient. Anaesthesia must be continued until full recovery from neuromuscular block is demonstrable.

As plasma cholinesterase activity is reduced by the presence of suxamethonium, a plasma sample to measure the patient's cholinesterase activity should not be taken for several days after prolonged block has been experienced, by which time new enzyme has been synthesised. A patient who is found to have reduced enzyme activity and structurally abnormal enzyme should be given a warning card or alarm bracelet, detailing his or her genetic status. Examining the plasma cholinesterase activity and genetic status of the patient's immediate relatives should be considered. Historically, testing for atypical plasma cholinesterases was done using the dibucaine number (see further reading).

Acquired factors

In these instances, the structure of plasma cholinesterase is normal but its activity is reduced. Thus neuromuscular block is prolonged by only minutes rather than hours. Causes of reduced plasma cholinesterase activity include the following:

- Liver disease, because of reduced enzyme synthesis.
- Carcinomatosis and starvation, also because of reduced enzyme synthesis.
- Pregnancy, for two reasons: an increased circulating volume (dilutional effect) and decreased enzyme synthesis.
- Anticholinesterases, including those used to reverse residual neuromuscular block after a non-depolarising NMBA (e.g. neostigmine); these drugs inhibit plasma cholinesterase in addition to acetylcholinesterase. The

organophosphorus compound *ecothiopate*, once used topically as a miotic in ophthalmology, is also an anticholinesterase.
- Other drugs which are metabolised by plasma cholinesterase and which therefore decrease its availability, including etomidate, ester local anaesthetics, anticancer drugs such as methotrexate, monoamine oxidase inhibitors and esmolol.
- Hypothyroidism.
- Cardiopulmonary bypass, plasmapheresis.
- Renal disease.

Adverse effects of suxamethonium

Although suxamethonium is a very useful drug for achieving tracheal intubation rapidly, it has several undesirable effects which may limit its use.

Muscle pains

Muscle pains occur especially in the patient who is ambulant soon after surgery, such as the day-case patient. The pains, thought possibly to be caused by the initial fasciculations, are more common in young, healthy patients with a large muscle mass. They occur in unusual sites, such as the diaphragm and between the scapulae, and are not relieved easily by conventional analgesics. The incidence and severity may be reduced by the use of a small dose of a non-depolarising NMBA given immediately before administration of suxamethonium (e.g. atracurium 0.05 mg kg^{-1}). However, this technique, termed *precurarisation* or *pretreatment*, reduces the potency of suxamethonium, necessitating administration of a larger dose to produce the same effect. Between 1 and 3 min have been recommended between administering the non-depolarising NMBA and the subsequent suxamethonium, which can lead to a period of partial curarisation in an awake patient. Many other drugs have been used in an attempt to reduce the muscle pains, including lidocaine, calcium, magnesium and repeated doses of thiopental, but none is completely reliable.

Increased intraocular pressure

Increased intraocular pressure is thought to be caused partly by the initial contraction of the external ocular muscles and contracture of the internal ocular muscles after administration of suxamethonium. It is not reduced by precurarisation. The effect lasts for as long as the neuromuscular block, and concern has been expressed that it may be sufficient to cause expulsion of the vitreous contents in the patient with an open eye injury. This is unlikely. Protection of the airway from gastric contents must take priority in the patient with a full stomach in addition to an eye injury, as inhalation of gastric contents may threaten life (see Chapter 38). It is also possible that suxamethonium may increase intracranial pressure, although this is less certain.

Increased intragastric pressure

In the presence of a normal lower oesophageal sphincter, the increase in intragastric pressure produced by suxamethonium should be insufficient to produce regurgitation of gastric contents. However, in the patient with incompetence of this sphincter from, for example, hiatus hernia, regurgitation may occur.

Hyperkalaemia

It has long been recognised that administration of suxamethonium during halothane anaesthesia increases serum potassium concentration by 0.5 mmol l^{-1}. This is thought to be caused by muscle fasciculation. It is probable that the effect is less marked with the newer potent inhalational agents isoflurane, sevoflurane and desflurane. A similar increase occurs in patients with renal failure, but as these patients may already have an elevated serum potassium concentration, such an increase may precipitate cardiac irregularities and even cardiac arrest.

In some conditions in which the muscle cells are swollen or damaged, or in which there is proliferation of extrajunctional receptors (see Table 8.1), this release of potassium may be exaggerated. This is most marked in the burned patient, in whom K$^+$ concentrations up to 13 mmol l^{-1} have been reported. Suxamethonium should be avoided in this condition. In diseases of the muscle cell or its nerve supply, hyperkalaemia after suxamethonium may also be exaggerated. These include the muscular dystrophies, dystrophia myotonica and paraplegia. Hyperkalaemia has been reported to cause death in such patients. Suxamethonium may also precipitate prolonged contracture of the masseter muscles in patients with these disorders, making tracheal intubation impossible. The drug should be avoided in any patient with a neuromuscular disorder, including the patient with *malignant hyperthermia*, in whom the drug is a recognised trigger factor.

Hyperkalaemia after suxamethonium has also been reported, albeit rarely, in patients with widespread intra-abdominal infection, severe trauma and closed head injury.

Cardiovascular effects

Suxamethonium has muscarinic, in addition to nicotinic, effects, as does acetylcholine. The direct vagal effect (muscarinic) produces sinus bradycardia, especially in patients with high vagal tone, such as children and the physically fit. It is also more common in the patient who has not received an anticholinergic agent (such as glycopyrronium bromide) or who is given repeated increments of suxamethonium. It is advisable to use an anticholinergic routinely if it is planned to administer more than one dose of suxamethonium. Nodal or ventricular escape beats may develop in extreme circumstances.

Allergic anaphylaxis

Immunoglobulin E (IgE)–mediated allergic reactions to suxamethonium are rare but may occur, especially after repeated exposure to the drug. They are more common after suxamethonium than any other neuromuscular blocking agent. A blood test is available to measure plasma suxamethonium IgE concentrations to aid in the diagnosis of allergic anaphylaxis to this agent. No such test is available commercially for the other NMBAs.

Characteristics of depolarising neuromuscular block

If neuromuscular block is monitored (see later), several differences between depolarising and non-depolarising block may be defined. In the presence of a small dose of suxamethonium:

- A decreased response to a single, low-voltage (1 Hz) twitch stimulus applied to a peripheral nerve is detected. Tetanic stimulation (e.g. at 50 Hz) produces a small but sustained response.
- If four twitch stimuli are applied at 2 Hz over 2 s (train-of-four stimulus), followed by a 10-s interval before the next train-of-four, no decrease in the height of successive stimuli is noted (Fig. 8.5).
- The application of a 5-s burst of tetanic stimulation after the application of single twitch stimuli, followed 3 s later by a further run of twitch stimuli, produces no potentiation of the twitch height; there is no *post-tetanic potentiation* (sometimes termed *facilitation*).
- Neuromuscular block is *potentiated* by the administration of an anticholinesterase such as neostigmine.
- If repeated doses of suxamethonium are given, the characteristics of this depolarising block alter; signs typical of a non-depolarising block develop (see later). Initially, such changes are demonstrable only at fast rates of stimulation, but with further increments of suxamethonium, they may occur at slower rates. This phenomenon is termed *dual block* or *phase 2 block*.
- Muscle fasciculation is typical of a depolarising block.

Non-depolarising neuromuscular blocking agents

Unlike suxamethonium, these drugs do not alter the structural conformity of the postsynaptic acetylcholine receptor and therefore do not produce an initial contraction. Instead, they compete with the neurotransmitter at this site, binding reversibly to one or two of the α receptors whenever these are not occupied by acetylcholine. The end-plate potential produced in the presence of a non-depolarising agent is therefore smaller; it does not reach the threshold necessary to initiate a propagating action potential to activate the

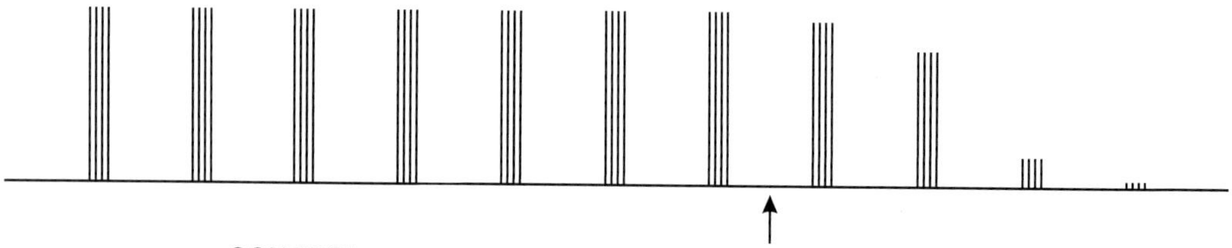

Fig. 8.5 The train-of-four twitch response recorded before (CONTROL) and after a dose of suxamethonium. Before administration of suxamethonium 1 mg kg^{-1}, four twitches of equal height are visible. After giving the drug (SUCC), the heights of all four twitches decrease equally; no fade of the train-of-four is seen. Within 1 min, the trace has been ablated.

sarcolemma and produce an initial muscle contraction. More than 75% of the postsynaptic receptors have to be blocked in this way before there is failure of muscle contraction – a large safety factor. However, in large doses, non-depolarising NMBAs impair neuromuscular transmission sufficiently to produce profound neuromuscular block.

Metabolism of NMBAs does not occur at the neuromuscular junction. By the end of surgery, the end-plate concentration of the NMBA is decreasing as the drug diffuses down a concentration gradient back into the plasma, from which it is cleared. Thus more receptors are stimulated by the neurotransmitter, allowing recovery from block. An anticholinesterase given at this time increases the half-life of acetylcholine at the neuromuscular junction, facilitating recovery.

Non-depolarising neuromuscular blocking agents are highly ionised, water-soluble drugs which are distributed mainly in plasma and extracellular fluid. Thus they have a relatively small volume of distribution. They are of two main types of chemical structure: either *benzylisoquinolinium compounds*, such as atracurium, mivacurium, cisatracurium, tubocurarine and alcuronium; or *aminosteroid compounds*, such as rocuronium, vecuronium, pancuronium and pipecuronium. All these drugs possess at least one quaternary ammonium group, $N^+(CH_3)_3$, to bind to an α subunit on the postsynaptic receptor. Some benzylisoquinolinium compounds consist of quaternary ammonium groups joined by a thin chain of methyl groups. They are therefore more liable to breakdown in the plasma than are the aminosteroids. They are also more likely to release histamine.

Benzylisoquinolinium compounds

Tubocurarine chloride is the only naturally occurring neuromuscular blocking agent. It is derived from the bark of the South American plant *chondrodendron tomentosum*, which has been used for centuries by South American Indians as an arrow poison. It was the first non-depolarising neuromuscular blocking agent to be used in humans. It has a marked propensity to produce histamine release and thus hypotension, with possibly a compensatory tachycardia.

Historically, tubocurarine, alcuronium and gallamine have been used in clinical practice, but they are no longer available in the UK. Alcuronium chloride is a semisynthetic derivative of toxiferin, an alkaloid of calabash curare. Gallamine triethiodide is a trisquaternary amine. It was first used in France in 1948. The only recent use of gallamine in the UK was as a small pretreatment dose (10 mg) before suxamethonium.

Atracurium besilate

Atracurium besilate, introduced into clinical practice in 1982, was developed by Stenlake at Strathclyde University. Quaternary ammonium compounds break down spontaneously at varying temperature and pH, a phenomenon recognised for more than 100 years and known as *Hofmann degradation*. Atracurium was developed in the search for such an agent which broke down at body temperature and pH. Hofmann degradation may be considered as a safety net in the sick patient with impaired liver or renal function as atracurium is still cleared. Some renal excretion occurs in the healthy patient (10%), as does ester hydrolysis in the plasma; probably only about 45% of the drug is eliminated by Hofmann degradation in the normal patient.

Atracurium (and vecuronium) was developed in an attempt to obtain a non-depolarising agent which had a more rapid onset, was shorter acting and had fewer cardiovascular effects than the older agents. Atracurium 0.5 mg kg^{-1} does not produce neuromuscular block as rapidly as suxamethonium; the onset time is 2.0–2.5 min (Table 8.2). However, recovery occurs more rapidly from it than after use of the older non-depolarising agents, and atracurium may be reversed easily 20–25 min after administration of a dose of $2 \times ED_{95}$ (0.45 mg kg^{-1}). The drug does not have any direct cardiovascular effect but may release histamine and may therefore produce a local wheal and flare around the injection site, especially if a small vein is used. This may be accompanied by a slight reduction in arterial pressure. Using $3 \times ED_{95}$ is associated with increased histamine release, and therefore rapid sequence with atracurium is not advised. It can produce anaphylaxis, but to a lesser degree than suxamethonium.

Table 8.2 Time to 95% depression of the twitch response after a dose of $2 \times ED_{95}$ of a neuromuscular blocking drug (when tracheal intubation should be possible), and time to 20%–25% recovery when an anticholinesterase may be used to reverse residual block produced by a non-depolarising drug

	95% Twitch depression (s)	20%–25% Recovery (min)
Depolarising		
Suxamethonium	60	10
Non-depolarising		
Benzylisoquinoliniums		
Atracurium	110	43
Cisatracurium	150	45
Mivacurium	170	16
Doxacurium	250	83
Aminosteroids		
Rocuronium	75	33
Vecuronium	180	33
Pancuronium	220	75
Pipecuronium	300	95
No longer used		
Tubocurarine	220	80+
Alcuronium	420	70
Gallamine	300	80
Rapacuronium	<75	15

A metabolite of Hofmann degradation, *laudanosine,* has epileptogenic properties, although fits have never been reported in humans. The plasma concentrations of laudanosine required to make animals convulse are much higher than those occurring during general anaesthesia, even if large doses of atracurium are given during a prolonged procedure, and there is little cause for concern about this metabolite in clinical practice. In patients with multiple organ failure, who may receive atracurium for several days in ICU, laudanosine concentrations are higher, but no reports of cerebral toxicity have occurred.

Cisatracurium
Cisatracurium is the most recently introduced benzylisoquinolinium neuromuscular blocking drug. It is of particular interest because it is an example of the development of a specific isomer of a drug to produce a clean substance with the desired clinical actions but with reduced side effects. Cisatracurium is the 1R-*cis* 1'R-*cis* isomer of atracurium and one of 10 isomers of the parent compound. It is three to four times more potent than atracurium ($ED_{95} = 0.05$ mg kg^{-1}) and has a slightly slower onset and longer duration of action. Its main advantage is that it does not release histamine and therefore is associated with greater cardiovascular stability. It undergoes even more Hofmann degradation than atracurium.

Doxacurium chloride
Doxacurium chloride, a bisquaternary ammonium compound, is only available in the United States. It undergoes a small amount of metabolism in the plasma by cholinesterase (6%) but is excreted mainly through the kidneys. It is the most potent non-depolarising neuromuscular blocking agent available; an intubating dose is only 0.05 mg kg^{-1}. It has a very slow onset of action (see Table 8.2) and a prolonged and unpredictable duration of effect. However, it has no cardiovascular effects and may therefore be of use during long surgical procedures in which cardiovascular stability is required, such as cardiac surgery.

Mivacurium chloride
Mivacurium chloride is metabolised by plasma cholinesterase at 88% of the rate of suxamethonium. An intubating dose ($2 \times ED_{95} = 0.15$ mg kg^{-1}) has a similar onset of action to an equipotent dose of atracurium, but in the presence of normal plasma cholinesterase, recovery after mivacurium is much faster (see Table 8.2), and administration of an anticholinesterase may not be necessary (if neuromuscular function is being monitored and good recovery can be demonstrated). Full recovery in such circumstances takes about 20–25 min, but the drug may be antagonised easily within 15 min. Mivacurium is useful particularly for surgical procedures requiring muscle relaxation in which even atracurium and vecuronium seem too long acting and when it is desirable to avoid the side effects of suxamethonium (e.g. for bronchoscopy, oesophagoscopy, laparoscopy or tonsillectomy). The drug produces a similar amount of histamine release to atracurium.

In the presence of reduced plasma cholinesterase activity, because of either inherited or acquired factors, the duration of action of mivacurium may be increased. The action of the drug may also be prolonged in patients with hepatic or renal disease, in whom plasma cholinesterase activity may be reduced.

Aminosteroid compounds

Aminosteroid compounds, non-depolarising NMBAs, possess at least one quaternary ammonium group, attached to a steroid nucleus. They produce fewer adverse cardiovascular effects than do the benzylisoquinolinium compounds and do not stimulate histamine release from mast cells to the same degree. They are excreted unchanged through the kidneys and also undergo deacetylation in the liver. The deacetylated metabolites may possess weak neuromuscular blocking properties. The parent compound may also be excreted unchanged in the bile.

Pancuronium bromide

Pancuronium bromide, a bisquaternary amine and the first steroid NMBA used clinically, was developed by Savege and Hewitt and marketed in 1964. The intubating dose is 0.1 mg kg^{-1}, which takes 3–4 min to reach its maximum effect (see Table 8.2). The clinical duration of action of the drug is long, especially in the presence of potent inhalational agents or renal dysfunction, as 60% of a dose of the drug is excreted unchanged through the kidneys. It is also deacetylated in the liver; some of the metabolites have neuromuscular blocking properties.

Pancuronium does not stimulate histamine release; however, it has direct vagolytic and sympathomimetic effects which may cause tachycardia and hypertension. It slightly inhibits plasma cholinesterase and therefore potentiates any drug metabolised by this enzyme, such as suxamethonium and mivacurium.

Vecuronium bromide

Vecuronium bromide is steroidal agent that was developed in an attempt to reduce the cardiovascular effects of pancuronium. It is similar in structure to the older drug, differing only in the loss of a methyl group from one quaternary ammonium radical. Thus it is a monoquaternary amine. An intubating dose of 0.1 mg kg^{-1} produces profound neuromuscular block within 3 min. This dose produces clinical block for about 30 min. Vecuronium rarely produces histamine release, nor does it have any direct cardiovascular effects, although it allows the cardiac effects of other anaesthetic agents, such as bradycardia produced by the opioids, to go unchallenged. Vecuronium is excreted through the kidneys (30%), although to a lesser extent than pancuronium, and undergoes hepatic deacetylation; the deacetylated metabolites have neuromuscular blocking properties. Repeated doses should be used with care in patients with renal or hepatic disease because they accumulate.

Pipecuronium bromide

Pipecuronium bromide, an analogue of pancuronium, was developed in Hungary in 1980 and is marketed in Eastern Europe and the United States. The intubating dose is 0.07 mg kg^{-1}. The onset time and time to recovery from block are similar to those of pancuronium (see Table 8.2), and excretion of the drug through the kidneys is significant (66%). In contrast to pancuronium, pipecuronium produces marked cardiovascular stability, having no vagolytic or sympathomimetic effects. It may therefore be useful during major surgery in patients with cardiac disease.

Rocuronium bromide

Rocuronium bromide, a monoquaternary amine, has a very rapid onset of action for a non-depolarising NMBA. It is six to eight times less potent than vecuronium but has approximately the same molecular weight; consequently, a greater number of drug molecules may reach the postjunctional receptors within the first few circulations, enabling faster development of neuromuscular block. In a dose of 0.6 mg kg^{-1}, good or excellent intubating conditions are achieved within 60–90 s; this is only slightly slower than the onset time of suxamethonium. The clinical duration is 30–45 min. At higher doses, such as 0.9 to 1.2 mg kg^{-1}, rocuronium has an onset time similar to suxamethonium, albeit with a greater range of effect. In such doses, however, rocuronium is a very long-acting drug, lasting about 90 min.

In most other respects, rocuronium resembles vecuronium. The drug stimulates little histamine release or cardiovascular disturbance, although in high doses it has a mild vagolytic property which sometimes results in an increase in heart rate. The drug is excreted unchanged in the urine and in the bile, and thus the duration of action may be increased by severe renal or hepatic dysfunction. Rocuronium has no metabolites with significant neuromuscular blocking activity.

Anaphylactic reactions are more common after rocuronium than after other aminosteroid neuromuscular blocking drugs. They occur at a similar rate to anaphylactic reactions to atracurium and mivacurium.

Rapacuronium bromide

Rapacuronium bromide was the last aminosteroid to become available. It is less potent than rocuronium ($2 \times ED_{95} = 1.5$ mg kg^{-1}) and in equipotent doses has an even more rapid onset of action (<75 s). After several reports to the US Food and Drug Administration of bronchospasm and hypoxaemia after administration of rapacuronium, especially in small children, the manufacturers voluntarily withdrew the drug from release in the United States in 2002. It has never been commercially available in the UK.

Factors affecting duration of non-depolarising neuromuscular block

The duration of action of non-depolarising NMBAs is affected by several factors. Effects are most marked with the longer-acting agents, such as pancuronium. Prior administration of suxamethonium potentiates the effect and prolongs the duration of action of non-depolarising drugs. Concomitant administration of a potent inhalational agent increases the duration of block. This is most marked with the ether anaesthetic agents such as isoflurane and sevoflurane but

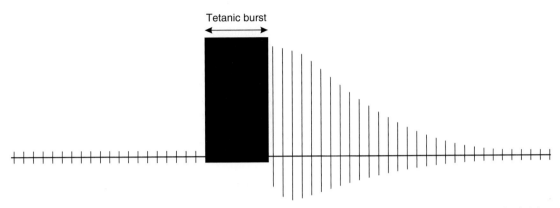

Fig. 8.6 A 5-s burst of tetanus (50 Hz), applied after a run of single twitch stimuli, causes a transient increase in the height of subsequent twitches, although they gradually decrease to their former height; this is post-tetanic potentiation (PTP) or facilitation (PTF). The number of twitches detectable after the burst of tetanus is referred to as the *post-tetanic count*.

occurs to a lesser extent with halothane. Other factors include the following:

- *pH changes.* Metabolic and, to a lesser extent, respiratory acidosis extend the duration of block. With monoquaternary amines such as vecuronium, this effect is produced by the ionisation, under acidic conditions, of a second nitrogen atom in the molecule, making the drug more potent.
- *Body temperature.* Hypothermia potentiates block because impairment of organ function delays metabolism and excretion of these drugs. Enzyme activity is also reduced. This may occur in patients undergoing cardiac surgery; reduced doses of NMBAs are required during cardiopulmonary bypass.
- *Age.* Non-depolarising NMBAs which depend on organ metabolism and excretion may be expected to have a prolonged effect in old age, as organ function deteriorates. In healthy neonates, who have a higher extracellular volume than adults, resistance may occur, but if the baby is sick or immature, then because of underdevelopment of the neuromuscular junction and other organ functions, increased sensitivity may be encountered. Children of school age tend to be relatively resistant to non-depolarising NMBAs when given on a per weight basis.
- *Electrolyte changes.* A low serum potassium concentration potentiates neuromuscular block by changing the value of the resting membrane potential of the postsynaptic membrane. A reduced ionised calcium concentration also potentiates block by impairing presynaptic acetylcholine release.
- *Myasthenia gravis.* In this disease, the number and half-life of the postsynaptic receptors are reduced by autoantibodies produced in the thymus gland. Thus the patient may be more sensitive to the effects of non-depolarising NMBAs. Resistance to suxamethonium may be encountered.
- *Other disease states.* Because of the altered pharmacokinetics of NMBAs in hepatic and renal disease, prolongation of action may be found in these conditions, especially if excretion of the drug is dependent upon these organs.

Characteristics of non-depolarising neuromuscular block

If a small, subparalysing dose of a non-depolarising neuromuscular blocking drug is administered, the following characteristics are recognised:

- Decreased response to a low-voltage twitch stimulus (e.g. 1 Hz) which, if repeated, decreases further in amplitude. This effect, which is in contrast to that produced by a depolarising drug, also occurs to a greater degree when the train-of-four (TOF) twitch response is applied, and even more so with higher, tetanic rates of stimulation. It is referred to as 'fade' or decrement.
- Post-tetanic potentiation (PTP) or facilitation (PTF) of the twitch response may be demonstrated (Fig. 8.6).
- Neuromuscular block is reversed by administration of an anticholinesterase.
- No muscle fasciculation is visible.

Reversal agents

Anticholinesterases

Anticholinesterases are used in clinical practice to inhibit the action of acetylcholinesterase at the neuromuscular

141

junction, thus prolonging the half-life of acetylcholine and potentiating its effect, especially in the presence of residual amounts of non-depolarising NMBA at the end of surgery. The most commonly used anticholinesterase during anaesthesia is neostigmine, but edrophonium and pyridostigmine are also available. These carbamate esters are water-soluble, quaternary ammonium compounds which are absorbed poorly from the gastrointestinal tract. The more lipid-soluble tertiary amine, physostigmine, has a similar effect and is more suitable for oral administration but crosses the blood–brain barrier. Organophosphorus compounds, which are used as poisons in farming and in nerve gas, also inhibit acetylcholinesterase, but unlike other agents, their effect is irreversible; recovery occurs only on generation of more enzyme, which takes some weeks.

Anticholinesterases are given orally to patients with *myasthenia gravis*. In this disease the patient possesses antibodies to the postsynaptic nicotinic receptor, reducing the efficacy of acetylcholine. The use of these drugs is thought to increase the amount and duration of action of acetylcholine at the neuromuscular junction, thus enhancing neuromuscular transmission.

Neostigmine
Neostigmine combines reversibly with acetylcholinesterase by formation of an ester linkage. Neostigmine is excreted largely unchanged through the kidneys and has a half-life of about 45 min. It is presented in brown vials, as it breaks down on exposure to light. Neostigmine potentiates the action of acetylcholine wherever it is a neurotransmitter, including all cholinergic nerve endings; thus it produces bradycardia, salivation, sweating, bronchospasm, increased intestinal motility and blurred vision. These cholinergic effects may be reduced by simultaneous administration of an anticholinergic agent such as atropine or glycopyrronium bromide. In the absence of a non-depolarising neuromuscular blocking agent, neostigmine can cause muscle fasciculation, fade of the TOF response and muscle weakness. The usual dose of neostigmine is between 0.035–0.05 mg kg^{-1}, in combination with either atropine 0.015 mg kg^{-1} or glycopyrronium bromide 0.01 mg kg^{-1}. It should only be administered after the spontaneous return of at least the second twitch of the TOF, and preferably the fourth twitch. It takes at least 2 min to have an initial effect, and recovery from neuromuscular block is maximally enhanced by 10 min.

Edrophonium
Edrophonium is an anticholinesterase that forms an ionic bond with the enzyme but does not undergo a chemical reaction with it. The effect is therefore more short lived than with neostigmine, of the order of only a few minutes. Edrophonium has a quicker onset of action than neostigmine, producing signs of recovery within 1 min. However, its effects are more evanescent; when edrophonium is given in the presence of profound neuromuscular block, the degree of neuromuscular block may *increase* after an initial period of recovery. It should only be used to reverse mivacurium and when all four twitches of the TOF are detectable. The dose of edrophonium is 0.5–1.0 mg kg^{-1}.

Pyridostigmine
Pyridostigmine has a slower onset time than neostigmine or edrophonium and also a longer duration of action. It is used more often as oral therapy in patients with myasthenia gravis than in anaesthesia.

Physostigmine
Physostigmine, an anticholinesterase also known as *eserine*, is a tertiary amine and is more lipid soluble than the other carbamate esters. It is therefore absorbed more easily from the gastrointestinal tract and also crosses the blood–brain barrier.

Organophosphorus compounds
Organophosphorus compounds are irreversible inhibitors of acetylcholinesterase; by phosphorylation of the enzyme, they produce a very stable complex which is resistant to reactivation or hydrolysis. Synthesis of new enzyme must occur before recovery. These agents, which include di-isopropylfluorophosphonate (DFP) and tetraethylpyrophosphate (TEPP), are used as insecticides and chemical warfare agents. They are absorbed readily through the lungs and skin. Poisoning is not uncommon among farm workers. Muscarinic effects such as salivation, sweating and bronchospasm are combined with nicotinic effects, such as muscle weakness. Central nervous effects such as tremor and convulsions may occur, as may unconsciousness and respiratory failure. Reactivators of acetylcholinesterase are used to treat this form of poisoning; they include *pralidoxime* and *obidoxime*. Atropine, anticonvulsants and artificial ventilation may be necessary. Chronic exposure may produce polyneuritis. Carbamates such as pyridostigmine are used prophylactically in those threatened by chemical warfare with these compounds.

Ecothiopate is an organophosphorus compound with a quaternary amine group; it was used as an eyedrop preparation in ophthalmology to produce miosis in narrow-angle glaucoma. It inhibits cholinesterase by phosphorylation and thus potentiates all esters metabolised by this enzyme. It has now been withdrawn from the UK market. A new generation of organophosphorus compounds may be beneficial in Alzheimer's disease, and clinical trials are in progress.

Cyclodextrins
Sugammadex
Anticholinesterases, although used routinely in anaesthetic practice, are recognised to have disadvantages. The most

important is that recovery from block must be established before they are given. Their muscarinic effects may be disadvantageous in patients with a history of nausea and vomiting or in the presence of cardiac arrhythmias or bronchospasm.

A novel approach to reversal of neuromuscular block was therefore developed. Sugammadex, a γ-cyclodextrin, was designed to encapsulate rocuronium (and to a lesser extent vecuronium) in the plasma, preventing its access to the nicotinic receptor and encouraging dissociation from it. Sugammadex consists of eight oligosaccharides arranged in a cylindrical structure to encapsulate all four steroidal rings of rocuronium completely (Fig. 8.7). This cylindrical structure is known as a toroid. The hydrophilic external tails on the toroid are negatively charged, attracting the quaternary nitrogen group on the NMBA and drawing it into the lipophilic core of sugammadex. The complex of sugammadex and rocuronium is excreted in the urine and has no muscarinic effect; the use of anticholinergic agents is unnecessary. Sugammadex has a low incidence of adverse effects, although hypersensitivity rashes, anaphylaxis and bradycardia have been reported. Full recovery of the TOF response is usually complete within 2–3 min.

Dose

The dose is adjusted according to the degree of residual block. If at least two twitches of the TOF response are detectable (when anticholinesterases can be used), 2 mg kg^{-1} should be given. If block is still profound, with no response to the TOF and a post-tetanic count of 1–2, 4 mg kg^{-1} should be used. If it is necessary to reverse block immediately in the case of, for instance, a 'cannot intubate, cannot oxygenate' scenario, sugammadex 16 mg kg^{-1} should be used.

Sugammadex does not antagonise neuromuscular block produced by the benzylisoquinoliniums or suxamethonium and has only a limited effect in reversing pancuronium. Sugammadex became available in the UK in 2008. Its relatively high cost has limited its use.

Neuromuscular monitoring

There is no clinical tool available to measure neuromuscular transmission accurately in a muscle group. Thus neither the amount of acetylcholine released in response to a given stimulus nor the number of postsynaptic receptors blocked

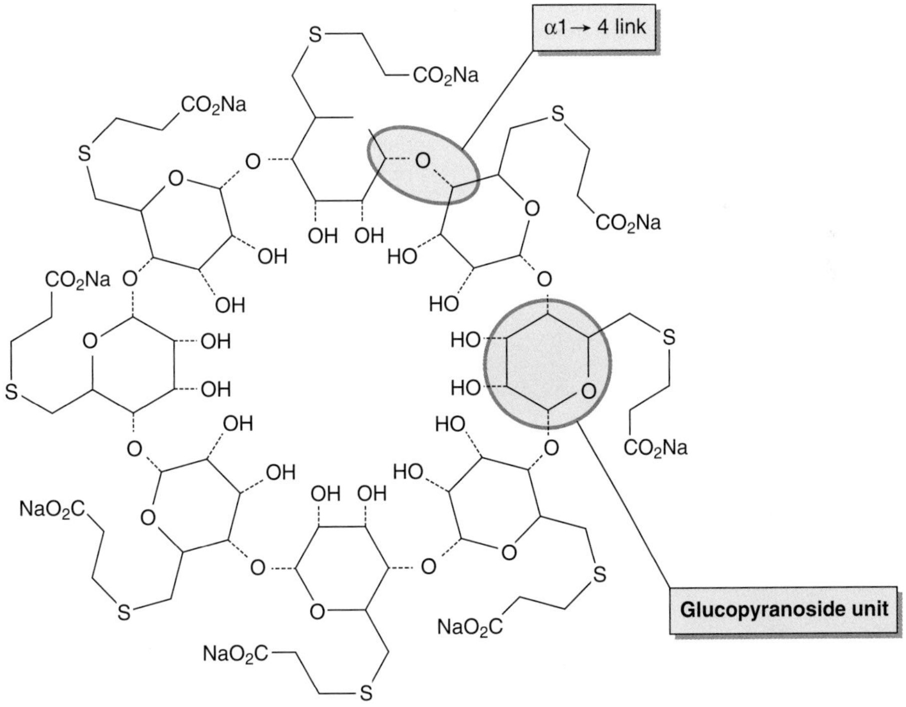

Fig. 8.7 The cyclical structure of sugammadex consisting of eight glucopyranoside units linked by oxygen radicals (example marked by *circle*). The negatively charged hydrophilic chains on the outside of the molecule attract rocuronium to the core of the toroid. (From Wikipedia.com.)

by a non-depolarising NMBA may be assessed. However, it is possible to obtain a crude estimate of muscle contraction during anaesthesia using a variety of techniques. All require the application to a peripheral nerve of a current of up to 60 mA for a fraction of a millisecond (often 0.2 ms), necessitating a voltage of up to 300 mV. Usually a nerve which is readily accessible to the anaesthetist, such as the ulnar, facial or common peroneal nerve, is used. The muscle response to the nerve stimulus may then be assessed by either *visual* or *tactile* means, or it may be recorded by more sophisticated methods.

Mechanomyography

A strain-gauge transducer may be used to measure the force of contraction of, for instance, the thumb, in response to stimulation of the ulnar nerve at the wrist. This measurement may then be charted using a recording device. Accurate measurements of the twitch or tetanic response may be made, although the hand must be splinted firmly for reproducible results. This technique is primarily a research tool.

Electromyography

The electromyographic response of a muscle is measured in response to the same electrical stimulus, using recording electrodes similar to ECG pads placed over the motor point of the stimulated muscle. For instance, if the ulnar nerve is stimulated, the recording electrodes are placed over the motor point of the adductor pollicis in the thumb (Fig. 8.8). A compound muscle action potential may be recorded. Although primarily a research tool, there are several simple clinical instruments which give a less accurate but similar

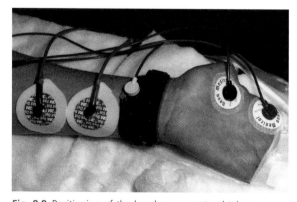

Fig. 8.8 Positioning of the hand necessary to obtain an electromyographic recording of the response of the adductor pollicis muscle to stimulation of the ulnar nerve is demonstrated. An earth electrode is placed round the wrist. Two recording electrodes are placed over the muscle on the hand; the distal one lies over the motor point.

recording. Maintaining the exact position of the hand is not as essential with electromyography as it is with mechanomyography.

Accelerography

In accelerography the acceleration of the thumb is measured in response to the nerve stimulus and the force of contraction derived (force = mass × acceleration). Clinical equipment is available (e.g. the TOF Watch SX, which is an accelerograph) that provide a quantitative assessment of, for instance, the twitch height compared with a control reading. The TOF Watch SX, in addition, gives a readout of the train-of-four ratio (TOFR). This is essential to determine if an anticholinesterase is to be avoided. The TOFR must have reached 0.9 before tracheal extubation can be effected safely.

Modes of stimulation

Several different rates of stimulation can be applied to the nerve in an attempt to produce a sensitive index of neuromuscular function. It is considered essential always to apply a *supramaximal* stimulus to the nerve; that is, the strength of the electrical stimulus (V) should be increased until the response no longer increases. It is then increased by an additional 25%.

Twitch

A square-wave stimulus of short duration (0.1–0.2 ms) is applied to a peripheral nerve. In isolation, such a stimulus is of limited value, although if applied repeatedly, before and after a dose of a neuromuscular blocking agent, it may be possible to assess crudely the effects of the drug. Such rates of stimulation have the benefit of being less painful than tetanic stimulation, with no untoward effects after recovery from anaesthesia.

Train-of-four twitch response

In an attempt to assess the degree of neuromuscular block clinically, Ali and colleagues (1971) described a development of the twitch response which would be more sensitive than repeated single twitches and did not require a control response. Four stimuli (at 2 Hz) are applied over 2 s, with at least a 10-s gap between each TOF. On administration of a small dose of a non-depolarising NMBA, *fade* of the amplitude of the TOF may be visible. The ratio of the amplitude of the fourth to the first twitch is called the *train-of-four ratio*. In the presence of a larger dose of such a drug, the fourth twitch disappears first, then the third, followed by the second and finally the first twitch (Fig. 8.9A). On recovery from neuromuscular block, the first twitch appears first, then the second (when the first twitch has

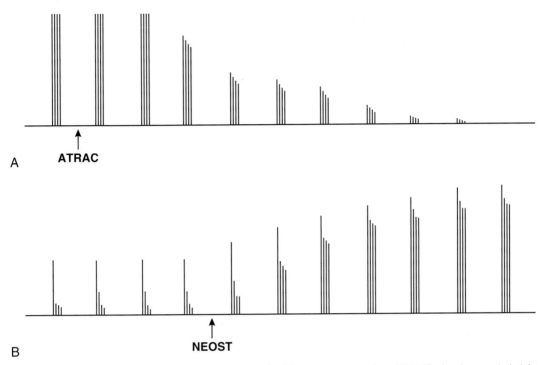

Fig. 8.9 (A) After administration of a non-depolarising NMBA (in this instance, atracurium *(ATRAC)*), the decrease in height of the fourth twitch of the TOF response is more marked than the decrease in height of the third twitch, which is more marked than the decrease in the second, which is greater than the decrease in the first. This effect is known as 'fade'. Within 2 min, the TOF response has been ablated completely. (B) On recovery, the first twitch response appears first, then the second, the third and, finally, the fourth. Marked fade is present, but after administration of an anticholinesterase (neostigmine *[NEOST]*), recovery of all four twitches occurs rapidly.

recovered to about 20% of control), then the third and finally the fourth (Fig. 8.9B).

It is thought that at least three of the four twitches must be absent to obtain adequate surgical access for upper abdominal surgery. Full reversal can only be relied upon if at least the second twitch is visible when an anticholinesterase is given. After reversal, good muscle tone – as assessed clinically by the patient being able to cough, raise his or her head from the pillow for at least 5 s, protrude the tongue and have good grip strength – may be anticipated when the TOFR has reached at least 0.7. However, recovery to a TOFR of 0.9 using acceleromyography has now been found to be necessary before extubation if the airway is to be protected completely. At TOF ratios of 0.7–0.9 there may still be an effect of NMBAs on the ventilatory response to hypoxaemia and also on the bulbar apparatus, with the potential for impairment of swallowing and pulmonary aspiration.

It is recognised that, although the number of twitches present in the TOF during neuromuscular block is easily counted by visual or tactile means, it is impossible, even for the expert, to assess the value of the TOFR accurately by these methods. Visual or tactile evaluation fails to detect

any fade of the TOF when the ratio is in excess of 40%. Thus failure to detect fade with a nerve stimulator does not always guarantee adequate reversal. Recording of the TOFR is essential for this purpose.

Tetanic stimulation

Tetanic stimulation is the most sensitive form of neuromuscular stimulation. Frequencies of 50–100 Hz are applied to a peripheral nerve to detect even minor degrees of residual neuromuscular block; thus tetanic fade may be present when the twitch response is normal. Tetanic rates of stimulation may be applied under anaesthesia, but in the awake patient, they are intolerably painful. Indeed, on recovery from anaesthesia in which tetanic stimulation has been applied, the patient may be aware of some discomfort in the area of application.

Post-tetanic potentiation or facilitation

Post-tetanic potentiation or facilitation is a method of monitoring developed in an attempt to assess more profound degrees of neuromuscular block produced by non-depolarising NMBAs. If a single twitch stimulus is applied to the nerve with little or no neuromuscular response, but after a 5-s delay, a burst of 50-Hz tetanus is given for 5 s, the effect of a further twitch stimulus 3 s later is enhanced (see Fig. 8.6). In the presence of profound block, the effect of repeated single twitches applied after the tetanus until the response disappears can be counted; this is termed the *post-tetanic count*. The augmentation of the twitch is thought to be caused by presynaptic mobilisation of acetylcholine as a result of the positive feedback effect of the run of tetanus.

Double-burst stimulation (DBS)

In an attempt to develop a clinical tool which would allow more accurate assessment of residual block by visual or tactile means than fade of the TOF response, Viby-Mogensen suggested the application of two or three short bursts of 50-Hz tetanus, each comprising two or three impulses, separated by a 750-ms interval. Each square-wave impulse lasts for 0.2 ms (Fig. 8.10). If records of the fade of the DBS and the TOF response are compared, they are very similar, but there is evidence to suggest that visual assessment of DBS in the later stages of recovery (TOFR <0.6), is more accurate. DBS is, however, an inadequate indicator of full recovery from neuromuscular block and cannot be used to determine sufficient recovery for tracheal extubation.

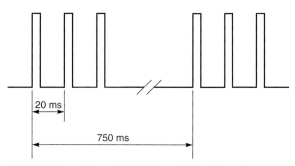

Fig. 8.10 The pattern of double-burst stimulation. Three bursts of 50-Hz tetanus, at 20-ms intervals, separated by a 750-ms gap, are shown.

Indications for neuromuscular monitoring

It is essential always to monitor neuromuscular function when a neuromuscular blocking agent is used during anaesthesia. There is evidence that if the TOFR is less than 0.7 on admission to the recovery room, duration of stay there is prolonged. There is also increasing evidence of a higher risk of postoperative pulmonary complications and increased duration of hospital stay in patients who have residual block detectable postoperatively.

References/Further reading

Ali, H.H., Utting, J.E., Gray, T.C., 1971. Quantitative assessment of residual antidepolarising block. II. Br. J. Anaesth. 43, 478–485.

Appiah-Ankam, J., Hunter, J.M., 2004. Pharmacology of neuromuscular blocking drugs. BJA CEACCP 4, 2–7.

Beecher, H.K., Todd, D.P., 1954. A study of the deaths associated with anesthesia and surgery. Ann. Surg. 140, 2–34.

Kalow, W., Genest, K., 1957. A method for the detection of atypical forms of human serum cholinesterase: determination of dibucaine numbers. Can. J. Biochem. 35, 339–346.

Khirwadkar, R., Hunter, J.M., 2012. Neuromuscular physiology and pharmacology: an update. BJA CEACCP. 12, 237–244.

King, J.M., Hunter, J.M., 2002. Physiology of the neuromuscular junction. BJA CEPD Reviews. 2, 129–133.

Srivastava, A., Hunter, J.M., 2009. Reversal of neuromuscular block. Br. J. Anaesth. 103, 115–129.

Chapter 9

Cardiovascular system

Hakeem Yusuff, Matthew Charlton

The autonomic nervous system

The term *autonomic nervous system* (ANS) refers to the nervous and humoral mechanisms that modify the function of the autonomous or automatic organs. These include heart rate (HR) and force of contraction; calibre of blood vessels; contraction and relaxation of smooth muscle in gut, bladder, bronchi; visual accommodation and pupillary size. Other functions include regulation of secretion from exocrine and other glands and aspects of metabolism (e.g. glycogenolysis and lipolysis) (Table 9.1). There is constant activity of both the sympathetic and parasympathetic nervous systems even at rest. This is termed sympathetic or parasympathetic tone and allows alterations in autonomic activity to produce rapid two-way regulation of physiological effect. The ANS is controlled by centres in the spinal cord, brainstem and hypothalamus, which are in turn influenced by higher centres in the cerebral and limbic cortices. The ANS is also influenced by visceral reflexes whereby afferent signals enter the autonomic ganglia, spinal cord, hypothalamus or brainstem and directly elicit appropriate reflex responses via the visceral organs. The efferent autonomic signals are transmitted through the body to two major subdivisions (separated by anatomical, physiological and pharmacological criteria), the sympathetic and the parasympathetic nervous systems.

Sympathetic nervous system

The sympathetic nervous system (SNS) includes nerves that originate in the spinal cord between the first thoracic and second lumbar segments (T1–L2) (Fig. 9.1). Fibres leave the spinal cord with the anterior nerve roots and then branch off as white *rami communicantes* to synapse in the bilateral paravertebral sympathetic ganglionic chains, although some preganglionic fibres synapse instead in the prevertebral ganglia (e.g. coeliac, mesenteric and hypogastric) in the abdomen before travelling to their effector organ with the relevant arteries. Postganglionic fibres travel from prevertebral and paravertebral ganglia in sympathetic nerves (to supply the internal viscera, including the heart) and spinal nerves (which innervate the peripheral vasculature and sweat glands). Sympathetic nerves throughout the circulation contain vasoconstrictor fibres, particularly in the kidneys, spleen, gut and skin; however, sympathetic vasodilator fibres predominate in skeletal muscle, coronary vessels and cerebral vessels. Sympathetic stimulation therefore causes predominantly vasoconstriction but also a redistribution of blood flow to skeletal muscle; constriction of venous capacitance vessels decreases their volume and thereby increases venous return.

Neurotransmitters of the sympathetic nervous system

Sympathetic preganglionic fibres release acetylcholine (ACh). They are therefore termed *cholinergic*, along with other neurons containing ACh. Acetylcholine activates nicotinic receptors on the postganglionic cell membrane, leading to the release of noradrenaline from the postganglionic fibre. All postganglionic sympathetic fibres release noradrenaline and are termed *adrenergic*, except for the postganglionic sympathetic fibres of the sweat glands, piloerector muscles and some blood vessels which are cholinergic. The adrenal medulla may be thought of as a modified postganglionic neuron, whose activation causes the release of adrenaline, released primarily as a circulating hormone (insignificant amounts being found in nerve endings).

Endogenous catecholamines (adrenaline, noradrenaline and dopamine) are synthesised from the essential amino acid phenylalanine (see Fig. 9.1). Their structure is based on a catechol ring (i.e. a benzene ring with ⁻OH groups

Table 9.1 Effects of the sympathetic and parasympathetic nervous systems on peripheral effector organs, and receptor subtypes mediating these functions (where known)

Organ	SYMPATHETIC Receptor subtype	Effect	PARASYMPATHETIC Receptor subtype	Effect
Heart	β_1, also β_2 ? also α and DA_1 α_1	↑ Heart rate ↑ Force of contraction ↑ Conduction velocity ↑ Automaticity (β_2) ↑ Excitability ↑ Force of contraction	M_2	↓ Heart rate ↓ Force of contraction Slight ↓ conduction velocity
Arteries	β_1 β_2 α_1, α_2 DA_1, β_2	Coronary vasodilatation Vasodilatation (skeletal muscle) Vasoconstriction (coronary, pulmonary, renal and splanchnic circulations, skin and skeletal muscle) Splanchnic and renal vasodilatation	M^a	Vasodilatation in skin, skeletal muscle, pulmonary and coronary circulations
Veins	α_1, also α_2 β_2	Vasoconstriction Vasodilatation		
Lung	β_2 α_1	Bronchodilation Inhibition of secretions Bronchoconstriction	M_1, M_3	Bronchoconstriction Stimulation of secretions
GI tract	α_1, α_2, β_2 α_1, α_2	Decreased motility Contraction of sphincters Inhibition of secretions	M_2, M_3	Increased motility Relaxation of sphincters Stimulation of secretions
Pancreas	β_2 α_1, α_2	Increased insulin release Decreased insulin release		
Kidney	β	Renin secretion		
Liver	β_2, α β_2, ?α	Glycogenolysis Gluconeogenesis	M	Glycogen synthesis
Bladder	β_2 α	Detrusor relaxation Sphincter contraction	M	Detrusor contraction Sphincter relaxation
Uterus	α_1 β_2	Myometrial contraction Myometrial relaxation		
Adipocytes	β_3	Lipolysis		
Eye	α_1	Mydriasis (radial muscle contraction) Ciliary muscle relaxation for far vision	M	Miosis Ciliary muscle contraction for near vision
Platelets	α_2	Promote platelet aggregation		
Sweat glands	M^b	Sweating		

All postganglionic parasympathetic fibres are muscarinic (M), but in many sites the subtype has not been identified.
[a]Muscarinic receptors are present on vascular smooth muscle, but they are independent of parasympathetic innervation and have little or no physiological role in the control of vasomotor tone.
[b]Sympathetic cholinergic fibres supply sweat glands and arterioles in some sites.

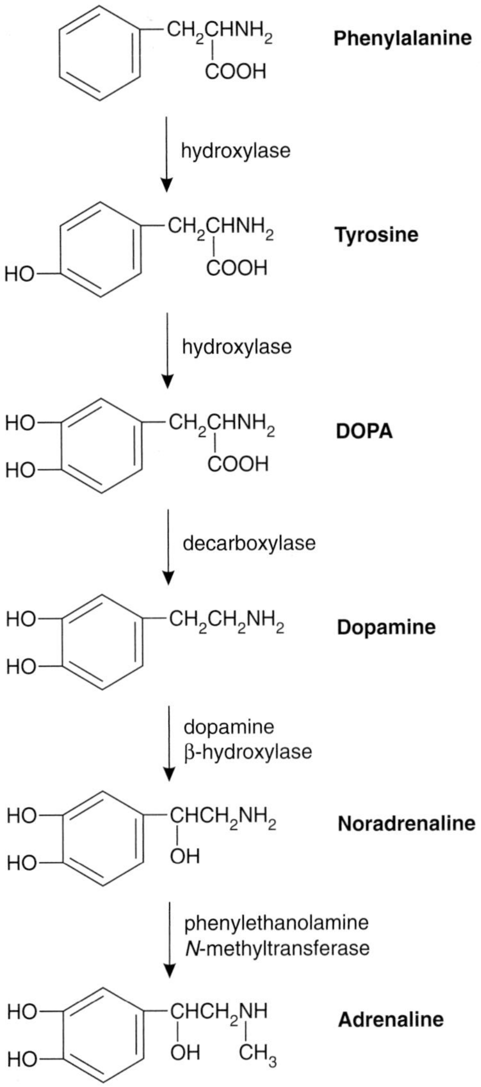

CH$_2$CHNH$_2$ COOH **Phenylalanine**

↓ hydroxylase

HO— CH$_2$CHNH$_2$ COOH **Tyrosine**

↓ hydroxylase

HO— HO— CH$_2$CHNH$_2$ COOH **DOPA**

↓ decarboxylase

HO— HO— CH$_2$CH$_2$NH$_2$ **Dopamine**

↓ dopamine β-hydroxylase

HO— HO— CHCH$_2$NH$_2$ OH **Noradrenaline**

↓ phenylethanolamine N-methyltransferase

HO— HO— CHCH$_2$NH OH CH$_3$ **Adrenaline**

Fig. 9.1 Synthesis of endogenous catecholamines.

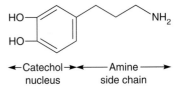

HO— HO— NH$_2$

←Catechol→ ←— Amine —→
nucleus side chain

Fig. 9.2 Standard molecular structure of catecholamines.

and subsequent reuse. Reuptake is by active transport back into the nerve terminal cytoplasm and then into cytoplasmic vesicles. This mechanism of presynaptic reuptake, termed *uptake₁*, is dependent on adenosine triphosphate (ATP) and Mg^{2+}, is enhanced by Li$^+$ and may be blocked by cocaine and tricyclic antidepressants. Endogenous catecholamines entering the circulation by diffusion from sympathetic nerve endings or by release from the adrenal gland are metabolised rapidly by the enzymes monoamine oxidase (MAO) and catechol O-methyltransferase (COMT) in the liver, kidneys, gut and many other tissues. The metabolites are conjugated before being excreted in urine as 3-methoxy-4-hydroxymandelic acid (VMA), metanephrine (from adrenaline) and norme-tanephrine (from noradrenaline). Noradrenaline taken up into the nerve terminal may also be deaminated by cytoplasmic MAO.

Another mechanism for the postsynaptic cellular reuptake of catecholamines, termed *uptake₂*, is present predominantly at the membrane of smooth muscle cells. It may be responsible for the termination of action of catecholamines released from the adrenal medulla.

Receptor pharmacology of the sympathetic nervous system

The actions of catecholamines are mediated by specific postsynaptic cell surface receptors, classified broadly into α- and β-adrenergic receptors (*adrenoceptors*) and dopamine receptors, each with a number of subtypes. Their location and function are summarised in Table 9.1. Two α- and β-receptor subtypes are well defined on functional, anatomical and pharmacological grounds (α$_1$ and α$_2$, β$_1$ and β$_2$). A third β-receptor subtype, β$_3$, is found in adipocytes, skeletal and ventricular muscle, and the vasculature. There are five subtypes of dopaminergic receptors (D$_1$–D$_5$), which are classified into two broader groups, D$_1$-like receptors (D$_1$ and D$_5$) and D$_2$-like receptors (D$_2$, D$_3$ and D$_4$). Modification of receptor activity is an important mechanism for modulating the function of effector organs.

Adrenergic receptors (and dopaminergic receptors) are proteins with a similar basic structure, comprising seven hydrophobic transmembrane domains and an intracellular chain. Differences in amino acid sequences of the intracellular chain differentiate α- and β-receptors. Both are linked to guanine nucleotide binding proteins (G-proteins) in the

in the 3 and 4 positions), and an ethylamine side chain (Fig. 9.2); substitutions in the side chain produce the different compounds. Dopamine may act as a precursor for both adrenaline and noradrenaline when administered exogenously.

The action of noradrenaline released from sympathetic nerve endings is terminated in one of three ways:
• Reuptake into the nerve terminal
• Diffusion into the circulation
• Enzymatic destruction

Most noradrenaline released from sympathetic nerves is taken back into the presynaptic nerve ending for storage

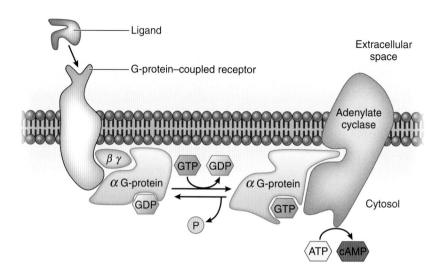

Fig. 9.3 G-protein–coupled receptor mechanism of action. *ATP,* Adenosine triphosphate; *cAMP,* cyclic adenosine monophosphate; *GDP,* guanosine diphosphate; *GTP,* guanosine triphosphate. (From Fletcher, A. (2017) The cell membrane and receptors. *Anaesthesia & Intensive Care Medicine,* 18 (6), 316–320.)

cell membrane. G-proteins are heterotrimeric proteins consisting of α, β and γ subunits. Binding of guanosine triphosphate (GTP) in response to receptor stimulation leads to dissociation of the α and βγ subunits. Gα plus GTP mediates the generation of second messengers that activate intracellular events. These second messenger systems include enzymes (adenylate cyclase, phospholipases) and ion channels (for calcium and potassium) (Fig. 9.3).

In addition to functional differences, adrenergic receptors differ in the intracellular mechanisms by which they act. Stimulation of β_1 and β_2 receptors activates G_s-proteins, which activate adenylate cyclase and cause the generation of intracellular cyclic adenosine monophosphate (cAMP). Cyclic adenosine monophosphate activates intracellular enzyme pathways (the third messengers) to produce the associated alteration in cell function (e.g. increased force of cardiac muscle contraction, liver glycogenolysis, bronchial smooth muscle relaxation). In cardiac myocytes the intracellular pathway involves the activation of protein kinases to phosphorylate intracellular proteins and increase intracellular Ca^{2+} concentrations. Intracellular cAMP concentration is modulated by the enzyme phosphodiesterase, which breaks down cAMP to inactive 5′ adenosine monophosphate (AMP). This is the site of action of phosphodiesterase inhibitor drugs. The balance between production and degradation of cAMP is an important regulatory system for cell function. α_2-Adrenoceptors interact with G_i-proteins to inhibit adenylate cyclase and Ca^{2+} channels but activate K^+ channels, phospholipase C and phospholipase A_2. Cholinergic M_2 receptors and somatostatin affect G_i-proteins in the same way.

In contrast, α_1-receptor stimulation does not directly affect intracellular cAMP concentrations but causes coupling with another G-protein, G_q, to activate membrane-bound phospholipase C. This in turn hydrolyses phosphatidylinositol bisphosphate (PIP2) to inositol triphosphate (IP_3), which produces changes in intracellular Ca^{2+} concentration and binding. These lead, for example, to smooth muscle contraction. Dopaminergic D_1-like receptors act via the G_s mechanism; D_2-like receptors act via the G_i mechanism.

Parasympathetic nervous system

The parasympathetic nervous system (PNS) controls vegetative functions, such as the digestion and absorption of nutrients, excretion of waste products and conservation and restoration of energy (see Table 9.1). Parasympathetic neurons arise from cell bodies of the motor nuclei of cranial nerves III, VII, IX and X in the brainstem and from the sacral segments of the spinal cord. The PNS is therefore described as having a craniosacral outflow. Long preganglionic fibres synapse in ganglia within or adjacent to the organ, giving rise to short postganglionic fibres which then supply the relevant tissues. The ganglion cells may be well organised (e.g. the myenteric plexus of the intestine) or diffuse (e.g. in the bladder or vasculature). As the majority of all parasympathetic nerves are contained in branches of the vagus nerve, which innervates the viscera of the thorax and abdomen, increased parasympathetic activity is characterised by signs of vagal overactivity. Parasympathetic fibres also pass to the eye via the oculomotor (IIIrd cranial) nerve and to the lacrimal, nasal and salivary glands via the facial (V^{th}) and glossopharyngeal (IXth) nerves. Fibres originating in the sacral portion of the spinal cord pass to the distal GI tract, bladder and reproductive organs.

Neurotransmitters of the parasympathetic nervous system

The chemical neurotransmitter at both pre- and postganglionic synapses is ACh, although transmission at postganglionic synapses may be modulated by other substances, including GABA, serotonin and opioid peptides. Acetylcholine is synthesised in the cytoplasm of cholinergic nerve terminals by the combination of choline and acetate (in the form of acetylcoenzyme A (acetyl-CoA), synthesised in the mitochondria as a product of normal cellular metabolism). Acetylcholine is stored in specific agranular vesicles and released from the presynaptic terminal in response to neuronal depolarisation to act at specific receptor sites on the postsynaptic membrane. It is rapidly metabolised by the enzyme acetylcholinesterase (AChE) to produce acetate and choline. Choline is then taken up into the presynaptic nerve ending for the regeneration of ACh. Acetylcholinesterase is synthesised locally at cholinergic synapses but is also present in erythrocytes and parts of the CNS.

Receptor pharmacology of the parasympathetic nervous system

Parasympathetic receptors are classified according to the actions of the alkaloids muscarine and nicotine. The actions of ACh at the postganglionic membrane are mimicked by muscarine and are termed muscarinic, whereas preganglionic transmission is termed nicotinic. Acetylcholine is also the neurotransmitter at the neuromuscular junction, acting via nicotinic receptors. Five subtypes of muscarinic receptors (M_1– M_5) have been characterised; all five subtypes exist in the CNS, but there are differences in their peripheral distribution and function. M_1 receptors are found in the stomach, where they mediate acid secretion, and in inflammatory cells in the lung (including mast cells and eosinophils), where they may have a role in airway inflammation. M_2 receptors predominate in the myocardium, where they modulate HR and impulse conduction. Prejunctional M_2 receptors are also involved in the regulation of synaptic noradrenaline and postganglionic ACh release. M_3 receptors are present in classic postsynaptic sites in glandular tissue (of the GI and respiratory tract) and bronchial smooth muscle, where they mediate most of the postjunctional effects of ACh. M_4 receptors have been isolated in cardiac and lung tissue in animal models and may have inhibitory effects. The distribution and functions of M_5 receptors are not yet defined. In common with adrenergic receptors, muscarinic receptors are coupled to membrane-bound G-proteins. M_1, M_3 and M_5 receptors are coupled to G_q-proteins and use IP_3 as a second messenger, whilst M_2 and M_4 receptors are coupled to G_i-proteins and use cAMP as a second messenger. Currently available anticholinergics probably act at all muscarinic receptor subtypes, but their clinical spectra differ, which suggests that they may have differential effects at different subtypes.

Cardiovascular physiology

Cardiovascular electrophysiology

The heart is a biomechanical pump required to ensure continued delivery of essential metabolic substrate to tissues and removal of by-products of metabolism. This mechanical function is the culmination of a process that links intrinsically generated electrical impulses with the mechanical deformation of cardiac muscles. Hence the generation of an effective and consistent electrical rhythm in the heart is crucial to its functioning.

Parts of the conduction system (pacemaker cells) have the property of automaticity. This is the intrinsic ability to generate electrical activity and act as a pacemaker when the impulse passes to other myocardial cells. The rate of impulse generation depends on the location of the pacemaker cell, with higher rates in the atria compared with the ventricles. The pacemaker cells consist of the sinoatrial (SA) node, the atrioventricular (AV) node, the bundle of His and the Purkinje fibres.

The normal cardiac impulse and its conduction

Under physiological conditions, the cardiac impulse is generated in the SA node, located at the intersection of the superior vena cava and the right atrium laterally. Impulse generation by the SA node supersedes the pacemaker cells below it in the conduction pathway, suppressing their automaticity.

Sinoatrial nodal impulses are propagated cell-to-cell throughout the atria, exiting via the AV node. At the AV node there is a delay of approximately 100 ms before the impulse is propagated onward, allowing the atria to depolarise fully before the ventricles. This is demonstrated as the *PR interval* of an ECG tracing. From the AV node the impulse passes into the bundle of His, which divides into right and left bundle branches, transmitting the cardiac impulse at a high velocity throughout the myocardium via the Purkinje fibre network.

Generation of the pacemaker action potential

The generation of an electrical impulse starts with the generation of an action potential. Pacemaker action potentials are divided into three phases characterised by the opening and closing of specific ion channels, Ca^{2+}, K^+ and to a lesser extent Na^+ (Fig. 9.4). Unlike other action potentials, pacemaker cells have no true resting membrane potential (RMP); they depolarise spontaneously at regular intervals, with the end of one action potential heralding the beginning of the next.

At the onset of the pacemaker action potential (the end of phase 3), membrane potential is –60 mV. Non-specific sodium and potassium channels open, causing the slow influx of positive ions into the cell and spontaneous depolarisation. The movement of positive ions is known as the 'funny current', abbreviated to I_f. Spontaneous depolarisation marks the onset of phase 4. At a membrane potential of approximately –50 mV, T-type Ca^{2+} channels open, followed by L-type Ca^{2+} channels (which open slowly) at around –40 mV. Upon reaching threshold potential (around –30 mV), all L-type Ca^{2+} channels are open, leading to more rapid depolarisation of the membrane (phase 0). Both I_f

and T-type Ca^{2+} channels close during phase 0. Repolarisation (phase 3) is initiated by closure of the L-type Ca^{2+} channels and opening of K^+ channels, causing an efflux of K^+ until the cell is hyperpolarised to –60 mV.

Cardiac myocyte action potential

Unlike pacemaker cells, cardiac myocytes possess a true RMP at around –90 mV as a result of K^+ conductance (efflux) through open K^+ channels. Depolarisation to threshold potential by an action potential in an adjacent cell causes rapid depolarisation because of opening of fast Na^+ channels and closure of K^+ channels (phase 0). Phase 1 represents an initial repolarisation caused by opening of K^+ channels and closure of fast Na^+ channels. At the same time, however, L-type Ca^{2+} channels open, with an influx of Ca^{2+} maintaining depolarisation, as demonstrated by the plateau phase of the action potential (phase 2). Repolarisation back to the RMP results from closure of L-type calcium channels and increased potassium conductance (phase 3) (see Fig. 9.4).

In contrast to the pacemaker action potential, the myocyte potential relies on fast Na^+ and Ca^{2+} channels. Sodium channels remain inactive after their closure during phase 1, being unable to be reactivated until after the membrane has repolarised. This is termed the *absolute refractory period* (ARP), where no matter how great the stimulus to the myocyte, it cannot be depolarised. This acts as a safety mechanism, preventing aberrant repeated depolarisations and tachyarrhythmias. After the ARP there is a period where

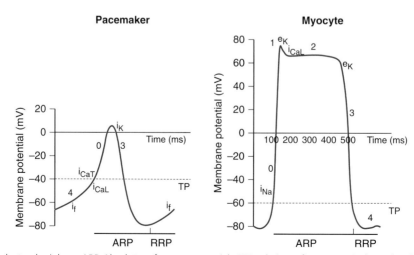

Fig. 9.4 Cardiac electrophysiology. *ARP,* Absolute refractory potential; *RRP,* relative refractory period; *TP,* threshold potential. (From Hebbes, C., & Thompson, P. (2015) Drugs acting on the heart: antiarrhythmics, *Anaesthesia & Intensive Care Medicine,* 16 (5), 232–236.)

the cardiac myocyte may be depolarised by a supranormal stimulus. This is the *relative refractory period*.

Control of heart rate

The control of HR occurs principally at the SA node. The rate produced by the SA node is dependent on the effects of the SNS and PNS. At rest, the SA node is under continual parasympathetic control via the vagus nerve (vagal stimulation), with the intrinsic rate (110–120 beats per min) being reduced to approximately 70 to 80 beats per min. In the denervated heart, such as after heart transplant, vagal stimulation is lost and the heart will therefore contract at the intrinsic SA nodal rate of 110–120 beats per min. Changes in the rate of impulse generation (and therefore HR) are achieved by altering the slope of phase 4 of the pacemaker action potential (Fig. 9.5). Increases in impulse generation are firstly brought about by a reduction in parasympathetic tone, followed by a sympathetically stimulated decrease in K^+ conductance and an increase in I_f and Ca^{2+} conductance, leading to a shortening of phase 4, therefore increasing HR (see Fig. 9.5B). Release of ACh by the PNS at the SA node increases potassium conductance whilst decreasing the I_f and Ca^{2+} currents. This causes a reduction in the angle of

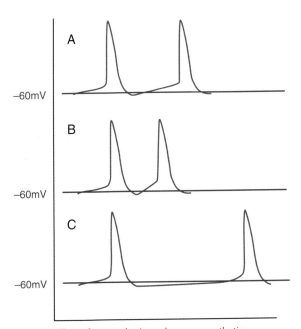

Fig. 9.5 Effect of sympathetic and parasympathetic stimulation on the membrane potential of the SA node. (A) Intrinsic rate; (B) sympathetic; (C) parasympathetic stimulation.

phase 4, prolonging the time to reach threshold, therefore reducing HR (see Fig. 9.5C).

Control of electrochemical gradients is essential to ensure the maintenance of membrane potential required for depolarisation and repolarisation to occur. Alterations in ion channel function and therefore the electrochemical gradient are the mechanisms of action of various antiarrhythmic medications (discussed later).

Cardiac muscle contraction

Cardiac muscle cells, although similar to striated skeletal muscle, are morphologically distinct. Cardiac myocytes have a branching structure and are attached end-to-end via a step-faced *intercalated disk*, containing two distinct junctions:

- *Desmosomes*. Transmembrane adhesion proteins of the cadherin family, providing structural support between myocytes, reducing the effect of shearing forces.
- *Gap junctions*. Containing connexons, which connect adjacent myocytes end-to-end to create a continuous membrane-spanning hollow tube. This allows rapid transmission of ionic currents and therefore electrical excitation from one cell to the next.

These features allow the rapid conduction of action potentials from cell to cell, with the myocardium therefore acting as one functional syncytium. Initiation of myocardial contraction originates from pacemaker cells within the heart, depolarisation then spreading from cell to cell. The ANS modulates this intrinsic function, controlling the force of contraction and rhythmicity of the heart (discussed later).

Influx of extracellular calcium via L-type Ca^{2+} channels is essential for successful myocyte contraction. Transverse (T) tubules are invaginations of the sarcolemma (myocyte cell membrane) and are in continuity with the extracellular space. Opening of L-type Ca^{2+} channels in response to depolarisation leads to the influx of Ca^{2+} from the extracellular space to the sarcoplasm. However, unlike in skeletal muscle, this is insufficient to generate myocyte contraction. The increase in intracellular calcium leads to opening of ryanodine receptor Ca^{2+} release channels present on the sarcoplasmic reticulum (SR). Calcium is subsequently released from the SR, significantly increasing the intracellular Ca^{2+} concentration, a process known as *calcium-induced calcium release* (CICR).

The sarcomere forms the functional unit of cardiac muscle consisting of interdigitating thick and thin filaments. The thick filament contains myosin, a large protein with two heads, with each possessing two binding sites, one for ATP and the other for actin. The thin filament is composed of three proteins: actin, tropomyosin and troponin. Actin forms a double-helix structure with regularly spaced myosin binding sites. Tropomyosin lies in the groove between the actin double helix, shielding the myosin binding sites. Troponin consists of three subunits: troponin T, binding the troponin complex to tropomyosin (hence T); troponin I which is thought to have an inhibitory function (hence I); and troponin C, which binds calcium (hence C).

The sarcomere can be described structurally from its microscopic appearance (Fig. 9.6). A Z-disk is present at the end of each sarcomere, to which thin filaments are joined, with the thick filament present in the centre of the sarcomere. The I-band (isotropic band), or light band, contains the area of thin filament not overlapped by thick filament; there are therefore two half I-bands per sarcomere. The A-band (anisotropic band), or dark band, comprises the entire length of the thick filament. The H-band (Heller band) encompasses the non-overlapped part of the A-band. The regular repeating pattern of dark and light bands leads to the striated muscle appearance.

After release of Ca^{2+} from the SR, actin-myosin cross-bridge formation follows a similar ATP-dependent process to that of skeletal muscle:

- Calcium binds to troponin C, leading to a conformational change in tropomyosin, rolling deeper into the groove between actin filaments and therefore exposing the myosin binding sites.
- Myosin heads bind ATP, which is rapidly hydrolysed to ADP and inactive phosphate (Pi), releasing energy.

- The energised myosin head is now able to bind to the actin filament, forming a cross-bridge.
- Myosin flexes on its actin-binding site, bringing the actin filament closer to the centre of the sarcomere, shortening the length of the sarcomere.
- Adenosine diphosphate and Pi dissociate from the myosin head, allowing ATP to once again bind to the myosin head.
- The myosin–ATP complex has a low affinity for the actin binding site and they dissociate, allowing this process to be repeated.

The whole process can be likened to a rowing motion, where myosin is the boat, myosin heads are the oars and the actin filaments are the water.

The process of cross-bridge cycling continues until the cytoplasmic calcium concentration decreases. As the sarcoplasmic calcium concentration falls, Ca^{2+} dissociates from troponin C. Tropomyosin recovers the myosin binding site on the actin filament. Myosin can no longer bind to actin, and relaxation occurs. There are three main mechanisms reducing intracellular calcium:

- *Plasma membrane Ca^{2+} adenosine triphosphatase* (ATPase) *pump*
    - Hydrolysis of ATP actively removes Ca^{2+} from the cell
    - Pump activity is regulated by phospholamban, an inhibitory protein
- *Na^+/Ca^{2+} exchanger*
    - Removes one Ca^{2+} ion from the cell in exchange for 3 Na^+ ions
    - Against concentration gradient, driven by low intracellular Na^+ concentrations
    - Responsible for about three quarters of Ca^{2+} expulsion
- *Sarcoplasmic/endoplasmic reticulum Ca^{2+} ATPase pump* (SERCA)
    - Hydrolysis of ATP to actively sequester Ca^{2+} in the SR

The Na^+/K^+ ATPase pump maintains the intracellular ionic concentration of Na^+, pumping 3 Na^+ out for every 2 K^+ in. This maintains the electrogenic gradient required for the successful functioning of the Na^+/Ca^{2+} exchanger. All these processes are energy-dependent. A continuous oxygen supply is required to fuel oxidative phosphorylation for them to continue.

Contractile force is dependent on the intracellular calcium concentration (alongside diastolic stretch). In skeletal muscle, troponin C is fully saturated by high sarcoplasmic calcium concentrations; cross-bridge formation is therefore maximal. This is not the case in cardiac muscle, where sarcoplasmic calcium concentrations are lower. Cross-bridge formation typically operates at approximately 40% of maximum, with increases in sarcoplasmic calcium concentration leading to increasing cross-bridge formation and therefore force of contraction. Factors governing the influx of extracellular Ca^{2+} during the plateau phase of contraction and its expulsion

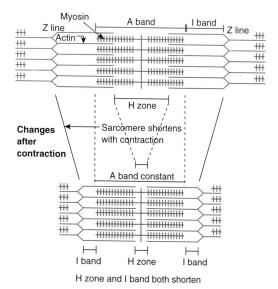

Fig. 9.6 The sarcomere. (From Wareham, A.C. (2014) Muscle. *Anaesthesia & Intensive Care Medicine*, 15 (6), 279–281.)

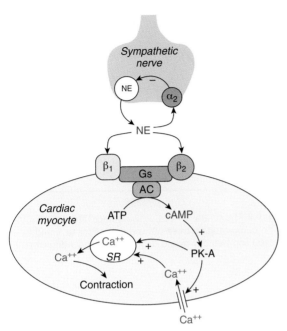

Fig. 9.7 The effect of sympathetic stimulation on inotropy. *AC*, Adenylate cyclase; *ATP*, adenosine triphosphate; *cAMP*; cyclic adenosine monophosphate; *NE*, norepinephrine; *PK-A*, protein kinase A; *SR*, sarcoplasmic reticulum. (From Klabunde, D.E. (2012) *Cardiovascular pharmacology concepts: Beta-adrenoreceptor agonists.* Available from: http://cvpharmacology.com/cardiostimulatory/beta-agonist.)

during diastole therefore determine the force of contraction (inotropy):

- Extracellular Ca^{2+} concentration
  - Higher concentrations lead to increased calcium flux and therefore more forceful contraction.
- Sympathetic stimulation (Fig. 9.7)
  - Release of noradrenaline, binding to β_1-adrenoceptors on the cardiac cell membrane, activates G_s G-protein–coupled receptors (GPCRs) (see also Chapter 1).
  - The G-protein α_s subunit activates membrane-bound adenylate cyclase, catalysing the conversion of ATP to cAMP.
  - Actions of cAMP include the following:
    - Activates the intracellular enzyme protein kinase A, which phosphorylates L-type calcium channels, increasing their open state probability and duration of opening.
    - This increases plateau Ca^{2+} and therefore positive inotropy.
    - Protein kinase A also phosphorylates phospholamban, increasing lusitropy (myocardial relaxation).

- Intracellular cAMP concentration relates to the rate of its production and the rate of its degradation (by phosphodiesterase).
  - Phosphodiesterase inhibitors (such as enoximone and milrinone) decrease the breakdown of cAMP, mimicking the effects of β_1-agonists.
- Parasympathetic stimulation
  - Parasympathetic stimulation of M_2 receptors by ACh leads to the activation of G_i.
  - The G_i subunit α_i inhibits adenylate cyclase, reducing the activation of L-type Ca^{2+} channels and therefore decreases calcium flux.
- Size of the plateau current
  - Increased by β_1-agonists.
  - Decreased by L-type Ca^{2+} channel blockers.
- Heart rate
  - Shorter diastolic times leads to decreased calcium efflux (and vice versa).
  - Force of contraction therefore generally increases with increasing HRs (the *Bowditch effect*).
  - The opposite can be seen with premature ectopic beats, even when conducted by the normal conduction pathway. The amount of calcium available for release from the SR is reduced, resulting in a reduced force of contraction.
  - After an ectopic beat there is a compensatory pause followed by a more forceful contraction (postextrasystolic potentiation), caused by both increased availability of Ca^{2+} from the SR and increased diastolic stretch.
- Digoxin
  - Raises sarcoplasmic calcium concentration via inhibition of the Na^+/K^+ ATPase pump and subsequent effects on the Na^+/Ca^{2+} exchanger (discussed in more detail later).

The cardiac cycle

The cardiac cycle describes the sequence of events occurring with every heartbeat. Its duration is the reciprocal of HR. The cycle can be divided into two phases – systole, when the ventricles are contracting, and diastole, when the ventricles are relaxing. Systole and diastole can be divided further into four distinct phases delineated by the position of the valves and the state of contraction of the ventricles:

1. Inflow phase – the AV valves are open and the aortic and pulmonary (outflow) valves are closed.
2. Isovolumetric contraction – both the AV and outflow valves are closed. The ventricles are contracting.
3. Outflow phase – the AV valves are closed and the outflow valves are open.
4. Isovolumetric relaxation – both the AV and outflow valves are closed. The ventricles are relaxing.

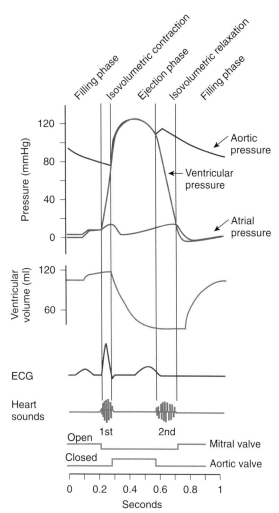

Fig. 9.8 The cardiac cycle, showing **blood pressures, ventricular volume, heart sounds and ECG.** (From Chan-Dewar, F. (2012) The cardiac cycle. *Anaesthesia & Intensive Care Medicine*, 13 (8), 391–396.)

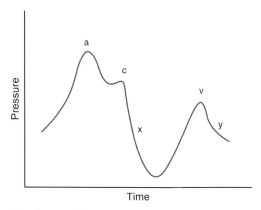

Fig. 9.9 The central venous pressure trace. The normal CVP trace demonstrating three upward deflections (a, c and v waves) and two downward deflections (x and y descents).

The cardiac cycle is traditionally described to start in late diastole, when the heart is relaxed, the AV valves are open and the outflow valves are closed (inflow phase). Fig. 9.8 demonstrates the cardiac cycle in its entirety. The following text explains the process in further detail.

1. Inflow phase

At the onset of the cardiac cycle the pressure within the atria is slightly higher than the pressure in the ventricles.

The AV valves are open. Blood flows slowly from the atria into the ventricles down the pressure gradient. Atrial depolarisation, corresponding to the P-wave of the ECG, denotes atrial systole. Contraction of the atria ejects the remaining blood into the ventricle. At rest this usually represents a relatively small amount of subsequent stroke volume, but this may be increased considerably during exercise. The volume of blood in the ventricles at the end of atrial systole (the end of diastole) is termed the *end-diastolic volume* (EDV). As there are no valves between the atria and the great veins, changes in atrial pressure are transmitted back along these vessels and can be seen as a characteristic *central venous pressure* (CVP) waveform (Fig. 9.9). Atrial contraction therefore causes a small rise in CVP corresponding to the a-wave of the CVP trace.

2. Isovolumetric contraction

Electrical depolarisation is propagated further via the AV node to the bundle of His and Purkinje network, leading to ventricular depolarisation and contraction. Ventricular contraction leads to a rapid rise in intraventricular pressure, exceeding the pressure in the atria and causing the AV valves to close. This can be heard on auscultation as the first heart sound (S1). As left-sided pressures are higher than right, the mitral valve closes slightly earlier than the tricuspid. This can be heard as a 'split' first heart sound. Electrical and mechanical abnormalities (such as right bundle branch block and Ebstein anomaly) can lead to prolonged splitting. The high intraventricular compared with atrial pressure leads to slight bulging of the AV valves back into the atrial cavity. Bulging of the tricuspid valve into the right atrium is seen as the C-wave of the CVP trace.

3. Ejection phase

Ongoing ventricular contraction continues to increase intraventricular pressure. When intraventricular pressure exceeds aortic/pulmonary artery pressure, the outflow valves open. Blood is rapidly ejected from the ventricle, causing a rise in aortic/pulmonary artery pressure.

Ongoing ejection causes intraventricular pressure to fall. Once the inertia of blood being ejected is overcome, the outflow valves close, generating the second heart sound (S2). This denotes the end of systole. The second heart sounds can be physiologically split during inspiration, with the pulmonary valve closing later than the aortic valve. Pathological splitting of S2 can result from a number of conditions, including valvular stenoses, bundle branch blocks and intraventricular shunts. Atrial septal defects lead to a 'fixed split' S2, which does not vary with the respiratory cycle. Closure of the aortic valve can be demonstrated on the arterial pressure trace as the dicrotic notch, caused by the elastic recoil of the aorta.

Right ventricular contraction pulls the tricuspid valve downwards towards the apex of the heart, increasing right atrial length. This causes the pressure within the atria to fall and blood to leave the central veins and enter the atria. This corresponds to the x descent of the CVP trace.

During ejection, approximately 55%–70% of ventricular blood is expelled (the ejection fraction). The volume of blood remaining in the left ventricle at the end of systole is termed the *end-systolic volume* (ESV).

4. Isovolumetric relaxation and rapid ventricular filling

After closure of the outflow valves, the ventricle is continuing to relax. It takes a small amount of time before the pressure in the ventricle drops below that of the atria, leading to opening once again of the AV valves. This is termed *isovolumetric relaxation* as all valves are closed and the ventricles are relaxing. The atria continue to fill during isovolumetric relaxation, leading to a small pressure rise corresponding to the V-wave of the CVP trace. When atrial pressure exceeds that of the ventricles, the AV valves open. As the ventricle is continuing to relax during this period, blood is rapidly ejected from the atria, corresponding to the y descent of the CVP trace.

Control of cardiac output

Stroke volume and cardiac output

Fundamentally the heart pumps out (cardiac output) the blood that arrives in it (venous return). Although there are beat-by-beat differences between systemic venous return (right atrium), right-sided cardiac output (pulmonary artery),

left-sided venous return (pulmonary veins) and systemic left-sided cardiac output (aorta), on average the heart must pump out what arrives.

Stroke volume (SV) describes the amount of blood ejected from the left ventricle per heartbeat. It can be calculated by subtracting the volume of the left ventricle at the end of systole (left ventricular end-systolic volume; LVESV) from the volume at the end of diastole (left ventricular end-diastolic volume; LVEDV). It is normally around 55–100 ml per beat.

$$SV = LVEDV - LVESV$$

Ejection fraction is a commonly quoted figure of left ventricular function, with a normal range between 55%–70%. *Ejection fraction* describes the stroke volume as a percentage of diastolic left ventricular volume.

$$EF = 100 \times \frac{SV}{LVEDV}$$

Cardiac output describes the volume of blood ejected from the left ventricle in a minute and is therefore the sum of SV and HR.

$$CO = SV \times HR$$

Control of cardiac output

Cardiac output can be controlled by altering its constituent elements, stroke volume and HR. Stroke volume is determined by three factors: preload, contractility and afterload.

Preload

Preload is defined as the initial stretching of the cardiac myocyte to its end-diastolic length. The Frank-Starling law dictates that the force of myocyte contraction is dependent on the preceding diastolic sarcomere length. If all other factors are kept constant, the force of contraction will increase non-linearly with increasing ventricular preload (i.e. increasing sarcomere length represented by left-ventricular end-diastolic pressure; LVEDP) (Fig. 9.10). This is also described as the length–tension relationship. The change in tension at differing sarcomere lengths is related to the number of actin-myosin cross-bridges formed. In cardiac muscle the maximum active tension possible (depending on the state of inotropy) corresponds to a sarcomere length of 2.2 μm. Sarcomere lengths less than this will demonstrate lower tension. At more than 2.2 μm, overlapping between actin and myosin filaments is reduced, decreasing the tension possible. Theoretically at sarcomere lengths greater than 3.6 μm there is no overlap, and the tension therefore falls to zero. This can be demonstrated in decompensated heart failure, where further increases in preload (e.g. from i.v. fluid administration) lead to further lengthening of the

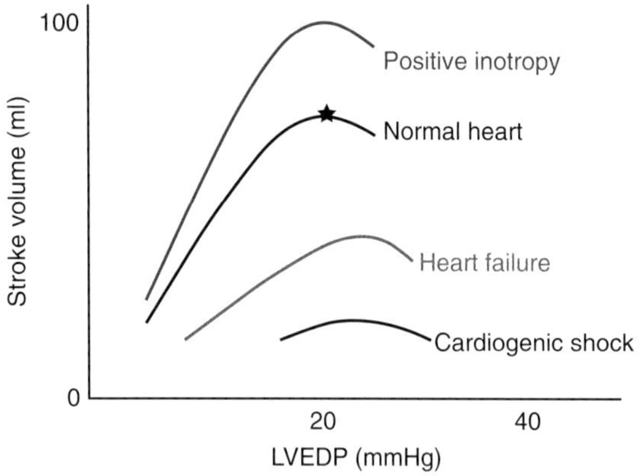

Fig. 9.10 The Frank–Starling curve. The effect of increasing sarcomere length (represented by left ventricular end-diastolic pressure; LVEDP) on the stroke volume at different states of cardiac function. (From Taylor, S., & Alexander, R. (2008) Optimization of the elective and emergency surgical patient. *Surgery*, 26 (9), 392–395.)

sarcomere, subsequently decreasing contractility and worsening SV. Preload is challenging to measure clinically. Central venous pressure can be used as an approximation of right ventricular preload, whereas pulmonary capillary wedge pressure (PCWP; measured using a pulmonary artery catheter) can be used to estimate left-sided filling pressures. It is important to understand that this is using pressure as a surrogate for sarcomere length; this involves several assumptions that may not be true in clinical practice.

Contractility

Contractility is the ability of the cardiac myocyte to increase (or decrease) the force of contraction as a result of changes in inotropy, a length-independent mechanism (as opposed to preload). The ANS plays a key role in regulating contractility. Contractility can also be manipulated pharmacologically (discussed later). Contractility is difficult to measure directly but can be estimated by the rate of pressure change during isovolumetric contraction.

Afterload

Afterload describes the force against which the ventricle must eject and equates to ventricular wall stress. It is determined by the pulmonary and systemic vascular resistances, aortic and main pulmonary arterial pressures and the force required to overcome any outflow valvular stenoses. Ventricular dilatation also increases ventricular wall stress and therefore afterload. All other things being equal, decreasing afterload will lead to increasing stroke volume and vice versa.

Control of blood pressure

Arterial pressure is normally tightly regulated to ensure adequate flow of blood to tissues whilst avoiding the harmful effects of high pressures on the vasculature and end-organs. Mean arterial pressure (MAP) is normally 65–100 mmHg, with normal systolic and diastolic blood pressures between 120–140 mmHg and 70–90 mmHg, respectively. Maintaining homeostasis relies on the modification of factors affecting MAP, namely systemic vascular resistance (SVR) and cardiac output (CO). Control of CO is described earlier. The relationship among blood flow, pressure difference and resistance is described in Darcy's law. This in turn can be used to determine SVR.

$$\text{Pressure difference} = \text{flow} \times \text{resistance}$$
$$MAP\text{-}RAP = CO \times SVR$$

where RAP is the right atrial pressure.
Rearranging this equation:

$$SVR = 80 \times \frac{(MAP\text{-}RAP)}{CO = SV \times HR = VR}$$
$$(80 = \textit{conversion factor between units})$$

and VR is venous return.

Systemic vascular resistance describes the resistance to blood flow offered by the systemic vasculature (excluding the pulmonary circulation) to the left side of the heart. It is sometimes referred to as total peripheral resistance (TPR). Mechanisms altering the vascular resistance principally rely on modification of luminal diameter by contraction and relaxation of vascular smooth muscle: Resistance to flow is inversely proportional to the fourth power of the radius and directly proportional to the length (Hagen–Poiseuille equation; see Chapter 15). *Vascular tone* describes the degree to which a blood vessel is constricted, with all vessels (both arterial and venous) demonstrating a concentration of vasoconstriction at rest (basal vascular tone). Vascular tone is determined by systemic neurohumoral mechanisms, such as sympathetic stimulation; local factors, such as myogenic mechanisms; and locally released vasoactive substances, such as nitric oxide, endothelin and eicosanoids.

Pulmonary vascular resistance (PVR) describes the resistance offered to blood flow by the pulmonary circulation to the right side of the heart. Under physiological conditions, the pulmonary vascular system is a low-resistance system. Pulmonary arterial pressures therefore remain low despite receiving the same CO as the systemic circulation. In addition to those factors described earlier, PVR is also influenced by total pulmonary blood flow, lung volumes and hypoxia.

Structure of vascular smooth muscle

Vascular smooth muscle (VSM), found in arteries, arterioles, venules and veins, is located in the middle layer of the vessel wall – the *tunica media*. Alterations in the tone of the tunica media lead to constriction or dilatation of the vessel; vessel radius is the most important factor determining resistance to flow (Hagen–Poiseuille formula; see Chapter 15). Changes in cross-sectional area are very important in determining SVR, particularly for arterioles, which contribute significantly to the overall resistance.

Vascular smooth muscle shares some similarities with cardiac myocytes but also many differences. As with cardiac myocytes, contractile tension is dependent on cytosolic calcium concentration. In VSM, contractile tension can also be regulated by altering the *sensitivity* of the contractile apparatus to calcium. The thin actin filament is longer in VSM than in cardiac muscle, allowing a significantly increased degree of shortening. Vascular smooth muscle lacks the troponin complex found in cardiac muscle, being replaced by two proteins, caldesmon and calponin. The SR provides a store of Ca^{2+} for muscular contraction, but this is smaller compared with that found in the cardiac myocyte. Vascular smooth muscle cells rely on the influx of extracellular calcium for contraction – hence the ability of L-type calcium channel blockers (particularly the dihydropyridines) to promote vasorelaxation. Calcium release from the SR is driven primarily by the opening of IP_3–Ca^{2+} release channels, in addition to the ryanodine receptor found in the SR of cardiac muscle.

Vascular smooth muscle contraction

Vascular smooth muscle contraction is slow but sustained compared with the short contractions (~300 ms) of cardiac muscle. In fact, VSM may be under constant basal tone throughout life. The process of VSM contraction is somewhat different to that of cardiac muscle, relying on the phosphorylation of a regulatory subunit called myosin light chains, found on the myosin heads. Only phosphorylated myosin light chains can bind with actin (and therefore contribute to contraction). Phosphorylation is dependent on the activity of the cytosolic enzyme *myosin light chain kinase* (MLCK) and the presence of ATP. The process is as follows:

- Cytosolic Ca^{2+} concentrations increase by release from the SR and entry through membrane-bound Ca^{2+} channels.
- Calcium binds to calmodulin, a cytosolic protein structurally similar to troponin C.
- The calcium–calmodulin complex activates MLCK.
- Myosin light chain kinase, in the presence of ATP, phosphorylates myosin light chains on the myosin head, activating them.

- Activated myosin heads bind with actin filaments and the ratcheting mechanisms of muscle contraction continue, similar to cardiac muscle.

In contrast to the short-lived contraction of cardiac muscle, the actin-myosin cross-bridges remain linked in a tense flexed state known as the 'latch state' because of the phosphorylated myosin light chains. This is an energy-efficient process requiring minimal ATP, and hence VSM can remain in this state for long periods (necessary to maintain the basal tone of the vasculature). Dissociation of the actin-myosin cross-bridges requires myosin light chains to be dephosphorylated by the enzyme *myosin light chain phosphatase* (MLCP). The activity of MLCP increases with decreasing cytosolic calcium concentrations.

Control of vascular tone

The degree of myosin light chain phosphorylation and therefore the tone of VSM is dependent on cytosolic calcium concentration and the activities of MLCK and MLCP (Fig. 9.11).

Ion channels and the maintenance of basal tone

The RMP of the vascular myocyte is less negative than the cardiac myocyte at around −50 to −60 mV. Vascular smooth muscle ion channels are complex and not uniform throughout the vascular system. The membrane potential is maintained by the outward flux of potassium and chloride and the inward flux of sodium. Influx of potassium caused by opening of membrane-bound potassium channels leads to depolarisation of the cell membrane and subsequent influx of calcium, thus leading to muscular contraction. There are four main potassium channels in the sarcolemmal membrane:

1. Inward-rectifier K^+ channels (K_{IR})
   - Open in response to high potassium (caused by exercising/respiring tissue) concentrations, leading to hyperpolarisation and vasodilatation.
   - Aim to maintain/increase flow in response to demand.
2. ATP-dependent K^+ channels (K_{ATP})
   - Open in response to falling concentrations of ATP and rising concentrations of ADP, guanosine diphosphate (GDP), adenosine and H^+ ions, leading to vasodilatation in response to falling energy supplies.
   - Nicorandil blocks K_{ATP}, leading to vasodilatation.
3. Voltage-dependent K^+ channels (K_V)
   - Contribute to the RMP and are involved in repolarisation.
4. Calcium-activated K^+ channels (K_{Ca})
   - As Ca^{2+} enters the cell, K_{Ca} channels open, making the membrane potential more negative.
   - Reduce vascular excitability and prevent vasospasm.

159

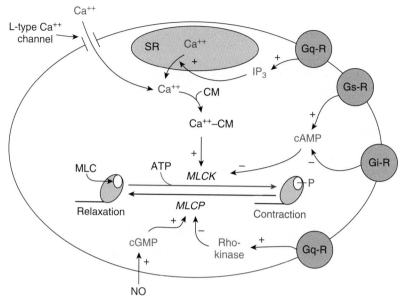

Fig. 9.11 Control of vascular tone. *ATP,* Adenosine triphosphate; *cAMP,* cyclic adenosine monophosphate; *CM,* calmodulin; *IP₃,* inositol triphosphate; *MLC,* myosin light chain; *MLCK,* myosin light chain kinase; *MLCP,* myosin light chain phosphatase; *NO,* nitric oxide; *P,* phosphate; *SR,* sarcoplasmic reticulum. (From Klabunde, D.E. (2014) *Cardiovascular pharmacology concepts: Vascular smooth muscle contraction and relaxation.* Available from: http://cvphysiology.com/Blood%20Pressure/BP026.)

Membrane-bound Ca^{2+} channels are the predominant means by which cytosolic Ca^{2+} concentrations are increased, promoting contraction, with relatively small calcium stores present in the SR. Unlike in myocardial contraction, depolarisation and smooth muscle contraction in the vasculature is not an all or nothing process. Increasing degrees of depolarisation lead to a graded response, with opening of Ca^{2+} channels and therefore increasing tone. Even at RMP of −50 mV, a number of Ca^{2+} channels will be open and therefore maintaining the basal tone of the vasculature. There are four main Ca^{2+} channels present:

1. Voltage-sensitive Ca^{2+} channels (VSCCs)
   - Mainly L-type, being abundant in arterioles
   - Open in response to membrane depolarisation
2. Receptor-operated channels (ROCs)
   - Non-selective cation conducting channels, with a preponderance for Ca^{2+} ions
   - Voltage *independent* – activated by binding of diacylglycerol (DAG) after activation of G_q G-protein–coupled receptors
   - Couples the stimulation of G-protein receptors by noradrenaline and other vasoactive compounds to VSM contraction
3. Store-operated cation channels (SOCs)
   - Present on the SR
   - Activated by IP₃, therefore G-protein activation leads to Ca^{2+} release by both ROCs and SOCs

4. Stretch-activated cation channels (SACs)
   - Mechanoreceptors activated by stretch
   - Involved in the autoregulation of blood flow as part of the myogenic response (see later)

Intrinsic control of vascular tone

Intrinsic control of vascular tone encompasses all of those mechanisms located within the tissue or organ itself.

Myogenic autoregulation

- Autoregulatory mechanism of arteriolar vessels maintaining constant flow of a range of pressures.
- As intraluminal pressure is increased, arteriolar VSM becomes stretched.
- Stretching leads to slight depolarisation of the cell membrane and graded opening of VSCCs, along with activation of SACs.
- Opening of these calcium channels leads to Ca^{2+} influx and vasoconstriction.
- The opposite occurs in response to decreased intraluminal pressure.
- Increased shear stress caused by flow and vasoconstriction leads to the release of vasodilatory compounds from the endothelium, avoiding excessive vasoconstriction.

Endothelial regulation

- The endothelium produces vasodilatory molecules, including nitric oxide (NO), endothelium-derived hyperpolarising factor (EDHF), prostacyclin (PGI_2) and endothelin, a vasoconstrictor.
- Shear stress stimulates the production of NO by the constitutive enzyme nitric oxide synthase (endothelial; eNOS).
- Hypoxia stimulates endothelin production, leading to pulmonary vasoconstriction, a contributing factor in high-altitude pulmonary hypertension.

Vasoactive factors

- Increasing metabolic rate leads to the production of vasodilatory metabolites aimed at increasing blood flow and oxygen delivery, the mechanism of reactive hyperaemia.
- Substances include K^+, H^+, lactate and adenosine.
- Hypoxia vasodilates systemic vessels via opening of K_{IR} and K_{ATP} channels and desensitisation.
- Adenosine is formed from the breakdown of AMP (formed from the metabolism of ATP), activating A_{2a} receptors which are coupled to the G-protein G_s pathway.

Autacoids

- Autacoids are hormones that act locally at the site of production.
- Vasodilator autacoids include bradykinin, histamine and prostaglandins.
- Vasoconstrictor autacoids include serotonin, thromboxane A_2, leukotrienes and platelet activating factor.

Extrinsic control

Extrinsic control encompasses the ANS and systemically released hormones.

Sympathetic nervous system

- The SNS provides innervation to the vast majority of arteries and arterioles and is responsible for maintaining basal vascular tone.
- Activation of the SNS leads to the release of noradrenaline from postganglionic neurons.
- Noradrenaline acts predominantly at α_1-adrenoceptors to cause vasoconstriction.
- Noradrenaline is quickly removed after its release via two mechanisms: 80% is transported back into the postganglionic neuron by a Na^+-Cl^--amine cotransporter (uptake$_1$), where it is recycled or metabolised by monamine oxidase. Smaller amounts are transported into non-neuronal tissue (uptake$_2$); some reaches the circulation where it

is degraded by catechol O-methyltransferase to inactive metabolites.

Control of vascular resistance is predominantly by decreasing or increasing sympathetic stimulation around the basal tone set point to cause vasodilatation or vasoconstriction, respectively.

Systemic hormonal control

Adrenaline, vasopressin, angiotensin II and the natriuretic peptides also play a role in modulating vascular resistance, with all apart from adrenaline also being involved in the control of extracellular fluid volume (and therefore blood pressure via the effect on cardiac output).

- Vasopressin (antidiuretic hormone; ADH), is released in response to low plasma volume and changes in plasma osmolarity (central osmoreceptors).
  - Stimulation of V_2 receptors on the collecting ducts leads to water reabsorption and increase in circulating volume. The V_1 receptors are coupled to G_q, leading to vasoconstriction.
  - In the coronary and cerebral circulations, vasopressin stimulates eNOS, leading to vasodilatation, redirecting blood to the heart and brain.
- Angiotensin II is produced in response to low blood pressure, leading to an increase in blood pressure via several mechanisms:
  - Aldosterone secretion by the zona glomerulosa of the adrenal cortex, which causes sodium and water retention, increasing circulating volume.
  - Arteriolar vasoconstriction via direct activation of AT_1 receptors on vascular myocytes (G_q mechanism) and indirectly by stimulating noradrenaline exocytosis.
  - Stimulation of thirst – to increase circulating volume.
- Natriuretic peptides
  - Atrial natriuretic peptide (ANP) and brain natriuretic peptide (BNP) are released in response to increased cardiac filling pressures by the atria and ventricles, respectively, stimulating renal salt excretion and moderate dilatation of resistance vessels.
  - They act as a counterbalance to the renin-angiotensin system.

Cardiovascular reflexes

Short-term control of arterial blood pressure is accomplished via several cardiovascular reflexes – the baroreceptor reflex, chemoreceptor reflex and Bainbridge reflex.

The baroreceptor reflex is the best known and most important cardiovascular reflex, minimising fluctuations in mean arterial pressure. The baroreceptors are mechano-stretch receptors located in the adventitia of the carotid sinus and aortic arch. Afferent fibres from the carotid sinus join the glossopharyngeal nerve (IXth cranial nerve) and terminate in the nucleus tractus solitarius in the medulla. Aortic arch baroreceptor fibres join the vagus nerve (X[th] cranial nerve) and terminate in the medulla.

Increases in carotid sinus and aortic arch pressure cause distension of the vessel wall and increased baroreceptor firing. Integration in the medulla leads to a decrease in sympathetic outflow and increase in parasympathetic outflow. Together these cause vasodilatation and a decrease in HR, reducing cardiac output, SVR and blood pressure. The opposite effects (decreased baroreceptor stimulation, increased sympathetic and decreased parasympathetic activity) occur in response to a fall in blood pressure. Chronic hypo- or hypertension leads to resetting of the baroreceptor set point.

Peripheral chemoreceptors, located in the carotid and aortic bodies, produce similar effects to baroreceptors in response to low oxygen tension, increased P_{CO_2} and acidosis (which occur when blood flow is insufficient). Peripheral chemoreceptors are also activated in severe hypotension.

The *Bainbridge reflex* describes an increase in HR in response to an increase in atrial pressure to prevent an overload of blood in the atria. The afferent arm of the reflex is transmitted via the vagus nerve to the medulla to increase HR by a combination of vagal inhibition and sympathetic stimulation of the SA node. The reflex is active during sinus arrhythmia, where thoracic pressure becomes more negative upon inspiration, increasing venous return and hence increasing HR.

Baroreflexes play a crucial role in the compensatory mechanism associated with acute haemorrhage. Hypovolaemia leads to a reduction in venous return, stroke volume and subsequently MAP, with an associated decrease in the rate of baroreceptor stretch and firing. Decreased afferent firing leads to a compensatory decrease in vagal parasympathetic activity and an increase in sympathetic activity. Heart rate, force of contraction and SVR all increase to restore cardiac output. Extensive blood loss (>30%) can have paradoxical effect of causing vasodilatation and worsening of the clinical picture, the cause of which is not fully understood.

Valsalva manoeuvre

The Valsalva manoeuvre (Fig. 9.12) is performed by forced expiration against a closed glottis for a period of 10 s. Intrathoracic pressure changes associated with forced expiration lead to a series of reflex cardiovascular responses, which occur in four distinct phases:

Phase 1

- Intrathoracic pressure becomes highly positive.
- Blood is forced from the intrathoracic vasculature into the heart, transiently increasing MAP.
- Increased MAP leads to a baroreceptor-mediated bradycardia.

Phase 2

- Ongoing high intrathoracic pressure reduces venous return to the heart.
- The accompanying low HR leads to a fall in MAP.
- The reduction in MAP is detected by the baroreceptors, producing an increase in HR and MAP towards normal.

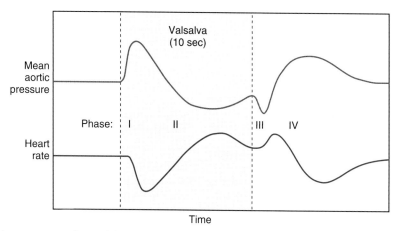

Fig. 9.12 The Valsalva manoeuvre. (From Klabunde, D.E. (2014) *Cardiovascular pharmacology concepts: Hemodynamics of a Valsalva maneuver.* Available from: http://www.cvphysiology.com/Hemodynamics/H014.)

Phase 3

- After airway pressure is released, intrathoracic pressure falls rapidly.
- Venous return rapidly fills the empty intrathoracic vessels, leading to a decrease in left ventricular preload and SV.
- MAP falls and is detected by the baroreceptors, leading to an increase in HR.

Phase 4

- Preload is restored but HR remains high, leading to an increased MAP.
- This is detected by the baroreceptors, causing a decreased HR. Mean arterial pressure and HR then return to their normal state.

Myocardial oxygen delivery

Oxygen delivery ($\dot{D}O_2$) to the myocardium is dependent on the arterial oxygen content of blood (CaO_2) and coronary blood flow (CBF).

$$\dot{D}O_2 = CBF \times CaO_2$$

Arterial oxygen content is determined by two factors: the oxygen bound to haemoglobin, and that dissolved in plasma.

$$CaO_2 = (1.34 \times [Hb] \times SaO_2) + (0.0225 \times PaO_2)$$

where 1.34 is *Hüfner's constant* (the theoretical maximum oxygen carrying capacity of 1 g of haemoglobin (Hb)) and 0.0225 is the amount of O_2 dissolved per 100 ml of plasma. The normal oxygen content of arterial blood is approximately 20 ml O_2 100 ml^{-1}. Oxygen consumption ($\dot{V}O_2$) can be determined by the Fick principle as the difference between arterial and venous oxygen contents (CvO_2).

$$\dot{V}O_2 = CBF(CaO_2 - CvO_2)$$

Under physiological conditions the oxygen content of arterial blood varies very little. The main determinant of myocardial oxygen delivery is therefore coronary blood flow, which is normally tightly matched to myocardial oxygen requirement, preventing hypoxia. In coronary arterial disease, stenosis of coronary vessels leads to a reduction in CBF and aerobic metabolism becomes flow dependent. Flow limitation during times of increased myocardial oxygen demand (such as exercise) leads to myocardial hypoxia, experienced as chest pain (angina). Diseased coronary vessels are more susceptible to vasospasm, again leading to myocardial

Table 9.2 Classification of myocardial infarction (MI)

Classification	Description
Type 1	Spontaneous MI (plaque rupture, thrombus, dissection)
Type 2	Ischaemia caused by imbalance between oxygen supply and demand
Type 3	MI resulting in death before biomarker values available
Type 4a	MI related to PCI
Type 4b	MI related to stent thrombosis
Type 5	MI related to CABG

CABG, Coronary artery bypass grafting; *PCI*, percutaneous coronary intervention.

ischaemia (unstable angina). Partial or complete occlusion of coronary blood flow, caused by thrombosis or rupture of an atherosclerotic plaque, can lead to myocardial infarction (classified in Table 9.2).

Therapies aimed at improving myocardial blood flow can be classified into surgical and medical interventions. Surgical interventions are aimed at increasing the intraluminal diameter of stenosed vessels, therefore increasing flow. These include balloon dilatation (angioplasty), the positioning of intraluminal stents, and the bypassing of stenotic lesions completely by means of coronary artery bypass grafting. Medical interventions may be subclassified into agents used to treat and manage clot formation (thrombolytics and antiplatelet drugs) and those used to prevent and treat coronary arterial vasospasm (vasodilators, calcium channel blockers).

Cardiovascular pharmacology

Drugs acting on the sympathetic nervous system

Sympathomimetic agents

Sympathomimetic drugs partially or completely mimic the effects of sympathetic nerve stimulation or adrenal medullary discharge. They may act:
- directly on the adrenergic receptor (e.g. the catecholamines, phenylephrine, methoxamine);
- indirectly causing release of noradrenaline from the adrenergic nerve ending (e.g. amphetamine); or

163

Table 9.3 Classification of inotropes and vasopressors

Pure vasopressor	Inoconstrictor	Inodilator
Phenylephrine	Noradrenaline	Dobutamine
Vasopressin	Adrenaline	Dopexamine
	Ephedrine	PDE inhibitors
	Dopamine[a]	Dopamine[a]
	Metaraminol	Levosimendan

[a]Dopamine is an inodilator at low doses and an inoconstrictor at high doses.
PDE, Phosphodiesterase.

- by both mechanisms (e.g. dopamine, ephedrine, metaraminol).

The drugs may be classified according to their structure (catecholamine/non-catecholamine), their origin (endogenous/synthetic) and their mechanism of action (via adrenergic receptors or via a non-adrenergic mechanism) (Table 9.3).

Inotropy

Drugs which affect myocardial contractility are termed inotropes, although this term is usually applied to those drugs that increase cardiac contractility (strictly 'positive inotropes'). Myocardial contractility may be increased by:
- increasing intracellular cAMP by activation of the adenylate cyclase system (e.g. catecholamines and other drugs acting via the adrenergic receptor);
- decreasing breakdown of cAMP (e.g. phosphodiesterase inhibitors);
- increasing intracellular calcium availability (e.g. digoxin, calcium salts, glucagon); or
- increasing the response of contractile proteins to calcium (e.g. levosimendan) (Fig. 9.13).

Inotropes may also be classified into positive inotropic drugs which also produce systemic vasoconstriction (inoconstrictors) and those which also produce systemic vasodilatation (inodilators) (see Table 9.3). Inoconstrictors include noradrenaline, adrenaline and ephedrine. Inodilators are dobutamine, dopexamine, isoprenaline and phosphodiesterase inhibitors. Dopamine is an inodilator at low dose and an inoconstrictor at higher doses.

Catecholamines

Catecholamines are organic monoamines consisting of a catechol molecule with a variable amine side chain.

Catecholamine drugs may be endogenous (adrenaline, noradrenaline and dopamine) or synthetic (dobutamine, dopexamine and isoprenaline). Several other drugs with a non-catecholamine structure produce sympathomimetic effects via adrenergic receptors (e.g. ephedrine and phenylephrine). All catecholamine drugs are inactivated in the gut by MAO and are usually only administered parenterally. They all have very short half-lives *in vivo*, and so, when given by intravenous infusion, their effects may be controlled by altering the infusion rate. The comparative effects of different inotropes and vasopressors are outlined next.

Endogenous catecholamines

Adrenaline

Adrenaline is the principle catecholamine synthesised by the adrenal medulla (80%–90%). It is a potent agonist at both α- and β-adrenergic receptors. It is the treatment of choice in anaphylactic reactions and is used in the management of cardiac arrest and shock and occasionally as a bronchodilator. Except in emergency situations, bolus i.v. injection is avoided because of the risk of inducing cardiac arrhythmias.

The effects of adrenaline on arterial pressure and CO are dose dependent. At lower doses, β effects predominate, increasing HR and contractility, CO and myocardial oxygen consumption. β_2-Mediated vasodilatation in skeletal muscle and splanchnic arterioles leads to a decrease in SVR with a decrease in diastolic pressure and widened pulse pressure. At higher doses, α-mediated vasoconstriction becomes more prominent in venous capacitance vessels (increasing venous return) and the precapillary resistance vessels of skin, mucosa and kidney (increasing peripheral resistance). Systolic pressure increases further, but CO may decrease. Adrenaline causes marked decreases in renal blood flow, but CBF is increased. In contrast to other sympathomimetics, adrenaline has significant metabolic effects. Hepatic glycogenolysis and lipolysis in adipose tissue increase (β_1 and β_3 effects), and insulin secretion is inhibited (α_1 effect) so that hyperglycaemia occurs. Unlike indirect-acting sympathomimetics which cause release of noradrenaline, tachyphylaxis should not occur with adrenaline.

In cardiac arrest, adrenaline is administered intravenously at a dose of 1 mg (10 ml of 1 : 10000) (see Chapter 28). In anaphylaxis it is usually administered intramuscularly at a dose of 500 μg (0.5 ml of 1 : 1000) or via i.v. aliquots of 50–100 μg (see Chapter 27). Adrenaline can be administered as an i.v. infusion for cardiogenic shock at a range of $0.01-0.5$ μg kg^{-1} min^{-1}.

Noradrenaline

Noradrenaline is a potent arteriolar and venous vasoconstrictor, acting predominantly at α-receptors, with a slightly

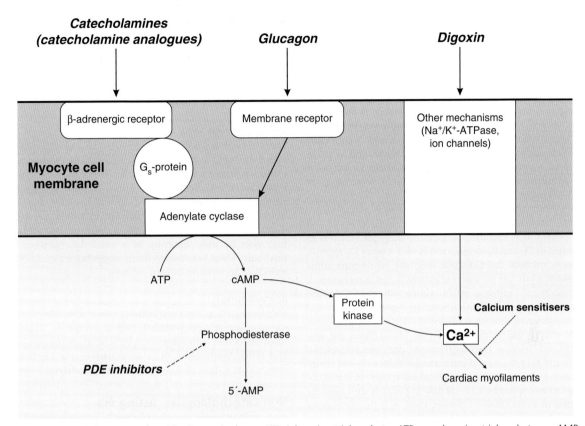

Fig. 9.13 Intracellular action of positive inotropic drugs. *ATP*, Adenosine triphosphate; *ATPase*, adenosine triphosphatase; *cAMP*, cyclic adenosine monophosphate; *PDE*, phosphodiesterase.

greater potency there than adrenaline. It is also a β-receptor agonist, but β_2 effects are not apparent in clinical use. Infusions of noradrenaline increase venous return, systolic and diastolic systemic and pulmonary arterial pressures and central venous pressure. Cardiac output increases alongside a baroreceptor-mediated reflex bradycardia. At higher doses, the α-mediated effects of widespread intense vasoconstriction overcome β_1 effects on cardiac contractility, leading to a decrease in CO at the cost of increased myocardial oxygen demand; renal blood flow and glomerular filtration rate also decrease. Its principal use is in the management of low SVR states such as septic shock and after cardiac bypass. Noradrenaline is administered as an i.v. infusion at a dose of 0.1–1 μg kg^{-1} min^{-1}.

Dopamine

Dopamine is the natural precursor of adrenaline and noradrenaline (see Fig. 9.1). It stimulates α- and β-adrenergic receptors and specific dopamine D_1 receptors in renal and mesenteric arteries. Dopamine has a direct positive inotropic action on the myocardium via β-receptors and by release of noradrenaline from adrenergic nerve terminals. The overall effects of dopamine are highly dose dependent. At low dosages (3 μg kg^{-1} min^{-1}), renal and mesenteric vascular resistances are reduced by an action on D_1 receptors, resulting in increased splanchnic and renal blood flows, glomerular filtration rate and sodium excretion. At doses of 5–10 μg kg^{-1} min^{-1}, β-mediated inotropic action predominates, increasing CO and systolic pressure, with little effect on diastolic pressure. At doses greater than 5–10 μg kg^{-1} min^{-1}, α-receptor activity predominates, with direct vasoconstriction. Renal and splanchnic blood flows decrease, and arrhythmias may occur. These are average doses when these effects occur; in clinical practice, interindividual variability makes the distinction between low- and high-dose dopamine rather blurred. Dopamine receptors are widely present in the CNS, particularly in the basal ganglia, the pituitary (where they mediate prolactin secretion) and the chemoreceptor trigger zone on the floor of the fourth ventricle (where they mediate nausea and vomiting).

Synthetic catecholamines

Dobutamine

Dobutamine is predominantly a β_1-agonist, with some activity at β_2-receptors. Its primary effect is an increase in cardiac output as a consequence of increased contractility and HR and decreased afterload. Systolic arterial pressure may therefore increase, but peripheral resistance is reduced or unchanged. It is primarily used as an inotrope (inodilator) in low CO states. Dobutamine increases SA node automaticity and conduction velocity in the atria, ventricles and AV node, with tachyarrhythmias occurring at higher doses. Dobutamine is administered as an i.v. infusion at a dose range of $0.5-40\ \mu g\ kg^{-1}\ min^{-1}$.

Dopexamine

Dopexamine is a synthetic dopamine analogue which is an agonist at D_1 and β_2-receptors. It is also a weak D_2 agonist, and it inhibits the neuronal reuptake of noradrenaline (uptake$_1$) but has no direct effects at β_1- or α-receptors. It produces mild increases in HR, contractility and CO (effects on β_2-receptors and noradrenaline uptake), renal and mesenteric vasodilatation (β_2 and D_1 effects) and natriuresis (D_1 effect). Coronary and cerebral blood flows are also increased. Systemic vascular resistance decreases and arterial pressure may decrease if intravascular volume is not maintained. Dopexamine has theoretical advantages in maintaining CO and splanchnic blood flow in patients with systemic sepsis or heart failure; however, there is little evidence of clinical benefit. It is administered as an i.v. infusion at a rate of $0.5-6\ \mu g\ kg^{-1}\ min^{-1}$.

Isoprenaline

Isoprenaline is a potent β-agonist primarily acting at the β_1-receptor. It is mainly used for the temporary emergency treatment of bradyarrhythmias. β_2 effects lead to broncho- and vasodilatation, with a decrease in SVR. Isoprenaline is only available in the UK via specialist importing companies. It is administered by i.v. infusion at a dose range of $0.5-20\ \mu g\ min^{-1}$.

Non-catecholamine sympathomimetics

Non-catecholamines: acting via adrenergic receptors

Ephedrine

Ephedrine is a naturally occurring sympathomimetic amine that possesses both direct (agonist at α- and β-receptors) and indirect activity via its potentiation of noradrenaline release from sympathetic nerve terminals. It causes an increase in HR, contractility, CO and arterial pressure (systolic > diastolic). Bronchodilation occurs via a β_2-mediated mechanism, and it is occasionally used for this purpose. Its duration

of action is longer than endogenous catecholamines as it is not metabolised by COMT or MAO. Tachyphylaxis can occur as a result of depletion of noradrenaline from nerve terminals and persistent occupation of adrenergic receptors. Ephedrine crosses the placenta and can increase fetal metabolic rate with a subsequent metabolic acidosis. It is usually administered by i.v. bolus at a dose of 3–9 mg.

Phenylephrine

Phenylephrine is a potent direct-acting α_1-agonist with clinical effects similar to those of noradrenaline. It causes widespread vasoconstriction with an increase in arterial pressure, reflex bradycardia and decrease in cardiac output. It may be administered by i.v. bolus (50–100 μg boluses) and i.v. infusion (50–150 μg min^{-1}) to maintain arterial pressure during general anaesthesia or other causes of low SVR. It may also be used topically as a nasal decongestant or mydriatic. There is some evidence suggesting a paradoxical reduction in cerebral oxygen delivery.

Metaraminol

Metaraminol is a direct and indirect non-specific adrenoceptor agonist. It acts primarily via α_1-receptors, causing vasoconstriction with subsequent increase in arterial pressure and reflex bradycardia. It is administered via i.v. bolus injection at a dose of 0.5–2 mg, titrated to effect.

Non-catecholamines: acting via non-adrenergic mechanisms

Phosphodiesterase inhibitors

Phosphodiesterase (PDE) inhibitors increase intracellular cAMP concentrations by inhibition of the enzyme responsible for cAMP breakdown (see Fig. 9.13). Increased intracellular cAMP concentrations promote the activation of protein kinases, which leads to an increase in intracellular Ca^{2+}. In cardiac muscle cells this causes a positive inotropic effect and facilitates diastolic relaxation and cardiac filling (positive lusitropy). In vascular smooth muscle, increased cAMP decreases intracellular Ca^{2+} and causes marked vasodilatation.

Several subtypes of phosphodiesterase isoenzyme exist in different tissues. Non-specific PDE inhibitors (e.g. aminophylline) are occasionally used to facilitate bronchodilation in the management of life-threatening asthma. An initial bolus dose of 5 mg kg^{-1} is administered (providing the patient is not receiving long-term oral theophylline therapy), followed by an i.v. infusion at a rate of $0.5-0.7$ mg kg^{-1} h^{-1}. Therapeutic drug monitoring is required because of its narrow therapeutic index. Adverse effects include tremors, tachyarrhythmia (including ventricular fibrillation), seizures and hypotension.

Phosphodiesterase III inhibitors (enoximone and milrinone) are selective for the isoenzyme present in myocardium, VSM and platelets. They are positive inotropes and potent arterial, coronary and venodilators. They decrease preload, afterload, PVR and PCWP, increasing cardiac index. Heart rate may increase or remain unchanged. In contrast to sympathomimetics, they improve myocardial function *without* increasing oxygen demand. Their effects are augmented by the coadministration of β_1-agonists (i.e. increases in cAMP production are synergistic with decreased cAMP breakdown). They have particular advantages in patients with chronic heart failure, in whom downregulation of myocardial β-adrenergic receptors occurs, so that there is a decreased inotropic response to β-sympathomimetic drugs. A similar phenomenon occurs with advanced age, prolonged (>72 h) catecholamine therapy and possibly with surgical stress. Phosphodiesterase III inhibitors are indicated for acute refractory heart failure, such as cardiogenic shock, or pre- or postcardiac surgery. All PDE III inhibitors may cause hypotension and are commonly coadministered with an α-agonist. Tachyarrhythmias may occur. Other adverse effects include nausea, vomiting and fever. Their half-life is prolonged markedly in patients with heart or renal failure, and they are commonly administered as an i.v. loading dose over 5 min with or without a subsequent i.v. infusion. Milrinone is a bipyridine derivative, whereas enoximone is an imidazole derivative. Enoximone undergoes substantial first-pass metabolism and is rapidly metabolised to an active sulphoxide metabolite that is excreted via the kidneys and which may accumulate in renal failure, prolonging the elimination half-life.

Vasopressin

Vasopressin is a peptide hormone secreted by the hypothalamus via the posterior pituitary. Its primary role is the regulation of body fluid balance. It is secreted in response to hypotension and promotes retention of water by action on specific cAMP-coupled V_2 receptors. It causes vasoconstriction by stimulating V_1 receptors in VSM and is particularly potent in hypotensive patients. It is increasingly used in the treatment of refractory vasodilatory shock which is resistant to catecholamines. The vasopressin analogue desmopressin is used to treat diabetes insipidus and in the management of von Willebrand's disease. Terlipressin (another analogue) is used to limit bleeding from oesophageal varices in patients with portal hypertension. When used for the management of low SVR states, vasopressin is administered as an i.v. infusion at a rate of 0.01–0.1 units min^{-1}.

Glucagon

Glucagon is a polypeptide secreted by the α cells of the pancreatic islets. Its physiological actions include stimulation of hepatic gluconeogenesis in response to hypoglycaemia and amino acids and as part of the stress response. These effects are mediated by increasing adenylate cyclase activity and intracellular cAMP by a mechanism independent of the β-adrenergic receptor (see Fig. 9.13). It increases cAMP in myocardial cells and so increases cardiac contractility. Glucagon causes nausea and vomiting, hyperglycaemia and hyperkalaemia and is not used as an inotrope except in the management of β-blocker poisoning.

Levosimendan

Levosimendan is a positive inotropic agent that acts by sensitising troponin C to Ca^{2+}, prolonging actin-myosin cross-bridge formation and therefore increasing contractility. This is an energy-independent process and therefore does not increase myocardial oxygen demand. Levosimendan also causes vasodilatation by opening ATP-sensitive K^+ channels in vascular smooth muscle, reducing pre- and afterload and improving myocardial oxygen supply. It may have a role in the management of acute heart failure and postresuscitation myocardial dysfunction.

Selective β-agonists

Selective β_2-receptor agonists (e.g. salbutamol, terbutaline, formoterol and salmeterol) relax bronchial muscle, uterine muscle and VSM while having much less effect on the heart than isoprenaline. These drugs are partial agonists (their maximal effect at β_2-receptors is less than that of isoprenaline) and are only partially selective for β_2-receptors. They are used widely in the treatment of bronchospasm. Although less cardiotoxic than isoprenaline, dose-related tremor, tachyarrhythmias, hyperglycaemia, hypokalaemia, hypomagnesaemia and hyperlactaemia may occur. β_2-Agonists are resistant to metabolism by COMT and therefore have a prolonged duration of action (mostly 3–5 h). Salmeterol is highly lipophilic, has a strong affinity for the β_2-adrenergic receptor, is longer acting than the other β_2-agonists and so is used for maintenance therapy in chronic asthma in combination with inhaled steroids. β_2-Agonists are usually administered by the inhaled route (metered dose inhaler or nebuliser) or intravenous route because of unpredictable oral absorption and a high hepatic extraction ratio. When inhaled, only 10%–20% of the administered dose reaches the lower airways; this proportion is reduced further when administered via a tracheal tube. Nevertheless, systemic absorption does occur, although adverse effects are less common during long-term therapy.

Salbutamol

Salbutamol is the β_2-agonist used most commonly for the prevention and treatment of bronchospasm. It is most commonly administered in its inhaled form by metered-dose inhaler (1–2 puffs of 100 μg each) or via nebuliser in more severe cases of bronchospasm (2.5–5 mg). In patients with life-threatening asthma it may be administered i.v. as both a bolus (250 μg) and infusion (3–20 μg min^{-1}). Intravenous administration requires cardiac monitoring as tachyarrhythmias may be significant. Salbutamol may also be used in the management of hyperkalaemia, temporarily driving K^+ intracellularly via stimulation of the Na^+–K^+ ATPase pump.

Sympatholytic agents

Sympatholytic drugs antagonise the effects of the SNS at either:
- central adrenergic neurons;
- peripheral autonomic ganglia/neurons; or
- postsynaptic α- or β-receptors.

These drugs are used largely for their effects in reducing blood pressure and HR, although there are other effects and indications.

Centrally acting sympatholytic drugs

Centrally acting sympatholytic agents act by agonism of central $α_2$-receptors to decrease sympathetic tone. They are also agonists at central imidazoline (I_1) receptors, which contributes to their hypotensive action. The I_1 receptors are present in several peripheral tissues, including the kidney. Central $α_2$ stimulation causes decreases in arterial pressure, peripheral resistance, venous return, myocardial contractility, CO and HR, but baroreceptor reflexes are preserved, and the pressor response to ephedrine or phenylephrine may be exaggerated. Stimulation of peripheral $α_2$-receptors on VSM causes direct arteriolar vasoconstriction, although the central effects of these drugs predominate overall. However, severe rebound hypertension may occur on stopping chronic oral therapy. $α_2$-Receptors in the dorsal horn of the spinal cord modulate upward transmission of nociceptive signals by modifying local release of substance P and calcitonin gene–related peptide. Centrally acting $α_2$-agonists produce analgesia by activation of descending spinal and supraspinal inhibitory pathways, these being greatest when administered by the epidural or spinal route. Other effects include dry mouth, sedation and anxiolysis.

Clonidine

Clonidine is a partial agonist at central and peripheral $α_2$-receptors and an I_1 receptor agonist. Clonidine has some effects at $α_1$-receptors ($α_2/α_1 > 200:1$). Clonidine reduces the MAC of inhalational anaesthetic agents by up to 50%. It has a synergistic analgesic effect with opioids which may be partly pharmacokinetic because the elimination half-life of opioids is also increased. Clonidine is well absorbed orally, with peak plasma concentrations after 60–90 min. It is highly lipid soluble, and approximately 50% is metabolised in the liver to inactive metabolites; the rest is excreted unchanged via the kidneys, with an elimination half-life of 9–12 h. Clonidine may be useful in the treatment of acute opioid withdrawal. Epidural clonidine 1–2 µg kg^{-1} increases the duration and potency of analgesia provided by epidural opioid or local anaesthetic drugs.

Dexmedetomidine

Dexmedetomidine has an eight times increased affinity for the $α_2$-receptor compared with clonidine and therefore produces less cardiovascular instability at comparable doses. It is principally used as a sedative in mechanically ventilated patients in ICU. It is particularly useful in those patients with delirium.

Methyldopa

Methyldopa easily crosses the blood–brain barrier, where it is converted to the active molecule, α-methyl noradrenaline, which is a full agonist at $α_2$-receptors. Its use is largely restricted to the management of pregnancy-associated hypertension.

Peripherally acting sympatholytic drugs

Adrenergic neuron blocking drugs

Guanethidine decreases peripheral SNS activity by competitively binding to noradrenaline binding sites in storage vesicles in the cytoplasm of postganglionic sympathetic nerve terminals. Further uptake of noradrenaline into the vesicles is inhibited, and it is metabolised by cytoplasmic MAO, so the nerve terminals become depleted of noradrenaline. Guanethidine has local anaesthetic properties and does not cross the blood–brain barrier. It is sometimes used to produce intravenous regional sympathetic blockade in the treatment of chronic limb pain associated with excessive autonomic activity (reflex sympathetic dystrophy or complex regional pain syndromes).

Ganglion blocking drugs

Nicotinic receptor antagonists (e.g. hexamethonium, pentolonium, trimetaphan) competitively inhibit the effects of ACh at autonomic ganglia and block both parasympathetic and sympathetic transmission. Sympathetic blockade produces venodilatation, decreased myocardial contractility and hypotension, but the effects vary depending on pre-existing sympathetic tone. Tachyphylaxis develops rapidly, and these drugs have now been superseded.

Adrenergic receptor antagonists

α-Receptor antagonists (α-blockers)

α-Blockers selectively inhibit the action of catecholamines at α-adrenergic receptors, diminishing vasoconstrictor tone and decreasing peripheral resistance. They are used mainly as second-line antihypertensive agents or for benign prostatic hyperplasia. They are important in the management of phaeochromocytoma. They may be classified according to their relative selectivity for $α_1$ and $α_2$-receptors.

Non-selective α-blockers

Non-selective α-blockers, such as phentolamine and phenoxybenzamine, produce more postural hypotension, reflex tachycardia and adverse GI effects (e.g. abdominal cramps, diarrhoea) than α1-selective drugs. *Phentolamine* 2–5 mg i.v. produces a rapid decrease in arterial pressure lasting 10–15 min and is used for the treatment of hypertensive crises. *Phenoxybenzamine* binds covalently (i.e. irreversibly and non-competitively) to α-receptors so that its effects last up to several days and may be cumulative on repeated dosing. It also reduces central sympathetic activity, which enhances vasodilatation, and has antagonist effects at 5-HT receptors. It is used for the preoperative preparation of patients with phaeochromocytoma.

Selective α-blockers

Selective α1-blockers include doxazosin and prazosin. *Doxazosin* has largely succeeded prazosin as it has a more prolonged duration of action. Reflex tachycardia and postural hypotension are less common than with direct-acting vasodilators (e.g. hydralazine) and the non-selective α-blockers but may still occur on initiating therapy. Nasal congestion, sedation and inhibition of ejaculation may occur.

β-Receptor antagonists (β-blockers)

Beta-blockers are structurally similar to the β-agonists. Variations in the molecular structure (primarily of the catechol ring) have produced compounds which do not activate adenylate cyclase and the second messenger system despite binding avidly to the β-adrenergic receptor. Beta-blockers are competitive antagonists with high receptor affinity, although their effects are attenuated by high concentrations of endogenous or exogenous agonists. They may be classified (Table 9.4) according to their:

- relative affinity for β1- or β2-receptors,
- agonist/antagonist activity,
- membrane-stabilising effect, or
- ancillary effects (e.g. action at other receptors).

First generation β-blockers (propranolol, timolol) are non-selective. Second-generation β-blockers (atenolol, metoprolol, bisoprolol) are selective for β1-receptors but have no ancillary effects, whereas third-generation agents are β1-selective but also have effects on other receptors. Labetalol and carvedilol are α1-antagonists, and celiprolol produces vasodilatation via an NO-mediated mechanism. Selective antagonists have theoretical advantages as some of the adverse effects of β-blockers are related to β2-antagonism (hyperglycaemia and bronchial tone).

Beta-blockers are used in the acute and chronic management of ischaemic heart disease, hypertension and arrhythmias. They reduce CO (decreased HR and contractility), central sympathetic nervous activity, plasma renin concentration and peripheral resistance. Secondary effects of β-blockage include reduction in myocardial oxygen demand and myocardial remodelling.

Labetalol

Labetalol is a competitive α1- and β-antagonist which is more active at β- than at α-receptors (1:3–1:7, depending on route). It may be administered orally or i.v. Intravenous bolus doses range from 50–200 mg, with infusion rates between 5–150 mg h^{-1}, titrated to effect. It reduces SVR whilst maintaining cerebral, renal and coronary blood flow.

Table 9.4 Pharmacological properties of β-blockers in common use

Drug	β1 selectivity	Partial agonist activity	Membrane stabilising effect	Terminal half-life (h)	Elimination
Atenolol	+	−	−	6–8	Renal
Bisoprolol	++	−	−	10–12	Hepatic, renal
Carvedilol	−	−	?	6–10	Hepatic
Celiprolol	+	+	?	5–6	Renal
Esmolol	+	−	−	0.15	Plasma hydrolysis
Labetalol	−	±	+	4	Hepatic
Metoprolol	+	−	±	4	Hepatic
Propranolol	−	−	++	5	Hepatic
Sotalol	−	+	+	8–15	Renal
Timolol	−	+	±	4	Hepatic, renal

Drugs acting on the parasympathetic nervous system

Parasympathetic antagonists

Parasympathetic antagonists block muscarinic ACh receptors and are either tertiary (atropine and hyoscine) or quaternary amine compounds (glycopyrronium bromide). Tertiary amines are more lipid soluble and cross biological membranes, such as the blood–brain barrier, affecting central ACh receptors and producing sedative or stimulatory effects.

Atropine

Atropine has widespread, dose-dependent antimuscarinic effects on parasympathetic functions. Salivary secretion, micturition, bradycardia and visual accommodation are impaired sequentially. Central nervous system effects (sedation or excitation, hallucinations and hyperthermia) may occur at high doses. Atropine is administered in doses of 0.6–3.0 mg i.v. to counteract bradycardia in the presence of hypotension and to prevent the bradycardia associated with vagal stimulation or the use of anticholinesterase drugs. Adverse cardiac effects of atropine include an increase in cardiac work and ventricular arrhythmias. Occasionally, atropine may produce an initial transient bradycardia, thought to be caused by increased ACh release, mediated by M_2 receptor antagonism. In therapeutic dosage, effects mediated by M_2 and M_3 receptors (tachycardia, bronchodilation, dry mouth, mydriasis) are both important.

Glycopyrronium bromide

Glycopyrronium bromide is a quaternary amine with similar anticholinergic actions to atropine but without central effects because it is a quaternary amine and does not cross the blood–brain barrier. It is used as an alternative to atropine during the reversal of neuromuscular blockade or as an antisialagogue during fibreoptic intubation. It is effective at a dose of 200 µg i.m./i.v., with minimal central or cardiovascular effects.

Parasympathetic agonists
Anticholinesterase drugs

Neostigmine and *pyridostigmine* antagonise AChE, thereby decreasing the breakdown of released ACh. They exert both nicotinic and muscarinic effects and are used in anaesthesia to reverse non-depolarising neuromuscular blockade, accompanied by an antimuscarinic drug to minimise the adverse vagal effects. Other anticholinesterases include edrophonium (short-acting) and pyridostigmine (long-acting), used for the diagnosis and symptomatic management of myasthenia gravis, respectively.

Vasodilators

Vasodilators dilate arteries or veins and may reduce afterload, preload or both. Acute and chronic heart failure are both associated with a reflex increase in sympathetic tone and an increase in SVR. By lowering this resistance (afterload), myocardial work and oxygen requirements are reduced. Vasodilators acting on the venous side of the circulation (e.g. nitrates) increase venous capacitance, reduce venous return to the heart and so decrease left ventricular filling pressure (preload), myocardial fibre length and myocardial oxygen consumption for the same degree of cardiac work performed. They have several clinical indications (Box 9.1).

Nitrates/nitric oxide donors

The organic nitrates (*glyceryl trinitrate* and *isosorbide mononitrate*) cause systemic and coronary vasodilatation. They act primarily on systemic veins, causing venodilatation, sequestration of blood in venous capacitance beds and a reduction in preload. Arteriolar dilatation occurs at higher doses, and afterload is reduced; tachycardia, hypotension and headaches may occur. Systolic pressure decreases more than diastolic pressure, so coronary perfusion pressure is preserved. In left ventricular failure, venodilatation is beneficial, reducing pulmonary congestion; cardiac dynamics may be improved so that stroke volume and CO increase.

Nitrates are used widely for the prevention and treatment of angina and myocardial infarction because they cause vasodilatation in stenotic coronary arteries and redistribution of myocardial blood flow. Glyceryl trinitrate (GTN) is a powerful myometrial relaxant. Nitrates also inhibit platelet aggregation *in vitro*. Nitrates are converted to the active compounds NO and nitrosothiols by a denitration mechanism involving reduced sulphydryl groups. Nitric oxide and nitrosothiols activate guanylate cyclase in the cytoplasm of VSM cells to increase intracellular cyclic guanosine monophosphate (cGMP). This leads to protein kinase phosphorylation and decreased intracellular Ca^{2+}, causing VSM relaxation and vasodilatation.

Sodium nitroprusside (SNP) is reduced to NO on exposure to reducing agents and in tissues, including VSM cell

---

Box 9.1 Indications for vasodilators

Acute and chronic left ventricular failure
Prophylaxis and treatment of unstable and stable angina
Treatment of acute myocardial ischaemia and infarction
Chronic hypertension
Acute hypertensive episodes
Elective controlled hypotensive anaesthesia

membranes. Its mechanism of action is ultimately similar to that of nitrates. Release of NO from SNP is accompanied by release of cyanide ions which are detoxified by the liver and kidney and excreted slowly in the urine. SNP is photodegraded to cyanide ions and must be protected from light before and during administration.

Potassium channel activators

Hydralazine, minoxidil and diazoxide are direct-acting arteriolar vasodilators which have largely been superseded. Minoxidil and diazoxide activate ATP-sensitive K^+ channels in VSM cells, causing K^+ efflux and membrane hyperpolarisation. This leads to closure of calcium channels, reduced intracellular calcium availability and consequently smooth muscle relaxation and arterial vasodilatation. Hydralazine may act via a similar mechanism. All these drugs reduce afterload, with little or no effect on preload. Their effects are limited by reflex tachycardia and a tendency to cause sodium and water retention (by activation of the renin-angiotensin system and a direct renal mechanism).

Hydralazine is the most widely used of these drugs. Its half-life is short (approximately 2.5 h) but its antihypertensive effect is relatively prolonged. It may be given as a slow i.v. bolus of 5–10 mg, with appropriate monitoring, for the treatment of hypertensive emergencies.

Nicorandil activates K^+ channels in VSM but also causes NO release and increases intracellular cGMP in vascular endothelium, causing venous dilatation. It therefore reduces preload as well as afterload and is a potent coronary vasodilator with no effect on HR or contractility. It is metabolised in the liver, excreted via the kidneys and does not cause tolerance. Nicorandil is used for the treatment of angina, e.g. in nitrate-tolerant patients or those unresponsive to β-blockers.

Calcium channel blockers

Calcium channel blockers (CCBs) are a diverse group of compounds that decrease Ca^{2+} entry into cardiac and VSM cells through the L-subtype of voltage-gated Ca^{2+} channels. Calcium channel blockers bind in several ways to the α_1 subunit of L-type channels to impede Ca^{2+} entry. Phenylalkylamines (verapamil) bind to the intracellular portion of the channel and physically occlude it, whereas dihydropyridines modify the extracellular allosteric structure of the channel. Benzothiazepines (diltiazem) act on the α_1 subunit, although the mechanism has not been fully elucidated, and may have further actions on Na^+/K^+ exchange and calcium–calmodulin binding.

Calcium channel blockers differ in their selectivity for cardiac muscle cells, conducting tissue and vascular smooth muscle, but they all decrease myocardial contractility and produce coronary and systemic vasodilatation with a con-

sequent decrease in arterial pressure. They have been used widely for the treatment of hypertension and angina but have been partly superseded by newer drugs. Other current indications include prevention of vasospasm in subarachnoid haemorrhage or Raynaud's disease.

Calcium channel blockers can be broadly classified into non-dihydropyridine drugs (verapamil and diltiazem) and the dihydropyridines (nifedipine, felodipine, nicardipine, nimodipine, amlodipine). Verapamil is used principally as an antiarrhythmic (discussed later). Diltiazem has a predominant effect on the coronary circulation and is mainly used in the treatment of hypertension and angina. The dihydropyridine drugs are more selective for VSM, with a slower onset and longer duration of action. They are therefore suited for use in the management of hypertension. *Nimodipine* is selective for cerebral vasculature and is used to prevent delayed cerebral ischaemia (DCI) after subarachnoid haemorrhage.

Antiarrhythmic drugs

Cardiac arrhythmias are irregular or abnormal heart rhythms and include bradycardias or tachycardias outside the physiological range. Patients may present for surgery with a pre-existing arrhythmia; alternatively, arrhythmias may be precipitated or accentuated during anaesthesia by several surgical, pharmacological or physiological factors (Box 9.2). Although several drugs (including anaesthetic drugs) have effects on HR and rhythm, the term *antiarrhythmic* is applied to drugs which primarily affect ionic currents within myocardial conducting tissue.

Box 9.2 Precipitants of arrhythmias during anaesthesia

Myocardial ischaemia/hypoxia
Hypercapnia
Halogenated hydrocarbons (volatile anaesthetic agents)
Catecholamines (endogenous or exogenous)
Electrolyte abnormalities (hypo- or hyperkalaemia, hypocalcaemia, hypomagnesaemia)
Hypotension
Autonomic effects (e.g. reflex vagal stimulation, brain tumours or trauma)
Acid–base abnormalities
Mechanical stimuli (e.g. during central venous cannulation)
Drugs (toxicity or adverse reactions)
Medical conditions (e.g. sepsis, myocarditis, pneumonia, alcohol abuse, thyrotoxicosis)

Arrhythmias are caused by abnormalities of impulse generation, conduction, or both via several mechanisms:

- Altered automaticity
  - Sympathetic/parasympathetic tone
  - Electrolyte abnormalities
- Unidirectional conduction block
  - Interruption of the normal conduction pathways caused by anatomical defects (congenital, ischaemia), alterations in refractory period or excitability
- Ectopic foci

Some arrhythmias are immediately life threatening, but all warrant attention because of their effects on CO and risk of degeneration to a dangerous tachyarrhythmia or bradyarrhythmia.

Mechanisms of action of antiarrhythmic drugs

An arrhythmia may be controlled either by slowing the primary mechanisms or, in the case of supraventricular arrhythmias, reducing the proportion of impulses transmitted through the AV node. The cardiac action potential may be pharmacologically manipulated in three ways:

- Reduction of automaticity
  - Reducing the I_f (and therefore the slope of phase 4)
  - Increasing the electronegativity of the membrane potential
  - Decreasing the electronegativity of the threshold potential
- Reduced speed of action potential conduction
  - Lowering the height and slope of phase 0
- Reduction in the rate of repolarisation
  - Prolonging the ARP

Antiarrhythmic drugs may be classified based on their effectiveness in particular arrhythmias (supraventricular vs ventricular arrhythmias) or on their effect on specific ion channels. The Vaughan Williams classification (Table 9.5) is based on electrophysiological mechanisms. This classification has limitations, with some drugs belonging to more than one class and some arrhythmias being caused by several mechanisms. In addition, some drugs (e.g. digoxin, adenosine and magnesium) do not fit into the classification, but it remains in use and is therefore described later. Indications for specific antiarrhythmic agents are given in Table 9.6.

Class I

Class I antiarrhythmic drugs block fast Na^+ channels, inhibiting Na^+ influx during depolarisation, decreasing the maximum rise of phase 0. In addition, class I agents decrease conduction velocity, excitability and automaticity to varying degrees. Some class I agents also have membrane stabilising

effects. Class I agents are subclassified based on their effect on the duration of the action potential.

- Class Ia (disopyramide, quinidine, procainamide) – lengthen the AP
- Class Ib (lidocaine, tocainide, mexiletine) – shorten the AP
- Class 1c (flecainide, propafenone) – do not alter AP length

Class II

Class II antiarrhythmic agents are β-blockers. Their antiarrhythmic effects are an intrinsic property of β-blockade – that is, reduced automaticity, prolonged AV node conduction and prolonged refractory period. Some β-blockers have class I (membrane-stabilising) activity at high doses (e.g. metoprolol, propranolol).

Class III

Class III antiarrhythmics prolong repolarisation of the AP in conducting tissues and myocardial muscle by K^+ channel blockade, decreasing outward K^+ conduction. All may prolong the QT interval and precipitate torsades de pointes, especially in high doses or in the presence of electrolyte disturbance. Sotalol possesses class II activity, and disopyramide possesses class I.

Amiodarone

Amiodarone is of particular interest for anaesthesia and intensive care medicine. Primarily a class III antiarrhythmic, inhibiting inward K^+ current, it also possesses class I, II and i.v. actions. It is a broad-spectrum antiarrhythmic, effective against a wide variety of supraventricular and ventricular arrhythmias, and is the preferred antiarrhythmic in the presence of left ventricular dysfunction. Amiodarone is an iodinated compound, and long-term oral therapy can lead to hypothyroidism and measurement errors in thyroid function tests, along with acute pneumonitis/pulmonary fibrosis, abnormal liver function and ataxia.

Class IV

Class IV agents are CCBs, preventing voltage-dependent calcium influx during depolarisation, particularly in the SA and AV nodes. The non-dihydropyridine CCB verapamil is the most selective for cardiac cells compared with diltiazem and the dihydropyridine CCBs.

Other antiarrhythmics

Other antiarrhythmic drugs have antiarrhythmic activity but cannot be classified into any of the groups described earlier.

Table 9.5 Vaughan Williams classification of antiarrhythmic drugs

Class	Examples	Mechanism	Effects	Indication
1a	Quinidine Disopyramide	Na^+ channel blockade (moderate) ↓ Conduction velocity Prolonged polarisation	Moderate ↓ V_{max} ↑ Action potential duration ↑ Refractory period QRS widened	Prevention of SVT, VT, atrial tachycardia WPW
1b	Lidocaine Mexiletine	Na^+ channel blockade (mild) ↓ Conduction velocity Shortened repolarisation	Mild ↓ V_{max} ↓ Action potential duration ↓ Refractory period QRS unchanged	Prevention of VT/VF during ischaemia
1c	Flecainide Propafenone	Na^+ channel blockade (marked) ↓ Conduction velocity No change in repolarisation	Marked ↓ V_{max} Minimal change in action potential duration and refractory period QRS widened	Conversion/prevention of SVT/VT/VF
2	Beta-blockers	β-Adrenergic receptor blockade	Decreased automaticity (SA and AV nodes)	Prevention of sympathetic-induced tachyarrhythmias, rate control in AF, 2° prevention after MI, prevention of AV node re-entrant tachycardia
3	Amiodarone Bretylium Sotalol	Inhibition of inward K^+ current	Markedly prolonged repolarisation ↑ Action potential duration ↑ Refractory period QRS unchanged	Prevention of SVT/VT/VF
4	Diltiazem	Ca^{2+} channel blockade	↓ Depolarisation and V_{max} of slow response cells in SA and AV nodes ↓ Action potential duration ↓ Refractory period of AV node	Rate control in AF Prevention of AV node re-entrant tachycardias
Other[a]	Digoxin	Inhibition of Na^+/K^+ ATPase pump ↑ Intracellular Ca^{2+}, vagal and sympathetic effects	Slows AV node conduction Positive inotropy	Rate control and treatment of AF and atrial flutter
	Adenosine	Agonist at A_1- & A_2-receptors	Suppresses SA and AV node conduction ↓ Automaticity	Conversion of paroxysmal SVT Diagnosis of conduction defects
	Magnesium	Blockade of atrial Ca^{2+} channels Blocks K^+ channels	↑ Refractory period Prolongs atrial conduction	Treatment of ventricular dysrhythmias including torsades de pointes

[a]The original Vaughan Williams classification included classes 1-4 only. Digoxin, adenosine and other drugs which do not fit into this classification are sometimes termed 'class 5' but are included here as 'Other'.
AF, Atrial fibrillation; *AV,* atrioventricular; *ATPase,* adenosine triphosphatase; *SA,* sinoatrial; *SVT,* supraventricular tachycardia; *VF,* ventricular fibrillation; *VT,* ventricular tachycardia; *WPW,* Wolff–Parkinson–White syndrome.

Table 9.6 Drug treatments for specific arrhythmias

Atrial Fibrillation	Paroxysmal atrial fibrillation	Atrial flutter	Paroxysmal SVT	WPW	Ventricular arrhythmias
Digoxin	Amiodarone	Digoxin	Adenosine	Amiodarone	Amiodarone
β-Blockers	Propafenone	Amiodarone	Verapamil	Disopyramide	Lidocaine
Verapamil	Flecainide	Sotalol	β-blockers	Flecainide	Disopyramide
Amiodarone	Dronedarone	Propafenone		β-blockers	Flecainide
Dronedarone					Propafenone
					Magnesium (torsades de pointes)

WPW, Wolff–Parkinson–White syndrome.

Digoxin

Digoxin is a cardiac glycoside derived from the plant species *digitalis* (foxglove). Although previously used in the management of heart failure, it has largely been superseded for this indication and is now mainly used in the management of supraventricular tachyarrhythmia, particularly atrial fibrillation. Digoxin has several actions, including direct effects on the myocardium and both direct and indirect actions on the ANS. It increases myocardial contractility and decreases conduction through the AV node and bundle of His (prolonging phase 4). Its mechanism of action is inhibition of membrane Na^+/K^+-ATPase activity. Intracellular Na^+ concentration increases, driving the Na^+/Ca^{2+} exchange towards Ca^{2+} influx, increasing intracellular Ca^{2+} and myocardial contractility. In addition to direct cardiac actions, digitalis compounds have direct and indirect vagal effects. Central vagal tone, cardiac sensitivity to vagal stimulation and local myocardial concentrations of ACh are all increased, and these effects may be partly antagonised by atropine. Digoxin has a low therapeutic index. Electrocardiographic changes can be demonstrated even at therapeutic concentrations, with downsloping ST-segment depression (reverse-tick) and T-wave inversion being misinterpreted as ischaemia. Toxicity is more common in patients with hypokalaemia, hypomagnesaemia, hypercalcaemia and renal impairment. Toxicity classically presents with cardiac (particularly ventricular arrhythmias), CNS, visual and GI disturbances. Digoxin-specific antibody fragments may be used to treat cases of severe toxicity, as they form complexes with the digoxin molecule that are subsequently excreted in the urine.

Adenosine

Adenosine is an endogenous purine nucleoside which mediates a variety of natural cellular functions via membrane-bound adenosine receptors, of which four subtypes (A_1, A_{2A}, A_{2B}, A_3) have been identified. Activation of A_1 receptors at the SA and AV nodes leads to activation of K^+ channels and increased K^+ conductance. Cell membranes become hyperpolarised and automaticity within the SA and AV nodes is reduced, blocking AV node conduction. Adenosine can be used to cardiovert paroxysmal supraventricular tachyarrhythmias and as an aid to the diagnosis of stable broad-complex tachyarrhythmias when the origin is unknown. Adenosine has a very short duration of action (<10 s) and is administered via rapid i.v. bolus injection. It causes brief but severe chest tightness and a feeling of impending doom; the patient should be warned of these before administration.

Magnesium sulphate

Magnesium is a cofactor for many enzyme systems, including myocardial Na^+/K^+ ATPase. It antagonises atrial L- and T-type Ca^{2+} channels so that it prolongs both atrial refractory periods and conduction. Intravenous magnesium sulphate is the treatment of choice for torsades de pointes. It is a second-line treatment for supraventricular and ventricular arrhythmias, particularly those associated with digoxin toxicity or hypokalaemia, and is used as an anticonvulsant in patients with pre-eclampsia.

References/Further reading

Klabunde, R.E., 2011. Cardiovascular Physiology Concepts, second ed. Lippincott Williams & Wilkins.

Levick, J.R., 2009. An introduction to cardiovascular physiology, fifth ed. CRC Press, London, United Kingdom.

Rang, H.P., Ritter, J.M., Flower, R.J., Henderson, G., 2015. Rang & Dale's Pharmacology, eighth ed. Churchill Livingstone.

Chapter | **10** |

Respiratory system

Andrew Lumb, Paramesh Kumara

Control of breathing

Breathing is primarily concerned with the homeostasis of blood O_2 and CO_2 to ensure that both remain at appropriate concentrations despite wide variations in the body's metabolic needs. Breathing control is also vital for speaking and singing; it must also be modified to allow protective reflexes such as coughing, sneezing and vomiting. Unusually for such a fundamental function, breathing can be voluntarily controlled for a short time.

Respiratory centre

Central pattern generator

Breathing is initiated in the CNS by the central pattern generator (CPG), an oscillatory neural network located mostly in the pre-Bötzinger complex of the medulla. Six distinct groups of neurons make up the CPG, each of which produce cyclical bursts of activity in response to the neurotransmitters glutamate and glycine. Their overall output is broadly divided into three phases: inspiration, passive expiration and active expiration when required.

CNS connections to the CPG

The pontine respiratory group of neurons, previously known as the pneumotaxic centre, exerts fine control over the CPG respiratory neurons by coordinating the (sometimes conflicting) influences on breathing from elsewhere in the CNS. For example, hypothalamic and limbic system connections give rise to changes secondary to emotions such as fear and anger. The cortex has powerful respiratory effects, in particular voluntary control such as breath-holding or hyperventilation. These activities are short lived, with the chemical control of breathing normally overriding the cortex before harm occurs, though mild hypoxia/hypercapnia from breath-holding and tetany secondary to respiratory alkalosis after hyperventilation are possible. Control of breathing is vital for speech, with the cortex performing complex calculations to ensure that gaps in speech for breathing occur in suitable places.

Physiological factors affecting breathing control
Peripheral reflexes

A variety of afferent nerves connect to the respiratory centre:
- Mechanoreceptors in the upper airway respond to negative pressures, activating a rapid reflex increase of pharyngeal dilator muscle activity. In patients with sleep-disordered breathing, there is increased activity of this reflex even when awake, so that airway obstruction worsens when sleep or drugs suppress the reflex.
- Nociceptors in the pharynx and upper airways respond to chemical or physical irritants (e.g. cold air) and initiate the protective sneeze, cough and expiration reflexes or, in more severe situations, laryngeal closure, apnoea or bronchoconstriction.
- Pulmonary stretch receptors called slowly adapting receptors (SARs) are found in airway walls and monitor lung volumes. Rapidly adapting receptors in the airway mucosa monitor changes in tidal volume, respiratory frequency and lung compliance. Increased activity of SARs inhibits inspiration in response to lung distension, known as the Hering-Breuer reflex.

Carbon dioxide

Arterial $P\text{CO}_2$ is an important regulator of respiration, and blood $P\text{CO}_2$ is tightly controlled. Hypercapnia produces a linear increase in ventilation by increasing both rate and depth of respiration (Fig. 10.1A). Alveolar ventilation rises

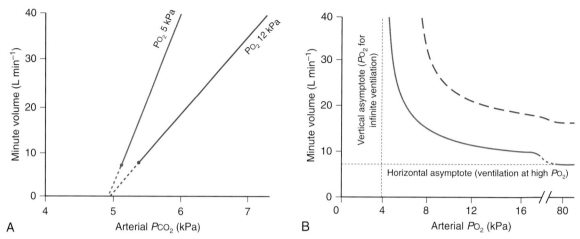

Fig. 10.1 Acute ventilatory responses to changes in blood gases. (A) Hypercapnic response showing the linear increase in ventilation from the resting point (*circle*). The *dotted lines* show the line extrapolated back to the theoretical point where ventilation would cease (apnoeic threshold). Note that when the subject is hypoxic the response is both steeper and shifted to the left. (B) Hypoxic response showing the hyperbolic increase in ventilation as hypoxia worsens. The *dashed line* shows the exaggerated response in a patient who is either hypercapnic or exercising.

1–2 L min^{-1} for each 0.1 kPa increase in $P\text{a}CO_2$, although there is wide variation between individuals depending on factors such as age, genetics, fitness, diurnal variation, hormones and drugs. High $P\text{a}CO_2$ causes respiratory fatigue, ultimately leading to respiratory depression, hypoventilation, worsening hypercapnia and CO_2 narcosis.

Hypocapnia produces a decrease in ventilation. There is no effect below a $P\text{a}CO_2$ of about 4 kPa when, in a conscious patient, the cerebral cortex is believed to be responsible for preventing apnoea. This response does not occur during general anaesthesia, so patients may develop prolonged apnoea when the apnoeic threshold is reached (see Fig. 10.1A).

The ventilatory response to CO_2 is mediated primarily by the central chemoreceptors, a collection of pH-sensitive glutaminergic neurons in the medulla. This provides an indirect measure of CO_2 as CSF is separated from the blood by the blood–brain barrier (BBB), which is impermeable to hydrogen and bicarbonate ions. Carbon dioxide diffuses easily across the BBB and reacts with water, forming carbonic acid, from which hydrogen ions are released. Hypercapnia also causes cerebral vasodilation, which further facilitates diffusion of CO_2 into the CSF. The normal pH of CSF is lower than blood (7.32) and CSF has less buffering capacity, and so for any change in PCO_2 the pH change in CSF is greater than in blood. If the PCO_2 of CSF is maintained, there will be a compensatory change in bicarbonate concentration with a return of CSF pH, and hence ventilation, back towards normal.

Oxygen

Peripheral chemoreceptors are situated in the carotid bodies at the bifurcation of the common carotid arteries and in the aortic arch. The carotid bodies contain chemoreceptors that respond to O_2, CO_2 and pH. Afferents travel in the glossopharyngeal nerve via Hering's nerve to the nucleus tractus solitarius. The aortic body contains chemoreceptors that sense O_2 and CO_2 but not pH with afferent fibres in the vagus nerve.

Peripheral chemoreceptors have a faster response than central chemoreceptors, and their mechanism of action remains incompletely understood. The carotid body has a large blood flow relative to its metabolic activity, so arterial PO_2 is the primary stimulus, and anaemia has no effect. Increased PO_2 produces minimal changes of ventilation, but a decrease to less than 8 kPa results in a hyperbolic rise (Fig. 10.1B) such that at 6 kPa ventilation is approximately doubled. This acute hypoxic ventilatory response is augmented by hypercapnia or exercise. With prolonged hypoxia the acute response reduces after only a few minutes, referred to as hypoxic ventilatory decline, which is mediated centrally.

Respiratory stimulants

Several classes of drug stimulate ventilation and have been used when ventilatory drive is inadequate. These agents increase respiratory drive through a variety of mechanisms. For example, acetazolamide increases H$^+$ concentration in

Table 10.1 Clinical pharmacology of doxapram

Mechanism of action	Indications	Administration	Adverse effects
Central nervous system stimulant, with particular efficacy on the respiratory centre	• Reverse postoperative respiratory depression • Short-term management of acute ventilatory failure	Intravenous injection or infusion	• Perianal warmth, dizziness and sweating • Hypertension and tachycardia • Rarely laryngospasm, confusion and seizures

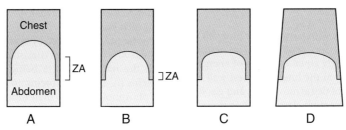

Fig. 10.2 'Piston in a cylinder' analogy of diaphragm activity and chest volume. (A) Resting end-expiratory position. (B) Inspiration with pure piston-like behaviour. (C) Inspiration with pure non–piston-like behaviour with flattening of the dome. (D) Combination of piston-like and non–piston-like behaviour in an expanding cylinder, which equates most closely with inspiration *in vivo* when supine. *ZA*, Zone of apposition. (With permission from Lumb, A. (2017) *Nunn's applied respiratory physiology.* 8th ed. London, Elsevier.)

extracellular fluid around the respiratory centre. Doxapram stimulates the respiratory centre directly and is sometimes used in anaesthetic practice (Table 10.1). Stimulants should not be used if muscle fatigue is thought to be contributing to respiratory failure. Non-invasive ventilation (NIV) has mostly replaced respiratory stimulants in the management of respiratory failure.

Respiratory muscles

Intercostal muscle contraction can increase or decrease the volume of the ribcage. The external intercostals are normally inspiratory and increase the volume of the ribcage in all directions by rotating the ribs posteriorly. The internal intercostal muscles normally have the opposite, expiratory effect by pulling the ribs downward and inward. Intercostal muscles also contribute to locomotion and posture, so their contribution to breathing is variable, but in the upright position they are thought to account for about two thirds of each breath, reducing to one third when supine.

The diaphragm is a dome-shaped musculotendinous structure separating the chest and abdominal cavities; it is innervated by the phrenic nerve. There are several ways the diaphragm can increase chest volume, and its activity is

clearly illustrated with the 'piston in a cylinder' analogy where the trunk represents the cylinder and the diaphragm a piston (Fig. 10.2). In the end-expiratory position (relaxed) much of the diaphragm is in direct contact with the ribcage, the zone of apposition (ZA). During contraction, the dome shape of the diaphragm can be maintained but the ZA shortened, like a piston, greatly increasing chest volume. There can also be non–piston-like behaviour when the ZA remains unchanged but contraction reduces the dome's curvature, expanding the lung. Third, piston-like and non–piston-like behaviour can occur together with expansion of the lower ribcage (a piston in an expanding cylinder), which occurs in the supine position. Piston-like behaviour is the most efficient as almost all muscular activity contributes to tidal volume, whereas in the other actions energy is wasted as, for example, when each side of the flattened dome simply pulls against the opposite side. This explains why the hyperexpanded chest seen in various lung diseases results in poor ventilatory capacity.

Accessory muscles, whose primary functions include neck movement and posture, can be used to aid inspiration when required. They include the scalene, sternocleidomastoid and platysma muscles.

Expiratory muscles contract when active expiration is required, usually above a minute volume of 30–40 L min^{-1}, and include the internal intercostal and abdominal wall muscles, the latter contracting to increase intra-abdominal pressure, causing cephalad displacement of the diaphragm.

Work of breathing

Work is defined as the force applied over a distance and is measured in Joules (Newton metres (see Chapter 15)). For breathing this equates to the volume of gas moved in response to the pressure applied with units of litre-kilopascal (volume × pressure). As *work of breathing* refers to the energy required for breathing over time – that is, the rate at which work is performed – *power* (joule-seconds = watts) is actually the more correct term.

During resting breathing with passive expiration, all the work of breathing is used for inspiration. This requires expenditure of approximately equal amounts of energy to overcome the elastic recoil of the lung and chest wall and the non-elastic resistance of tissue movement and gas flow in the airway. Energy overcoming elastic recoil is stored as potential energy in the elastic tissue of the lungs and chest wall for use during expiration; the remainder is dissipated as heat. During slow and deep breathing, the work done against elastic forces is increased, whereas during quick and shallow breaths, the work against airway and tissue resistance is increased.

Respiratory system mechanics

Elastic recoil

The respiratory system has two main components, the lungs and the chest wall, which move together as a single unit. They are both elastic; at the end of expiration the lung has inward elastic recoil, which is exactly balanced by the outward elastic recoil of the chest wall. This results in a negative intrapleural pressure.

Lung parenchyma and chest wall tissues contain elastin, a molecule whose structure opposes efforts to stretch it and which immediately returns to its resting shape when tension is removed. With ageing, repeated episodes of inflammation cause replacement of elastin by the inelastic molecule collagen, so tissue elasticity reduces. This leads to the slow deterioration of respiratory function seen with age, changes that are accelerated by repeated molecular insults, such as by smoking.

Although elastin accounts for most of the elasticity of the chest wall, an approximately equal contribution in the lung originates from surface forces between liquid and gas. Surface forces develop at the air–water interface of the alveoli and encourage alveoli to collapse, a situation which is prevented from occurring by surfactant.

Surfactant

Surface forces in lung are reduced by the presence of a mixture of molecules known as surfactant. Surfactant reduces elastic recoil of the lungs overall but also changes surface forces within alveoli according to their size. As alveoli become smaller, their surface forces reduce so they become more compliant – as a result, gas will flow from larger alveoli into small alveoli, so all alveoli tend towards the same size, stabilising the lung tissue. Without surfactant, smaller alveoli would rapidly collapse. How surfactant does this at a molecular level is poorly understood, but it probably involves layers or 'rafts' of phospholipid of various thickness on the liquid surface of the alveoli forming and breaking apart with each breath.

Surfactant is produced by type II alveolar epithelial cells. Around 90% of surfactant consists of phospholipid molecules, with the remaining 10% being four different surfactant proteins (A–D). The proteins are important for organising the phospholipids into their functional layers in surfactant production and release from epithelial cells, and have important immunological and antioxidant roles.

Artificial surfactant may be used to treat conditions where surfactant is lacking, such as neonatal respiratory distress syndrome. Surfactant proteins are required to facilitate spreading of the surfactant in the lung after intratracheal instillation, and natural surfactants are therefore more effective as therapeutic agents than synthetic surfactants.

Time dependence of respiratory system elasticity

If a lung is expanded by a given volume and held constant for a few seconds, the initial higher pressure required for inflation falls to a lower pressure that still maintains lung volume. The same mechanism gives rise to hysteresis on a pressure–volume curve when the inflation and deflation curves are different (Fig. 10.3). The lung volume at any given pressure during deflation is larger than during inflation because of time dependency.

Time dependency results from surfactant activity, stress relaxation of elastin and redistribution of gas within the lung. The first two of these are inherent properties of the molecules concerned.

Redistribution of gas occurs in the lung as a result of differing resistance and compliance of nearby lung regions. A 'fast alveolus' functional unit has low resistance and/or low compliance and will fill quickly, whereas a 'slow alveolus' has high resistance and/or high compliance and so will fill slowly. With an inspiratory pause, the fast alveoli will redistribute some of their volume to slow alveoli. Gas redistribution is minimal in healthy lungs but becomes important in diseased lungs with varying regional resistance

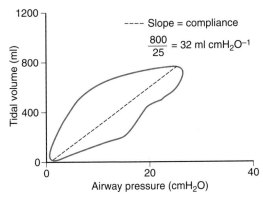

Fig. 10.3 Using a pressure–volume curve to measure dynamic compliance. End-expiratory and end-inspiratory no-flow points occur when the trace is horizontal. At this point, airway pressure and alveolar pressure are equal, so the pressure gradient is the difference between alveolar and atmospheric pressure. Total respiratory system dynamic compliance is therefore the slope of the line between these points. In this patient, compliance is low. (With permission from Lumb, A. (2017) *Nunn's applied respiratory physiology.* 8th ed. London, Elsevier.)

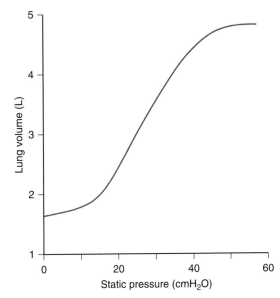

Fig. 10.4 Static compliance curve of the respiratory system, including contributions from both lungs and chest wall. Note the reduced compliance at both high and low lung volumes.

and compliance, which can be easily identified in theatre from the sloping phase III of a capnogram.

Compliance

Defined as the change in lung volume per unit pressure change, compliance can be measured for the lungs, chest wall or both depending on which pressure gradient is used:

- lung: alveolar–intrapleural (transpulmonary pressure);
- chest wall: intrapleural–atmospheric; or
- total (respiratory system): alveolar–atmospheric.

When measured together, lung and chest wall compliance are in series (analogous to capacitance) and therefore addition of the reciprocals of lung and chest wall compliance equals the reciprocal of total compliance.

Compliance is measured when no gas is flowing, at which point mouth pressure equals alveolar pressure. Intrapleural pressure is difficult to measure, so most compliance measurements are of the respiratory system. Static compliance is measured by inflating the lungs in volume increments, allowing the pressure to stabilise at each volume, and plotting this as a graph over the whole lung volume (Fig. 10.4).

Dynamic compliance is measured during normal breathing by recording the no-flow points on a flow–volume curve (see Fig. 10.3). Static compliance is always greater than dynamic compliance as the latter removes the time dependency of the respiratory system.

Lung compliance is affected by lung volume (see Fig. 10.4). This effect can be excluded by calculating the specific compliance,

which is equal to compliance/functional residual capacity (FRC) and is independent of age and sex. Lung compliance is also affected by posture, pulmonary blood volume, age, bronchial muscle tone and disease; it is reduced in restrictive lung disease and increased in emphysema. Increasing compliance with age and emphysema both result from loss of total alveolar surface area, illustrating the importance of surface forces in lung recoil.

Chest wall compliance is affected by the mobility of the ribcage (e.g. the ossification of cartilage with increasing age). It is also reduced by obesity or pathological skin conditions such as chest wall burns. Posture has a major effect, with reduced chest wall compliance in the supine position (by 30%) and prone position (by 60%) compared with the sitting position.

Static lung volumes

Static lung volumes are volumes of gas contained within the lung when no gas is flowing. Combinations of two or more volumes are known as capacities (Fig. 10.5; normal values in Table 10.2) and include the following:

- Tidal volume (V_T): volume inspired with each breath.
- Inspiratory reserve volume (IRV): volume that can be inspired above a normal V_T; IRV + V_T is therefore inspiratory capacity.
- Expiratory reserve volume (ERV): volume that can be expired after a normal tidal expiration.
- Vital capacity (VC) = IRV + V_T + ERV: volume exhaled after maximal inspiration and maximal expiration.

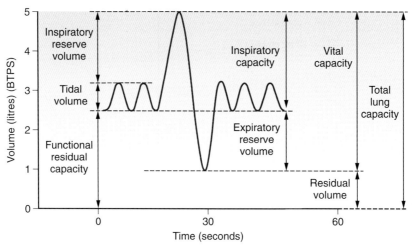

Fig. 10.5 Static lung volumes. The spirometer curve shows lung volumes measured by simple bedside spirometry. These are tidal volume, inspiratory reserve volume, inspiratory capacity, expiratory reserve volume and vital capacity. The residual volume, total lung capacity and functional residual capacity can only be measured with more complex techniques. Normal values are shown in Table 10.2. *BTPS,* Body temperature and pressure, saturated. (With permission from Lumb, A. (2017) *Nunn's applied respiratory physiology.* 8th ed. London, Elsevier.)

- Residual volume (RV): volume remaining after a maximal expiration.
- FRC = ERV + RV: volume remaining after a normal expiration.
- Total lung capacity (TLC) = VC + RV: volume of gas in the lungs after a maximal inspiration.

The V_T IRV, ERV and VC can be measured by simple bedside spirometry, but RV requires a gas dilution or plethysmographical technique, and both FRC and TLC depend on RV.

Static lung volumes are affected by height, sex, age and ethnicity, so calculating a normal value for an individual requires inclusion of these factors. Consequently, in clinical use lung volumes are best expressed as a percentage of predicted value for the individual (see Table 10.2).

Respiratory system resistance

Resistance to flow of gas into the lungs results from airway resistance, tissue resistance and inertance. Tissue resistance originates from the elasticity of lungs and chest wall and describes their reluctance to change shape with breathing. Inertance is the resistance caused during the change in direction of gas and tissues when they move with respiration. Inertance is negligible except for the unusual situation of high-frequency artificial ventilation.

Airway resistance results from frictional resistance to gas flow through airways. In laminar flow, from Hagen–Poiseuille's law, resistance is inversely proportional to the fourth power of the radius and dependent on viscosity of the gas and the length of the tube. For turbulent flow resistance

varies with flow rate, and the relationship is not linear. Reynolds' number (= gas density × velocity × diameter / viscosity) determines which type of flow will occur, with a high number (approximately >2000) resulting in turbulent flow (see Chapter 15). Gas flow is generally turbulent in the upper airway and large bronchi, becoming laminar in bronchioles (1 mm diameter, generation 11) and beyond, but this varies with the speed of air flow. With a doubling of the number of airways with each generation beyond the trachea, the cross-sectional area of the combined airways increases exponentially and so gas velocity rapidly reduces, favouring laminar flow. Airway resistance therefore depends greatly on changes in small airway diameter.

Passive control of airway size

Bronchioles lack cartilaginous support and depend entirely on traction by elastic recoil of surrounding lung tissue to remain open. Lung volume therefore has a significant effect on airway resistance (Fig. 10.6). This explains why, in patients with chronic small airway obstruction, hyperinflation of the lungs helps alleviate obstruction, but the hyperinflation also impairs respiratory muscle function (see earlier).

Airway collapse

The reliance of small airways on lung tissue to remain open means there will be regional variation in airway size. In dependent lung regions, particularly when upright, compression of lung by gravity may reduce airway size to the point

Table 10.2 Lung function: normal values

Static and dynamic spirometry values (L) for average male and female subjects in an upright posture. See Fig. 10.5 for spirometer trace.

	Male	Female
IRC	3.09	2.72
ERV	1.56	1.98
FRC[a]	3.76	4.14
RV	1.96	2.00
VC	4.62	4.12
TLC	6.68	6.12
FEV$_1$	3.77	3.18
FVC	4.62	4.12
FEV$_1$/FVC (%)	76.9	77.6
PEFR (L min^{-1})	586	457

[a]FRC is reduced by approximately 0.5 L in the supine position.
Values shown are based on an average 40-year-old European with height and ideal body weight of 1.75 m/69 kg (male) and 1.62 m/55 kg (female).

Other values relevant to anaesthetists

Measurement	Symbol	Adult (65 kg)
Tidal volume	V_T	7–10 ml kg^{-1}
Dead space	V_D	2.2 ml kg^{-1}
Minute ventilation (expired)	$\dot{V}_E$	85–100 ml kg^{-1} min^{-1}
Respiratory rate	RR	12–18 breath min^{-1}
Arterial O$_2$ partial pressure	PaO_2	12.6 kPa[b]
Arterial CO$_2$ partial pressure	$PaCO_2$	5.1 ± 1.0 kPa

[b]Declines with age, so may be calculated using formula $PaO_2 = 13.6 - (0.044 \times age)$ (years) kPa

Respiratory mechanics

Compliance (supine position)	L kPa^{-1}	ml cmH$_2$O^{-1}
Total respiratory system	0.85	83
Lung	2.00	196
Chest wall	1.50	147
Resistance	**kPa L^{-1} s**	
Total respiratory system	0.26	
Airways	0.12	
Lung tissue	0.02	
Chest wall tissue	0.12	

ERV, Expiratory reserve volume; *FEV$_1$*, forced expiratory volume in one second; *FRC*, functional residual capacity; *FVC*, forced vital capacity; *IRC*, inspiratory reserve capacity; *PEFR*, peak expiratory flow rate; *RV*, residual volume; *TLC*, total lung capacity; *VC*, vital capacity.

that airway closure occurs. This will be exacerbated as lung volume is reduced towards residual volume. The volume of the lungs when dependent airways begin to close is known as closing capacity; closing volume is the closing capacity minus RV.

Closing capacity increases linearly with age and is less than FRC in young adults; it increases to become equal to FRC at a mean age of 44 years in the supine position and 75 years when upright. When the FRC is less than the closing capacity, some of the pulmonary blood flow will be distributed to alveoli with closed airways, causing a shunt and deterioration of oxygenation.

In addition to this volume-related collapse, high expiratory airway flow rates can cause flow-related collapse. During normal resting breathing or a rapid inspiration, chest expansion maintains a subatmospheric pressure in the pleura while the airways are at atmospheric pressure, so the transmural pressure gradient keeps the airways open. However, with a forced expiration the intrapleural pressure becomes positive, the transmural pressure gradient reverses and small airways close. This is known as dynamic airway compression and is easily demonstrated with a vital capacity manoeuvre on a flow–volume curve (Fig. 10.7).

Active control of airway size

There are four pathways involved in controlling muscle tone in small airways:

1. Neural pathways in the lung are primarily parasympathetic, with acetylcholine acting on M_3 muscarinic receptors to cause bronchoconstriction. Stimulation of M_3 receptors activates a G_q protein to activate phospholipase to produce inositol triphosphate, which binds to sarcoplasmic reticulum, releasing calcium and causing smooth muscle contraction. There is no significant sympathetic innervation of airways, but a non-cholinergic parasympathetic bronchodilator system exists, acting via vasoactive intestinal peptide and nitric oxide (NO) release.

2. Humoral control results from the presence of numerous β_2-adrenergic receptors on bronchial smooth muscle that cause bronchodilatation in response to circulating adrenaline. The β_2-receptor stimulation activates a Gs protein to activate adenylate cyclase to produce cyclic adenosine monophosphate (cAMP), which inhibits Ca^{2+} release from intracellular stores, causing smooth muscle relaxation. The cAMP produced is rapidly inactivated by phosphodiesterase.

3. Direct physical and chemical stimulation of parasympathetic afferents in the respiratory epithelium induces reflex bronchoconstriction and can result in laryngospasm or bronchospasm.

4. Cellular mechanisms include activation of mast cells, eosinophils and other immune cells, releasing inflammatory mediators in response to physical stimulation or pathogens. Histamine, leukotrienes, bradykinin and substance P may be released, and all cause bronchoconstriction.

Abnormalities of airway resistance are most easily observed with dynamic lung volume recordings (Fig. 10.8), which can be performed at the bedside.

Bronchodilator drugs

The increasing prevalence of both asthma and chronic obstructive pulmonary disease (COPD) worldwide has stimulated the search for effective bronchodilators. There are three groups:

1. *Selective β_2-receptor agonists.* These are highly effective drugs normally used by inhalation in the treatment of acute and chronic asthma and COPD. They act by binding to the transmembrane domains of the β_2-receptor, stabilising it in its active state. They are available as either short-acting agents (e.g. salbutamol) or long-acting (e.g. salmeterol), the latter always being administered with an inhaled steroid for chronic treatment.

2. *M_3 acetylcholine receptor antagonists.* These inhaled drugs also exist as short-acting (e.g. ipratropium) and long-acting (e.g. tiotropium) agents and are used more for managing COPD patients in whom overactivity of the parasympathetic system is common. They act by competitively antagonising M_3 receptors in the airway and by using the inhaled route avoid most of the systemic side effects of anticholinergics.

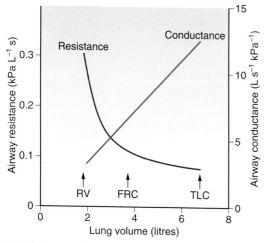

Fig. 10.6 Airway resistance and conductance (= 1/resistance) as a function of lung volume in the upright position. Specific conductance (sGaw) is the gradient of the conductance line. *FRC,* Functional residual capacity; *RV,* residual volume; *TLC,* total lung capacity. (With permission from Lumb, A. (2017) *Nunn's applied respiratory physiology.* 8th ed. London, Elsevier.)

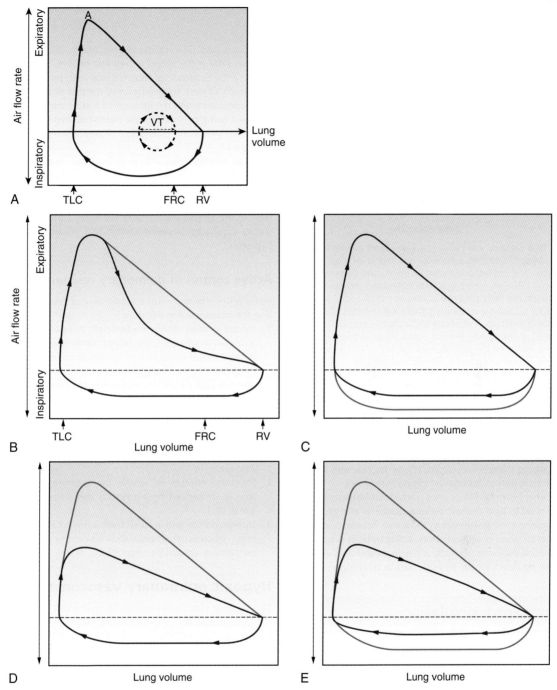

Fig. 10.7 Flow–volume curves. Instantaneous air flow rate (y axis) is plotted against lung volume (x axis). (A) Normal subject. Tidal volume is the small loop. The large loop shows exhalation to residual volume *(RV)*, then inhalation to total lung capacity *(TLC)*, followed by maximal expiration back to RV. Peak expiratory flow rate (point A) depends on effort, but flow rate soon becomes limited by airway collapse, and the line becomes linear, however hard the subject tries to exhale. Parts B–E show abnormal traces, with the normal loop in grey. (B) Small airway obstructive disease such as chronic obstructive pulmonary disease with a concave expiratory phase caused by early closure of small airways. (C) Variable extrathoracic obstruction with a flattened inspiratory phase and normal expiratory loop. (D) Variable intrathoracic obstruction in which the inspiratory phase is normal but flow limitation occurs early on expiration. (E) Fixed large airway obstruction, either intrathoracic or extrathoracic, causes flow limitation in both phases of respiration. *FRC,* Functional residual capacity. (Parts B–E with permission from Lumb, A. (2017) *Nunn's applied respiratory physiology.* 8th ed. London, Elsevier.)

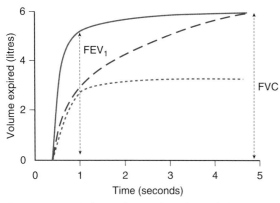

Fig. 10.8 Dynamic lung volumes. The subject inhales to total lung capacity and then exhales as fast and as long as possible. The *dashed line* shows an obstructive pattern, with reduced FEV_1/FVC ratio suggesting obstructed airways slowing expiration but with a normal volume eventually achieved. The *dotted line* shows a restrictive pattern with normal FEV_1/FVC ratio and a reduced FVC. Note that in both cases FEV_1 is reduced, showing why this is a useful single test for lung disease whatever the pathophysiology. *FEV_1*, Forced expiratory volume in one second; *FVC*, forced vital capacity.

3. *Phosphodiesterase (PDE) inhibitors.* Non-specific PDE inhibitors such as theophylline block several different PDE isoenzymes, prolonging the effects of cAMP. Their lack of specificity means many biological systems are affected, causing a range of severe side effects. They are also believed to have anti-inflammatory effects in the lung.

Other bronchodilator drugs include leukotriene antagonists used to treat chronic asthma caused by allergy, as they antagonise some inflammatory mediators. Inhaled anaesthetic agents are good bronchodilators, acting by both suppressing the neural pathways normally active in asthma and, at higher doses, by direct airway smooth muscle relaxation.

Pulmonary circulation

The pulmonary circulation differs from the systemic by being a high-flow, low-pressure system that can accommodate a high cardiac output (CO) without a significant pressure increase. Pulmonary blood volume can vary widely as changes in body position and systemic vascular tone displace blood to and from the chest.

Pulmonary vascular resistance

Mean pulmonary arterial pressure (PAP) is only 22 cmH_2O, and at such low pressures, gravity influences blood flow, with increased flow in dependent areas. In the upright posture, flow at the apices is very low or even absent. As a result of the existence of lung regions with low perfusion, increased CO leads to distension of the thin-walled pulmonary vasculature and recruitment of further capillaries that were not being perfused. These passive changes occur with barely any measurable change in PAP even when CO increases severalfold.

Lung volume also affects pulmonary vascular resistance (PVR), which increases when the lungs are either inflated or deflated away from FRC. The former results from compression of the alveolar capillaries in the alveolar wall as the alveoli expand and the latter from kinking of corner capillaries between alveoli and possibly localised hypoxia.

Active control of pulmonary resistance

As for active airway control there are several systems controlling the pulmonary vasculature.

1. Neural control involves adrenergic sympathetic nerves acting on α_1 adrenergic receptors causing vasoconstriction, but this system seems to have no significant role in health. Parasympathetic fibres cause vasodilatation acting via acetylcholine release, M_3 muscarinic receptor stimulation and an NO-mediated pathway. Non-cholinergic parasympathetic nerves exist and are vasodilatory. In patients after lung transplantation, when all these pathways are disconnected, there are no major changes to the pulmonary circulation, so their physiological significance is unclear.
2. Humoral control in which the pulmonary vasculature is influenced by numerous molecules shown in Table 10.3.
3. Increased P_{CO_2} and acidosis have a slight vasoconstrictor effect, whereas hypocapnia/alkalosis cause a more reliable pulmonary vasodilator response.

Hypoxic pulmonary vasoconstriction

The hypoxic pulmonary vasoconstriction reflex represents a fundamental difference between pulmonary and systemic circulations: The former constricts when hypoxic; the latter dilates. Hypoxic pulmonary vasoconstriction (HPV) begins *in utero* to minimise blood flow through the non-ventilated developing lung. After birth, HPV is the principal way we match ventilation and perfusion of the lungs by diverting blood away from hypoxic lung regions.

Pulmonary oxygen sensing is similar to that in the carotid body. It involves K^+ channels and several poorly understood modulators such as reactive oxygen species, the cellular energy state and hypoxia-inducible factor (HIF) activity. Hypoxic pulmonary vasoconstriction intensity varies among

Table 10.3 Receptors and agonists involved in active control of pulmonary vascular tone

Receptor group	Subtypes	Principal agonists	Responses	Endothelium-dependent?
Adrenergic	α_1	Noradrenaline	Constriction	No
	α_2	Noradrenaline	Dilatation	Yes
	β_2	Adrenaline	Dilatation	Yes
Cholinergic	M_3	Acetylcholine	Dilatation	Yes
Amines	H_1	Histamine	Variable	Yes
	H_2	Histamine	Dilatation	No
	$5\text{-}HT_1$	5-HT	Variable	Variable
Purines	P_{2x}	ATP	Constriction	No
	P_{2y}	ATP	Dilatation	Yes
	A_1	Adenosine	Constriction	No
	A_2	Adenosine	Dilatation	No
Eicosanoids	TP	thromboxane A_2	Constriction	No
	IP	prostacyclin (PGI_2)	Dilatation	?
Peptides	NK_1	Substance P	Dilatation	Yes
	NK_2	Neurokinin A	Constriction	No
	?	VIP	Relaxation	Variable
	AT	angiotensin	Constriction	No
	ANP	ANP	Dilatation	No
	B_2	Bradykinin	Dilatation	Yes
	ET_A	Endothelin	Constriction	No
	ET_B	Endothelin	Dilatation	Yes
	?	Adrenomedullin	Dilatation	?
	V_1	Vasopressin	Dilatation	Yes

The existence of many of the substances listed is at present only established in animals, and their physiological or pathological relevance in humans therefore remains uncertain.
5-HT, 5-Hydroxytryptamine; *ANP*, atrial natriuretic peptide; *ATP*, adenosine triphosphate; *VIP*, vasoactive intestinal peptide.
(With permission from Lumb, A. (2017) *Nunn's applied respiratory physiology.* 8th ed. London, Elsevier.)

individuals, normally occurs in a patchy distribution to avoid excessive pulmonary hypertension and is biphasic (Fig. 10.9). The second, more intense, phase develops after 40 min and is mediated by the release from endothelial cells of a paracrine peptide hormone, endothelin.

In addition to its physiological role, HPV has major implications when a patient becomes globally hypoxic, for example at altitude, and some patients develop pulmonary oedema. Hypoxic pulmonary vasoconstriction also plays an important role in pathological conditions of the lung, helping to maintain adequate PO_2 while also sometimes causing pulmonary hypertension.

Pulmonary vasodilators

With multiple physiological systems affecting PVR, involving a multitude of receptors and agonists (see Table 10.3), it is unsurprising that drugs acting on the pulmonary circulation have unpredictable effects. For example, almost all pulmonary vasodilators (Table 10.4) attenuate HPV and so reducing

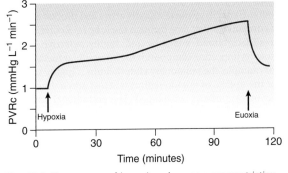

Fig. 10.9 Time course of hypoxic pulmonary vasoconstriction with prolonged hypoxia (end-tidal PO_2 6.7 kPa). Phase 1 of the response is complete within a few minutes, and phase 2 occurs approximately 40 min later. Note that after prolonged hypoxia, PVRc does not return to baseline immediately. *PVRc*, Pulmonary vascular resistance corrected for cardiac output. (With permission from Lumb, A. (2017) *Nunn's applied respiratory physiology.* 8th ed. London, Elsevier.)

Table 10.4 Clinical pharmacology of pulmonary vasodilators

Mechanism of action	Example	Route of administration	Indications	Adverse effects
Direct relaxation of pulmonary arteriolar smooth muscle cells	Nitric oxide	Inhaled	Management of critically ill patient with PHT	Toxicity from production of NO_2 and methaemoglobin
Prostacyclin receptor stimulation	Iloprost	Inhaled	Primary PHT	Systemic vascular effects
Prostacyclin receptor stimulation	Epoprostenol (prostacyclin)	Intravenous	Management of critically ill patient with PHT	Need for intravenous access; flushing and hypotension
Calcium channel blockade	Nifedipine	Oral	Primary PHT	Systemic effects (e.g. hypotension)
Endothelin receptor blockade[a]	Bosentan	Oral	Primary PHT	Liver dysfunction
Phosphodiesterase 5 inhibition	Sildenafil	Oral	Primary PHT	Few and minor
Angiotensin receptor antagonism[a]	Ramipril	Oral	Primary PHT	Systemic effects (e.g. hypotension)

[a]These agents also slow the rate of vascular remodelling and so the progress and irreversibility of PHT.
PHT, Pulmonary hypertension.

pulmonary hypertension may be at the cost of worsening hypoxaemia in patients with respiratory disease.

Processing of endogenous compounds by the pulmonary circulation

Endothelial cells are metabolically active and process a variety of compounds that pass through the lung by a combination of surface-bound enzymes and highly selective uptake proteins importing compounds for intracellular metabolism. For example, the pulmonary endothelium is highly selective for the uptake of noradrenaline, whereas adrenaline passes through capillaries unchanged. The endothelial surface is rich in angiotensin-converting enzyme for activating angiotensin I into the vasoactive octapeptide angiotensin I. The same enzyme also completely inactivates circulating bradykinin. The fate of hormones passing through the lung is shown in Table 10.5.

Many drugs are also removed from blood on passing through the lungs, though for most this occurs by retention of the drug in lung tissue rather than metabolism. The highly specific uptake mechanisms seem to prevent drugs entering endothelial cells where the metabolic enzymes reside. Basic ($pKa >8$) and lipophilic drugs tend to be taken up in the pulmonary circulation, whereas acidic

drugs remain bound to plasma proteins. Drug binding in the pulmonary circulation may act as a drug reservoir within the lung, with drugs then being released slowly, or occasionally rapidly returned to the plasma when binding sites either become saturated or when the drug is displaced by a molecule with greater affinity for the binding site.

Regional ventilation and perfusion

Ventilation

Distribution of gas during inspiration is not uniform throughout the lung, with increased ventilation of dependent regions irrespective of posture. Most of this variation is caused by gravity: Dependent regions are compressed by the weight of lung above and therefore the alveoli are less expanded and thus more compliant (see Fig. 10.4), leading to greater ventilation. There is also a smaller contribution to non-uniform ventilation because of unequal branching patterns of the airways causing preferential ventilation of central versus peripheral lung regions. Inspiratory flow rate also affects ventilation as different functional units have differing compliance and resistance and hence different filling rates, as described earlier.

Table 10.5 Metabolic changes to hormones passing through the pulmonary circulation

	EFFECT OF PASSING THROUGH PULMONARY CIRCULATION		
Group	Activated	No change	Inactivated
Amines		Dopamine Adrenaline Histamine	5-hydroxy-tryptamine (5-HT) Noradrenaline
Peptides	Angiotensin I	Angiotensin II Atrial natriuretic peptide Oxytocin Vasopressin	Bradykinin Endothelins
Arachidonic acid derivatives	Arachidonic acid	PGI_2 (prostacyclin) PGA_2	PGD_2 PGE_2 $PGF_2\alpha$ Leukotrienes
Purine derivatives			Adenosine ATP, ADP, AMP

ADP, Adenosine diphosphate; *AMP*, adenosine monophosphate; *ATP*, adenosine triphosphate.

Perfusion

Lung perfusion is affected by gravity in a similar way to ventilation, but to an even larger extent because of the greater weight of blood relative to lung tissue. This increases the driving pressure across the lung in dependent regions. Compression of lung tissue in dependent areas also results in greater numbers of smaller alveoli per unit lung volume and so perfusion is increased. As for distribution of ventilation, perfusion of central regions is greater than in peripheral regions because of the branching patterns of pulmonary arteries, irrespective of body position.

Effect of alveolar pressure on lung perfusion

In addition to gravity, alveolar pressure has a regional effect on PVR. First described by West in 1965 using a Starling resistor model and the analogy of a river flowing over a weir, it soon became traditional to divide the lung into three West zones (Fig. 10.10) showing the relationship between alveolar, pulmonary arterial and pulmonary venous pressures.

In zone 1, non-dependent lung areas, alveolar pressure exceeds arterial pressure, which always exceeds pulmonary venous pressure; therefore there is no perfusion (the Starling resistor is closed; no water flows over the weir). In zone 2, PAP exceeds the alveolar pressure, which exceeds the pulmonary venous pressure, and flow is therefore determined by alveolar pressure (the Starling resistor is partially open; some water

flows over the weir, but the downstream level is still below the weir). In zone 3, dependent lung regions, both the pulmonary arterial and venous pressure exceed alveolar pressure; therefore flow is independent of alveolar pressure (the Starling resistor is fully open; the weir is totally submerged).

Positive pressure ventilation has profound effects on these relationships by increasing alveolar pressure throughout the lung, increasing the amount of lung in zone 1.

$\dot{V}/\dot{Q}$ relationships

Overall, ventilation ($\dot{V}$) and perfusion ($\dot{Q}$) are closely matched in the lung, with typical values of 4 L min^{-1} for alveolar ventilation and 5 L min^{-1} for perfusion, giving a $\dot{V}/\dot{Q}$ ratio of 0.8. However, as already described, both $\dot{V}$ and $\dot{Q}$ increase progressively on moving from non-dependent to dependent areas, more so for $\dot{Q}$. As a result, in a healthy person in the upright position, the $\dot{V}/\dot{Q}$ ratio at the lung apices is around 2.0 and 0.6 at the bases. In horizontal positions there is no major difference in $\dot{V}/\dot{Q}$ ratios in different lung regions. In healthy patients, most areas of the lung therefore have similar $\dot{V}/\dot{Q}$ ratios, between 0.8 and 1.0, but increasing age and the effects of general anaesthesia both cause an increase in $\dot{V}/\dot{Q}$ scatter (i.e. parts of the lung with abnormally high or low $\dot{V}/\dot{Q}$ ratios).

A helpful way to understand the effects of $\dot{V}/\dot{Q}$ scattering is the three-compartment Riley model of gas exchange (Fig. 10.11). This divides the lung into only three functional areas: 'ideal' alveoli ($\dot{V}/\dot{Q} = 1$) where all gas exchange occurs; an area which has no perfusion ($\dot{V}/\dot{Q} = \infty$), which is alveolar

187

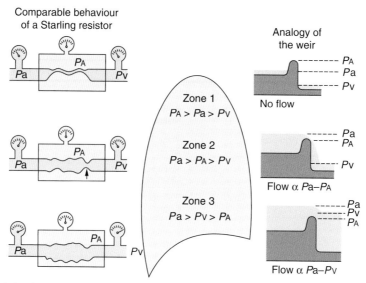

Fig. 10.10 The effect of alveolar pressure and gravity on pulmonary vascular resistance illustrated by a Starling resistor *(left)*, a river flowing over a weir *(right)* and West zones *(central)*. See text for full discussion. *Pa*, Pulmonary artery pressure; *PA*, alveolar pressure; *Pv*, pulmonary venous pressure. (With permission from Lumb, A. (2017) *Nunn's applied respiratory physiology.* 8th ed. London, Elsevier.)

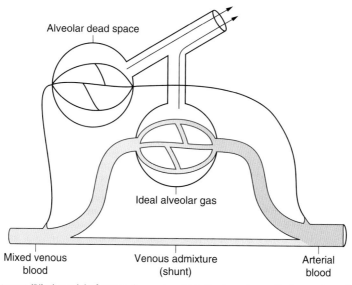

Fig. 10.11 Three-compartment (Riley) model of gas exchange in which the lung theoretically consists of only three functional units comprising alveolar dead space, ideal alveoli and venous admixture (shunt). Gas exchange occurs only in the ideal alveoli. In reality the measured alveolar dead space consists of true alveolar dead space together with a component caused by areas with high $\dot{V}/\dot{Q}$ ratios, and the measured venous admixture consists of true venous admixture (shunt) together with a component caused by areas with low $\dot{V}/\dot{Q}$ ratios. Note that ideal alveolar gas is always exhaled contaminated with alveolar dead space gas so impossible to sample. (With permission from Lumb, A. (2017) *Nunn's applied respiratory physiology.* 8th ed. London, Elsevier.)

dead space; and an area with no ventilation ($\dot{V}/\dot{Q} = 0$), which is pulmonary shunt.

In vivo there are of course an infinite number of compartments with differing $\dot{V}/\dot{Q}$ ratios anywhere between 0 and ∞. But all areas with $\dot{V}/\dot{Q}$ <1 will still result in inadequate oxygenation of venous blood, leading to arterial hypoxaemia, and all areas with $\dot{V}/\dot{Q}$ >1 will contribute to alveolar dead space and impair CO_2 excretion. Thus a widening of the range of $\dot{V}/\dot{Q}$ ratios in a patient quickly leads to inadequate gas exchange.

Alveolar air equation

It is impossible to measure oxygen concentration in an ideal alveolus, and therefore it must be calculated using the alveolar air equation. Alveolar PO_2 (P_{AO_2}) can be useful for identifying where an impairment of oxygenation may be occurring by, for example, calculating alveolar–arterial oxygen difference (A-a)dO_2, which is usually less than 2 kPa. The alveolar air equation assumes that the alveolar concentration of any gas is related to its inspired concentration and uptake/output between the alveolus and pulmonary circulation. Provided F_{IO_2} has not recently changed, the concentrations of N_2 and water vapour in the alveolus will be constant; therefore P_{AO_2} depends only on inspired O_2, P_{ACO_2} and the respiratory quotient (ratio of CO_2 excretion:oxygen consumption). Because of its high solubility P_{ACO_2} can be assumed to equal P_{aCO_2}. On this basis many versions of the alveolar oxygen equation exist, a simple version being:

$$\text{Alveolar } PO_2 = P_{IO_2} - \frac{P_{aCO_2}\left(1 - F_{IO_2}\left(1 - RQ\right)\right)}{RQ}$$

Shunt

Shunt simply describes blood entering the left side of the systemic circulation without passing through ventilated lung. Venous admixture is the amount of mixing of venous blood with pulmonary end-capillary blood that would be required to produce the observed arterial oxygenation and so includes

shunt and a component from blood passing through lung areas with $0 > \dot{V}/\dot{Q} < 1$ which is incompletely oxygenated. Different causes of shunt are shown in Table 10.6.

Venous admixture is calculated using the shunt equation and based on the assumption that the total oxygen carried by the systemic circulation must equal that carried by the oxygenated blood passing through the lungs and the mixed venous blood passing through the shunt. In equation form:

$$\dot{Q}_T \times CaO_2 = \dot{Q}_S \times C\bar{v}O_2 + (\dot{Q}_T - \dot{Q}_S) \times Cc'O_2$$

This can be rearranged to:

$$\frac{\dot{Q}_T}{\dot{Q}_S} = \frac{(Cc'O_2 - CaO_2)}{(Cc'O_2 - C\bar{v}O_2)}$$

$\dot{Q}_T$ = total flow (= CO)
$\dot{Q}_S$ = shunt flow
$C\bar{v}O_2$ = mixed venous O_2 content
CaO_2 = arterial O_2 content
$Cc'O_2$ = pulmonary end-capillary O_2 content (i.e. blood passing the ideal alveolus). This cannot be measured but may be estimated from calculated P_{aO_2}.

Dead space

This is the volume of inspired air that does not take part in gas exchange. There are three types of dead space:
1. *Anatomical.* This is the volume of the conducting airways where gas exchange does not take place. It is dependent on body size and approximately 2 ml kg^{-1}. It is affected by posture, with less anatomical dead space in the supine position and an increased volume in the 'sniffing the morning air' position. Clinical factors affecting anatomical dead space are the type of airway (e.g. tracheostomy or tracheal tube), drugs acting on the bronchi and tidal volume. It can be measured using Fowler's method with a nitrogen or CO_2 washout technique.
2. *Alveolar.* This is inspired gas which passes through the anatomical dead space and mixes with gas at the alveolar

Table 10.6 Classification and common causes of shunt

Type of shunt	Intrapulmonary	Extrapulmonary
Physiological	Bronchial veins: originate from systemic circulation and drain into the pulmonary vein Arteriovenous anastomosis of pulmonary arterioles; normally closed but may open with high cardiac output	Venae cordis minimae (Thebesian veins): small veins of the heart draining into the chambers of the left heart
Pathological	Pulmonary pathological conditions (e.g. atelectasis, consolidation, alveolar oedema, venous drainage from tumours)	Congenital heart disease with a right-to-left shunt (e.g. Fallot's tetrad, Eisenmenger's syndrome)

level but does not take part in gas exchange (i.e. air from lung regions with $\dot{V}/\dot{Q} >1$). Situations where alveolar dead space increases include:

- low CO resulting in poor perfusion of non-dependent lung regions,
- pulmonary embolism, and
- artificial ventilation when increased alveolar pressure and PVR increase zone 1 conditions. This is particularly important in the lateral position when the upper lung develops significant alveolar dead space, which will be further worsened by an open chest.

3. *Physiological.* This equals the sum of anatomical and alveolar dead spaces. Physiological dead space is measured using the Bohr equation, which is based on the assumption that the volume of expired CO_2 must equal the volume of CO_2 breathed out from ventilation of ideal alveoli (assuming inspired CO_2 is negligible). In equation form:

$$P_{ACO_2} \times (V_T - V_D) = P_{\overline{E}CO_2} \times V_T$$

rearranged into the Bohr equation:

$$\frac{V_D}{V_T} = \frac{(P_{ACO_2} - P_{\overline{E}CO_2})}{P_{ACO_2}}$$

V_D = dead space volume

$P_{\overline{E}CO_2}$ = mixed expired P_{CO_2} (note that this is not the same as end-expiratory P_{CO_2}, which approximates to alveolar P_{CO_2})

P_{ACO_2} = ideal alveolar P_{CO_2}, which may be assumed to equal arterial P_{CO_2} except when a large shunt exists.

In clinical situations changes in physiological dead space are usually as a result of altered alveolar dead space as anatomical dead space is approximately fixed provided any artificial airway is unchanged.

Oxygen and carbon dioxide transport

The movement of O_2 and CO_2 from the atmosphere to their site of use and production in the mitochondria involves three physical processes:

1. Mass movement of gas in response to pressure changes (tidal breathing)
2. Facilitated mass movement by binding to haemoglobin, which is physically moved around the body
3. Diffusion down a concentration gradient

The various barriers to oxygen movement on this path are best illustrated by the oxygen cascade (Fig. 10.12).

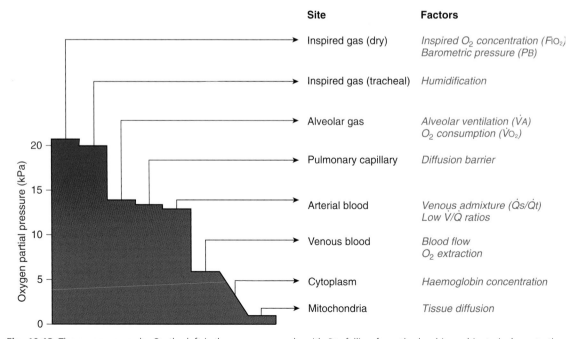

Fig. 10.12 The oxygen cascade. On the left is the oxygen cascade with P_{O_2} falling from the level in ambient air down to the low concentration in mitochondria, estimated to be about 0.15 kPa (referred to as the Pasteur point), below which there is a switch to anaerobic metabolism. On the right is a summary of the factors influencing oxygenation at each site down the cascade. (Adapted with permission from Lumb, A. (2017) *Nunn's applied respiratory physiology.* 8th ed. London, Elsevier.)

Diffusion

Many factors affect the ability of gases to diffuse between the pulmonary capillary and alveolus (in either direction):

- *Size of the molecule.*
- *Partial pressure of the gas in the alveolus.*
- *Solubility of the gas in water as it moves from the gas phase into the tissues.* This is affected by temperature.
- *Surface area available for diffusion.* In the lungs this may be affected by pathological conditions (e.g. emphysema) where total alveolar surface area is reduced.
- *The physical barrier between alveolus and haemoglobin.* This includes the alveolar epithelial cell, basement membrane, interstitial space, endothelial cell, plasma, red blood cell (RBC) membrane and cytoplasm. Despite this long list of structures, diffusion of O_2 and CO_2 is rapid with no significant barrier. Equilibration of both gases is normally complete within the time blood spends in a pulmonary capillary (0.8 s on average). A diffusion barrier only exists in elite athletes, at very high altitude or in diseased lung such as with pulmonary oedema.

In the tissues there is a more significant diffusion barrier between the haemoglobin and the mitochondria, with some cells lying some distance from their source of oxygen. As a result, in muscle cells, with their high oxygen requirement, myoglobin assists with this process.

O_2 carriage in blood

Oxygen is carried in the blood in two forms – dissolved and bound to haemoglobin. The amount of dissolved oxygen is 0.023 ml dl^{-1} kPa^{-1} at 37°C, which equates to about 0.25 ml per 100 ml of blood at normal arterial PO_2. The amount of O_2 bound to haemoglobin is given by:

$$CO_2 = 1.34 \times [Hb] \times SO_2$$

where
1.34 = binding capacity of haemoglobin in ml per gram (the Hüfner constant),
[Hb] = haemoglobin concentration in g dl^{-1}, and
SO_2 = oxygen saturation of the haemoglobin.

Under normal circumstances this results in approximately 19 ml dl^{-1}, giving a total oxygen carriage in blood of about 20 ml dl^{-1}.

Haemoglobin

Different forms of haemoglobin are present as the O_2 carrying molecule throughout most of the animal kingdom. In humans the molecule consists of four globin chains, each containing a crevice at the base of which is a haem molecule with an iron atom to which O_2 binds. Adult haemoglobin (HbA) contains two α- and two β-globin chains; foetal haemoglobin (HbF) has two α and two γ chains.

Haemoglobin binding to O_2 is an example of molecular cooperativity in that when one chain binds an O_2 molecule, this changes the shape of the whole protein, including the other globin chains. This shape change makes it easier for the next chain to bind an O_2 and so on with subsequent O_2 molecules. In deoxyhaemoglobin (HHb) the bonds within the protein are strong, and this form is referred to as tense Hb or THb. As successive O_2 molecules bind the bonds become more relaxed, the crevice binding sites open slightly until, when fully oxygenated, the molecule is described as in its relaxed, or R, state. This molecular interaction explains the characteristic shape of the oxygen–haemoglobin dissociation curve (Fig. 10.13).

A similar mechanism – that is, subtle changes to the bonds within the molecule – also explains the various factors that alter haemoglobin O_2 binding affinity (see Fig. 10.13). For example, the Bohr effect is the right shift of the curve with decreased pH. This is critical for unloading of O_2 in systemic capillaries when the rising CO_2 decreases pH and facilitates the dissociation of O_2 from the haemoglobin.

Many abnormal forms of haemoglobin exist, resulting from abnormalities of the globin chain (thalassaemia or sickle cell disease), the Fe ion (methaemoglobin) or the binding site (carboxyhaemoglobin). Most other oxygen-carrying molecules (Fig. 10.14) are shifted to the left of HbA to operate effectively at lower PO_2 values.

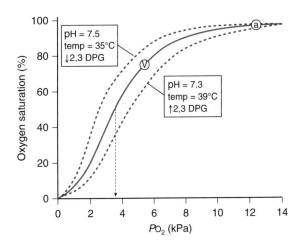

Fig. 10.13 Oxygen dissociation curves for normal human adult haemoglobin (HbA). The *dashed arrow* shows the P50 for this curve, which is the oxygen partial pressure at which the Hb saturation is 50% (normally 3.5 kPa). The normal values for arterial *(a)* and venous *(v)* blood are also shown. The *dashed lines* show the changes in curve shape resulting from alterations of pH, temperature or red cell 2,3-diphosphoglycerate (2,3 DPG) concentration.

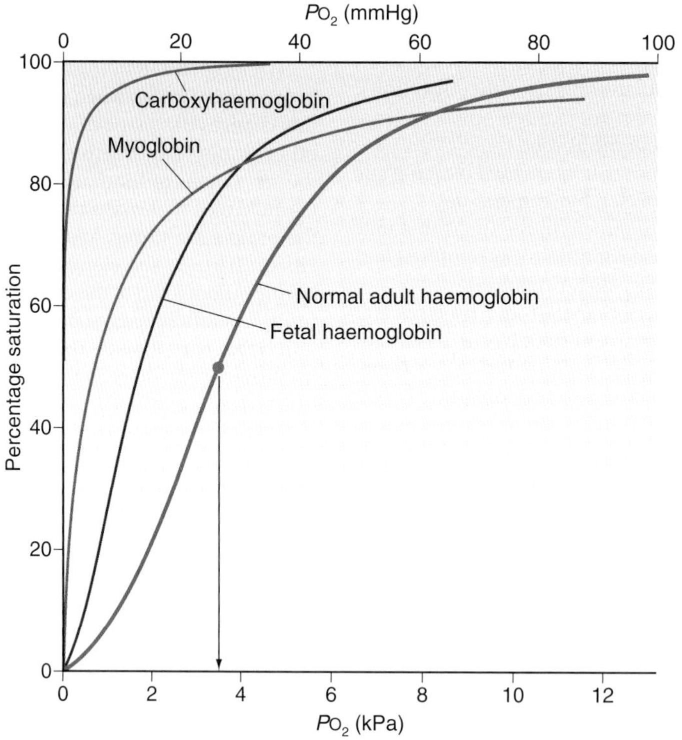

Fig. 10.14 Oxygen dissociation curves for other forms of haemoglobin and myoglobin. The normal adult haemoglobin (HbA) curve (see Fig. 10.12) is shown in blue. Foetal haemoglobin is adapted to operate at a lower PO_2 than adult blood to facilitate placental oxygen transport and so is shifted considerably to the left. Myoglobin approaches full saturation at PO_2 concentrations normally found in skeletal muscle (2–4 kPa), so its oxygen is only released at very low PO_2 during exercise. Carboxyhaemoglobin can be dissociated only by the maintenance of very low concentrations of PCO. (With permission from Lumb, A. (2017) *Nunn's applied respiratory physiology*. 8th ed. London, Elsevier.)

Cellular hypoxia

It is clear from the preceding section that there are numerous ways O_2 transport could fail. When considering why tissue may be hypoxic, the classification described by Barcroft in 1920 remains useful in that it is important to consider all three aspects of oxygen delivery shown in Fig. 10.15. This also illustrates how physiological compensation can improve O_2 delivery – for example, increased CO in anaemic patients or polycythaemia at altitude.

Oxygen therapy

Increasing inspired O_2 for therapeutic reasons is widespread and often undertaken without due consideration of the physiology. If used to treat hypoxaemia, there are only two ways that increasing FIO_2 will help. First, if there is alveolar hypoventilation of any cause leading to hypercapnia, then, based on the alveolar air equation, increased FIO_2 will easily

counteract this by maintaining alveolar PO_2. Second, in any lung regions with $0 > \dot{V}/\dot{Q} < 1$ the blood will be better oxygenated with modest increases in FIO_2. Areas of shunt ($\dot{V}/\dot{Q} = 0$) will not be affected as there is no ventilation. Thus the potential benefit of using O_2 in hypoxaemia depends on the underlying pathophysiology.

When using O_2 therapy it is important to be aware of some adverse effects. These include respiratory depression in patients who are using the hypoxic ventilatory response to stimulate their breathing. Increasing FIO_2 abolishes HPV in poorly ventilated lung regions, increasing the blood flow to those regions. This may improve oxygenation, but by diverting blood away from other lung regions will increase areas of high $\dot{V}/\dot{Q}$ and so alveolar dead space. Some patients with acute exacerbations of COPD are susceptible to developing hypercapnia with O_2 therapy; this was previously thought to be due to respiratory depression, but recent work suggests the effects on HPV and $\dot{V}/\dot{Q}$ relationships are a more likely

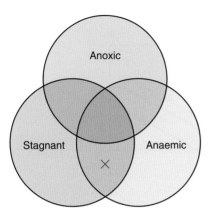

Fig. 10.15 Barcroft's classification of causes of hypoxia displayed on a Venn diagram to illustrate the possibility of combinations of more than one source of cellular hypoxia. The lowest overlap, marked with a cross, represents coexistent anaemia and low cardiac output. The central area illustrates a combination of all three types of hypoxia (e.g. a patient with sepsis resulting in anaemia, circulatory failure and lung injury). (With permission from Lumb, A. (2017) *Nunn's applied respiratory physiology.* 8th ed. London, Elsevier.)

explanation. Irrespective of the cause, O_2 therapy in patients with COPD should always be guided by measuring SpO_2 and appropriate targets agreed based on the clinical situation.

Use of O_2 for stagnant hypoxia in patients who are not hypoxaemic (e.g. stroke or myocardial ischaemia) has little effect as the additional dissolved oxygen will be small compared with the total oxygen carriage. More importantly, high PO_2 has been found to be a systemic vasoconstrictor, particularly in diseased blood vessels, so giving extra O_2 may actually do harm. Oxygen therapy is therefore now only indicated in these conditions if the patient is hypoxaemic.

CO_2 carriage in blood

CO_2 is carried in blood in three forms:
1. *Physical solution.* CO_2 is more soluble than O_2, and at 37 °C has a solubility of 0.23 mmol l^{-1}, which equates to around 2.8 ml dl^{-1} in venous blood.
2. *As bicarbonate ion.* When CO_2 dissolves in water, it hydrates to carbonic acid, which then ionises to bicarbonate and a hydrogen ion:

$$CO_2 + H_2O \rightleftharpoons H_2CO_3 \rightleftharpoons H^+ + HCO_3^-$$

The first stage of this reaction is slow and in biological systems is catalysed by the enzyme carbonic anhydrase (CA), which is abundant in RBCs. Carbonic anhydrase is one of the fastest enzymes known, using a central zinc atom to hydrolyse water before a nearby histidine residue removes the H^+ ion, allowing the Zn-OH molecule to react with CO_2.

Large quantities of H^+ ions are produced by this reaction in the RBC, much of which is buffered by intracellular buffer systems, including haemoglobin, and the remainder is exported from the RBC in exchange for a chloride ion. This transfer, known as the Hamburger shift, is facilitated by a membrane-bound protein named band 3, which is unusual in that it acts by a ping-pong mechanism, unlike most other ion transporters which simultaneously exchange the two ions.
3. *Carbamino carriage.* Amino groups ($R\text{-}NH_2$) on proteins combine directly with CO_2 to form carbamino compounds. Suitable groups only occur at the amino end of protein chains and as side groups on lysine and arginine, and haemoglobin has many such binding sites. Furthermore HHb, with the molecule in the T state, has more suitable binding sites, partly explaining the Haldane effect by which deoxygenated blood carries more CO_2 than oxygenated. The remainder of the Haldane effect is due to the greater buffering capacity of HHb.

Fig. 10.16 shows a CO_2 dissociation curve for blood. It is clear that most of the CO_2 content of blood is in the form of bicarbonate, but the differences between arterial and venous blood mean that carbamino carriage is the most important component in terms of transport in the body.

Respiratory effects of general anaesthesia

Control of breathing

There is reduced ventilation during general anaesthesia, partly because of low metabolic demand, but mostly from direct respiratory depression by anaesthetic drugs (see Chapters 3 and 4), and hypercapnia is usual unless ventilation is supported. The ventilatory response to CO_2 is depressed in a linear fashion by all current inhaled anaesthetics to the same degree at equal minimum alveolar concentration (MAC) values. The ventilatory response to hypoxia is exquisitely sensitive to inhaled anaesthetics, being abolished at 1 MAC and still reduced by about 50% at 0.2 MAC, the concentration at which many patients will be waking up but therefore not be protected by this reflex.

Respiratory muscle activity is abnormal during general anaesthesia. Airway muscles relax and cause obstruction soon after induction of anaesthesia. With spontaneous breathing, intercostal activity is depressed and diaphragm contraction is preserved. This leads to uncoordinated activity, with diaphragm contraction causing indrawing of the upper ribcage in early inspiration, particularly if airway resistance is increased. Phasic activity of the normally inactive expiratory

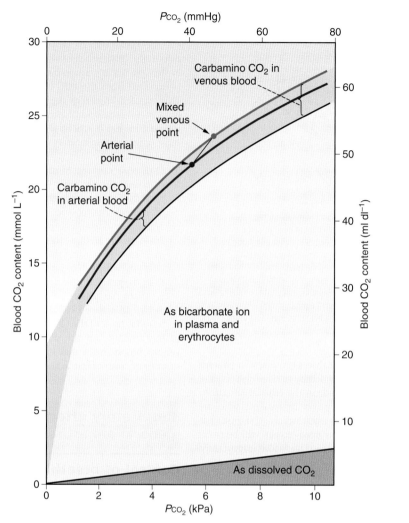

Fig. 10.16 Components of the CO_2 dissociation curve for whole blood. Dissolved CO_2 and bicarbonate ion vary with PCO_2 but are only minimally affected by the state of oxygenation of the haemoglobin and so do not differ greatly between arterial and venous blood. Carbamino carriage of CO_2 is strongly influenced by the state of oxygenation of haemoglobin, so the CO_2 dissociation curves for arterial *(red)* and venous *(blue)* blood are different. (With permission from Lumb, A. (2017) *Nunn's applied respiratory physiology.* 8th ed. London, Elsevier.)

(abdominal) muscles develops, giving an appearance of the patient straining to exhale.

Effects of general anaesthesia on FRC and gas exchange

In addition to the abnormal phasic activity of respiratory muscles during general anaesthesia, there are also changes to resting muscle tone with reduced size of the ribcage, cephalad

displacement of the diaphragm in dependent areas and increased spinal curvature. Together these changes decrease thoracic volume and FRC by 15%–20%. This exacerbates the normal regional variation in ventilation described earlier, and areas of collapse (atelectasis) develop in dependent regions in most patients during general anaesthesia, which is easily demonstrated on CT scans (Fig. 10.17).

Atelectasis forms within minutes of induction, and the amount that develops is increased by using 100% O_2 or zero expiratory airway pressure (ZEEP). Use of moderate positive end-expiratory pressure (PEEP) concentrations of 5–10 cmH_2O and only using 100% O_2 when justified clinically can help prevent atelectasis forming. Once formed, atelectasis requires high airway pressures to re-expand, the so-called opening pressure being 40 cmH_2O, or higher in severely obese patients. Two recruitment manoeuvres described for achieving this are shown in Fig. 10.18.

The reduced FRC, in combination with an abnormal breathing pattern or artificial ventilation, leads to significant abnormalities of $\dot{V}/\dot{Q}$ relationships. Irrespective of the mode of ventilation used, there are increases in areas of both high and low $\dot{V}/\dot{Q}$ ratio, with the former increasing alveolar dead space and so impairing CO_2 excretion and the latter increasing venous admixture and so challenging oxygenation. As a result, in all but the most young and healthy patients, FIO_2 must be increased to better oxygenate blood in areas with $0 > \dot{V}/\dot{Q} < 1$ and ventilatory support provided if severe hypercapnia is not acceptable.

Positive pressure ventilation

Intermittent positive pressure ventilation (IPPV) is usually delivered via a tracheal or tracheostomy tube. During inspiration the airway pressure is intermittently raised above ambient pressure and gas flows into the lungs by overcoming the elastic and non-elastic resistances.

Many different ventilation modes are available, as shown in Fig. 10.19.

In pressure-controlled ventilation, as the lung inflates, non-elastic resistance to flow is high initially and reduces exponentially, and as the lung expands, the elastic resistance increases; flow rate is therefore initially high and declines during inspiration. In volume-controlled ventilation, with a constant flow, elastic resistance increases as the lung inflates, whereas non-elastic resistance remains unchanged and so inflation pressure rises throughout inspiration.

Expiration is usually passive by allowing the airway pressure to fall to ambient unless PEEP is applied. This increases the FRC, reduces airway resistance and may prevent atelectasis. Intrinsic or auto-PEEP occurs when expiratory time is inadequate for complete lung deflation, resulting in

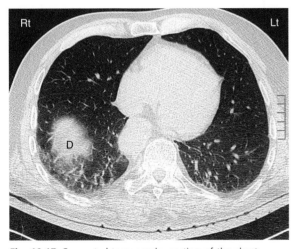

Fig. 10.17 Computed tomography section of the chest during general anaesthesia in a supine patient. Increased lung density as a result of atelectasis is seen in the dependent regions of both lungs. *D*, Dome of the right diaphragm. (With permission from Lumb, A. (2017) *Nunn's applied respiratory physiology.* 8th ed. London, Elsevier.)

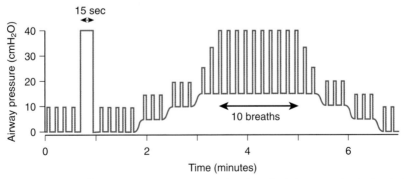

Fig. 10.18 Schematic representation of two manoeuvres to re-expand atelectasis during anaesthesia. On the left is a vital capacity manoeuvre involving a single large breath to an airway pressure of 40 cmH_2O sustained for 15 s. To the right, the PEEP and large tidal volume strategy show progressive application of PEEP up to 15 cmH_2O, followed by increased tidal volume until a peak airway pressure of 40 cmH_2O or tidal volume of 18 ml kg^{-1} is achieved, which is then maintained for 10 breaths before a stepwise return to normal ventilator settings.

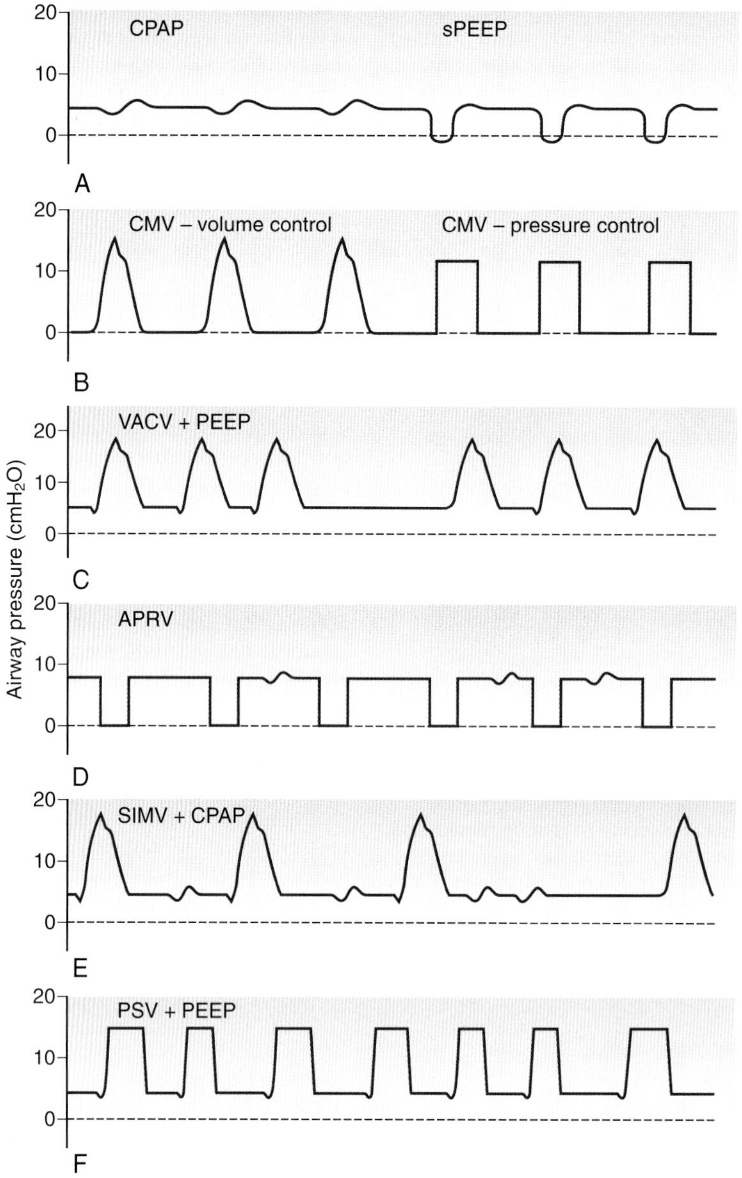

Fig. 10.19 Airway pressure during some common modes of artificial ventilation. (A) Continuous positive airway pressure (CPAP) and true positive end-expiratory pressure applied during spontaneous breathing (sPEEP). (B) Control mode ventilation (CMV) showing volume and pressure-controlled inspiration. (C) Volume assist–control ventilation (VACV), where breaths are triggered by a fall in circuit pressure. When apnoea occurs, ventilator breaths occur without triggering. (D) Airway pressure release ventilation (APRV) with an upper airway pressure (P_{high}) of 8 cmH$_2$O and simultaneous spontaneous breathing. (E) Synchronised intermittent mandatory ventilation (SIMV), as for VACV except that spontaneous breathing can occur between ventilator breaths. (F) Pressure support ventilation (PSV) in which pressure-controlled breaths are triggered by the patient, who also controls the duration of each breath. When this mode of ventilation is used during non-invasive ventilation, it may be referred to as bilevel (inspiratory and expiratory) positive airway pressure (BiPAP). In practice, many ventilators allow combinations of these modes, for example, SIMV, PSV and PEEP together. (With permission from Lumb, A. (2017) *Nunn's applied respiratory physiology.* 8th ed. London, Elsevier.)

breath 'stacking', and when severe can exacerbate the cardiovascular effects of IPPV.

The inspiratory to expiratory (I:E) ratio is usually set between $1:2–1:4$ with a respiratory rate of 12–20 breaths per min. Reduction of inspiratory time to less than 1 s may cause an increase in dead space. Inverse I:E ratio further increases the FRC but may result in intrinsic PEEP, as outlined earlier.

Effects of IPPV on the lungs

Physiologically a positive pressure in the chest only occurs transiently with coughing or straining, though pressures achieved may be quite high, or for more prolonged periods such as during the second stage of labour. Positive pressure ventilation raises intrathoracic pressure during each inspiration or throughout the whole respiratory cycle if PEEP is used. Changes to the mean intrathoracic pressure determine most of the physiological effects, and this is influenced by all the different ventilator settings chosen.

Respiratory effects

Artificial ventilation effectively rests the respiratory muscles that are designed to work permanently. Diaphragmatic atrophic muscular changes can be seen after less than 24 h of artificial ventilation and result in substantially reduced diaphragmatic strength. Therefore ventilatory *support,* in which the diaphragm continues to function, is much preferred to replacing respiratory muscle activity entirely.

During IPPV the $\dot{V}/\dot{Q}$ ratio distribution is widened because pulmonary blood flow is reduced by impaired venous return and increased PVR. This normally causes increased $\dot{V}/\dot{Q}$ ratios in non-dependent regions and so greater alveolar dead space. PEEP will exacerbate these effects by further reducing CO, adding to alveolar dead space, but PEEP may also improve ventilation in dependent areas that remain adequately perfused. In healthy patients IPPV and PEEP do not significantly improve oxygenation, but in diseased lungs their effects of increasing FRC may decrease venous admixture and so improve oxygenation.

Much of the anatomical dead space in the upper airway is bypassed by tracheal or tracheostomy tubes, but the addition of catheter mounts and filters, as well as expansion of corrugated ventilator tubing during inspiration, partially counteracts this. Overall, therefore, IPPV has little effect on the physiological dead space, with reduced anatomical and increased alveolar dead space counteracting each other.

Ventilator-induced lung injury

Prolonged artificial ventilation can cause lung injury by several mechanisms:
• In *oxygen toxicity,* elevated F_{IO_2} exposes alveolar epithelial to high P_{O_2} values, which can, through the production

of reactive oxygen species, lead to cellular damage and lung inflammation.
• *Barotrauma* describes high airway pressures damaging airway epithelial cells, allowing air to enter lung tissue, causing pneumothorax or pneumomediastinum.
• *Volutrauma* describes overdistension of lung tissue, which again disrupts epithelial cells, resulting in inflammation, oedema and airway collapse.
• *Atelectrauma* describes cyclical collapse and reopening of small airways and alveoli, impairing surfactant function.
• *Biotrauma* describes release of inflammatory mediators as a result of all of the previous mechanisms. This leads to local and systemic inflammatory responses and may be exacerbated by bacterial translocation from lung tissue to the systemic circulation.

Respiratory physiology at high altitude

Ascent from sea level involves a progressive reduction in the density of the air, and although the fractional concentration of O_2 remains 0.21, the partial pressure decreases (Table 10.7). Further challenges to breathing at altitude result from low temperature and humidity.

Symptoms and signs of high-altitude exposure depend on the altitude attained and the rate of ascent, with rapid ascent being hazardous. Visual impairment occurs first, particularly night vision, followed by reduced mental performance and ataxia. Headache, fatigue, dizziness and difficulty sleeping are common symptoms of early acute mountain sickness, which in severe cases can progress to life-threatening pulmonary or cerebral oedema, requiring rapid descent. An individual's likelihood of developing pulmonary oedema is closely related to their HPV reflex.

Respiratory effects of altitude

Hypoxia is the main respiratory challenge at altitude. The acute ventilatory response and hypoxic ventilatory decline occur within the first 30 min (Fig. 10.20), leaving the subject with an almost normal minute volume and P_{CO_2} but very hypoxic. Acclimatisation then occurs over the course of several days by increasing ventilation, resulting in hypocapnia, which, from the alveolar air equation, will increase alveolar P_{O_2} by the same amount (see Fig. 10.20). Concentrations of P_{O_2} will never return to sea-level values, but symptoms improve considerably with this acclimatisation. The mechanism of acclimatisation remains incompletely understood. Changes to CSF pH were previously believed to be responsible, but this is no

Table 10.7 Barometric pressure and oxygen availability and altitude

ALTITUDE		Barometric pressure	Inspired P_{O_2}	Equivalent F_{IO_2} at sea level	F_{IO_2} required to give sea level inspired P_{O_2}
feet	metres	kPa	kPa	%	%
0	0	101	19.9	20.9	20.9
4000	1220	87.8	16.9	17.8	24.5
8000	2440	75.2	14.4	15.1	28.8
12,000	3660	64.4	12.1	12.8	34.2
16,000	4880	54.9	10.1	10.7	40.8
20,000	6100	46.5	8.4	8.8	49.3
24,000	7320	39.2	6.9	7.3	60.3
28,000	8540	32.9	5.6	5.9	74.5
35,000	10,700	23.7	3.7	3.8	—
63,000	19,200	6.3	0	0	—

Commercial aircraft cabins are pressurised to a maximum cabin altitude of 8000 feet, equivalent to 15% O_2 at sea level. Above 33,000 feet, where most commercial aircraft fly, 100% O_2 is required to achieve normal sea-level inspired P_{O_2}. At 63,000 feet, barometric pressure equals the saturated vapour pressure of water at 37°C, so water boils and survival is not possible.

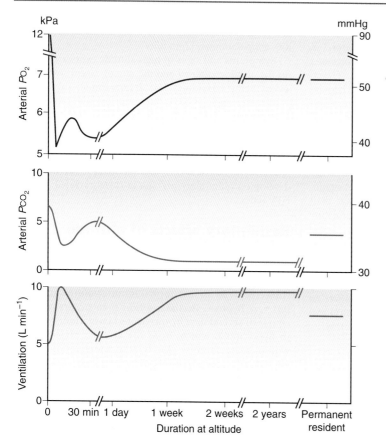

Fig. 10.20 Changes in ventilation and blood gases with a prolonged stay at altitude. See text for explanation. (With permission from Lumb, A. (2017) *Nunn's applied respiratory physiology.* 8th ed. London, Elsevier.)

longer accepted, and direct changes of the O_2 sensitivity of both central and peripheral chemoreceptors are now thought more likely.

Adaptation describes the different responses of residents rather than visitors at high altitude and has both genetic and physiological origins. Permanent residents at high altitude have lower ventilation and higher P_{CO_2} than visitors but still maintain equivalent P_{O_2} (see Fig. 10.20) because they develop comparatively more alveoli during childhood and so oxygen uptake is improved.

Chapter | **11**

Renal physiology: function and anatomy

Jonathan Barratt, Ricky Bell

The kidneys have a number of diverse functions. The main roles are as follows:

- Filtration and elimination of metabolic waste products
- Maintenance of fluid and electrolyte homeostasis
- Control of acid–base status
- Production of erythropoietin to stimulate red cell synthesis
- Hydroxylation of circulating calcifediol (25-hydroxyvitamin D3) to calcitriol (1,25-dihydroxyvitamin D3), the active form of vitamin D, for calcium homeostasis
- Blood pressure maintenance and control of sodium and water retention or elimination through the renin–angiotensin–aldosterone system

Renal anatomy

Each kidney is 10–12 cm in length (depending on patient size), weighs approximately 150 g and is located retroperitoneally either side of the spinal column. They are covered in a layer of fascia and fat, and each has an adrenal gland lying at their upper pole. The right kidney lies slightly lower than the left as it is pushed downwards by the liver. The kidneys move gently with respiration and excursion of the diaphragm. Renal blood supply arises directly from the descending aorta through the renal artery, which leaves the aorta inferior to the origin of the superior mesenteric artery at the level of L1–2. The right renal artery passes posteriorly to the inferior vena cava, and the right renal vein to reach the renal hilum. The left renal artery is shorter than the right because the descending aorta lies to the left of the vena cava. Correspondingly the left renal vein is longer than the right renal vein. The renal arteries are 4–6 cm in length and around 0.5–0.6 cm in diameter. Each renal artery

branches to an anterior and posterior branch and splits further to supply the kidney. Around 30% of the population have one or more accessory renal arteries, and there may be early branching in 10% of the population; this is important for successful anastomosis in renal transplantation. The branches ultimately divide into arterioles and form the capillary network of the glomerulus. These capillaries reform into arterioles and branch off smaller arteries which bring oxygenated blood to the functioning unit of the kidney, the nephron. The blood then passes through the nephron and into the renal vein, back to the inferior vena cava and returns to the right side of the heart (Fig. 11.1).

The kidneys receive 20%–25% of cardiac output, which is a very large proportion compared with their relatively small size; this reflects their importance and function as filtering units of the circulation.

The kidney is separated into an outer cortex and inner medulla, surrounded by a capsule of fibrous tissue overlying the cortex. This outer cortex contains the majority of nephrons. The nephron is the functional unit of the kidney and comprises the glomerulus and Bowman's capsule; proximal convoluted tubule; descending then ascending loop of Henle, which in turn becomes the thick ascending limb; distal convoluted tubule; and finally the collecting duct, which progresses down into the renal papilla.

Glomerular anatomy, filtration and tubular feedback

A typical adult kidney contains between 800,000 and 1,000,000 nephrons. Within the nephron renal blood flow divides down to the afferent arterioles that become the

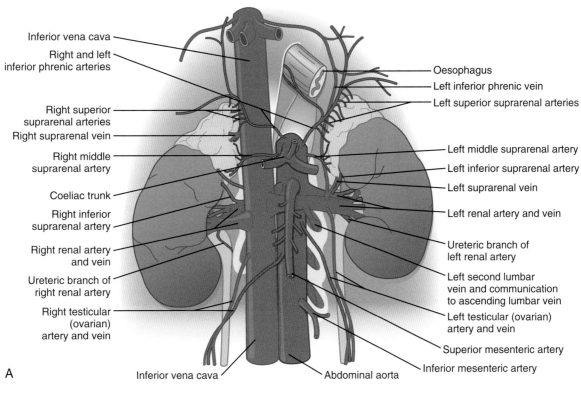

A

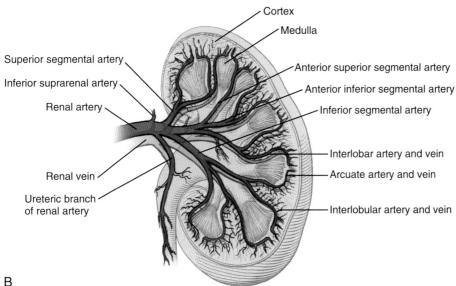

B

Fig. 11.1 Anatomical position of the kidneys and great vessels and blood supply of the kidney. (From Netter, F.H. (2014). *Atlas of human anatomy.* 6th ed. Philadelphia, Saunders Elsevier; and Raissian, Y. & Grande, J.P. (2013) Embryology and normal anatomy of the kidney. In: Lager, D., & Abrahams, N. (eds.) *Practical renal pathology.* Philadelphia, Saunders Elsevier.)

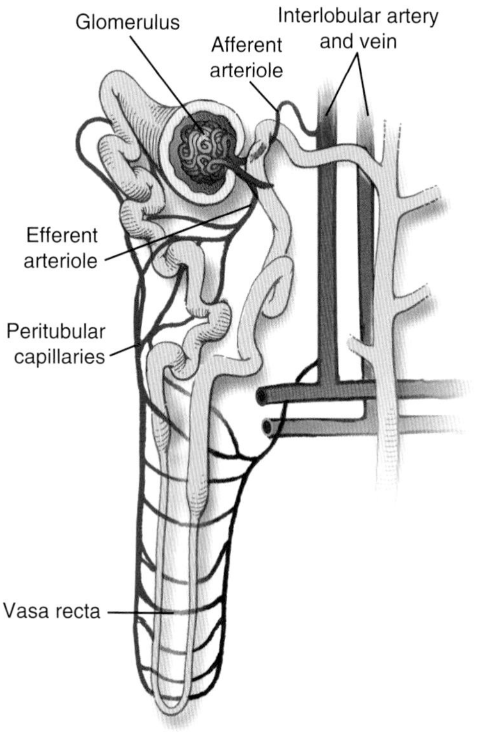

Fig. 11.2 Microcirculation of the kidney. Note two capillary beds in series is an almost unique feature of the renal circulation (it also occurs in the hypothalamus). First blood passes through the glomerulus removing fluid and solutes. Next blood flows through the peritubular capillaries where required water and solutes are reabsorbed. (From Raissian, Y. & Grande, J.P. (2013) Embryology and normal anatomy of the kidney. In: Lager, D., & Abrahams, N. (eds.) *Practical renal pathology*. Philadelphia, Saunders Elsevier.)

capillary network of the glomerulus (Fig. 11.2). After this, instead of forming a venous system they become the efferent arterioles. The efferent arterioles divide to become a second set of capillaries, the vasa recta. These serve to supply oxygenated blood to the renal medulla, descending with the loop of Henle, and also to maintain the solute gradients of the medulla necessary for the countercurrent multiplier and concentration of urine. This configuration results in the bulk of the blood supply directed towards the cortex but leaves delivery of oxygen to the tubules in the medullary region, with limited reserve if there is decreased perfusion, even in health. Small alterations in this renal perfusion can lead to tubular ischaemia.

Blood enters each glomerulus via an afferent arteriole and on into a network of capillaries that form the bulk of the glomerulus. These capillaries are lined by fenestrated

endothelial cells with pores 50–100 nm in diameter. Glomerular filtration of blood into the tubule occurs as a result of the high hydrostatic pressure within the glomerular capillaries, which is maintained by tonic differential vasoconstriction of the afferent and efferent arterioles, compared with the relatively low pressure in Bowman's space. The endothelial pores allow free filtration of fluid, solutes and small proteins less than 70 kDa in size but prevent the passage of blood cells and larger proteins. The glomerular basement membrane (GBM) is the next barrier to filtration. The GBM is synthesised predominantly of type IV collagen (which contains the autoantigen responsible for antiglomerular basement membrane disease) and contains ultrastructural pores approximately 3.5 nm in diameter that prevent the passage of most proteins. The final barrier to filtration is specialised epithelial cells called podocytes, which are attached to the GBM and face into Bowman's space. The podocytes synthesise a negatively charged glycocalyx, which forms an integral component of the glomerular filtration barrier and limits the filtration of proteins with a negative charge. Albumin, the most abundant plasma protein, is able to traverse the endothelial pores and GBM because of its flexibility and epilipsoid shape, but the negative charge of this glycocalyx prevents significant filtration of albumin in health. The ultrafiltrate in Bowman's space contains fluid of the same composition and osmolality as plasma but lacking the majority of dissolved proteins. Two healthy kidneys generate a glomerular filtration rate (GFR) of 125 ml min^{-1}, equivalent to the production of 180 L of urine per day.

Tubuloglomerular feedback is the mechanism by which the kidney autoregulates blood flow and filtration pressure to maintain an optimal GFR. The key components of this process are the macula densa and granular cells within the juxtaglomerular apparatus. Within each nephron the distal collecting tubule folds back upon itself to bring a portion, the macula densa, to lie adjacent to the glomerulus and to the afferent and efferent arterioles. The macula densa detects the tubular sodium and chloride concentrations in the thick ascending limb and distal convoluted tubule. High sodium or chloride concentrations are interpreted as signifying an increased GFR, which leads to increased activity of the apical Na-K-2Cl cotransporter, causing increased intracellular Na$^+$, cell swelling and release of adenosine triphosphate (ATP). This ultimately results in afferent arteriolar vasoconstriction, reducing glomerular blood flow; contraction of glomerular mesangial cells, reducing the area for filtration; and inhibition of renin release by granular cells, which collectively decrease GFR. In the setting of a decreased GFR, less Na$^+$ or Cl$^-$ is detected by the macula densa, and the opposite occurs.

The myogenic mechanism of renal autoregulation is more straightforward. When the perfusion pressure of the kidney increases, the afferent arterioles detect this increased pressure through stretch receptors: The smooth muscle of the arteriole contracts, increasing resistance to flow to the glomerulus. When pressure drops, the afferent arteriole relaxes to allow increased flow so that overall blood flow is relatively constant.

Renin–angiotensin–aldosterone system and vasopressin

The renin–angiotensin–aldosterone system (RAAS) is activated either by low tubular flow rates at the macula densa or low systemic blood pressure detected by baroreceptors in the carotid sinus (Fig. 11.3). Causes include hypotension secondary to heart failure, hypovolaemia or vasodilatory states such as sepsis. Specifically, low pressure in the afferent arterioles, reduced Na^+ and Cl^- in tubular fluid at the juxtaglomerular apparatus or renal sympathetic activation (β_1-mediated) stimulates release of the proteolytic enzyme renin from the juxtaglomerular cells. This cleaves the plasma protein angiotensinogen into the decapeptide angiotensin I. Angiotensin-converting enzyme (ACE) then cleaves two amino acids from angiotensin I to produce an octapeptide,

angiotensin II, which acts to increase arterial blood pressure and renal perfusion. Within the kidney there is vasoconstriction of both the afferent and efferent arterioles (more pronounced on the efferent arteriole), resulting in increased vascular resistance and preservation of GFR. Angiotensin II also causes constriction of systemic arterial resistance vessels and venoconstriction. It triggers the release of aldosterone from the zona glomerulosa of the adrenal cortex, which promotes Na^+ reabsorption in exchange for K^+ and water in the distal tubule to expand intravascular volume. Angiotensin-converting enzyme is the target of ACE inhibitors (e.g. ramipril, lisinopril, perindopril) used in the control of hypertension and heart failure. Inhibition of ACE leads to lower arteriolar resistance and dilation of both arteries and veins, thus deceasing preload and afterload on the heart. Increased urinary Na^+ and water excretion decreases blood volume. Angiotensin-converting enzyme inhibitors (ACEIs) also inhibit cardiac and vascular remodelling.

Angiotensin II receptor blockers (ARBs, e.g. losartan, candesartan) have similar pharmacological effects; these drugs are used for the same indications in patients intolerant of ACEIs.

Renin–angiotensin–aldosterone system

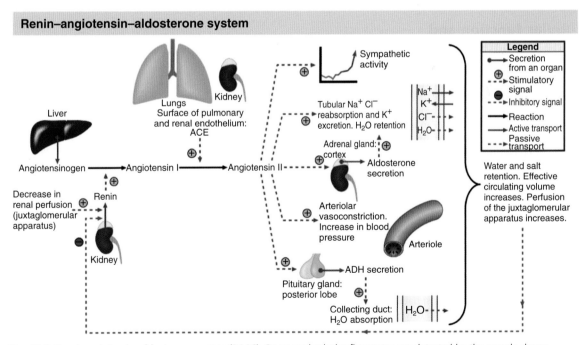

Fig. 11.3 Renal–angiotensin–aldosterone system (RAAS). Decreased tubular flow rates are detected by the macula densa, stimulating juxtaglomerular cells to release renin, which converts angiotensinogen to angiotensin I. This is then converted by angiotensin-converting enzyme *(ACE)* to angiotensin II and exerts systemic effects to increase blood pressure. *ADH*, Antidiuretic hormone. (From Melzer, J. (2013) Renal physiology. In: Hemmings, H., & Egan, T. (eds.) *Pharmacology and physiology for anesthesia.* Philadelphia, Saunders Elsevier.)

Vasopressin

Vasopressin, also called antidiuretic hormone (ADH) or arginine vasopressin (AVP), is another hormone key to water homeostasis and blood pressure regulation. Arginine vasopressin is produced in the neurones of the hypothalamus and stored in vesicles within the posterior pituitary. Vasopressin is released in response to increased blood osmolality detected by hypothalamic osmoreceptors; systemic hypotension or hypovolaemia detected by cardiopulmonary baroreceptors of the great veins and atria; or angiotensin II acting on the hypothalamus. Arginine vasopressin acts on the V_2 receptors on the collecting ducts of the kidneys through promotion of increased transcription and insertion of aquaporin-2 channels into the apical membrane of the collecting duct. These channels allow the movement of water out of the collecting duct to the surrounding interstitial fluid, which has higher osmolarity, leading to retention of free water. Vasopressin also acts on blood vessels by stimulating V_1 receptors present on vascular smooth muscle to cause potent vasoconstriction. This is the rationale for the use of vasopressin in vasodilatory shock (see Chapter 9).

Vasopressin release is also stimulated by pain, vomiting, acidosis, hypoxia and hypercapnia. Ethanol reduces the secretion of vasopressin, leading to increased diuresis and free water loss.

Tubular function and urine formation

Normal GFR is around 125 ml min^{-1}. This is usually indexed to body surface area (BSA) of 1.73 m^2 (the estimated BSA of 25-year-old Americans in the 1920s). This is equivalent to the production of 180 L of urine per day, but the vast majority of this ultrafiltrate (99.5%) is reabsorbed as it passes along the nephron. The bulk of this reabsorption occurs in the proximal convoluted tubule (PCT).

Proximal convoluted tubule

The PCT is the segment of the nephron where the majority of water and solute reabsorption occurs. The surface area over which this reabsorption occurs is significantly increased by the presence of densely packed microvilli forming a brush border on the luminal surface of the proximal tubule. The cytoplasm of the proximal tubule epithelial cells (PTEC) is densely packed with mitochondria to supply the ATP needed for the Na/K–adenosine triphosphatase (ATPase) pump, situated basolaterally. This pump drives active transport of Na$^+$ ions across the basolateral surface of the PTEC, thereby creating the necessary concentration gradient to drive Na$^+$ (and water) reabsorption from the early urine into the PTEC. This process enables the proximal tubule to reabsorb approximately two thirds of the Na$^+$ and water in the early ultrafiltrate (Fig. 11.4).

Reabsorption of glucose, amino acids and phosphate from the filtrate occurs via cell membrane cotransporters, which rely on the same Na$^+$ gradient and are therefore similarly ATP dependent. The threshold for glucose reabsorption by the proximal tubule is 9–10 mmol L^{-1}, or 160–180 mg dl^{-1}. Above this concentration the capacity of the PCT to reabsorb glucose is exceeded, and glucose will appear in the urine. This threshold is lower in pregnant women – typically around 7 mmol L^{-1} or 125 mg dl^{-1}, hence the finding of non-diabetic glycosuria in pregnant women.

Approximately 65% of the filtered K$^+$ is resorbed by solvent drag and simple diffusion in the proximal tubule. Bicarbonate reabsorption occurs in exchange for hydrogen ions. A failure of proximal tubule bicarbonate reabsorption leads to proximal (type 2) renal tubular acidosis.

A small quantity of creatinine is secreted into the filtrate in the PCT.

Carbonic anhydrase inhibitors such as acetazolamide have their site of action in the PCT.

Loop of Henle

The loop of Henle is responsible for reabsorption of 25% of filtered solutes and 20% of filtered water. Most of the processes responsible for concentration of urine and its final composition occur in the loop of Henle. The structure of the loop of Henle is specifically designed to generate and maintain a concentration gradient between the tubular fluid and the surrounding medulla to promote water reabsorption by means of the countercurrent multiplier. It comprises three main sections.

Thin descending limb of the loop of Henle

The first part is the thin descending limb, which has a low permeability to solutes whilst being permeable to water because of the presence of aquaporin I channels. On passage through the thin descending limb the osmolarity of the filtrate increases as water is removed. The filtrate typically has an osmolarity of 300 mOsm L^{-1} when it enters from the PCT, but as it descends the osmolarity increases as the water diffuses from the tubule into the higher osmolarity of the interstitial fluid of the medullary space (Fig. 11.5). As the tubule descends deeper into the medulla, the medullary space osmolarity gradually increases from 600 mOsm L^{-1} in the outer medulla to a maximum of 1200 mOsm L^{-1} in the inner medulla. This causes movement of water but not solutes (because the epithelial cells are relatively impermeable) from the lumen of the thin descending limb into the surrounding interstitial fluid of the medulla. The tip of the loop represents the highest concentrating ability of the nephron. The loop then reflects upwards and becomes the thin ascending limb of the loop of Henle.

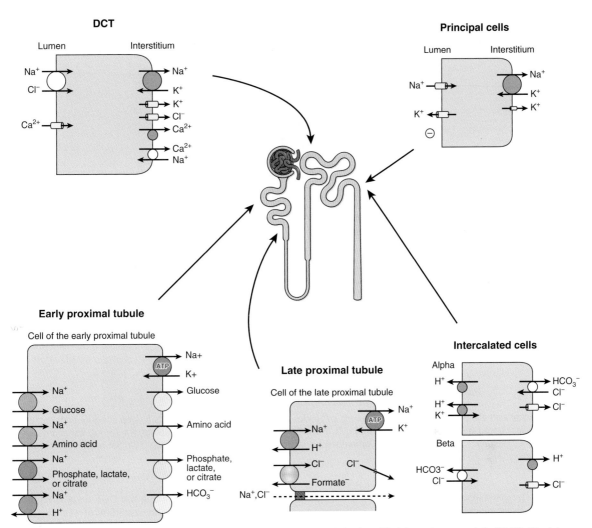

Fig. 11.4 Electrolyte transport in the nephron. *DCT,* Distal convoluted tubule. (Modified from Costanzo, L.S. (2018). *Physiology.* 6th ed. St. Louis, Elsevier; and Bailey, M.A., Shirley, D.G., & Unwin, R.J. (2014) Renal physiology. In: Johnson, R., Feehally, J., & Floege, J. (eds.) *Comprehensive clinical nephrology.* 5th ed. Philadelphia, Saunders Elsevier.)

Thin ascending limb of the loop of Henle

In contrast to the thin descending limb, the thin ascending limb of the loop of Henle is relatively impermeable to water, whereas permeability for solutes is increased, and solutes are reabsorbed principally via the Na-K-2Cl symporter and the Na-H antiporter. As a consequence of solute reabsorption, the osmolarity of the tubular fluid falls from 1200 mOsm L^{-1} to 100–150 mOsm L^{-1}.

Thick ascending limb of the loop of Henle

Unlike the thin descending and ascending limbs of the loop of Henle, where movement of water and solutes is through passive diffusion down concentration gradients, the thick ascending limb of the loop of Henle utilises ATP-dependent active transport to drive reabsorption of water and solutes. The main stimulus for active transport is the Na/K ATPase transporter situated in the basolateral membrane of the tubular epithelial cells. The Na/K ATPase generates ion gradients within the tubular epithelial cells as a consequence of movement of 3 Na$^+$ ions out of the cell into the peritubular fluid and movement of 2 K$^+$ ions into the cell. This provides the necessary intracellular driver for Na$^+$, K$^+$ and Cl$^-$ reabsorption by secondary active transport via the luminal Na-K-2Cl symporter and Na$^+$ reabsorption via the luminal Na-H antiporter, as a means of maintaining electrochemical

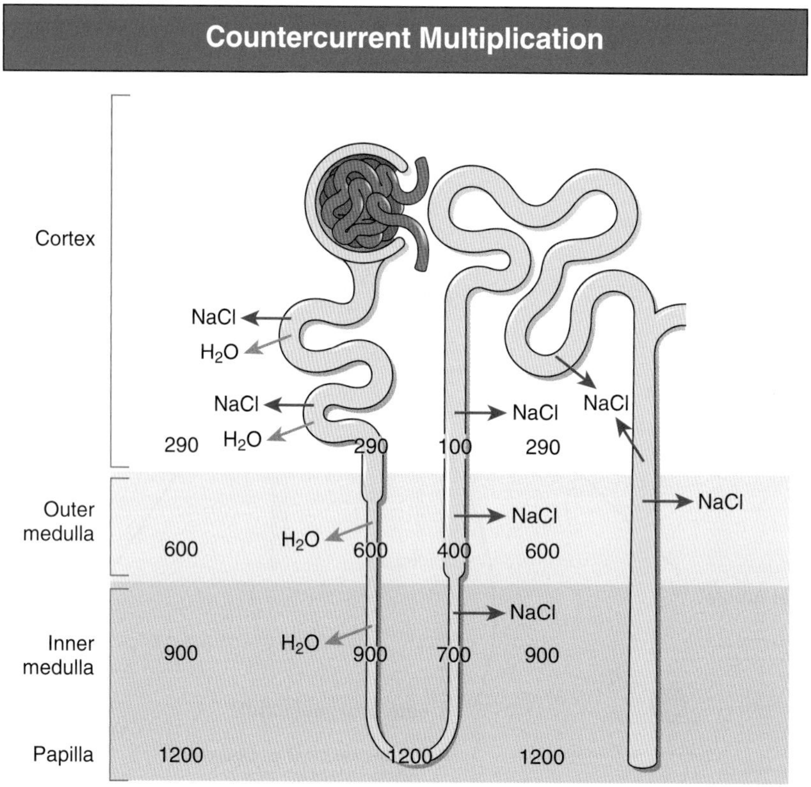

Fig. 11.5 Water and electrolyte movement in the loop of Henle. The nephron drawn represents a deep (long-looped) nephron. Figures represent approximate osmolalities (mOsm kg⁻¹). (From Bailey, M.A., Shirley, D.G., & Unwin, R.J. (2014) Renal physiology. In: Johnson, R., Feehally, J., & Floege, J. (eds.) *Comprehensive clinical nephrology.* 5th ed. Philadelphia, Saunders Elsevier.)

neutrality. The generated electrical and concentration gradients also drive magnesium and calcium reabsorption through specific membrane-bound transporters.

Loop diuretics inhibit the luminal Na-K-2Cl cotransporter in the thick ascending limb, thereby preventing reabsorption of Na^+, K^+ and Cl^-, promoting natriuresis, kaliuresis and diuresis.

The cortical thick ascending limb transitions into the distal convoluted tubule.

Distal convoluted tubule

The distal convoluted tubule (DCT) is largely impermeable to water and is principally responsible for the regulation of K^+, Na^+, HCO_3^- and Ca^{2+} excretion (see Fig. 11.4). At the junction of the thick ascending limb of the loop of Henle and the DCT lies the macula densa, a group of specialised epithelial cells whose function is to monitor the osmolality of tubular filtrate, principally sensing the tubular concentration of Na^+ and Cl^- and providing tubuloglomerular feedback.

As the filtrate passes along the DCT there is regulated reabsorption of HCO_3^- and secretion of H^+, the extent to which this occurs being dependent on body pH. Na^+ reabsorption is regulated by aldosterone, which increases Na^+ reabsorption in exchange for K^+ (See Figs 11.4 and 11.6). Ca^{2+} reabsorption in the DCT is regulated by parathyroid hormone, secreted in response to decreased serum Ca^{2+} concentrations detected by the calcium-sensing receptors on the surface of parathyroid cells.

The DCT contains the thiazide-sensitive Na-Cl cotransporter.

Collecting tubule

The collecting tubule is the final component of the nephron and is where the final concentration of urine occurs as it passes onwards through the medulla into the renal calyces. Each tubule is approximately 20 mm in length and 20–50 μm in diameter. The collecting tubule is lined with two types of cells: the principal cells and the intercalated cells.

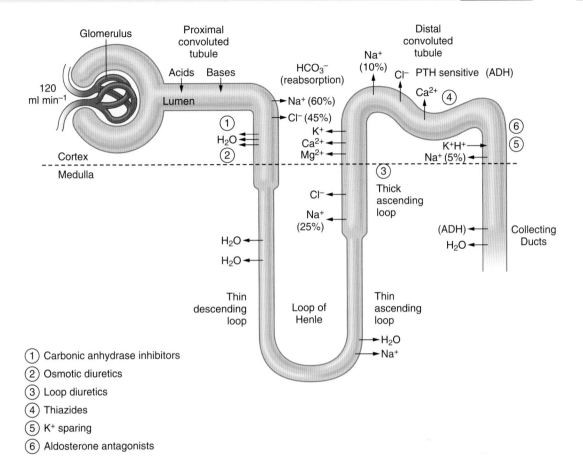

Fig. 11.6 Sites of action of diuretics along the nephron. *ADH,* Antidiuretic hormone; *PTH,* parathyroid hormone. (From Svensén, C. (2013) Electrolytes and diuretics. In: Hemmings, H., & Egan, T. (eds.) *Pharmacology and physiology for anesthesia.* Philadelphia, Saunders Elsevier.)

① Carbonic anhydrase inhibitors
② Osmotic diuretics
③ Loop diuretics
④ Thiazides
⑤ K⁺ sparing
⑥ Aldosterone antagonists

The principal cells contain a basolateral Na/K ATPase which generates a low intracellular Na⁺ and high intracellular K⁺ concentration; this is used to generate luminal gradient to promote reabsorption of Na⁺ and excretion of K⁺ through specific ion channels. Water reabsorption occurs in this part of the tubule via aquaporin channels under the influence of ADH (vasopressin). The aquaporin channels lie within vesicles in the cell cytoplasm and insert into the luminal membrane of the principal cell in response to ADH, allowing water to be reabsorbed and tubular filtrate to be further concentrated.

The intercalated cell plays an important role in acid–base balance by secreting H⁺ via active transport using a luminal H⁺ ATPase. Defects in these cells can lead to an inability to lower urine pH beyond 5.3 and the development of type 1, or distal, renal tubular acidosis.

Pharmacology of drugs acting on the kidney

Diuretics

Diuretics cause an increase in the excretion of water and electrolytes. They are widely prescribed for hypertension, heart failure and clinical situations associated with fluid overload. When used on a long-term basis, they not only change the body's sodium and fluid balance but also act as mild vasodilators. When diuretics are prescribed for the treatment of fluid retention and oedema, three important principles have to be kept in mind. First, although a dramatic diuretic response may be required in pulmonary oedema and acute cardiac failure, a mild sustained diuresis is more appropriate in the majority of patients and will minimise adverse effects. Second, plasma K^+ concentration and hydration status must always be monitored. Third, diuretic therapy only treats the symptoms and does not influence the underlying cause or change the outcome of a patient with oedema.

Diuretics are classified according to their mechanism and site of action on the nephron (see Fig. 11.6):

- Glomerulus and proximal renal tubule (e.g. osmotic diuretics, carbonic anhydrase inhibitors)
- Ascending limb of the loop of Henle (e.g. loop diuretics)
- Distal tubule (e.g. thiazides, potassium-sparing diuretics, aldosterone antagonists)

Site of action: whole nephron

Osmotic diuretics

Mannitol

Mannitol is an alcohol produced by the reduction of mannose. It is absorbed unreliably from the GI tract and therefore has to be given by i.v. injection; bolus doses of $0.25-1$ g kg^{-1} are used. Initially it stays within the intra-vascular space but is then slowly redistributed into the extravascular compartment. Mannitol does not undergo metabolism and is excreted unchanged through the kidneys. Mannitol expands intravascular volume and then undergoes free glomerular filtration with almost no reabsorption in the proximal tubule. This leads to an osmotic force that retains water and Na^+ in the tubule, with a consequent osmotic diuresis – that is, increased urinary excretion of Na^+, water, HCO_3^- and Cl^-. Mannitol does not alter urinary pH. The increased renal blood flow reduces the rate of renin secretion; this decreases the urine-concentrating capacity of the kidney.

It is primarily used as rescue therapy in the setting of raised intracranial pressure to draw fluid by osmosis from swollen brain cells. It is also used for reduction of intraocular pressure. It takes 15–30 min to have maximal effect and is given as a bolus dose as mannitol molecules may cross the blood–brain barrier and continuous infusion is thought to worsen raised intracranial hypertension. Mannitol may have other effects when given for raised intracranial pressure, including reduction in blood viscosity and free radical scavenging. It is osmotically active and will act as an unmeasured osmole and increase the osmolar gap if calculated.

Site of action: proximal convoluted tubule

Carbonic anhydrase inhibitors

Acetazolamide

Acetazolamide is a carbonic anhydrase inhibitor. Under normal physiological conditions, the enzyme carbonic anhydrase is responsible for reabsorption of Na^+ and excretion of H^+ in the PCT of the nephron. Inhibition of carbonic anhydrase decreases H^+ excretion, and therefore Na^+ and HCO_3^- ions stay in the renal tubule. This results in the production of alkaline urine with high Na^+ and HCO_3^- content. Delivery to the collecting tubules of this Na^+ HCO_3^- load will enhance K^+ secretion, causing a resultant kaliuresis, and can worsen hypokalaemia. The increased Na^+ excretion leads to a modest diuresis. Cl^- is retained instead of HCO_3^- to maintain an ionic balance. All these changes result in a hyperchloraemic metabolic acidosis.

Acetazolamide is well absorbed, not metabolised, and is excreted almost unchanged by the kidney within 24 h. Toxicity is very rare. The adult oral and intravenous dose is $250-1000$ mg day^{-1} in divided doses.

Carbonic anhydrase inhibitors are seldom used as primary diuretics because of their weak diuretic effect. They are mainly used in the setting of prevention and management of acute mountain sickness or treatment of raised intraocular pressure. They are occasionally used in the setting of intensive care to promote urinary HCO_3^- loss in patients with metabolic alkalosis and raised HCO_3^-.

Site of action: loop of Henle

Loop diuretics

Loop diuretics act primarily on the medullary part of the ascending limb of the loop of Henle. After initial glomerular filtration and proximal tubular secretion, they inhibit the active reabsorption of Cl^- in the thick portion of the ascending limb. This leads to Cl^-, Na^+, K^+ and H^+ remaining in the tubule to maintain electrical neutrality and their increased excretion in the urine. The extent of the following diuresis is determined by the concentration of active drug in this part of the tubule. Because the ascending limb plays an important role in the reabsorption of sodium chloride in the kidney, these drugs produce a potent diuretic response. The decrease in sodium chloride reabsorption leads to a reduced urine-concentrating ability of the normally hypertonic medullary interstitium. Furosemide, bumetanide and torsemide are classified as loop diuretics because of their common site of action. Furosemide is the most commonly used.

Furosemide

Furosemide is the diuretic of choice in acute pulmonary oedema or other states of fluid overload (e.g. cardiac, renal or liver failure). It reduces intravascular fluid volume by promoting a rapid, powerful diuresis even in the presence of a low GFR and also causes pulmonary vasodilatation. The latter precedes the diuretic effect to produce rapid symptomatic relief of dyspnoea occurred. In hypertensive patients, vasodilatation and preload reduction lead to a decrease in arterial pressure. Approximately 96% of the drug is bound to plasma proteins, with a relatively low volume of distribution; it is therefore not filtered by the glomerulus but instead is excreted in the PCT. In hypoalbuminaemia furosemide is less bound to albumin. Instead it diffuses into tissues and has a resultant larger volume of distribution, necessitating a significantly increased dosage to elicit the same effects. Metabolism and excretion into the GI tract contribute to about 30% of the elimination of a dose of furosemide. The remainder is excreted unchanged through glomerular filtration and tubular secretion. Impaired renal function affects the elimination process, but liver disease does not seem to influence this. The elimination half-life of furosemide is 1–1.5 h.

Furosemide increases renal artery blood flow as long as intravascular fluid volume is maintained. It causes redistribution so that flow to the outer part of the cortex remains unchanged while inner cortex and medullary flow is increased. It leads to an improved renal tissue oxygen tension, and though it may be of clinical benefit in the setting of oliguric AKI to promote or maintain a diuresis to avoid fluid overload, it has no overall effect on duration or severity of AKI or the need for renal replacement therapy.

Excessive doses of furosemide can lead to fluid or electrolyte abnormalities and ototoxicity. Severe hypokalaemia may precipitate dangerous cardiac arrhythmias, especially in the presence of high concentrations of digoxin. It may also enhance the effect of non-depolarising neuromuscular blocking drugs. Hyperuricaemia and prerenal uraemia may develop and may precipitate acute gout in a patient with pre-existing gout.

Furosemide may cause high intrarenal concentrations of aminoglycosides and cephalosporins; this may enhance the nephrotoxic effects of these drugs. This effect of furosemide is dose dependent, and continuous i.v. infusions may be used to reduce peak furosemide concentrations. Prolonged high blood concentrations of furosemide may have a direct toxic action, resulting in interstitial nephritis. It may also cause transient or permanent deafness because of changes in the endolymph electrolyte composition.

Bolus furosemide is usually administered intravenously (0.1–1 mg kg^{-1}) or orally (0.75–3 mg kg^{-1}). Intravenous furosemide is usually started as a slow 20–40 mg injection in adults, and increased to effect, but higher doses or even an infusion may be required in the elderly, in patients with renal failure or severe congestive cardiac failure, or those in intensive care. Typical infusion doses used in ICU patients are 2–10 mg/h.

Bumetanide

The mechanism of action and effects of bumetanide and furosemide are similar, but bumetanide has greater bioavailability, so smaller doses are needed, and elimination is less dependent on renal function. Ototoxicity may be slightly less common than with furosemide, but renal toxicity is more of a problem. Hypokalaemia occurs with both drugs. In clinical practice there is no clear advantage or disadvantage over furosemide, providing equivalent doses are administered. The normal adult dose is 0.5–3 mg i.v. over 1–2 min. The onset of diuresis is within 30 min, and this usually lasts for about 4 h.

Site of action: distal convoluted tubule

Thiazide diuretics

Many thiazides are available, all with similar dose–response curves and diuretic effects. Bendroflumethiazide is most commonly used; alternatives include chlorothiazide, hydrochlorothiazide and chlorthalidone. Compared with loop diuretics, thiazides have a longer duration of action (6–12 h), act at a different site, have a low ceiling effect and are less effective in chronic kidney disease.

Thiazides inhibit the active pump for Na$^+$ and Cl$^-$ reabsorption in the cortical ascending part of the loop of Henle and the DCT. Therefore the urine-concentrating ability of the kidney is not impaired, as normally this area is responsible for less than 5% of Na$^+$ reabsorption. The diuresis achieved by the thiazides is therefore never as effective as that of the loop diuretics. It is mild but sustained. In contrast with loop diuretics, the excretion of Ca^{2+} is decreased and hypercalcaemia may occur. In the presence of high aldosterone activity, the increase in Na$^+$ delivery to the distal renal tubules is associated with increased K$^+$ loss, similar to that of the loop diuretics. The reduced clearance of uric acid by thiazides may cause hyperuricaemia.

Thiazides are used extensively in low doses and often combined with a low-sodium diet for the management of essential hypertension. A reduction in extracellular fluid volume and mild peripheral vasodilatation are responsible for the sustained antihypertensive effect. The full antihypertensive effect may take up to 12 weeks to become established. Higher doses of thiazides are used for the management of congestive cardiac failure and other oedematous conditions such as nephrotic syndrome and liver cirrhosis.

The most common adverse effects of the thiazides are dehydration and hypovolaemia, which may present as orthostatic hypotension. During chronic therapy, thiazides typically cause hyponatraemic, hypokalaemic, hypochloraemic, metabolic alkalosis. In combination with magnesium depletion, the hypokalaemia may trigger serious cardiac arrhythmias, digoxin toxicity, muscle weakness and the potentiation of non-depolarising neuromuscular blocking agents.

Thiazides decrease the tubular secretion of urate, which may lead to hyperuricaemia and gout. They are sulphonamide derivatives and may therefore cause inhibition of insulin release from the pancreas and blockade of peripheral glucose utilisation. This may precipitate hyperglycaemia or an increase in insulin requirements in a patient with diabetes mellitus.

They also lead to an increase in total blood cholesterol. Indapamide is a commonly used thiazide-like diuretic with similar properties and is recommended as an antihypertensive agent. At lower doses, indapamide has vasodilatory effects, with the diuretic effect becoming more apparent with higher doses.

Site of action: distal convoluted tubule

Potassium-sparing diuretics

Only a small part of Na^+ reabsorption into the renal cells takes place via the sodium–potassium exchange mechanism in the distal tubules. The K^+-retaining diuretics act on the DCTs and the collecting ducts and therefore cause only a limited diuresis. There are two subgroups in this category: drugs acting independently of the aldosterone mechanism (e.g. triamterene and amiloride) and aldosterone antagonists (e.g. spironolactone or eplerenone).

These drugs increase the urinary excretion of Na^+, Cl^- and HCO_3^- and lead to an increase in urinary pH. They prevent excessive loss of K^+ that occurs with the loop and thiazide diuretics by reducing the sodium–potassium exchange. K^+-sparing drugs do, however, augment the diuretic response of these drugs when given in combination.

Amiloride and triamterene

Amiloride acts directly on the distal tubule and collecting duct. It causes K^+ retention and an increase in Na^+ loss. Amiloride is almost always used in combination with thiazide or loop diuretics. It then has a synergistic action in terms of diuresis, although it opposes the K^+ loss. Amiloride has few side effects. Hyperkalaemia and acidosis may occur, and it is therefore contraindicated in patients with advanced chronic kidney disease.

Triamterene has characteristics similar to those of amiloride.

Spironolactone and eplerenone

Aldosterone causes Na^+ reabsorption and K^+ loss in the DCT. Spironolactone has a steroid molecular structure, acts as a competitive antagonist on the aldosterone receptors and inhibits Na^+ reabsorption and K^+ loss. In the absence of aldosterone, it has no effect.

After oral absorption, spironolactone is immediately metabolised to a number of metabolites, some of which are active.

Heart failure leads to a decreased cardiac output state, whereas liver cirrhosis leads to decreased vascular resistance and loss of oncotic pressure, with leak of intravascular fluid. Both of these conditions lead to decreased renal perfusion. This prompts release of renin, and subsequent production of aldosterone, and salt and water retention. Spironolactone is an important adjunct in the diuretic management of heart failure as well as in liver cirrhosis, ascites and secondary hyperaldosteronism. Spironolactone is used late in the stepwise management of hypertension but has an important role in the presence of high mineralocorticoid levels such as in Conn's syndrome or prednisone therapy. Spironolactone is often combined with thiazides to maximise the diuretic effect and prevent K^+ loss.

Hyperkalaemia may develop if spironolactone is used in the presence of renal dysfunction. If used in high doses, it may cause gynaecomastia and impotence as a result of inhibition of androgen production as well as antagonism of androgen signalling and weak agonism at oestrogen receptors.

Eplerenone is a selective aldosterone receptor antagonist that is more specific for the mineralocorticoid receptor than spironolactone and without antiandrogenic side effects. It is mainly used in the management of heart failure in the setting of ischaemic heart disease.

Desmopressin

Desmopressin (trade name DDAVP) is a synthetic analogue of vasopressin; it is not a diuretic but has important effects on water handling. Desmopressin is used in the setting of central diabetes insipidus as a replacement for absent vasopressin. It is also used in haemophilia and von Willebrand's disease, as well as platelet dysfunction caused by uraemia, where it is used to promote the release of von Willebrand's factor to promote coagulation. As an analogue of vasopressin, its effects are identical. It promotes aquaporin channel insertion to the collecting duct, increasing permeability to free water and movement of water from the collecting duct to the interstitium and bloodstream, which leads to further concentration of urine. Side effects of administration include acute hyponatraemia as free water is resorbed and serum Na^+ is diluted, which can lead to seizures and cerebral oedema. Omission of desmopressin in patients already established on the drug for central diabetes insipidus can lead to dehydration and rapid rises in serum Na^+ as urinary concentrating ability is lost, and to the potentially devastating side effects of central pontine myelinolysis if this is not recognised. Guidelines suggest serum Na^+ concentration should raise by no more than 12 mmol L^{-1} per day. Desmopressin can be given acutely intravenously 1–4 µg day^{-1} or more chronically by mouth or intranasal spray.

Assessment of renal function

Renal function is measured as a GFR to reflect the quantity of blood filtered by the kidneys each minute

(Tables 11.1–11.3). It is the filtration product of the average filtration rate of single nephrons and the total number of nephrons in both kidneys:

$$GFR = Urine\ flow \times \frac{[S]_U}{[S]_P}$$

where $[S]_{U/P}$ are concentrations of a substance in the urine and plasma, respectively.

Normal GFR is 80–120 ml min^{-1} 1.73 m^{-2}. Despite the importance of accurate knowledge of GFR for the anaesthetist, common practice is to use a calculated or estimated GFR (eGFR) based on the serum creatinine concentration rather

Table 11.1 Normal serum/plasma values

Osmolality	280–300 mOsm kg^{-1}
Creatinine	45–120 µmol L^{-1}
Urea	2.7–7.0 mmol L^{-1}

Table 11.2 Normal urinary chemistry

Osmolality	300–1200 mOsm kg^{-1}	
Creatinine excretion	8.8–17.6 mmol per 24 h (men) 7.0–15.8 mmol per 24 h (women)	
pH	4.5–8.0	
Na$^+$ excretion	40–220 mmol per 24 h	Na$^+$ concentration <20 mmol L^{-1} = appropriate conservation of sodium in the context of hypovolemia
K$^+$ excretion	25–125 mmol per 24h	

Table 11.3 Measurement of renal function

Endogenous	Pros	Cons
Serum creatinine	Cheap Easy Endogenous	Affected by muscle mass, ethnic origin and some medications Inaccurate in mild renal impairment
Creatinine (Cr) clearance	Endogenous	24-h urine collection needed Overestimates GFR because of Cr secretion by tubules
Cystatin C	Endogenous Adds accuracy to serum creatinine measurement	
Exogenous markers		
Inulin	Highly accurate UK reference standard	Requires intravenous access Requires urine collection Slightly overestimates GFR
^{51}Chromium EDTA	Highly accurate UK reference standard Undergoes only glomerular filtration	Requires intravenous access Repeated blood sampling Radioactive
^{125}I-iothalamate	Highly accurate UK reference standard	Requires intravenous access Repeated blood sampling Radioactive
Iohexol	Highly accurate UK reference standard Not radioactive	Requires intravenous access Repeated blood sampling
Tc-99m DTPA	Highly accurate	Requires intravenous access Repeated blood sampling Radioactive

GFR, Glomerular filtration rate; *Tc-99m DPTA*, technetium 99 diethylene-triamine-pentaacetate acid.

than an actual measured GFR. Creatinine is the most commonly used metabolite for calculation of an eGFR. Serum creatinine is derived from muscle catabolism or protein intake, and in the absence of changes in GFR the serum concentration of creatinine is generally stable for an individual. It is freely filtered by the glomerulus but is also secreted by the PCT, which accounts for 10%–20% of excreted creatinine. Serum creatinine varies inversely with GFR, but this relationship is not directly linear. Furthermore in acute illness a significant deterioration in renal function has often occurred before serum creatinine increases. Metabolites other than creatinine have been proposed as more suitable markers of GFR. In particular cystatin C has generated some interest, but creatinine is currently the most widely used in clinical practice.

Estimated GFR can be calculated from a serum creatinine concentration using a number of different formulae, but the most commonly used formula is the Modification of Diet in Renal Disease (MDRD) study formula, which incorporates a correction for patient race, age and sex. An alternative is the Cockcroft-Gault formula, which incorporates age, sex and body weight but overestimates GFR in the overweight and oedematous and underestimates in those of African origin. It is worth noting that both these commonly used measures are accurate enough for the majority of clinical situations but are only valid in steady states of creatinine concentration, and rapidly changing creatinine such as in the setting of acute kidney injury or after renal transplant will not translate accurately to changes in GFR.

Measured serum creatinine values can be misleading. Serum creatinine concentrations can be increased by high muscle mass and protein-rich diets, as well as by drugs impairing tubular secretion of creatinine such as trimethoprim, cimetidine and certain fibrates. In all these instances a creatinine-based eGFR may incorrectly suggest impairment of renal function. By contrast, low serum creatinine concentrations may be present in patients with reduced muscle mass, such as those with neurodegenerative disease or severe wasting, or after limb amputation; these lead to a high creatinine-based eGFR which can be falsely interpreted as equating to preserved renal function. Age-related variation in muscle mass and turnover can also affect estimations of GFR to a clinically important degree.

Glomerular filtration rate can be more accurately measured (a measured GFR vs. an estimated GFR) using clearance methods, with the gold standard being an inulin clearance. Inulin is a small inert molecule, is freely filtered and is not reabsorbed or secreted by the renal tubules. Conducting a measured GFR (mGFR) is laborious and time consuming: Inulin is infused until a steady plasma concentration is achieved and then the infusion stopped and the rate at which inulin is cleared from the blood and appears in the urine is measured. The mGFR can then be calculated. Alternatively, and more commonly, [51]chromium EDTA clearance is used to measure GFR. This only requires a single injection and blood tests 2, 3 and 4 h after injection to calculate mGFR. More recently urinary iothalamate clearance and plasma clearance of iohexol have been used, particularly in clinical studies, to calculate mGFR.

Acute kidney injury and contrast nephropathy

Acute kidney injury (formerly known as acute renal failure) is defined as the abrupt (occurring over hours to days) and sustained decline in GFR, urine output or both. *Acute kidney injury* (AKI) describes a continuum of renal damage ranging from decreased urine output or small elevations in creatinine to complete anuria and the need for renal replacement therapy. It is common, with one in five emergency admissions to hospital having some degree of AKI, occurs often in patients undergoing emergency surgery and occurs in more than 60% of those admitted to the intensive care. There are multiple staging systems for AKI. The Kidney Disease: Improving Global Outcomes (KDIGO) system (Table 11.4) is most commonly used, and increasing grade of AKI is associated with increasing mortality. Despite extensive research no specific therapies have been found to improve recovery and treatment of AKI, and current treatment strategies remain the identification and removal of the initial insult and good supportive care.

The aetiology of AKI is often categorised as prerenal, renal (intrinsic) and postrenal. Prerenal AKI is caused by a decrease in the effective blood flow and oxygen delivery to the kidney and can be due to decreased mean arterial pressure but also due to a decreased cardiac output with preserved MAP, as in the setting of cardiogenic shock. In the initial phase of prerenal AKI, renal blood flow decreases, and there is decreased delivery of blood to the glomerulus and filtration pressure falls. An immediate consequence of this is activation of autoregulatory mechanisms within the kidney in an attempt to preserve glomerular filtration pressure and promote Na^+ and water reabsorption, such as activation of the RAAS and release of ADH. This will be reflected clinically in decreased urine output and increased urine osmolality with a low urinary Na^+ concentration. While this is occurring, the blood concentrations of nitrogen-containing compounds increases, often termed prerenal azotaemia. At this point restoration of adequate renal blood flow should rapidly reverse these changes.

As a consequence of autoregulation, renal perfusion remains stable over a relatively wide range of MAP in healthy kidneys (Fig. 11.7). However, if the limits of autoregulation are exceeded, renal perfusion and oxygen delivery will fall, oxygen uptake will outstrip oxygen delivery and renal ischaemia will develop. The glomeruli are relatively protected

Table 11.4 Kidney Disease: Improving Global Outcomes (KDIGO) diagnostic criteria for acute kidney injury		
Stage	**Serum creatinine criteria**	**Urine output criteria**
1	1.5–1.9 times baseline OR ≥26.4 µmol L^{-1} increase	< 0.5 ml kg^{-1} h^{-1} for 6–12 h
2	2.0–2.9 times baseline	<0.5 ml kg^{-1} h^{-1} for ≥12 h
3	≥3.0 times baseline OR Increase in serum creatinine to ≥354 µmol L^{-1} OR Initiation of renal replacement therapy OR in patients aged <18 years, decrease in eGFR to <35 ml min^{-1} 1.73 m^{-2}	<0.3 ml kg^{-1} h^{-1} for ≥24 h OR anuria for ≥12 h
eGFR, Estimated glomerular filtration rate.		

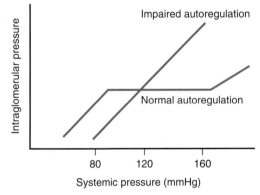

Fig. 11.7 Renal autoregulation. Relationship of systemic to glomerular pressure in the setting of normal or abnormal renal autoregulation. (From Sarafidis, V., Pantelis, A., & Bakris, G.L. Evaluation and treatment of hypertensive urgencies and emergencies. In: Johnson, R., Feehally, J., & Floege, J. (eds.) *Comprehensive clinical nephrology.* 5th ed. Philadelphia, Saunders Elsevier.)

from ischaemia because of their large flow of blood, but as a result of the relatively poorly vascularised inner medulla and the high oxygen requirements of the tubules, even a limited period of hypoxia can lead to tubular ischaemia and subsequent acute tubular necrosis (ATN). Acute tubular necrosis is thought of as the most common intrinsic renal injury encountered in clinical practice but is a histological term and typically only occurs in AKI of low cardiac output states.

Sepsis is the most common cause of AKI and is classically thought of as prerenal, with hypoperfusion and subsequent ATN as the cause of renal impairment. Evidence suggests septic AKI can occur in the setting of increased or maintained renal perfusion, as in the setting of hyperdynamic sepsis, with ATN a relatively uncommon feature. Sepsis is thought to lead to kidney injury by a combination of microcirculatory dysfunction and filtered inflammatory mediators such as cytokines, chemokines and complement fragments that have toxic effects on tubular cells, leading to tubular cell vacuolisation, swelling, apoptosis and loss of tubular function.

Established AKI is treated with supportive care, including renal replacement therapy (RRT) and early removal of the underlying cause whilst the kidney recovers. There are currently no specific treatments for AKI that have been found to hasten renal recovery.

Intrinsic renal injury

Intrinsic renal disease, caused by direct injury to the glomeruli or tubules, as a cause of AKI is far less common than prerenal AKI. Glomerular injury may be ischaemic in origin but often requires profound periods of hypoperfusion, leading to renal infarction. Glomerular injury is more often autoimmune in origin and marked by focal necrotising lesions, capillaritis and formation of cellular crescents in Bowman's space. Clinically this is associated with haematuria and proteinuria as a result of immune-mediated damage to the GBM and is termed rapidly progressive glomerulonephritis (RPGN). When untreated this can lead to irreversible sclerosis of the glomeruli and marked tubulointerstitial scarring. Causes of

RPGN include antiglomerular basement membrane disease (Goodpasture syndrome) caused by development of autoantibodies to type IV collagen in the GBM and alveoli, leading to rapid development of irreversible renal failure and in some cases life-threatening pulmonary haemorrhage. A more common cause of RPGN is antineutrophil cytoplasmic antibody (ANCA)–associated vasculitis, often associated with systemic symptoms commonly affecting the respiratory tract and ear, nose and throat. The first investigation in any case of AKI should be a urine dipstick analysis, ideally before placement of a urinary catheter. Haematuria or proteinuria should raise the suspicion of RPGN and prompt discussion with a nephrologist.

Other causes of intrinsic AKI include exposure to tubular toxins such as myoglobin as a consequence of large-volume muscle breakdown. During rhabdomyolysis the damaged muscle releases large quantities of myoglobin, which is freely filtered by the glomerulus and both binds to Tamm-Horsfall protein in the tubules to form casts and leads to production of free radicals, causing direct cellular injury within the tubule. At high concentrations the aminoglycoside antibiotics, such as gentamicin, tobramycin and neomycin, can cause AKI because of their disruption of protein synthesis within the tubular cells. Careful pharmacokinetic monitoring of these antibiotics is required to prevent this toxicity.

Radiological contrast agents can also cause AKI, principally as a result of ischaemia secondary to reactive renal vasoconstriction and medullary hypoxia in response to the contrast agent, as well as direct tubular toxicity. The risk of contrast-induced nephropathy (CIN) is increased in those patients with concomitant AKI or chronic kidney disease, diabetes, dehydration or increasing age and after administration of large-volume, high-viscosity contrast agents. High osmolar contrast agents have largely been replaced by iso-osmolar agents, and the incidence of CIN has reduced significantly. Preventative hydration strategies are effective in preventing CIN. Current KDIGO guidelines suggest volume expansion before contrast administration with 0.9% sodium chloride or sodium bicarbonate solution should be considered; there is no convincing evidence for the prophylactic use of either fenoldopam or theophyllines. The mainstay of treatment is supportive, and most patients recover quickly without requiring renal replacement therapy. Temporary RRT is required in <1% of healthy patients receiving contrast; the proportion is slightly higher (3%) in those with underlying chronic kidney disease (CKD) or undergoing percutaneous coronary intervention.

Postrenal causes of AKI are those where drainage of both kidneys is blocked, resulting in increased intrarenal pressure, hydronephrosis and, if left unchecked, tubular injury. Typical causes of renal tract obstruction include renal stones, renal or bladder tumour, and bladder obstruction from enlarged prostate, urethral stricture and pelvic malignancy. Renal tract ultrasound or CT are the investigations of choice to identify hydronephrosis and the level of obstruction. Bypassing the obstruction is the immediate goal, either with a bladder catheter (urethral/suprapubic), nephrostomy or ureteric stenting. Estimated GFR can be normal with a single kidney or unilateral renal tract obstruction. Therefore an abnormal eGFR indicates bilateral renal disease. Urine output may appear within normal limits in cases of unilateral obstruction but causes irreparable damage to the obstructed kidney if not rectified. After relief of any renal tract obstruction there can be a significant postobstructive diuresis as a result of loss of the concentrating ability of the kidney, and this can place the patient at significant risk of profound electrolyte losses and dehydration.

Some decrease in urine output is to be expected after major surgery. This is a consequence of the adaptive physiological stress response to trauma leading to activation of the sympathetic nervous system, RAAS and release of ADH (see Chapter 13). These mechanisms combine to maintain MAP by vasoconstriction and conserve both sodium and water, leading to a reduced urine output and potentially oliguria. This is a normal response and requires careful monitoring for the development of AKI. However this ADH-mediated oliguria should not be mistaken for oliguria as a consequence of hypovolaemia (postoperative bleeding) or inflammatory mediators (postoperative sepsis). Unfortunately there is still no reliable way to differentiate these causes of oliguria, and clinical judgement must be used.

The clinical consequences and management implications of acute and CKD are discussed further in Chapters 19 and 20.

References/Further reading

Bagshaw, S.M., George, C., Bellomo, R., et al., 2008. Early acute kidney injury and sepsis: a multicentre evaluation. Crit. Care 12, R47.

Basile, D., Anderson, M., Sutton, T.A., 2012. Pathophysiology of acute kidney injury. Compr. Physiol. 2 (2), 1303–1353. doi:10.1002/cphy.c110041.

Bellomo, R., Kellum, J., Ronco, C., et al., 2017. Acute kidney injury in sepsis. Int. Care Med. 43 (6), 816–828.

Clinical Practice Guidelines for Acute Kidney Injury, 2012. Available from: http://www.kdigo.org/clinical_practice_guidelines/AKI.php.

Cruz, D.N., Ricci, Z., Ronco, C., 2009. Clinical review: RIFLE and AKIN – time for reappraisal. Crit. Care 13, 211.

Fähling, M., Seeliger, E., Patzak, A., Persson, P.B., 2017. Understanding and preventing contrast-induced acute kidney injury. Nat. Rev. Nephrol. 13 (3), 169–180. doi:10.1038/nrneph.2016.196.

McCormick, J.A., Ellison, D.H., 2015. Distal convoluted tubule. Compr. Physiol. 5 (1), 45–98. doi:10.1002/cphy.c140002.

Shirley, D.G., Unwin, R.J., 2010. Renal physiology. In: Floege, J., Johnson, R., Feehally, J. (Eds.), Comprehensive Clinical

Nephrology, fourth ed. Elsevier, Missouri, pp. 15–28.

Tojo, A., Kinugasa, S., 2012. Mechanisms of glomerular albumin filtration and tubular reabsorption. Int. J. Nephrol. 2012. doi:10.1155/2012/481520.

Chapter | **12** |

Fluid, electrolyte and acid–base balance

Gareth Williams

The realisation that the enzyme systems and metabolic processes responsible for the maintenance of cellular function are dependent on an environment with stable electrolyte and hydrogen ion concentrations led Claude Bernard to describe the *milieu interieur* more than 100 years ago. Complex homeostatic mechanisms have evolved to maintain the constancy of this internal environment and thus prevent cellular dysfunction.

role within the cell membrane and the subsequent control of movement of substances in and out of cells.

The concentration and distribution of these substances is fundamental to the maintenance of normal cellular function; systems to regulate water and sodium balance are particularly vital. The homeostasis of this environment occurs through both passive (non-energy consuming) and active transport processes.

Physiology of electrolytes and water balance

Mammalian intracellular and extracellular fluids (plasma) comprise about 70% *water*, containing a large variety of *ions* (electrolytes) and *organic molecules* (predominantly formed from carbon and hydrogen).

Water (H_2O), the biological solvent, is a polar molecule – that is, it carries a non-uniform distribution of charge because of the greater positivity of the oxygen nucleus. This means as a solvent it only dissolves other polar molecules such as ions.

An ion is any charged molecule or atom. These may be small monoatomic structures such as sodium and potassium or much larger organic molecules such as proteins. The term *electrolyte* refers to any substance that produces an electrically conducting solution when dissolved in a polar solvent such as water. They can be divided into cations (+ve) and anions (–ve). pH is a determinant of the ionised state of some molecules (see later). Electrolytes have very diverse biological roles and in particular are a major source of osmotic pressure within body fluids.

Organic molecules are generally non-polar and therefore do not dissolve in water – that is, they are hydrophobic but lipophilic. These properties play an important biological

Basic definitions

Osmosis refers to the movement of *solvent* molecules across a membrane into a region in which there is a higher concentration of *solute*. This movement may be prevented by applying a pressure to the more concentrated solution – the effective osmotic pressure. This is a colligative property: The magnitude of effective osmotic pressure exerted by a solution depends on the number rather than the type of particles present.

The amounts of osmotically active particles present in solution are expressed in *osmoles*. One osmole of a substance is equal to its molecular weight in grams (1 mol) divided by the number of freely moving particles which each molecule liberates in solution. Thus 180 g of glucose in 1 L of water represents a solution with a molar concentration of 1 mol L^{-1} and an *osmolarity* of 1 mOsm L^{-1}. Sodium chloride ionises in solution, and each ion represents an osmotically active particle. Assuming complete dissociation into Na^+ and Cl^-, 58.5 g of NaCl dissolved in 1 L of water has a molar concentration of 1 mol L^{-1} and an osmolarity of 2 osm L^{-1}. In body fluids, solute concentrations are much lower (mmol L^{-1}) and dissociation is incomplete. Consequently a solution of NaCl containing 1 mmol L^{-1} contributes slightly less than 2 mOsm L^{-1}.

The term *osmolality* refers to the number of osmoles per unit of total weight of solvent, whereas *osmolarity* refers to the number of osmoles per litre of solvent. Osmolality (unlike osmolarity), is not affected by the volume of various solutes in solution. Confusion regarding the apparently interchangeable use of the terms *osmolarity* (measured in osm L^{-1}) and *osmolality* (measured in osm kg^{-1}) is caused by their numerical equivalence in body fluids; plasma osmolarity is 280–310 mOsm L^{-1} and plasma osmolality is also 280–310 mOsm kg^{-1}. This equivalence is explained by the almost negligible solute volume contained in biological fluids and the fact that most osmotically active particles are dissolved in water, which has a density of 1 (i.e. osm L^{-1} = osm kg^{-1}). As the number of osmoles in plasma is estimated by measurement of the magnitude of freezing point depression, the more accurate term in clinical practice is osmolality.

Cations (principally Na^+) and anions (Cl^- and HCO_3^-) are the major osmotically active particles in plasma. Glucose and urea make a smaller contribution. Plasma osmolality (P_{OSM}) may be estimated from the formula:

$$P_{OSM} = 2[Na^+](mmol\ L^{-1}) + blood\ glucose\,(mmol\ L^{-1})$$
$$+ blood\ urea(mmol\ L^{-1}) = 290\ mOsm\ kg^{-1}$$

Osmolality is a chemical term and may be confused with the physiological term *tonicity*. *Tonicity* is used to describe the effective osmotic pressure of a solution relative to that of plasma; that is, it is the osmotic pressure gradient between two solutions. The critical difference between osmolality and tonicity is that *all* solutes contribute to osmolality, but only solutes that do not cross the cell membrane contribute to tonicity. Thus tonicity expresses the osmolal activity of solutes restricted to the extracellular compartment – that is, those which exert an osmotic force affecting the distribution of water between intracellular fluid (ICF) and extracellular fluid (ECF). As urea diffuses freely across cell membranes, it does not alter the distribution of water between these two body fluid compartments and does not contribute to tonicity. Other solutes that contribute to plasma osmolality but not tonicity include ethanol and methanol, both of which distribute rapidly throughout the total body water. In contrast, mannitol and sorbitol are restricted to the ECF and contribute to both osmolality and tonicity. The tonicity of plasma may be estimated from the formula:

$$plasma\ tonicity = 2[Na^+](mmol\ L^{-1})$$
$$+ blood\ glucose\,(mmol\ L^{-1})$$
$$= 285\ mOsm\ kg^{-1}$$

Compartmental distribution of total body water

The volume of total body water (TBW) may be measured using radioactive dilution techniques involving either deuterium or tritium, both of which cross all membranes freely and equilibrate rapidly with hydrogen atoms in body water. Such measurements show that approximately 60% of lean body mass (LBM) is water in the average 70-kg male adult. As fat contains little water, females have proportionately less TBW (55%) relative to LBM. Total body water decreases with age, decreasing to 45%–50% in later life.

The distribution of TBW between the main body compartments is illustrated in Fig. 12.1. One third of TBW

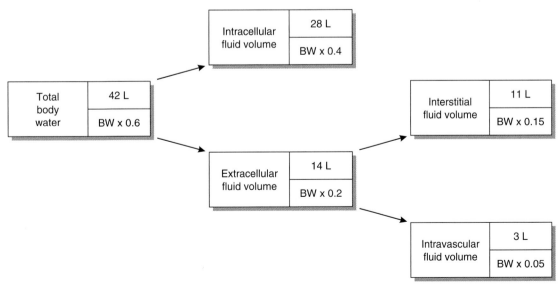

Fig. 12.1 Distribution of total body water in a 70-kg male and related to body weight (BW).

is contained in the extracellular fluid volume (ECFV) and two thirds in the intracellular fluid volume (ICFV). The ECFV is subdivided further into the interstitial and intravascular compartments. In addition to the absolute volumes of each compartment, Fig. 12.1 shows the relative size of each compartment compared with body weight.

Solute composition of body fluid compartments

Extracellular fluid

The capillary endothelium behaves as a freely permeable membrane to water, cations, anions and many soluble substances such as glucose and urea (but not protein). As a result the solute compositions of interstitial fluid and plasma are similar. Each contains sodium as the principal cation and chloride as the principal anion. Protein behaves as a non-diffusible anion and is present in a higher concentration in plasma. The concentration of Cl^- is slightly higher in interstitial fluid to maintain electrical neutrality (Gibbs–Donnan equilibrium).

Intracellular fluid

Intracellular fluid differs from ECF in that the principal cation is potassium and the principal anion is phosphate. In addition, there is a high protein content. In contrast to the capillary endothelium, the cell membrane is *selectively* permeable to different ions and freely permeable to water. Thus equalisation of osmotic forces occurs continuously and is achieved by the movement of water across the cell membrane. The osmolalities of ICF and ECF at equilibrium must be equal. Water moves rapidly between ICF and ECF to eliminate any induced osmolal gradient. This principle is fundamental to an understanding of fluid and electrolyte physiology.

Fig. 12.2 shows the solute composition of the main body fluid compartments. Although the total concentration of intracellular ions exceeds that of extracellular ions, the numbers of osmotically active particles (and thus the osmolalities) are the same on each side of the cell membrane (290 mOsm kg^{-1} of solution).

Water homeostasis

Normal day-to-day fluctuations in TBW are small (<0.2%) because of a fine balance between input and output. Fig. 12.3 depicts daily water balance in a healthy 70-kg adult under normal conditions, in whom input and output balance. Normal total water requirement in a 70-kg adult is 2.5 L from all sources. The principal sources of water are ingested fluid, water content of food and metabolic water. Intravenously administered fluid in the hospitalised patient may be a key source. Fluid losses are classified as *insensible* or *sensible*. Insensible losses emanate from the skin and lungs; sensible losses occur mainly from the kidneys and GI tract. It is important to be aware of increased potential losses secondary to pathological processes such as pyrexia.

In health, two key interrelated processes govern water balance: *osmoregulation* and *volume regulation*. Osmoregulation (the control of plasma osmolality) is vital in maintaining cell volume and preventing the serious ramifications of alterations of this, such as cerebral oedema. Plasma osmolality is principally determined by sodium concentration, but it is actually water balance (in *vs.* out) that regulates this rather than alteration in sodium excretion/retention. Osmoreceptors (adapted neurons) situated within the supraoptic nuclei of the hypothalamus but outside the blood–brain barrier are

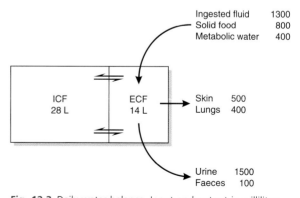

Fig. 12.3 Daily water balance. Input and output in millilitres. Note the contributions of water from metabolism and solid food to water intake. Losses from skin and lungs may vary widely (e.g. fever, hyperventilation). Urinary water excretion also varies under the influence of antidiuretic hormone (ADH), aldosterone and other hormones.

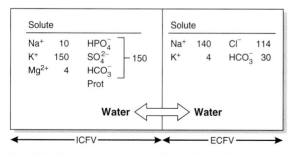

Fig. 12.2 Principal solute composition of body fluid compartments. All concentrations are expressed in mmol L^{-1}.

Table 12.1 Electrolyte contents of commonly used intravenous fluids

Solution	Electrolyte content (mmol L^{-1})				Osmolality (mOsm kg^{-1})
Saline 0.9% (normal saline)	Na$^+$	154	Cl$^-$	154	308
Saline 0.45% (half-normal saline)	Na$^+$	77	Cl$^-$	77	154
Glucose 4%/saline 0.18% (glucose–saline)	Na$^+$	31	Cl$^-$	31	284
Glucose 5%		Nil			278
Compound sodium lactate (Hartmann's solution)	Na$^+$	131	Cl$^-$	112	281
	K$^+$	5	HCO$_3^-$	29	
	Ca^{2+}	4	(as lactate)		

sensitive to changes in plasma osmolality more or less than that of 290 mOsm L^{-1}. An increase of only 1% triggers the release of antidiuretic hormone (ADH), stimulating thirst and renal water retention. By comparison volume regulation is controlled by alterations in renal sodium excretion. This is mediated through numerous systems, including baroreceptors in the carotid sinuses, aortic arch, and cardiac atria and within the juxtaglomerular apparatus of the kidney (see Chapters 9 and 11). As the name suggests, baroreceptors do not detect volume, but rather they respond to changes in pressure via stretch. This brings about stimulation of the sympathetic nervous system and the renin–angiotensin–aldosterone system, causing alterations in release of ADH, renin, angiotensin and natriuretic peptides. This process is fundamental in the biological response to hypovolaemia.

Practical fluid balance

Calculation of the daily prescription of fluid is an arithmetic exercise to balance the input and output of water and electrolytes.

Table 12.1 shows the electrolyte contents of five solutions used commonly for intravenous therapy in the UK. These solutions are adequate for most clinical situations. Two self-evident but important generalisations may be made regarding solutions for intravenous infusion:

Rule 1

All infused Na$^+$ remains in the ECF; Na$^+$ cannot gain access to the ICF because of the sodium pump. Thus if saline 0.9% is infused, all Na$^+$ remains in the ECF. As this is an isotonic solution, there is no change in ECF osmolality and therefore no water exchange occurs across the cell membrane. Thus saline 0.9% expands ECFV only. However, if saline 0.45% is given, ECF osmolality decreases; this causes a shift of

Table 12.2 Compartmental expansion resulting from infusion of 1 litre of saline 0.9%, saline 0.45% or glucose 5%

Intravenous infusion of 1000 ml	Change in volume (ml)		Remarks
	ECF	ICF	
Saline 0.9%	+1000	0	Na$^+$ remains in ECF
Glucose 5%	+333	+666	66% of TBW is ICF
Saline 0.45%	+666	+333	33% of TBW is ECF

ECF, Extracellular fluid; ICF, intracellular fluid; TBW, total body water.

water from ECF to ICF. If saline 1.8% is administered all Na$^+$ remains in the ECF, its osmolality increases and water moves from ICF to ECF to maintain osmotic equality.

Rule 2

Water without sodium expands the TBW. After infusion of a solution of glucose 5%, the glucose enters cells and is metabolised. The infused water enters both ICF and ECF in proportion to their initial volumes.

Table 12.2 illustrates the results of infusion of 1 litre of saline 0.9%, saline 0.45% or glucose 5% in a 70-kg adult.

Intravenous fluids are widely and regularly prescribed and administered. In recent years there has been a growing realisation that poor fluid prescription can lead to harm. There is still much uncertainty as to optimal fluid types and regimens. In 2013 the National Institute for Health and Care Excellence (NICE) published guidelines to address this (Intravenous fluid therapy in adults in hospital;

nice.org.uk/guidance/cg174). This introduced the concept of the 5 Rs:
- Resuscitation: crystalloids preferred with sodium content between 130–154 mmol and i.v. boluses of 250–500 ml over 15 min
- Replacement: consider ongoing fluid and electrolyte abnormalities and losses (Fig. 12.4)
- Routine maintenance: consider patient's normal maintenance needs (Table 12.3)

- Redistribution: depends on fluid given and ongoing pathological conditions (e.g. sepsis)
- Reassessment: ABCDE (airway, breathing, circulation, disability, exposure), indicators of perfusion such as urine output, lactate.

This guidance emphasises the need to 'assess the patient's likely fluid and electrolyte needs from their history, clinical examination, current medications, clinical monitoring and laboratory investigations'. Tables 12.3 and 12.4 and

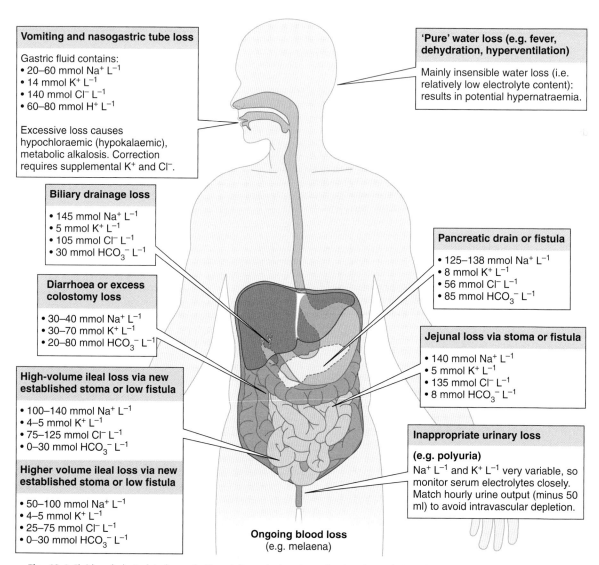

Vomiting and nasogastric tube loss

Gastric fluid contains:
- 20–60 mmol Na^+ L^{-1}
- 14 mmol K^+ L^{-1}
- 140 mmol Cl^- L^{-1}
- 60–80 mmol H^+ L^{-1}

Excessive loss causes hypochloraemic (hypokalaemic), metabolic alkalosis. Correction requires supplemental K^+ and Cl^-.

'Pure' water loss (e.g. fever, dehydration, hyperventilation)

Mainly insensible water loss (i.e. relatively low electrolyte content): results in potential hypernatraemia.

Biliary drainage loss
- 145 mmol Na^+ L^{-1}
- 5 mmol K^+ L^{-1}
- 105 mmol Cl^- L^{-1}
- 30 mmol HCO_3^- L^{-1}

Pancreatic drain or fistula
- 125–138 mmol Na^+ L^{-1}
- 8 mmol K^+ L^{-1}
- 56 mmol Cl^- L^{-1}
- 85 mmol HCO_3^- L^{-1}

Diarrhoea or excess colostomy loss
- 30–40 mmol Na^+ L^{-1}
- 30–70 mmol K^+ L^{-1}
- 20–80 mmol HCO_3^- L^{-1}

Jejunal loss via stoma or fistula
- 140 mmol Na^+ L^{-1}
- 5 mmol K^+ L^{-1}
- 135 mmol Cl^- L^{-1}
- 8 mmol HCO_3^- L^{-1}

High-volume ileal loss via new established stoma or low fistula
- 100–140 mmol Na^+ L^{-1}
- 4–5 mmol K^+ L^{-1}
- 75–125 mmol Cl^- L^{-1}
- 0–30 mmol HCO_3^- L^{-1}

Inappropriate urinary loss

(e.g. polyuria)
Na^+ L^{-1} and K^+ L^{-1} very variable, so monitor serum electrolytes closely. Match hourly urine output (minus 50 ml) to avoid intravascular depletion.

Higher volume ileal loss via new established stoma or low fistula
- 50–100 mmol Na^+ L^{-1}
- 4–5 mmol K^+ L^{-1}
- 25–75 mmol Cl^- L^{-1}
- 0–30 mmol HCO_3^- L^{-1}

Ongoing blood loss
(e.g. melaena)

Fig. 12.4 Fluid and electrolyte losses in the adult surgical patient, absolute losses being dependent on measured volumes.

Table 12.3 Normal daily maintenance needs per kg ideal body weight

Water	30–35 ml kg^{-1}
Sodium	1–2 mmol kg^{-1}
Potassium	1 mmol kg^{-1}
Chloride	1.5 mmol kg^{-1}
Phosphate	0.2–0.5 mmol kg^{-1}
Calcium	0.1–0.2 mmol kg^{-1}
Magnesium	0.1–0.2 mmol kg^{-1}

Fig. 12.4 summarise some of the key elements of practical fluid management.

Dehydration

Dehydration with accompanying salt loss is a common disorder in the acutely ill surgical patient.

Assessment of dehydration

Assessment of dehydration is a clinical assessment based upon the following:

History. How long has the patient had abnormal loss of fluid? How much has occurred (e.g. volume and frequency of vomiting)?

Examination. Specific features are thirst, dryness of mucous membranes, loss of skin turgor, orthostatic hypotension or tachycardia, reduced jugular venous pressure (JVP) or central venous pressure (CVP) and decreased urine output. In the presence of normal renal function, dehydration is associated usually with a urine output of <0.5 ml kg^{-1} h^{-1}. The severity of dehydration may be described clinically as mild, moderate or severe, and each category is associated with the following water loss relative to body weight:

- *Mild:* loss of 4% body weight (approximately 3 L in a 70-kg patient) – reduced skin turgor, sunken eyes, dry mucous membranes
- *Moderate:* loss of 5%–8% body weight (approximately 4–6 L in a 70-kg patient) – oliguria, orthostatic hypotension and tachycardia in addition to the above
- *Severe:* loss of 8%–10% body weight (approximately 7 L in a 70-kg patient) – profound oliguria and compromised cardiovascular function.

Laboratory assessment

The degree of haemoconcentration and increase in albumin concentration may be helpful if the patient was not previously

Table 12.4 Practical fluid balance

Fluid composition of body compartments	Typical blood volume
Infant	90 ml kg^{-1}
Child	80 ml kg^{-1}
Adult male	70 ml kg^{-1}
Adult female	60 ml kg^{-1}
Total water content (TWC)	
60% male (55% female) of body weight (18–40 years)	
55% male (46% female) of body weight (>60 years)	
Volume of ECF 35% TWC	
Volume of ICF 65% TWC	
Intraoperative fluid requirements – adult	
Initial volume	1.5 ml kg^{-1} h^{-1} for duration of preoperative starvation
+ (2) Maintenance	1.5 ml kg^{-1} h^{-1}
+ (3) Operative insensible losses	Guided by intraoperative monitoring (e.g. cardiac output); aim for neutral fluid balance.
+ (4) Blood loss	Consider replacement with blood and appropriate clotting products when blood loss exceeds 20% of estimated blood volume or [Hb] <80 g L^{-1}

ECF, Extracellular fluid; *ICF*, intracellular fluid; *Hb*, haemoglobin.

anaemic. Increased blood urea concentration and urine osmolality (>650 mOsm kg^{-1}) confirm the clinical diagnosis.

Perioperative fluid therapy, optimisation and enhanced recovery

The perioperative period is associated with significant alteration in fluid balance. It is practical to think in terms of preoperative dehydration secondary to nil by mouth status, which should be minimised where possible; intraoperative losses, whole blood loss in particular; and postoperative losses, often referred to as 'third-space' losses. Failure to maintain adequate fluid therapy during these periods results in reduced ECFV and circulating volume, reduced cardiac output and tissue oxygen delivery. This in turn is associated with increased perioperative morbidity and mortality. There is some evidence for the role of intraoperative fluid optimisation (or 'goal-directed' fluid therapy) during major surgical procedures. These approaches rely on manipulation of monitored physiological variables such as left ventricular stroke volume using appropriate monitors of cardiac output such as the oesophageal Doppler probe or pulse contour analysis (see Chapter 17) to optimise stroke volume and tissue perfusion. This has been associated with reduced duration of hospital stay and postoperative complications (see Chapter 30).

In slight contrast to the concept of fluid optimisation there is the concept of enhanced recovery after surgery (ERAS), particularly for major elective GI surgery (see also Chapter 30). The aims of ERAS protocols are to attenuate the surgical stress response and reduce end-organ dysfunction through an integrated pathway before, during and after surgery. Enhanced recovery after surgery relies upon the application of a series of evidence-based interventions. The perioperative fluid strategy aims to minimise preoperative dehydration (e.g. limiting bowel preparation before bowel surgery), optimise intraoperative fluid therapy with goal-directed techniques and reduce the need for postoperative i.v. fluids with early commencement of oral intake, thus allowing return of normal gut function and early mobilisation. Some evidence suggests reduced duration of hospital stay and healthcare costs.

Normally potassium is not administered in the first 24 h after surgery as endogenous release of potassium from tissue trauma and catabolism warrants restriction. The postoperative patient differs from the 'normal' patient in that the stress reaction modifies homeostatic mechanisms; stress-induced release of ADH, aldosterone and cortisol cause retention of Na^+ and water and increased renal K^+ excretion (see Chapter 13). However, restriction of fluid and sodium in the postoperative period must be balanced with increased losses by evaporation and 'third-spacing', on one hand, and the common tendency for excessive i.v. fluid administration on the other.

This syndrome of *inappropriate ADH secretion* (see later) may persist for several days in elderly patients, who are at risk of symptomatic hyponatraemia if given hypotonic fluids in the postoperative period. Elderly patients, those undergoing orthopaedic surgery or taking long-term thiazide diuretics are especially at risk if given 5% glucose postoperatively. Such patients may develop water intoxication and permanent brain damage as a result of relatively modest reductions in serum sodium concentration.

After major surgery, assessment of fluid and electrolyte requirements involves clinical assessment of the patient, accurate fluid balance, blood tests and sometimes urinary electrolytes. Measurement of cardiac output surrogates such as stroke volume variability may also be needed in critically ill patients. Fluid and electrolyte requirements in infants and small children differ from those in the adult (see Chapter 33).

Patients with renal failure require fluid replacement for abnormal losses, although the total volume of fluid infused should be reduced to a degree determined by the urine output.

Crystalloids or colloids

The debate over whether to administer a crystalloid solution (e.g. saline 0.9%, Hartmann's/Ringer's lactate) or a colloid solution (e.g. gelatines, starches, albumin) to patients has been ongoing for many years. However, few high-quality studies have demonstrated any advantage for the administration of colloids over crystalloids. Theoretical advantages of colloids include rapid and sustained plasma volume expansion for a given administered dose (ml kg^{-1}) with a smaller concomitant expansion of the ECFV, thereby limiting tissue oedema. However, there are some associated adverse effects with some colloids such as platelet dysfunction, acute kidney injury (particularly in sepsis), allergy and cost. Consequently the use of synthetic colloids is decreasing, with crystalloids recommended as first-line by most authorities. Albumin may have a role in certain circumstances.

Sodium, potassium, chloride, phosphate and magnesium

Sodium balance

Daily ingestion amounts to 50–300 mmol. Losses in sweat and faeces are minimal (approximately 10 mmol day^{-1}), and the kidney makes final adjustments. Urine sodium excretion may be as little as 2 mmol day^{-1} during salt restriction or may exceed 700 mmol day^{-1} after salt loading. Sodium balance is related intimately to ECFV and water balance.

Disorders of sodium and water balance
Hypernatraemia

Hypernatraemia is defined as a plasma sodium concentration of >150 mmol L^{-1} and may result from pure water loss, hypotonic fluid loss or salt gain. In the first two conditions, ECFV is reduced, whereas salt gain is associated with an expanded ECFV. For this reason the clinical assessment of volaemic status is important in the diagnosis

Table 12.5 Causes of hypernatraemia	
Pure water depletion	
Extrarenal loss	Failure of water intake (coma, elderly, postoperative) Mucocutaneous loss Fever, hyperventilation, thyrotoxicosis
Renal loss	Diabetes insipidus (cranial, nephrogenic) Chronic renal failure
Hypotonic fluid loss	
Extrarenal loss	Gastrointestinal (vomiting, diarrhoea) Skin (excessive sweating)
Renal loss	Osmotic diuresis (glucose, urea, mannitol)
Salt gain	
	Iatrogenic ($NaHCO_3$, hypertonic saline) Salt ingestion Steroid excess

and management of hypernatraemic states. The common causes of hypernatraemia are summarised in Table 12.5. The abnormality common to all hypernatraemic states is intracellular dehydration secondary to ECF hyperosmolality. Primary water loss resulting in hypernatraemia may occur during prolonged fever, hyperventilation or severe exercise in hot, dry climates. However, a more common cause is the renal water loss that occurs when there is a defect in either the production or release of ADH (cranial diabetes insipidus) or an abnormality in response to ADH (nephrogenic diabetes insipidus).

The administration of osmotic diuretics results temporarily in plasma hyperosmolality. An osmotic diuresis may occur also in hyperglycaemia. During an osmotic diuresis, the solute causing the diuresis (e.g. glucose, mannitol) constitutes a significant fraction of urine solute, and the sodium content of the urine becomes hypotonic relative to plasma sodium. Thus osmotic diuretics cause hypotonic urine losses, which may result in hypernatraemic dehydration.

Hypertonic dehydration may occur also in paediatric patients. Diarrhoea, vomiting and anorexia lead to loss of water in excess of solute (hypotonic loss). Concomitant fever, hyperventilation and the use of high-solute feeds may combine to exaggerate the problem. Extracellular fluid volume is maintained by movement of water from ICF to ECF to equalise osmolality, and clinical evidence of dehydration may not be apparent until 10%–15% of body weight has been lost. Rehydration must be undertaken gradually to prevent the development of cerebral oedema.

Measurement of urine and plasma osmolalities and assessment of urine output help in the diagnosis of hypernatraemic, volume-depleted states. If urine output is low and urine osmolality exceeds 800 mOsm kg^{-1}, then both ADH secretion and the renal response to ADH are present. The most likely causes are extrarenal water loss (e.g. diarrhoea, vomiting or evaporation) or insufficient intake. High urine output and high urine osmolality suggest an osmotic diuresis. If urine osmolality is less than plasma osmolality, reduced ADH secretion or impairment of the renal response to ADH should be suspected; in both cases, urine output is high.

Hypernatraemia caused by salt gain is usually iatrogenic in origin. It occurs when excessive amounts of hypertonic sodium bicarbonate are administered during resuscitation or when isotonic fluids are given to patients who have only insensible losses. Treatment comprises induction of a diuresis with a loop diuretic if renal function is normal; urine output is replaced in part with glucose 5%. Dialysis or haemofiltration may be necessary in patients with renal dysfunction.

Consequences of hypernatraemia

The major clinical manifestations of hypernatraemia involve the central nervous system. Severity depends on the rapidity with which hyperosmolality develops. Acute hypernatraemia is associated with a prompt osmotic shift of water from the intracellular compartment, causing a reduction in cell volume and water content of the brain. This results in increased permeability and even rupture of the capillaries in the brain and subarachnoid space. The patient may present with pyrexia (a manifestation of impaired thermoregulation), nausea, vomiting, convulsions, coma and virtually any type of focal neurological syndrome. The mortality and long-term morbidity of sustained hypernatraemia (Na^+ >160 mmol L^{-1} for over 48 h) is high irrespective of the underlying cause. In many cases the development of hypernatraemia can be anticipated and prevented (e.g. cranial diabetes insipidus associated with head injury), but in situations where preventative strategies have failed, treatment should be instituted without delay.

Treatment of hypernatraemia

The magnitude of the water deficit can be estimated from the measured plasma sodium concentration and calculated TBW:

$$\text{water deficit} = (\text{measured}[Na^+]/140 \times TBW) - TBW$$

Thus in a 75-kg patient with a serum sodium of 170 mmol L^{-1}:

$$\text{water deficit} = (170/140 \times 0.6 \times 75) - (0.6 \times 75)$$
$$= 54.6 - 45$$
$$= 9.6 \, L$$

223

For hypernatraemic patients *without* volume depletion, 5% glucose is sufficient to correct the water deficit. However, the majority of hypernatraemic patients are frankly hypovolaemic, and intravenous fluids should be prescribed to repair both the sodium and the water deficits. Regardless of the severity of the condition, isotonic saline is the initial treatment of choice in the volume-depleted, hypernatraemic patient, as even this fluid is *relatively* hypotonic in patients with severe hypernatraemia. When volume depletion has been corrected, further repair of any water deficit may be accomplished with hypotonic fluids. Fluid therapy should be prescribed with the intention of correcting hypernatraemia over a period of 48–72 h to prevent the onset of cerebral oedema.

Hyponatraemia

Hyponatraemia is defined as a plasma sodium concentration <135 mmol L^{-1}. Hyponatraemia is a common finding in hospitalised patients. It may occur as a result of water retention, sodium loss or both; consequently it may be associated with an expanded, normal or contracted ECFV. As in hypernatraemia, the state of ECFV is important in determining the cause of the electrolyte imbalance.

As plasma osmolality decreases, an osmolality gradient is created across the cell membrane and results in movement of water into the ICF. The resulting expansion of brain cells is responsible for the symptoms of hyponatraemia, or water intoxication: nausea, vomiting, lethargy, weakness and obtundation. In severe cases (plasma Na^+ <115 mmol L^{-1}), seizures and coma may result.

A scheme depicting the causes of hyponatraemia is shown in Fig. 12.5. True hyponatraemia must be distinguished from pseudohyponatraemia. Sodium ions are present only in plasma water, which constitutes 93% of normal plasma. In the laboratory the concentration of sodium in plasma is measured in an aliquot of whole plasma, and the concentration is expressed in terms of plasma volume (mmol L^{-1} of whole plasma). If the percentage of water present in plasma is decreased, as in hyperlipidaemia or hyperproteinaemia, the amount of Na^+ in each aliquot of plasma is also decreased even if its concentration in plasma water is normal. A clue to this cause of hyponatraemia is the finding of a normal plasma osmolality. Pseudohyponatraemia is not encountered when plasma sodium concentration is measured by increasingly used ion-specific electrodes, because this method assesses directly the sodium concentration in the aqueous phase of plasma.

True hyponatraemic states may be classified conveniently into *depletional* and *dilutional* types. Depletional hyponatraemia occurs when a deficit in TBW is associated with an even greater deficit of total body sodium. Assessment of volaemic status reveals hypovolaemia. Losses may be *renal* or *extrarenal*. Excessive renal loss of sodium occurs in Addison's disease, diuretic administration, renal tubular acidosis and salt-losing nephropathies; usually urine sodium concentration exceeds 20 mmol L^{-1}. Extrarenal losses occur usually from the GI tract (e.g. diarrhoea, vomiting) or from sequestration into the 'third-space' (e.g. peritonitis, surgery). Normal kidneys respond by conserving sodium and water to produce a urine that is hyperosmolal and low in sodium. In both situations, treatment should be directed at expanding the ECFV with saline 0.9%.

Dilutional hyponatraemic states may be associated with hypervolaemia and oedema or with normovolaemia. Again, assessment of volaemic status is important. If oedema is present, there is an excess of total body sodium with a proportionately greater excess of TBW. This is seen in congestive heart failure, cirrhosis and the nephrotic syndrome and is caused by secondary hyperaldosteronism. Treatment comprises salt and water restriction and spironolactone.

In normovolaemic hyponatraemia there is a modest excess of TBW and a modest increase in ECFV associated with normal total body sodium. Pseudohyponatraemia is excluded by finding high protein or lipid concentrations and a normal plasma osmolality. True normovolaemic hyponatraemia is commonly iatrogenic in origin. The syndrome of inappropriate intravenous therapy (SIIVT) is caused usually by administration of intravenous fluids with a low sodium content to patients with isotonic losses.

A more chronic water overload may occur in patients with hypothyroidism and in conditions associated with an inappropriately elevated concentration of ADH. The syndrome of inappropriate ADH secretion (SIADH) is characterised by hyponatraemia, low plasma osmolality and an inappropriate antidiuresis – that is, a urine osmolality higher than anticipated for the degree of hyponatraemia. It occurs in the presence of malignant tumours (e.g. lung, prostate, pancreas), which produce ADH-like substances; in neurological disorders (e.g. head injury, tumours, infections); and in some severe pneumonias. A number of drugs are associated with increased ADH secretion or potentiate the effects of ADH (Box 12.1). In patients with SIADH, the urine is concentrated in spite of hyponatraemia. Management comprises restriction of fluid intake to encourage a negative fluid balance. In severe or refractory cases, demeclocycline or lithium may result in improvement. Both drugs induce a state of functional diabetes insipidus and have been used effectively in SIADH if the primary disease cannot be treated.

Consequences of hyponatraemia. Symptoms vary with the underlying cause, the magnitude of the reduction of plasma sodium and the rapidity with which the plasma sodium concentration decreases. Serious consequences involve the central nervous system and result from intracellular overhydration, cerebral oedema and raised intracranial pressure. Nausea, vomiting, delirium, convulsions and coma result.

Treatment of hyponatraemia. Acute symptomatic hyponatraemia is a medical emergency and requires prompt

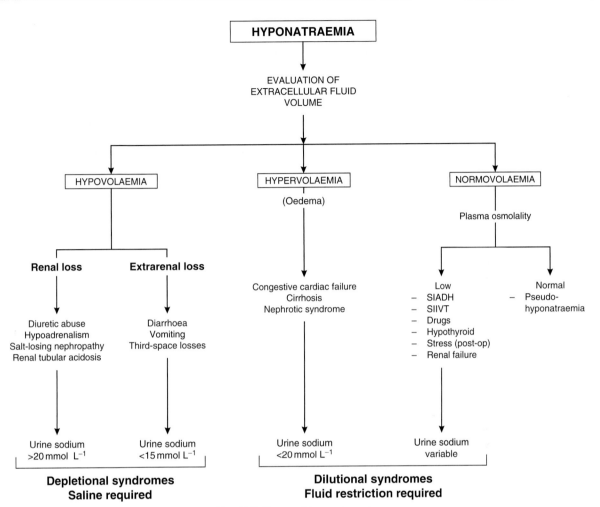

Fig. 12.5 Causes of hyponatraemia.

Box 12.1 **Drugs associated with antidiuresis and hyponatraemia**

Increased ADH secretion

Hypnotics – barbiturates
Analgesics – opioids
Hypoglycaemics – chlorpropamide, tolbutamide
Anticonvulsants – carbamazepine
Miscellaneous – phenothiazines, tricyclics

Potentiation of ADH at distal tubule

Paracetamol
Indometacin
Chlorpropamide

ADH, Antidiuretic hormone.

intervention using hypertonic saline. The rapidity with which hyponatraemia should be corrected is the subject of controversy because of observations that rapid correction may cause central pontine myelinolysis, a disorder characterised by paralysis, coma and death. As a causal relationship between this syndrome and the rate of increase of plasma sodium has not been established and it is clear that there is a prohibitive mortality associated with inadequately treated water intoxication, rapid correction of the symptomatic hyponatraemic state is warranted. Sufficient sodium should be given to return the plasma concentration to 125 mmol L⁻¹ only, and this should be administered over a period of no less than 12 h. The amount of sodium needed to cause the desired correction in the plasma sodium can be calculated as follows:

$$Na^+ \text{ required (mmol)} = TBW$$
$$\times (\text{desired } [Na^+] - \text{measured } [Na^+])$$

Hypertonic saline (3%) contains 514 mmol L^{-1} of Na^+, and administration poses the risk of pulmonary oedema, especially in oedematous patients, in whom renal dialysis is preferable.

Potassium balance

The normal daily intake of potassium is 50–200 mmol. Minimal amounts are lost via the skin and faeces; the kidney is the primary regulator. However, the mechanisms for the retention of potassium are less efficient than those for sodium. In periods of K^+ depletion, daily urinary excretion cannot decrease to less than 5–10 mmol. A considerable deficit of total body potassium occurs if intake is not restored. Hypokalaemia is a more common abnormality than hyperkalaemia.

Hypokalaemia

Hypokalaemia is defined as a plasma potassium concentration <3.5 mmol L^{-1}. Non-specific symptoms of hypokalaemia include anorexia and nausea, effects on skeletal and smooth muscle (muscle weakness, paralytic ileus) and abnormal cardiac conduction (delayed repolarisation with ST-segment depression, reduced height of the T wave, increased height of the U wave and a widened QRS complex).

The causes of hypokalaemia are summarised in Table 12.6. Management includes diagnosis and treatment of the underlying disorder in addition to repletion of total body potassium stores. As a general rule a reduction in plasma K^+ concentration by 1 mmol L^{-1} reflects a total body K^+ deficit of approximately 100 mmol. Potassium supplements may be given orally or intravenously. The maximum infusion rate should not exceed 0.5 mmol kg^{-1} h^{-1} to allow equilibration with the intracellular compartment; much slower rates are generally used.

The potassium salt used for replacement therapy is important. In most situations, and especially in the presence of alkalosis, potassium should be replaced as the chloride salt. Supplements are available also as the bicarbonate and phosphate salts. Hypokalaemia is usually associated with magnesium deficiency, and magnesium may need replacement as well.

Hyperkalaemia

Hyperkalaemia is defined as a plasma potassium concentration >5 mmol L^{-1}. Vague muscle weakness progressing to flaccid paralysis may occur. However, the major clinical feature of an increasing plasma potassium concentration is the characteristic sequence of ECG abnormalities. The earliest change is the development of tall, peaked T waves and a shortened QT interval, reflecting more rapid repolarisation (6–7 mmol L^{-1}). As plasma K^+ increases (8–10 mmol L^{-1}) abnormalities in depolarisation manifest as widened QRS complexes and widening, and eventually loss, of the P wave; the widened QRS complexes merge finally into the T waves (sine wave pattern). Plasma concentrations in excess of 10 mmol L^{-1} are associated with ventricular fibrillation and asystole. The cardiac toxicity of K^+ is enhanced by hypocalcaemia, hyponatraemia or acidaemia. The causes of hyperkalaemia are summarised in Box 12.2.

Immediate treatment in keeping with current guidelines is necessary if the plasma potassium concentration exceeds 6.5 mmol L^{-1} or if there are any serious ECG abnormalities. Specific treatment may be achieved by four mechanisms:
- Chemical antagonism of the membrane effects.
- Enhanced cellular uptake of K^+.
- Dilution of ECF.
- Removal of K^+ from the body.

Methods for the immediate management of severe hyperkalaemia are summarised in Box 12.3.

Chloride balance

Along with sodium, chloride is the major determinant of ECF osmolality. Chloride homeostasis is maintained largely by the kidney, with 99% of the filtered Cl^- being reabsorbed in the distal tubule. As discussed later, chloride plays an important role in acid–base balance, isolated changes in chloride concentration being a key determinant of the strong ion difference (SID) and therefore hydrogen ion concentration. Changes in Cl^- concentration must always be evaluated in conjunction with Na^+ concentration.

Hyperchloraemia. This is defined as a plasma chloride concentration >110 mmol L^{-1}. The most common cause of hyperchloraemia is the administration of chloride-rich

Table 12.6 Causes of hypokalaemia	
Cause	**Comments**
Reduced intake	Usually only contributory
Tissue redistribution	Insulin therapy, alkalaemia, β_2-adrenergic agonists, familial periodic paralysis, vitamin B_{12} therapy
Increased loss	
Gastrointestinal (urine K^+ <20 mmol L^{-1})	Diarrhoea, vomiting, fistulae, nasogastric suction, colonic villous adenoma
Renal	Diuretic therapy, primary or secondary hyperaldosteronism, malignant hypertension, renal artery stenosis (high renin), renal tubular acidosis, hypomagnesaemia, renal failure (diuretic phase)

Box 12.2 Causes of hyperkalaemia

Factitious (pseudo-hyperkalaemia)

In vitro haemolysis
Thrombocytosis
Leukocytosis
Tourniquet
Exercise

Impaired excretion

Renal failure
Acute or chronic hyperaldosteronism
Addison's disease
K^+-sparing diuretics
Indomethacin

Tissue redistribution

Tissue damage (burns, trauma)
Rhabdomyolysis
Tumour necrosis
Hyperkalaemic periodic paralysis
Massive intravascular haemolysis
Suxamethonium

Excessive intake

Blood transfusion
Excessive i.v. administration

Box 12.3 Immediate management of hyperkalaemia

In the presence of ECG changes: 10 ml calcium gluconate 10% i.v. (or equivalent dose of calcium chloride) over 5 min. May be repeated to maximum of 30 ml. No change in plasma [K^+]. Effect immediate but transient.
Fast-acting insulin (e.g. *Actrapid*) 10 units in 50 ml glucose 50% (25 g) via infusion pump (monitor blood glucose) over 10–30 min. May be repeated and/or followed by an insulin/glucose infusion.
Nebulised salbutamol 5 mg repeated to a maximum of 20 mg (caution in patients with significant ischaemic heart disease).
Renal replacement therapy (haemodialysis or continuous haemofiltration)

intravenous fluid, particularly 0.9% saline. Excessive extracellular Cl^- concentration leads to a hyperchloraemic metabolic acidosis (HCMA). This occurs secondary to a decrease in the SID (see later) and subsequent release of H^+ through hydrolysis of water to maintain physiological electrical neutrality. Some studies have suggested that HCMA leads to decreased renal blood flow and might therefore exacerbate acute kidney injury, although there is no clear evidence of an increase in mortality or morbidity. However, the observed acidaemia is at best a clinical distraction. HCMA is best avoided by using balance salt solutions such as Hartmann's. Correction with loop diuretics or sodium bicarbonate is also effective.

Hypochloraemia. Hypochloraemia is defined as plasma chloride <98 mmol L^{-1}. Hypochloraemia occurs when there is excessive loss of Cl^- (e.g. upper GI fluid loss) or excess extracellular water (e.g. hypotonic fluid administration, SIADH). Concomitant deficiency of the cations Na^+ and K^+ often accompany hypochloraemia. Effective treatment can usually be achieved with the administration of sodium chloride, plus or minus potassium.

Phosphate balance

Inorganic phosphate (PO_4^{3-}) is a predominantly intracellular anion (ICF concentration = 100 mmol L^{-1} and ECF concentration = 1.0 mmol L^{-1}). It is fundamental in intracellular metabolic processes such as formation of ATP, DNA and cell membranes. Approximately 85% of the body's phosphate is found in bone and teeth as calcium phosphate. The GI and renal tracts regulate total body phosphate. Measured plasma phosphate therefore reflects a balance between intra- and extracellular flux, rather than alterations in total body phosphate, and is influenced by pH, fluid balance and intracellular aerobic metabolism.

Hyperphosphataemia. Hyperphosphataemia is defined as plasma [PO_4^{3-}] >1.4 mmol L^{-1}. It is caused either by failure of renal phosphate excretion (or increased renal reabsorption) or excessive release (redistribution) of intracellular phosphate (e.g. cellular necrosis from rhabdomyolysis or other conditions, metabolic acidosis, lactic acidosis and ketoacidosis) and cytotoxic therapy (tumour lysis syndrome, particularly lymphoma and leukaemia). It is commonly associated with hypocalcaemia. Hyperphosphataemia is usually short lived in the presence of normal renal function but may require saline diuresis or renal replacement therapy in severe cases.

Hypophosphataemia. Hypophosphataemia is defined as a plasma [PO_4^{3-}] <0.8 mmol L^{-1}. Chronic hypophosphataemia usually reflects failure of GI absorption secondary to vitamin D deficiency or renal loss. In the acute care setting, however, it predominantly resultant from transcellular shifts. This is seen in alkalaemia (particularly respiratory) and commonly in ICU patients suffering with refeeding syndrome. Asymptomatic patients require little or no management. Patients with severe hypophosphataemia (<0.3 mmol L^{-1}) and symptomatic patients (muscle weakness and/or confusion) require intravenous phosphate replacement therapy.

Magnesium balance

After potassium, magnesium is the most abundant intracellular cation, 99% of total Mg^{2+} being intracellular. Like phosphate it is fundamental to many intracellular metabolic processes, including hundreds of enzyme-dependent reactions, DNA and RNA synthesis and protein manufacture.

Hypermagnesaemia. Hypermagnesaemia is defined as plasma $[Mg^{2+}]$ >1.1 mmol L^{-1}. Acute hypermagnesaemia is uncommon but may be seen in acute renal failure or from excessive administration of Mg^{2+} salts. Symptoms include muscle weakness, hypercapnic respiratory failure and hypotension. Treatment includes renal replacement therapy if renal failure is present, cessation of exogenous magnesium, diuresis in the presence of normal renal function and calcium gluconate if cardiac symptoms are present.

Hypomagnesaemia. Hypomagnesaemia is defined as plasma $[Mg^{2+}]$ <0.6 mmol L^{-1}. In contrast to hypermagnesaemia, hypomagnesaemia is common in critical illness. Like many acute electrolyte disturbances, hypomagnesaemia does not usually represent true magnesium deficiency. If severe, symptoms include weakness, muscle cramps, tremor and cardiac dysrhythmias such as atrial fibrillation. Symptomatic patients should be managed with intravenous magnesium sulphate, 20–60 mmol over 24 h. Hypomagnesaemia is associated with hypokalaemia.

Table 12.7 Comparison of logarithmic and arithmetic methods of expressing hydrogen ion concentration in the range of blood $[H^+]$ compatible with life

pH	$[H^+]$ (nmol L^{-1})	
7.8	16	
7.7	20	
7.6	25	Alkalaemia
7.5	32	
7.4	**40**	Normal
7.3	50	
7.2	63	
7.1	80	
7.0	100	Acidaemia
6.9	125	
6.8	160	

Acid–base balance

Hydrogen ion homeostasis is a fundamental prerequisite to virtually all biochemical processes; hydrogen ion concentration $[H^+]$ significantly influences protein, including enzyme, structure and function, and therefore nearly all biochemical pathways and many drug mechanisms. Unlike the majority of ions, $[H^+]$ is controlled at the nanomolar rather than millimolar level. Total body H^+ turnover per day is in the order of 150 mmol, although most of this is 'trapped' within metabolic pathways (particularly ATP hydrolysis). The resultant acids may be considered as volatile (from metabolic CO_2 production) and non-volatile (from carbohydrate, fat and protein metabolism). Although the lungs and kidneys play a primary role in $[H^+]$ homeostasis, the liver and GI tract are also important particularly in relation to ammonium metabolism.

Because of the very low concentration of hydrogen ions in body fluids, the pH notation was adopted for the sake of practicality. This system expresses $[H^+]$ on a logarithmic scale:

$$pH = -log_{10}[H^+]$$

A more logical arithmetic convention which expresses $[H^+]$ in nmol L^{-1} is gaining popularity. Table 12.7 compares values of $[H^+]$ expressed as pH and nmol L^{-1} and reveals several disadvantages of the pH notation. The most obvious disadvantage is that it moves in the opposite direction to $[H^+]$; a decrease in pH is associated with increased $[H^+]$ and

vice versa. It is also apparent that the logarithmic scale distorts the quantitative estimate of change in $[H^+]$; for example, twice as many hydrogen ions are required to reduce pH from 7.1 to 7.0 as are needed to reduce it from 7.4 to 7.3. The pH scale gives the false impression that there is relatively little difference in the sensitivity of biological systems to an equivalent increase or decrease in $[H^+]$. However, when $[H^+]$ is expressed in nmol L^{-1}, it becomes apparent that tolerance is limited to a reduction in $[H^+]$ of only 24 nmol L^{-1} from normal but to an increase of up to 120 nmol L^{-1}. Nevertheless, the pH notation remains the most widely used system and is used in the remainder of this chapter.

Basic definitions

An *acid* is a substance that dissociates in water to produce H^+; a *base* is a substance that can accept H^+. Strong acids dissociate completely in aqueous solution, whereas weak acids (e.g. carbonic acid, H_2CO_3) dissociate only partially. The *conjugate base* of an acid is its dissociated anionic product. For example, bicarbonate ion (HCO_3^-) is the conjugate base of carbonic acid:

$$H_2CO_3 \rightleftharpoons H^+ + HCO_3^-$$

A *buffer* is a combination of a weak acid and its conjugate base (usually as a salt), which acts to minimise any change in $[H^+]$ that would occur if a strong acid or base were added to it. Buffers in body fluids represent an important defence against $[H^+]$ change. The carbonic acid/bicarbonate system is an important buffer in blood and has historically been

Table 12.8 Compensatory mechanisms in acid–base disturbances

Primary disorder	pH	HCO_3^-	$PaCO_2$	Compensation
Metabolic acidosis	↓	↓↓		Hyperventilation ↓ $PaCO_2$
Metabolic alkalosis	↑	↑↑		Hypoventilation ↑ $PaCO_2$
Respiratory acidosis	↓		↑↑	Renal retention of HCO_3^-
Respiratory alkalosis	↑		↓↓	Renal elimination of HCO_3^-

↓↓ or ↑↑ denotes the primary abnormality.
The final pH depends on the degree of compensation. Respiratory compensation for metabolic disorders is rapid; renal compensation for respiratory disorders is slow.

used as the principal determinant of physiological pH (this in no small part is due to the relationship this system has with $PaCO_2$). However, it is important to appreciate the existence of other buffer systems such as plasma proteins, haemoglobin and phosphate. The pH of a buffer system may be determined from the Henderson–Hasselbalch equation, which for the carbonic acid/bicarbonate system relates pH, $[H_2CO_3]$ and $[HCO_3^-]$:

$$pH = pK + log_{10} HCO_3^- - H_2CO_3$$

where K = dissociation constant and $pK = -log_{10}K$.

This equation shows that $[H^+]$ in body fluids is a function of the *ratio* of base to acid. For the bicarbonate buffer system pK is 6.1. As most of the carbonic acid pool exists as dissolved CO_2, the equation may be rewritten:

$$pH = 6.1 + log_{10} HCO_3 - 0.225 \times PCO_2$$

The value 0.225 represents the solubility coefficient of CO_2 in blood (ml kPa^{-1}). Normally, $[HCO_3^-]$ is 24 mmol L^{-1} and $PaCO_2$ is 5.3 kPa. Thus:

$$pH = 6.1 + log_{10} \left(\frac{[24]}{[0.225 \times 5.3]} \right) = 7.4$$

Most acid–base disorders may be formulated in terms of the Henderson–Hasselbalch equation. The pH of plasma is kept remarkably constant at 7.36–7.44 (i.e. a hydrogen ion concentration of 40 ± 5 nmol L^{-1}). This is achieved by:

- regulation of H^+ excretion and bicarbonate regeneration by the kidney and
- regulation of CO_2 by the alveolar ventilation of the lungs.

Cellular metabolism poses a constant threat to buffer systems by the production of volatile and non-volatile acids. Thus the acid–base status of body fluids reflects the metabolism of both H^+ and CO_2.

Acid–base disorders

Conventional acid–base nomenclature involves the following definitions:

- *Acidosis* – a process that causes acid to accumulate
- *Acidaemia* – present if pH <7.36
- *Alkalosis* – a process that causes base to accumulate
- *Alkalaemia* – present if pH >7.44

Simple acid–base disorders are common in clinical practice, and their successful management can usually be achieved by analysis of the carbonic acid/bicarbonate system as outlined earlier. In particular, determination of pH, $[HCO_3^-]$ and $PaCO_2$, along with calculation of *standard bicarbonate, base excess* and *anion gap* (see later), will enable meaningful diagnosis and treatment. The first step involves diagnosis of the primary disorder; this is followed by an assessment of the extent and appropriateness of any compensation.

Primary acid–base disorders are either *respiratory* or *metabolic*. The disorder is respiratory if the primary disturbance involves CO_2 and metabolic if it involves $[HCO_3^-]$. Thus four potential primary disturbances exist (Table 12.8) and each may be identified by analysis of pH, $[HCO_3^-]$ and $PaCO_2$. Both pH and $PaCO_2$ are measured directly by the blood gas machine. $[HCO_3^-]$ is measured directly on the electrolyte profile but is derived in most blood gas machines. Other derived variables include *standard bicarbonate* and *base excess*. The standard bicarbonate is not the actual bicarbonate of the sample but an estimate of bicarbonate concentration after elimination of any abnormal respiratory contribution to $[HCO_3^-]$ (i.e. an estimate of $[HCO_3^-]$ at a $PaCO_2$ of 5.3 kPa). The base excess (in alkalosis) or base deficit (in acidosis) is the amount of acid or base (in mmol) required to return the pH of 1 litre of blood to normal at a $PaCO_2$ of 5.3 kPa; it is a measure of the magnitude of the metabolic component of the acid–base disorder.

After the primary disorder has been identified it is necessary to consider if it is acute or chronic and if any compensation has occurred. The body defends itself against changes in pH by compensatory mechanisms, which *tend* to return pH towards normal. Primary respiratory disorders are compensated by a metabolic mechanism and vice versa. For example, a primary respiratory acidosis is compensated for by renal retention of HCO_3^-, whereas a primary metabolic acidosis is compensated for by hyperventilation and a decrease in $PaCO_2$. Thus in each case the *acidaemia* produced by the primary acidosis is reduced by a compensatory alkalosis. The response to respiratory alkalosis is increased renal elimination of HCO_3^-, and metabolic alkalosis results in hypoventilation and increased $PaCO_2$, pH being restored towards normal by the compensatory respiratory acidosis. In each case the efficiency of compensatory mechanisms is limited; compensation is usually only partial and rarely complete. Overcompensation does not occur.

Metabolic acidosis

The cardinal features of metabolic acidosis are decreased $[HCO_3^-]$, low pH and an appropriately low $PaCO_2$. The extent of the acidaemia depends upon the nature, severity and duration of the initiating pathological condition in addition to the efficiency of compensatory mechanisms. The magnitude of the compensatory response is proportional to the decrease in $[HCO_3^-]$. The lower limit of the respiratory response is a $PaCO_2$ of 1.3 kPa. In a steady state:

- predicted $PaCO_2 = (0.2 \times$ observed bicarbonate$) + 1.1$ (kPa); and
- if the observed $PaCO_2$ differs from the predicted value, then an independent respiratory disturbance is present.

In most instances establishing the presence and the cause of a metabolic acidosis is straightforward. In difficult cases an important clue to the nature of the abnormality is given by the measurement of the *anion gap* in plasma:

$$\text{anion gap} = ([Na^+] + [K^+]) - ([Cl^-] + [HCO_3^-])$$

In reality the numbers of cations and anions in plasma are the same, and an anion gap exists because negatively charged proteins, together with phosphate, lactate and organic anions (which maintain electrical neutrality), are not measured. The normal anion gap is 12–18 mmol L^{-1}. In the critically ill population, adjustments for hypoalbuminaemia (albumin itself being an anion) and hypophosphataemia should be made as follows:

$$\text{corrected anion gap} = ([Na^+] + [K^+])$$
$$- ([Cl^-] + [HCO_3^-])$$
$$- (0.2 \times [\text{albumin}] \text{g dl}^{-1} + 1.5$$
$$\times [\text{phosphate}] \text{mmol L}^{-1})$$

Table 12.9 Types and causes of metabolic acidosis

High anion gap	
Overproduction of acid	Diabetic ketoacidosis Lactic acidosis: Type A – ↓$\dot{D}O_2$ (e.g. shock, hypoxaemia) Type B – Normal $\dot{D}O_2$ but impaired tissue O_2 utilisation or lactate clearance (e.g. metformin, hepatic failure) Starvation
Exogenous acid	Salicylates Methanol Ethylene glycol
Reduced excretion	Renal failure
Normal anion gap	
Bicarbonate loss	*Extrarenal* Diarrhoea Biliary/pancreatic fistula Ileostomy Ureterosigmoidostomy *Renal* Renal tubular acidosis Carbonic anhydrase inhibitors
Addition of acid (with chloride)	HCl, NH_4Cl, arginine or lysine hydrochloride

Clinically it is useful to divide the metabolic acidoses into those associated with a normal anion gap and those with an increased anion gap. The former are caused by loss of HCO_3^- from the body and replacement with chloride. In acidoses associated with an increased anion gap HCO_3^- has been titrated by either endogenous (e.g. lactic acidosis, diabetic ketoacidosis) or exogenous acids (e.g. poisons), thus increasing the number of unmeasured plasma anions without altering the plasma chloride concentration (Table 12.9). Another useful concept is the *osmolal / osmolar* (depending on units used) *gap*:

Osmolal gap = measured osmolality – calculated osmolality

The concept is similar to the anion gap. A raised osmolal gap implies unrecognised or unmeasured osmotically active molecules within the plasma. A raised osmolal gap in conjunction with metabolic acidosis should immediately raise concern of methanol, ethylene glycol, paraldehyde or formaldehyde poisoning requiring urgent treatment. Other causes of raised osmolal gap in the absence of acidaemia include hyperglycaemia, hyperlipidaemias and paraproteinaemias.

Clinical effects and treatment

Metabolic acidosis results in widespread physiological disturbances, including reduced cardiac output, pulmonary hypertension, arrhythmias, Kussmaul respiration and hyperkalaemia; the severity of the disturbances is related to the extent of the *acidaemia*. Treatment should be directed initially at identifying and reversing the cause. If acidaemia is considered to be life threatening (pH <7.2, [HCO_3^-] <10 mmol L^{-1}), measures may be required to restore blood pH to normal. Overzealous use of sodium bicarbonate may lead to rapid correction of blood pH, with the risks of tetany and convulsions in the short term and volume overload and hypernatraemia in the longer term. The required quantity of bicarbonate should be calculated:

Bicarbonate requirement (mmol)

= body weight (kg) × base deficit (mmol L^{-1}) × 0.3

Administration of sodium bicarbonate should be followed by repeated measurements of plasma [HCO_3^-] and pH. Sodium bicarbonate is available as isotonic (1.4%; 163 mmol L^{-1}) and hypertonic (8.4%; 1000 mmol L^{-1}) solutions. Slow infusion of the hypertonic solution is advisable to minimise adverse effects.

When considering the use of sodium bicarbonate in the context of metabolic acidaemia it is important to realise that carbon dioxide is generated during the buffering process. This may result in a superimposed respiratory acidosis, especially in those patients with impaired ventilatory reserve or at the limit of compensation. It is also important to distinguish those acidoses associated with tissue hypoxia (e.g. cardiac arrest, septic shock) from those where tissue hypoxia is not a factor. It appears that therapy with sodium bicarbonate often exacerbates the acidosis if tissue hypoxia is present. For example, in patients with type A lactic acidosis, $NaHCO_3$ increases mixed venous $PaCO_2$, which rapidly crosses cell membranes, resulting in an intracellular acidosis, particularly in cardiac and hepatic cells. Theoretically this could result in decreased myocardial contractility and cardiac output and decreased lactate extraction by the liver, aggravating the lactic acidosis. Current guidelines for the management of cardiopulmonary arrest no longer recommend the routine use of sodium bicarbonate. However, if the acidosis is not associated with tissue hypoxaemia (e.g. uraemic acidosis), then the use of sodium bicarbonate results in a potentially beneficial increase in arterial pH.

Metabolic alkalosis

The cardinal features of a metabolic alkalosis are an increased plasma [HCO_3^-], a high pH and an appropriately raised $PaCO_2$. The compensatory response of hypoventilation is

---

> **Box 12.4 Types and causes of metabolic alkalosis**
>
> ### Chloride responsive (urine chloride <20 mmol L^{-1})
>
> Loss of acid
> Vomiting
> Nasogastric suction
> Gastrocolic fistula
> Chloride depletion
> Diarrhoea
> Diuretic abuse
> Excessive alkali
> $NaHCO_3$ administration
> Antacid abuse
>
> ### Chloride resistant (urine chloride >20 mmol L^{-1})
>
> Primary or secondary hyperaldosteronism
> Cushing's syndrome
> Severe hypokalaemia

---

limited and not very effective. For diagnostic and therapeutic reasons, it is usual to subdivide metabolic alkalosis into the chloride-responsive and chloride-resistant varieties (Box 12.4). The differential diagnosis of metabolic alkalosis, and in particular the classification of patients on the basis of the urinary chloride concentration, is important because of the differences in treatment of the two groups. In chloride-responsive alkalosis the administration of saline causes volume expansion and results in the excretion of excess bicarbonate; if potassium is required it should be given as the chloride salt. In patients in whom volume administration is contraindicated the use of acetazolamide results in renal loss of HCO_3^- and an improvement in pH. H_2-receptor antagonists may be helpful if nasogastric suction is contributing to hydrogen ion loss.

Severe alkalaemia with compensatory hypoventilation may result in seizures or CNS depression. In life-threatening metabolic alkalosis rapid correction is necessary and may be achieved by administration of hydrogen ions in the form of dilute hydrochloric acid. Acid administration requires central vein cannulation, as peripheral infusion causes sclerosis of veins. Acid is given as 0.1 mol L^{-1} HCl in glucose 5% at a rate no greater than 0.2 mmol kg^{-1} h^{-1}.

Respiratory acidosis

The cardinal features of respiratory acidosis are a primary increase in $PaCO_2$, a low pH and an appropriate increase in plasma bicarbonate concentration. The extent of the acidaemia is proportional to the degree of hypercapnia. Buffering

<table>
<tr><td>

Box 12.5 Causes of respiratory acidosis

Central nervous system

Drug overdose
Trauma
Tumour
Degeneration or infection
Stroke
Cervical cord trauma

Peripheral nervous system

Polyneuropathy
Myasthenia gravis
Poliomyelitis
Botulism
Tetanus
Organophosphorus poisoning

Primary pulmonary disease

Airway obstruction
Asthma
Laryngospasm
Chronic obstructive airways disease
Parenchymal disease
ARDS
Pneumonia
Severe pulmonary oedema
Chronic obstructive airways disease
Loss of mechanical integrity
Flail chest

ARDS, Acute respiratory distress syndrome.

</td><td>

Box 12.6 Causes of respiratory alkalosis

Voluntary control

Voluntary hyperventilation
Pain, anxiety, distress

Specific conditions

CNS disease
    Meningitis/encephalitis
    Stroke
    Tumour
    Trauma
Respiratory disease
    Pneumonia
    Pulmonary embolism
    Early pulmonary oedema or ARDS
    High altitude
Shock
    Cardiogenic
    Hypovolaemic
    Septic
Miscellaneous
    Cirrhosis
    Gram-negative septicaemia
    Pregnancy
    IPPV
Drugs/hormones
    Salicylates
    Aminophylline
    Progesterone

ARDS, Acute respiratory distress syndrome; *CNS*, central nervous system; *IPPV*, intermittent positive-pressure ventilation.

</td></tr>
</table>

processes are activated rapidly in acute hypercapnia and may remove enough H^+ from the ECF to result in a secondary increase in plasma $[HCO_3^-]$.

Usually hypoxaemia and the manifestations of the underlying disease dominate the clinical picture, but hypercapnia *per se* may result in coma, raised intracranial pressure and a hyperdynamic cardiovascular system (tachycardia, vasodilatation, ventricular arrhythmias) resulting from release of catecholamines. There are many causes of respiratory acidosis, the most important of which are classified in Box 12.5. Treatment consists of reversing the underlying pathology if possible and mechanical ventilatory support if required.

Respiratory alkalosis

The cardinal features of respiratory alkalosis are a primary decrease in $PaCO_2$ (alveolar ventilation in excess of metabolic needs), an increase in pH and an appropriate decrease in plasma bicarbonate concentration. Usually hypocapnia

indicates a disturbance of ventilatory control (in patients not receiving mechanical ventilation). As in respiratory acidosis, the manifestations of the underlying disease usually dominate the clinical picture. Acute hypocapnia results in cerebral vasoconstriction and reduced cerebral blood flow and may cause light-headedness, confusion and, in severe cases, seizures. Circumoral paraesthesia, hyperreflexia and tetany are common. Cardiovascular manifestations include tachycardia and ventricular arrhythmias secondary to the alkalaemia.

The causes of respiratory alkalosis are summarised in Box 12.6. Treatment comprises correction of the underlying cause and thus differential diagnosis is important.

Stewart's physicochemical theory of acid–base balance

The 'traditional' model based on carbonic acid/bicarbonate chemistry with renal and pulmonary regulation of hydrogen ion concentration is relatively easy to understand and apply in common clinical situations. However, it is at best a simplified model of a much more complex reality and as such has some limitations. It struggles to explain the phenomena of hyperchloraemic acidosis, the effect of other acids not buffered by the bicarbonate system and the important role of plasma proteins. In the 1980s, Stewart, a Canadian physiologist, suggested that the bicarbonate system could not be viewed in isolation but rather that the effect of fundamental physicochemical laws (mass action and electrochemical neutrality) on multiple biochemical reactions had to be considered, the bicarbonate system just being one of these, which in turn set $[H^+]$. He went on to theorise three independent variables which determine water dissociation, which is the major source of protons and therefore determinant of pH:

- *The strong ion difference* = $([Na^+] + [K^+] + [Mg^{2+}] + [Ca^{2+}])$ + $([Cl^-] - [lactate])$ – that is, the total concentration of fully dissociated cations minus the total concentration of fully dissociated anions
- *Total weak acid concentration* (A_{TOT}) = $2.43 \times$ [total protein] – this includes associated and dissociated ions (predominantly albumin)
- $\alpha \times P_{CO_2}$

where α is the solubility coefficient for carbon dioxide.

These three variables come together to form the Stewart equation:

$$pH = \frac{pKa + \log[SID] - Kb\,[A_{TOT}]/[Kb + 10 - pH]}{\alpha + PaCO_2}$$

If albumin is removed from this equation it is remarkably similar to the Henderson–Hasselbalch equation. In humans the SID equates to about 40 mmol L^{-1} (i.e. a net positive charge). This is the *apparent* SID (SIDa). However, we know plasma cannot be charged, and SIDa is offset by the *effective* SID (SIDe), which is generated by poorly dissociated weak acids (albumin, phosphate and sulphate). The difference between SIDa and SIDe is the *strong ion gap* (SIG), which is analogous but superior to the anion gap as it accounts for total weak acid, and in particular albumin. Within this theory it is not just the function of the lungs (CO_2) and the kidneys (SID) being modelled but also the organs determining A_{TOT}, namely the GI tract and liver. The Stewart equation also emphasises the importance of $[Cl^-]$ as a key determinant of SID and therefore pH. An increasing $[Cl^-]$ in relation to $[Na^+]$, say after excessive 0.9% saline administration, will decrease SID (with a normal SIG) and thereby decrease pH. This explains the common clinical phenomenon of hyperchloraemic acidosis. It is also worthy of note that Stewart's theory rejects HCO_3^- as an independent variable and therefore a determinant of pH, as in the classical model, being altered by both changes in $PaCO_2$ and SID.

This physicochemical approach does not fundamentally alter our clinical classification or management of acid–base disturbance but may, in the view of some, improve our diagnostic resolution and understanding, such as in hyperchloraemic acidosis and hypoalbuminaemic alkalosis. It is, however, a relatively cumbersome equation and as such has not entered into common bedside usage. These different approaches to acid–base balance are not in themselves right or wrong but rather different viewpoints of the same scenario.

Chapter 13

Metabolism, the stress response to surgery and perioperative thermoregulation

John Andrzejowski, Catherine Riley

Metabolism

Metabolism may be defined as the chemical processes that enable cells to function. Basal metabolic rate (BMR) is the minimum amount of energy required to maintain basic autonomic function and normal homeostasis at rest. In a healthy resting adult, BMR is in the region of 2000 kcal day^{-1} (equivalent to 40 kcal m^{-2} h^{-1}). One calorie is the energy to raise the temperature of 1 g of water from 15°C to 16°C. A more practical measure in human physiology is the kcal or calorie (Cal).

Cellular respiration pathway

The *cellular respiration pathway* describes how adenosine triphosphate (ATP) is produced from carbohydrates, fats and proteins. Amino acids, lipids, and other carbohydrates (see later for details of each) are converted to various intermediates, allowing them to enter the cellular respiration pathway through a variety of routes The main two intermediates are nicotinamide adenine dinucleotide (NAD$^+$) and flavin adenine dinucleotide (FAD$^+$). These molecules are present in high concentrations and can accept electrons to become negatively charged. They combine with a hydrogen atom to become their reduced forms, namely NADH and FADH$_2$. These reduced molecules act as shuttles for electrons in the process known as oxidative phosphorylation, in which they give up their electrons in the mitochondrial electron transport chain to create ATP, which the body can then use to drive energy-consuming processes (e.g. Na$^+$ transport or signalling).

Adenosine triphosphate is present in all cells and contains two high-energy phosphate bonds. It can be thought of as the energy currency of the body. Hydrolysis of 1 mole of ATP to adenosine diphosphate (ADP) releases 8 kcal of energy. Additional hydrolysis of the phosphate bond from ADP to adenosine monophosphate (AMP) also releases 8 kcal (Fig. 13.1).

Once these molecules enter the pathways, it makes no difference where they came from; they simply go through the remaining steps, yielding NADH, FADH$_2$ and ATP (Fig. 13.2).

Let us consider the oxidation of 1 mole of glucose in the cellular respiration pathway in the presence of oxygen. Cellular respiration in the presence of oxygen consists of what can be considered as three distinct processes.

1. The glycolytic pathway *(glycolysis)* takes place in the cell cytoplasm and is not reliant on the presence of oxygen. Glycolysis results in the splitting of each 6-carbon glucose molecule into two 3-carbon molecules of *pyruvate*. This results in the net formation of two molecules of ATP anaerobically but also generates two pairs of NADH for entry into the electron transport chain (see Fig. 13.2).

2. *Oxidation* of each of the pyruvic acid (3-carbon) molecules to produce the 2-carbon acetyl–coenzyme A (*acetyl-CoA*) takes place in the mitochondria and results in the production of two pairs of NADH molecules for entry into the electron transport chain. Acetyl-CoA then combines with the 4-carbon molecule, oxaloacetic acid to form the 6-carbon molecule, *citric acid*. Citric acid enters the Krebs (or tricarboxylic acid; TCA) cycle. In this process, for each molecule of glucose that is metabolised, a further six pairs of NADH, two pairs of FADH$_2$ and two molecules of ATP as well as six molecules CO$_2$ are produced (see Fig. 13.2).

3. *Oxidative phosphorylation* also takes place in the mitochondrial matrix. This process is also known as the *electron transport chain*. Each molecule of NADH and FADH$_2$ yields three and two molecules of ATP, respectively. Thus in perfect conditions, oxidative phosphorylation results in 38 molecules of ATP per molecule of glucose when the products of glycolysis are included. The total yield may be lower in certain circumstances.

The complete oxidation of 1 mole of glucose (180 g) in a calorimeter releases 686 kcal of heat energy (3.8 kcal g^{-1}). However, because each of the 38 molecules of ATP releases 8 kcal, a maximum of 304 kcal of energy is synthesised from each mole of glucose. The efficiency of the glycolytic pathway is therefore 44%; the remainder of the energy is released as heat. Extra heat can be generated if required by uncoupling of oxidative phosphorylation. Protein and fat can potentially release 4.1 and 9.3 kcal g^{-1} of energy, respectively.

Anaerobic glycolysis

This is the process of ATP formation in the absence of oxygen and is possible because the first two steps of glycolysis do not require oxygen. Oxygen is needed for pyruvate to be converted to acetyl-CoA. Thus, in anaerobic conditions (e.g. hypoperfusion) the accumulation of pyruvic acid and hydrogen ions would stop the glycolytic reaction. However, pyruvic acid and hydrogen ions can combine in the presence of *lactic dehydrogenase* to form lactic acid, which diffuses easily out of cells, allowing anaerobic glycolysis to continue (see Fig. 13.2). This is a highly inefficient use of the energy within glucose since only two ATP molecules are produced. When oxygen is again available to the cells, lactic acid is reconverted to glucose or used directly for energy.

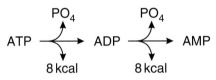

Fig. 13.1 Hydrolysis of adenosine triphosphate (ATP). *ADP,* Adenosine diphosphate; *AMP,* adenosine monophosphate.

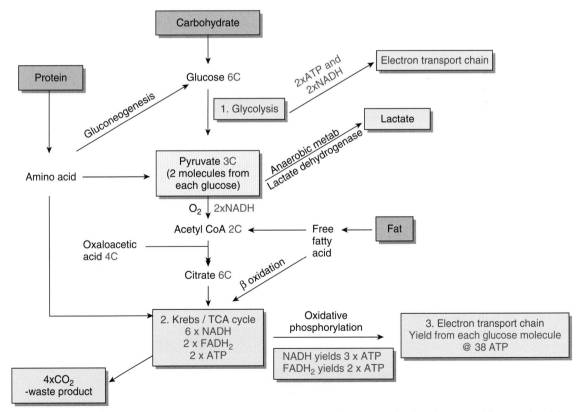

Fig. 13.2 Summary of the glycolytic pathway. Krebs citric acid cycle. Note that two molecules of pyruvic acid are produced for each molecule of glucose metabolised. Each pyruvic acid molecule enters the Krebs citric acid cycle. *FFA,* Free fatty acid.

The pentose phosphate pathway

The glycolytic pathway metabolises 70% of glucose. A second mechanism, the pentose phosphate pathway (also known as the hexose monophosphate shunt), is responsible for metabolism of the remaining 30%, although ATP is neither consumed nor produced. An enzymatic abnormality in the glycolytic pathway therefore does not completely inhibit energy metabolism.

In the irreversible, oxidative part of the pentose phosphate pathway, glucose-6-phosphate (which is one of the first products of glycolysis) is shunted away from the glycolytic pathway to produce:

1. ribose-5-phosphate (a 5-carbon sugar), which is needed for nucleic acid (DNA and RNA) production, and
2. NADPH. This is an electron donor that is important for anabolism and as an antioxidant for the control of potentially toxic oxygen free radicals.

In the non-oxidative phase, the pathway allows for the interconversion of a variety of sugars, such as fructose and glyceraldehyde produced by glycolysis, to form ribose-5-phosphate (see earlier).

Gluconeogenesis

This is the formation of glucose from non-carbohydrate carbon substrates such as glucogenic amino acids, triglycerides (TGs), pyruvate and lactate. It occurs when stores of glycogen are depleted and is mediated by the release of glucagon triggered by hypoglycaemia. It occurs mostly in the liver and kidneys, although the intestine, muscles and even astrocytes are also capable of gluconeogenesis.

Carbohydrates

Cell membranes are impermeable to glucose, so it is transported by a carrier protein (GLUT4) across the membrane in a process termed *facilitated diffusion,* a passive process that does not require energy expenditure by the cell. Facilitated diffusion of glucose is increased tenfold by the action of insulin, which speeds the translocation of GLUT4-containing endosomes into the cell membrane. In contrast, glucose absorption in the GI tract and reabsorption in the renal tubule are both active (energy-consuming) processes involving cotransport with sodium ions via sodium-dependent glucose transporters (SGLT). The final product of carbohydrate digestion is glucose.

After absorption into cells, glucose may be used immediately or stored in the form of glycogen, particularly in the liver and muscles. The process of releasing glucose molecules from the glycogen molecule in times of high metabolic demand is termed *glycogenolysis.* This process is initiated by the enzyme *phosphorylase,* which is activated in the presence of adrenaline and glucagon (released from the α cells of the pancreas in response to hypoglycaemia).

Proteins

Proteins may be synthesised from the 22 amino acids found in all cells of the body. The type of protein depends on the genetic material in the DNA, which determines the sequence of amino acids formed and the nature of the synthesised proteins.

There is equilibrium between the amino acids in plasma, plasma proteins and tissue proteins. The nine essential amino acids (Box 13.1) must be ingested as they cannot be synthesised in the body. Others are *non-essential* (i.e. may be synthesised in the cells). Synthesis occurs by *transamination,* whereby an amine radical ($^-NH_2$) is transferred to the corresponding α-keto acid. Amino acids have a weak carboxylic acidic group (^-COOH) and an amine group ($^-NH_2$). Their entry into cells requires facilitated or active transport using carrier mechanisms. They are conjugated into proteins by the formation of peptide linkages using energy derived from ATP. Large proteins may be composed of several peptide chains wrapped around each other (secondary structure) and bound by weaker links, such as hydrogen bonds, electrostatic forces and sulfhydryl bonds (tertiary structure).

Breakdown of excess amino acids into glucose (gluconeogenesis) generates energy or storage as fat, both of which occur in the liver. The breakdown of amino acids occurs by the process of *deamination,* which takes place in the liver. It involves the removal of the amine group with the formation of the corresponding keto acid. The amine radical may be recycled to other molecules or released as ammonia. In the liver, two molecules of ammonia are combined to form urea (Fig. 13.3). Amino acids may also take up ammonia to form the corresponding amide.

Several hormones influence protein metabolism. Growth hormone, insulin and testosterone are anabolic (i.e. they increase the rate of cellular protein synthesis). Other hormones, such as glucocorticoids, are catabolic (i.e. they decrease the amount of protein in most tissues, except the liver). Glucagon promotes gluconeogenesis and protein

Box 13.1 **Essential amino acids**	
Histidine	Phenylalanine
Leucine	Threonine
Isoleucine	Tryptophan
Lysine	Valine
Methionine	

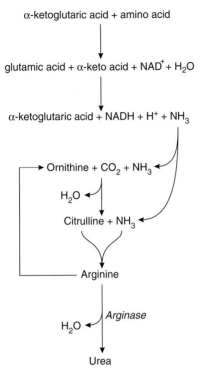

α-ketoglutaric acid + amino acid

↓

glutamic acid + α-keto acid + NAD^+ + H_2O

↓

α-ketoglutaric acid + NADH + H^+ + NH_3

Ornithine + CO_2 + NH_3

H_2O

Citrulline + NH_3

Arginine

Arginase

H_2O

Urea

Fig. 13.3 Deamination is the process of metabolising amino acids. Ammonia is the end product. Two molecules of ammonia combine as shown to form urea. This occurs in the liver.

breakdown. Thyroxine indirectly affects protein metabolism by affecting metabolic rate. If insufficient energy sources are available to cells, thyroxine may contribute to excess protein breakdown. Conversely, if adequate amino acid and energy sources are available, thyroxine may increase the rate of protein synthesis.

Lipids

Lipids are a diverse group of compounds characterised by their insolubility in water and solubility in non-polar solvents. The three main lipid groups are the TGs, phospholipids (PLs) and cholesterol. Functions of lipids include the following:
- Storage of energy for long-term use (e.g. TGs)
- Hormonal roles (e.g. steroids such as oestrogen)
- Insulation – thermal (TGs) and electrical (sphingolipids)
- Protection of internal organs (e.g. TGs and waxes)
- Structural components of cells (e.g. PL membranes and cholesterol)

The basic structure of both TGs and PLs is the fatty acid, which is a carboxylic acid with a long aliphatic chain. This chain can be either saturated (with no C-C double bonds) or unsaturated (one or more double bonds). Triglycerides are composed of three long-chain fatty acids bound with one molecule of glycerol. Phospholipids differ in that the third fatty acid is replaced by a compound such as inositol, choline or ethanolamine. Cholesterol has a sterol nucleus that is formed from fatty acid molecules.

After absorption in the GI tract, lipids are aggregated into chylomicrons (diameter 90–1000 nm). These molecules are too large to pass the endothelial cells of the portal system and so enter the circulation via the thoracic duct. Chylomicrons transport lipids to adipose, cardiac, and skeletal muscle tissue, where their TG components are hydrolysed by the activity of the lipoprotein lipase, allowing the released *free fatty acids* (FFAs) to be absorbed by the tissues. The remnants (e.g. cholesterol) are taken up by the liver.

Alpha-linolenic (omega-3) and linoleic (omega-6) acids are the essential polyunsaturated fatty acids that cannot be synthesised in humans and must be acquired from plant and fish sources. Together with their derivative arachidonic acid, they form prostaglandins, lipoxins and leukotrienes (collectively termed eicosanoids).

Transport of lipids from the liver or adipose cells to other tissues as an energy source occurs by binding to plasma albumin. The fatty acids are then referred to as FFAs, to distinguish them from other fatty acids in the plasma. After 12 h of fasting, all chylomicrons have been removed from the blood, and circulating lipids then occur in the form of *lipoproteins*. Lipoproteins are smaller particles than chylomicrons but are also composed of TGs, PLs and cholesterol. They may be classified as:
- very low-density lipoproteins (VLDLs), consisting mainly of TGs;
- low-density lipoproteins (LDLs), consisting mainly of cholesterol; or
- high-density lipoproteins (HDLs), consisting mainly of protein.

Cholesterol

Cholesterol is a lipid with a sterol nucleus and is formed from acetyl-CoA. It may be absorbed from food (animal sources only) but is also synthesised in the liver and, to a lesser extent, other tissue (Fig. 13.4). Its primary function is in the formation of bile salts in the liver, which promote the digestion and absorption of lipids. Other functions include the formation of adrenocortical and sex hormones and as part of the water-resisting properties of skin.

HMG-CoA reductase is the rate-controlling enzyme in the production of cholesterol. It is inhibited by LDL and cholesterol. This enzyme is the target for statins used in the prevention of hypercholesterolaemia and atherosclerosis.

High thyroid-stimulating hormone (TSH) (e.g. hypothyroidism) and low insulin levels result in higher cholesterol levels. Oestrogen reduces cholesterol concentrations.

High serum cholesterol concentrations are correlated with increased incidences of atherosclerosis and coronary artery disease. Prolonged increases in VLDL, LDL and chylomicron remnants are associated with atherosclerosis. Conversely, HDL is protective.

Lipids may be stored in the liver or adipose cells for later use or used immediately as an energy source. Triglyceride is hydrolysed to its constituent glycerol and three fatty acids; glycerol is then conjugated to glycerol 3-phosphate and enters the glycolytic pathway, which generates ATP as described earlier. Fatty acids need *carnitine* as a carrier agent to enter mitochondria, where they undergo β oxidation. The precise number of ATP molecules formed from a molecule of TG depends on the length of the fatty acid chain; longer chains provide more acetyl-CoA and hence more molecules of ATP.

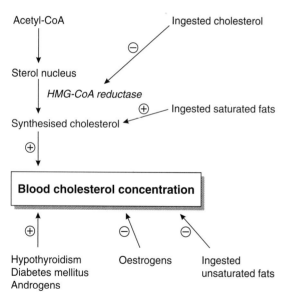

Fig. 13.4 Factors affecting blood cholesterol concentration.

Newborns have a special type of fat, termed brown fat, which on exposure to a cold stressor is stimulated to break down into FFAs and glycerol. In brown adipose tissue, oxidation and phosphorylation are not coupled, and therefore the metabolism of brown fat is especially thermogenic.

Ketones

Initial degradation of fatty acids occurs in the liver, but the acetyl-CoA may not be used either immediately or completely. Ketones, or keto acids, are *acetoacetic acid*, formed from two molecules of acetyl-CoA; β-*hydroxybutyric acid*, formed from the reduction of acetoacetic acid; or *acetone*, formed when a smaller quantity of acetoacetic acid is decarboxylated (Fig. 13.5). Ketones are organic acids that diffuse from their site of production in the liver into the circulation for transport to peripheral tissues, where they are available for oxidisation to acetyl-CoA to produce energy as ATP. Ketones are produced in response to prolonged fasting, starvation, intense exercise and diabetes. In these conditions, carbohydrate metabolism is absent or minimal, leading to intense gluconeogenesis. In diabetes, decreased insulin results in a reduction in intracellular glucose, and in starvation, carbohydrates are lacking simply because they are not being ingested. The ensuing fat breakdown results in large quantities of ketone release from the liver. Ketones can cross the blood–brain barrier and are an important energy source when glucose is lacking. There is a limit to the rate of tissue ketone utilisation because depletion of essential carbohydrate intermediate metabolites slows the rate at which acetyl-CoA can enter the Krebs cycle. Hence blood ketone concentration may increase rapidly, causing metabolic acidosis and ketonuria. Acetone may be discharged on the breath, giving a characteristic sweet odour.

Measuring metabolic rate

Basal metabolic rate is determined at complete mental and physical rest 12–14 h after food ingestion if body temperature is within the normal range. Metabolic rate increases by approximately 8% for every 1°C rise of body temperature. Basal metabolic rate may be measured by indirect calorimetry, which involves the measurement of water, CO_2 or protein

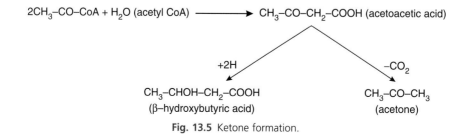

Fig. 13.5 Ketone formation.

Box 13.2 Factors influencing metabolic rate

Malnutrition (20%)
Sleep (15%)
Exercise (up to 2000 × increase BMR)
Protein ingestion
Age: <5 years has × 2 BMR of >70
Thyroid hormone imbalance (↑ or ↓ by 50%)
Sympathetic stimulation
Testosterone (by 15%)
Temperature
Anaesthesia (20% ↓) (regional anaesthesia – no effect)

BMR, Basal metabolic rate.

Table 13.1 Daily water and electrolyte requirement

	Daily requirement (kg^{-1} day^{-1})
Water (ml)	30–35
Sodium (mmol)	1–2
Potassium (mmol)	1
Magnesium (mmol)	0.1–0.2
Calcium (mmol)	0.1–0.2
Phosphate (mmol)	–.2–0.5

breakdown products produced. Alternatively, O_2 consumption can be measured. A total of 4.82 kcal of energy is produced per litre of O_2 consumed, although accurate assessment depends on information about the type of food ingested. Factors influencing BMR are listed in Box 13.2. An estimate of the BMR can be made using a validated method such as the Schofield equation. This equation estimates the BMR from the body weight, age and sex with additional factors such as physical activity and current illness.

Basic nutritional requirements

Exercise, metabolic stress or illness will require additional calories above basal metabolic requirements. When prescribing nutrition in critical care, catabolism, muscle wasting and nitrogen loss are inevitable regardless of caloric input, and trying to match the calorie requirement can lead to very large amounts of energy being prescribed. This could lead to overfeeding, which is associated with poor outcomes. The European Society for Clinical Nutrition and Metabolism (ESPEN) recommends starting at 25–30 kcal kg^{-1} day^{-1} with a protein intake of 1 g kg^{-1} day^{-1}. Protein gives approximately 4 kcal g^{-1}; the remaining calorie requirement should be provided by carbohydrates and lipids in a ratio of 1:1. Carbohydrates also provide approximately 4 kcal g^{-1} and lipids 9 kcal g^{-1}.

The lipid content of total parenteral nutrition (TPN) is increasingly in the form of olive oil–based preparations, which are well tolerated in the critically ill. The protein requirement includes nitrogen 0.15–0.2 g kg^{-1} day^{-1} with the addition of 0.35 g kg^{-1} day^{-1} glutamine in critically ill patients. The electrolyte content of TPN should be guided by serum concentrations and ongoing losses. Typical daily requirements are shown in Table 13.1 (see also Chapter 12). A typical TPN prescription is shown in Table 13.2.

Table 13.2 Example of a daily TPN prescription for a healthy 70-kg patient

Total kcal/day	2100
Protein (g)	70 g = 280 kcal
Nitrogen (g)	10.5
Glutamine (g)	24.5
Carbohydrate	2100 – 280 = 1820 / 2 = 900 kcal = 225 g glucose
Fat	2100 – 280 = 1820 / 2 = 900 kcal = 100 g lipids
Sodium (mmol)	100
Potassium (mmol)	70
Calcium (mmol)	7
Magnesium (mmol)	7
Phosphate (mmol)	28
Volume (ml)	2000
Trace elements (e.g. copper, selenium) and vitamins (e.g. thiamine, vitamin B)	Standard in TPN

TPN, Total parenteral nutrition.

Starvation

Starvation is defined as a severe deficiency in calorie intake to less than that required for maintenance of metabolic requirements. Initially glycogenolysis provides the brain with its primary energy substrate, glucose, until depletion of glycogen occurs after approximately 24 h. Blood glucose concentrations are then maintained by gluconeogenesis, with a peak effect at around 2 days. Gluconeogenesis uses products from lipolysis and muscle breakdown to produce glucose and acetyl-CoA; this increases the formation of ketone bodies. The clinical consequence of starvation is the progressive loss of tissue fat and protein. The average adult has sufficient stores to sustain life for about 3 months.

During starvation or when no protein is ingested (e.g. after major surgery), 20–30 g day^{-1} of protein is catabolised for energy purposes. This occurs despite the continuing availability of some stored carbohydrates and fats. When carbohydrate and fat stores are exhausted, the rate of protein catabolism is increased to >100 g day^{-1}, resulting in a rapid decline in tissue function. During marked systemic inflammation or after major surgery, functional catabolism also occurs.

Nutritional status can be assessed by history (weight loss, recent dietary intake, relevant gastrointestinal (GI) disease and comorbidities such as neoplasia). Examination reveals consequences of vitamin and mineral deficiencies (e.g. bruising, gum disease, osteomalacia) and evidence of soft tissue wasting and dehydration. Body mass index (BMI, kg m^{-2}) is a crude measurement and does not account for body composition (e.g. fat vs. muscle). Body mass index categories are as follows:
- Underweight (<18.5)
- Ideal (18.5–24.9)
- Overweight (25–29.9)
- Obese (>30)
- Severely obese (>35)
- Very severely obese (>40)

Body density and fat percentage can be estimated using anthropometric measurements to estimate nutritional status. These include mid-upper-arm circumference and skin fold thickness to indirectly measure subcutaneous adipose tissue at specified anatomical sites such as the triceps or iliac crest. A functional measurement of nutritional status can also be made by fist grip strength.

Other than a subjective global assessment, severe malnutrition is defined by ESPEN criteria for severe undernutrition as including one of the following:
- Weight loss >10%–15% over the preceding 6 months
- BMI <18.5 kg m^{-2}
- Serum albumin <30 g L^{-1} (with no hepatic or renal dysfunction)

Patients who are malnourished or at risk of undernutrition can be identified using screening tools such as the MUST (Malnutrition Universal Screening Tool). This comprises five steps:
1. Assess BMI.
2. Calculate percentage of unplanned weight loss.
3. Add acute disease effect.
4. Use tables to generate a score of overall risk of malnutrition.
5. Use this score to guide the plan of care.

The effects of chronic malnutrition on anaesthesia

Malnourished patients have increased risks of inadvertent perioperative hypothermia, increased susceptibility to infection with greater risk of wound infection and anastomotic breakdown, and increased risk of pressure ulceration. Malnutrition is associated with increased duration of hospital stay and duration of mechanical ventilation in the critically ill. Patients with decreased serum albumin have altered volume of distribution and altered fraction of protein-bound and unbound drug, potentially leading to unpredictable drug effects (see Chapter 1). Altered drug metabolism may also occur because of decreased microsomal enzyme activity and protein deficiency.

Malnourished patients are at risk of refeeding syndrome when feeding is re-established in hospital, either enterally or parenterally. This is associated with hypophosphataemia, as phosphate ions are taken intracellularly when a glucose substrate is restored. Adenosine triphosphate depletion and muscle weakness follow, with potential tissue hypoxia, seizures and cardiorespiratory arrest in severe cases. To avoid this, feeding should be started slowly in the malnourished patient, with 50% of calorie requirement given for the first 48 h before increasing to full feed.

Many elderly patients have nutritional deficits as well as being classed as frail. Some clinicians prescribe iron, folate and vitamin B12 replacement in the perioperative period to correct anaemia as well as protein and vitamin D supplements to minimise loss of muscle mass (sarcopenia) (see Chapter 31). Some units have instigated exercise programs sometimes known as prehabilitation to improve functional capacity before surgery.

The stress response to surgery

The physiological syndrome known as the stress response has evolved to enable humans to enter a catabolic state that mobilises energy stores and conserves water to enhance chances of survival in times of danger. The perioperative stress response to surgery varies in size and duration in proportion to the extent of injury or metabolic insult. If left unmodified in the perioperative period, it results in little benefit and much potential harm (Fig. 13.6).

The two principal components of the stress response are the *neuroendocrine* response and the *cytokine* response (Table 13.3). The neuroendocrine response is stimulated by painful afferent neural stimuli reaching the CNS. From baseline, serum cortisol concentrations reach a peak at around 4–6 h

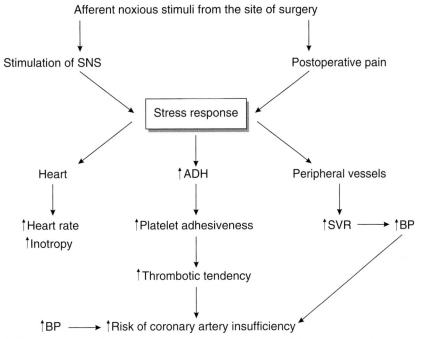

Fig. 13.6 Potential effect of the surgical stress response on coronary arterial blood flow. *ADH*, Antidiuretic hormone; *SNS*, sympathetic nervous system; *SVR*, systemic vascular resistance.

from the start of surgery. The stress response may be diminished by the use of a regional anaesthetic technique such as epidural or high-dose opioids (see later).

The cytokine (e.g. interleukin-6 and tumour necrosis factor) component of the stress response is stimulated by *local tissue damage* at the site of the surgery itself and is not inhibited by regional anaesthesia. It is diminished by minimally invasive surgery, especially laparoscopic techniques. Triggers are listed in Box 13.3.

Carbohydrate mobilisation

Shortly after any surgical stress, the body becomes relatively insulin resistant. Peripheral insulin resistance leads to reduced glucose uptake, whereas hepatic resistance leads to gluconeogenesis. It is thought that injured tissue lacks this insulin resistance, and the higher glucose concentrations may promote wound healing. Hyperglycaemia however is pro-inflammatory and may lead to glycosuria and osmotic diuresis. It also increases the risk of wound infection, myocardial infarction and renal failure as well as leading to increased hospital stay. The NICE-SUGAR study suggested that outcomes are best when blood glucose levels are kept to less than 10 mmol l^{-1} using an insulin infusion.

> **Box 13.3 Triggers of the neuroendocrine and cytokine response in patients after surgery**
>
> Noxious afferent stimuli (especially pain)
> Local inflammatory tissue factors, especially cytokines
> Pain and anxiety
> Starvation
> Hypothermia and shivering
> Haemorrhage
> Acidosis
> Hypoxaemia
> Infection

Protein catabolism

Major surgery results in a net excretion of nitrogen-containing compounds (negative nitrogen balance; measured by increased nitrogen excretion in the urine), reflecting catabolism of protein into amino acids for gluconeogenesis or to form acute-phase proteins. This is partly because of perioperative starvation but mainly because of the stress response, which causes decreased total protein synthesis in addition

241

Table 13.3 Components of the stress response to surgery

Component	Response	Physiological change	Effect
Neuroendocrine response	**Hypothalamic-pituitary-adrenal:** • ↑ ACTH, ↑ GH, ↑ ADH, • ↑ β-endorphin, ↑ prolactin • Activation of renin-angiotensin-aldosterone system **Sympathetic nervous system:** • ↑ catecholamines • ↓ insulin • ↑ glucagon	• Lipolysis • Na⁺ retention • K⁺ excretion • ↑ heart rate • ↑ cardiac output • ↑ SVR • ↑ arterial pressure • Insulin resistance • ↑ acute phase proteins (liver) • Proteolysis	• ↑ free fatty acids, which can be used as energy by peripheral tissues and brain • Myocardial ischaemia • Arrhythmias • Vasoconstriction • Hyperglycaemia • ↓ hepatic synthesis of albumin • Release amino acids for acute phase proteins and for gluconeogenesis
Cytokine response	**Cytokine and inflammatory mediator release:** • ↑ IL-1, ↑ IL-6, ↑ TNF-α • ↑ prostaglandins • ↑ neutrophils ↓ lymphocytes	• Platelet adhesion • ↑ coagulation • Local inflammation • ↑ metabolic rate • Pyrexia • ↑ demand on cardiovascular system	• Thromboembolic disease • Pain • Sweating • ↑ insensible fluid loss • Myocardial ischaemia

ACTH, Adrenocorticotropic hormone; *ADH*, antidiuretic hormone; *GH*, growth hormone; *IL*, interleukin; *SVR*, systemic vascular resistance; *TNF*, tumour necrosis factor.

to protein breakdown. Up to 0.5 kg day⁻¹ of lean muscle mass may be lost postoperatively, with peripheral skeletal muscle predominantly affected, but visceral protein may also be catabolised. To minimise protein catabolism contributing to weight loss and impaired wound healing, ESPEN recommends the following:

• Daily protein intake of 1.5 g kg⁻¹ ideal body weight in surgical patients to limit nitrogen losses. This is double the usual daily requirement.
• Carbohydrate loading before surgery and nutritional support (enteral route where possible) in the perioperative period for patients at high nutritional risk.
• Addition of immunonutrition (the ingestion of amino acids such as glutamine and arginine, omega-3 fatty acids, and nucleotides) after trauma or burns.

Such a regimen is best commenced 5–7 days before major surgery and can continue for a similar period after operation in the malnourished.

Severely undernourished patients (see earlier) may require up to 14 days of parenteral nutrition in the perioperative period.

Fat Metabolism

The net effect of the hormonal alterations listed in Table 13.3 is lipolysis, stimulated by catecholamines acting at α₁-adrenoreceptors to increase plasma concentrations of FFAs. Free fatty acids may be oxidised in the liver to form ketones (e.g. acetoacetate), which may be used as a source of energy by peripheral tissues.

Cardiovascular effects

The stress response to surgery and postoperative pain activates the sympathetic nervous system (SNS), which, by increasing heart rate and arterial pressure, increases myocardial oxygen demand. Activation of the SNS may also cause coronary artery vasoconstriction, reducing the supply of oxygen to the myocardium, predisposing to myocardial ischaemia. Increased antidiuretic hormone (ADH) release from the posterior pituitary leads to water retention and contributes to increased platelet adhesiveness and thromboembolic disease (see Fig. 13.6).

Gastrointestinal effects

The stress response to surgery and afferent nociceptive input results in a relative imbalance between the sympathetic and parasympathetic nervous systems, resulting in ileus, which delays resumption of an enteral diet, prolonging the stress response.

Renal effects

Part of the stress response includes protective mechanisms to maintain intravascular volume, with activation of the renin–angiotensin–aldosterone pathway and increased secretion of antidiuretic hormone. This results in retention of both salt and water and the loss of potassium ions for up to 5 days postoperatively.

Acute kidney injury (AKI) results in an increase in serum creatinine and a decrease in urine output (see Chapter 11). Most postoperative AKI is caused by acute tubular injury secondary to renal hypoperfusion or direct tubular insult, and microvascular dysfunction caused by the inflammatory response of major surgery or sepsis. Elderly patients and those with comorbidities such as chronic kidney disease or diabetes mellitus are at high risk. Surgical factors (emergency, cardiac or vascular surgery) and pharmacological factors (NSAIDs, ACE inhibitors, radiocontrast) also increase the risk of AKI. Renal risk can be minimised using surgical techniques that avoid cross-clamping major vessels and by limiting time spent on cardiopulmonary bypass.

Immunological system effects

Many mediators of the stress response (cortisol, interleukins, prostaglandins, etc.) are cellular and humoral immunosuppressants. It is not known if stress response–mediated immunosuppression, lasting for several days after surgery, influences patient outcome.

Local factors and the immunological (cytokine) response

Severe injury in a denervated limb can elicit the stress response, confirming that non-neural stimuli are also involved. Cytokines and mediators of inflammation are released in response to local tissue destruction or trauma, increasing peripheral nociceptive activity. The LAFA (LAparoscopy and/or FAst track) trial confirmed that the magnitude of this response is proportional to the extent of tissue damage. Laparoscopic techniques and the enhanced recovery protocol (nutrition, analgesia and fluid) resulted in less stress response activation and preserved immune function.

Effect of anaesthesia on the stress response

There is no evidence that limiting the endocrine and metabolic responses to surgery is beneficial in all patients, but it is considered advantageous to decrease the stress response in patients with cardiovascular disease. Most intravenous and inhalational anaesthetic agents have no appreciable effect on either the neuroendocrine or the cytokine elements of the stress response. Etomidate infusions are associated with reduced cortisol concentrations secondary to inhibition of the 11β-hydroxylase enzyme associated with increased mortality. At much higher doses, adrenal 18β-hydroxylase and cholesterol side chain cleavage enzymes are inhibited, thus reducing aldosterone and other steroid hormone synthesis. There is some evidence that inhibition of 11β-hydroxylase occurs after a single induction dose of etomidate, reducing plasma cortisol concentrations for several hours, but the clinical significance of this is unclear (see Chapter 4). High-dose opioid analgesia (e.g. 2 fentanyl 50–100 µg kg^{-1}) may completely inhibit the neuroendocrine element (apart from that triggered by cardiopulmonary bypass) if given *before* surgical incision. These high doses of opioids are impractical for most operations because they would cause postoperative respiratory depression. Epidural analgesia using local anaesthetic drugs commenced before the surgical incision and continued postoperatively significantly reduces the stress response to upper abdominal surgery and can completely supprkess the response to lower limb or pelvic surgery.

Thermoregulation and anaesthesia

Humans are homeothermic, requiring a nearly constant core temperature that never deviates more than a few tenths of a degree either side of normal. Anaesthesia and surgery have dramatic effects on temperature regulation, such that postoperative hypothermia is the rule rather than the exception. Hypothermia results in significant morbidity, including coagulopathy, prolonged duration of drug action, increased risk of surgical wound infection and shivering.

Physiology

It is useful to consider thermoregulatory physiology in terms of a two-compartment model. A central core compartment, comprising the major trunk organs and the brain (the main sources of heat production), accounts for two thirds of body heat content. Core body temperature is maintained within a narrow interthreshold range (36.8°C–37.2°C), which facilitates optimal cellular enzyme function. The peripheral compartment consists of the limbs and skin and subcutaneous tissues over the body surface. It amounts to about one third of total body heat content. In contrast with the core, peripheral tissues have wide variation in temperature, ranging from 2 °C–3 °C below to more than 20 °C below core temperature in extreme conditions. Peripheral tissue acts as a heat sink to absorb or give up heat to maintain core temperature within its narrow range.

Heat balance

Thermogenesis

Maintaining core temperature within a narrow range requires balancing heat production and loss. It is achieved by a control system consisting of afferent thermal receptors, central integrating systems and efferent control mechanisms (Fig. 13.7). Thermoregulation is a multilevel, multiple-input system with the spinal cord, nucleus raphe magnus and locus subcoeruleus involved in both generating afferent thermal signals and modulating efferent thermoregulatory responses.

Body heat is produced by metabolism, shivering and exercise. Basal metabolic rate cannot be manipulated by thermoregulatory mechanisms. Vasoconstriction and shivering are the principal autonomic mechanisms of preserving body heat and increasing heat production.

Adjacent to the centre in the posterior hypothalamus on which the impulses from cold receptors impinge, there is a motor centre for shivering. It is normally inhibited by impulses from the heat-sensitive area in the anterior hypothalamus, but when cold impulses exceed a certain rate, the motor centre for shivering becomes activated by spillover of signals, and it sends impulses bilaterally into the spinal cord. Initially this increases the tone of skeletal muscles throughout the body, but when this muscle tone increases above a specific level, shivering is observed. Shivering may increase heat production sixfold.

Non-shivering thermogenesis is also an important mechanism in increasing heat production. Its role in adult thermogenesis is thought to be minimal, increasing the rate of heat production by less than 10%–15%, compared with the doubling seen in neonates. Non-shivering thermogenesis occurs mainly in brown adipose tissue (BAT). This subtype of adipose tissue contains large numbers of mitochondria in its cells, supplied by extensive SNS innervation, stimulation of which leads to oxidative metabolism of the mitochondria which is *uncoupled* from phosphorylation, so that heat is produced instead of generating ATP. Exercise may increase heat production by as much as twentyfold for a short time at maximal intensity.

Heat loss

Perioperative heat loss occurs predominantly by radiation (50%–60%), convection (25%–30%), evaporation (10%–20%) and conduction (5%). Radiation is the major route of heat loss and is proportional to the difference in temperature between the patient and environment to the power of four. Conductive and convective heat losses are proportional to the difference between skin temperature and ambient temperature. Unwarmed fluid infusion is a form of conductive heat loss. Air flow accelerates cooling at a rate proportional to the square root of the air velocity. Evaporative heat loss from skin is usually minimal (<5% of overall heat loss) in a warm operating theatre or when using a heat and moisture filter in the circuit. Evaporative losses may become significant in surgery in which warm moist viscera are exposed to the air, such as laparotomy, and after the application of cleaning fluids (particularly alcoholic), when the latent heat of vaporisation draws heat from the body to lower core temperature by as much as 0.2 °C–0.4 °C m^{-2}.

Thermoregulation

Thermoregulation is achieved by a physiological control system consisting of peripheral and central thermoreceptors, an integrating control centre and efferent response systems (see Fig. 13.7).

Thermoreceptors

Afferent thermal input comes from anatomically distinct cold and heat receptors, located predominantly in the skin

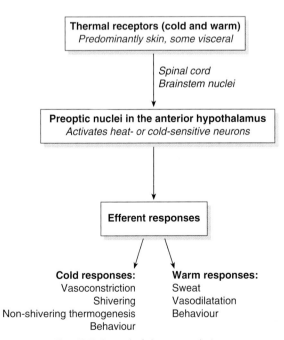

Fig. 13.7 Control of thermoregulation.

but also centrally. The afferent thermal input comes from both core (80%) and peripheral (20%) compartments. The peripheral input is from thermally sensitive receptors located in the skin and mucous membranes, whereas core input occurs from thermoreceptors located in the hypothalamus itself, brain, spinal cord and thoracic and abdominal tissue. Cold-specific receptors are innervated by Aδ fibres. Heat receptors are innervated by C fibres. Cold receptors in the skin outnumber heat receptors tenfold and are the major mechanism by which the body protects itself against cold temperatures. Afferent input from these cold receptors in the skin is transmitted to the posterior hypothalamus.

Afferent thermal signals provide feedback to temperature-regulating centres in the hypothalamus. The preoptic area of the hypothalamus contains temperature-sensitive and temperature-insensitive neurons. The temperature-sensitive neurons, which predominate by 4:1, increase their discharge rate in response to increased local heat, and this activates heat loss mechanisms. Conversely, cold-sensitive neurons increase their rate of discharge in response to cooling. Detection of cold differs from detection of heat in that the principal mechanism of detection of cold is input from cutaneous cold receptors. At normothermia, most afferent input comes from cold receptors. Blockade of this afferent input by regional anaesthesia explains why the lower limbs are often perceived by the patient as feeling warm when epidural or spinal anaesthesia are established.

Central control

The central control mechanism, situated in the hypothalamus, determines mean body temperature by integrating thermal signals from peripheral and core structures and comparing mean body temperature with a predetermined set point temperature. The set point or physiological thermostat of the thermoregulatory system is the temperature at which the system requires zero action to maintain that temperature (36.8°C–37.2°C). The limits of this range represent the thresholds at which cold or heat responses are instigated, and hence it has been termed the interthreshold range. Normally it is less than 1°C, but this increases to 4°C during general anaesthesia (Fig. 13.8).

Effector mechanisms

In extreme cold conditions, vasoconstriction and shivering are of limited effect compared with behavioural measures such as taking shelter and wearing protective clothing.

Physiological responses to heat result in vasodilatation and sweating, which are the major autonomic mechanisms of increasing heat loss. Maximal sweating rates may reach over 1 litre h^{-1} for a short time, resulting in heat loss of up to 15 times BMR.

Physiological responses to cold are generally of more relevance to anaesthesia because hypothermia is common during most procedures. In normal adults the first response to a decrease in core temperature below the normal range (36.5°C–37.5°C) is peripheral vasoconstriction. If core

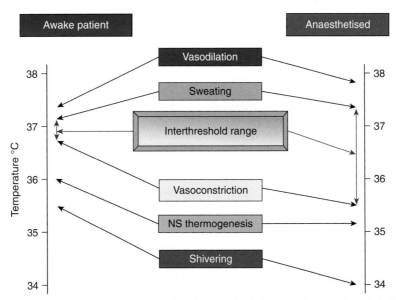

Fig. 13.8 Thresholds for thermoregulatory effectors. **Awake:** The interthreshold range is approximately 0.5°C. **Anaesthetised:** Thresholds for vasoconstriction and shivering are now much lower, leading to unabated heat loss.

temperature continues to decrease, shivering commences. Vasoconstriction and shivering are characterised by *threshold onset, gain* and *maximal response intensity. Threshold* is the temperature at which the effector is activated. *Gain* is the rate of response to a given decrease in core temperature. Normally the threshold core temperature for thermoregulatory vasoconstriction is 36.5°C, with shivering commencing at 36.0°C–36.2°C.

Measurement of temperature

The site that gives the most accurate, direct measurement of core temperature is the pulmonary artery. Many studies have compared other measurement sites and technologies with this core measurement site. The most accurate are those from thermocouples placed in the distal oesophagus (approximately 40 cm from the teeth), bladder and *directly* at the tympanic membrane (under direct vision; mainly for research purposes). Nasopharyngeal probes also perform very well when inserted approximately 10 cm into the nares (shallow placement can result in interference from ambient temperatures). Invasive measurements such as these are of limited use in conscious patients, in whom surrogate estimates of core temperature are used instead. The easiest and most accurate device is a digital oral thermometer. Other indirect measurements include infrared aural, forehead or axillary sites. The accuracy of infrared forehead and axillary readings are hampered by the algorithm programmed into the device that adjusts the temperature readout; they are not generally used as first-line monitors. Indirect aural thermometers are quick and easy to use but can give inaccurately low readings as a result of user error or from debris in the ear canal preventing the tympanum being accessed. If a second reading taken from the opposite ear still demonstrates hypothermia, then a check using a more accurate device such as a digital oral thermometer (readings within ±0.25°C of core) is recommended before delaying discharge from recovery until normothermia is achieved. The relatively new zero heat flux forehead thermometer is promising but takes approximately 5 min to obtain the first reading. The physical principles of thermometers are detailed in Chapter 17.

Effect of general anaesthesia on thermoregulation

Anaesthesia affects the homeostatic mechanisms controlling thermoregulation and impairs the mechanisms which would normally limit the associated heat loss.

Widening of the interthreshold range

General anaesthesia causes a dose-dependent widening of the interthreshold range, with an increase in the temperature at which thermoregulatory responses to heat are activated and an even greater reduction in the temperature at which thermoregulatory responses to cold are activated. Typically the interthreshold range widens by 2°C–4°C, with the body becoming poikilothermic within this temperature range (Fig. 13.8). However, once core temperature falls outside this range, the gain (the rate of response to a given decrease in core temperature) and maximal response intensity of homeostatic mechanisms are unaffected. Volatile and intravenous anaesthetic agents impair thermoregulation to a similar extent.

Stages of hypothermia

Mild hypothermia during general anaesthesia follows a distinctive pattern and occurs in three phases (see Fig. 13.9):

Phase 1 (redistribution stage)
Under normal conditions, the temperature gradient between core and peripheral compartments is maintained by tonic vasoconstriction. On induction of anaesthesia, normal vasoconstrictor tone is reduced and vasodilatation occurs, allowing heat to flow down its concentration gradient from the warm core to the cooler periphery, resulting in a mild core hypothermia (core temperature about 35.5°C–36.0°C). This core hypothermia occurs because of *redistribution* of body heat on induction of anaesthesia, and *overall* heat loss from the body is minimal. Peripheral temperature increases during this phase (Fig. 13.10; upper picture). Redistribution hypothermia results in an initial rapid decrease in core temperature of approximately 1°C over the first 30 min, but mean body temperature and body heat content remain constant during this 30 min.

A number of factors affect the magnitude of this initial phase 1 hypothermia:

* A greater temperature gradient between the core and periphery results in a greater decrease in core temperature. Patients who have been left in a cold reception room will have a relatively cold peripheral compartment and will suffer a greater degree of redistribution hypothermia.
* Obese patients tend to be chronically vasodilated and have a warm peripheral compartment. Vasodilatation on induction of anaesthesia and redistribution hypothermia both occur to a lesser extent in the obese.
* Neonates, and to a lesser extent children, have a much smaller peripheral compartment than adults, and any decrease in core temperature on induction of anaesthesia is likely to be true heat loss rather than redistribution hypothermia.

Phase 2 (heat loss > heat production)
Phase 2 is a slower linear decrease in core temperature to 34°C–35°C over the next 2 h and is due to heat loss exceeding heat production. General anaesthesia reduces metabolic

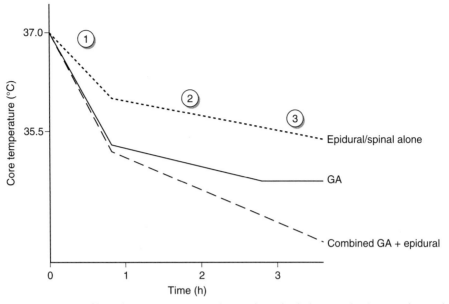

Fig. 13.9 Characteristic patterns of hypothermia during general anaesthesia (GA) alone, epidural or spinal anaesthesia alone and combined general and epidural anaesthesia. Patients in this last category are more likely to develop profound hypothermia than others (see text).

heat production by 15%–40%, particularly through decreased brain metabolism and reduced respiratory muscle activity. Increased heat loss occurs through peripheral vasodilatation, through evaporative heat loss from the body surface and from exposed body cavities (some animal studies have shown that as much as 50% of total heat loss can come from exposed bowel). Convective losses are increased because of air currents, and the use of unwarmed fluids contributes to conductive losses.

Phase 3 (plateau phase)

Phase 3 is a core temperature plateau (or thermal equilibrium), where heat loss equals heat production (either metabolic or warming devices) (see Fig. 13.9). This core temperature plateau results largely from thermoregulatory vasoconstriction, triggered by a core temperature of 33°C–35°C. Patients with impaired autonomic responses (e.g. elderly patients and those with diabetes, Parkinson's disease, Shy–Drager syndrome, etc.) are less able to establish effective vasoconstriction, and in these patients, establishment of a plateau phase may be delayed.

Effect of regional anaesthesia on thermoregulation

Regional anaesthesia widens the interthreshold range, resulting in a redistribution of body heat in a similar manner to general anaesthesia. Because redistribution during spinal or epidural anaesthesia is confined usually to the lower half of the body, the initial core hypothermia is not as pronounced as in general anaesthesia (approximately 0.5°C). There are some effects above the block level, probably related to a blockade of afferent input to the hypothalamus. The major difference for spinal or epidural anaesthesia is that the plateau phase does not emerge because vasoconstriction is blocked (see Fig. 13.9). Heat loss continues unabated during epidural anaesthesia despite the activation of effector mechanisms above the level of the block. Therefore patients undergoing long procedures with combined general and epidural anaesthesia are at greater risk of hypothermia.

Consequences of perioperative hypothermia

The reduction in BMR secondary to hypothermia may have a protective effect in certain circumstances. Moderate hypothermia is routine practice in many centres during cardiopulmonary bypass. In most situations the deleterious adverse postoperative consequences of mild hypothermia outweigh the potential benefits. Wound infections are inversely proportional to tissue oxygen tension for 4 h after exposure; inadvertent intraoperative hypothermia leads to decreased tissue oxygen tension and directly impairs T cell and neutrophil function, thereby further increasing the risk of surgical site infection. Platelet function is impaired by a decrease in the release of thromboxane, though fibrinolytic

247

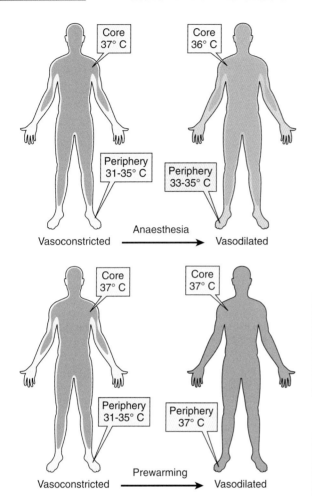

Fig. 13.10 Effect of anaesthesia *(upper)* and prewarming *(lower)* on core–periphery temperature gradients.

Table 13.4 Consequences of perioperative hypothermia	
Cardiac	CO ↓, HR ↓, BP ↓ PR duration ↑, QRS duration ↑, QT interval prolonged, J waves Blood viscosity ↑ Cardiac work ↑ MI risk ↑
Wound infection	Caused by vasoconstriction and hence low tissue oxygen tension (P_tO_2)
Prolonged drug action	
Negative nitrogen balance, metabolism ↓, 8% per 1°C below normal temperature	
Prolonged coagulation. Blood loss and risk of blood transfusion increased	
DVT/PE risk ↑	
Oxyhaemoglobin dissociation curve shifted to right	
Stress response ↑	
Patient discomfort/shivering	

BP, Blood pressure; CO, cardiac output; DVT, deep vein thrombosis; HR, heart rate; MI, myocardial infarction; PE, pulmonary embolism.

activity is preserved. Both the intrinsic and extrinsic coagulation cascade are impaired, resulting in increased blood loss and need for perioperative transfusion.

Hypothermia can significantly prolong the action of drugs such as propofol, fentanyl and neuromuscular blockers and can decrease the minimum alveolar concentration (MAC) of volatile anaesthetic agents. Postoperatively, circulating endogenous concentrations of noradrenaline may be higher in hypothermic patients, causing vasoconstriction and increased arterial pressure. This can potentially cause cardiovascular morbidity, especially because oxygen consumption is further increased by shivering. Shivering also aggravates pain, raises intracranial and intraocular pressure and impedes monitoring. Perioperative thermal discomfort is often remembered by patients as the worst aspect of their perioperative experience (Table 13.4).

Box 13.4 **Strategies for prevention of perioperative hypothermia**

Accurate temperature measurement
Keeping patients warm preoperatively: consider active prewarming
Intraoperative use of forced air convective warming device
Underbody pressure relieving warming mattress
Heating and humidifying inspired gases
Increased ambient temperature to 21°C
Infusing warmed i.v. fluids

Physical, active and passive strategies for avoiding perioperative hypothermia

Preventing redistribution-induced hypothermia may be achieved by physical and pharmacological means (Box 13.4). Passive insulation with a single layer of any insulating material is relatively ineffective. Warm blankets, although comforting for patients in the short term, become mere insulators as they rapidly cool to ambient temperature. Heat and moisture exchange filters retain significant amounts of moisture and heat within the respiratory system. Once forced air warming is commenced, ambient temperature has little effect on the incidence of hypothermia; however, while the patient is exposed, theatre temperature should be kept above 21 °C.

Active forced air warming systems are the best way to minimise hypothermia and are particularly effective when used intraoperatively for vasodilated patients, allowing heat applied peripherally to be transferred rapidly to the core.

Resistive, pressure relieving heat mattresses (e.g. Inditherm) are less effective at preventing heat loss, possibly because relatively little heat is lost from the back; however, they can be of additional benefit when used in combination with forced air warming.

Forced air warmers should be used for anaesthesia longer than 30 min and for all patients at high risk of perioperative hypothermia. It should be started on the ward 30 min before induction if the patient's core temperature is less than 36.0 °C.

Pre-emptive skin surface warming does not increase core temperature but increases total body heat content, particularly in the arms and legs, and removes the gradient for heat loss via the skin. Thus if a human is prewarmed, the arms and legs become warmer and appear the same dark shade as the core compartment (as shown in the lower picture of Fig. 13.10). Even 10 min of prewarming can help prevent inadvertent perioperative hypothermia caused by initial vasodilatation and heat redistribution. It should be considered in all patients preoperatively but will be of most benefit for patients at high risk of hypothermia and in situations where intraoperative forced air warming is impractical (e.g. in obstetrics or where disruption of laminar air flow might present a perceived risk). To save costs, unsoiled forced air warming blankets can be left *in situ* and used in the postanaesthetic care unit if necessary. Infusion of 1 litre of i.v. fluids at room temperature can cool an average adult by up to 0.25 °C, so fluids should be warmed before (e.g. from a warming cabinet) or during administration using an inline warmer.

References/Further reading

Buggy, D.J., Crossley, A.W.A., 2000. Thermoregulation, mild perioperative hypothermia and post-anaesthetic shivering. Br. J. Anaesth. 84, 615–628.

Burton, D., Nicholson, G., Hall, G., 2004. Endocrine and metabolic response to surgery. Continuing Ed Anaesthesia Crit Care Pain 4 (5), 144–147.

Desborough, J.P., 2000. The stress response to trauma and surgery. Br. J. Anaesth. 85, 109–117.

Weimann, A., Braga, M., Carli, F., et al., 2017. ESPEN guideline: clinical nutrition in surgery. Clin. Nutr. 36 (3), 623–650.

Hall, J.E., 2015. Metabolism and temperature regulation. In: Guyton, A.C., Hall, J.E. (Eds.), Textbook of medical physiology, thirteenth ed. WB Saunders, Philadelphia.

Horn, E.P., Bein, B., Böhm, R., et al., 2012. The effect of short time periods

of pre-operative warming in the prevention of peri-operative hypothermia. Anaesthesia 67 (6), 612–617.

KDIGO Guidelines: Acute Kidney Injury. http://kdigo.org/guidelines/acute-kidney-injury/.

NICE 2016 Clinical Guideline 65 Hypothermia: prevention and management in adults having surgery https://www.nice.org.uk/guidance/cg65.

Chapter | **14** |

Blood, coagulation and transfusion

Pamela Wake

Haematological conditions and drugs can have a significant impact on the conduct of anaesthesia. Anaesthetists need to have an understanding of the pathophysiology associated with various haematological diseases and drugs that are known to increase the risk of thrombosis, infection, or haemorrhage. In addition, as one of the largest groups of clinicians responsible for the transfusion of various blood products, anaesthetists need to be familiar with the rationale for their safe use and the impact of major haemorrhage and blood transfusion.

The physiology of blood

Blood cells and plasma

Red blood cells (RBCs, or erythrocytes) typically survive for about 120 days after their release into the circulation. They are created in bone marrow and are released as reticulocytes, which mature over 2 days into adult RBCs. In healthy adults, 1%–2% of RBCs present in the circulation are reticulocytes. Reticulocytes and RBCs do not have nuclei, but residual RNA can still be found in reticulocytes as they mature into erythrocytes.

The classic shape of an erythrocyte is a biconcave disk 8 μm in diameter, but because they deform easily, erythrocytes can pass through capillaries smaller than this.

At the end of their 120-day lifespan, old red cells are destroyed by macrophages in the liver, spleen and bone marrow. The iron contained within is made available for further RBC production, whilst the porphyrins are converted into unconjugated bilirubin.

The primary function of RBCs is to carry oxygen, bound to haemoglobin, to body tissues. In adults the majority of haemoglobin present is HbA (comprising two α- and two β-globin chains: $\alpha_2\beta_2$). A small amount of HbA_2 is also present ($\alpha_2\delta_2$), as is an even smaller amount of fetal haemoglobin, HbF ($\alpha_2\gamma_2$). Fetal haemoglobin and HbA_2 typically represent less than 4% of the total amount of haemoglobin. Each globin chain contains a pocket of haem in which iron is held in its ferrous state, allowing it to bind reversibly with oxygen. As oxygen binds to each haem pocket in turn, the whole haemoglobin molecule changes shape, increasing its overall affinity for oxygen. When the haemoglobin molecule unloads oxygen, the overall affinity for oxygen decreases because 2,3-diphosphoglycerate (2,3-DPG) displaces the two β chains. These changes account for the sigmoid shape of the oxygen–haemoglobin dissociation curve. Increased concentrations of carbon dioxide, hydrogen ions, 2,3-DPG, and sickle haemoglobin (HbS) shift the oxygen–haemoglobin dissociation curve to the right. Fetal haemoglobin does not bind with 2,3-DPG and so its dissociation curve is shifted to the left.

White blood cells (leukocytes) present in the circulation include granulocytes (neutrophils, eosinophils, basophils), lymphocytes and monocytes. The main purpose of white cells is to defend against infection from micro-organisms, and to do this they must be able to pass out of the vasculature into the interstitial space. Once present in tissues, monocytes may differentiate into macrophages.

Neutrophils, monocytes and macrophages are the three major phagocytic cells responsible for the destruction of bacteria, fungi or damaged cells. Phagocytic cells respond to foreign substances in three stages: chemotaxis, whereby phagocytes are attracted to sites of inflammation by chemical signals; phagocytosis, which is where the phagocyte ingests the material in question (often aided by a process called opsonisation, in which particles are tagged by immunoglobulins or complement); and destruction, which is achieved by the release of reactive oxygen species within the cell.

Eosinophils are involved in both allergic reactions and the response to parasitic infections. Lymphocytes are subdivided into B cells, T cells and natural killer (NK) cells. B and T cells release immunoglobulins in response to antigens derived from bacteria, viruses and other foreign particles. Many of these antigens are processed and presented to the lymphocytes by specialist macrophages, termed antigen presenting cells (APC). Lymphocytes that recognise specific antigens can proliferate and produce clones of themselves in response to a specific threat. This threat response is effectively memorised by the organism, resulting in an *adaptive immune response*. Natural killer lymphocytes do not need prior activation by antigens and are therefore part of an *innate immune response*, which is responsible for identifying tumour cells or cells invaded by some viruses.

Platelets have a lifespan of approximately 5 days and are produced by the natural breaking apart of megakaryocytes to form cell fragments with no nucleus. Their primary role is haemostasis, but they are also involved in the release of mediators such as fibroblast growth factor.

All the cells within the circulation are suspended in plasma: a mixture of water, electrolytes, proteins such as albumin and globulins, various nutrients such as glucose, and clotting factors.

Blood coagulation

The physiology of haemostasis involves a complex interaction among the endothelium, clotting factors and platelets. Normally the subendothelial matrix and tissue factor (TF) are separated from platelets and clotting factors by an intact endothelium. However, blood vessel damage leads to vasospasm, which reduces initial bleeding and slows blood flow, increasing contact time between the blood and the area of injury. Initial haemostasis occurs through the action of platelets. Circulating platelets bind directly to exposed collagen with specific glycoprotein Ia/IIa receptors. von Willebrand's factor, released from both endothelium and activated platelets, strengthens this adhesion. Platelet activation results in a shape change, increasing platelet surface area, allowing the development of extensions which can connect to other platelets (pseudopods). Activated platelets secrete a variety of substances from storage granules, including calcium ions, adenosine diphosphate (ADP), platelet activating factor, von Willebrand's factor, serotonin, factor V and protein S. Activated platelets also undergo a change in a surface receptor, glycoprotein GIIb/IIIa, which allows them to cross-link with fibrinogen. In parallel with all these changes the coagulation pathway is activated, and further platelets adhere and aggregate (Fig. 14.1).

The classical description of coagulation pathways includes an *intrinsic* pathway and an *extrinsic* pathway in which clotting factors are designated with Roman numerals (see Fig. 14.1). Each pathway consists of a cascade in which a clotting factor is activated and in turn catalyses the activation of another pathway. The intrinsic pathway involves the sequential activation of factors XII, XI and IX. The extrinsic pathway involves the activation of factor VII by TF and is sometimes called the *tissue factor pathway*. Of the two pathways, the extrinsic pathway is considered to be the more important because abnormal expression of the intrinsic pathway does not necessarily result in abnormal clotting. The intrinsic pathway may have an additional role in the inflammatory response.

Both the intrinsic and extrinsic pathways result in a *final common pathway* which involves the activation of factor X. Activated factor X in turn converts prothrombin to thrombin (factor II to IIa), which allows the conversion of fibrinogen to fibrin (factor I to Ia). Fibrin then becomes cross-linked to form a clot.

It is important to note that this description of intrinsic and extrinsic pathways is essentially a description of what happens in laboratory *in vitro* conditions. The *in vivo* process is much more of an interplay among platelets, circulating factors and the endothelium.

The following steps can be conceptualised (see Fig. 14.1):

- *Initiation*. Damaged cells express TF, which, after activation by binding with circulating factor VIIa, initiates the coagulation process by activating factor IX to factor IXa and factor X to factor Xa. Rapid binding of factor Xa to factor II occurs, producing small amounts of thrombin (factor IIa).
- *Amplification*. The amount of thrombin produced by these initiation reactions is insufficient to form adequate fibrin, so a series of amplification steps occurs. Activated factors IX, X and VII promote the activation of factor VII bound to TF. Without this step, there are only very small amounts of activated factor VII present. In addition, thrombin generates activated factors V and VIII.

There is a parallel system of anticoagulation, involving antithrombins and proteins C and S, which helps prevent an uncontrolled cascade of thrombosis. Thrombin binds to thrombomodulin on the endothelium. This prevents the procoagulant action of thrombin. In addition, the thrombin–thrombomodulin complex activates protein C. Along with its cofactor, protein S, activated protein C proteolyzes factor Va and factor VIIIa. Factor Va increases the rate of conversion of prothrombin to thrombin, and factor VIIIa is a cofactor in the generation of activated factor X. Inactivation of these two factors therefore leads to a marked reduction in thrombin production. Activated protein C also has effects on endothelial cells and leukocytes independent of its anticoagulant properties, including anti-inflammatory properties, reduction of leukocyte adhesion and chemotaxis and inhibition of apoptosis.

Antithrombin is a serine protease inhibitor found in high concentrations in plasma. It inhibits the action of activated factors Xa, iXa, XIa, XIIa and thrombin and also factor VIIa from the extrinsic (tissue factor) pathway. Heparin binds to antithrombin to increase the inactivation of thrombin by a factor of more than 2000. Antithrombin deficiency states predispose to thrombosis.

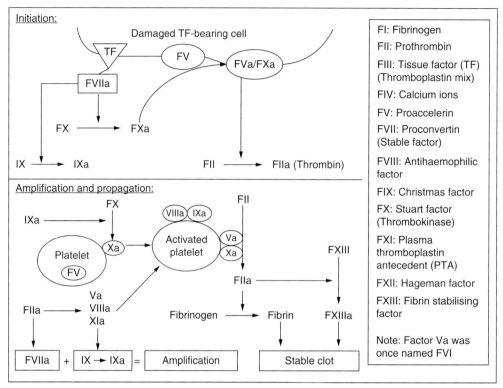

Fig. 14.1 Clotting processes. (From Curry, A.N.G., & Pierce, J.M.T. (2007) *Continuing education in anaesthesia critical care & pain.* 2(2), 45–50.)

In addition, platelet adhesion and aggregation are normally inhibited in intact blood vessels by the negative charge present on the endothelium, which prevents platelet adhesion, and by substances which inhibit aggregation, such as nitric oxide and prostacyclin.

Controlled fibrinolysis occurs naturally, involving the conversion of plasminogen to plasmin, which in turn degrades fibrin. Plasminogen can be activated by a naturally occurring tissue plasminogen activator and urokinase.

Common laboratory tests used to investigate coagulation include the following:

- Activated prothrombin time (PT), which tests for factors involved in the extrinsic coagulation pathway (prothrombin, factors V, VII, X); normal range 12–14 s, but often expressed as a ratio (the international normalised ratio, INR)
- Activated partial thromboplastin time (APTT, also known as the kaolin cephalin clotting time, KCCT), which tests for factors present within the intrinsic pathway (including factors I, II, V, VIII, IX and X); normal range 26–33.5 s, often also expressed as a ratio (APTTR)

- Thromboplastin time (TT), which tests for the presence of fibrinogen and the function of platelets; normal range 14–16 s
- Fibrinogen assay; normal range 1.5–4 g L^{-1}

Coagulopathies and their impact on anaesthesia and surgery

Various conditions and drugs are known to be associated with increased blood loss during surgery (Tables 14.1 and 14.2).

Monitoring of coagulation

If a patient presents with a known condition or with a history of abnormal bleeding (e.g. menorrhagia or excessive bleeding after previous minor injuries), a coagulation profile including platelet count, PT, TT and APTT is indicated. A platelet count is part of the full blood count considered routine before major surgery. In contrast, coagulation screens should not be considered routine. They are designed for

Table 14.1 Conditions known to increase blood loss

Coagulopathies	Anticoagulant drugs	See Table 14.2
	Auto-antibodies	Antibodies to individual factors, associated with haemophilia treatment
	Congenital diseases	Common disorders include: • Factor XI deficiency • Haemophilia A and haemophilia B (Christmas disease) • von Willebrand's disease
	Disseminated intravascular coagulation (DIC)	Common causes include: • Allergy • Embolism (e.g. pulmonary embolism, fat embolism) • Extracorporeal circulation • Infection • Malignancy • Pregnancy complications (e.g. abruption, amniotic fluid embolism, fetal death, pre-eclampsia) • Transfusion reactions • Trauma and burns
	Haemodilution	Massive transfusion
	Liver disease	As a result of thrombocytopaenia or reduced coagulation factor synthesis
	Vitamin K deficiency	Biliary tract or bowel disorders Inadequate diet
	Envenomation	Various snake venoms have the ability to cause hypofibrinogenaemia, DIC or platelet antagonism
Platelet disorders	Decreased production	Aplastic anaemia Congenital (e.g. Fanconi's) anaemia Folate deficiency Liver disease Malignancy with marrow infiltration Marrow fibrosis or myelodysplastic syndrome Radiation poisoning Toxins (drug or chemical reactions, including alcohol) Tuberculosis with marrow infiltration Vitamin B12 deficiency Viral infections (e.g. HIV)
	Increased consumption	Autoimmune thrombocytopaenic purpura DIC Drugs causing immune-mediated reactions (e.g. heparin/HIT) HELLP syndrome (in pregnancy) Hypersplenism Infections causing immune-mediated reactions (e.g. HIV, mononucleosis) Paroxysmal nocturnal haemoglobinuria Post-transfusion purpura Sepsis TTP/HUS
	Impaired function	Congenital (e.g. Glanzmann thrombasthenia) Drugs (see Table 14.2) Hypergammaglobulinaemia Myeloproliferative diseases Uraemia

Continued

Table 14.1 Conditions known to increase blood loss—cont'd

Vascular disorders	Acquired	Henoch–Schönlein purpura Vitamin C deficiency (scurvy)
	Congenital	Hereditary haemorrhagic telangiectasia Ehlers–Danlos syndrome

HELLP, Haemolysis, elevated liver enzymes, low platelets; *HIT,* heparin-induced thrombocytopaenia; *HUS,* haemolytic uraemic syndrome; *TTP,* thrombotic thrombocytopaenic purpura.

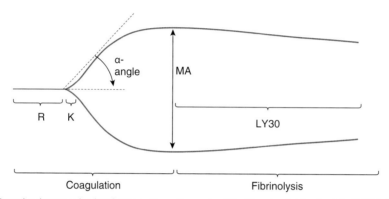

Fig. 14.2 A typical thromboelastography (TEG) trace. (From Gempeler, F.E., Diaz, L., & Murcia, P.C. (2009) Evaluating coagulation in prostatectomy. *Revista Colombiana de Anestiologia,* 37, 202–211.)

specific investigation of patients with bleeding disorders, not as screening tests (see Chapters 19 and 20). They have a low probability of detecting a clinically important abnormality in the absence of any relevant history. During surgery or major haemorrhage, point-of-care viscoelastic monitors such as the thromboelastograph or rotational thromboelastograph measure blood coagulation at the bedside and help aid decision making about which blood products should be given. Unlike other tests of coagulation, thromboelastography (TEG) and rotational thromboelastometry (ROTEM) assess platelet function, clot strength and fibrinolysis. In TEG a small sample of the patient's blood is gently rotated through an angle of 4 degrees and 25 mins, repeated six times a minute to imitate sluggish venous blood flow. A pin is suspended from a torsion wire into the blood sample. Development of fibrin strands couple the motion of the cup to the pin. This coupling is directly proportional to the clot strength. Increased tension in the wire is detected by the electromagnetic transducer, and the electrical signal is amplified to create a trace. From the shape of the trace produced, various measurements indicate the time to clot formation, speed of clot formation, clot strength and fibrinolysis (Fig. 14.2). These values can be used to help decision making about which blood products or antifibrinolytics are required to correct coagulation.

Four values are produced that represent clot formation. The R value represents the time until the clot is first detected. K value is the time from the end of R until the clot reaches 20 mm (speed of clot formation). Alpha angle gives similar information to K. Maximum amplitude (MA) reflects clot strength. LY30 is the percentage decrease in amplitude 30 after MA; it reflects the degree of fibrinolysis. A prolonged R time is usually treated with fresh frozen plasma. The α-angle represents the conversion of fibrinogen to fibrin, and therefore a depressed α-angle is often treated with cryoprecipitate. Most of the MA is derived from platelet function, and therefore a reduced MA is usually treated with platelet transfusions or drugs that improve platelet function such as desmopressin (DDAVP). Rotational thromboelastometry uses a modification of TEG. A disposable pin is attached to a shaft which is connected to a thin spring and slowly oscillates back and forth. Movement originates from the pin and not the cup, and the signal is transmitted using an optical detector instead of a torsion wire. Because of its design, ROTEM is more robust, and it is relatively insensitive to mechanical shocks or vibrations. By using differing activators and inhibitors it is possible to obtain differential information about specific aspects of the coagulation process such as heparin, platelets, coagulation factors, fibrinogen and fibrinolysis. The advantage of these monitors over formal

Table 14.2 Drugs known to increase or reduce blood loss

Commonly used drugs that increase blood loss		
Antiplatelet agents	ADP receptor inhibitors	Clopidogrel, prasugrel, ticagrelor, ticlopidine
	cAMP inhibitors	Dipyridamole
	Cyclo-oxygenase inhibitors	Aspirin, non-steroidal anti-inflammatory drugs (NSAIDs)
	Glycoprotein IIb/IIIa antagonists	Abciximab, eptifibatide, tirofiban
	Phosphodiesterase inhibitors	Cilostazol
	Thromboxane inhibitors	Terutroban
	Thromboxane & PDGF inhibition	Prostacyclin (e.g. epoprostenol)
Anticoagulants	Factor Xa inhibitor	Rivaroxaban, apixaban, fondaparinux
	Heparins (factors II, Xa)	Heparin (unfractionated), low molecular weight heparins (LMWHs), heparinoids (e.g. danaparoid)
	Thrombin (factor II) inhibitors	Dabigatran, argatroban, hirudins (e.g. lepirudin, bivalirudin)
	Vitamin K antagonists (factors II, VII, IX, X)	Coumarins (e.g. warfarin), phenindione
Fibrinolytic drugs	Plasminogen activation	Alteplase, reteplase, streptokinase, tenecteplase, urokinase
Miscellaneous	Calcium (factor IV) antagonism	Citrate[a]
	Inhibition of factor conversion (V–Va; VIII–VIIIa)	Activated protein C[b]
		Drug-eluting stents[c]
Drugs that reduce blood loss		
Aminocaproic acid	Plasminogen activation inhibitor	
Aprotinin	Inhibitor of plasmin, trypsin, chymotrypsin, kallikrein, thrombin and activated protein C	
Conjugated oestrogens	Stimulate factors VII, XII and von Willebrand's factor release	
DDAVP (desmopressin)	Stimulates factor VIII and von Willebrand's factor release	
Etamsylate	Increased platelet aggregation, possible inhibition of prostacyclin metabolites	
Protamine	Reverses the effects of heparin	
Tranexamic acid	Plasminogen activation inhibitor (and plasmin inhibitor at high doses)	
Vitamin K	Required for the production of factors II, VII, IX and X; therefore can reverse the effects of vitamin K antagonists	
Miscellaneous	Topical haemostatic agents (e.g. oxidised cellulose, thrombin sealants, fibrin sealants, chitin dressings, platelet gels, cyanoacrylates) Various blood components (see Table 14.5)	

[a]Citrate may be used to anticoagulate some dialysis machines and may be used to 'lock' CVCs (i.e. keep them from becoming blocked with blood clot).
[b]Activated protein C has been used in the treatment of severe sepsis.
[c]Used in various angioplasty procedures; mechanism of action depends on drug being released by the stent.
PDGF, Platelet-derived growth factor.

laboratory tests of coagulation is the speed at which the results are obtained, allowing correction of coagulopathies more promptly and with the correct products. Regular calibration, correct use and understanding of results are key to their safe and effective use.

Diseases affecting coagulation

Patients known to have inherited abnormalities of coagulation, such as haemophilias A and B and von Willebrand's disease, need specialist input from a haematologist because they are likely to need supplementation of specific factor concentrates before surgery, guided by factor assays. This is particularly true of patients known to have antibodies (inhibitors) to the factor in question. Because spontaneous joint or muscle haemorrhage is common, it is rare for patients with severe disease to present for unrelated surgery with an occult diagnosis of haemophilia. Less severe disease (e.g. patients who are heterozygous for haemophilia with abnormally low factor concentrations) or acquired disease (e.g. acquired von Willebrand's disease) may occasionally present unexpectedly during surgery, and a suspicion of abnormal clotting during surgery should prompt urgent blood samples to assess the coagulation profile.

In the past the use of factor concentrates from pooled donor units meant that many patients with haemophilia were infected with HIV or hepatitis viruses, and older patients may therefore be infected.

Depending on the type of haemophilia, tranexamic acid (an antifibrinolytic), desmopressin (DDAVP) or repeated factor infusions may need to be given intraoperatively. The use of desmopressin may be associated with water retention and, potentially, acute hyponatraemia.

Thrombocytopenia

Thrombocytopenia is usually defined as a platelet count $< 100 \times 10^9$ L^{-1}; however, the point at which thrombocytopenia becomes important clinically depends upon the scenario. It can be caused by a reduction in platelet production (or increased platelet breakdown; see Table 14.1). Immune thrombocytopenia (ITP) is a relatively common cause of a low platelet count, and these patients need referral to a haematologist preoperatively as in most cases the platelet count increases to a level considered safe for surgery in response to a short course of corticosteroids. Some thrombocytopenic patients may require perioperative platelet transfusions if they do not respond.

It is not clear exactly what level of platelet count is acceptable for any given procedure, but the following guidance has been suggested:
- Platelet count $> 50 \times 10^9$ L^{-1} for most types of surgery, gastroscopy, insertion of invasive lines and liver biopsy.
- $>75 \times 10^9$ L^{-1} for neuraxial anaesthesia.
- 100×10^9 L^{-1} for neurosurgery and ophthalmic surgery.

It should be noted that platelet transfusions are relatively contraindicated in haemolytic-uraemic syndrome/thrombotic thrombocytopenic purpura (TTP), where their use may precipitate further thrombosis. In such cases the risks of transfusion should be weighed against the risks of bleeding.

One notable cause of perioperative thrombocytopaenia is heparin-induced thrombocytopaenia (HIT), an antibody-mediated reaction thought to occur after exposure to heparin concurrent with a physiological insult such as surgery or critical illness. Heparin-induced thrombocytopaenia is more strongly associated with unfractionated heparin than low molecular weight heparins (LMWHs), usually occurs 4–6 days after exposure and results in the platelet count decreasing to values up to 50% less than the patient's normal value. Heparin-induced thrombocytopaenia rarely results in acute haemorrhage; it is thought to be associated with a prothrombotic tendency requiring cessation of heparin and sometimes treatment with an alternative anticoagulant such as danaparoid (warfarin is not suitable in this situation). Several scoring systems exist to evaluate the likelihood of HIT, and a laboratory enzyme-linked immunosorbant assay (ELISA) can be used for confirmation.

Acquired coagulopathies

Acquired coagulopathy can also occur as an acute event, such as after major trauma, during major haemorrhage or in the presence of disseminated intravascular coagulopathy (DIC). In major haemorrhage, clotting factors can become depleted if not replaced promptly. The management of coagulopathy in major haemorrhage should be guided by clinical urgency and laboratory tests.

Trauma-induced coagulopathy

Bleeding accounts for 30%–40% of all trauma-related deaths and usually occurs within hours after injury. In almost half of haemorrhagic deaths after trauma, coagulopathy is implicated and is highly preventable. The aetiology of trauma-induced coagulopathy is multifactorial (Box 14.1) and complex but certainly appears before administration of intravenous fluids or blood products, so is not solely a consequence of haemodilution. An acute endogenous coagulopathy (i.e. acute traumatic coagulopathy; ATC) occurs within minutes after injury, before and independent of iatrogenic factors; this is now accepted as the primary cause of impaired coagulation after injury. In ATC there is immediate activation of multiple haemostatic pathways, with increased fibrinolysis. Acute traumatic coagulopathy presents immediately after injury and continues throughout the resuscitation phase. Resuscitation-associated coagulopathy which involves hypothermia, metabolic acidosis and dilutional coagulopathy aggravates ATC. Genetic factors, tissue inflammation and existing comorbidities also contribute to

Box 14.1 **Factors associated with coagulopathy in trauma**

Physiological dilution of clotting factors
Hypothermia
Acidosis
Red cell loss
Trauma-induced fibrinolysis
Injury-related inflammation
Hypoperfusion
Hypocalcaemia
Genetic predispositions
Iatrogenic – dilution by fluids, anticoagulant effects of
  intravenous fluids

Table 14.3 Diagnostic scoring system for disseminated intravascular coagulation (DIC)

If the patient has an underlying disorder known to be associated with overt DIC, score as below.	
Platelet count	
■ $>100 \times 10^9 \text{ L}^{-1}$	
	0 points
■ $50–100 \times 10^9 \text{ L}^{-1}$	
	1
■ $<50 \times 10^9 \text{ L}^{-1}$	
	2
Increased fibrin marker (e.g. D-dimer or fibrin degradation products)	
■ No increase	
	0
■ Moderate increase	
	1
■ Strong increase	
	2
Prolonged PT	
■ <3 s more than normal	
	0
■ $3–6$ s more than normal	
	1
■ >6 s more than normal	
	2
Fibrinogen level	
■ $>1 \text{ g L}^{-1}$	
	0
■ $<1 \text{ g L}^{-1}$	
	1
A calculated score ≥5 is compatible with overt DIC. The score should be repeated daily.	
A calculated score <5 may be suggestive of non-overt DIC. The score should be repeated every 1–2 days.	

(Reproduced from Levi, M., Toh, C.H., Thachil, J., & Watson, H.G. (2009) Guidelines for the diagnosis and management of disseminated intravascular coagulation. British Committee for Standards in Haematology. *British Journal of Haematology.* 145(1), 24–33. © Blackwell Publishing.)

the coagulopathy. Together they are referred to as trauma-induced coagulopathy.

Most trauma centres have well-defined policies for managing major blood loss (see later). After publication of the CRASH-2 study, tranexamic acid (1 g as soon as possible after injury, followed by 1 g given over 8 h) is recommended for patients presenting with major trauma.

Disseminated intravascular coagulation

In DIC the microcirculation of different organs becomes damaged by fibrin clots generated by hyperactive coagulation pathways. The pathophysiological production of so many fibrin clots results in a consumptive coagulopathy, rendering the patient susceptible to haemorrhage as a result of surgery or other invasive procedures. Disseminated intravascular coagulation has several causes (Table 14.3), and these should be identified and corrected wherever possible. The diagnosis of DIC can be difficult to make and relies upon evaluating the results of several aspects of a coagulation profile; a haematologist should be consulted if DIC is suspected. A scoring system exists to evaluate the likelihood of DIC (see Table 14.3). Patients who develop DIC in the perioperative period, or who require surgery to treat the cause of DIC (e.g. patients with intra-abdominal sepsis), are at increased risk of major haemorrhage. They are likely to need replacement of consumed coagulation factors in the form of platelets, fresh frozen plasma and cryoprecipitate.

Occasionally, DIC may present as a predominantly thrombotic condition, and in these cases, heparin may be indicated.

Drug-induced coagulopathies

The increase in numbers of interventional cardiology procedures has been accompanied by an ever-increasing number of available anticoagulant drugs. As well as the traditional anticoagulants such as unfractionated heparin and warfarin, many newer direct oral anticoagulants (DOACs) are prescribed. These drugs act on different aspects of coagulation (see Table 14.2) and have different half-lives, so the times required for discontinuation before surgery also differ. Factor Xa inhibitors are named with Xa in the drug name – api*xa*ban, rivaro*xa*ban. In addition, the clearance of some DOACs is affected by renal function, and creatinine clearance should be considered when advising patients when to stop their medication (see Table 19.3; Chapter 19).

If surgery is required urgently, it may be necessary to reverse the effects of anticoagulant therapy acutely. This should be done under the guidance of a haematologist, but in the case of heparin may involve the use of protamine. Rapid reversal of vitamin K–dependent coagulopathy can be achieved safely with prothrombin complex concentrates (PCCs). Vitamin K takes hours to work and should be given at the same time to reduce the risk of postoperative coagulopathy. In less urgent situations, vitamin K can be given alone or the warfarin simply stopped for a few days. Many of the DOACs are irreversible, and close coordination with a haematologist is required. Dabigatran is an exception as a reversal agent (idarucizumab) is available; this may be given if serious bleeding occurs or if urgent surgery is required. In acute circumstances where drugs are thought to be affecting platelet function, platelet transfusions may be considered.

Interventional procedures and regional anaesthesia in coagulopathic patients

Interventional procedures such as the insertion of central venous catheters, epidural block or regional nerve blocks constitute a significant risk of haemorrhage or haematoma formation in coagulopathic patients. Of particular note are the risks of airway obstruction from failed jugular venous catheter insertion and paralysis caused by epidural haematoma formation.

It is likely that the routine use of ultrasound imaging has reduced the risks associated with many procedures, but in profoundly coagulopathic patients it may still be advisable to resort to alternative, safer techniques; for example, central venous catheterisation of the femoral vein may be preferable to the subclavian or internal jugular routes.

The level of coagulopathy at which various procedures can be considered safe is far from clear. Suggested thresholds for minimum platelet counts are discussed above, whilst INR and APTT ratios of ≤1.4 have been considered *relatively* safe for most procedures undertaken by anaesthetists.

There are specific problems when the effect of a drug on coagulation is difficult to measure directly. There are several consensus statements on the safety of neuraxial blockade

in differing circumstances. These typically include the following:
- LMWH (*thromboprophylaxis* dose): needle insertion should be delayed until 12 h after last dose; epidural catheters should be removed at least 12 h after the last dose and at least 4 h before the next dose
- Subcutaneous unfractionated heparin thromboprophylaxis: needle insertion should be delayed until 4 h after the last dose; epidural catheters should be removed at least 1 h before the next dose
- NSAID therapy, including low-dose aspirin: can be continued and does not seem to represent an increased risk
- Ticlopidine: should be discontinued 14 days before neuraxial blockade
- Clopidogrel: should be discontinued 7 days before neuraxial blockade
- GIIb/IIIa inhibitors: should be discontinued 9–48 h before neuraxial blockade

It should be noted that evidence in this area is sparse, and these guidelines are largely based on evidence from case series. Available guidelines are incomplete, difficult to extrapolate to different settings (e.g. regional anaesthetic techniques with lower associated risk) and may not represent best practice. When in doubt, senior anaesthetic and/or specialist haematology advice should be sought.

Thrombosis and acute ischaemic events

All hospital patients should undergo an assessment of their risk of developing venous thromboembolism (VTE) (see Table 19.12; Chapter 19) to ensure that appropriate prophylactic measures are taken. Reassessment should be undertaken after 24 h and at any time that the patient's clinical condition changes. Any assessment should weigh the risk of developing VTE against the risk of bleeding which might occur when pharmacological prophylaxis is prescribed. There are also a number of congenital and acquired conditions which are associated with an increased risk of VTE (Table 14.4). Methods of pharmacological prophylaxis include subcutaneous LMWHs, subcutaneous unfractionated heparin and newer anticoagulants such as fondaparinux, dabigatran and rivaroxaban. Antiplatelet agents such as aspirin are not considered to provide adequate protection against VTE when used in isolation.

Mechanical methods of VTE prophylaxis are often also used, either as an adjunct to pharmacological methods or as an alternative to them where the bleeding risk is considered high. Mechanical methods include antiembolism stockings and foot-impulse or pneumatic compression devices (both stockings and compression devices may be thigh or knee

Table 14.4 Conditions known to increase the risk of thrombosis

Acquired	Antiphospholipid syndrome
	Cardiac failure
	Diabetes
	Heparin-induced thrombocytopaenia
	Hyperlipidaemia
	Malignancy
	Myeloproliferative disorders
	Nephrotic syndrome
	Oral contraceptive pill (oestrogen therapies)
	Paroxysmal nocturnal haemoglobinuria
	Polycythaemia
	TTP/HUS
Congenital	Antithrombin deficiency
	Dysfibrinogenaemia
	Factor V Leiden variant (activated protein C resistance)
	Hyperhomocysteinaemia
	Protein C deficiency
	Protein S deficiency
	Prothrombin genetic variant

HUS, Haemolytic uraemic syndrome; *TTP*, thrombotic thrombocytopaenia purpura.

length). There is very little evidence to support the use of any one mechanical device rather than the alternatives. Mechanical methods may not be appropriate in patients with damaged skin, peripheral neuropathy, oedema, peripheral arterial disease or other conditions in which fitting the devices might be problematic or cause damage.

In patients who are at very high risk of both bleeding and thromboembolic events, the pre-emptive insertion of a vena cava filter may be required.

Blood products and blood transfusion

The transfusion of whole blood is relatively uncommon, and donated blood is usually separated into its constituent components, which are then available for transfusion. A wide range of blood products are available, the most common of which are listed in Table 14.5 along with their indications. Units of packed red cells are most commonly transfused during the resuscitation of acute haemorrhage or as a treatment of symptomatic anaemia.

Red cell concentrates are commonly leukocyte depleted and resuspended to a haematocrit of 0.6. In the UK the red cells are usually suspended in an additive solution: SAGM

(saline to maintain isotonicity; adenine as an adenosine triphosphate (ATP) precursor to maintain red cell viability; glucose for red cell metabolism; mannitol to reduce red cell lysis). These additives are designed to extend the safe storage period, and packed red cells are kept refrigerated at 4 °C. Currently, red cells can be stored for up to 5–6 weeks. There is ongoing debate as to whether the storage lesion which occurs during this time is clinically relevant, with some studies suggesting that outcomes are worse for patients who have had 'old' blood transfused.

Red cell storage lesion

A variety of biochemical and immunological changes occur during red cell storage which may have clinical impact.
- Concentrations of 2,3-DPG fall rapidly (undetectable within 2 weeks). The clinical consequence is less clear, probably because 2,3-DPG concentrations are restored to normal very rapidly after transfusion.
- Adenosine triphosphate depletion occurs, particularly beyond 5 weeks, and is associated with morphological changes. As with 2,3-DPG, ATP normalises promptly after transfusion, and the morphological changes reverse.
- Haemoglobin has been found to be an important part of the control of regional blood flow because of its interaction with nitric oxide. This ability is lost early (days) after blood storage, but the clinical impact of this is not yet clear.
- Morphological changes during storage are complex, but in general, red cells become less deformable; these changes may be only partly reversible.
- It has long been recognised that red cell transfusion can have systemic immunological effects, including effects on organ transplants, infection and malignancy. The causes of these effects are not clear but may involve residual leukocytes and immunological mediators released by red cells.

In patients who are asymptomatic and not actively bleeding, current evidence suggests that there is no benefit in transfusion provided that the haemoglobin concentration is 70 g L⁻¹ or greater. This 'trigger' of 70 g L⁻¹ is derived from the Transfusion Requirements in Critical Care (TRICC) trial. Despite the publication of this study, there remains doubt as to what the 'safe' level of anaemia is for patients with some specific conditions, including ischaemic heart disease, head injury and acute burns. For patients who are symptomatic or who are actively bleeding, a higher target haemoglobin concentration of 90–100 g L⁻¹ is often adopted. More information on patient blood management is provided in Chapter 20.

Packed red cells must be checked before they are transfused to ensure that the donated blood is compatible with the recipient's blood, the most important aspect of which is ABO and Rhesus D (RhD) compatibility.

Table 14.5 Indications and uses of blood products

Blood product	Indication	Presentation and/or dose
Albumin (human albumin solution; HAS)	• Fluid resuscitation/correction of hypovolaemia[a] • Therapeutic plasma exchange • Ascites and large volume paracentesis • Spontaneous bacterial peritonitis • Hepatorenal syndrome • Correction of hypoalbuminaemia[b]	Iso-oncotic (4.5%) Hyperoncotic (20%) Volume depends upon product
Cryoprecipitate	*Correction of hypofibrinogenaemia* • Coagulopathy caused by major haemorrhage • Disseminated intravascular coagulopathy • Hereditary hypofibrinogenaemia	Typically issued as $10 \times 20–40$ ml bags or $1 \times \approx$ 300 ml bag 300 ml contains 1.5–3 g fibrinogen In haemorrhage, maintain fibrinogen >1 g L^{-1}
Fresh frozen plasma (FFP)	*Correction of coagulation factor deficiencies* • Coagulopathy caused by major haemorrhage • Liver disease • Inherited coagulation deficiencies if specific factor concentrates not available • Warfarin overdose if prothrombin complex concentrate not available • Therapeutic plasma exchange	Issued in bags of approximately 300 ml Dose is 12–15 ml kg^{-1} (typically 1000 ml for an adult) In haemorrhage, transfuse to maintain prothrombin time and activate partial thromboplastin time at $<1.5 \times$ normal ranges
Platelets	*Correction of thrombocytopaenia, or where there is evidence of platelet dysfunction* • Thrombocytopaenia caused by major haemorrhage • Haematological malignancies and their treatment • Idiopathic or thrombotic thrombocytopaenic purpura • Disseminated intravascular coagulopathy	Issued in bags of 250–300 ml Each bag increases platelet count by approximately 20×10^9 L^{-1} In haemorrhage associated with multiple trauma or CNS trauma, maintain platelet count $>100 \times 10^9$ L^{-1} In other situations, triggers may vary (see text)
Red cells (packed red cells; PRC)	• Resuscitation of major haemorrhage • Correction of symptomatic anaemia • Treatment of sickle-cell crises	Packed red cells are issued in bags of approximately 300 ml^{-1}, which will raise the haemoglobin concentration in adults by approximately 10 g L^{-1} Transfusion triggers vary according to context (see text) Suspended in SAGM (saline, adenine, glucose, mannitol)

[a]Albumin may be used safely for volume resuscitation, but there is little evidence to suggest that it is associated with improved outcomes compared with other resuscitation fluids. It may be associated with worse outcomes when used in certain conditions such as traumatic brain injury.
[b]The use of human albumin solution to correct hypoalbuminaemia is contentious. Hypoalbuminaemia is associated with increased mortality in critically ill patients, but actively correcting it is not clearly associated with improved outcome. Hyperoncotic albumin has also been used in the management of acute respiratory distress syndrome (ARDS).
CNS, Central nervous system.

- Patients of blood group O can receive only group O donated blood.
- Patients of blood group A can receive group O or group A donated blood.
- Patients of blood group B can receive group O or group B donated blood.
- Patients of blood group AB can receive groups O, A, B or AB donated blood.
- Patients with RhD-positive blood can receive RhD-positive or RhD-negative blood.
- Patients with RhD negative blood will preferentially be given RhD-negative blood but occasionally may be transfused RhD-positive blood unless they are an RhD-negative female patient with childbearing potential, in which case they should only ever receive RhD-negative blood.

Other, less common, RBC antibody/antigen reactions may also occur, and if time allows, a full cross-match should be undertaken. In more urgent situations a more limited approach may be necessary.

Fresh frozen plasma (FFP) is derived from whole blood plasma and is frozen to −35 °C. It is a rich source of clotting factors. Once thawed to room temperature it must be transfused within 4 h; however, it may be stored at 4 °C for 24 h. Each bag of FFP is derived from a single donor. The transfusion of FFP also depends upon ABO grouping but is more complex. Group O FFP may only be given to group O patients, whilst FFP of groups A, B and AB may be given to any recipient, but only if it does not contain a high titre of anti-A or anti-B activity. If possible, the transfused unit of FFP should be of the same group as the recipient.

Cryoprecipitate is prepared from plasma and contains fibrinogen, von Willebrand's factor, factor VIII, factor XIII and fibronectin. It is usually given in prepooled concentrates of five units; each individual unit is from a separate donor. Cryoprecipitate is stored frozen and defrosted for use, and pooled concentrates should be transfused within 4 h of thawing.

Platelet transfusions may either be pooled from several donors or obtained from a single donor by apheresis. They are stored in temperature-controlled incubators at 20 °C–24 °C with constant agitation. The shelf life of a bag of platelets is 5 days (7 days if bacterial screening has been performed).

The transfusion of blood products is not without risk (Table 14.6), and whenever possible, informed consent should be obtained from the recipient first. Of particular note are the risks associated with the transfusion of incompatible blood products, which are considered to be Never Events within the UK (the equivalent to No Pay events within the US system). A zero-tolerance approach to pretransfusion sampling, blood product checking and administration is recommended. In Europe there is a legal obligation to keep a permanent record of all blood products that have been transfused.

Major haemorrhage and massive transfusion protocols

Successful management of major haemorrhage requires a protocol–driven multidisciplinary team approach with involvement of medical, anaesthetic and surgical staff of sufficient seniority underpinned by clear lines of communication between clinicians and the transfusion laboratory. It should result in the immediate release and administration of blood components for initial resuscitation without prior approval from a haematologist. Such protocols work best when specific to clinical areas such as the emergency department, maternity unit, or in clinical scenarios such as trauma or major intraoperative haemorrhage. Their activation should also mobilise other resources such as additional staff such as porters, blood warmers, pressure infusers and cell salvage devices.

Most major haemorrhage packs contain four units of RBCs and four of FFP (equivalent to the standard dose of 15–20 ml kg^{-1}). Depending on the situation, platelets may also be provided, and PCCs may be substituted for FFP.

Group O red cells should be readily available and transfused if group-specific or cross-matched blood is not yet available. Children and women of childbearing age must receive O Rh-negative blood, whilst men and older women can also receive O Rh-positive. If possible, the transfusion of red cells and clotting products should be guided by laboratory results or by near-patient testing (e.g. near-patient haemoglobinometers or TEG). However, waiting for confirmation of coagulopathy before administering appropriate therapy is likely to lead to greater blood loss, use of more blood products and worse outcome.

In the initial resuscitation phase in trauma, administration of RBCs and FFP in a ratio of 1:1 should be used to replace fluid volume. The administration of two pools of cryoprecipitate and one adult dose of platelets should be considered until test results are available and bleeding controlled. The management of major haemorrhage is discussed further in Chapter 27 (Management of Critical Incidents).

Blood management for elective surgery

If large volumes of blood loss (>1000 ml or >20% of estimated total blood volume) are anticipated, such as during major elective surgery, it should be planned for in advance.

- *Preoperatively:*
  - In patients who are known to be anaemic, the cause of the anaemia should be investigated and, if possible, corrected before surgery.

Table 14.6 Risks and complications of blood transfusion

Acute

	Clinical Signs	Pathophysiology
Acute haemolytic reaction	Fever and other symptoms/signs of haemolysis within 24 hours of transfusion, with by one or more of: • decrease in Hb • increase in LDH or bilirubin • positive direct antiglobulin test (DAT) • positive crossmatch	Oligosaccharide antigens present on donor red cell membranes react with antibodies in the recipient's plasma leading to degranulation of mast cells, inflammation, increased vascular permeability and hypotension.
Transfusion-related acute lung injury (TRALI)	Acute dyspnoea with hypoxia and bilateral pulmonary infiltrates on chest radiograph, occurring within 6 h of transfusion and not associated with TACO or other likely causes.	Immune-mediated leucocyte agglutinating antibodies from the donor react with white cells of the recipient. The leucoagglutinates are trapped in the lungs causing capillary leak, neutrophil extravasation and activation. Non-immune mediated. An initial insult e.g. sepsis primes the vascular endothelium to attract neutrophils which are then activated by biologically active compounds in stored blood.
Transfusion-related circulatory overload (TACO)	Circulatory overload within six hours of transfusion resulting in four of: • tachycardia • hypertension • acute respiratory distress • pulmonary oedema • evidence of positive fluid balance	Acute left ventricular or congestive cardiac failure
Acute transfusion reactions	Febrile, allergic or hypotensive reactions occurring within 24 hours of a transfusion (excluding incorrect component transfusion, haemolytic reactions, TRALI, TACO or bacterial contamination).	Either donor leucocyte antigens react with recipient white cell antibodies or soluble donor antigens react in an already sensitised patient.
Coagulopathy/massive transfusion		Dilution of clotting factors and platelets if large volumes of red blood cells are given.
Delayed		
Delayed haemolytic reaction	Fever and other symptoms or signs of haemolysis more than 24 hours after transfusion; confirmed by one of the following: • decrease in Hb or failure of increment • increase in bilirubin • incompatible crossmatch not detectable before transfusion More common in patients with sickle cell disease	The recipient is already alloimmunised (e.g. to Rh and Kidd). They respond to the repeated presentation of antigen-positive red cells, which leads to degranulation of mast cells.
Iron overload	Recurrent transfusions cause progressive tissue injury, cirrhosis and cardiomyopathy.	Circulating iron from recurrent transfusions exceeds the binding capacity of transferrin and becomes deposited in organs including the heart and the liver.

Table 14.6 Risks and complications of blood transfusion—cont'd

Delayed		
Transfusion-related graft versus host disease	Characterised by fever, rash, liver dysfunction, diarrhoea, pancytopenia, and bone marrow hypoplasia occurring less than 30 days following transfusion.	Lymphocytes from the donor proliferate within an immunocompromised recipient, or an immune competent recipient with a very similar HLA type to the donor.
Purpuric reactions	Thrombocytopenia 5–12 days after red cell transfusion.	A previously sensitised recipient produces alloantibodies that attack donor platelet antigens and also destroy the patient's own platelets.
Infection transmitted by transfusion	Requires evidence of infection after transfusion and infection in either the donor or transfused product.	Potential agents: • Bacteria • Malaria • HIV • Hepatitis viruses • HTLV • New-variant CJD

- The management of patients with a known coagulopathy should be discussed with a haematologist before surgery because clotting factor replacement may be required. If patients are prescribed medication that is known to affect blood clotting, consideration should be given to stopping this before anaesthesia if possible (see earlier).
- *Intraoperatively:*
  - Blood conservation strategies should be employed whenever possible. These can involve the proactive or reactive use of pharmacological treatments such as tranexamic acid, or topical fibrin sealants (see Table 14.2). Alternatively, mechanical methods of blood conservation may be employed – for example, tourniquets in lower limb surgery.

Intraoperative cell salvage (ICS) is a method of blood conservation in which blood which is lost during surgery is collected by surgical suction, mixed with fluid containing an anticoagulant (usually citrate or heparin) and then centrifuged to create an autologous red cell concentrate which can be transfused back into the patient. The whole procedure is performed in the operating theatre, with an almost continuous circuit between surgical suction and transfusion (Fig. 14.3).

Cell salvage is particularly useful for patients in whom transfusion is complicated by a refusal to accept allogeneic blood or by the lack of availability of a rare blood type. Cell salvage has been used successfully in a wide variety of surgical operations, including Caesarean section and operations for malignancy. When used during obstetric haemorrhage, there is no evidence to suggest that the risk of amniotic fluid embolism is increased, despite the theoretical risk. The

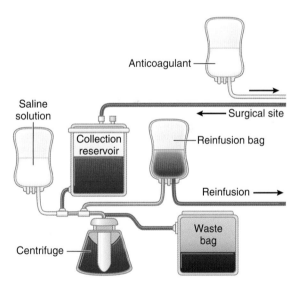

Fig. 14.3 Components of an intraoperative cell salvage system.

use of cell salvage during operations for malignancy remains controversial because of the potential risk of metastatic spread, which may be present even if salvaged blood is transfused through a leukocyte filter. At present there is no evidence to support these concerns; and in the case of surgery for urological malignancy, there are case series which suggest no increased risk to survival if cell salvage is used in conjunction with a leukocyte filter. Cell salvage should not be used in procedures in which there is the potential for blood to become contaminated by faecal contents, pus, iodine, orthopaedic cement or topical clotting agents.

Jehovah's Witnesses

Blood transfusion is not acceptable to most patients who are Jehovah's Witnesses, even if refusal may increase their risk of death. In most cases this principle also extends to blood products such as FFP and platelets, although this should be checked with each individual because each may interpret differently the definition of what constitutes a blood transfusion. If an adult Jehovah's Witness has clearly indicated that he or she will not accept a blood transfusion and it is evident that the patient has the mental capacity to make such a decision, it is unethical to proceed with a transfusion. This remains true even if at some later point the patient loses capacity, for example, by becoming unconscious.

Many hospitals provide specific consent forms for Jehovah's Witnesses that cover the risks associated with transfusion refusal, and many hospitals also have a Jehovah's Witness liaison who may be able to advise on acceptable alternative strategies. For example, intraoperative cell-salvaged blood is often acceptable, as is the use of cardiopulmonary bypass technology where there has been no priming with autologous blood.

The general principles of blood conservation outlined earlier are the same in Jehovah's Witnesses as in other patients. However, when haemorrhage becomes extreme, it is likely that the patient will need extended postoperative critical care management; this may include elective mechanical ventilation and measures to stimulate haemoglobin recovery such as iron supplementation and the administration of erythropoietin.

References/Further reading

Anaesthesia and perioperative care for Jehovah's Witnesses and patients who refuse blood, 2018. Association of Anaesthetists. Available from: https://www.aagbi.org/sites/default/files/JW_Guideline_2018.pdf.

Cell salvage for perioperative blood conservation, 2018. Association of Anaesthetists. Available from: https://www.aagbi.org/sites/default/files/cell%20salvage.pdf.

Gando, S., Levi, M.M., Toh, C.H., 2016. Disseminated intravascular coagulation. Nat. Rev. Dis. Primers. 2, 16037.

Hébert, P.C., Wells, G., Tweeddale, M., et al., 1997. Does transfusion practice affect mortality in critically ill patients? Transfusion requirements in critical care (TRICC) investigators and the Canadian Critical Care Trials Group. Am. J. Respir. Crit. Care Med. 155(5), 1618–1623.

Horlocker, T.T., Vandermeulen, E., Kopp, S.L., 2018. Regional Anesthesia in the Patient Receiving Antithrombotic or Thrombolytic Therapy: American Society of Regional Anesthesia and Pain Medicine Evidence-Based Guidelines (4th ed). Reg. Anesth. Pain Med. 43, 263–309.

Joint United Kingdom Blood Transfusion and Tissue Transplantation Services Professional Advisory Committee. Transfusion Management of Major Haemorrhage. http://www.transfusionguidelines.org/transfusion-handbook.

Klein, A.A., Arnold, P., Bingham, R.M., et al., 2016. AAGBI: the use of blood components and alternatives 2016. Anaesthesia 71(7), 829–842.

National Institute for Health and Care Excellence (UK), 2015. Blood transfusion. Available from: https://www.nice.org.uk/guidance/ng24.

National Institute for Health and Care Excellence (UK), 2015. Venous thromboembolic diseases: diagnosis, management and thrombophilia testing. Available from: https://www.nice.org.uk/guidance/cg144.

Section |2|

Physics and apparatus

Chapter | **15** |

Basic physics for the anaesthetist

Patrick Magee

Knowledge of some physics is required to understand the function of many items of apparatus for anaesthesia delivery and physiological monitoring. This chapter emphasises aspects of physical principles, but the reader should expand on this by further reading (Davey & Diba 2012; Magee & Tooley 2011) and by reading relevant chapters on equipment. Sophisticated measurement techniques may be required for more complex types of anaesthesia in intensive care and during anaesthesia for severely ill patients; an understanding of the principles and limitations involved in performing such measurements is required.

Basic definitions

It is now customary in medical practice to employ the International System (Système Internationale; SI) of units. Common exceptions to the use of the SI system include measurement of arterial pressure and, to a lesser extent, gas pressure. The mercury column is used to calibrate electronic arterial pressure measuring devices and so 'mmHg' is retained. Sea-level atmospheric pressure is often referred to as 760 mmHg or 1.013 bar (or approximately 1 bar). Low pressures are expressed usually in kilopascals (kPa), whilst higher pressures are referred to in bar (100 kPa = 1 bar).

The fundamental quantities in physics are mass, length and time, from which other measures can be derived (Table 15.1). Expressed in basic SI units they are as follows:

Mass (m). The unit of mass is the kilogram (kg).
Length (l). The unit is the metre (m).
Time (t). Measured in seconds (s).

From these basic definitions, several units of measurement may be expressed as derived units:

Volume has units of m^3.

Density is defined as mass per unit volume:

$$density\ (\rho) = \frac{mass}{volume}\ kg\ m^{-3}$$

Velocity is defined as the distance travelled per unit time:

$$velocity\ v = \frac{distance}{time}\ m\ s^{-1}$$

Acceleration is defined as the rate of change of velocity:

$$acceleration\ a = \frac{velocity}{time}\ m\ s^{-2}$$

Force is that which is required to give mass an acceleration:

$$force\ (F) = mass \times acceleration$$
$$= ma$$

The SI unit of force is the newton (N). One newton is the force required to give a mass of 1 kg an acceleration of $1\ m\ s^{-1}$:

$$1\ N = 1\ kg\ m\ s^{-2}$$

Weight is the force of the earth's attraction for a body, even if we incorrectly express it as mass. When a body falls freely under the influence of gravity, it accelerates at a rate of $9.81\ m\ s^{-2}$ (*g*):

$$weight\ (W) = mass \times g$$
$$= m \times 9.81\ kg\ m\ s^{-2}$$

Momentum is defined as mass multiplied by velocity:

$$momentum = m \times v\ kg\ m\ s^{-1}$$

Note that force is also the rate of change of momentum.

Table 15.1 Physical quantities

The fundamental physical quantities are mass, length time, flow of electric current, chemical amount of a substance, thermodynamic temperature and luminous intensity. The other measures are derived from these.

Quantity	Definition	Symbol	SI unit
Length	Unit of distance	l	metre (m)
Mass	Amount of matter	m	kilogram (kg)
Mole	Chemical amount of substance	mol	mol
Density	Mass per unit volume (m/V)	ρ	kg m^{-3}
Time		t	second (s)
Velocity	Distance per unit time (l/t)	v	m s^{-1}
Acceleration	Rate of change of velocity (v/t)	a	m s^{-2}
Force	Gives acceleration to a mass (ma)	F	newton (N) (kg m s^{-2})
Weight	Force exerted by gravity on a mass (mg)	W	kg $\times$ 9.81 m s^{-2}
Pressure	Force per unit area (F/A)	P	N m^{-2}
Temperature	Tendency to gain or lose heat	T	kelvin (K) or degree Celsius (°C)
Work	Performed when a force moves an object (force $\times$ distance)	U	joule (J) (N m)
Energy	Capacity for doing work (force $\times$ distance)	U	joule (J) (N m)
Power	Rate of performing work (joules per second)	P	watt (W) (J s^{-1})
Current	Flow of electric charge	I	ampere (A)
Luminous intensity	Luminous intensity	cd	candela

Work is undertaken when a force moves an object:

$$work = force\ F \times distance\ l\ \text{N m or joules (J)}$$

Energy is the capacity for undertaking work. Thus it has the same units as those of work. Energy can exist in several forms, such as mechanical (kinetic energy (KE) or potential energy (PE)), thermal or electrical, and all have the same units.

Power (*P*) is the rate of doing work. The SI unit of power is the watt:

$$power = \frac{work}{time}\ \text{J s}^{-1}\ \text{or watts (W)}$$
$$= \text{watt (W)}$$

Pressure is defined as force per unit area:

$$pressure\ P = \frac{force\ F}{area}\ a\ \text{N m}^{-2}\ \text{or pascal (P)}$$

As 1 Pa is a rather small unit, it is more common in medical practice to use the kilopascal (kPa): 1 kPa ≈ 7.5 mmHg.

Basic mathematical functions

The following mathematical functions relevant to anaesthetic practice are described:
- The straight line
- The rectangular hyperbola
- The exponential
- Rate of change, differentiation
- Area under a curve, integration

For clarity mathematical notation often uses the period as the symbol for product (multiplication). This is used in this chapter when necessary.

$$A.B.C = A \times B \times C = ABC$$

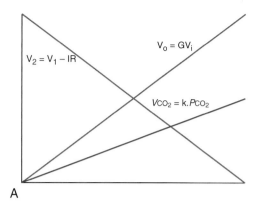

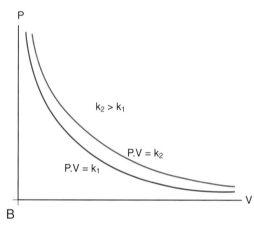

Fig. 15.1. (A) Different straight line relationships of the form $y = mx + c$. (B) Rectangular hyperbola of the type: $PV = k$.

The straight line (Fig. 15.1A) is a direct relationship between two variables with a constant slope. A relevant example is:

$$VCO_2 = K.PCO_2$$

CO_2 volume production is directly proportional to its partial pressure. Similarly,

$$V_{out} = G.V_{in}$$

where the output voltage from an amplifier is directly proportional to the input voltage, multiplied by the gain, G. These lines go through the origin, but there may be an offset on either axis, for the line

$$y = mx + c$$

where m is the slope and c is the offset value of y when x = 0; an example here might be a version of Ohm's law:

$$V_2 = V_1 - IR$$

where the voltage drop across a resistor R carrying a current I is $V_1 - V_2$.

The rectangular hyperbola (Fig. 15.1B) occurs when the product of two variables is constant. A relevant example is Boyle's law at a given temperature T:

$$PV = nRT$$

Note the curve does not cross either axis, but approaches them asymptotically at each extreme. If the temperature of the gas is raised, the curve is shifted upwards and outwards, indicating greater thermal energy.

An exponential function is one where the magnitude of a variable is proportional to the rate of change of that variable:

$$y = k\frac{dy}{dt}$$

and represents many natural and engineering processes. A tear-away exponential, representing bacterial growth for example, is shown in Fig. 15.2A, and a negative exponential (Fig. 15.2B) is one where the magnitude of the variable is decreasing; a relevant example here is plasma drug concentration after a bolus injection:

$$C = C_0 e^{-kt}$$

It touches the y-axis and does not touch the x-axis. Useful time values to characterise the behaviour of the variable include the half-life $t_{1/2}$ when $C = C_0/2$, and the time constant τ (tau) when $C = C_0/e$. A third variation on the exponential is shown in Fig. 15.2C and represents lung filling, for example.

If we want to express the rate of change of a process using a function of time f(t) (as earlier to define an exponential function for example), calculus allows us to perform a mathematical procedure of differentiation to give df(t)/dt. The differential of velocity (ms^{-1}) with respect to time is acceleration (ms^{-2}) The reader is referred to other texts (Cruikshank 1998; Magee & Tooley 2011) for more detail.

Sometimes it is useful to know the area under a curve, and the opposite mathematical procedure is integration. Examples include calculation of energy of a gas by the area under the P–V curve in Fig. 15.1B or the area under a thermal dilution curve in the calculation of cardiac output.

Fluids

Substances may commonly exist in solid, liquid or gaseous form. Other states exist and may be encountered directly

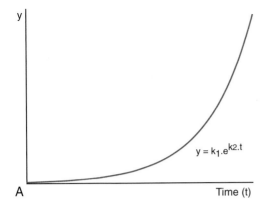

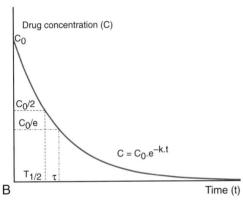

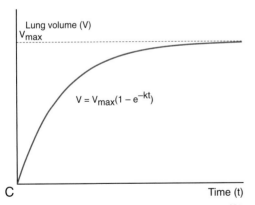

Fig. 15.2. (A) Positive exponential of the form $y = k_1.e^{k2.t}$.
(B) Negative exponential of the form $C = C_o.e^{-k.t}$.
(C) A variant of an exponential of the form $V = V_{max}(1 - e^{-kt})$.

or indirectly by anaesthetists, including plasma and non-classical states such as glass and liquid-crystal. These forms or phases differ from each other according to the random movement of their constituent atoms or molecules. In solids,

molecules oscillate about a fixed point, whereas in liquids the molecules possess higher velocities and therefore higher KE; they move more freely and thus do not bear a constant relationship in space to other molecules. The molecules of gases possess even higher KE and move freely to an even greater extent.

Both gases and liquids are termed fluids. Liquids are incompressible and at constant temperature occupy a fixed volume, conforming to the shape of a container; gases have no fixed volume but expand to occupy the total space of a container. Nevertheless, the techniques for analysing the behaviour of liquids and gases (or fluids in general) in terms of their hydraulic and thermodynamic properties are very similar.

In the process of vaporisation, random loss of liquid molecules with higher kinetic (thermal) energies from the liquid, occurs while vapour molecules randomly lose thermal (kinetic) energy and return to the liquid state. Heating a liquid increases the KE of its molecules, permitting a higher proportion to escape from the surface into the vapour phase. The acquisition by these molecules of higher KE requires an energy source, and this usually comes from the thermal energy of the liquid itself, which leads to a reduction in its thermal energy as vaporisation occurs and hence the liquid cools. Vaporisation is discussed in more detail later.

Collision of randomly moving molecules in the gaseous phase with the walls of a container is responsible for the pressure exerted by a gas. The difference between a gas and a vapour will also be discussed later.

Behaviour of gases

There are three gas laws that determine the behaviour of gases and which are important to anaesthetists. These are derived from the kinetic theory of gases; they depend on the assumption that the substances concerned are perfect gases (rather than vapours), and they assume a fixed mass of gas.

Boyle's law states that, at constant temperature, the volume (*V*) of a given mass of gas varies inversely with its absolute pressure (*P*):

$$PV = k_1$$

Charles' law states that, at constant pressure, the volume of a given mass of gas varies directly with its absolute temperature (*T*):

$$V = k_2T$$

The third gas law (sometimes known as Gay-Lussac's law) states that, at constant volume, the absolute pressure

269

of a given mass of gas varies directly with its absolute temperature:

$$P = k_3 T$$

Combining these three gas laws:

$$PV = kT$$

or

$$\frac{P_1 V_1}{T_1} = \frac{P_2 V_2}{T_2}$$

where suffixes 1 and 2 represent two conditions different in P, V and T of the gas. Note that where a change of conditions occurs slowly enough for $T_1 = T_2$, conditions are said to be *isothermal*, and the combined gas law could be thought of as another form of Boyle's law.

Boyle's law can be used to derive *Dalton's law of partial pressures* to describe a mixture of gases in a container. This states that in such a mixture the pressure exerted by each gas is the same as that which it would exert if it alone occupied the container. Dalton's law can be used to compare volumetric fractions (concentrations) to calculate partial pressures, which are an important concept in anaesthesia. Thus in a cylinder of air at an absolute pressure of 100 bar, the pressure exerted by nitrogen is equal to 79 bar, as the fractional concentration of nitrogen is 0.79.

Avogadro's hypothesis, also deduced from the kinetic theory of gases, states that equal volumes of gases at the same temperature and pressure contain equal numbers of molecules.

Avogadro's number is the number of molecules in 1 g molecular weight of a substance and is equal to 6.022×10^{23}.

Under conditions of standard temperature and pressure (STP) (0°C and 1.013 bar), 1 g molecular weight (i.e. 28 g of nitrogen or 44 g of carbon dioxide) of any gas occupies a volume of 22.4 litres (L).

These data are useful in calculating, for example, the quantity of gas produced from liquid nitrous oxide. The molecular weight of nitrous oxide is 44. Thus 44 g of N_2O occupy a volume of 22.4 L at STP. If a full cylinder of N_2O contains 3.0 kg of liquid, then vaporisation of all the liquid would yield:

$$\frac{22.4 \times 3.0 \times 1000\,L}{44}$$
$$= 1527\,L \text{ at STP}$$

The gas laws can be applied to calculate its volume at, say, room temperature, bearing in mind that the Kelvin scale of temperature should be used for such calculations.

If the temperature of a vapour is low enough, then sufficient application of pressure to it will result in its liquefaction. If the vapour has a higher temperature, implying greater molecular KE, no amount of compression liquefies it. The critical temperature of such a substance is the temperature above which that substance cannot be liquefied by compression alone because the molecules have too much KE to allow liquefaction. A substance in such a state is considered a gas, whereas a substance in 'gaseous' form below its critical temperature is a vapour. The critical pressure is that which must be applied to the substance to liquefy it at the critical temperature.

The critical temperature of oxygen is −118°C, that of nitrogen is −147°C, and that of air is −141°C. Thus at room temperature, cylinders of these substances contain gases. In contrast, the critical temperature of carbon dioxide is 31°C and that of nitrous oxide is 36.4°C. The critical pressures are 73.8 and 72.5 bar, respectively; at higher pressures, cylinders of these substances at UK room temperature contain a mixture of gas and liquid. Fig. 15.3 shows the pressure-volume isotherms for a substance at, below and above its critical temperature.

A 'full' cylinder of oxygen on an anaesthetic machine contains compressed gaseous oxygen at a pressure of 137 bar gauge pressure. If the cylinder of oxygen slowly empties and the temperature remains constant, the volume of gas

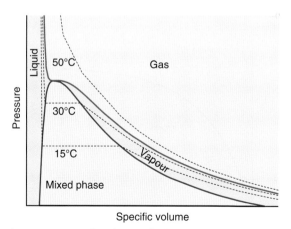

Fig. **15.3** Curves of isotherms of a liquid/vapour/gas showing the isotherms greater than, less than, and at the critical temperature. Above critical temperature nitrous oxide exists as a gas and cannot be converted to a liquid by pressure alone. Within the mixed phase region, the vapour is in equilibrium with its liquid. Hence as a nitrous oxide cylinder empties, pressure remains constant, provided temperature remains constant. Between the isobaric region and the critical temperature nitrous oxide is a vapour. Note also that nitrous oxide does not behave as an ideal gas – the curve of pressure against volume is not a rectangular hyperbola.

contained is related linearly to its absolute pressure (by Boyle's law). In practice, linearity is not followed because temperature falls as a result of adiabatic expansion of the compressed gas; the term *adiabatic* implies a change in the condition (pressure, volume and temperature) of a gas without exchange of heat energy with its surroundings.

By contrast, a nitrous oxide cylinder contains liquid nitrous oxide in equilibrium with its vapour. The pressure in the cylinder remains relatively constant at the saturated vapour pressure for that temperature as the cylinder empties to the point at which liquid has totally vaporised. Rapid emptying of the cylinder will reduce the cylinder temperature and hence the vapour pressure. Subsequently, there is a linear decline (linear assumes constant temperature) in pressure proportional to the decline in volume of gas remaining within the cylinder.

Filling ratio

The degree of filling of a nitrous oxide cylinder is expressed as the mass of nitrous oxide in the cylinder divided by the mass of water that the cylinder could hold. Normally a cylinder of nitrous oxide is filled to a ratio of 0.75 in a temperate climate. This should not be confused with the volume of liquid nitrous oxide in a cylinder. A 'full' cylinder of nitrous oxide at room temperature is filled to the point at which approximately 90% of the interior of the cylinder is occupied by liquid, the remaining 10% being occupied by nitrous oxide vapour. Incomplete filling of a cylinder is necessary because thermally induced expansion of the liquid in a totally full cylinder may cause cylinder rupture. Because vapour pressure increases with temperature, it is necessary to have a lower filling ratio in tropical climates (0.67) than in temperate climates.

Entonox

Entonox is the trade name for a compressed gas mixture containing 50% oxygen and 50% nitrous oxide. The mixture is compressed into cylinders containing gas at a pressure of 137 bar gauge pressure (see later). The nitrous oxide does not liquefy because the two gases in this mixture dissolve in each other at high pressure. In other words, the presence of oxygen reduces the critical temperature of nitrous oxide. The critical temperature of the mixture is −7°C, the 'pseudocritical temperature'. Cooling of a cylinder of Entonox to a temperature below −7°C results in separation of liquid nitrous oxide, and its use results in oxygen-rich gas being released initially, followed by a hypoxic nitrous oxide-rich gas. Consequently it is recommended that when an Entonox cylinder may have been exposed to low temperatures, it should be stored horizontally for a period of not less than 24 h at a temperature of 5°C or above. In addition, the cylinder should be inverted several times before use.

Pressure

Although the use of SI units of measurement is generally accepted in medicine, a variety of ways of expressing pressure are still used, reflecting custom and practice. Arterial pressure is still referred to universally in terms of mmHg because a column of mercury is still used occasionally to measure arterial pressure and to calibrate electronic devices.

Measurement of central venous pressure is sometimes referred to in cmH_2O because it can be measured using a manometer filled with saline, but it is more commonly described in mmHg when using an electronic transducer system. Note that, although we speak colloquially of cmH_2O or mmHg, the actual expression for pressure measured by a column of fluid is $P = \rho.g.H$, where ρ is fluid density, g is acceleration as a result of gravity and H is the height of the column. Because mercury is 13.6 times more dense than water, a mercury manometer can measure a given pressure with a much shorter length of column of fluid. For example, atmospheric pressure (P_B) exerts a pressure sufficient to support a column of mercury of height 760 mm (Fig. 15.4):

$$1 \text{ atmospheric pressure} = 760 \text{ mmHg}$$
$$= 1.01325 \text{ bar}$$
$$= 760 \text{ torr}$$
$$= 1 \text{ atmosphere absolute (ata)}$$
$$= 14.7 \text{ lb in}^{-2}$$
$$= 101.325 \text{ kPa}$$
$$= 10.33 \text{ metres of } H_2O$$

In considering pressure, it is necessary to indicate whether or not atmospheric pressure is taken into account. Thus a diver working 10 m below the surface of the sea may be described as compressed to a depth of 1 atmosphere or working at a pressure of 2 atmospheres absolute (2 ata).

To avoid confusion when discussing compressed cylinders of gases, the term *gauge pressure* is used. *Gauge pressure* describes the pressure of the contents above ambient pressure. Thus a full cylinder of oxygen has a gauge pressure of 137 bar, but the contents are at a pressure of 138 bar absolute.

Gas regulators

Pressure relief valves

The Heidbrink valve is a common component of many anaesthesia breathing systems. In the Magill breathing system, the anaesthetist may vary the force in the spring(s), thereby controlling the pressure within the breathing system (Fig. 15.5). At equilibrium the force exerted by the spring is equal to the force exerted by gas within the system:

Force (F) = gas pressure (P) × disc area (A)

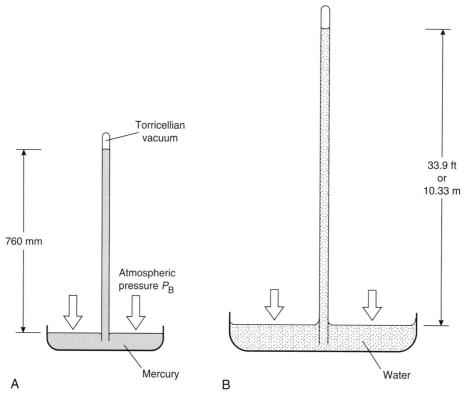

Fig. 15.4 The simple barometer described by Torricelli (not to scale). (A) Filled with mercury. (B) Filled with water.

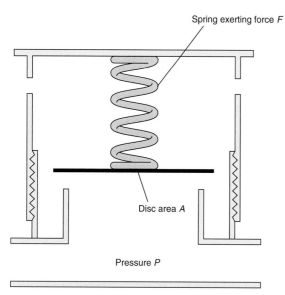

Fig. 15.5 A pressure relief valve.

Modern anaesthesia systems contain a variety of pressure relief valves, in each of which the force is fixed so as to provide a gas escape mechanism when pressure reaches a preset level. Thus an anaesthetic machine may contain a pressure relief valve operating at 35 kPa situated on the back bar of the machine between the vaporisers and the breathing system to protect the flowmeters and vaporisers from excessive pressures. Modern ventilators contain a pressure relief valve set at 7 kPa to protect the patient from barotrauma. A much lower pressure is set in relief valves which form part of anaesthetic scavenging systems, and these may operate at pressures of 0.2–0.3 kPa to protect the patient from negative pressure applied to the lungs.

Pressure-reducing valves (pressure regulators)

Pressure regulators have two important functions in anaesthetic machines:
- They reduce high pressures of compressed gases to manageable levels (acting as pressure-reducing valves).

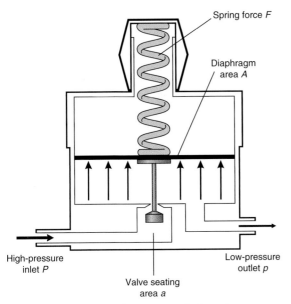

Fig. 15.6 A simple pressure-reducing valve.

- They minimise fluctuations in the pressure within an anaesthetic machine, which would necessitate frequent manipulations of flowmeter controls.

Modern anaesthetic machines are designed to operate with an inlet gas supply at a pressure of 3–4 bar (usually 4 bar in the UK), as do hospital pipelines, and therefore no pressure regulators are required between them. In contrast, the contents of cylinders of all medical gases (i.e. oxygen, nitrous oxide, air and Entonox) are at much higher pressures. Thus a pressure-reducing valve is required between the cylinder and the anaesthetic machine flowmeter.

The principle on which the simplest type of pressure-reducing valve operates is shown in Fig. 15.6. High-pressure gas enters through the valve and forces the flexible diaphragm upwards, tending to close the valve and prevent further ingress of high-pressure gas.

If there is no tension in the spring, the relationship between the reduced pressure (p) and the high pressure (P) is very approximately equal to the ratio of the areas of the valve seating (a) and the diaphragm (A):

$$pA = Pa$$

or

$$\frac{p}{P} = \frac{a}{A}$$

By tensing the spring, a force F is produced which offsets the closing effect of the valve. Thus p may be increased by increasing the force in the spring.

Without the spring, the simple pressure regulator has the disadvantage that reduced pressure decreases proportionally with the decrease in cylinder pressure. The addition of a force from the spring considerably reduces but does not eliminate this problem. During high flows, the input to the valve may not be able to keep pace with the output. This can cause the regulated pressure to fall. A two-stage regulator can be employed to overcome this.

Pressure demand regulators

These are regulators in which gas flow occurs when an inspiratory effort is applied to the outlet port. The Entonox valve is a two-stage regulator, and its mode of action is demonstrated in Fig. 15.7. The first stage is identical to the reducing valve described earlier. The second-stage valve contains a diaphragm. Movement of this diaphragm tilts a rod, which controls the flow of gas from the first-stage valve. The second stage is adjusted so that gas flows only when pressure is below atmospheric.

Flow of fluids

Viscosity (η) is the constant of proportionality relating the stress (τ) between layers of flowing fluid (or between the fluid and the vessel wall) and the velocity gradient across the tube or vessel, dv/dr.

Hence:

$$\tau = \eta \frac{dv}{dr}$$

or

$$\eta = \frac{shear\ stress}{velocity\ gradient}$$

In this context, velocity gradient is equal to the difference between velocities of different fluid layers divided by the distance between layers (Fig. 15.8A). The units of the coefficient of viscosity are Pascal seconds (Pa s).

Fluids for which η is constant are referred to as Newtonian fluids. However, most biological fluids are non-Newtonian, an example of which is blood; viscosity changes with the rate of flow of blood (as a result of change in distribution of cells) and, in stored blood, with time.

Viscosity of liquids diminishes with increase in temperature, whereas viscosity of a gas increases with increase in temperature. An increase in temperature is due to an increase of KE of fluid molecules. This can be thought of as causing a freeing up of intermolecular bonds in liquids and an increase in intermolecular collisions in gases.

Laminar flow through a tube is illustrated in Fig. 15.8B. In this situation there is a smooth, orderly flow of fluid

273

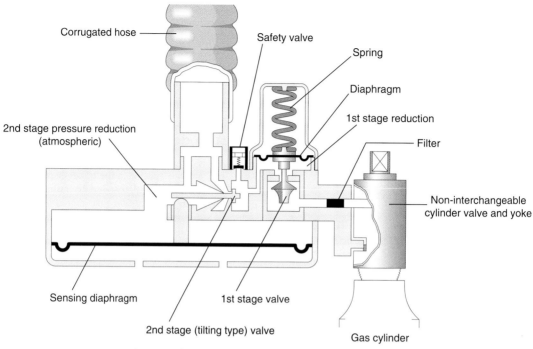

Fig. 15.7 The Entonox two-stage pressure demand regulator.

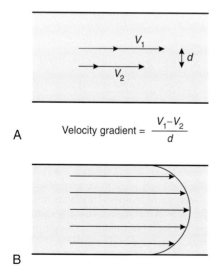

Fig. 15.8 (A) Velocity gradient. (B) Diagrammatic illustration of laminar flow.

such that molecules travel with the greatest velocity in the central axial stream, whilst the velocity of those in contact with the wall of the tube may be virtually zero. The linear velocity of axial flow is twice the average linear velocity of flow.

In a tube in which laminar flow occurs, the relationship between flow and pressure is given by the Hagen–Poiseuille formula:

$$\dot{Q} = \frac{\pi \Delta P r^4}{8\eta l}$$

where $\dot{Q}$ is the flow, ΔP is the pressure gradient along the tube, r is the radius of the tube, η is the viscosity of fluid and l is the length of the tube.

The Hagen–Poiseuille formula applies only to Newtonian fluids and to laminar flow. In non-Newtonian fluids such as blood, increase in velocity of flow may alter viscosity because of variation in the dispersion of cells within plasma.

In turbulent flow, fluid no longer moves in orderly planes but swirls and eddies around in a haphazard manner as illustrated in Fig. 15.9. Essentially, turbulent flow is less efficient in the transport of fluids because energy is wasted in the eddies, in friction and in sound (bruits). Although viscosity is the important physical variable in relation to

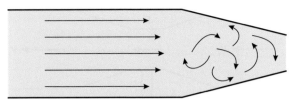

Fig. 15.9 Diagrammatic illustration of turbulent flow.

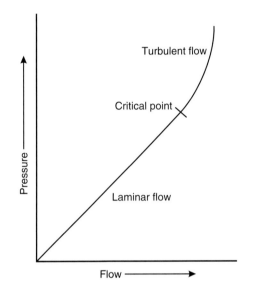

Fig. 15.10 The relationship between pressure and flow in a fluid is linear up to the critical point, above which flow becomes turbulent.

the behaviour of fluids in laminar flow, turbulent flow is more markedly affected by changes in fluid density.

The relationship between pressure and flow is linear in the laminar region, but as velocity increases, a point is reached (the critical point or critical velocity) at which the flow becomes turbulent (Fig. 15.10). The critical point depends upon several factors, which are related by the formula used for calculation of (the dimensionless) Reynolds' number:

$$Reynold's\ number = \frac{v\rho r}{\eta}$$

where v is the fluid linear velocity, r is the radius of the tube, ρ is the fluid density and η is its viscosity.

Studies with cylindrical tubes have shown that if Reynolds' number exceeds 2000, flow is likely to be turbulent, whereas if less than 2000, flow is usually laminar. However, localised areas of turbulent flow can occur at lower Reynolds' numbers when there are changes in fluid direction or changes in cross-sectional area of the tube.

The flow rate in turbulent flow ($\dot{Q}$) is dependent on the following:

- Square root of the pressure difference driving the flow (ΔP)
- Square of the radius of the vessel (r)
- Square root of density (ρ) of the fluid – that is:

$$\dot{Q} \propto \frac{\sqrt{\Delta P}.r^2}{\sqrt{\rho}}$$

A tube typically has a length many times its diameter, whereas in an orifice the diameter of the fluid pathway exceeds the length. Flow through an orifice is much more likely to be turbulent.

Turbulence and flow resistance in physiology and anaesthetic practice

In the upper respiratory tract there is often turbulent flow at high flow rates in the trachea, with flow gradually becoming laminar as branching of airways occurs and airway diameter and flow velocity reduce. In addition an obstruction in the upper respiratory tract causes downstream turbulence; thus for the same respiratory effort (driving pressure), a lower tidal volume is achieved than when flow is laminar. The extent of turbulent flow may be reduced by reducing gas density; clinically this is sometimes achieved by administration of oxygen-enriched helium rather than oxygen alone (the density of oxygen is 1.31 kg m^{-3} and that of helium is 0.16 kg m^{-3}). This reduces the likelihood of turbulent flow and reduces the respiratory effort required.

In anaesthetic breathing systems a sudden change in diameter of tubing or irregularity of the wall may be responsible for a change from laminar to turbulent flow. Thus tracheal and other breathing tubes should possess smooth internal surfaces, gradual bends and no constrictions. Resistance to breathing is much greater when a tracheal tube of small diameter is used (Fig. 15.11). Tubes should be of as large a diameter and as short as possible.

In the circulation, high-velocity pulsatile flow from the left ventricle to the aorta, a large diameter vessel, predisposes to turbulent blood flow. Similarly in the bronchial tree, as the vessels bifurcate and become smaller and the velocity of flow diminishes as the cardiac output is divided, flow becomes laminar.

The Venturi, the injector and Bernoulli

A Venturi is a tube with a section of smaller diameter than either the upstream or the downstream parts of the tube.

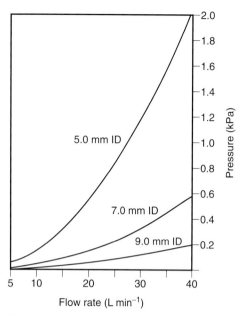

Fig. 15.11 Resistance to gas flow through tracheal tubes of different internal diameter *(ID)*.

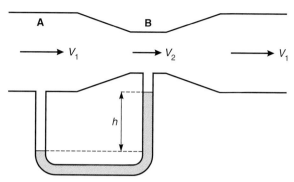

Fig. 15.12 The Bernoulli principle. See text for full details.

The principles governing the behaviour of fluids flowing through a Venturi were formulated by Bernoulli in 1778, some 60 years earlier than described by Venturi himself. In any continuum the energy of the fluid may be described by the Bernoulli equation, which suggests that the sum of energies (potential (PE) and kinetic (KE)) possessed by the fluid is constant – that is:

$$KE + PE = \frac{\rho v^2}{2} + P = constant$$

assuming that the predominant fluid flow is horizontal, such that gravitational PE can be ignored.

In a Venturi (Fig. 15.12), in order that fluid flow be continuous, its velocity must increase through its narrowed throat ($v_2 > v_1$). This is associated with an increase in KE and Bernoulli's equation shows that there is an associated reduction in PE and therefore in pressure. Beyond the constriction, velocity decreases back to the initial value and the pressure rises again. In Fig. 15.12, at point A, the energy in the fluid energy consists of potential (pressure) and kinetic (velocity), but at point B the amount of KE has increased because of the increased velocity, and the pressure is reduced here. A Venturi has a number of uses, including that of a flow measurement device. For optimum performance of a Venturi, it is desirable for fluid flow to remain laminar, and this is achieved by gradual opening of the tube beyond the constriction. In this way, if a U tube manometer is placed

with one limb sampling the pressure at point A and the other at point B, then if the flow remains laminar, the Hagen–Poiseuille equation suggests a linear relationship between the pressure difference and the flow, hence the device can be used as a flowmeter. This contrasts with an orifice, at the outflow of which the flow is usually turbulent. Although an orifice can also be used as a flowmeter, the relationship between pressure difference and flow is non-linear, and it must be carefully calibrated. Another use of a Venturi is as a device for entraining fluid from without. If a flow of oxygen is fed into a Venturi through a nozzle, the low pressure induced at the throat may be used to entrain air, thus giving a metered supply of oxygen-enriched air or acting as an injector by multiplying the amount of air flowing through the Venturi towards the patient's lungs. If, instead, a hole is made in the side of the Venturi at the throat, then the low pressure at that point may form the basis of a suction device (Fig. 15.13).

The injector principle may be seen in anaesthetic practice in several types of Venturi oxygen masks which provide oxygen-enriched air. With an appropriate flow of oxygen (usually exceeding 4 L min⁻¹), there is a large degree of entrainment of air. This results in a total gas flow that exceeds the patient's peak inspiratory flow rate, thus ensuring that the inspired oxygen concentration remains relatively constant, and it prevents an increase in apparatus dead space which always accompanies the use of low-flow oxygen devices. The same principle is used in:

- *Nebulisers.* These are used to entrain water from a reservoir. If the water inlet is suitably positioned, the entrained water may be broken up into a fine mist by the high gas velocity.
- *Ventilators.* It can also be used as the principle of a driving gas in a ventilator (Fig. 15.14).

The Coanda effect

The Coanda effect describes a phenomenon whereby when a jet of fluid (gas or liquid) flows across a flat surface it will

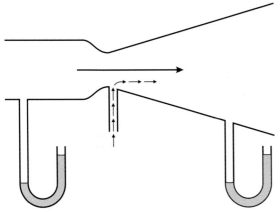

Fig. 15.13 Fluid entrainment by a Venturi injector.

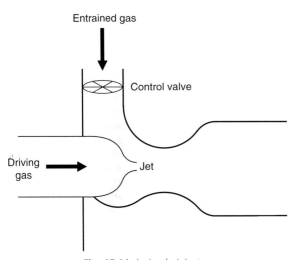

Entrained gas

Control valve

Driving gas

Jet

Fig. 15.14 A simple injector.

tend to cling either to the surface. This occurs because of the lower pressure occurring around the jet (see earlier). If this pressure is balanced (by ambient surrounding pressure), then the jet carries on in a straight line. However, if an object (surface) reduces the rate at which this pressure is balanced, an effective negative pressure exists between the jet and the surface, leading to the clinging effect. The most visible demonstration of this is the way water from a tap clings to the surface of a sink. If the jet is passing through a Y junction, the flow tends to be bi-stable – it flows down one or other limb, not both. This is exploited in fluid-logic ventilators – small pressures applied perpendicular to the jet distal to the restriction may enable gas flow to be switched from one side to another (Fig. 15.15). The effect is also of relevance to echocardiography as intracardiac jets may follow

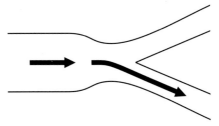

Fig. 15.15 The Coanda effect.

more discrete paths than otherwise expected, thereby altering jet sizes and Doppler-based measurements.

Heat

Heat is the energy that may be transferred from a body at a hotter temperature to one at a colder temperature. Its units are therefore joules. As discussed earlier, energy takes a number of forms and, if account is taken of energy losses, they are interchangeable. For example, if heat energy is applied to an engine, mechanical energy is the output. In a refrigeration cycle, mechanical energy is put in and heat is extracted from the cold compartment to the environment. Temperature is a measure of the tendency of an object to gain or lose heat.

Temperature and its measurement

The Kelvin scale was adopted as an international temperature scale. The triple point of water is chosen as one reference point for the temperature scale; this is the point at which all three phases of water (ice, water, steam) are in equilibrium with each other, and although the pressure at which this occurs is very low (0.006 bar), the temperature at which this occurs is only fractionally greater than that of the ice point at atmospheric pressure (1.013 bar). The internationally agreed temperature number of the triple point of water is 273.16, because it is this number of units above the recognised absolute zero of temperature which was deduced from extrapolations of the relationships between pressure, volume and temperature of gases. Hence the unit of thermodynamic temperature (the Kelvin; K) is the fraction 1/273.16 of the thermodynamic temperature of the triple point of water. The difference in temperature between the ice point for water and the steam point remains 100 units, which makes the range almost identical to the earlier empirically derived Celsius scale. It is not precisely the same, because this scale has its datum at 273.15 K (i.e. 0.01 K below the triple point). Although the unit on the thermodynamic Celsius scale is identical to that on the Kelvin scale, it is usual to denote 273.15 K as 0°C.

Consequently the intervals on the Celsius scale are identical to those on the Kelvin scale and the relationship between the two scales is as follows:

$$temperature \ K = temperature \ °C + 273.15$$

Several methods are used to measure temperature in clinical practice. These are detailed in Chapter 17.

The specific heat capacity of a substance is the energy required to raise the temperature of 1 kg of the substance by 1 K – that is:

$$heat \ energy \ required \ (J) \\ = m \ (kg) \times specific \ heat \ capacity \times \Delta T \ (K)$$

Its units are J kg^{-1} K^{-1}. For gases there are slight differences in specific heat capacities depending on whether the thermodynamic process being undergone is at constant pressure or at constant volume. The specific heat capacity of different substances is of interest because anaesthetists are often concerned with maintenance of body temperature in unconscious patients.

Heat is lost from patients by the processes of:

- conduction;
- convection;
- radiation, which is the most common mode of heat loss; and
- evaporation.

The specific heat capacity of gases is up to 1000 times lower than that of liquids. Consequently, humidification of inspired gases is a more important method of conserving heat than warming dry gases; in addition, the use of humidified gases minimises the very large energy loss produced by evaporation of fluid from the respiratory tract.

The skin acts as an almost perfect radiator; radiant losses in susceptible patients may be reduced by the use of reflective aluminium foil (space blanket).

Vaporisation

In a liquid, molecules are in a state of continuous motion because of their KE and are held in the liquid state because of intermolecular attraction by van der Waal's forces. Some molecules may develop velocities sufficient to escape from these forces, and if they are close to the surface of a liquid, these molecules may escape to enter the vapour phase. Increasing the temperature of a liquid increases its KE and a greater number of molecules escape. As the faster moving molecules escape into the vapour phase, the net velocity of the remaining molecules reduces; thus the energy state and therefore temperature of the liquid phase are eventually reduced. The amount of heat required to convert a unit

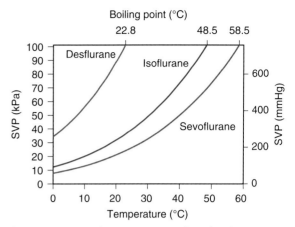

Fig. 15.16 Curves of vapour pressure plotted against temperature for a number of volatile anaesthetic agents and water. The values on the upper part of the x-axis refer to the boiling point, the temperature at which the saturated vapour pressure *(SVP)* equals ambient pressure.

mass of liquid into a vapour without a change in temperature of the liquid is termed the latent heat of vaporisation.

In a closed vessel containing liquid and gas, a state of equilibrium is reached when the number of molecules escaping from the liquid is equal to the number of molecules re-entering the liquid phase. The vapour concentration is then said to be saturated at the specified temperature. *Saturated vapour pressure* of liquids is independent of the ambient pressure but increases with increasing temperature.

The boiling point of a liquid is the temperature at which its saturated vapour pressure becomes equal to the ambient pressure. Thus on the graph in Fig. 15.16 the boiling point of each liquid at 1 atmosphere is the temperature at which its saturated vapour pressure is 101.3 kPa.

If we consider the simplest form of vaporiser (Fig. 15.17), the concentration (C) of anaesthetic in the gas mixture emerging from the outlet port is dependent upon:

- *The saturated vapour pressure* of the anaesthetic liquid in the vaporiser. A highly volatile agent such as desflurane is present in a much higher concentration than a less volatile agent (i.e. with a lower saturated vapour pressure) such as halothane or isoflurane.
- *The temperature* of the liquid anaesthetic agent, as this determines its saturated vapour pressure.
- *The splitting ratio* – that is, the flow rate of gas through the vaporising chamber (F_v) in comparison with that through the bypass ($F - F_v$). Regulation of the splitting ratio is the usual mechanism whereby the anaesthetist controls the output concentration from a vaporiser.
- *The surface area* of the anaesthetic agent in the vaporiser, which must be maximised using baffles and wicks to maximise gas exposure to liquid agent.

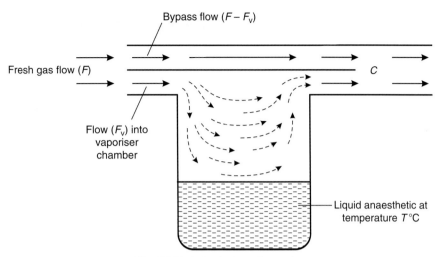

Fig. 15.17 A simple type of vaporiser.

- *Duration of use.* As the liquid in the vaporising chamber evaporates, its temperature and thus its saturated vapour pressure decrease. This leads to a reduction in concentration of anaesthetic in the mixture leaving the exit port unless temperature compensation methods are used. Classically, this is a bimetallic strip acting as a partial valve at the point where the flow splits to reduce bypass flow as temperature falls. (This is where the name TEC originates – TEmperature Compensated.)
- *The flow characteristics* through the vaporising chamber. In the simple vaporiser illustrated, gas passing through the vaporising chamber may fail to mix completely with vapour as a result of streaming because of poor design. This lack of mixing is flow dependent.
- *Altitude.* If the saturated vapour pressure (SVP) of the agent in the vaporising chamber is P_S, and the ambient pressure is P_A, then the concentration of the agent in the chamber is P_S/P_A according to Dalton's law of pressures (see Fig. 15.17). The addition of the bypass gas makes the output a fraction f of this concentration, and the output is $f.P_S/P_A$. If the vaporiser is used at altitude, because of a reduced ambient pressure. the output concentration is higher than at sea level. However, the pharmacological effect of the agent is dependent on its partial pressure $f.P_S$, so no vaporiser recalibration is required.
- *Back pressure (pumping effect).* Some gas-driven mechanical ventilators produce an increase in pressure in the outlet port and back bar of the anaesthetic machine. The increased pressure during inspiration compresses the gas in the vaporiser; some gas in the region of the inlet port of the vaporiser is forced into the vaporising

chamber, where more vapour is added to it. Subsequently there is a temporary surge in anaesthetic concentration when the pressure decreases at the end of the inspiratory cycle. This effect does not occur with efficient vaporisers because gas in the outlet port is already saturated with vapour. However, when pressure reduces at the end of inspiration, some saturated gas passes in retrograde fashion out of the inspiratory port and mixes with the bypass gas. Thus a temporary increase in total vapour concentration may still occur in the gas supplied to the patient. Methods of overcoming this problem include the following:

- Incorporation of a one-way valve in the outlet port
- Construction of a bypass chamber and vaporising chamber which are of equal volumes so that the gas in each is compressed or expanded equally
- Construction of a long inlet tube to the vaporising chamber so that retrograde flow from the vaporising chamber does not reach the bypass channel

Humidity and humidification

Absolute and relative humidity

Absolute humidity (g m^{-3} or mg L^{-1}) is the mass of water vapour present in a given volume of air (or any other gas). Relative humidity (RH) is the ratio of mass of water vapour in a given volume of air to the mass required to saturate that volume of gas at the same temperature.

Because a mass of water vapour in a sample of air has an associated temperature-dependent vapour pressure, RH may also be expressed as:

$$RH = \frac{actual\ vapour\ pressure}{saturated\ vapour\ pressure}$$

In normal practice, RH may be measured using:

- *The hair hygrometer.* This operates on the principle that a hair elongates if humidity increases; the hair length controls a pointer. It is reasonably accurate only in the range of 15%–85% relative humidity.
- *The wet and dry bulb hygrometer.* The dry bulb measures the actual temperature, whereas the wet bulb measures a lower temperature as a result of the cooling effect of evaporation of water. The rate of vaporisation is related to the humidity of the ambient gas, and the difference between the two temperatures is a measure of ambient humidity; the RH is obtained from a set of tables.
- *Regnault hygrometer.* This consists of a thin silver tube containing ether and a thermometer to show the temperature of the ether. Air is pumped through the ether to produce evaporation, thereby cooling the silver tube. When gas in contact with the tube is saturated with water vapour, it condenses as a mist on the bright silver. The temperature at which this takes place is known as the *dew point,* from which RH is obtained from tables.

Humidification of the respiratory tract

Air drawn into the respiratory tract becomes fully saturated with water in the trachea at a temperature of 37 °C. Under these conditions, the SVP of water is 6.3 kPa (47 mmHg); this represents a fractional concentration of 6.2%. The concentration of water is 44 mg L^{-1}. At 21 °C, saturated water vapour contains 2.4% water vapour or 18 mg L^{-1}. Thus there is a considerable capacity for patients to lose both water and heat when the lungs are ventilated with dry gases.

There are various means of humidifying inspired gas:

- Heat and moisture exchanging (HME) humidifiers are made of a material, wire mesh or rolled corrugated paper, which cools and condenses the water vapour of the expired breath and absorbs this water; this leaves it available to humidify the gas aliquot of the next inspired breath. They are about 70% efficient.
- Venturi systems are used in some nebulisers; a gas supply entrains water, which is broken up into a large number of droplets. The ultrasonic nebuliser operates by dropping water onto a surface, which is vibrated at a frequency of 2 MHz. This breaks up the water particles into extremely small droplets. The main problem with these nebulisers is the possibility that supersaturation of inspired gas may occur and the patient may be overloaded with water.

Solubility of gases

Henry's law states that, at a given temperature, the amount of a gas dissolved in a liquid is directly proportional to the partial pressure of the gas in equilibrium with the liquid. If a liquid is heated and its temperature rises, the partial pressure of its saturated vapour increases. This will result in gas molecules coming out of solution and a lesser amount of gas remaining dissolved in the liquid. This is exemplified by the carbon dioxide bubbles in a bottle of tonic water becoming more apparent as time elapses from its removal from the refrigerator.

It is customary to confine the term *tension* to the partial pressure of a gas exerted by gas molecules in solution, but the terms are synonymous. The tension of the gas in solution is in equilibrium with the partial pressure of the gas above it. A relatively insoluble gas will reach equilibrium more quickly than a soluble one.

Solubility coefficients

The Bunsen solubility coefficient is the volume of gas which dissolves in a unit volume of liquid at a given temperature when the gas in equilibrium with the liquid is at a pressure of 1 atmosphere. The Ostwald solubility coefficient is the volume of gas which dissolves in a unit volume of liquid at a given temperature independent of pressure.

The partition coefficient is the ratio of the amount of substance in one phase compared with a second phase, each phase being of equal volume and in equilibrium, e.g. the amount of carbon dioxide in the gas phase compared with the amount of carbon dioxide dissolved in blood. As with the Ostwald coefficient, it is necessary to define the temperature but not the pressure. The partition coefficient may be applied to two liquids, but the Ostwald coefficient applies to partition between gas and liquid. The blood/gas partition coefficient of an anaesthetic agent is an indicator of the speed with which the alveolar gas concentration equilibrates with the inspired concentration, a low coefficient (e.g. desflurane 0.42) leading to rapid equilibration. The oil/gas partition coefficient is a measure of its potency, a high coefficient (e.g. isoflurane 98.5) indicating an agent highly soluble in cerebral tissue, leading to high anaesthetic potency and low minimum alveolar concentration (MAC). The Overton–Meyer correlation shows an inverse relationship between the logarithms of MAC and oil/gas partition coefficients (for some but not all molecules).

Diffusion

If two different gases or liquids are separated in a container by an impermeable partition which is then removed, gradual mixing of the two different substances occurs as a result of the kinetic activity of each species of molecule. This is illustrated in Fig. 15.18. The principle governing this process is described by Fick's law of diffusion, which states that the rate of diffusion of a substance across unit area is proportional to the concentration gradient. Graham's law (which applies to gases only) states that the rate of diffusion of a gas is inversely proportional to the square root of its molecular weight or density.

In the example shown in Fig. 15.18B, the interface between fluids X and Y immediately after removal of the

partition would be the interface between the two species of fluid. In biology, however, there is normally a membrane separating gases or separating gas and liquids.

The rate of diffusion of gases may be affected by the nature of the membrane. In the lungs the alveolar membrane is moist and may be regarded as a water film. Thus diffusion of gases through the alveolar membrane is dependent not only on the properties of diffusion described earlier but also on the solubility of gas in the water film. As carbon dioxide is more highly soluble in water than oxygen, it diffuses more rapidly across the alveolar membrane, despite the larger partial pressure gradient for oxygen.

Osmosis

In the examples given earlier, the membranes are permeable to all substances. However, in biology, membranes are often semipermeable – that is, they allow the passage of some substances but are impermeable to others. This is illustrated in Fig. 15.19. In Fig. 15.19A, initially equal volumes of water and glucose solution are separated by a semipermeable membrane. Water molecules pass freely through the membrane to dilute the glucose solution This process continues until the volume of the diluted glucose solution supports a significantly greater head of fluid pressure than the water volume on the other side of the membrane. This hydrostatic pressure opposes the flow of water molecules through the membrane into the glucose solution, driven by the difference in solution constituents. This driving pressure is termed the osmotic pressure. Note that, depending on the membrane properties, the glucose molecules are probably too large to allow significant flow in the opposite direction. By application of a hydrostatic pressure on the glucose side (Fig. 15.19C),

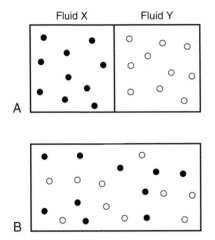

Fig. 15.18 Illustration of diffusion in fluids. (A) Fluids X and Y separated by partition. (B) Mixing of fluids after removal of partition.

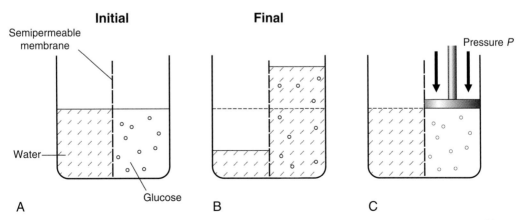

Fig. 15.19 Diagram to illustrate osmotic pressure. (A) Water and glucose placed into two compartments separated by a semipermeable membrane. (B) At equilibrium, water has passed into the glucose compartment to balance the pressure. (C) The magnitude of osmotic pressure of the glucose is denoted by a hydraulic pressure *P* applied to the glucose to prevent any movement of water into the glucose compartment.

the process of further transfer of water molecules can be prevented or even reversed; this pressure (P) is equal to the osmotic pressure exerted by the glucose solution.

Substances in dilute solution behave in accordance with the gas laws. Thus 1 g molecular weight of a dissolved substance occupying 22.4 L of solvent exerts an osmotic pressure of 1 bar at 273 K. Dalton's law also applies; the total osmotic pressure of a mixture of solutes is equal to the sum of osmotic pressures exerted independently by each substance.

The osmotic pressure of a solution depends on the number of dissolved particles per litre. Thus a molar solution of a substance which ionises into two particles (e.g. NaCl) exerts twice the osmotic pressure exerted by a molar solution of a non-ionising substance (e.g. glucose). The osmotic pressure may be produced by all of a mixture of substances in a fluid. Thus it is the sum of the individual molarities of each particle.

Whereas osmolarity is the number of osmoles per litre of solution, the term *osmolality* refers to the number of osmoles per kilogram of water or other solvent. Thus osmolarity may vary slightly from osmolality as a result of changes in density because of the effect of temperature on volume, although in biological terms the difference is extremely small.

Another effect of particles in a solvent is the lowering of its freezing point, and the extent to which this occurs is used to calculate its osmolarity. It is the basis of road gritting in icy conditions. In addition, the boiling point of a solution is raised in proportion to osmolarity.

In the circulation, water and the majority of ions are freely permeable across the endothelial membrane, but plasma proteins do not traverse into the interstitial fluid. The term oncotic pressure is used to describe the osmotic pressure exerted by the plasma proteins alone. Plasma oncotic pressure is relatively small (approximately 1 mOsm L^{-1} equivalent to 25 mmHg) in relation to total osmotic pressure exerted by plasma (approximately 300 mOsm L^{-1} equivalent to 6.5 bar).

Electricity

Basic elements and circuits

The ampere (A) is the unit of electric current in the SI system. It represents the flow of 6.24×10^{18} electrons per second. The ampere is defined as the current which, if flowing in two parallel wires of infinite length placed 1 m apart in a vacuum, produces a force of 2×10^{-7} N m^{-1} on each of the wires.

Electric charge is the measure of the amount of electricity, and its SI unit is the coulomb (C). The coulomb is the quantity of electric charge that passes a point when a current of 1 A flows for a period of 1 s:

$$coulombs\ (C) = current\ (A) \times time\ (s)$$

Electrical potential exists when one point in an electric circuit has more positive charge than another. Electrical potential is analogous to height in a gravitational field where a mass possesses PE because of its height; another analogy might be the pressure at the bottom of a water reservoir to drive a turbine. The electrical potential of the earth is regarded as the reference point for zero potential and is referred to as 'earth' or 'ground'. When a potential difference is applied across a conductor, it produces an electric current; current flows from an area of higher potential to one of lower potential.

The unit for potential difference is the volt. One volt is defined as the potential difference which produces a current of 1 ampere in a substance when the rate of energy dissipation is 1 watt (W), as demonstrated in the equation:

$$potential\ difference\ \mathrm{V} = \frac{power\ (\mathrm{W})}{current\ (\mathrm{I})}$$

A volt can also be defined as a potential difference producing a change in energy of 1 J when 1 coulomb is moved across it. This definition is often used in connection with defibrillators.

Ohm's law states that the current (I) flowing through a resistance (R) is proportional to the potential difference (V) across it. The unit for electrical resistance is the ohm (Ω). The ohm is that resistance which will allow 1 A of current to flow under the influence of a potential difference of 1 volt.

$$resistance\ \mathrm{R} = \frac{potential\ (\mathrm{V})}{current\ (\mathrm{I})}$$

$$\Omega = \frac{\mathrm{V}}{\mathrm{A}}$$

An electric circuit with several resistances in series has the same current flowing in each, and a different voltage drop across each one; total circuit resistance is the sum of all resistances. A circuit with several resistances in parallel has the same voltage drop across each of them, and the current is divided between each; the inverse of the circuit resistance is the sum of the inverse of all resistances.

A total understanding of anaesthetic monitoring equipment and other equipment supplied by electricity and its mode of action depends upon a detailed knowledge of electronics. However, the equipment can usually be used safely by the anaesthetist as a type of black box; that is, the inside of the box may be a mystery, but the anaesthetist must be familiar with the operating controls and the ways in which the apparatus may malfunction or adversely affect the patient or give an erroneous output.

In the UK the mains electricity is supplied at a voltage of 240 V with a frequency of 50 Hz, and in the United States at a voltage of 110 V and a frequency of 60 Hz. These voltages are potentially dangerous, although the danger is related predominantly to the current which flows through the patient as governed by Ohm's law.

For a resistor in a circuit, Ohm's law tells us that the voltage drop across it is equal to the product of current and resistance, with no relationship to voltage frequency. When dealing with alternating current, it is necessary to use the term *impedance* in place of resistance as impedance takes into account the frequency relationship between current and voltage, which is important in the presence of capacitors and inductors. The impedance offered to flowing current by a capacitor is inversely proportional to the current frequency. Hence a capacitor blocks direct current and is used to store charge in a DC circuit. Appropriate combinations of capacitors and resistances form the basis of high and low pass signal filters, useful for reducing signal noise in various monitors. For an inductance, the impedance is proportional to the current frequency. A magnetic field is induced around any current carrying wire and is very much stronger around a coiled wire such as an inductor; this magnetic field induces a voltage in the coil, proportional to current frequency, which opposes the driving voltage; this is useful for modifying the output from a defibrillator. Two separate coils of wire wrapped around two sides of an iron core use mutual inductance to produce an electrical output from an input which is not electrically connected to it; by differing the number of coils between the two sides, the output voltage can be increased or decreased from the input side, and this is the basis of a transformer.

Biological electrical signals

Biological signals are often in the micro- or millivolt range, with frequency bandwidths which are highly variable, from Hz to MHz. There is plenty of scope for swamping and obliterating these signals with others, such as mains electricity (230 V at 50 Hz), or diathermy (high current in MHz range). As mentioned earlier, capacitor circuits are used to produce high-pass and low-pass signal filters, to allow through wanted signals to monitors and block others. In addition, electronic amplifiers use two inputs (a differential input), one of which inverts the incoming signal so that signals common to both inputs, such as mains noise, are cancelled out, and only signals differential to both inputs, such as from ECG leads, are amplified; this is called common mode rejection. An amplifier must be calibrated for the signals it is designed to process to ensure a linear relationship between the input signal and the amplified output.

Sometimes a rising signal (e.g. lung volume on inspiration) does not follow the same path as the diminishing signal (lung volume on expiration), and this is hysteresis. (Further detail is provided in Chapter 17.)

Electrical safety

If an increasing magnitude of electrical current at 50 Hz passes through the body, there is initially a tingling sensation at a current of 1 mA. An increase in the current produces increasing pain and muscle spasm until, at 80–100 mA, arrhythmias and ventricular fibrillation may occur. The electrical disturbance that current can cause to biological tissue is related to the current frequency, the greatest sensitivity occurring at mains frequencies of 50–60 Hz, with increasing resilience to such damage at lower and higher frequencies. The choice of 50–60 Hz for mains current is due to the lower energy losses which occur in transmission lines; the unfortunate side effect is the danger to life.

The damage to tissue by electrical current is related also to the current density; a current passing through a small area is more dangerous than the same current passing through a much larger area. Other factors relating to the likelihood of ventricular fibrillation are the duration of passage of the current and its frequency. Radiofrequencies in the megahertz range (such as those used in diathermy) have no potential for fibrillating the heart but do cause burns, the basis of their use in diathermy.

It is clear from Ohm's law that the size of the current is dependent upon the size of the impedance to current flow. A common way of reducing the risk of a large current injuring the anaesthetist in the operating theatre is to wear high-impedance shoes.

Mains electricity supplies may induce currents in other circuits or on cases of instruments. The resulting induced currents are termed leakage currents and may pass through either the patient or anaesthetist to earth. There are three classes of electrical insulation which are designed to minimise the risk of a patient or anaesthetist forming part of an electrical circuit between the live conductor of a piece of equipment and earth:

- *Class I equipment* (fully earthed). The main supply lead has three cores (live, neutral and earth). The earth is connected to all exposed conductive parts, and in the event of a fault developing which short-circuits current to the casing of the equipment, current flows from the case to earth. If the current flow is small enough, the casing is rendered safe; if large enough, the fuse on the live input to the device is blown and the equipment is rendered unusable but safe.
- *Class II equipment* (double insulated). This has no protective earth. The power cable has only live and neutral

conductors, and these are double insulated. The casing is normally made of non-conductive material.

- *Class III equipment* (low voltage). This relies on a power supply at a very low voltage produced from a secondary transformer situated some distance away from the device. Potentials do not exceed 24 V (AC) or 50 V (DC). Electric heating blankets, for example, are rendered safer in this way.

Isolation circuits

All modern patient-monitoring equipment uses an isolation transformer so that the patient is connected only to the secondary circuit of the transformer, which is not earthed. Thus even if the patient makes contact between the live circuit of the secondary transformer and earth, no current is transmitted to earth. If the part of a circuit applied to the patient is not earthed, it is said to be floating, designated by F in its safety classification.

Microshock

Induced currents and leakage currents can also occur in electromedical equipment which has a component within the patient, such as a cardiac pacemaker or a saline-filled catheter connected to a transducer. With the skin breached as the first defence against shock, it only takes very small currents to cause manifestations of electrical shock, and this is termed *microshock*. A current of 100 μA is enough to cause ventricular fibrillation under these circumstances.

Safety testing

The International Electrotechnical Commission has produced recommendations (adopted by the British Standards Institute) defining the levels of permitted leakage currents and patient currents from different types of electromedical equipment. Whenever new equipment is bought for a hospital, it should be subjected to tests which verify that the leakage currents and other electrical safety characteristics are within the allowed specifications. Equipment is labelled according to whether it is suitable for external (B, BF) or internal (CF) application to the patient, with testing to appropriate levels of leakage current. Regular servicing of equipment should be carried out by qualified engineers to ensure that these safe characteristics are maintained.

The defibrillator

Capacitance is the ability to store electric charge. The defibrillator is an instrument in which electric charge is stored

in a capacitor and then released in a controlled fashion. Direct current (DC) rather than alternating current (AC) energy is used. Direct current energy is more effective, causes less myocardial damage and is less arrhythmogenic than AC energy. Biphasic defibrillators are now available, as they use a lower energy level, potentially resulting in less cardiac damage. Defibrillators are set according to the amount of energy stored and this depends on both the stored charge and the potential:

$$available\ energy\ (J) = stored\ charge\ (C) \times potential\ (V)$$

To defibrillate a heart, two electrodes are placed on the patient's chest. When the defibrillator is discharged, the energy stored in the capacitor is released as a current pulse through the patient's chest and heart. This current pulse gives a synchronous contraction of the myocardium after which a refractory period and normal or near-normal beats may follow. The voltage may be up to 5000 V with a stored energy of up to 400 J. In practice an inductor is included in the output circuit to ensure that the electric pulse has an optimum shape and duration. The inductor absorbs some of the energy which is discharged by the capacitor.

Diathermy

The severity of the effects described earlier of passing current through the body depends on the amplitude and frequency of the current. These effects diminish as the frequency of the current increases, being small above 1 kHz and negligible above 1 MHz. However, the heating and burning effects of electric current can occur at all frequencies.

A diathermy machine is used to pass electric current of high frequency (about 1–2 MHz) through the body to cause cutting and/or coagulation by burning local tissue where the current density is high. In the electrical circuit involving diathermy equipment, there are two connections with the patient. In unipolar diathermy these are the patient plate and the active electrode used by the surgeon (Fig. 15.20A). The current travels from the active electrode through the patient and exits through the patient plate. The current density is high at the active end where burning or cutting occurs, but it is low at the plate end, where no injury occurs. If for any reason (e.g. a faulty or poorly connected plate) the current flows from the patient through a small area of contact between the patient and earth, then a burn may occur at the point of contact.

In bipolar diathermy there is no patient plate, but the current travels down one side of the diathermy forceps and out through the other side (Fig. 15.20B). This type of diathermy uses low power and, because the current does not travel through the patient, it is advisable to use this in patients with a cardiac pacemaker.

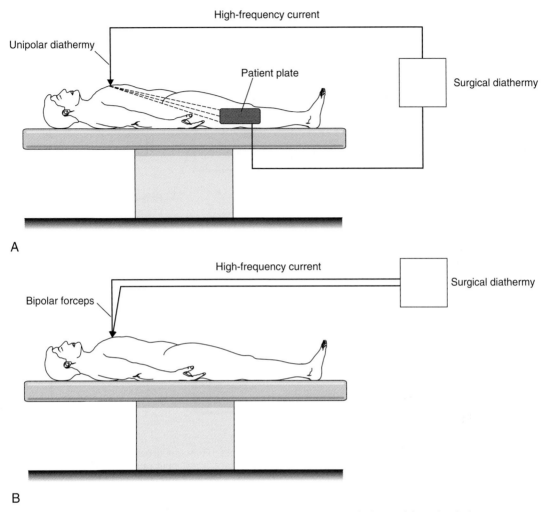

Fig. 15.20 Principle of the surgical diathermy system. (A) Unipolar diathermy. (B) Bipolar diathermy.

Radiation

X-rays

X-rays are electromagnetic radiation produced when a beam of electrons is accelerated from a cathode to strike an anode (often made of tungsten). They are used for imaging purposes.

Radiation safety

Exposure to radioisotopes and X-rays should be kept to a minimum because of the risks of tissue damage and chromosomal changes. Guidelines regarding the use of ionising radiation were issued in the UK by the Department of Health in May 2000 in a document called Ionising Radiation

(Medical Exposure) Regulations 2000 (IRMER 2000). The aims of that document are to protect patients against unnecessary exposure to radiation and to set standards for practitioners using ionising radiation. Lead absorbs X-rays, and so it is incorporated into aprons worn by staff who are exposed to radiation. The X-ray dose reduces according to the inverse square law – so moving twice as far away from the beam reduces exposure fourfold.

Magnetic resonance imaging

Nuclear magnetic resonance (NMR) is a phenomenon that was first described by Bloch and Purcell in 1945 and has been used widely in chemistry and biochemistry. The more recent application of NMR to imaging came to be known as magnetic resonance imaging (MRI).

Physical principles of MRI

Because of the presence of protons, all atomic nuclei possess a charge and they spin; this combination results in a local magnetic field. An MRI scanner produces images from hydrogen atoms because of their widespread presence in the body. When placed in a powerful static magnetic field of 1–3 Tesla, the atoms align themselves longitudinally with the field. Approximately half of the nuclei are aligned parallel to the field and the other half antiparallel to it. When aligned in this way, the atoms also precess about their spinning axis; that is, they wobble like a spinning top, and they do so out of phase with one another, at a frequency, the Larmor frequency, characteristic of the hydrogen atom and proportional to the applied magnetic field. When such a population of nuclei is subjected intermittently to a second magnetic field which is oscillating at the Larmor frequency (usually in the radiofrequency range), at right angles to the static field, they all turn to the higher energy, antiparallel direction, and they precess in phase; this is magnetic resonance (Magee 2018). The signal from the precessing atoms is resonant, and its vector is perpendicular to the main magnetic field, so it is detectable by the radiofrequency receivers. After 1 ms the radiofrequency field is removed and the atoms relax and revert to their lower energy, parallel alignment with the main field. As they do so, they release energy, from which images are made at different phases of relaxation known as T1 and T2.

To maintain such a large magnetic field, the magnets are supercooled to become superconductors of electrical current.

The presence of a strong magnetic field means that MRI-compatible anaesthetic equipment is essential. Ferromagnetic equipment may become projectiles, and pacemakers may fail.

Ultrasound

Ultrasonic vibration is defined as between 20 kHz and the MHz range. An ultrasound probe or transmitter consists of a piezo-electric crystal which generates mechanical vibration, a vibrating pressure wave, in response to an electrical input (Fig. 15.21A). Conversely, it can also produce an electrical output in response to a mechanical pressure wave input (Fig. 15.21B).

The wavelength (λ) and the transmission frequency (f) are related to the propagation velocity c by the formula

$$c = f\lambda$$

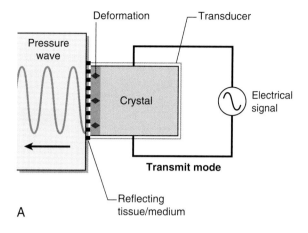

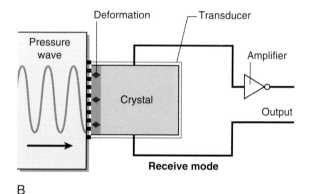

Fig. 15.21 Ultrasound generated from a piezo-electric crystal. An electrical signal input causes the crystal to deform (A), creating a pressure wave. Air conducts ultrasound poorly, so coupling between probe and surface requires gel. In (B) the reverse process occurs and a reflected pressure wave induces an electrical signal, which can be used to create an image. (Adapted from Magee, P., & Tooley, M. (2011) *Physics, clinical measurement and equipment of anaesthetic practice for the FRCA*. Oxford, Oxford University Press. By permission of Oxford University Press.)

Ultrasound velocity in a tissue and the attenuation of the wave varies depending on the tissue it is travelling through. In soft tissues the wave velocity is between 1460 and 1630 m s^{-1}, whereas in bone it is 2700–4100 m s^{-1}. Bone attenuates the waveform about 10 times as quickly as soft tissue. The greatest penetration is achieved with the lowest frequency but with poor resolution, whereas the converse holds for high-frequency waves. The clinical compromise is to use a frequency that will give good resolution, with adequate penetration of the tissues being investigated. It is the reflection of the ultrasound wave at the interface between two tissues or at tissue–fluid (air) interfaces, which provides a diagnostic image. The same piezo-electric crystal is usually used as the receiver, with the transmission mode switched off. The induced pressure changes coupled to the transducer induce electrical signals, which produce an image (see Fig. 15.21B). A real-time two-dimensional image, using multiple probes, can be produced; this is known as a *B* scan.

Ultrasound can also be used in Doppler mode. When an ultrasonic wave reflects off a stationary object, the reflected wave has the same frequency as the transmitted wave. When the object (such as a collection of red blood cells) is moving towards the transmitter, however, it encounters more oscillations per unit time than its stationary equivalent, so the frequency of the reflected wave is increased. Conversely, when the object is moving away from the ultrasound wave, the frequency of the reflected wave is reduced. This property can be used as a non-invasive technique for measurement of blood velocity (not flow) within the body.

For a transmitted frequency f_t, of wavelength λ, and the velocity of sound in the medium c:

$$f_t = \frac{c}{\lambda}$$

If the beam hits an object which is moving directly towards the transmitter at velocity v, the frequency of the waves arriving at the reflector (f_r) will now be:

$$f_r = \frac{c + v}{\lambda}$$

The reflector will now act as a source which is moving towards the transmitter, and the actual frequency sensed by the transmitter (in receiver mode) will be:

$$f_r = \frac{c + 2v}{\lambda}$$

The apparent increase in frequency is given by:

$$f_d = (f_r - f_t) = \frac{c + 2v}{\lambda} - \frac{c}{\lambda}$$

$$= \frac{2v}{\lambda}$$

$$= 2vf_t c$$

The frequency difference can be transduced into an audible signal or used to calculate the velocity of the blood cells. Normally the Doppler beam is applied non-invasively, from outside the blood vessel, at an angle θ to it. The resulting frequency shift must be multiplied by cosθ. Thus, rearranging the equations:

$$v = fd \times c2 f_t \times \cos\theta$$

Clearly the greatest accuracy in measuring blood velocity (e.g. to derive cardiac output) is achieved by having the probe aligned as far as is possible with the vessel (e.g. the aorta). Having measured mean velocity of the blood in a vessel to calculate blood flow, the mean diameter of the vessel must also be measured and its cross-sectional area calculated using the formula *flow = velocity × area*. The use of ultrasound in clinical practice is discussed further in Chapter 17.

Lasers

A laser produces an intense beam of light which results from stimulation of atoms (the laser medium) by electrical or thermal energy. Laser light has three defining characteristics: coherence (all waves are in phase both in time and in space), collimation (all waves travel in parallel directions) and monochromaticity (all waves have the same wavelength). The term *laser* is an acronym for light amplification by stimulated emission of radiation.

Physical principles of lasers

When atoms of the lasing medium are excited from a normal ground state into a high-energy state by a pumping source, this is known as the excited state (Magee 2018). When the atoms return from the excited state to the normal state, the energy is often dissipated as light or radiation of a specific wavelength characteristic of the atom (spontaneous emission). In normal circumstances, when this change from higher to lower energy state occurs, the light emitted is more likely to be absorbed by an atom in the lower energy state rather than meet an atom in a higher energy. In a laser the number of excited atoms is raised significantly so that the light emitted strikes another high-energy atom, and as a result, two light particles with the same phase and frequency are emitted (stimulated emission). These stages are summarised as follows:

- *Excitation*: stable atom + energy → high-energy atom
- *Spontaneous emission*: high-energy atom → stable atom + a photon of light
- *Stimulated emission*: photon of light + high-energy atom → stable atom + 2 photons of light

The light emitted is reflected back and forth many times between mirrored surfaces, giving rise to further stimulation. This amplification continues as long as there are more atoms in the excited state than in the normal state.

A laser system has four components (Fig. 15.22).

- *The laser medium* may be gas, liquid or solid. Common surgical lasers are CO_2, argon gas and neodymium:yttrium-aluminium-garnet (Nd:YAG) crystal. This determines the wavelength of the radiation emitted. The Nd-YAG and CO_2 lasers emit invisible infrared radiation, and argon gives blue-green radiation.

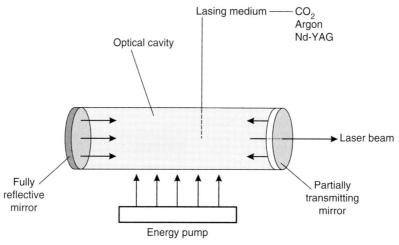

Fig. 15.22 Principle of a laser system.

- *The pumping source* supplies energy to the laser medium, and this may be either an intense flash of light or electric discharge.
- *An optical cavity* is the container in which the laser medium is encased. It also contains mirrors used to reflect light to increase the energy of the stimulated emission. One of the mirrors is a partially transmitting mirror, which allows the laser beam to escape.
- *The light guide* directs the laser light to the intended site. This may be in the form of a hollow tube or a flexible fibreoptic guide.

The longer the wavelength of the laser light, the more strongly it is absorbed, and the power of the light is converted to heat in shallower tissues (e.g. CO_2). The shorter the wavelength, the more scattered is the light, and the light energy is converted to heat in deeper tissues (e.g. Nd:YAG).

Lasers are categorised into four classes according to the degree of hazard they afford: class 1 is the least dangerous, and class 4 the most dangerous. Surgical lasers which are specifically designed to damage tissue are class 4.

Optical fibres

Optical fibres are used in the design of endoscopes and bronchoscopes to be able to see around corners. Optical fibres use the principle of total internal reflection, and this allows transmission of the light along the optical fibres (Fig. 15.23). As a result, if light passes into one end of a fibre of glass or other transparent material, it may pass along the fibre by being continually reflected from the glass/air boundary. Endoscopes and bronchoscopes contain bundles of flexible transparent fibres.

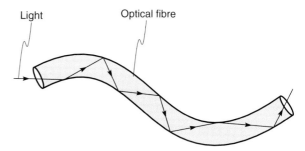

Fig. 15.23 Principle of the optical fibre.

Fires and explosions

Although the use of inflammable anaesthetic agents has declined greatly over the last two to three decades, other inflammable agents may be used in the operating theatre, such as alcohol for skin sterilisation.

Fires are produced when fuels undergo combustion. A fire becomes an explosion if the combustion is sufficiently rapid to cause pressure waves that, in turn, cause sound waves. If these pressure waves possess sufficient energy to ignite adjacent fuels, the combustion is extremely violent.

Fires require three ingredients:
- fuel;
- oxygen or other substance capable of supporting combustion, including nitrous oxide; and
- a source of ignition – that is, a source of heat sufficient to raise the fuel temperature to its ignition temperature.

Fuels

The modern volatile anaesthetic agents are non-flammable and non-explosive at room temperature in either air or oxygen.

Oils and greases form excellent fuels. In the presence of high pressures of oxygen, nitrous oxide or compressed air, these fuels may ignite spontaneously, as in the diesel engine. Thus oil or grease must not be used in supplies of these gases.

Ethanol, used as a disinfectant (see Chapter 18), burns readily in air, and the risk is increased in the presence of oxygen or nitrous oxide. Other non-anaesthetic flammable substances include methane in the gut (which may be ignited by diathermy when the gut is opened), paper dressings and plastics found in the operating theatre suite.

The stoichiometric concentration of a fuel and oxidising agent is the concentration at which all combustible vapour and agent are completely utilised. Thus the most violent reactions take place in stoichiometric mixtures, and as the concentration of the fuel moves away from the stoichiometric range, the reaction gradually declines until a point is reached (the flammability limit) at which ignition does not occur.

Support of combustion

It should always be remembered that as the concentration of oxygen increases, so does the likelihood of ignition of a fuel and the conversion of the reaction from fire to explosion.

Nitrous oxide supports combustion. During laparoscopy, there is a risk of perforation of the bowel and escape of methane or hydrogen into the peritoneal cavity. Consequently carbon dioxide is preferred to produce the pneumoperitoneum for this procedure, as it does not support combustion; in addition, it has a much greater solubility in blood than nitrous oxide, thereby diminishing the risk of gas embolism.

Sources of ignition

The two main sources of ignition in the operating theatre are static electricity and diathermy.

Electrostatic charge occurs when two substances are rubbed together and one of the substances has an excess of electrons while the other has a deficit. Electrostatic charges are produced on non-conductive material, such as rubber mattresses, plastic pillowcases and sheets, woollen blankets, some synthetic fabrics, rubber tops of stools and non-conducting parts of anaesthetic machines and breathing systems.

Diathermy equipment has now become an essential element of most surgical practices. However, it should not be used in the presence of inflammable agents. Other sources include the following:

- Electric sparks from switches, X-ray machines, and so on
- Faulty electrical equipment
- Heat from endoscopes
- Laser (particular risk in the airway; see Chapter 37)

Where possible, antistatic conducting material should be used in place of non-conductors. The resistance of antistatic material should be between 50 kΩ cm^{-1} and 10 MΩ cm^{-1}.

All material should be allowed to leak static charges through the floor of the operating theatre. However, if the conductivity of the floor is too high, there is a risk of electrocution if an individual forms a contact between mains voltage and ground. Consequently the floor of the operating theatre is designed to have a resistance of 25–50 kΩ when measured between two electrodes placed 1 m apart. This allows the gradual discharge of static electricity to earth. Personnel should wear conducting shoes, each with a resistance of between 0.1 and 1 Ω.

Moisture encourages the leakage of static charges along surfaces to the floor. The risk of sparks from accumulated static electricity charges is reduced if the RH of the atmosphere is kept to more than 50%.

References/Further reading

Brown, B., Smallwood, R., Barber, D.C., et al., 1999. Medical physics and biomedical engineering. Taylor & Francis, New York.

Cruikshank, S., 1998. Mathematics and statistics in anaesthesia. Oxford University Press, New York.

Davey, A., Diba, A., 2012. Ward's anaesthetic equipment, 6th ed. Saunders, Edinburgh.

Davis, P., Kenny, G., 2003. Basic physics and measurement in anaesthesia. Butterworth-Heinemann, Philadelphia.

Magee, P., 2018. Physics for anaesthesia: Magnetic resonance imaging; depth of anaesthesia monitoring; LASER; and light spectroscopy. BJA Education 18 (4), 102–108.

Magee, P., Tooley, M., 2011. The physics, clinical measurement and equipment of anaesthetic practice for the FRCA, 2nd edition. Oxford University Press, Oxford.

Chapter | **16** |

Anaesthetic apparatus

Mary Mushambi, Satya Francis

Anaesthetists must have a sound understanding and knowledge of the functioning of all the anaesthetic equipment they use. Failure to understand the use of or check equipment before use is an important recognised cause of complications and death. This is especially true of ventilators, where lack of knowledge may result in a patient being subjected to hypoxaemia, hypercapnia, pulmonary barotrauma and volutrauma. It is essential that anaesthetists check that all equipment is functioning correctly before anaesthesia (see Chapter 22). The routine of testing anaesthetic equipment may be compared to an aircraft pilot's checklist, an essential preliminary before every flight.

This chapter summarises the principles of anaesthetic equipment in routine use (Box 16.1) with the exception of airway devices, which are discussed in Chapter 23.

Gas supplies

Bulk supply of anaesthetic gases

In most modern hospitals, piped medical gases and vacuum (PMGV) systems have been installed. These obviate the requirement to hold large numbers of cylinders in the operating theatre suite. Normally only a few cylinders are kept in reserve, usually attached directly to the anaesthetic machine and for patient transport.

The advantages of the PMGV system are reductions in costs, the need to transport cylinders and accidents caused by cylinder contents being exhausted. However, there have been several occurrences where critical incidents or death have resulted from incorrect connections between the components of piped medical gas supplies.

The PMGV system comprises five sections:
- Bulk store
- Distribution pipelines in the hospital
- Terminal outlets, situated usually on the walls or ceilings of the operating theatre suite and other sites
- Flexible hoses connecting the terminal outlets to the anaesthetic machine
- Connections between flexible hoses and anaesthetic machines

Responsibility for the first three items lies with hospital engineering and pharmacy departments. Ultimately the anaesthetist is responsible for checking the correct functioning of the last two components within the operating theatre.

Bulk store

Oxygen

In small hospitals, oxygen may be supplied to the PMGV from a bank of several oxygen cylinders attached to a manifold. Oxygen cylinder manifolds consist of two groups of large cylinders (size J). The two groups alternate in supplying oxygen to the pipelines. In both groups, all cylinder valves are open so that they empty simultaneously. All cylinders have non-return valves. The supply automatically changes from one group to the other when the first group of cylinders is nearly empty. The changeover also activates an electrical signalling system, which alerts staff of the need to change the empty cylinders.

In larger hospitals, pipeline oxygen originates from a liquid oxygen store. Liquid oxygen is stored at a temperature of approximately $-165\,°C$ at 10.5 bar in a vacuum-insulated evaporator (VIE) (Fig. 16.1). The VIE consists of an inner stainless steel tank and an outer steel jacket, and a vacuum is maintained between the inner tank and the outer jacket. Some heat passes from the environment through the insulating layer between the two shells of the flask, increasing the tendency to evaporation and pressure increase within the chamber. Pressure is maintained constant by transfer of gaseous oxygen into the pipeline system (via a warming device). However, if the pressure increases to more than 17 bar (1700 kPa), a safety valve opens and oxygen runs to waste. During periods of high demand when the supply of oxygen from the VIE is inadequate, the pressure decreases and a valve opens to allow liquid oxygen to pass into an evaporator, from which gas vents into the pipeline system.

Liquid oxygen plants are housed some distance away from hospital buildings because of the risk of fire. Even when a hospital possesses a liquid oxygen plant, reserve banks of oxygen cylinders are necessary in case of liquid oxygen supply failure.

Box 16.1 **Classification of anaesthetic equipment described in this chapter**

Supply of gases:
    From outside the operating theatre
    From cylinders within the operating theatre, together
        with the connections involved
The anaesthetic machine:
    Unions
    Cylinders
    Reducing valves
    Flowmeters
    Vaporisers
Safety features of the anaesthetic machine
Anaesthetic breathing systems
Ventilators
Apparatus used in scavenging waste anaesthetic gases
    Suction apparatus
    Infusion devices
    Warming devices
    Decontamination of equipment

Oxygen concentrators
Recently, oxygen concentrators have been used to supply hospitals, and the use of these devices is likely to increase. The oxygen concentrator depends upon the ability of an artificial zeolite to entrap molecules of nitrogen. These devices cannot produce pure oxygen, but the concentration usually exceeds 90%; the remainder comprises nitrogen, argon and other inert gases. Small oxygen concentrators are available for domiciliary use. Oxygen concentrators are described in Chapter 45.

Nitrous oxide

Nitrous oxide and Entonox may be supplied from banks of cylinders connected to manifolds similar to those used for oxygen.

Medical compressed air

Compressed air is supplied from a bank of cylinders into the PMGV system. Air of medical quality is required,

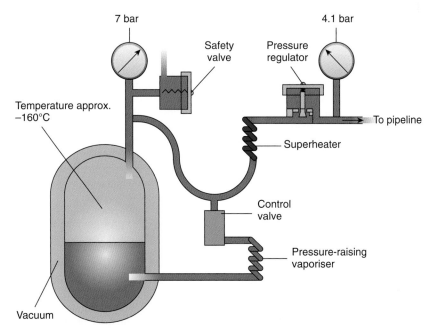

Fig. 16.1 Schematic diagram of a vacuum-insulated evaporator for liquid oxygen supply system.

as industrial compressed air may contain fine particles of oil.

Piped medical vacuum

Piped medical vacuum is provided by large vacuum pumps which discharge via a filter and silencer to a suitable point, usually at roof level, where gases are vented to atmosphere. Although concern has been expressed regarding the possibility of volatile anaesthetic agents dissolving in the lubricating oil of vacuum pumps and causing malfunction, this fear has not been realised.

Terminal outlets

Terminal outlets have been standardised in the UK since 1978, but there is no universal specification. Six types of terminal outlet are found commonly in the operating theatre. The terminals are colour-coded and also have non-interchangeable connections specific to each gas:

- *Vacuum (yellow)*. A vacuum of at least 53 kPa (400 mmHg) should be maintained at the outlet, which should be able to accommodate a free gas flow of at least 40 L min^{-1}.
- *Compressed air (white/black)* at 4 bar. Used for anaesthetic breathing systems and ventilators.
- *Air (white/black)* at 7 bar. To be used only for powering compressed air tools used, for example during orthopaedic surgery.
- *Nitrous oxide (blue)* at 4 bar.
- *Oxygen (white)* at 4 bar.
- *Scavenging*. There are a variety of scavenging outlets from the operating theatre. The passive systems are designed to accept a standard 30-mm connection.

Whenever a new pipeline system has been installed or servicing of an existing pipeline system undertaken, a designated member of the pharmacy staff should test the gas obtained from the sockets using an oxygen or other gas analyser. Malfunction of an oxygen/air mixing device may result in entry of compressed air into the oxygen pipeline, rendering an anaesthetic gas mixture hypoxic. Because of this and other potential mishaps, oxygen analysers should be used routinely during anaesthesia.

Gas supplies

Gas supplies to the anaesthetic machine should be checked at the beginning of each session to ensure the gas that issues from the pipeline or cylinder is the same as that passing through the appropriate flowmeter. This ensures that pipelines are not connected incorrectly. Anaesthetic machines in both the operating theatre and the anaesthetic room should be checked. Checking of anaesthetic machine and medical gas supplies is detailed in Chapter 22.

Cylinders

Cylinders are constructed from molybdenum steel, aluminium or composites (e.g. carbon-fibre wrapped aluminium). They are checked periodically by the manufacturer to ensure that they can withstand hydraulic pressures considerably higher than those during normal use. One cylinder in every 100 is cut into strips to test the metal for tensile strength, flattening impact and bend tests. Medical gas cylinders are tested hydraulically every 10 (steel) or 5 (composite) years and the tests recorded by a mark stamped on the neck of the cylinder: this includes test pressure, date performed, chemical formula of the cylinder's content and the tare weight. Cylinders may also be inspected endoscopically or using ultrasound for cracks or defects on their inner surfaces.

The cylinders are provided in a variety of sizes (A to J) and colour coded according to the gas supplied. Modern CD (460 L) and HX (2300 L) cylinders have similar dimensions to their counterparts but are filled to 23,000 kPa rather than 13,700 kPa. Cylinders attached to the anaesthetic machine are usually size E. The cylinders comprise a body and a shoulder containing threads into which are fitted a pin index valve block, a bull-nosed valve or a hand-wheel valve.

The pin index system was devised to prevent interchangeability of cylinders of different gases. Pin index systems are provided for the smaller cylinders of oxygen and nitrous oxide (and also carbon dioxide) which may be attached to anaesthetic machines. The pegs on the inlet connection slot into corresponding holes on the cylinder valve.

Full cylinders are usually supplied with a plastic dust cover to prevent contamination by dirt. This cover should not be removed until immediately before the cylinder is fitted to the anaesthetic machine. When fitting the cylinder to a machine, the yoke is positioned and tightened with the handle of the yoke spindle. After fitting, the cylinder should be opened to make sure that it is full and that there are no leaks at the gland nut or the pin index valve junction, caused, for example, by absence of or damage to the washer. The washer used is normally a Bodok seal, which has a metal periphery designed to keep the seal in good condition for a long period.

Cylinder valves should be opened slowly to prevent sudden surges of pressure and should be closed with no more force than is necessary, otherwise the valve seating may be damaged.

The sealing material between the valve and the neck of the cylinder may be constructed from a fusible material which melts in the event of fire and allows the contents of the cylinder to escape around the threads of the joint.

The primary method of cylinder identification is the cylinder label. Colour coding is a secondary method. The

Table 16.1 Medical gas cylinders used in the UK

| | COLOUR | | PRESSURE AT 15°C | |
	Body	Shoulder	kPa	Bar
Oxygen	Black	White	13,700	137
Nitrous oxide	Blue	Blue	4400	44
CO_2	Grey	Grey	5000	50
Helium	Brown	Brown	13,700	137
Air	Grey	White/black quarters	13,700	137
O_2/helium	Black	White/brown quarters	13,700	137
N_2O/O_2 (Entonox)	Blue	White/blue quarters	13,700	137

Table 16.2 Medical gas cylinder sizes and capacities by cylinder size (A–J) and height (inches)

| | CAPACITIES (L) | | | | | | | | |
	A/10 in	B/10 in	C/14 in	D/18 in	CD/20 in	E/31 in	F/34 in	G/49 in	J/57 in
Oxygen			170	340	460	680	1360	3400	6800
Nitrous oxide			450	900		1800	3600	9000	
CO_2			450	900		1800			
Helium				300			1200		
Air								3200	6400
O_2/helium						600	1200		
O_2/CO_2							1360	3400	
Entonox								3200	6400

colour codes used for medical gas cylinders in the UK are shown in Table 16.1. Different colours are used for some gases in other countries. A proposal was agreed to in 2013 to harmonise cylinder colours throughout Europe. The body will be painted white and only the shoulders will be colour coded. The shoulder colours for medical gases will correspond to the current UK colours but will be horizontal rings rather than quarters. The conversion will be complete by 2025. Cylinder sizes and capacities are shown in Table 16.2.

Oxygen, air and helium are stored as gases in cylinders and the cylinder contents can be estimated from the cylinder pressure. The pressure gradually decreases as the cylinder empties. According to the universal gas law, the mass of the gas is directly proportional to the pressure, and the volume of gas that would be available at atmospheric pressure can be calculated using Boyle's law.

Nitrous oxide (N_2O) and carbon dioxide (CO_2) cylinders contain liquid and vapour and the cylinders are filled to a known filling ratio (see Chapter 15). The cylinder pressure cannot be used to estimate its contents because the pressure remains relatively constant until after all the liquid has evaporated and the cylinder is almost empty, though cylinder pressure may change slightly because of temperature changes during use. The contents of N_2O and CO_2 cylinders can be estimated from the weight of the cylinder.

The anaesthetic machine

The anaesthetic machine comprises:
- a means of supplying gases either from attached cylinders or from piped medical supplies via appropriate unions on the machine;
- methods of measuring flow rate of gases;
- apparatus for vaporising volatile anaesthetic agents;

293

- breathing systems and a ventilator for delivery of gases and vapours from the machine to the patient; and
- apparatus for scavenging anaesthetic gases to minimise environmental pollution.

Supply of gases

In the UK, gases are supplied at a pipeline pressure of 4 bar (400 kPa), and this pressure is transferred directly to the bank of flowmeters and back bar of the anaesthetic machine. Flexible colour-coded hoses connect the pipeline outlets to the anaesthetic machine. The anaesthetic machine end of the hoses should be permanently fixed using a nut and liner union where the thread is gas specific and non-interchangeable. The non-interchangeable screw thread (NIST) is the British standard.

The gas issuing from medical gas cylinders is at a much higher pressure, necessitating the interposition of a pressure regulator between the cylinder and the bank of flowmeters. In some older anaesthetic machines (and in some other countries), the pressure in the pipelines of the anaesthetic machine may be 3 bar (300 kPa).

Pressure gauges

Pressure gauges (Bourdon gauges) measure the pressure in the cylinders or pipeline. Anaesthetic machines have pressure gauges for oxygen, air and N_2O. These are mounted usually on the front panel of the anaesthetic machine.

Pressure regulators

Pressure regulators are used on anaesthetic machines for three purposes:
- They help to reduce the high pressure of gas in a cylinder to a safe working level.
- They are used to prevent damage to equipment on the anaesthetic machine (e.g. flow control valves).
- As the contents of the cylinder are used, the pressure within the cylinder decreases and the regulating mechanism maintains a constant outlet pressure, obviating the necessity to make continuous adjustments to the flowmeter controls.

The operating principles of pressure regulators are discussed in Chapter 15.

Flow restrictors

Pressure regulators usually are omitted when anaesthetic machines are supplied directly from a pipeline at a pressure of 4 bar. Changes in pipeline pressure would cause changes in flow rate, necessitating adjustment of the flow control valves. This is prevented by the use of a flow restrictor upstream of the flowmeter (flow restrictors are simply constrictions in the low-pressure circuit).

A different type of flow restrictor may be fitted also to the downstream end of the vaporisers to prevent back-pressure effects (see Chapter 15).

Pressure relief valves on regulators

Pressure relief valves are often fitted on the downstream side of regulators to allow escape of gas if the regulators were to fail (thereby causing a high output pressure). Relief valves are set usually at approximately 7 bar for regulators designed to give an output pressure of 4 bar.

Flowmeters

The principles of flowmeters and some different types are described in Chapter 17.

Problems with flowmeters

- *Non-vertical tube.* This causes a change in shape of the annulus and therefore variation in flow. If the bobbin touches the side of the tube, resulting friction causes an even more inaccurate reading.
- *Static electricity.* This may cause inaccuracy (by as much as 35%) and sticking of the bobbin, especially at low flows. This may be reduced by coating the inside of the tube with a transparent film of gold or tin.
- *Dirt* on the bobbin may cause sticking or alteration in size of the annulus and therefore inaccuracies.
- *Back-pressure.* Changes in accuracy may be produced by back-pressure. For example, the Manley ventilator may exert a back-pressure and depress the bobbin; there may be as much as 10% more gas flow than that indicated on the flowmeter. Similar problems may be produced by the insertion of any equipment which restricts flow downstream (e.g. Selectatec head, vaporiser).
- *Leakage.* This results usually from defects in the top sealing washer of a flowmeter.

It is unfortunate that in the UK the standard position of the oxygen flowmeters is on the left, followed by either nitrous oxide or air (if all three gases are supplied). On several recorded occasions, patients have suffered hypoxia because of leakage from a broken flowmeter tube in this type of arrangement, as oxygen, being at the upstream end, passes out to the atmosphere through any leak. This problem is reduced if the oxygen flowmeter is placed downstream (i.e. on the right-hand side of the bank of flowmeters) as is standard practice in the United States. In the UK this problem is now avoided by designing the outlet from the oxygen flowmeter to enter the back bar downstream from the outlets of other flowmeters (Fig. 16.2). Modern anaesthetic machines do not have a flowmeter for CO_2. Some newer anaesthetic machines such as the Primus Dräger (Fig. 16.3A) do not have the traditional flowmeters which are used in machines such as the Blease Frontline (Fig. 16.3B);

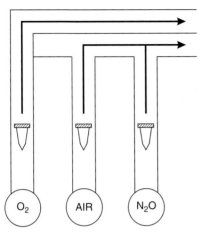

Fig. 16.2 Oxygen is the last gas to be added to the gas mixture being delivered to the back bar.

gas delivery is under electronic control, and there is an integrated heater within a leak-tight breathing system. The gas flow is indicated electronically by a numerical display. In the event of an electrical failure, there is a pneumatic backup which continues the delivery of fresh gas. These machines are particularly well suited to low and minimal flow anaesthesia, and they use standard vaporisers.

The emergency oxygen flush is a non-locking button which, when pressed, delivers pure oxygen from the anaesthetic outlet. On modern anaesthetic machines, the emergency oxygen flush lever is situated downstream from the flowmeters and vaporisers. A flow of about 35–45 L min^{-1} at pipeline pressure is delivered. This may lead to dilution of the anaesthetic mixture with excess oxygen if the emergency oxygen tap is opened partially by mistake and may result in awareness. There is also a risk of pulmonary barotrauma if the high pressure is accidentally delivered directly to the patient's lungs.

Quantiflex

The Quantiflex mixer flowmeter (Fig. 16.4) eliminates the possibility of reducing the oxygen supply inadvertently. One dial is set to the desired percentage of oxygen, and the total

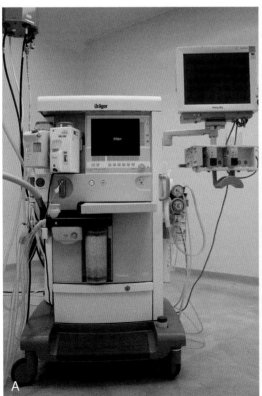

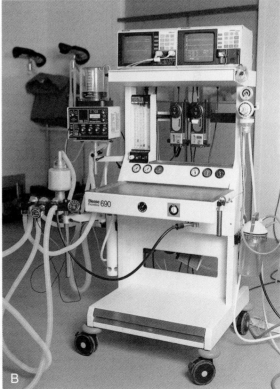

Fig. 16.3 (A) The Primus Dräger anaesthetic machine. (B) Blease Frontline anaesthetic machine.

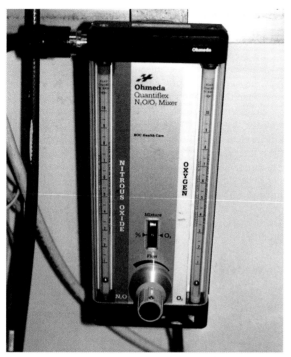

Fig. 16.4 A Quantiflex flowmeter. The required oxygen percentage is selected using the dial, and total flow of the oxygen/nitrous oxide mixture is adjusted using the grey knob.

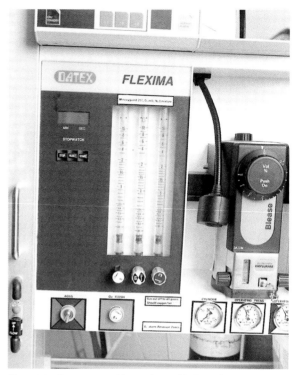

Fig. 16.5 Flowmeters with mechanical linkage between nitrous oxide and oxygen.

flow rate is adjusted independently. The oxygen passes through a flowmeter to provide evidence of correct functioning of the linked valves. Both gases arrive via linked pressure-reducing regulators. The Quantiflex is useful in particular for varying the volume of fresh gas flow (FGF) from moment to moment whilst keeping the proportions constant. In addition, the oxygen flowmeter is situated downstream of the N_2O flowmeter.

Hypoxic guard

The majority of modern anaesthetic machines such as that shown in Fig. 16.3B possess a mechanical linkage between the N_2O and oxygen flowmeters. This causes the N_2O flow to decrease if the oxygen flowmeter is adjusted to give less than 25%–30% O_2 (Fig. 16.5).

Vaporisers

The principles of vaporisers are detailed in Chapter 15.
Modern vaporisers may be classified as:
• *Drawover vaporisers*. These have a very low resistance to gas flow and may be used for emergency use in the field (e.g. Oxford miniature vaporiser; OMV (see Chapter 45))

• *Plenum vaporisers*. These are intended for unidirectional gas flow, have a relatively high resistance to flow and are unsuitable for use either as drawover vaporisers or within a circle system. Examples include the TEC type in which there is a variable bypass flow.

Temperature regulation in the TEC vaporisers is achieved using a bimetallic strip.

There have been several models of the TEC vaporiser. The TEC Mark 3 included several advances from the Mark 2 (now obsolete), including improved vaporisation resulting from increased area of the wicks, reduced pumping effect by having a long tube through which the vaporised gas leaves the vaporising chamber, improved accuracy at low gas flows and a bimetallic strip situated in the bypass channel and not the vaporising chamber. The Mark 4 incorporated mechanisms to prevent both spillage into the bypass channel if the vaporiser was accidentally inverted and the possibility of two vaporisers being turned on at the same time when connected to the back bar of the anaesthetic machine (see later). The TEC Mark 5 vaporiser (Fig. 16.6) has improved surface area for vaporisation in the chamber, improved key-filling action and an easier mechanism for switching on the rotary valve and lock with one hand. The TEC 5 is still used but no longer produced by the manufacturer and has been superseded by the TEC 7; differences are relatively

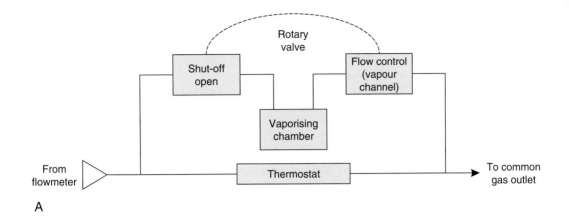

A

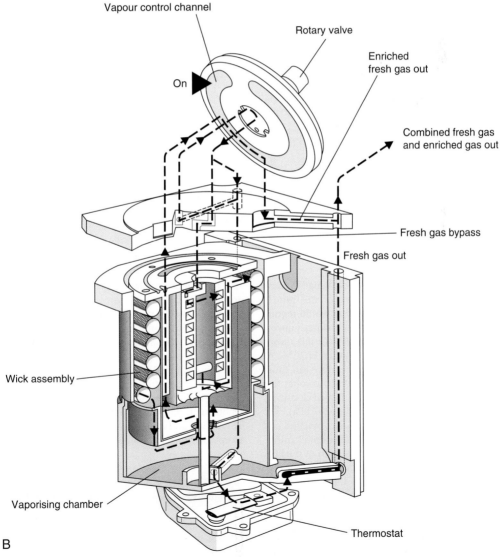

B

Fig. 16.6 (A) Working principles of a vaporiser. (B) Schematic diagram of the TEC 5 vaporiser.

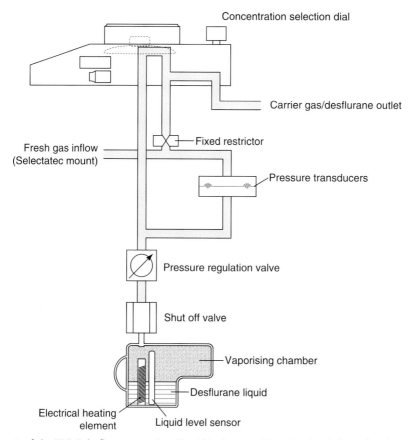

Fig. 16.7 Components of the TEC 6 desflurane vaporiser. Liquid in the vaporising chamber is heated and mixed with fresh gas; the pressure-regulating valve balances both fresh gas pressure and anaesthetic vapour pressure.

minor. Desflurane presents a particular challenge because it has a high saturated vapour pressure of 664 mmHg (89 kPa) at 20°C. A conventional vaporiser would require high FGF for useful clinical concentrations, making it uneconomical. It has a low boiling point of 23.5°C; this means that it is almost boiling at a room temperature of 20°C. As a result, small changes in ambient temperature can cause large swings in saturated vapour pressure. To combat this problem, the TEC 6 (Figs 16.7 and 16.8) is heated electrically to 39°C with a pressure of 1550 mmHg (207 kPa). The vaporiser has electronic monitors of vaporiser function and alarms. The FGF does not enter the vaporisation chamber. Instead, desflurane vapour enters into the path of the FGF. A control dial regulates the flow of desflurane vapour into the FGF. The dial calibration is from 1% to 18%. The vaporiser has a backup 9-volt battery in case of mains failure.

Anaesthetic-specific connections are available to link the supply bottle (container of liquid anaesthetic agent) to the appropriate vaporiser (Fig. 16.9). These connections reduce the extent of spillage (and thus atmospheric pollution) and

also the likelihood of filling the vaporiser with an inappropriate liquid. In addition to being designed specifically for each liquid, the connections themselves are colour coded (e.g. purple for isoflurane, yellow for sevoflurane).

Halothane contains a stabilising agent, 0.01% thymol, to prevent breakdown of halothane by heat and ultraviolet light (see Chapter 3). Thymol is less volatile than halothane, and its concentration may increase during use. This can impair the vaporisation of halothane, and thymol inhalation is potentially harmful. Therefore halothane vaporisers should be emptied and refilled every 2 weeks. Longer intervals are acceptable for other volatile agents.

Safety features of modern anaesthetic machines

Safety features of modern anaesthetic machines include the following:

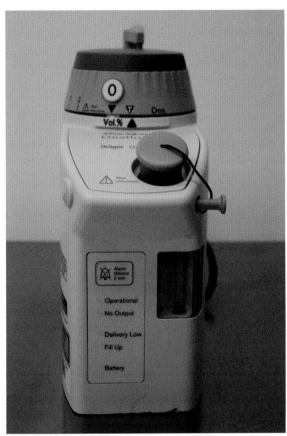

Fig. 16.8 A TEC 6 desflurane vaporiser. Note it is set at the 'T' transport setting for safe transport, and an electrical supply is required to heat the vaporising chamber.

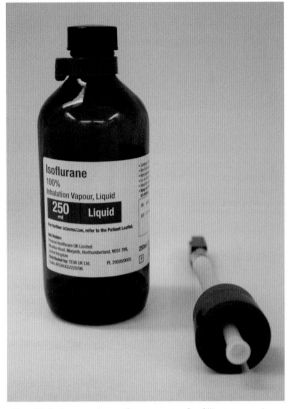

Fig. 16.9 An agent-specific connector for filling a vaporiser.

- The flexible hoses are colour coded and have non-interchangeable screw-threaded connectors to the anaesthetic machine.
- The pin index system prevents incorrect attachment of gas cylinders to an anaesthetic machine. Cylinders are colour coded, and they are labelled with the name of the gas that they contain.
- Pressure relief valves are present on the downstream side of pressure regulators.
- Flow restrictors are present on the upstream side of flowmeters.
- The bank of flowmeters are arranged whereby the oxygen flowmeter is on the right (i.e. downstream) or oxygen is the last gas to be added to the gas mixture being delivered to the back bar (see Fig. 16.2).
- Sometimes a single regulator and contents meter is used both for cylinders in use and for the reserve cylinder. When one cylinder runs out, the presence of a non-return valve prevents the empty cylinder from being refilled by

the reserve cylinder and also enables the empty cylinder to be removed and replaced without interrupting the supply of gas to the patient.
- Pressure gauges indicate the pressures in the pipelines and the cylinders.
- An oxygen bypass valve (emergency oxygen) delivers oxygen directly to a point downstream of the vaporisers. When operated, the oxygen bypass should give a flow rate of at least 35 L min^{-1}.
- The TEC vaporisers (Mark 4 and later) have the interlocking Selectatec system (Fig. 16.10), which has locking rods to prevent more than one vaporiser being used at the same time. The locking lever must be engaged when a vaporiser is mounted on the back bar, as otherwise the control dial cannot be moved.
- Modern anaesthetic machines have a mechanical linkage between the N$_2$O and oxygen flowmeters that prevents the delivery of less than 25%–30% oxygen.
- The oxygen flowmeter is always in the same position (left) on UK anaesthetic machines and is of larger dimensions and ridged to clearly differentiate it from the other flowmeters.

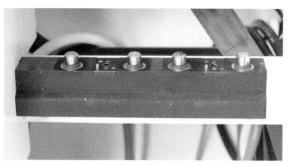

Fig. 16.10 A Selectatec block on the back bar of an anaesthetic machine. This permits the vaporiser to be changed rapidly without interrupting the flow of carrier gas to the patient.

- All flow meters have written labels and are usually colour coded as well.
- A pressure relief valve may be situated downstream of the vaporiser, opening at 34 kPa to prevent damage to the flowmeters or vaporisers if the gas outlet from the anaesthetic machine is obstructed.
- A pressure relief valve set to open at a low pressure of 5 kPa may be fitted to prevent the patient's lungs from being damaged by high pressure.
- All anaesthetic machines should incorporate an oxygen failure device. The ideal warning device should have the following characteristics:
  - Activation depends on the pressure of oxygen alone, independent of any other gas pressures.
  - Does not use a battery or mains power.
  - Gives an audible signal of sufficient duration and distinctive character.
  - Give a warning of impending failure and a further warning that failure has occurred.
  - Interrupts the flow of all other gases when it comes into operation.
  - The breathing system should open to the atmosphere, the inspired oxygen concentration should be at least equal to that of air, and accumulation of CO_2 should not occur. In addition, it should be impossible to resume anaesthesia until the oxygen supply has been restored.
- The reservoir bag in a breathing system is highly distensible and seldom reaches pressures exceeding 3.9 kPa or 40 cmH$_2$O (see later).

In the event of power failure, there is battery backup in all modern anaesthetic machines.

Magnetic resonance imaging compatible anaesthetic machines are available such as the Prima SP Anaesthetic machine (Penlon), which is made from non-ferrous metals and can be used up to the 1000 Gauss line.

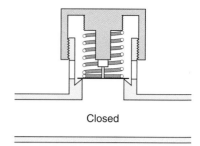

Closed

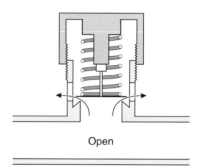

Open

Fig. 16.11 Diagram of a spill valve. See text for details.

Breathing systems

The delivery system that conducts anaesthetic gases from the machine to the patient is often referred to as a circuit but is described more accurately as a breathing system. Terms such as *open circuits, semi-open circuits* or *semi-closed circuits* should be avoided. The closed circuit, or circle system, is the only true circuit, as anaesthetic gases are recycled.

Adjustable pressure-limiting valve

Most breathing systems incorporate an adjustable pressure-limiting valve (APL valve, spill valve, pop-off valve, expiratory valve), which is designed to vent gas when there is a positive pressure within the system. During spontaneous ventilation, the valve opens when the patient generates positive pressure within the system during expiration; during positive pressure ventilation, the valve is adjusted to produce a controlled leak during the inspiratory phase.

Several valves of this type are available. They comprise a lightweight disc (Fig. 16.11) which rests on a knife-edge seating to minimise the area of contact and reduce the risk of adhesion resulting from surface tension of condensed water. The disc has a guiding stem to position it correctly. A light spring is incorporated in the valve so that the pressure required to open it may be adjusted. During spontaneous breathing, the tension of the spring is low so that the resistance to expiration is minimised. During controlled

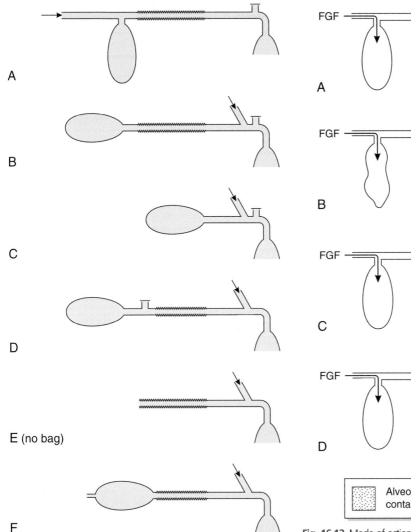

Fig. 16.12 Mapleson classification of anaesthetic breathing systems. (A) Mapleson A (Magill). (B) Mapleson B. (C) Mapleson C. (D) Mapleson D. (E) Mapleson E. (F) Mapleson F. The *arrow* indicates entry of fresh gas to the system.

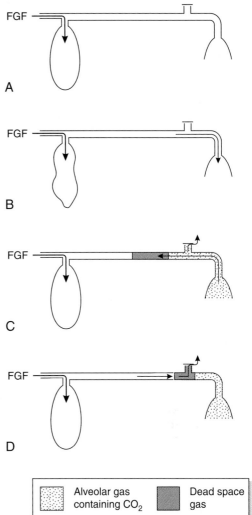

| Alveolar gas containing CO_2 | Dead space gas |

Fig. 16.13 Mode of action of Magill attachment during spontaneous ventilation. (A) Before insipration. (B) Inspiration. (C) Expiration. (D) Expiratory pause. See text for details. *FGF*, Fresh gas flow.

F system. The systems differ considerably in their efficiency, which is measured in terms of the FGF rate required to prevent rebreathing of alveolar gas during ventilation (Table 16.3).

Mapleson A systems

The most commonly used Mapleson A system is the Magill attachment. The corrugated hose should be of adequate length (usually approximately 110 cm). It is the most efficient system during spontaneous ventilation but one of the least efficient when ventilation is controlled.

During spontaneous ventilation (Fig. 16.13), there are three phases in the ventilatory cycle: inspiration, expiration

ventilation, the valve top is screwed down to increase the tension in the spring so that gas leaves the system at a higher pressure than during spontaneous ventilation. Modern valves, even when screwed down fully, open at a pressure of 60 cmH₂O. Most valves are encased in a hood for scavenging.

Classification of breathing systems

In 1954, Mapleson classified anaesthetic breathing systems into five types, A–E (Fig. 16.12); the Mapleson E system was modified subsequently by Rees but is classified as the Mapleson

Table 16.3 Mapleson classification of anaesthetic breathing systems

Mapleson	Systems	Uses	FGF SV	FGF IPPV
A	Magill Lack	Spontaneous ventilation	70–100 ml kg^{-1} min^{-1}	Minimum 3 × MV
B		Very uncommon, not in use today		
C		Resuscitation Bagging		Minimum 15 L min^{-1}
D	Bain	Spontaneous, IPPV ventilation	150–200 ml kg^{-1} min^{-1}	70–100 ml kg^{-1} min^{-1}
E	Ayre's T-piece	Very uncommon, not in use today		
F	Jackson Rees	Paediatric <25 kg	2.5–3 × MV Minimum 4 L min^{-1}	

FGF, Fresh gas flow; *IPPV,* intermittent positive pressure ventilation; *MV,* minute ventilation; *SV,* spontaneous ventilation.

and the expiratory pause. Gas is inhaled from the system during inspiration (Fig. 16.13B). During the initial part of expiration, the reservoir bag is not full and thus the pressure in the system does not increase; exhaled gas (the initial portion of which is dead space gas) passes along the corrugated tubing towards the bag (Fig. 16.13C), which is filled also by fresh gas from the anaesthetic machine. During the latter part of expiration, the bag becomes full; the pressure in the system increases and the spill valve opens, venting all subsequent exhaled gas to atmosphere. During the expiratory pause, continued flow of fresh gas from the machine pushes exhaled gas distally along the corrugated tube to be vented through the spill valve (Fig. 16.13D). Provided that the FGF rate is sufficiently high to vent all *alveolar* gas before the next inspiration, no rebreathing takes place from the corrugated tube. If the system is functioning correctly and no leaks are present, an FGF rate equal to the patient's alveolar minute ventilation is sufficient to prevent rebreathing. In practice, a higher FGF is selected to compensate for leaks; the rate selected is usually equal to the patient's total minute volume (approximately 6 L min^{-1} for a 70-kg adult).

The system increases dead space to the extent of the volume of the anaesthetic face mask and angle piece to the spill valve. The volume of this dead space may amount to 100 ml or more for an adult face mask. Paediatric face masks reduce the extent of dead space, but it remains too high to allow use of the system in infants or small children (<4 years old).

The characteristics of the Mapleson A system are different during controlled ventilation (Fig. 16.14). At the end of inspiration (produced by the anaesthetist squeezing the reservoir bag), the bag is usually less than half full (see later). During expiration, dead space and alveolar gas

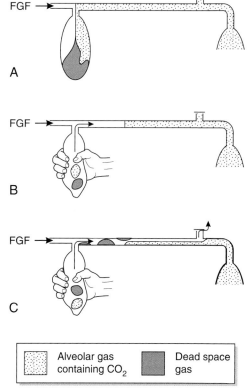

Alveolar gas containing CO_2		Dead space gas

Fig. 16.14 Mode of action of Magill attachment during controlled ventilation. (A) Expiration. (B and C) Inspiration. See text for details. *FGF,* Fresh gas flow.

pass along the corrugated tube and are likely to reach the reservoir bag, which therefore contains some CO_2 (Fig. 16.14A). During inspiration, the valve does not open initially because its opening pressure has been increased by the anaesthetist to generate a sufficient pressure within the system to inflate the lungs. Thus alveolar gas re-enters the patient's lungs and is followed by a mixture of fresh dead space and alveolar gases (Fig. 16.14B). When the valve does open, it is this mixture which is vented (Fig. 16.14C). Consequently, the FGF rate must be very high (at least three times alveolar minute volume) to prevent rebreathing. The volume of gas squeezed from the reservoir bag must be sufficient both to inflate the lungs and to vent gas from the system.

The major disadvantage of the Magill attachment during surgery is that the spill valve is attached close to the mask. This makes the system heavy, particularly when a scavenging system is used, and it is inconvenient during head or neck surgery. The Lack system (Fig. 16.15) is a modification of the Mapleson A system with a coaxial arrangement of tubing. This permits positioning of the spill valve at the proximal end of the system. The inner tube must be of sufficiently wide bore to allow the patient to exhale with minimal resistance. The Lack system is not quite as efficient as the Magill attachment.

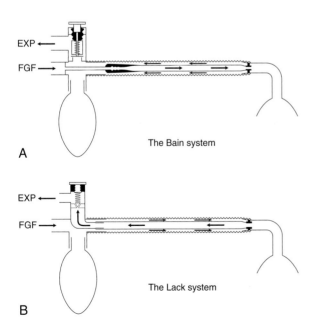

EXP ←
FGF →

The Bain system

A

EXP ←
FGF →

The Lack system

B

Fig. 16.15 Coaxial anaesthetic breathing systems. (A) Bain system (Mapleson D). (B) Lack system (Mapleson A). *EXP,* Expired gas; *FGF,* fresh gas flow.

Mapleson B and C systems

These systems produce mixing of alveolar and fresh gas during spontaneous or controlled ventilation. Very high FGF rates are required to prevent rebreathing. There is no clinical role for the Mapleson B system. The Mapleson C system is used in some hospitals to ventilate the lungs with oxygen during patient transport, but a self-inflating bag with a non-rebreathing valve is often used instead.

Mapleson D system

The Mapleson D arrangement is inefficient during spontaneous breathing (Fig. 16.16). During expiration, exhaled gas and fresh gas mix in the corrugated tube and travel towards the reservoir bag (Fig. 16.16B). When the reservoir bag is full, the pressure in the system increases, the spill valve opens and a mixture of fresh and exhaled gas is vented; this includes the dead space gas, which reaches the reservoir bag first (Fig. 16.16C). Although fresh gas pushes alveolar gas towards the valve during the expiratory pause, a mixture of alveolar and fresh gases is inhaled from the corrugated tube unless the FGF rate is at least twice the patient's minute volume (i.e. at least 12 L min^{-1} in the adult); in some patients, an FGF rate of 250 ml kg^{-1} min^{-1} is required to prevent rebreathing.

However, the Mapleson D system is more efficient than the Mapleson A during controlled ventilation (Fig. 16.17), especially if an expiratory pause is incorporated into the ventilatory cycle. During expiration, the corrugated tubing and reservoir bag fill with a mixture of fresh and alveolar gas (Fig. 16.17A). Fresh gas fills the distal part of the corrugated tube during the expiratory pause (Fig. 16.17B). When the reservoir bag is squeezed, this fresh gas enters the lungs, and when the spill valve opens a mixture of fresh and alveolar gas is vented. The degree of rebreathing may thus be controlled by adjustment of the FGF rate, but this should always exceed the patient's minute volume.

The Bain coaxial system (see Fig. 16.15) is the most commonly used version of the Mapleson D system. Fresh gas flow is supplied through a narrow inner tube. This tube may become disconnected, resulting in hypoxaemia and hypercapnia. Before use, the system should be tested by occluding the distal end of the inner tube transiently with a finger or the plunger of a 2 ml syringe; there should be a reduction in the flowmeter bobbin reading during occlusion and an audible release of pressure when occlusion is discontinued. Movement of the reservoir bag during anaesthesia does not necessarily indicate that fresh gas is being delivered to the patient.

The Bain system may be used to ventilate the patient's lungs with some types of automatic ventilator (e.g. Penlon Nuffield 200; Fig. 16.18). A 1 m length of corrugated tubing is interposed between the patient valve of the ventilator and

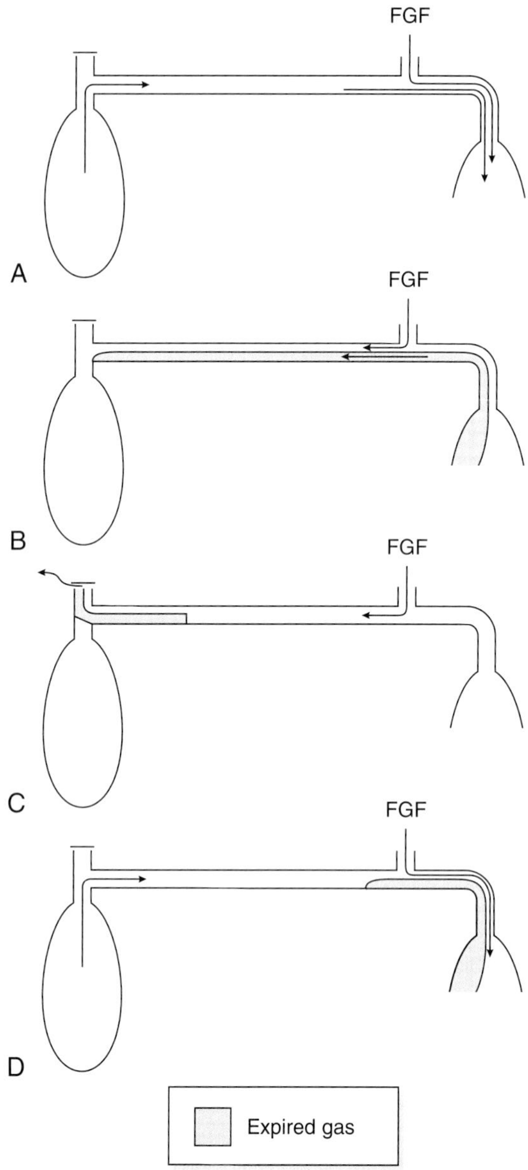

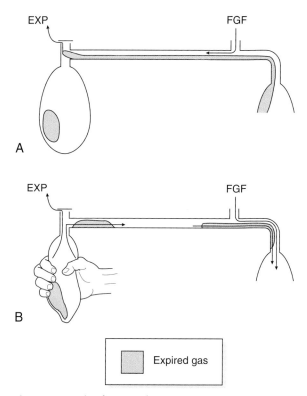

A

B

C

D

Expired gas

Fig. 16.16 Mode of action of Mapleson D breathing system during spontaneous ventilation. (A and D) Inspiration. (B and C) Expiration. See text for details. *FGF,* Fresh gas flow.

EXP · FGF

A

EXP · FGF

B

Expired gas

Fig. 16.17 Mode of action of Mapleson D breathing system during controlled ventilation. (A) Expiration. (B) Inspiration. See text for details. *EXP,* Expired gas; *FGF,* fresh gas flow.

some of the alveolar gas are vented through the exhaust valve of the ventilator. The degree of rebreathing is regulated by the anaesthetic gas flow rate; a flow of 70–80 ml kg^{-1} min^{-1} should result in normocapnia and a flow of 100 ml kg^{-1} min^{-1} in moderate hypocapnia. A secure connection between the Bain system and the anaesthetic machine must be ensured. If this connection is loose, a leak of fresh gas occurs; this causes rebreathing of ventilator gas and results in awareness, hypoxaemia and hypercapnia.

Mapleson E and F systems

The Mapleson E system, or Ayre's T-piece, has virtually no resistance to expiration. It was used extensively in paediatric anaesthesia before the advantages of continuous positive airways pressure (CPAP) were recognised, but is now obsolete. It functions in a manner similar to the Mapleson D system in that the corrugated tube fills with a mixture of exhaled and fresh gas during expiration and with fresh gas during the expiratory pause. Rebreathing is prevented if the FGF rate is 2.5–3 times the patient's minute volume. If the volume of the corrugated tube is less than the patient's tidal volume,

the reservoir bag mount (Fig. 16.19); the spill valve *must* be closed completely. An appropriate tidal volume and ventilatory rate are selected on the ventilator, and anaesthetic gases are supplied to the Bain system. During inspiration, the gas from the ventilator pushes a mixture of anaesthetic and alveolar gas from the corrugated outer tube into the patient's lungs; during expiration, the ventilator gas and

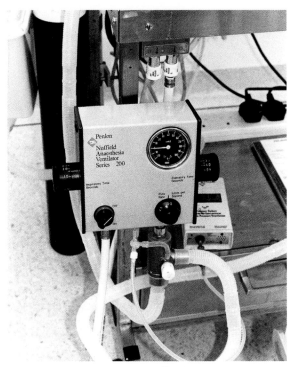

Fig. 16.18 The Penlon Nuffield 200 ventilator.

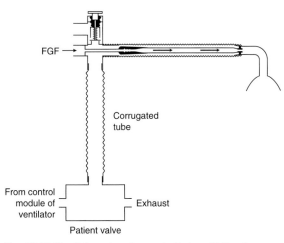

Fig. 16.19 The Bain system for controlled ventilation by a mechanical ventilator (e.g. Penlon Nuffield 200). A 1 m length of corrugated tubing with a capacity of at least 500 ml is required to prevent gas from the ventilator reaching the patient's lungs. $PaCO_2$ is controlled by varying the fresh gas flow *(FGF)* rate.

some air may be inhaled at the end of inspiration; consequently, an FGF rate of at least 4 L min^{-1} is recommended with a paediatric Mapleson E system.

During spontaneous ventilation, there is no indication of the presence or the adequacy of ventilation. It is possible to attach a visual indicator, such as a piece of tissue paper or a feather, at the end of the corrugated tube, but this is not very satisfactory.

Intermittent positive pressure ventilation (IPPV) may be applied by occluding the end of the corrugated tube with a finger. However, there is no way of assessing the pressure in the system and there is a possibility of exposing the patient's lungs to excessive volumes and pressures.

The Mapleson F system, or Rees' modification of the Ayre's T-piece, includes an open-ended bag attached to the end of the corrugated tube. This confers several advantages:

- It provides visual evidence of breathing during spontaneous ventilation.
- By occluding the open end of the bag temporarily, it is possible to confirm that fresh gas is entering the system.
- It provides a degree of CPAP during spontaneous ventilation and positive end-expiratory pressure (PEEP) during IPPV.
- It provides a convenient method of assisting or controlling ventilation. The open end of the reservoir bag is occluded between the fourth and fifth fingers and the bag is squeezed between the thumb and index finger; the fourth and fifth fingers are relaxed during expiration to allow gas to escape from the bag. It is possible with experience to assess (approximately) the inflation pressure and to detect changes in lung and chest wall compliance.

However, one main disadvantage of the Mapleson F system is that efficient scavenging is unsatisfactory and is non-standard.

Mapleson ADE system

This system provides the advantages of the Mapleson A, D and E systems. It can be used efficiently for spontaneous and controlled ventilation in both children and adults.

It consists of two parallel lengths of 15-mm-bore tubing; one delivers fresh gas, and the other carries exhaled gas. One end of the tubing connects to the patient via a Y-connection and the other end contains the Humphrey block (Fig. 16.20). The Humphrey block (Fig. 16.21) comprises an APL valve, a lever to select spontaneous or controlled ventilation, a reservoir bag, a port to connect a ventilator and a safety pressure relief valve that opens at a pressure above 6 kPa.

When the lever is in the A mode (up), the reservoir bag is connected to the breathing system as it would be in the Mapleson A system. The breathing hose connecting the bag to the patient is the inspiratory limb. The expired gases travel along the other tubing back to the APL valve, which is connected to the scavenging system.

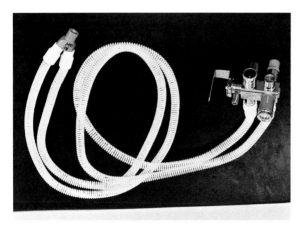

Fig. 16.20 The ADE system.

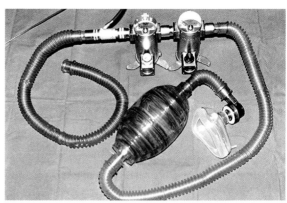

Fig. 16.22 The Triservice apparatus. (Courtesy Dr S. Kidd.)

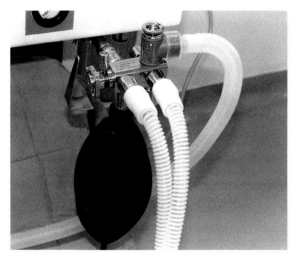

Fig. 16.21 The Humphrey block. This consists of an APL valve, a lever to select spontaneous or controlled ventilation, a reservoir bag, a port to connect to the ventilator and a safety pressure relief valve.

With the lever in the D/E mode (down), the reservoir bag and the APL valve are isolated from the breathing system. What was the expiratory limb in the A mode now delivers gas to the patient. The hose returning gas to the Humphrey block now functions as a reservoir to the T-piece. This hose would open to atmosphere via a port adjacent to the bag mount, but in practice this port is connected to a ventilator such as the Penlon Nuffield.

In adults, an appropriate FGF is 50–60 ml kg^{-1} min^{-1} in spontaneously breathing patients and 70 ml kg^{-1} min^{-1} in ventilated patients.

Drawover systems

Occasionally it is necessary to administer inhalational anaesthesia outside the hospital; this requires simple, portable equipment. The Triservice apparatus was designed by the British armed forces for use in battlefield conditions (Fig. 16.22). It comprises a self-inflating bag, a non-rebreathing valve (e.g. Ambu E, Rubens), which vents all expired gases to atmosphere, one or two OMVs (which have a low internal resistance), an oxygen supply and a length of corrugated tubing that serves as an oxygen reservoir. It can be used for either spontaneous or controlled ventilation. The practical use of drawover vaporisers is discussed further in Chapter 45.

Rebreathing systems

Anaesthetic breathing systems in which some gas is rebreathed by the patient were designed originally to economise on the use of cyclopropane. In addition, they reduce the risk of atmospheric pollution and increase the humidity of inspired gases, thereby reducing heat loss from the patient. Rebreathing systems may be used as closed systems, in which fresh gas is introduced only to replace oxygen and anaesthetic agents absorbed by the patient. More commonly the system is used with a small leak through a spill valve, and the fresh gas supply exceeds basal oxygen requirements. Because rebreathing occurs, these systems must incorporate a means of absorbing CO_2 from exhaled alveolar gas.

Soda lime

Soda lime (Table 16.4) is the substance used most commonly for absorption of CO_2 in rebreathing systems. The major constituent is calcium hydroxide, but sodium and potassium

Table 16.4 Composition of soda lime

$Ca(OH)_2$	94%
NaOH	5%
KOH	<1% or nil
Silica	0.2%
Moisture content	14%–19%

hydroxides may also be present. Absorption of carbon dioxide occurs by the following chemical reactions:

$$CO_2 + 2NaOH \rightarrow Na_2CO_3 + H_2O + heat$$

$$Na_2CO_3 + Ca(OH)_2 \rightarrow 2NaOH + CaCO_3$$

Water is required for efficient absorption. There is some water in soda lime and more is added from the patient's expired gas and from the chemical reaction. The reaction generates heat, and the temperature in the centre of a soda lime canister may exceed 60°C. Sevoflurane interacts with soda lime to produce substances that are toxic in animals, but there is no significant risk in humans (see Chapter 3). There is new evidence suggesting that the presence of strong alkalis such as sodium and potassium hydroxides could be the trigger of the interaction between volatile agents and soda lime. CO_2 absorbers such as Amsorb Plus do not contain these hydroxides.

The size of soda lime granules is important. If granules are too large, the surface area for absorption is insufficient; if they are too small, the narrow space between granules results in a high resistance to breathing. Granule size is measured by a mesh number. Soda lime consists of granules in the range of 4–8 mesh. (A 4-mesh strainer has four openings per square inch and an 8-mesh strainer has eight openings.) Silica is added to soda lime to reduce the tendency of the granules to disintegrate into powder. In addition, soda lime contains an indicator which changes colour as the active constituents become exhausted. The rate at which soda lime becomes exhausted depends on the capacity of the canister, the FGF rate and the rate of CO_2 production. In a completely closed system, a standard 450 g canister becomes inefficient after approximately 2 h.

Baralyme

Baralyme is another carbon dioxide absorber. It is a mixture of approximately 20% barium hydroxide and 80% calcium hydroxide. It may also contain some potassium hydroxide, an indicator and moisture. Barium hydroxide contains eight molecules of water of crystallisation, which help to fuse the mixture so that it retains the granular structure under various conditions of heat and moisture. The granules of baralyme are similar to those of soda lime.

Circle system

The circle system has many advantages and is in widespread use for induction and maintenance of anaesthesia. In this system the soda lime canister is mounted on the anaesthetic machine, and inspiratory and expiratory corrugated tubing conducts gas to and from the patient. The system incorporates a reservoir bag and spill valve and two low-resistance one-way valves to ensure unidirectional movement of gas (Fig. 16.23). These valves are normally mounted in glass domes so that they may be observed to be functioning correctly. The spill valve may be mounted close to the patient or beside the absorber; it is generally more convenient to use a valve near the absorber. Fresh gas enters the system between the absorber and the inspiratory tubing.

The soda lime canister is mounted vertically and thus channelling of gas through unfilled areas is not possible. The canister cannot contribute to dead space; consequently a large canister may be used, and the soda lime needs to be changed less often.

The major disadvantage of the circle system arises from its volume. If the system is filled with air initially, low flow rates of anaesthetic gases are diluted substantially and adequate concentrations cannot be achieved. Even if the system is primed with a mixture of anaesthetic gases, the initial rapid uptake by the patient results in a marked decrease in concentrations of anaesthetic agents in the system, resulting in light anaesthesia. Consequently it is necessary usually to provide a total FGF rate of 3–4 L min^{-1} to the system initially. This flow rate may be reduced subsequently, but it must be remembered that dilution of fresh gas continues at low flow rates and that rapid changes in depth of anaesthesia cannot be achieved.

Volatile anaesthetic agents may be delivered to a circle system in two ways:

• *Vaporiser outside the circle (VOC)* (Fig. 16.24A). If a standard vaporiser (e.g. TEC series) is used, it must be placed on the back bar of the anaesthetic machine because of its high internal resistance. If low FGF rates (<1 L min^{-1}) are used, the change in concentration of volatile anaesthetic agent achieved in the circle system is very small because of dilution, even if the vaporiser is set to deliver a high concentration (Fig. 16.25A). It may be necessary to change FGF rate rather than the vaporiser setting to achieve a rapid change in depth of anaesthesia. The concentration of volatile agent in the system depends on the patient's expired concentration (which is recycled), the rate of uptake by the patient (which decreases with time and is lower with agents of low blood/gas solubility coefficient), the concentration of agent supplied and the FGF rate.

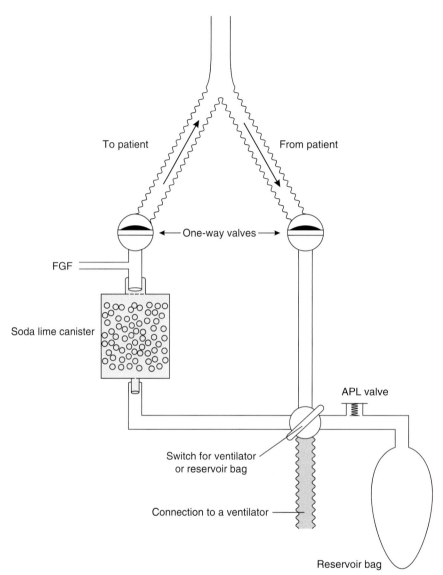

Fig. 16.23 Mechanism of the circle system. The direction of gas flow is controlled via the unidirectional valves. A lever allows the ventilation to be either spontaneous through the reservoir bag and APL valve or controlled by a ventilator. *APL,* Adjustable pressure-limiting valve; *FGF,* fresh gas flow.

- *Vaporiser inside the circle (VIC)* (Fig. 16.24B). Drawover vaporisers with a low internal resistance (e.g. Goldman) may be placed within the circle system. During each inspiration, vapour is added to the inspired gas mixture. In contrast to a VOC system, the inspired concentration is higher at low FGF rates because the expired concentration is diluted to a lesser extent (Fig. 16.25B), and the vaporiser *adds* to the concentration present in the expired gas. VIC systems are rarely used now.

If FGF rate is low, the use of the circle system by the inexperienced anaesthetist may result either in inadequate anaesthesia or in severe cardiovascular and respiratory depression. In addition, a hypoxic gas mixture may be delivered if low flow rates of a nitrous oxide/oxygen mixture are supplied, because after 10–15 min, oxygen is taken up in larger volumes than N_2O. These difficulties can be overcome by continuous monitoring of the inspired concentrations of oxygen, CO_2 and volatile anaesthetic agent

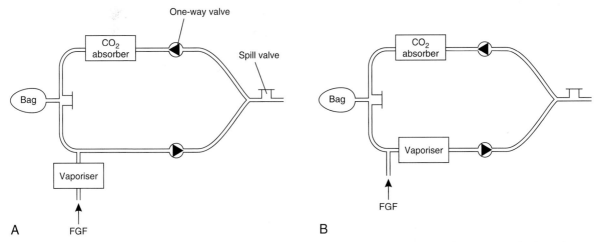

Fig. 16.24 Diagrammatic representation of circle system. (A) Vaporiser outside the circle (VOC). (B) Vaporiser inside the circle (VIC). *FGF,* Fresh gas flow.

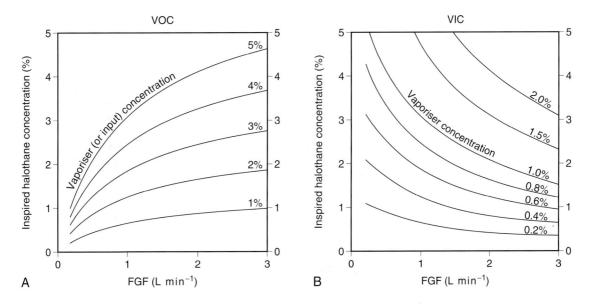

Fig. 16.25 Variation of inspired concentration of halothane with fresh gas flow *(FGF)* rate. Total minute ventilation is 5 L min⁻¹. (A) Vaporiser outside the circle *(VOC)*; note that dilution of the fresh gas results in much lower concentrations in the circle system than the concentration set on the vaporiser unless FGF rate approaches 3 L min⁻¹. (B) Vaporiser inside the circle *(VIC)*; at low flow rates lack of dilution of expired halothane concentration, with additional halothane vaporised during each inspiration, results in inspired concentrations much higher than those set on the vaporiser. Even at an FGF rate of 3 L min⁻¹, inspired concentration is approximately 50% higher than the vaporiser setting.

(see Chapter 17). The anaesthetist *must* be aware that one-way valves may stick and therefore these should be checked both at the preanaesthetic check of the machine and during anaesthesia. Rebreathing can occur if the valves stick in the open position, and total occlusion of the circuit can occur if the expiratory valve is stuck in the closed position, barotrauma or volutrauma can result. Obstructed filters located in the expiratory limb of the circle breathing system have caused increased airway pressure, haemodynamic collapse and bilateral tension pneumothorax. Because the circle system has many connections, the anaesthetist should be vigilant about checking for any leak or

Table 16.5 Advantages and disadvantages of the circle system

Advantages	Disadvantages
Inspired gases are humidified and warmed	More components than simpler systems such as the Bain system
Economical	*Risk of delivering hypoxic mixture
Minimal atmospheric pollution	Increased resistance to breathing Slow change in the depth of anaesthesia *Risk of awareness *Risk of a rise in end-tidal CO_2 if soda lime exhausted Risk of unidirectional valves sticking Not ideal for paediatric patients breathing spontaneously Some inhalational agents may interact with soda lime

*Risks reduced by adequate monitoring of inspired oxygen, end-tidal carbon dioxide and inhalational agent concentration.

disconnection. Common source of leaks include points of connection within the breathing circuit and at the carbon dioxide absorber canister. Breathing circuit pressure sensors, workstation tidal volume sensors and capnography can help to identify leaks and misconnections.

The advantages and disadvantages of the circle system are summarised in Table 16.5.

Manual resuscitation breathing systems

Occasionally a patient may require emergency ventilatory support using a source that does not rely on pressurised gas or electricity. It is recommended that such a breathing system is readily available in all areas where anaesthetics are administered in case of emergency.

Many different types of manual resuscitation breathing systems are available. They all comprise the following:
• Self-inflating bag
• Non-rebreathing valve
• Fresh gas input with or without an oxygen reservoir bag
The self-inflating bag has a volume of approximately 1500 ml, 500 ml and 250 ml for the adult, child and infant sizes, respectively. The non-rebreathing valve has several components which ensure that, during the inspiratory phase, gas flows out of the bag into the patient and, during the expiratory phase, the valve ensures that exhaled gas escapes through the expiratory port without mixing with fresh gas. Three types of non-rebreathing systems are available, the

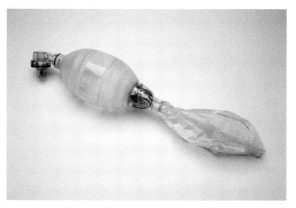

Fig. 16.26 The Laerdal manual resuscitation breathing system.

Ruben, Ambu and Laerdal systems (Fig. 16.26). Functionally they are very similar but with some minor differences. The Ruben valve has a spring-loaded bobbin within the valve housing. The Ambu system has several series of valves which have either a single valve or double-leaf valves to control unidirectional flow. The Laerdal system has three components: a duck-billed inspiratory/expiratory valve, a valve body housing inspiratory and expiratory ports and a non-return flap valve in the expiratory port.

Ventilators

Mechanical ventilation of the lung may be achieved by several mechanisms, including the generation of a negative pressure around the whole of the patient's body except the head and neck (cabinet ventilator or iron lung), a negative pressure over the thorax and abdomen (cuirass ventilators) or a positive pressure over the thorax and abdomen (inflatable cuirass ventilators). However, during anaesthesia, and in the majority of patients who require mechanical ventilation in ICU, ventilation is achieved by the application of positive pressure to the lungs through a supraglottic airway, tracheal tube or tracheostomy tube. Only positive pressure ventilation is described here.

Many different ventilators are available and this section discusses only the principles of use. Before using any ventilator, it is *essential* that the anaesthetist understands its functions fully; failure to do so may result in the delivery of a hypoxic gas mixture, rebreathing of CO_2 and/or delivery of a mixture that contains no anaesthetic gases. If an unfamiliar ventilator is encountered, it may be helpful to use a dummy lung (a small reservoir bag on the patient connection) and to discuss the capabilities and limitations of the machine with a senior colleague. In addition, the manufacturer's user handbook may be consulted or details may be obtained from a specialist book.

The principles of operation of ventilators are described best by considering each phase of the ventilatory cycle: inspiration, change from inspiration to expiration, expiration, and change from expiration to inspiration.

Inspiration

The patterns of volume and pressure change in the lung are determined by the characteristics of the ventilator (Fig. 16.27). Ventilators may deliver a predetermined flow rate of gas *(constant flow generators)* or exert a predetermined pressure

(constant pressure generators), although some machines produce a pattern that does not conform precisely to either category. Most flow generators produce a constant flow of gas during inspiration, although a few generate a sinusoidal flow pattern if the ventilator bellows is driven via a crank.

Constant pressure generator

Constant pressure-generating ventilators produce inspiration by generating a constant, predetermined pressure. If airway resistance increases or if compliance decreases, these ventilators deliver a reduced tidal volume at the preset cycling pressure (Fig. 16.28). Consequently their performance is variable.

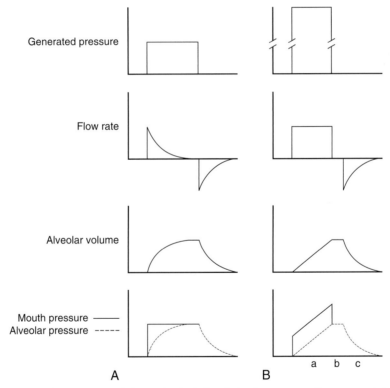

Fig. 16.27 Graphs of generated pressure, mouth (or tracheal tube) and alveolar pressures, flow rate and alveolar volume changes during inspiration and subsequent expiration produced by a constant pressure generator (A) and a constant flow generator (B). A constant pressure generator exerts a low pressure (e.g. 1.5 kPa, 15 cmH$_2$O). At the start of inspiration, the pressure in the alveoli is zero. Gas flows rapidly into the alveoli at a rate determined by airway resistance, resulting in rapid increases in alveolar volume and pressure. The mouth–alveolar pressure gradient decreases and flow rate, and consequently the rate of increase of alveolar volume and pressure decreases also. When the alveolar pressure equals the ventilator pressure, flow ceases. A constant flow generator generates a very high internal pressure (e.g. 400 kPa) but has a high internal resistance to limit flow rate. The pressure gradient between machine and alveoli remains virtually constant throughout inspiration, and thus flow rate is constant. The increases in alveolar volume and (assuming constant compliance) pressure are linear. Because flow rate is constant, the pressure gradient between mouth and alveoli is constant throughout inspiration (a). Mouth pressure decreases to equal alveolar pressure during the inspiratory pause when flow ceases (b). Gas flow out of the lung during expiration (c) is passive.

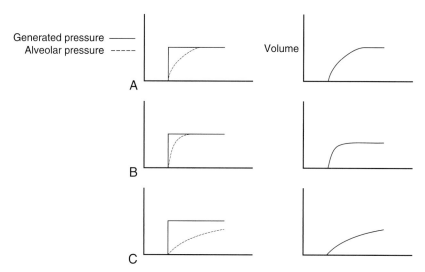

Fig. 16.28 Generated and alveolar pressures and alveolar volume during inspiration with a constant pressure generator. (A) Normal. (B) Decreased compliance. (C) Increased airway resistance. Note that both abnormalities reduce alveolar volume.

Constant flow generator

Constant flow ventilators produce inspiration by delivering a predetermined constant flow rate of gas during inspiration. Changes in resistance or compliance make little difference to the volume delivered (unless the ventilator is pressure cycled; see later), although airway and alveolar pressures may change (Fig. 16.29). For example, decreased compliance results in delivery of a normal tidal volume; however, the rate of increase of alveolar pressure is greater than normal (i.e. the slope is greater), and airway pressure is correspondingly higher to maintain an appropriate pressure gradient between the tracheal tube and the alveoli. If airway resistance increases, the pressure at the tracheal tube (and the gradient between tracheal tube and alveolar pressures) is higher than normal throughout inspiration, but alveolar pressure and the slopes of both pressure curves are normal. Constant flow generators do not compensate for leaks; the tidal volume delivered to the lungs decreases.

Some ventilators generate a pressure rather higher than that required to inflate the lungs but not high enough to maintain constant flow throughout inspiration. The flow, volume and pressure changes within the lung are shown in Fig. 16.30.

Change from inspiration to expiration

The change from inspiration to expiration is termed *cycling* and may be achieved in one of three ways:

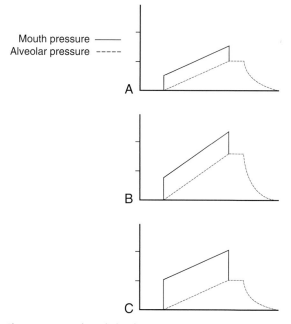

Fig. 16.29 Mouth and alveolar pressures during inspiration with a constant flow generator. (A) Normal. (B) Decreased compliance. (C) Increased airway resistance. Alveolar volume remains constant because flow rate is constant. Decreased compliance results in an increased rate of increase of alveolar pressure; mouth pressure also increases more steeply, but the gradient between mouth and alveolar pressures remains normal. Increased airway resistance increases the mouth–alveolar pressure gradient.

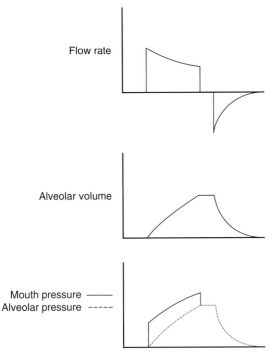

Fig. 16.30 Pressure, flow and alveolar volume characteristics during inspiration with a ventilator with a moderately high internal pressure. At higher bellows pressures, and in a patient with normal compliance and airway resistance, the characteristics approximate to those of a constant flow generator (see Fig. 16.27B). At low bellows pressures, if compliance decreases or if airway resistance increases, the pattern is similar to that of a constant pressure generator.

- *Volume cycling.* The ventilator cycles into expiration whenever a predetermined tidal volume has been delivered. The duration of inspiration is determined by the inspiratory flow rate.
- *Pressure cycling.* The ventilator cycles into expiration when a preset airway pressure is achieved. This allows compensation for small leaks but, in common with a constant pressure generator, a pressure-cycled ventilator delivers a different tidal volume if compliance or resistance change. In addition, inspiratory time varies with changes in compliance and resistance.
- *Time cycling.* This is the method used most commonly by modern ventilators. The duration of inspiration is predetermined. With a constant flow generator, it may be desirable to preset a tidal volume; when this has been delivered, there is a short inspiratory pause (which improves gas distribution within the lung) before the inspiratory cycle ends. The use of this volume-preset mechanism must be differentiated from volume cycling, in which the ventilator cycles into expiration whenever

the preset tidal volume has been delivered (and therefore the respiratory rate may be variable). When a constant pressure generator is time cycled, the tidal volume delivered depends on the compliance and resistance of the lungs and on the pressure within the bellows.

Expiration

Usually the patient is allowed to exhale to atmospheric pressure; flow rate decreases exponentially. Subatmospheric pressure should not be used during expiration as it induces closure of small airways and air trapping. PEEP may be applied (see Chapter 48).

Change from expiration to inspiration

On most ventilators, the change from expiration to inspiration is achieved by time cycling. However, it may be desirable occasionally to use pressure cycling in response to a subatmospheric pressure generated by the patient's inspiratory effort.

Delivery of anaesthetic gas

Some ventilators deliver a minute volume determined by a preset tidal volume and rate. When used in anaesthesia, these machines must be supplied with a flow rate of anaesthetic gases which equals or exceeds the minute volume delivered; otherwise air, or gas used to drive the ventilator, is entrained and delivered to the patient. Older ventilators such as the Blease Manley are driven by the anaesthetic gas supply, can deliver only that gas, and divide it into predetermined tidal volumes (*minute volume dividers*).

Ventilators may be used to compress bellows in a separate system which contains anaesthetic gases (bag-in-a-bottle); it is possible to provide IPPV in a circle system in this way. The bag-in-a-bottle ventilator (Fig. 16.31) consists of a chamber with a tidal volume range of 0–1500 ml (adult mode) or 0–400 ml (paediatric mode) and ascending bellows that accommodate FGF. The control unit has controls, displays and alarms, and these may include tidal volume, respiratory rate, inspiratory to expiratory (I/E) ratio, airway pressure and an on/off/standby switch. Compressed air or oxygen is used as the driving gas. On entering the chamber, the compressed gas forces the bellows down, delivering the FGF within the bellows to the patient. The driving gas in the chamber and the FGF in the bellows remain separate.

The Penlon Nuffield 200 ventilator (see Fig. 16.18) is an intermittent blower. It is a very versatile ventilator which may be used in different age groups and using different breathing systems. The control unit consists of an airway pressure gauge

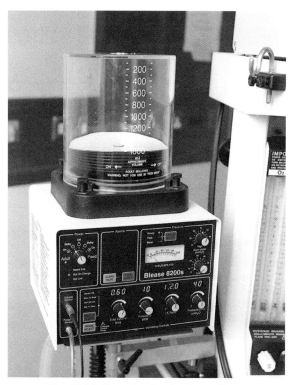

Fig. 16.31 Blease bag-in-a-bottle ventilator.

(cmH$_2$O), an on/off switch and controls to set inspiratory and expiratory time (seconds) and inspiratory flow rate (L s^{-1}). Below the control unit, there is a connection for the driving gas (oxygen or air) and the valve block. A small tube connects the valve block to an airway pressure monitor and to a ventilator alarm. The valve block consists of a port for tubing to connect to the breathing system reservoir bag mount (Bain system) or the ventilator port (Mapleson ADE system), an exhaust port which can be connected to the scavenging system and a pressure relief valve which opens at 6–7 kPa. With this standard valve, the ventilator is a time-cycled flow generator. The valve block can be changed to a paediatric Newton valve, and this then converts the ventilator to a time-cycled pressure generator.

Older anaesthetic machine ventilators had a minimal number of controls, usually for minute volume, tidal volume, ventilator frequency and I/E ratio. Modern anaesthetic machine ventilators are highly efficient; they are electrically powered, single-circuit, microprocessor-controlled gas flow and piston driven with no need for drive gas. They have the advantages of a compact, heated breathing circuit. Fresh gas decoupling is a safety feature incorporated in both piston ventilators and descending bellows ventilators to prevent barotrauma. These ventilators use electronic gas mixers rather than conventional rotameters. Inclusion of a reservoir

bag during mechanical ventilation is an additional safety feature. The visual movement is proof that the ventilator is functioning. They have the facility for complex integrated monitoring and data-recording systems and include adjustable, audible and visual alarms. The newer models resemble critical care ventilators in the settings that are available. When switched on, they perform automatic self-tests using dual processor technology, they have volume- or pressure-controlled ventilation modes, assisted spontaneous ventilation and electronically adjusted PEEP. Sophisticated internal spirometry compensates for factors such as leaks and patient compliance. They are suitable for a wider range of patients and weights and can deliver tidal volumes as low as 20 ml. The ventilator in the Primus Dräger (see Fig. 16.3A) anaesthetic machine is an electronically controlled piston ventilator which provides several modes of ventilation, including volume control, pressure control, pressure support and volume mode autoflow. All these modes can be synchronised with patient effort and can have additional pressure support.

Monitoring of ventilator function

Continuous clinical monitoring is essential when any ventilator is used, even those which incorporate sophisticated measurement and warning devices. In addition to standard clinical monitoring (see Chapter 17), ventilator function must be monitored by measurement of expired tidal volume, airway pressure, inspired oxygen concentration and detection of ventilator disconnection. Disconnection alarms are the most important, and anaesthetic machines should have at least three: low peak inspiration pressure, low exhaled tidal volume and low exhaled CO$_2$. Other built-in alarms include high peak airway pressure, high PEEP, low oxygen supply pressure and negative pressure.

Humidification and bacterial filters

The incorporation of a humidifier in the inspiratory limb, or of a condenser humidifier at the connection with the tracheal tube, is essential during long-term ventilation in the ITU. Bacterial filters (Fig. 16.32) are recommended for all patients undergoing anaesthesia.

Portable ventilators

Several types of portable ventilator are available for use during the transport of critically ill patients, such as the Pneupac VR1 and the Oxylog. The Oxylog 3000 (Fig. 16.33) and 3000Plus ventilators offer sophisticated ventilation in emergency situations and during transport. Portable gas-powered ventilators use pneumatic energy to provide inspiratory gas flow and regulate the respiratory cycle. A microprocessor-controlled ventilator uses electrical power to regulate the respiratory cycle, but inspiratory flow may be driven either pneumatically or by an electrical compressor. They are time-cycled, constant volume and pressure-controlled ventilators and deliver tidal volumes of 50 ml or more. They incorporate various modes of ventilation suitable for critically ill patients, including IPPV, synchronised intermittent mandatory ventilation (SIMV) with adjustable pressure assist during spontaneous breathing, CPAP and biphasic positive airway pressure (BIPAP), apnoea ventilation for switching over automatically to volume-controlled ventilation if breathing stops, and non-invasive ventilation (NIV). Other features include monitoring of airway pressure and expiratory minute volume, integrated capnography and enhanced data connectivity.

The characteristics of several common ventilators are summarised in Table 16.6.

High-frequency ventilation

High-frequency ventilation (HFV) may be defined as ventilation at a respiratory rate of greater than four times the patient's resting respiratory rate. Of the three types of HFV (Table 16.7), high-frequency jet ventilation (HFJV) is most commonly used. The tidal volume used in HFJV is small compared with conventional ventilation. This is delivered at high pressure (up to 5 bar) through a tracheal cannula or catheter. Inspiratory flow rates of up to 100 L min^{-1} may be required. The inspiratory time is adjustable from 20% to 50% of the cycle. The mechanism by which HFV is able to maintain gas exchange is not clear. Typical values for adult ventilation are as follows:

- Ventilation rate 100–150 cycles min^{-1}
- Driving pressure 100–200 kPa
- Inspiratory cycle 20%–40%

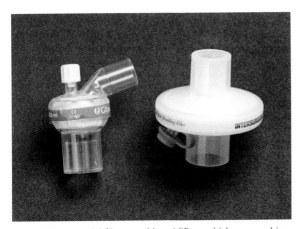

Fig. 16.32 Bacterial filters and humidifiers which are used in breathing systems: *Left,* a paediatric filter incorporated into an angle piece; *right,* an adult filter.

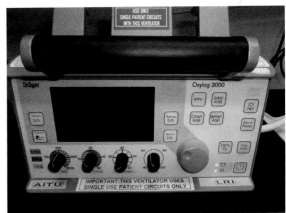

Fig. 16.33 The Oxylog 3000, an emergency ventilator.

Table 16.6 Classification of some common ventilators used during anaesthesia

Ventilator	Driven by	Cycling to expiration	Cycling to inspiration	Pressure/flow generator	Minute volume divider	Volume preset
Manley MP3, MP5	Anaesthetic gases	Time/volume	Time	Pressure	Yes	Yes
Nuffield 200	Compressed air or oxygen	Time	Time	Flow	No	No
Bag-in-bottle	Compressed air or oxygen	Time	Time	Flow	No	Yes
Single circuit Piston ventilators	Electrical	Time	Time	Flow	No	Yes
Oxylog 3000 transport ventilator	Gas powered	Time	Time	Flow	No	Yes

Table 16.7 Types of high-frequency ventilation

Type of ventilation	Rate of ventilation (cycles min^{-1})
High-frequency positive pressure ventilation (HFPPV)	60–100
High-frequency jet ventilation (HFJV)	100–400
High-frequency oscillation ventilation (HFOV)	400–2400

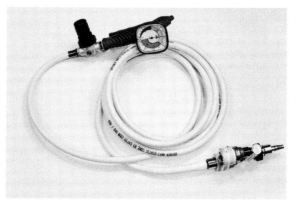

Fig. 16.34 Manually controlled Venturi injector.

High-frequency jet ventilation is used during some operations on the larynx, trachea or lung and in a small number of patients in intensive care. Gases should be humidified when using HFJV. Gas exchange may be unpredictable, and the technique should not be used by the trainee without supervision.

Venturi injector device

The Venturi injector consists of a high-pressure oxygen source (at about 400 kPa from either the anaesthetic machine or direct from a pipeline), on/off trigger and connection tubing that can withstand high pressure. The Manujet (Fig. 16.34) is a newer design of a manually controlled Venturi injector device. It can be connected to a rigid bronchoscope or tracheal tube or to a transtracheal or transcricothyroid cannula (Fig. 16.35). The driving pressure can be altered according to patient size from neonate to adult. A Venturi effect is created, which entrains atmospheric air and allows intermittent insufflation of the lungs with oxygen-enriched air at airway pressures of 2.5–3.0 kPa. It can be used in laryngeal or tracheobronchial surgery or for difficult airway situations such as fibreoptic intubation, upper airway obstruction or a 'can't intubate, can't oxygenate' scenario (see Chapter 23). Possible complications include barotrauma, gastric distension and awareness if inadequate quantities of intravenous anaesthetic drugs are administered. When Venturi injector devices are employed, it is essential to ensure that gas is able to leave the lungs though the upper airway during expiration.

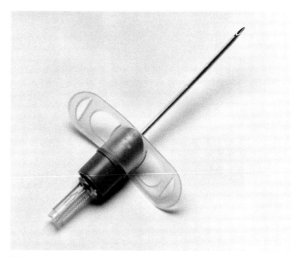

Fig. 16.35 Cricothyroid cannula to use with a Venturi injector device.

Scavenging

There are regulatory requirements for installation and correct functioning of anaesthetic gas scavenging equipment. There is little evidence that exposure to waste anaesthetic agents has deleterious effects on staff at the concentrations commonly encountered, but international guidance is to reduce these to as low as practical (Table 16.8).

The principal sources of pollution by anaesthetic gases and vapours are as follows:

- Discharge of anaesthetic gases from ventilators
- Expired gas vented from the spill valve of anaesthetic breathing systems
- Leaks from equipment (e.g. from an ill-fitting face mask)
- Gas exhaled by the patient after anaesthesia; may occur in the operating theatre and recovery rooms
- Spillage during filling of vaporisers

Most attention has been paid to ways of removing gas from the expiratory ports of breathing systems and ventilators, but other methods of reducing pollution include the following:

Table 16.8 Workplace exposure limits for anaesthetic agents

Agent	Long-term exposure limit (ppm) (8-h time-weighted average reference period)	
	UK	US
Nitrous oxide	100	25
Isoflurane	50	2
Sevoflurane	—	2
Desflurane	—	2

The limit of 2 parts per million (ppm) in the United States is based on the lowest detectable level at the time the standards were first introduced. The US recommendations apply to all halogenated anaesthetic agents.

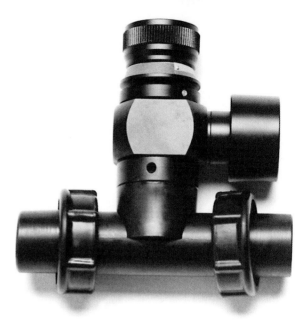

Fig. 16.36 An adjustable pressure-limiting (APL) valve with scavenging attachment.

- *Reduced use of anaesthetic gases and vapours.* The circle system reduces the potential for atmospheric pollution. The use of inhalational anaesthetics may be avoided by using total intravenous anaesthesia or local anaesthetic techniques.
- *Air conditioning.* Air conditioning units that produce a rapid change of air in the operating theatre reduce pollution substantially. However, some systems recycle air, and older operating theatres, dental surgeries and obstetric delivery suites may not be equipped with air conditioning.
- *Care in filling vaporisers.* Great care should be taken not to spill volatile anaesthetic agent when a vaporiser is filled. The use of agent-specific connections (see Fig. 16.9) reduces the risk of spillage. In some countries, vaporisers must be filled only in a portable fume cupboard.

Scavenging apparatus

Modern scavenging has four components for collecting, transferring, receiving and disposal of waste gases from the breathing circuit. The collecting system comprises a purpose-built, gas-tight shroud enclosing an APL valve (Fig. 16.36) of the breathing circuit. Waste gases from ventilators are collected by attaching the scavenging system to the expiratory port of the ventilator. Connectors on scavenging systems have a diameter of 30 mm to prevent inappropriate connections to other anaesthetic apparatus. The transfer system comprises wide-bore tubing leading from the collecting system to the receiving system (Fig. 16.37). The receiving system comprises a reservoir, air brake, flow indicator and filter. Disposal systems may be active, semiactive or passive.

Active systems

Active systems employ apparatus to generate a negative pressure within the scavenging system to propel waste gases to the outside atmosphere. The system may be powered by a vacuum pump (see Fig. 16.37) or a Venturi system (Fig. 16.38). The exhaust should be capable of accommodating 75 L min^{-1} continuous flow with a peak of 130 L min^{-1}. Usually a reservoir system is used to permit high peak flow rates to be accommodated. In addition, there must be a pressure-limiting device within the system to prevent the application of negative pressure to the patient's lungs.

Semi-active systems

The waste gases may be conducted to the extraction side of the air-conditioning system, which generates a small negative pressure within the scavenging tubing. These systems have variable performance and efficiency.

Passive systems

Passive systems vent the expired gas to the outside atmosphere via a wide-bore pipe (Fig. 16.39). Gas movement is generated by the patient. Consequently the total length of tubing must not be excessive or resistance to expiration is high. The pressure within the system may be altered by wind conditions at the external terminal; on occasions, these may generate

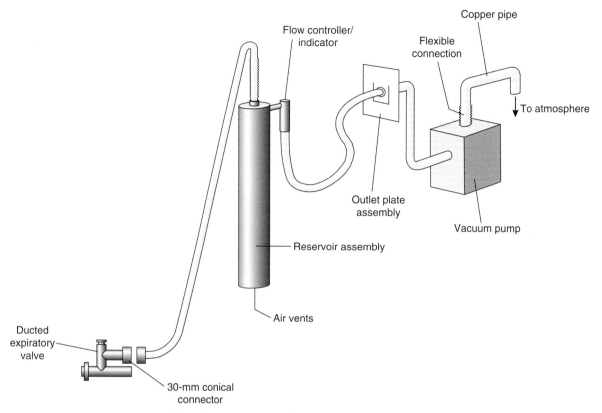

Fig. 16.37 Components of an active scavenging system.

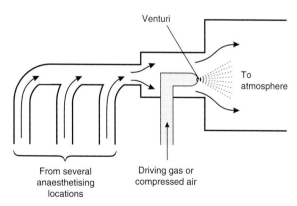

Fig. 16.38 A Venturi system for active scavenging of anaesthetic gases.

a negative pressure, but they may also generate high positive pressures. Each scavenging location should have a separate external terminal to prevent gases being vented into adjacent locations. Two spring-loaded valves to guard against excessive negative (−50 Pa) and positive (1000 Pa) pressures must be incorporated within the system.

Irrespective of the type of disposal system, tubing used for scavenging must not be allowed to lie on the floor of the operating theatre, as compression (e.g. by feet or by items of equipment) results in increased resistance to expiration and may generate dangerously high pressure within the patient's lungs.

Reservoir bags

Reservoir bags are used in breathing systems; they are made of either rubber or plastic and can be single use or reusable. The International Standards Organisation (ISO) specifies requirements for reservoir bags which include design, size

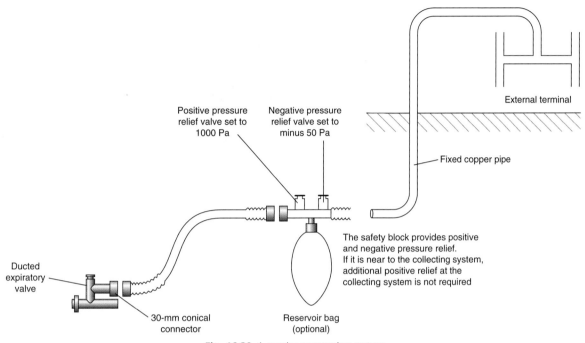

Positive pressure
relief valve set to
1000 Pa

Negative pressure
relief valve set to
minus 50 Pa

External terminal

Fixed copper pipe

The safety block provides positive
and negative pressure relief.
If it is near to the collecting system,
additional positive relief at the
collecting system is not required

Ducted
expiratory
valve

30-mm conical
connector

Reservoir bag
(optional)

Fig. 16.39 A passive scavenging system.

and distension. When made of latex rubber, the bag is highly distensible, which means that the pressure in the breathing system seldom exceeds 3.9 kPa (40 cmH$_2$O), preventing the patient's lungs from damage by high pressure, even when the APL valve is inadvertently left closed. The increasing prevalence of latex allergy means that latex-free reservoir bags are routinely used. Latex-free bags have been found to be less distensible and pressures in the breathing system can exceed 4.4 kPa (45 cmH$_2$O).

Reservoir bags range in size from 0.5 to 6 L. Standard sizes are 2 L for adults and 0.5 L for paediatrics.

The functions of the reservoir bag include:
- serving as a reservoir of inspired gases;
- providing a means of manual ventilation of the lungs;
- serving as a visual or tactile observation to monitor the patient's spontaneous respiration; and
- protecting the patient from excessive pressure in the breathing system.

Protecting the breathing system in anaesthesia

After fatal incidents in which anaesthetic tubing became blocked, the UK Department of Health recommended several measures to minimise the risk of recurrence. These include training, increasing awareness of the potential for anaesthetic tubing to become blocked accidentally and protecting vulnerable components of the breathing system by keeping the components individually wrapped until use. The Department of Health recommends the use of the Association of Anaesthetists' document 'Checking Anaesthetic Equipment' and that all trainees should be trained in the correct procedure for checking anaesthetic equipment.

Suction apparatus

Suction apparatus is vital during anaesthesia and resuscitation to clear the airway of any mucus, blood or debris. It is also used during surgery to clear the operating field of either blood or fluid.

Suction apparatus consists of a source of vacuum, a suction unit and suction tubing. The source of vacuum can be either piped vacuum or electrically or manually operated units. Piped vacuum is the most commonly used source in many operating theatres.

The suction unit consists of a reservoir jar, bacterial filter, vacuum control regulator and vacuum gauge. The reservoir jar is graduated so that the volume of aspirate may be estimated. It contains a cut-off valve. The cut-off valve has a float that rises as the fluid level increases and shuts off the valve when the reservoir jar is full. This prevents liquid from the suction jar entering the suction system. There is a

319

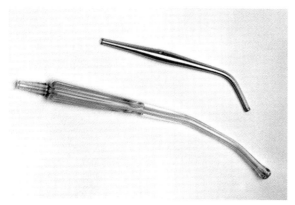

Fig. 16.40 Yankauer suction connectors. Adult and paediatric apparatus.

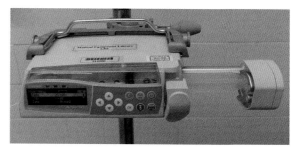

Fig. 16.41 A syringe driver. An electric motor drives a plastic syringe plunger to infuse the contents of a syringe.

bacterial filter between the cut-off valve and the suction control unit to prevent air that has been contaminated during passage through the apparatus infecting the atmosphere when it is blown out. The filter also traps any particulate or nebulised matter. Filters should be changed at regular intervals.

The vacuum regulator adjusts the degree of vacuum. The vacuum is indicated on the pressure gauge. This is normally marked in mmHg or kPa. The needle on the gauge goes in an anticlockwise direction as the vacuum increases. Suction units can achieve flows of greater than 25 L min^{-1} and a vacuum of greater than 67 kPa. However, flows and vacuum as high as these are seldom necessary and can cause harm if used inappropriately, particularly in children.

The suction reservoir jar is connected to the patient via a suction tubing and either a Yankauer hand piece (Fig. 16.40) or suction catheters.

Infusion pumps

Infusion pumps are programmable devices that can be adjusted to give variable rates of infusion or bolus administration. Many pumps operate from battery and/or mains electricity. They incorporate warnings and alarms such as excessive downstream and upstream pressure, air in the tube, syringe/bag empty or nearly empty and low battery. Categories of infusion devices include volumetric pumps, syringe drivers, patient-controlled analgesia (PCA) pumps and target-controlled infusion (TCI) anaesthetic pumps.

Volumetric pumps

Volumetric pumps utilise either liner or rotary peristaltic action or a piston cassette pump inset to control the prescribed infusion volume. They are generally used to deliver large volumes of fluids such as intravascular fluids, blood and blood products.

Syringe drivers

Syringe drivers utilise an electronically controlled electric motor to drive a plastic syringe plunger to infuse the contents of a syringe into the patient (Fig. 16.41). Some devices can accept different sizes of syringes. Syringe drivers should not be positioned above the level of the patient as gravitational pressure can be generated, especially if the pump is more than 100 cm above the patient. Antisiphon valves should be used to prevent free flow from the syringe pump. Antireflux valves should be used in any other line to prevent backflow up a low-pressure line and avoid subsequent inadvertent bolus.

Patient-controlled analgesia pump

Patient-controlled analgesia pumps allow patients, within defined limits, to control their own drug delivery. A demand button delivers a preset bolus of analgesic drug when activated by the patient. The preset bolus size and lockout time with or without a background infusion and dose limits are preprogrammed by the doctor.

Target-controlled infusion pumps

Target-controlled infusion pumps use advanced software technology to administer anaesthetic drugs such as remifentanil or propofol, and estimate plasma and effect (brain) concentration levels based on patient's weight and age.

Key specific additional features of a TCI infusion pump (Fig. 16.42) include the following:
- A safe, usable interface, featuring a clear display of necessary data
- Ability to enter patient details and target plasma or effector site drug concentration.
- Software with pharmacokinetic model to provide a variety of TCI algorithms, such as Schnider, Marsh or Minto, which are validated for a specific drug to control the infusion rate

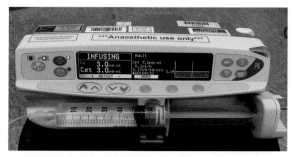

Fig. 16.42 A target-controlled infusion (TCI) pump using advanced software technology to administer remifentanil, and estimated effect (brain) concentration levels, based on patient's weight and age.

- A straightforward method for controlling the infusion
- A clear alarm system to indicate problems
- Ability to accept and automatically sense the size of syringes from major manufacturers

Perioperative warming devices

Accidental perioperative hypothermia can be prevented by the use of perioperative intravenous fluids and body warming devices. The use of these devices in clinical practice is discussed in Chapter 13.

Intravenous fluid warming devices

Many fluid warming devices are available. The heating methods used include passing intravenous fluid tubing through heating blocks (dry warming system), countercurrent heat exchange, water baths, convection air system, heated cabinets and insulators. The ability of these devices to deliver heated fluid depends on the flow rate, the length of the tubing between the warmer and the patient and the heating method.

Simple in-line fluid warmers have a plate warming system and a disposable device specific administration set. The cassette within the disposable set acts as a heat exchanger (Fig. 16.43). Level 1 infuser systems incorporate a countercurrent water heat exchanger designed to maximise heat transfer without compromising flow.

Safety issues associated with the use of intravenous fluid warmers include:
- Risk of air embolism, particularly during rapid infusion with the Level 1 infusers.
- Delivery of contaminated fluids with devices which use a countercurrent warming system.
- Potential thermal damage to transfused blood cells. A maximum operating temperature of 43 °C for blood

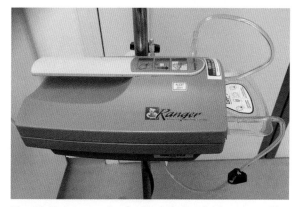

Fig. 16.43 An example of a simple in-line fluid warmer with a plate warming system and a disposable administration set. (Image copyright 3M.)

warmers has been recommended. All devices should have an audiovisual over- and under-temperature alarm.

Body warming devices

A number of devices are available to provide convective or direct contact thermal warming.

Forced air warmers operate by distributing heated air generated by a power unit (Fig. 16.44) through a specifically designed downstream blanket. Heat is transferred to the body area covered; convective and radiant heat losses from the skin under the warmer are also reduced. They incorporate 0.2-µm filters to reduce the risk of contamination. These require maintenance.

Warmers that principally provide heat by conduction use either a mattress or blanket. Their performance depends on the surface area available for warming by direct contact. Resistive heating uses a low-voltage electric current that passes through a semiconductive polymer or carbon-fibre system to generate heat. These systems are reusable, energy efficient and easily cleaned and hence are quite economical.

Circulating water devices operate by passing heated water in a mattress, blanket or garment which is in contact with the patient. Water has a greater specific heat capacity and thermal conductivity than air and is therefore a more efficient medium for heat transfer.

Safety issues related to body warmers include the following:
- They are a potential cause of burns (especially if used on limbs without blood flow (e.g. tourniquet, cross-clamps).
- Forced air warmers can potentially disrupt laminar flow systems in the operating theatre.
- There is no good evidence that properly used forced air warmers are a source of infection; hypothermia is a risk factor for surgical infection.

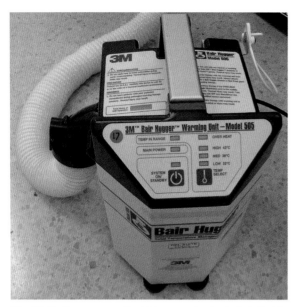

Fig. 16.44 The power unit which generates heated air that is forced through a hose connected to a disposable blanket. (Image copyright 3M.)

Decontamination of anaesthetic equipment

Anaesthetic equipment is a potential vector for transmission of diseases (see Chapter 18). Concerns have been raised about the possibility that multiple-use devices may transfer bloodborne infections between patients, including prions thought to be responsible for causing variant Creutzfeldt-Jakob disease (vCJD). The Association of Anaesthetists' guidelines state that single-use, disposable anaesthetic equipment should always be used when possible. For reusable anaesthetic equipment, compliance with local hospital control policies and awareness of decontamination practices are important to minimise the risk of cross-infection.

Decontamination processes are a combination of either cleaning and disinfection or cleaning and sterilisation.

- *Cleaning* is the physical removal of foreign material, and it is an essential first step in decontamination as it reduces the bioburden (the population of viable infectious agents contaminating a device).
- *Disinfection* is the killing of non-sporing organisms (bacteria and most viruses) using heat (pasteurisation) or chemicals.
- *Sterilisation* is the killing of all micro-organisms, including viruses, fungi and spores. It is usually achieved by steam sterilisation (autoclave), dry hot air, ethylene oxide or γ irradiation.

Hospital equipment is classified into three categories (the Spalding classification) based on the degree of risk of infection associated with its use: critical, semicritical and non-critical items.

- Critical items are those that enter sterile tissue or the bloodstream such as surgical instruments and intravascular catheters. These are required to be sterilised before use.
- Semicritical items are those which come in contact with mucous membranes and non-intact skin but do not break the blood barrier. Such equipment includes anaesthetic breathing systems, laryngoscopes and fibreoptic endoscopes. They present an intermediate risk of transmitting infection, and it is recommended that these should have a high level of disinfection with high concentrations of disinfectants such as glutaraldehyde 2%, stabilised hydrogen peroxide, peracetic acid, superoxidised water, chlorine and chlorine-releasing compounds. Prolonged exposure to some high-level disinfectants can also destroy bacterial spores and can therefore be used for sterilisation.
- Non-critical items come into contact with intact skin but not mucous membranes; such equipment includes blood pressure cuffs and pulse oximeter. They present a low risk of transmission, and cleaning or low-level disinfection of these items is sufficient. Low-level disinfectants include 70% alcohol, 0.5% chlorhexidine and 10% sodium hypochlorite.

References/Further reading

Al-Shaikh, B., Stacey, S., 2013. Essentials of anaesthetic equipment, 4th ed. Churchill Livingstone, London.

Association of Anaesthetists of Great Britain and Ireland. 2008. Infection control in anaesthesia 2 Association of Anaesthetists, London.

Association of Anaesthetists of Great Britain and Ireland, 2012. Checking anaesthetic equipment. Anaesthesia 67, 660–668.

Davey, A., Diba, A., 2012. Anaesthetic equipment, 6th ed. W B Saunders, London.

Dorsch, J.A., Dorsch, S.E., 2008. Understanding anaesthetic equipment, 5th ed. Williams and Wilkins, London.

John, M., Ford, J., Harper, M., 2014. Peri-operative warming devices: performance and clinical application. Anaesthesia 69, 623–638.

Sinclair, C., Thadsad, M.K., Barker, I., 2006. Modern anaesthetic machines. Continuing Education in Anaesthesia Critical Care and Pain 6, 75–78.

Wilson, A.J., Nayak, S., 2016. Disinfection, sterilization and disposables. Anaesthesia Intensive Care 17(10), 475–479.

Chapter | 17 |

Clinical measurement and monitoring

Simon Scott

The ability to measure and monitor patients' physiology is fundamental to modern anaesthetic practice, and a variety of sophisticated instruments are available. It is crucial that the anaesthetist understands not only the data being generated but also the limitations of any equipment and potential sources of error. Furthermore, the anaesthetist must have the knowledge and experience to integrate multiple clinical measurements. A comprehensive understanding of each monitoring system is therefore crucial to ensure optimal patient care and avoid potentially harmful mistakes.

Clinical measurement is limited by four major constraints:

- *Feasibility.* It is often technically difficult to record a physiological variable (e.g. stroke volume) reliably or accurately.
- *Reliability.* This depends on the device being calibrated and used correctly (e.g. proper placement of ECG electrodes, appropriate sizing of the NIBP cuff). Delicate equipment, such as a blood gas analyser, requires regular maintenance and calibration.
- *Interpretation.* Any measurement must be understood correctly as part of a complex physiological system. Arterial pressure may be within the normal range despite severe hypovolaemia; global measurements of end-tidal carbon dioxide tension or oxygen saturation are influenced by many factors other than ventilation. Anaesthetists must integrate all this information when assessing a patient's physiology.
- *Value* in improving patient care. This includes the ease, convenience and usefulness of a measurement and evidence of improvement in patient safety and outcome.

Monitoring represents the assessment and use of measurements to direct therapy. Monitors usually comprise four components (Box 17.1):

- A device that connects to the patient
- A measuring device (often a transducer that converts a measurement into electrical signals)

- A computer, which amplifies and filters the signal, then integrates it with other variables to produce useful information
- A display showing the results as a wave, number or combination

Note that monitors often do not directly measure the displayed variable and that the displayed variable may not reflect the underlying physiology. For example, an ECG does not measure cardiac function; therefore a normal ECG trace does not indicate that the heart is pumping effectively. When interpreting measurements the following questions should be asked:

- *What is being measured?* Whilst arterial pressure is a direct measurement, 'depth of anaesthesia' is less obvious. Furthermore, a monitor may display a variable (e.g. heart rate) using different sources (e.g. pulse oximeter, ECG, arterial waveform) and so can change in the absence of any physiological derangement.
- *How is it measured?* Arterial pressure is often measured by either a transducer attached to an arterial cannula or an automated oscillometer. The values between each can differ, and this difference should be accounted for when monitoring the patient.
- *Is the environment appropriate?* Many monitors are designed for use in operating theatres and may not function correctly if exposed to cold and vibration (e.g. in an ambulance or helicopter). The magnetic field of an MRI scanner is also a hostile environment.
- *Is the patient appropriate?* Monitors designed for adults may be inaccurate when used on small children. Obese adults may require a large blood pressure cuff, and ECG readings may be of low quality.
- *Has the monitor been applied to the correct part of the patient?* For example, in aortic coarctation, arterial pressure may be markedly different in each arm. Pulse oximeters also fail to operate reliably if placed distal to a blood pressure cuff.

- *Is the variable within the range of the monitor?* Most monitors are validated on healthy patients in laboratories. They are not necessarily accurate at physiological extremes such as in anaphylaxis or septic shock or outside the limits of a healthy individual (e.g. low saturations in pulse oximetry).
- *Has the monitor been checked, serviced and calibrated at the correct intervals?* Regular servicing and calibration are expensive and time consuming. All equipment should be tagged with a service sticker that identifies the service date, when the next service is due and who to contact in case of malfunction. Equipment should not be used if it has not been serviced or is past its service date.

Box 17.2 shows the checks that the anaesthetist should follow before using a patient monitor.

Process of clinical measurement

Stages of clinical measurement

There are four stages of clinical measurement:

- Detection of the biological signal by a sensor
- Transduction, which is conversion from one form of energy (the sensor output) to another (usually electrical)
- Amplification and signal processing to extract and magnify the signal and reduce unwanted noise
- Display and storage of the output; whilst commonly the electronic representation of a biological signal, this also includes the height of a fluid-column manometer for pressure measurement, expansion of alcohol in a thin glass column for temperature measurement, or a mechanical recording for peak-flow measurements

Essential requirements for clinical measurement

Clinical measurement devices detect a biological signal and reproduce it in a convenient display or recording. The conversion of a biological signal into an electrical recording introduces some key concepts: linearity, drift, hysteresis, signal-to-noise ratio, static and dynamic response, and accuracy and precision.

Linearity describes the response of a measurement system to changes in the biological input signal; for example, if the true mean arterial pressure of a patient increases by a factor of 0.5 (MAP from 60–90 mmHg) the measurement device will respond by a factor of 0.5. In practice there is a limited range in which the relationship is linear; this is usually provided by the manufacturer.

Hysteresis occurs where the response of the measurement device has some dependence on previous measurements, thereby altering linearity. For example, temperature measurement can be affected in some systems by whether the patient's temperature is increasing or decreasing, resulting in measurements that under or overread the true temperature. Bimetallic strips used for temperature compensation in vaporisers are particularly prone to hysteresis; the rate of deformation of the strip on heating is different to the rate of deformation when the strip then starts to cool.

Drift describes the slow increase or decrease of measurement values when there is no change in the underlying biological value. Pressure transducers often show drift, with the zero-point changing over time, caused by heating of the electrical components affecting their resistance. Regular calibration in the form of setting the zero point against atmospheric pressure minimises the clinical impact of drift. Two-point calibration – calibrating against zero and another point at the maximum value in the device's operating range – further protects against drift affecting the linearity of response. More points can be used to ensure accuracy (Fig. 17.1).

Signal-to-noise ratio (SNR) reflects the degree by which the measured signal is affected by other patient or environmental signals. For example, the EEG measures tiny neuronal voltages and can easily be overwhelmed by larger voltages from the patient (muscle electrical activity) or environment (mains electricity). Increasing the SNR using filters, signal processing and isolation devices ensures that the measured EEG potentials accurately reflect the biological neuronal electrical signals.

Response can be either dynamic or static. Most medical devices display a dynamic response, which is a changing measurement to a rapidly changing underlying signal, as seen with arterial pressure transduction. A static response is commonly seen for single values or values that change very slowly over time, such as temperature. Importantly, in static systems there is time for the measurement device to

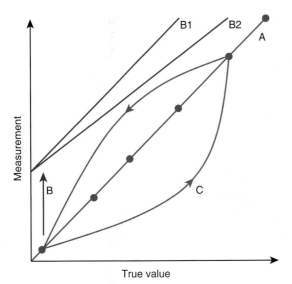

Fig. 17.1 A linear response is seen in *A* where a change in the true value is matched by a proportional change in the measured value. *B* demonstrates zero drift, with *B1* being a proportional change to the whole linear response, and *B2* demonstrating drift affecting zero more than the higher values. A 2-point or greater calibration protects against *B2*. Hysteresis is seen in *C*; true values being underread non-linearly in the ascent, with true values being overread in the descent. This pattern is seen with bimetallic strips in temperature measurement.

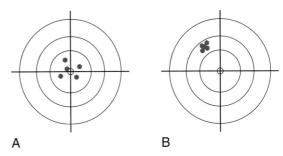

A   B

Fig. 17.2 (A) Accuracy is represented by this target; the dots group round a centre (true) point, but not to each other. (B) Precision is represented by this target; the dots are grouped together but not on the centre point.

settle around the true value, unlike dynamic systems where a slow response can lead to inaccurate measurements.

Accuracy is the difference between a measurement and the actual physiological variable, usually determined by a gold standard measurement. Calibration enhances accuracy, usually tested against a known value, such as the zero-reference point for direct arterial pressure measurement.

Precision is the reproducibility of repeated measurements. Single recordings are unreliable for imprecise measurements, particularly when a test requires patient cooperation, practice or effort, such as peak expiratory flow rate. Repeated measurements demonstrate the variability in response (Fig. 17.2).

There are no perfect monitors. Even if the reported value is 'true', it must be interpreted in the context of the patient and their environment. *Treat the patient, not the monitor* is an old adage that remains true.

The importance of repeated measurements

Differences in repeated clinical measurements arise from three causes:

- Change within the patient
- Inherent variability in the signal or its measurement
- Confounding errors – the recorded measurement does not reflect the signal

Consistent repeated measurements ensure precision but not accuracy (e.g. invasive blood pressure recordings may be consistent but inaccurate if the transducer is not correctly calibrated). In general calibrated instruments are accurate but not necessarily precise (e.g. cardiac output monitors are generally either accurate but imprecise if they require calibration or inaccurate but precise if they do not). Therefore anaesthetists should be aware of the accuracy and precision of measurement systems, and when a measurement does not fit the clinical picture, use a different technique to confirm or refute the initial reading.

Measurement of continuous signals over time

Continuous signals (as used in most modern measurement devices) also need an assessment of the response of the system to a changing biological signal. The reliability of such signals is determined by their input–output relationship. Accuracy requires good zero and gain stability, a linear amplitude response and minimal hysteresis, and an adequate frequency response. These concepts will be explored later, but it is important to realise environmental changes can influence the response of a measurement device to a changing biological signal (e.g. humidity may affect capnography measurements).

Analogue and digital measurement

Modern measurements usually transduce an analogue biological signal to an electrical signal, but mechanical devices still have an important role. For example, peak flow meters, which are convenient and need no electrical source, use the physics of gas flow to move a calibrated indicator. Analogue computers, comprising electronic circuits and operational amplifiers, are also still in use, primarily in the electronics industry in the form of oscilloscopes. However, modern high-powered digital computers have overtaken most of the roles previously undertaken by analogue systems.

Digital signal processing

Digitisation is the process of converting a continuous analogue signal into discrete values, achieved by sampling the signal at regular intervals. A waveform can be broken up into a series of separate points; the frequency of sampling determines how close together these points are and represents the resolution of the digital device (see later). The advantage of digital processing is that the digitised signal can be manipulated and analysed using sophisticated software calculations.

Analogue-to-digital conversion

Computers process information in discrete form, operating on data expressed as either 0 or 1 (i.e. binary code). The resolving power of a computer is limited by the maximum number of digits that can be represented in binary code. For example, an 8-bit computer processor can use binary code to represent 2^8 decimal numbers from 00000000 (or 0 as a decimal number) to 11111111 (equivalent to 255 as a decimal number). An analogue signal can be resolved by an 8-bit converter with an accuracy of 1 part in 255, or 0.4%. More modern processors capable of 32-bit conversion therefore can represent 2^{32} decimal numbers, giving a resolving power of 0.00000002%. In the domestic market 64-bit computing is now common. This accuracy comes at a cost in terms of hardware, power consumption and storage requirements.

Sampling frequency is an important part of signal resolution. A low sampling frequency may be adequate for a slowly changing waveform, but it may not be representative of high-frequency components. This introduces an aliasing error in which different signals become indistinguishable. According to the Nyquist theorem, the sampling frequency should be at least twice the component of the input signal waveform with the highest frequency and sufficient amplitude; for example, a sampling frequency of 100 Hz would adequately capture the fastest rate of change in a physiological pressure signal.

Data display

Data can be presented in either analogue or digital form. A type of analogue display is a mechanical spirometer that records flow on a dial driven by gears. The cathode ray oscilloscope is an effective screen-based display for continuous analogue electrical signals.

Modern monitors can integrate various physiological measurements and display information in a variety of formats

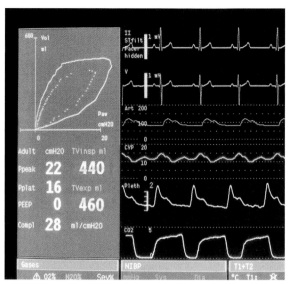

Fig. 17.3 Standard anaesthetic monitoring screen.

(e.g. discrete numbers, tables or waveforms). Most monitoring systems follow good ergonomic principles, with different variables separated consistently by position on the screen and by colour. Important information can be displayed in a variety of formats, much of which is modifiable by the user to display relevant information (Fig. 17.3).

Despite many attempts to simplify patient data into geometric shapes or bar graphs, data continue to be displayed most often as simple numbers supported by waveforms (e.g. invasive pressures) and graphical or tabular (numeric) display of time trends. Trends are particularly useful when clinical problems may produce gradual change. For example, in neurosurgery a gradual decrease in end-tidal carbon dioxide concentration may indicate multiple air emboli.

Biological electrical signals

The detection and recording of biological electrical potentials are important clinical measurements that incorporate many of the key principles of clinical measurement.

Depolarisation of the cell membrane of excitable cells is fundamental to their action and generates a transient potential difference between the active cell and surrounding tissues. The summation of synchronous extracellular potentials from many excitable cells generates a widespread electric field detectable by electrodes on the body surface. The ECG and EEG are two well-established measures of biological electrical activity. Nerve conduction studies may be used to diagnose potential iatrogenic nerve injury.

Biological electrical signals are detected using electrodes constructed of silver and coated with silver chloride. Low, stable impedance (the resistance to alternating current) between skin and electrode minimises mains interference. Symmetrical electrode impedance and insignificant polarisation control drift. The electrolytic silver chloride layer is however very thin, prone to deterioration and only suitable for single use. Movement artefacts are minimised by separating the electrode surface from the skin with a foam pad impregnated with electrolyte gel. Degreasing with alcohol before applying the electrode helps reduce skin impedance and ensure satisfactory adhesion.

Biological electrical signals are recorded as waveforms. All complex waveforms can be described as a mixture of simple sine waves of varying amplitude, frequency and phase – Fourier analysis. These consist of a fundamental wave (the slowest sine wave in the waveform) and a series of harmonics that are multiples of the frequency of the fundamental wave and shifted in phase. The lower harmonics tend to have the greatest amplitude. For all continuous biological signals (including mechanical, e.g. arterial pressure waveform), a reasonable approximation may be obtained by accurate reproduction of the fundamental frequency and first 10 harmonics. It is important, however, that both the amplitude and phase difference of each harmonic are faithfully reproduced through the transduction system.

Amplification and gain stability

The amplitude of tiny bioelectrical signals must be increased by amplification and unwanted noise and interference minimised. The degree of amplification is termed *gain* and, whilst often user defined, should remain constant over the recording period. Calibration voltages may also be incorporated for correct adjustment of gain. The amplification of the signal should be constant across the whole range of signal amplitudes, and this amplitude linearity is often specified by equipment manufacturers for a specific amplitude range.

Input impedance and common mode rejection

Amplifiers for biological signals require high common mode rejection and high input impedance. The input and electrode impedances act as a potential divider: High electrode impedance and low amplifier input impedance are undesirable as they result in an attenuated electrical signal across the amplifier. The input impedance of modern amplifiers exceeds 5 MΩ to avoid problems, and careful attention must be paid to minimising electrode impedance, particularly for EEG recordings.

Pure amplification increases unwanted signals (noise) as much as the wanted – essentially it is the equivalent of

SINGLE-ENDED AND DIFFERENTIAL AMPLIFIERS

Single-ended amplifier. Amplifies input signal and any noise present

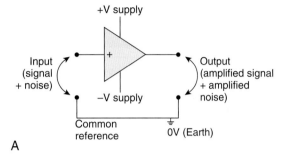

A

Differential amplifier. Input signal is applied to inputs 1 and 2. One of these inputs inverts the signal so that random noise which is common to both inputs is cancelled out before being amplified (**common mode rejection**)

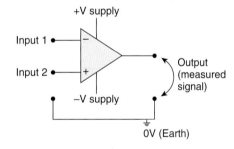

B

Fig. 17.4 Two types of amplifier; common mode rejection is particularly useful for minimising mains electricity interference. (A) Single-ended amplifier. (B) Differential amplifier.

the volume control on a radio. Differential amplification reduces unwanted noise. The potential difference between two input signals is amplified, but electrical signals common to both are attenuated. This feature is termed *common mode rejection* and effectively reduces mains interference in all biological signals and electrocardiographic contamination of smaller electroencephalographic signals. The common mode rejection ratio (CMRR) for a typical differential amplifier exceeds 10,000:1. In other words, a signal applied equally to both input terminals would need to be 10,000 times larger than a signal applied between them for the same change in output (Fig. 17.4).

Frequency response

The bandwidth of the amplifier describes the range of frequencies that it can accurately reproduce. It must cover the range of frequencies which are important in the signal. In

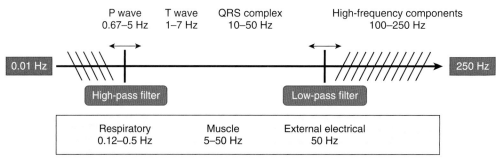

Fig. 17.5 Both high- and low-pass filters can be positioned to minimise interference depending on the clinical requirements. The ECG components often overlap with noise from other sources, and attempting to filter these sources will necessarily affect the accuracy of the ECG recording.

practice, amplifiers require a flat frequency response for ECG from 0.14 to 50 Hz, for EEG from 0.5 to 100 Hz and for EMG from 20 Hz to at least 2 kHz.

Ideally, when there is no input signal, any measurement should be zero (zero stability). However, low-frequency interference, largely caused by slow fluctuating potentials generated in the electrodes, produces baseline instability and drift. This is removed through a network of resistors and capacitors functioning as a high-pass filter which allows higher frequency biological signals to pass but attenuates low-frequency noise. Whilst this reduces the bandwidth of the amplifier, such a compromise allows an interpretable signal free of baseline instability. For example, ECG monitoring requires a continuous recording with a stable baseline, which is achieved at the expense of waveform reproduction. High-pass filtering removes movement artefact, but attenuation of the low-frequency elements of the ECG, such as the T-wave, may cause distortion. Conversely, diagnostic ECGs require accurate reproduction of the waveform, but the long time constants of the amplifiers result in baseline instability, with movement artefact being a particular issue. Other filters can attenuate particular frequencies. Highly selective band-reject filters attenuate 50 Hz interference (main voltage) from the signal. Low-pass filters are used to eliminate higher-frequency artefacts from an EEG signal. The purpose of filtering is to reduce unwanted noise relative to the signal. When the frequency range of signal and noise overlap, some degree of signal degradation is inevitable (Fig. 17.5).

Noise and interference

Electrical noise arising from the patient, the patient–electrode interface or the surroundings may interfere with accurate recording of biological potentials.

Noise originating from the patient
Millivolt ECG potentials on the body surface are hundreds of times larger than microvolt EEG signals on the scalp.

Electromyographic signals may be even larger, and muscular activity, especially shivering, causes marked interference. Two features of electronic amplifier design substantially improve the EEG SNR. Electrocardiographic potentials are essentially the same across the scalp and are ignored by amplifiers with a high common mode rejection. Electromyographic activity has a higher frequency content than the EEG signal and may be minimised by a low-pass filter which attenuates the higher-frequency response of the amplifier to a level which attenuates the EMG signals and does not interfere with the characteristics of the EEG.

Noise originating from the patient–electrode interface
Recording electrodes do not behave as passive conductors. All skin–metal electrode systems employ a metal surface in contact with an electrolyte solution. *Polarisation* describes the interaction between metal and electrolyte which generates a small electrical gradient. Electrodes comprising a metal that is plated with one of its own salts (e.g. silver–silver chloride) avoid this problem because current in each direction does not significantly change the electrolyte composition. Mechanical movement of recording electrodes may also cause significant potential gradients – alteration in the physical dimensions of the electrode changes the cell potential and skin–electrode impedance. Differences in potential between two electrodes connected to a differential amplifier are amplified, and asymmetry of electrode impedance seriously impairs the CMRR of the recording amplifier.

Noise originating outside the patient
Electrical interference. Mains frequency interference with the recording of biological potentials may be troublesome, particularly in electromagnetically noisy clinical environments. Patients function physically as large unscreened conductors and interact with nearby electrical sources through the processes of capacitive coupling and electromagnetic induction.

Capacitance permits alternating current to pass across an air gap. A live mains conductor and nearby patient behave as the two plates of a capacitor. The very small mains frequency current which flows through the patient is of no clinical significance but confounds the detection and amplification of biological potentials, creating unwanted interference in the recording. Capacitive coupled interference is minimised by reducing the capacitance and the alternating potential difference. This is achieved by moving the patient away from the source of interference and by screening mains-powered equipment with a conductive surround which is maintained at earth potential by a low-resistance earth connection and by surrounding leads with a braided copper screen – stray capacitances couple with the screen instead of the lead.

Alternating currents in a conductor generate a magnetic flux. This induces voltages in any nearby conductors which lie in the changing magnetic flux, including the patient or signal leads to the amplifier, which function as inefficient secondary transformers. This source of interference is minimised by keeping patients as far as possible from powerful sources of electromagnetic flux, especially mains transformers. Electromagnetic inductance may be minimised by ensuring that all patient leads are the same length, closely bound or twisted together until very close to the electrodes. This ensures that the induced signals are identical in all leads and therefore susceptible to common mode rejection.

The importance of low electrode impedance. High electrode impedance may exaggerate the effects of surrounding electrical interference. Capacitive and inductive coupling produce very small currents in the recording leads. If the electrode impedance is low, the potential at the amplifier input must remain close to the potential at the skin surface so that minimal interference results. If electrode impedance is high the small induced currents may create a significant potential difference across that impedance, leading to severe 50-Hz interference.

Radio frequency interference from diathermy is a significant problem for the recording of biological potentials. Electrocardiographic amplifiers may be provided with some protection by filtering the signal before it enters the isolated input circuit, filtering the power supply to block mains-borne radio frequencies and enclosing the electronic components in a double screen, the outer earthed and the inner at amplifier potential.

Biological mechanical signals

Pressure measurements are employed widely in anaesthesia and critical care, using several physical principles and a range of instruments. Liquid column manometers display pressure relative to a predefined zero point using specific fluids of known density. Mechanical pressure gauges, used particularly in high-pressure gas supplies, rely on pressure-dependent mechanical movement being amplified by a gearing mechanism, which drives a pointer across a scale.

For most physiological pressure measurements, diaphragm gauges are used: a flexible diaphragm moves according to the applied pressure. Modern diaphragm gauges are sensed by a transducer that converts the diaphragm's mechanical energy into electrical energy. This is often displayed as a waveform and is subject to the same principles of waveform acquisition and amplification as described previously.

Electromechanical transducers

The first step is movement of the diaphragm proportional to applied pressure. This depends on the stiffness of the diaphragm and substantially determines the operating characteristics of the transducer. Linearity of amplitude and frequency response are improved by using small stiff diaphragms, but this requires a more sensitive mechanism for sensing diaphragm movement.

Wire or silicon-crystal strain gauges are based on the principle that stretching or compression of a wire or silicon changes the electrical resistance, capacitance or inductance. They are very sensitive and display an excellent frequency response, but non-linearity and temperature dependence are difficult technical problems.

Optical transduction senses movement of the diaphragm by reflecting light from the silvered back of the convex diaphragm onto a photocell. Applied pressure causes the silvered surface to become more convex. This causes the reflected light beam to diverge, reducing the intensity of reflected light sensed by the photoelectric cell. This design is used in fibreoptic cardiac catheters for intravascular pressure measurement. These miniature pressure transducers are expensive but have a high-frequency response, and fibreoptic light sources eliminate the risk of microshock.

The cardiovascular system

A core role for the anaesthetist is ensuring adequate oxygen supply to the patient's tissues. This can be estimated clinically: Capillary refill time, urine output and pulse volume are all clinical measurements that act as surrogates for tissue perfusion. Such clinical observations remain crucial despite the wide availability of electronic monitoring systems.

Electrocardiography

The electrocardiogram measures myocardial electrical activity and allows identification of heart rate, rhythm and abnormalities such as myocardial ischaemia or infarction. The

329

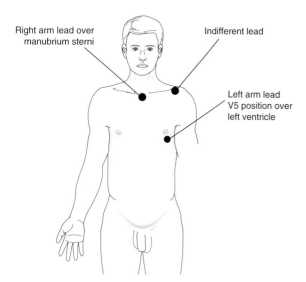

Right arm lead over manubrium sterni

Indifferent lead

Left arm lead V5 position over left ventricle

Fig. 17.6 The CM5 configuration for electrocardiograph monitoring.

synchronous depolarisation and prolonged action potentials in cardiac muscle summate to generate a potential field of relatively higher amplitude. This potential difference is detected between two electrodes placed on the body surface, and the third lead is used as a reference electrode. The very small absolute voltage changes (1 mV in amplitude with a frequency response of 0.05–100 Hz) require amplification before being displayed as a waveform.

Different lead positions detect electrical activity from different parts of the myocardium. The commonest position of the electrodes is the CM5 arrangement as this is the best position to detect ischaemia of the left ventricle (Fig. 17.6).

Alarms may be set to identify arrhythmias, bradycardia and tachycardia. Most monitors display the heart rate and, in addition, a measure of ST segment depression and elevation produced by cardiac ischaemia or infarction. This may be displayed as a trend over time. Unfortunately the relatively small voltages measured are easily swamped by skeletal muscle activity or surgical diathermy, leading to false alarms. The signal may also be severely degraded if the electrode gel has been allowed to dry out or if the weight of the leads pulls on the electrodes. The monitor only identifies ischaemia in a single area; multiple lead systems are required to monitor the whole myocardium.

Arterial pressure

Indirect methods

Aside from palpating the pulse, the majority of measurements of arterial pressure depend on signals generated by the occlusion of a major artery using a cuff, known as the Riva–Rocci method. Systolic pressure can be estimated by the return of a palpable distal pulse; auscultation of the Korotkoff sounds can determine systolic and diastolic pressures. These methods, however, are too time consuming during anaesthesia and difficult because of poor access to the patient's arm.

Oscillometric measurement of arterial pressure

Oscillometric measurement estimates arterial pressure by analysing the pressure oscillations produced by a cuff occluding pulsatile blood flow in an artery during cuff deflation. Modern machines use a single cuff with two tubes for inflation and measurement (commonly referred to as a DINAMAP – device for indirect non-invasive automatic mean arterial pressure). During slow deflation, each pulse generates a pressure change in the cuff distinguishable from the slowly decreasing cuff pressure. Above systolic pressure, these changes are small but suddenly increase in magnitude when the cuff pressure reaches the systolic point. As the cuff pressure decreases further, the amplitude reaches a peak and then starts to diminish. The point of maximal amplitude correlates closely with the mean arterial pressure. As the cuff pressure reaches diastolic pressure, the amplitude falls abruptly (Fig. 17.7). To avoid high cuff pressures and long deflation times, monitors inflate the cuff to just above a normal systolic pressure and then slowly decrease the pressure until a pulse is detected. Consequently, estimates of diastolic pressure can be unreliable. If a pulse is not detected, the cuff is then inflated to a higher pressure. This process may be repeated several times before a measurement is made.

Commercial instruments attempt to improve the reliability of the measurement. For example, at each successive plateau pressure during the controlled deflation, successive pressure fluctuations are compared and accepted only if they are similar. All automatic instruments require a regular cardiac cycle with no great differences between successive pulses. Accurate and consistent readings may be impossible in patients with an irregular rhythm, particularly atrial fibrillation. Furthermore, mechanical interference (e.g. patient shivering or movement of the arm) can prevent accurate measurement.

Clinical studies comparing automatic oscillometric instruments with direct arterial pressure have demonstrated good correlation for systolic and mean pressure with a tendency to overestimate at low pressures and underestimate at high pressures. Diastolic pressures are less reliable. The 95% confidence intervals approximate to 15 mmHg. The disadvantages of automated oscillometry are shown in Box 17.3.

Other techniques

Alternative techniques use pressure, low-frequency sound, Doppler shift of an ultrasound signal or plethysmography.

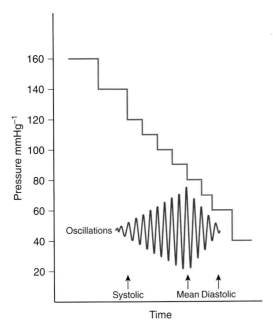

Fig. 17.7 The NIBP measurement uses a cuff that deflates in steps *(line on graph)*; pressure oscillations from the vessels opening and closing increase in amplitude towards the mean arterial pressure, then cease when the cuff pressure is below diastolic.

Box 17.3 **Disadvantages of automated oscillometry**

Delayed measurement with arrhythmias or patient movement
Inaccuracy with systolic pressure <60 mmHg
Inaccurate if the wrong size cuff used
May be inaccurate in obese patients
Discomfort in awake patients
Skin and nerve damage in prolonged use
Delay in injected drugs reaching the circulation
Backflow of blood into i.v. cannulae
Pulse oximeter malfunction as cuff is inflated

Most common amongst these in perioperative practice is the Penaz technique, which measures the effect of external pressure on the blood flow through a finger (e.g. Finometer, Nexfin, CNAP). The principle is of a control loop. The volume of the finger is measured using light absorption. A feedback loop to an encircling cuff provides counterpressure to the arterial pulsation to keep the volume constant. The pressure required to keep the volume constant is equivalent to arterial pressure. With improvements in technology, these devices

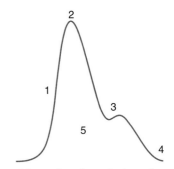

Fig. 17.8 Arterial waveform for a single cardiac cycle; the slope of *1* approximates to cardiac contractility, *2* represents systolic pressure, *3* is the dichrotic notch (aortic valve closure), *4* is diastolic pressure and the area of *5* approximates stroke volume.

are increasingly used for continuous non-invasive arterial pressure measurement. Some systems incorporate an automated recalibration process to counter issues of drift. Direct arterial cannulation is avoided, and accuracy is generally good.

Direct measurement

Direct arterial pressure measurement requires insertion of a cannula (20–22G) into an artery (usually radial because the ulnar artery may compensate for occluded radial flow) connected via a fluid column to the transducer. As fluids are incompressible, the pressure in the artery is transmitted to a transducer, which converts pressure into an electrical signal for display by the monitor. The transducer should be at the level of the left ventricle and the transducer opened to the atmosphere to provide a zero reading before use. Monitors usually display the waveform and systolic and diastolic pressures as well as the mean pressure, calculated by integration of the waveform to derive the average pressure across one cardiac cycle. The waveform provides useful additional information: visual estimates of pressure, frequency response and damping, and relative hypovolaemia during positive pressure seen as variability or swing in the waveform. Furthermore, it provides a visual approximation of contractility, vascular resistance and stroke volume (Fig. 17.8).

The main advantages of direct arterial pressure systems are that they provide accurate real-time measurement (essential when administering drugs such as vasopressors) and permit convenient blood sampling (Box 17.4). Invasive arterial pressure monitoring has become standard practice for high-risk and severely ill patients, both in the operating theatre and ICU.

However, malpositioning of the transducer, failure to zero the transducer or problems with damping (see later) introduce error. For example, if the operating table is moved upwards while the transducer remains static, the difference

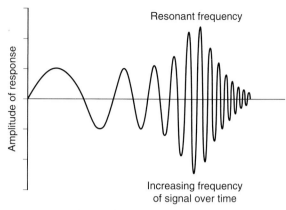

Fig. 17.9 Stimulation of the output of a catheter-transducer system with increasing frequency of a constant amplitude input signal. The linearity of response is lost as the frequency approaches the resonant frequency of the system.

in height artificially increases the pressure reading. Unusual readings should be checked against a reading from a non-invasive monitor. Problems relating to arterial cannulation are shown in Box 17.5.

Resonant frequency and damping
As previously described, Fourier analysis converts complex waveforms into a series of sine waves. For an arterial waveform, the pulse frequency represents the fundamental frequency, with accurate reproduction of the waveform requiring transduction up to the 10th harmonic; that is, for a pulse of 120 bpm, transduction requires a linear frequency of up to (120 × 10) / 60 = 20 Hz. To ensure that the amplitude and phase difference of each harmonic is accurately reproduced, the transduction system must have a natural frequency greater than the frequency components of the waveform, as well as sufficient damping. The fluid and diaphragm of an arterial pressure transducer constitute a mechanical system which oscillates in simple harmonic motion at its natural resonant frequency. This determines the frequency response of the measurement system (Fig. 17.9). If the resonant frequency of the measurement system overlaps any sine-wave component of the measured waveform, the entire system will have increased resonance (in this case, inaccurately elevated systolic pressure). The resonant frequency of a catheter-transducer measuring system is highest, and the damping effect of frictional resistance to fluid flow is lowest,

when the velocity of movement of fluid in the catheter is minimised. This is achieved with a stiff, low-volume displacement diaphragm and a short, wide, rigid catheter.

Determination of the resonant frequency and damping
The resonant frequency and the effects of damping may be estimated by applying a step change in pressure to the catheter-transducer system and recording the response (Fig. 17.10). An underdamped system responds rapidly but overshoots and oscillates close to the natural resonant frequency of the system; frequency components of the pressure wave close to the resonant frequency are exaggerated. By contrast, an overdamped system responds slowly, and the recorded signal decreases slowly to reach the baseline, with no overshoot. High-frequency oscillations are damped, underestimating the true pressure changes. These extremes are undesirable. In general, MAP is least affected by damping, but an underdamped system will overestimate systolic pressure and underestimate diastolic pressure. The converse is true for an overdamped system: The systolic pressure will be an underestimate, and the diastolic will be an overestimate.

Optimal damping
Optimal damping maximises the frequency response of the system, minimises resonance and represents the best compromise between speed of response and accuracy of transduction. A small overshoot represents approximately 7% of the step change in pressure, with the pressure then following the arterial waveform (see Fig. 17.10).

Damping is relatively unimportant when the frequencies being recorded are less than two thirds of the natural frequency of the catheter-transducer system. Modern transducer

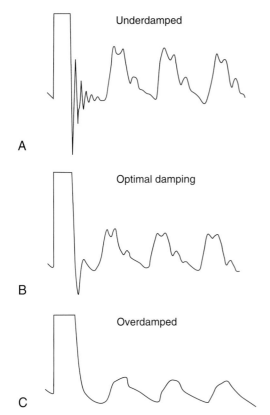

Fig. 17.10 Damping of arterial pressure waves and the response to a square wave signal from the fast flush device. (A) Underdamped. (B) Optimal damping. (C) Overdamped.

systems using small compliance transducers connected to a short, stiff catheter with a minimum of constrictions or connections approximate to this ideal. The system also includes a pressurised bag of 0.9% saline producing a flow of 1–3 ml h^{-1} through a restrictor to prevent clot formation, as well as allowing a higher flow rate to flush the system, such as after blood sampling. Air bubbles in the system, clotting or kinking in the vascular catheter and arterial spasm lower the natural resonant frequency and increase the damping.

Accuracy of arterial pressure measurements

Invasive devices provide the accepted gold standard for arterial pressure measurement. However, the catheter-transducer system requires careful setup, and arterial pressure varies throughout the arterial tree. As the pulse wave travels from the ventricle to peripheral arteries, changes in vessel diameter and elasticity affect the pressure waveform, which becomes shorter with increased amplitude. Differences in

arterial pressure between limbs are common, particularly in patients with arterial disease.

Indirect methods using an occluding cuff make intermittent measurements, with the systolic and diastolic readings reflecting the conditions in the artery at the time they are measured. By contrast, direct pressure measurements are the average of several cycles, more precisely reflecting mean pressure. Indirect measurements may be compromised by taking a small number of infrequent samples from a variable signal.

Central venous pressure

Central venous pressure represents the pressure of blood entering the right atrium, usually 2–3 mmHg. Whilst often considered a measure of central venous blood volume, it is notoriously unreliable in the critically ill or those with abnormal right-sided cardiac function, and alone it rarely provides an accurate reflection of a patient's circulating fluid volume. However, access to the central venous system is useful for the administration of vasoactive or irritant drugs or for central venous sampling.

There are four common routes for central venous catheterisation.

- Internal jugular catheters are used most commonly because the vein is superficial, of larger diameter and easily managed. This is often the most appropriate route for use in an emergency. However, the insertion point is adjacent to several vital structures, including the carotid artery, pleura, brachial plexus and cervical spine, risking direct needle trauma to these structures. Ultrasound guidance is recommended for internal jugular catheterisation.
- Catheters inserted into the subclavian vein offer similar problems to internal jugular venous catheters, and if accidental arterial puncture occurs, the overlying clavicle obscures bleeding and makes direct compression of the artery impossible. The proximity of the pleura increases the risk of accidental lung puncture. The subclavian route should therefore be used only after first considering the internal jugular approach. The insertion point under the clavicle may make it easier to anchor the catheter to the skin, which is an advantage for longer term use. Ultrasound guidance can assist insertion but is technically more challenging than for internal jugular access.
- Long, small-diameter catheters inserted via the antecubital fossa are relatively easy and safe to insert. However, catheters inserted via the basilic or cephalic vein are sometimes difficult to advance past the shoulder. X-ray imaging is required to confirm placement, and thrombosis of the veins is common after 24 h. The length of the narrow catheter reduces frequency responsiveness.
- Femoral venous catheters are inserted just below the inguinal ligament. They are relatively easy to insert and may be of large gauge to allow rapid transfusion of fluids.

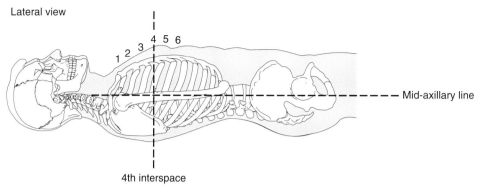

Lateral view

4 5 6

1 2 3

Mid-axillary line

4th interspace

Fig. 17.11 Surface markings used to identify the position of the right atrium.

Box 17.6 **Complications of central venous catheterisation**

Acute

Arrhythmias
Bleeding
Air embolus – on insertion or removal
Pneumothorax
Damage to thoracic duct, oesophagus, carotid artery, stellate ganglion
Cardiac puncture
Catheter embolisation
Misplaced (retained) guidewire

Delayed

Bacteraemia/sepsis
Thrombosis
Cardiac rupture

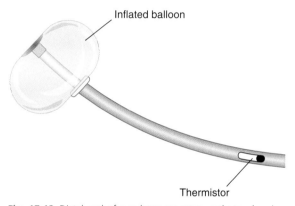

Inflated balloon

Thermistor

Fig. 17.12 Distal end of a pulmonary artery catheter showing inflated balloon and thermistor.

Pulmonary artery pressure

Cardiac output and systemic arterial pressure are determined by the filling pressure of the left side of the heart. The pulmonary artery flotation catheter (PAFC, or Swan-Ganz catheter) (Fig. 17.12) enables measurement of left-sided pressures, imperfect surrogates for left ventricular end-diastolic volume. It is rarely used now because of frequent complications, a lack of evidence of improved survival and the introduction of non-invasive techniques to estimate cardiac output.

A PAFC is a long catheter with three or four lumens and a thermistor near the tip. It is inserted into the internal or subclavian vein through a large cannula. A flexible plastic sheath allows the catheter to be inserted, withdrawn and rotated after insertion without desterilising it. After insertion into the superior vena cava, saline is injected to inflate a balloon at the tip. The pressure at the tip is measured via a transducer and displayed on a monitor. The catheter is then advanced slowly so that the blood flow directs the

This route is often chosen in children. However, the site of insertion is often within a skin fold, making skin flora contamination more likely.

Central venous catheters are usually connected to the same type of transducer and flush system described for arterial cannulae. This provides a continuous pressure reading. However, because central venous pressure (CVP) is low, great care is required to ensure that the pressure is measured relative to the correct zero point (fourth intercostal space in the midaxillary line) on the patient (Fig. 17.11). Single readings may help diagnose right-sided cardiac failure such as after acute pulmonary embolus or cardiac tamponade. Repeat measurements were traditionally used to guide fluid therapy, but this should be discouraged as there is little correlation between CVP and cardiac output in response to fluid challenges. Complications (Box 17.6) are infrequent but potentially serious.

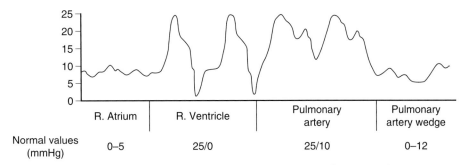

Fig. 17.13 Diagrammatic representation of pressure waveforms. *R*, Right.

catheter towards the pulmonary artery. As the catheter is advanced, a series of changes in pressure is observed, marking the progression through the right atrium and right ventricle into the pulmonary artery (Fig. 17.13). Eventually the balloon wedges into a pulmonary artery. At this point, the tip is isolated from the pulmonary artery and measures the pressure in the pulmonary capillaries, a reflection of left atrial pressure. Although the ability to estimate left atrial pressure is useful, repeat measurements after a circulatory challenge are more informative than a single reading.

The PAFC has led to many advances in our understanding of cardiac physiology and the mechanisms and treatments of diseases such as sepsis. However, catheter placement may be difficult, and prolonged manipulation may be needed to direct the catheter into the pulmonary artery. Arrhythmias are extremely common during catheter insertion, and the technique carries specific risks (Box 17.7) in addition to all those of central venous catheterisation (see Box 17.6).

Cardiac output

Cardiac output is closely linked to oxygen delivery; in clinical practice, low cardiac output is linked to increased mortality. However, factors such as the pressure changes caused by positive pressure ventilation, changes in heart rate and arrhythmias introduce complexities in measurement and interpretation. Therefore monitors do not produce consistent results even when synchronised with the heartbeat and respiratory cycle. Dilution techniques have been regarded as the gold standard against which other methods are compared.

The Fick principle
The Fick principle defines flow by the ratio of the uptake or clearance of a tracer within an organ to the arteriovenous difference in tracer concentration. It may be used to measure cardiac output (oxygen uptake or indicator dilution) and regional blood flow (e.g. cerebral blood flow using the uptake of nitrous oxide) and renal blood flow from the excretion of compounds cleared totally by the kidney, such as para-aminohippuric acid.

In patients with minimal cardiac shunt and reasonable pulmonary function, pulmonary blood flow may be calculated from the ratio of the oxygen consumption and the difference in oxygen content between arterial and mixed venous blood, as follows:

$$Pulmonary\ blood\ flow = \frac{oxygen\ consumption}{arteriovenous\ oxygen\ content\ difference}$$

Oxygen consumption from a reservoir is measured using an accurate spirometer and oxygen content measured with a co-oximeter. Measurements should be made at steady-state situations, with constant inspired oxygen concentration and blood samples obtained slowly whilst the oxygen consumption is being determined. True mixed-venous blood samples must be obtained from a pulmonary artery catheter. Alternative indicator dilution techniques described here are less demanding. The effects of ventilation and beat-to-beat variation in cardiac output are averaged over the long period of measurement of oxygen consumption. Errors in measurement of oxygen consumption limit the accuracy of this technique (±10%).

Indicator dilution
An indicator is injected as a bolus into the right side of the heart, and the concentration reaching the systemic side of

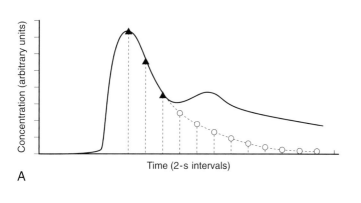

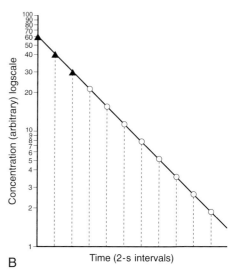

Fig. 17.14 (A) Single injection indicator dilution curve showing distortion of downslope produced by recirculation. (B) Replot on semilogarithmic paper. ▲, Points taken from the downslope in A to establish the slope of the replot in B; ○, points taken from B to plot tail of curve in A. (Reproduced with permission from Sykes, M.K., Vickers, M.D., & Hull, C.J. (1991) *Principles of clinical measurement*. 3rd ed. Oxford, Blackwell Scientific.)

the circulation is plotted against time (Fig. 17.14). The average concentration is calculated from the area under the concentration–time curve divided by the duration of the curve. The cardiac output during the period of this measurement is the ratio of the dose of indicator to the average concentration.

The general formula is:

$$Cardiac\ output\ (litres\ min^{-1})$$
$$= \frac{indicator\ dose\ (units) \times 60}{average\ concentration\ (units\ litre^{-1}) \times time\ (s)}$$

The main problem with this technique is that when the dye has been measured at the artery, it passes back to the heart and then back to the arteries (known as recirculation), making the calculations more complex. This may be circumvented by extrapolation of the early exponential downslope to define the tail of the curve which would have been recorded if recirculation had not occurred (see Fig. 17.14). The area under the curve is calculated by integration.

Chemical indicator dilution

Original studies used indocyanine green, a non-toxic chemical indicator with a relatively short half-life. It also has a peak spectral absorption at 800 nm, the wavelength at which absorption of oxygenated haemoglobin is identical to that of reduced haemoglobin. The measurement is therefore not affected by arterial saturation. However, because the dye is cleared from the circulation only slowly, recirculation makes repeated measurements impossible. More recent monitors use an injection of lithium as a marker, which is detected with a modified arterial catheter.

Thermal indicator dilution

This technique requires a PAFC to be in the pulmonary artery. The principle is similar to other indicator dilution methods. A bolus of 10 ml cold saline is injected into the right atrium, and a thermistor at the tip of the PAFC measures the temperature change. The smaller the temperature drop, the larger the cardiac output. The recorded temperatures generate an exponential dilution curve with no recirculation. The heat dose is the difference in temperature between the injectate and blood multiplied by the density, specific heat and volume of the injectate. The average change in heat content is the area under the temperature–time graph multiplied by the density and specific heat of blood. However, errors occur where mixing of the fluid bolus with venous blood is incomplete, and correction values are necessary, such as for changes in injectate temperature during injection through the catheter. The average of three separate readings is taken as a reliable cardiac output measurement and should be repeated, particularly after changes in therapy.

The measurement of cardiac output using both dye and thermodilution is now automated with computer-controlled sampling, calculation of indicator dilution curves, rejection algorithms for artefacts or curves which are not exponential and online calculation of cardiac output.

Continuous cardiac output monitors have also been introduced. These use a similar principle, but instead of using a bolus of cold saline, the catheter has an electrical coil which is heated at intervals, creating a bolus of warm blood that passes into the pulmonary artery. This eliminates much of the operator error and produces frequently updated measurements of cardiac output, allowing the effect of interventions to be observed.

Monitors have also been developed that do not require a pulmonary artery catheter but use a bolus of iced saline injected into a modified central venous catheter and a peripheral arterial catheter with a built-in thermistor (e.g. the PiCCO (pulse index continuous cardiac output) monitor).

Most of the current monitors allow cardiac output data to be integrated with other measurements such as arterial and venous pressure to provide calculated values of, for example, systemic vascular resistance and stroke volume. This aids the choice and administration of vasoactive drugs.

Pulse contour analysis

The shape of the arterial pulse (the pulse contour) is a product of the rate of ejection of blood into the aorta and the elasticity of the arterial tree. Therefore, if some assumptions are made about the arterial tree, the volume ejected at each heartbeat (stroke volume) may be calculated from the shape of the arterial pulse contour. Multiplying this by the heart rate provides an estimate of cardiac output. This approach has the advantage of being able to calculate the cardiac output in near real-time using an arterial cannula alone.

However, the technique relies on assumptions on arterial tree elasticity which may not always be true in every patient. Therefore these systems may require calibration by another method such as thermodilution every 8–12 h to ensure accuracy (e.g. PiCCO and LiDCO (lithium dilution cardiac output) use thermodilution and lithium, respectively, for calibration)). Recently developed devices use complex algorithms linked with sensor measurements to make estimates of arterial elasticity and vascular tone and are promoted as not requiring calibration (e.g. FloTrac). Both the calibrated and uncalibrated systems also give a value for the variation of stroke volume with respiration, comparable to the arterial pressure swing described earlier. Higher values predict fluid responsiveness, provided certain conditions are met (e.g. closed chest, mandatory ventilation, tidal volumes of 8 ml kg^{-1}). However, the effects of critical illness and vasopressor use influence the accuracy and precision of these pulse contour analysis systems, and in general they are inferior to PAFC thermodilution techniques. These systems are commonly used as part of goal-directed fluid therapy (see Chapter 30).

Doppler ultrasonography

Ultrasound techniques can detect the shape, size and movement of tissue interfaces, especially soft tissues and blood, including the echocardiographic measurement of blood flow and the structure and function of the heart. Sound waves are transmitted by the oscillation of particles in the direction of wave transmission, defined by amplitude (the difference between ambient and peak pressures) and the wavelength (distance between successive peaks) or frequency (the number of cycles per second) (see Chapter 15). These characteristics are measured by a pressure transducer placed in the path of an oncoming wave. The human ear detects frequencies within the range of 20–20,000 Hz. Diagnostic ultrasound uses frequencies in the range of 1–10 MHz. Short-term diagnostic use of ultrasound appears to be free from hazard.

Generation and detection of ultrasound

The physics of ultrasound and Doppler effects are explained in Chapter 15.

Properties of ultrasound

Shorter wavelengths and higher frequencies improve resolution but reduce tissue penetration. Amplitude determines the intensity of the ultrasound beam, the number and size of echoes recorded and therefore sensitivity. Ultrasound is absorbed by tissues and reflected back at the junction between two tissues, tissue–fluid or tissue–air. This reflection at interfaces is the basis for diagnostic use of ultrasound. The intensity of the beam decreases exponentially as it passes through tissue. Attenuation depends on the nature and temperature of the tissue and is related linearly to the frequency of the ultrasound.

Reflections at most soft-tissue interfaces are weak, but bone–fat and tissue–air interfaces reflect the majority of incident energy. Structures lying behind a bone or air interface cannot be studied using ultrasound. Various ultrasound techniques are suited to different applications and have extremely sophisticated two-dimensional, real-time, brightness- and colour-modulated displays under microprocessor control.

Detection of motion by the Doppler effect: cardiac output

When ultrasound waves reflect off an object moving towards the transmitter, there is an apparent increase in frequency as the object encounters more oscillations per unit time. This is termed the Doppler effect. The change in frequency is proportional to the velocity of the object and two constants: the frequency of the transmitted ultrasound and the velocity of ultrasound in the medium. The velocity (v) of the object can be calculated using the Doppler equation:

$$v = \frac{cf_d}{2f_t \cos\theta}$$

where f_d is change in Doppler frequency, c is *speed of sound in medium*, f_t is transmitted frequency, and θ is angle of probe relative to the flow of blood.

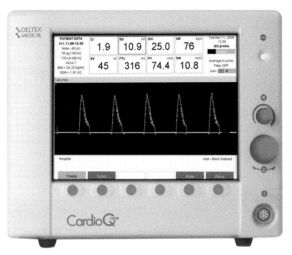

Fig. 17.15 Display of an oesophageal Doppler cardiac output monitor showing the pulse waveform from which a variety of haemodynamic variables are derived.

In practice a beam of ultrasonic waves is focused on the descending aorta, and reflections from red cells are measured by a transducer in the same probe. Probes may be transthoracic (usually placed in the sternal notch) or placed in the oesophagus. The signal obtained is displayed on the screen and indicates peak velocity and flow time. By making a number of assumptions about the nature of flow in the aorta, the cross-sectional area of the aorta (estimated from body surface area and age with a nomogram) and the percentage of CO passing down the thoracic aorta, SV and CO can be estimated. The internal algorithm for these calculations is based on calibration of total left ventricular stroke volume (measured by a PAFC) against descending aortic blood flow velocity and stroke distance as measured by the ODM (Fig. 17.15).

The advantages of these monitors are that they produce an almost real-time estimate of cardiac output, stroke volume and other calculated cardiovascular variables. Disadvantages include that they rely on the ultrasound beam being directed at the centre of the aorta and assume the aorta is a smooth tube. In practice, even small movements of the sensor may lead to marked changes in readings because the speed of red cells near the aortic wall is measured. Furthermore, the aorta is not completely circular and may contain atheroma, and the diameter (an estimate) can change by as much as 12% during systole. The Doppler shift also depends on the direction of the ultrasound beam relative to the axis. Provided that the angle is less than 20 degrees, the error in cardiac output is only about 6%. Conscious patients do not always tolerate the more accurate oesophageal probes, and certain surgical procedures preclude their use (e.g. oesophagectomy). Most systems provide a visual (and audible) measure of signal strength to assist in focussing the probe.

Despite these limitations, the ODM may be useful in high-risk patients undergoing relatively minor surgery or in patients undergoing surgery requiring cardiovascular control (see Chapter 30). However, whilst useful for monitoring responses to treatment, they are unable to provide reliable estimates of actual cardiac output. Complications are few.

Transoesophageal echocardiography

Transoesophageal echocardiography (TOE) uses a miniaturised ultrasound probe inserted into the oesophagus under anaesthesia. It provides a real-time picture of all four cardiac chambers and valves. Advantages are that it can identify any malfunctioning valves, any ischaemia-induced wall motion abnormalities and whether therapy has been successful (e.g. valve surgery). However, the equipment is expensive and requires an operator trained in use and interpretation of the data. In cardiac surgery they can demonstrate adequate cardiac function and valve competence at weaning from cardiopulmonary off bypass. They can also measure cardiac output using Doppler. However, they are only suitable for anaesthetised or sedated patients, cannot provide prolonged continuous measurements and are rarely used in non-cardiac surgery. Transthoracic echocardiography is increasingly employed in ICU to answer specific haemodynamic questions, such as cardiac contractility, identification of regional wall motion abnormalities and ejection fraction. Additional information about the lungs and pleura can be obtained at the same sitting. However, accurate results are operator dependent, and continuous cardiac output monitoring is not possible.

Thoracic electrical bioimpedance

Tissue impedance depends on blood volume. Measurement of thoracic impedance provides an index of stroke volume. Two circumferential electrodes are placed around the neck and two around the upper abdomen. A small (<1 mA), constant, high-frequency (>1 kHz) alternating current is passed between the outer electrodes, and the resulting potential difference is detected by the inner pair. This potential is rectified, smoothed and filtered to record voltage fluctuations which reflect changes in impedance as a result of ventilation and cardiac activity. The cardiac activity is extracted by signal averaging relative to the ECG R-wave. This represents changes in thoracic blood volume and clearly resembles the pulse waveform.

Modern instruments show a modest agreement with invasive measurements of cardiac output, although trends and rapid changes in cardiac output are reliably demonstrated. This method is inaccurate when there are intracardiac shunts or arrhythmias and underestimates cardiac output in a vasodilated circulation.

The respiratory system

Clinical

Clinical signs are important for the safe conduct of anaesthesia. Airway obstruction is often more rapidly recognised through signs such as tugging, paradoxical chest movement and poor movement of the reservoir bag than it is by monitoring devices. Auscultation can confirm normal breath sounds (although it does not reliably exclude oesophageal intubation) and detect abnormalities such as bronchospasm or excess secretions.

Respiratory rate

Respiratory rate may be timed clinically or derived from a capnograph. Also, many ECG monitors can pass a very small high-frequency alternating current through the leads; the increase in electrical impedance (resistance to an alternating current) across the chest during inhalation is measured and the respiratory rate calculated.

Oesophageal stethoscope

An oesophageal stethoscope comprises a balloon-tipped catheter with or without a temperature probe inserted into the patient's oesophagus and connected to an earpiece or stethoscope. The catheter is advanced until the heart sounds are maximal and then taped at the nose. It provides a constant monitor of both heart rate and ventilation and may identify the characteristic millwheel murmur of an air embolus. It is inexpensive, and it carries little morbidity. However, with the advent of monitors such as end-tidal capnography, it is rarely used.

Airway pressure

The lungs are damaged easily, and although anaesthetic machines incorporate pressure relief valves, these are designed to protect the machine rather than the patient. Ventilators usually allow a maximum airway pressure to be set to protect the patient, but excessive pressure may still be exerted by manual compression of the reservoir or self-inflating resuscitation bag. Pressure monitors should therefore be used during any positive pressure ventilation. All modern ventilators have pressure monitors, commonly a transducer in the form of a piezoelectric crystal that converts pressure to an electrical potential, which is then measured by the monitor and displayed.

Such pressure monitors are accurate and reliable but do not directly measure pressure within the lungs. Therefore the measured pressure may not be reliable if a narrow tracheal tube, long breathing circuit or high-frequency ventilation is used. High lung pressures may be a problem in obese patients or those with bronchospasm or in the head down position. There are also regional variations in pressure throughout the lung, particularly when inflamed or damaged.

In devices without electronic components, such as some transport ventilators, pressure can be measured by deformation of bellows or a metal tube. The deformation is linked to a needle with the pressure read from a scale. These simple devices are usually reliable but are susceptible to damage by excess pressure.

Measurement of gas flow and volume

The relationships among volume, flow and velocity are central to understanding gas flow and volume. Flow rate is defined as the volume passing a fixed point per unit time – that is, volume per second. Velocity is the distance moved by gas molecules in unit time. These are related directly and depend upon the cross-sectional area of flow:

$$Velocity = \frac{flow\ rate}{area}$$

The velocities of all molecules in a gas or liquid are not the same. Many devices measure velocity of gas flow rather than the flow rate and so are usually calibrated to a specific gas or liquid. Axial streaming is characteristic of laminar flow (Fig. 17.16).

Measuring volume

Measurements of gas volume depend on collecting the gases in a calibrated spirometer or passing the gases through some type of gas meter. However, volume can also be derived mathematically by integration of gas flow over time.

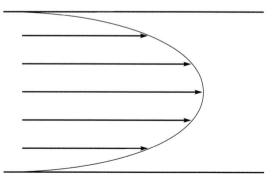

Fig. 17.16 Velocity profile during laminar flow. Velocity is zero at the walls of the containing tube and maximal in the axial stream.

Spirometers

Wet spirometers consist of a rigid cylinder suspended over an underwater seal and counterbalanced. Gas entering the bell causes it to rise. This linear displacement is proportional to the volume of gas. Wet spirometers are accurate at steady state and have been used to calibrate other volume-measuring devices. However, they are bulky and inconvenient, and the frequency response is damped by friction between the moving parts, causing the instrument to underread with rapidly changing rates of flow.

Dry spirometers are more convenient. Gas displaces a rolling diaphragm or bellows, and the expansion is recorded and related to gas volume. The original Vitalograph was a type of bellows spirometer used for lung function testing. The patient makes a maximal forced exhalation into the spirometer through a wide-bore tube. The expansion of the wedge-shaped bellows is recorded by a stylus on a pressure-sensitive chart. The stylus moves across the x-axis (time) at a constant rate. The resultant plot represents the volume–time plot of the patient's expiration (Fig. 17.17). The forced vital capacity (FVC) is the maximal volume expired. Understanding of technique and active cooperation of the patient are essential for accurate and precise recordings. The patient must make an airtight seal with the mouthpiece, with the nose occluded by a clip. Expiration should be as forcible and rapid as possible. Several attempts are recorded. The highest value measured is recorded because of the technique being effort dependent, which improves with practice.

Modern spirometers now use technology based on measuring flow and integrating the signal over time (see 'Measuring gas flow' later). These electronic devices are more portable and increasingly integrate with computers to allow personal monitoring and analysis of data.

Spirometry forms part of pulmonary function testing, alongside measurement of lung diffusion. In testing lung diffusion, the patient is asked to exhale to residual volume and then inhale completely a mixture of carbon monoxide (usually 0.3% CO), an inert gas such as helium or methane that will not cross the alveolar membrane, and air. The patient then holds their breath for 10 s and then exhales. Carbon monoxide readily crosses the alveolar membrane and binds to haemoglobin. As there is a negligible partial pressure of CO in the pulmonary capillaries, the difference between inhaled and exhaled gas over time relates to the ability of gas to diffuse across alveolar membranes. The role of the inert gas is to measure alveolar volume. The test estimates the thickness of the alveolar membrane, the pulmonary capillary volume and overall pulmonary surface area available for gas transfer. Limitations are that carbon monoxide is not a physiological gas so its relevance is uncertain, haemoglobin concentrations influence the result and testing is effort dependent.

Gas meters

Dry gas meters are widely used in the gas industry and are used also in medicine (e.g. in some mechanical ventilators to measure large volumes of gas). Displacement of bellows controls valves which alternately direct gas flow to fill and empty the bellows and also drives the pointer on a calibrated recording dial. Irregularities within each cycle disappear when the meter has returned to the same position in the cycle; hence, accuracy of measurements improves with increasing multiples of meter volume.

The Dräger volumeter

The volume of gas which flows through the Dräger volumeter is related to the rotation of two light, interlocking, dumbbell–shaped rotors. It is a simple meter and accurate but affected by moisture.

The Wright respirometer

The Wright respirometer contains a light mica vane which rotates within a small cylinder (Fig. 17.18). Inflowing air is directed onto the vane by tangential slits. Rotation of the vane drives a gear chain and pointer on a dial. This mechanism is inferential because it does not measure either the volume or the flow of total gas flowing through the device. It is calibrated for normal tidal volumes and breathing rates by a sine wave pump. However, the meter overreads at high tidal volumes and underreads at low tidal volumes because of the inertia of the moving parts.

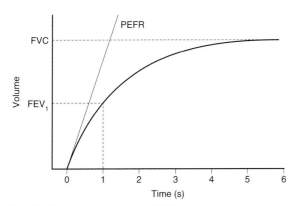

Fig. 17.17 Forced vital capacity *(FVC)*, forced expiratory volume in 1 s *(FEV₁)* and peak expiratory flow rate *(PEFR)* can all be derived from the volume–time plot of the Vitalograph (Sykes et al. 1991).

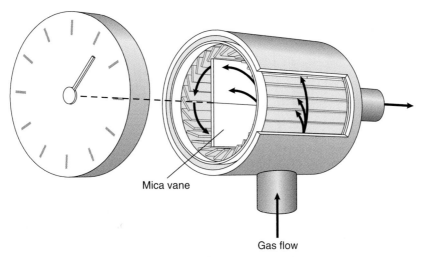

Fig. 17.18 Diagrammatic representation of the mechanism of the Wright Respirometer.

Integration of the flow signal

The flow signal from a rapidly responding flowmeter may be integrated electronically over time to calculate volume. However, integration exaggerates the effect of baseline drift; a small and insignificant change in the baseline of the flow signal produces substantial and increasing error in the volume signal. This effect is minimised by limiting the duration of integration (e.g. to a single tidal volume).

Indirect methods of measuring tidal volume

Methods that depend on measuring inspired or expired gases require a leak-free connection. This is feasible with tracheal intubation, but connecting an awake patient to the system may influence their pattern of breathing. There are indirect methods which derive tidal volume from measurements of chest wall movement. An example of this is respiratory inductance plethysmography. This device uses a wire coil sewn into an elasticated strap. Expansion of the chest or abdomen increases the space between the coils and so alters the inductance generated by a high-frequency alternating current (AC). The change in inductance depends on the cross-sectional area enclosed by the coil, which is closely related to change in volume. Inductance plethysmography has been used in physiological studies of postoperative respiratory depression and to detect apnoea.

Measuring gas flow
Volume–time methods

Flow rate may be calculated from spirometric measurements of volume of gas per unit time. These methods are accurate when corrected for temperature and pressure and are used widely to calibrate other flowmeters but are slow, cumbersome and have limited clinical application.

Most clinical methods are based on the relationship between pressure decrease and flow across a resistance – either a fixed pressure decrease across a variable orifice or a variable pressure change across a fixed orifice.

Variable orifice (constant pressure change) flowmeters

The orifice through which gas flows enlarges with the flow rate so that the pressure difference across the orifice remains constant. This is the physical principle of the rotameter.

Rotameter

The rotameter consists of a vertical glass tube inside which rotates a light metal alloy bobbin (Fig. 17.19). A fine-adjustment valve at the bottom of the rotameter controls flow, and when opened, the pressure of the gas forces the bobbin up the tube. The inside of the tube is an inverted cone, so that the cross-sectional area of the annular space exactly opposes the downward pressure resulting from the weight of the bobbin. The pressure decrease remains constant throughout the range of flows for which the tube is calibrated, and the bobbin rotates freely in the steady stream of gas. Laminar flow predominates at low flow rates, dependent on gas viscosity (see Chapter 15). Turbulent flow predominates at higher flow rates and so gas density becomes the important factor. Both gas density and viscosity vary with temperature and pressure, and each rotameter must be calibrated for one specific gas in appropriate conditions.

341

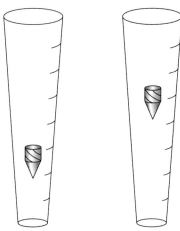

Fig. 17.19 Physical principle of the Rotameter flowmeter. The weight of the bobbin is exactly opposed by the pressure drop across the cross-sectional area of the annular space around the bobbin.

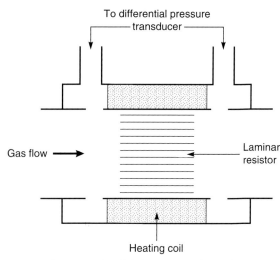

Fig. 17.20 The Fleisch pneumotachograph.

The peak flowmeter

Peak flowmeters may measure flow rates up to 1000 litres min^{-1}. Air flow causes a vane to rotate or a piston to move against the constant force of a light spring. This opens orifices which permit air to escape. The position adopted by the vane or piston depends primarily on the flow rate and on the area of the orifice required to maintain a constant pressure. The light moving vane or piston rapidly attains a maximum position in response to the peak expiratory flow and is held in this position by a ratchet. The reading is obtained from a mechanical pointer attached to the vane or piston.

Accurate results demand good technique. These devices must be held horizontally to minimise the effects of gravity on the moving parts. The patient must be encouraged to exhale as rapidly as possible. Values increase with practice, so maximum readings are recorded.

Variable pressure change (fixed orifice) flowmeters

In variable pressure change flowmeters the resistance is maintained constant so that changes of flow are accompanied by changes in pressure across the resistance element.

Bourdon gauge flowmeter

A Bourdon gauge is used to sense the pressure change across an orifice and is calibrated to the gas flow rate. These rugged meters are not affected by changes in position and are useful for metering the flow from gas cylinders at high

ambient pressure. Back-pressure causes overreading of the actual flow rate.

Pneumotachograph

The pneumotachograph measures flow rate by sensing the pressure change across a small but laminar resistance. Careful design ensures that the differential manometer senses the true lateral pressure exerted by the gas on each side of the resistance element (Fig. 17.20). The manometer is very sensitive, as pressure changes are tiny, and must have good zero and gain stability. Integration enables calculation of gas volume.

Pneumotachographs are sensitive instruments with a rapid response to changing gas flow, are used widely for clinical measurement of gas flows in respiratory and anaesthetic practice and are found in bedside spirometers. Their use in the operating theatre is limited by the need for frequent calibration, correction or compensation for changes in temperature, humidity, gas composition and pressure during mechanical ventilation. They are also susceptible to blockage, particularly by water condensation.

Other devices for measuring gas flow

Measurements other than pressure change across an orifice have been used to measure flow.

Hot-wire flowmeters

A fast-flowing gas cools a heated wire more quickly than a slow-flowing gas. Measuring temperature differences therefore enables calculation of gas flow. Whilst affected by changes in gas thermal conductivity (e.g. by water vapour), this method is inexpensive, robust, reliable and works over a wide range of flows. However, it is unable to determine direction of flow.

Ultrasonic flowmeters

These flowmeters use the vortex-shedding technique. Gas is passed through a tube containing a rod 1–2 mm in diameter, mounted at right angles to the direction of gas flow. Vortices form downstream of the rod, the number of vortices formed being directly related to the flow rate. The vortices are detected using ultrasound and integrated to give a volume signal. Measurement is not affected greatly by temperature, humidity or changes in gas composition. A critical flow rate is required for the formation of vortices, and the flowmeter is most accurate when the tidal volume is large.

Gas and vapour analysis

Chemical methods

Chemical methods are important historically for measurement of oxygen and carbon dioxide concentrations. A fractional volume of gas is changed to a different state via a chemical reaction; the fractional concentration is determined by the reduction in volume which occurs:

$$Fractional\ concentration = \frac{reduction\ in\ gas\ volume}{original\ volume}$$

Several types of apparatus have been described (e.g. the Haldane). Carbon dioxide is absorbed in a strongly alkaline potassium hydroxide solution; oxygen is absorbed in alkaline pyrogallol or sodium anthraquinone.

Physical methods

Instruments based on the physical properties of a gas or vapour are convenient, responsive and more suitable for continuous operation.

Speed of response is determined by two components:
- *Transit time* required for the sample to flow along the sampling catheter. This is minimised by using a narrow and short sampling catheter with a rapid sampling flow rate.
- *Response time* of the instrument to react to a change in gas concentration. It consists of the washout time of the analysis cell and sensing delays.

Zero drift and variations in gain are common problems, and most gas analysers require frequent calibration, ideally against gas mixtures of known composition.

Non-specific methods

Non-specific methods use a property of the gas that is common to all gases, but which is possessed by each gas to a differing degree.

Thermal conductivity

The ability of a gas to conduct heat is the basis of a katharometer. Gas is passed over a heated wire and the degree of cooling of the wire depends on the temperature of the gas, the rate of gas flow and the thermal conductivity of the gas. The reduction in temperature of the wire reduces its resistance, producing an electrical signal related to the gas concentration. In clinical practice, katharometers are usually used for the measurement of CO_2 and He and as detectors in gas chromatography systems.

Refractive index: interference refractometers

The refractive index is the ability of a substance to slow the speed of light. The delay through a gas depends on the number of gas molecules present; hence the refractive index also depends on the pressure and temperature of the gas. Light waves from a common source focussed on a screen via two linear slits in an opaque sheet generate an interference pattern. Areas where light passes through the two slits in phase are bright; light paths differing in length by half a wavelength, being out of phase, generate dark bands. When a gas is introduced into one light path, it delays transmission of the light waves, reducing the wavelength and altering the position of the dark bands. This change in position corresponds to the number of gas molecules in the light path, and if the refractive index of the gas is known, it is used to acquire its partial pressure. Interference refractometers are calibrated using known concentrations of gas or vapour. The response is essentially linear and remains stable after calibration.

This method of analysis is used to calibrate flowmeters and vaporisers accurately. Portable devices are useful for monitoring pollution by anaesthetic gases and vapours.

Specific methods

Specific methods identify and measure a gas using some unique property and are particularly suitable for complex mixtures of gases. These methods include the following:
- Magnetic susceptibility
- Absorption of radiation
- Mass spectrometry
- Gas–liquid chromatography

Their principles are explored further by reference to specific gases.

Oxygen

Oxygen concentration in a breathing system is measured using either a fuel cell or a paramagnetic analyser.

The fuel cell is the more common device. It contains a lead anode within a small container of electrode gel. When exposed to oxygen, the lead is converted to lead oxide, producing a small voltage which may be measured and amplified. Fuel cells are small, robust and reliable, although they require regular calibration. After around 6 months, they require replacement because the lead becomes oxidised. Accuracy is better than ±1% with a response time of <10 s.

The principle of the paramagnetic analyser is that oxygen molecules are attracted weakly to a magnetic field (paramagnetic). Most other anaesthetic gases are repelled by a magnetic field (diamagnetic). In the original analysers, a powerful magnetic field was passed across a chamber which contained two nitrogen-containing spheres suspended on a wire. When oxygen was introduced into the chamber, it tended to displace the spheres, causing them to rotate. The degree of rotation was measured to estimate the oxygen concentration.

A fast differential paramagnetic oxygen sensor uses the pneumatic bridge principle. The sample and reference gas are drawn by a common pump through two tubes surrounded by an electromagnet alternating at 110 Hz. Pressure differences between the two tubes are related to the paramagnetic properties of the sample and reference gases. The phasic changes in pressure are extremely small and measured with a miniature microphone. The output of the device is linear, very stable and has a fast response time of less than 150 ms (Fig. 17.21).

These monitors are accurate, reliable and do not need frequent maintenance. However, they overestimate oxygen concentration when pressure in the circuit is increased.

Carbon dioxide and anaesthetic gases

Absorption of radiation

Infrared radiation (1–15 μm) is absorbed by all gases with two or more dissimilar atoms in the molecule. Carbon dioxide, nitrous oxide and anaesthetic vapours absorb light at different wavelengths. Measurement of such gases is via an infrared light source that emits light at different wavelengths towards a photoelectric detector. The test gas absorbs the relevant wavelength of light, and any non-absorbed light passes to an optical filter. Only light with the wavelength corresponding to the test gas passes through to the detector. As per the Beer–Lambert laws (see 'Oximetry'), the amount of light absorbed is proportional to the concentration of the gas (Fig. 17.22). The test chamber is also heated to avoid condensation. Accuracy is around 0.5%, with a response time of <0.5 s.

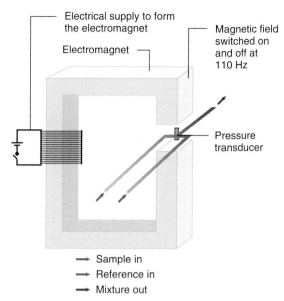

Datex paramagnetic analyser

Electrical supply to form the electromagnet

Electromagnet

Magnetic field switched on and off at 110 Hz

Pressure transducer

→ Sample in
→ Reference in
→ Mixture out

Fig. 17.21 Schematic of a paramagnetic analyser using the pneumatic bridge principle.

There are several sources of error with infrared analysis:

- Overlap of absorption spectra occurs between different gases. For instance, peak absorption for carbon dioxide, nitrous oxide and carbon monoxide is 4.3, 4.5 and 4.7 μm, respectively. Error is minimised by narrowing the band of infrared light.
- 'Collision broadening' is the apparent widening of the absorption spectrum of CO_2 by the physical presence of certain other gases, notably N_2 and N_2O. Whilst there are correction factors, calibration with a similar background gas mixture minimises error.
- Environment influences measurement because absorption is related to the partial pressure of the gas being analysed. Changes in atmospheric pressure, pressure in the breathing system and changes in resistance of the sampling line can introduce error.
- Unexpected vapours, such as ethanol from an intoxicated patient, may introduce errors.
- Modern gas analysers are very stable but require regular calibration. Accuracy at normal breathing frequencies also requires a satisfactory response time, typically a 90% or 95% rise time of less than 150 ms. Slow response is usually caused by blockage of the sampling line with condensation or sputum or by failure of the suction pump.

Most analysers are side stream systems: a small sample of gas is pumped into the analyser that necessarily involves

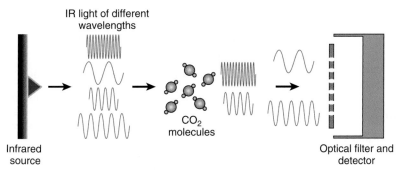

Fig. 17.22 Schematic representation of a CO_2 infrared analyser. The infrared source emits infrared light at different wavelengths through a sample containing CO_2. The CO_2 molecules absorb infrared of specific wavelengths proportional to the concentration of CO_2, whilst other wavelengths are unaffected. An optical filter then selects only the wavelengths absorbed by CO_2. The difference between light of the correct wavelength that reaches the detector and the light emitted from the infrared source is a measure of infrared light absorption by the test gas. This relates to the concentration of CO_2 in the test gas. *IR*, Infrared.

some delay. In most cases the sampled gas is passed into the scavenging system, but when low flows are required, it may be returned to the breathing system, although this can cause errors because of the mixing of inspiratory and expiratory gases. This arrangement allows the sensing chamber to be housed within a monitor, making it more robust.

The alternative main stream system places the sensing chamber in a connector within the patient breathing system and so reduces any delay in measurement. However, it also makes the sensor more prone to accidental damage.

Carbon dioxide concentration is usually displayed as a graph of concentration against time (capnograph). This provides visual confirmation that the airway is patent and that ventilation is occurring. It also provides the only reliable guarantee after tracheal intubation that the tube is not in the oesophagus.

At the start of expiration, the carbon dioxide concentration is zero (dead space gas). The concentration then increases to a plateau level (alveolar gas). The end-tidal value of carbon dioxide concentration approximates to alveolar, and therefore arterial, carbon dioxide partial pressure. However, when the respiratory rate is high, if tidal volume is low, if the sampling point is distant from the airway or if the gases tend to mix in the circuit, the end-tidal value tends to be artificially low. This may give the impression that the lungs are being hyperventilated. For these reasons, it is difficult to measure end-tidal carbon dioxide meaningfully in small children. This is also true in patients, often smokers, who have marked ventilation/perfusion mismatch; there is often a prolonged upstroke on the capnograph trace, and the relationship between end-tidal and arterial carbon dioxide tensions becomes less reliable (Fig. 17.23).

Low cardiac output states (e.g. air embolus, pulmonary embolism, ischaemia) reduce carbon dioxide delivery to the lung. This results in low end-tidal carbon dioxide readings

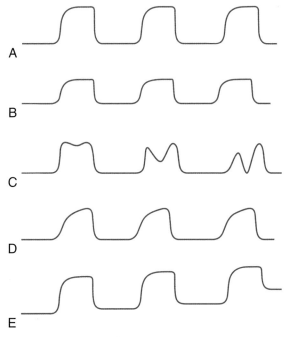

Fig. 17.23 A selection of capnograph traces, where A is that seen typically during anaesthesia, B represents a low cardiac output, C represents spontaneous respiratory efforts during mandatory ventilation (e.g. during recovery from muscle relaxation), D shows a trace often associated with bronchoconstriction (e.g. COPD), and E is what might be seen during rebreathing or exhaustion of soda lime in a circle breathing circuit.

and an increased arterial carbon dioxide tension. This is a useful sign in ICU or during surgery associated with an increased risk of blood or air emboli (e.g. neurosurgery). Infrared analysers are used predominately for measuring anaesthetic gases. Other methods are used occasionally either for calibration or for complex analyses.

Mass spectrometry

Mass spectrometers separate the components of complex gas mixtures according to their mass and charge by deflecting the charged ions in a magnetic field. When a sample is introduced into a mass spectrometer, it passes into a vacuum where it is bombarded with high-energy electrons. These break up larger molecules and strip off their outer electrons. The resulting positively charged ions are then accelerated by a negatively charged plate into a magnetic field. The magnetic field causes the moving particles to curve depending on their mass-to-charge ratio. A row of sensors then measures the number of molecules and their sizes in proportion to the partial pressure of the sampled gas (Fig. 17.24). A mass spectrum is produced by relating the detector output on the y-axis (calibrated to concentration of gas) to the accelerating voltage on the x-axis (calibrated to molecular weight).

Some molecules may lose two electrons and become doubly charged – they behave like ions with half the mass. Some fragmentation of molecules also occurs in the ionisation process, resulting in the production of a mass spectrum rather than a single peak for each molecule. These secondary peaks may be used to advantage, such as in the identification and quantification of CO_2 and N_2O, both of which share a parent peak at 44 Da but produce secondary peaks at 12 and 30 Da, respectively.

Mass spectrometers are expensive to purchase and maintain but are extremely accurate, have a very short response time, use very small sample flow rates (approx. 20 ml min^{-1}) and can identify a wide range of compounds. They may be sited centrally within large theatre complexes as part of a calibration and quality control system.

Gas–liquid chromatography

A gas chromatograph consists of two components: a column packed with inert beads covered in a thin film of oil (the stationary phase) and a constant stream of inert gas which passes through the column. When a sample of gas is introduced at one end, the mixture passes into the column and past the oil. Insoluble gases tend to stay in the carrier gas and move through the column quickly, whereas soluble gases tend to dissolve in the oil, slowing their progress. At the other end of the column is a non-specific detector unit which yields an electronic signal proportional to the quantity of each substance present. Commonly used detectors include katharometers, flame ionisation and electron capture detectors. Identification of a gas is determined by the duration of passage through the column and the quantity measured by the detector unit. Their chief advantage is the ability to identify the components in a mixture of unknown compounds.

In addition to gas analysis, the gas–liquid chromatograph may be used to analyse blood samples containing volatile or local anaesthetic agents, anticonvulsants and intravenous anaesthetic drugs.

Raman scattering

Passing a high-powered laser through a sample of gas causes a scattering of light of different wavelengths in a process known as the Raman effect. The change in wavelength is characteristic of the molecule under study. Sensors placed at the side of the chamber may detect this radiation and identify the gases present. The size and complexity of this technique have restricted its use.

Blood gas analysis

The glass pH electrode

A potential difference is generated across hydrogen ion-sensitive glass depending on the gradient of hydrogen ions. The hydrogen ion concentration within the pH electrode is fixed by a buffer solution so that the potential across the glass is dependent on the hydrogen ion concentration in the sample (Fig. 17.25).

Two silver–silver chloride electrodes generate a constant electrode potential at a fixed temperature. This provides a stable electrical connection with the buffer solution in the pH electrode and with a potassium chloride solution in the reference electrode separated from the test sample by a

Principle of mass spectrometer

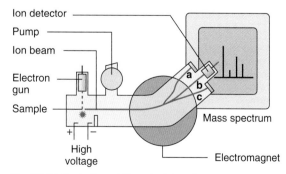

Fig. 17.24 Illustration of the principles of mass spectrometry.

pH electrode

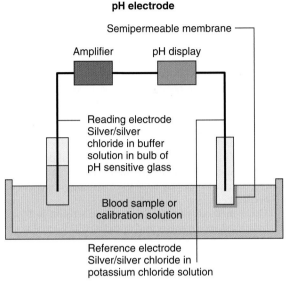

Fig. 17.25 Component parts of the pH electrode.

semipermeable membrane. The potential difference between the electrodes is determined by the pH of the test solution and the temperature; it is calibrated using two phosphate buffers of known fixed pH. Careful daily calibration is required to maintain accuracy, and the electrodes must be regularly cleaned of protein deposits. Reliable measurement of blood pH also depends on the quality of the blood sample, which must be free from air bubbles, heparinised and analysed promptly.

Dissociation of acids and bases is temperature dependent, and the electrodes and blood sampling channel are maintained at 37°C. Although the reference ranges for pH are only valid for 37°C, some clinicians still prefer to use temperature corrected values (pH-stat). This view is countered by proponents of alpha-stat interpretation (pH at 37°C irrespective of the patient's actual temperature), one argument being that the reference range should also be corrected if pH-stat interpretation is to be used, which is usually unknown.

The CO₂ electrode (Severinghaus electrode)

This is a modified glass pH electrode in contact with a thin layer of bicarbonate buffer solution. The buffer is trapped in a nylon mesh spacer and separated from the blood sample by a thin Teflon or silicone membrane which is permeable to CO_2 but not to blood cells, plasma or charged ions. The whole unit is maintained at 37°C. Carbon dioxide diffuses from the blood into the buffer and so increases the hydrogen

ion concentration in proportion to the $P\text{CO}_2$, according to the carbonic acid dissociation equation:

$$CO_2 + H_2O \rightleftharpoons H_2CO_3 \rightleftharpoons H^+ + HCO_3^-$$

The electrode must be calibrated by equilibrating the buffer with two known CO_2 concentrations. The response time is 2–3 min because of the time CO_2 takes to diffuse into the buffer solution and equilibrate.

Oxygenation

Oxygenation may be assessed by measuring the tension, saturation or content of oxygen, the relationship among these three measurements being determined by the shape and position of the oxyhaemoglobin dissociation curve. There are many causes of variations in both the shape and position of the curve, and it is usually necessary to measure the oxygen tension or saturation directly. Tension measurements are required for most respiratory problems, although saturation or content may be required for calculation of the percentage shunt.

Oxygen tension is usually measured using an oxygen electrode. Content is measured by vacuum extraction and chemical absorption, by driving the O_2 into solution and measuring the increase in $P\text{O}_2$ or by a galvanic cell analyser. Saturation is determined by photometric techniques involving the transmission or reflection of light at certain wavelengths.

Oxygen tension

Oxygen electrode: the polarographic method
The oxygen electrode (Clark) consists of a platinum wire, nominally 2 nm in diameter, embedded in a rough-surfaced glass rod. This is immersed in a phosphate buffer which is stabilised with KCl and contained in an outer jacket which incorporates an oxygen-permeable polyethylene or polypropylene membrane (Fig. 17.26). A polarising voltage of between 600 and 800 mV is applied to the platinum wire, and as oxygen diffuses through the membrane electrooxidoreduction occurs at the cathode:

$$O_2 + 2H_2O + 2e^- \rightarrow H_2O_2 + 2OH^-$$

Corresponding oxidation occurs at the Ag–AgCl anode:

$$4Ag \rightarrow 4Ag^+ + 4e^-$$

$$4Ag^+ + 4Cl^- \rightarrow 4AgCl$$

Thus a half cell is set up and a measurable current is generated, with electrons flowing from the silver anode to the platinum cathode. Higher tensions of oxygen increase the rate of reduction at the cathode, generating a higher measurable current between the anode and cathode. The

347

The pO₂ electrode

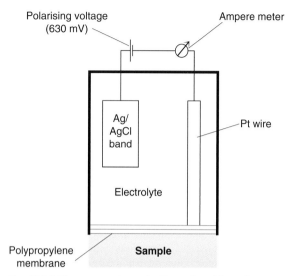

Fig. 17.26 The oxygen electrode. (Reproduced from the Radiometer Reference Manual. Permission from Radiometer A/S, Åkandevej 21, DK-2700 Brønshøj, Denmark.)

oxygen electrode may be used with gas mixtures or blood. Two-point calibration includes zero (electronic or oxygen-free gas) and 21% O_2, with measurements made at 37 °C. Errors occur when the electrode is contaminated by protein deposits, the plastic membrane is damaged or there is a delay in analysing the heparinised blood sample.

Galvanic or fuel cell
Galvanic cells convert energy from an oxidation-reduction chemical process into electrical energy. The potential generated is dependent on the oxygen concentration.

A gold mesh cathode catalyses the reduction of oxygen by reaction with water to hydroxyl ions, whereas lead is oxidised at the anode. Unlike the oxygen electrode, no battery is required. The reaction in the fuel cell generates a potential gradient. The chemical reaction uses up the components of the cell so that its life depends on the concentration of oxygen to which it is exposed and on the duration of exposure: in practice, 6–12 months. Fuel cells are widely used in reliable and portable oxygen analysers, which incorporate a digital readout and audible alarms. These are cheap and require little maintenance. Inaccurate responses to calibration with oxygen and air suggest that the fuel cell is exhausted and should be replaced.

Transcutaneous electrodes
Transcutaneous electrodes are non-invasive and used for monitoring neonatal blood gas tensions. The electrode is attached to the skin to form an airtight seal using a contact liquid, and the area is heated to 43 °C. At this temperature the blood flow to the skin increases and the capillary oxygen diffuses through the skin, allowing measurement of the diffused gases by the attached electrode. The values obtained from the transcutaneous electrode are lower than those from a simultaneous arterial specimen. Many factors affect the transcutaneous measurement of oxygen tension, including the skin site and thickness. Most importantly, the electrode depends on local capillary blood flow and under-reads in the presence of hypotension and microcirculatory perfusion failure. Problems occur with surgical diathermy; the heating current circuit provides a return path for the cutting current, which may cause the transcutaneous electrode to overheat.

Other methods of measuring oxygen tension in blood include mass spectrometry and optodes, which employ the quenching of fluorescence from illuminated dye.

Oxygen content

The total amount of oxygen in blood may be measured directly, but this is technically demanding and rarely used. The van Slyke technique uses a chemical and volumetric or manometric analysis of oxygen content. Oxygen is driven from a small sample by denaturing the haemoglobin with acid. The volume of gas at atmospheric pressure, or the pressure at constant volume, is recorded before and after the chemical absorption of oxygen. The change is related directly to the oxygen content of the fixed volume of blood. Alternative detectors have been used to measure oxygen displaced from haemoglobin (e.g. a galvanic cell).

These time-consuming and operator-dependent laboratory techniques have been replaced by calculation of oxygen content from measurements of the oxygen saturation of haemoglobin, haemoglobin concentration and the tension of oxygen in blood:

$$Oxygen\ content\ of\ blood\ \mathrm{ml\ dl^{-1}} = S_{O_2}\% \times Hb\ \mathrm{g\ dl^{-1}} \times 1.34 + 0.0225 \times P_{O_2}\ \mathrm{(kPa)}$$

where 1.34 is the Huffner constant and 0.0225 is the solubility of oxygen in blood.

Accurate estimates require that the oxygen saturation of haemoglobin is measured directly, not calculated from oxygen tension and an arbitrary but unmeasured oxyhaemoglobin dissociation curve.

Oximetry: measurement of oxygen saturation

In vitro oximetry
Oximetry relies on the differing absorption of light at different wavelengths by the various states of haemoglobin.

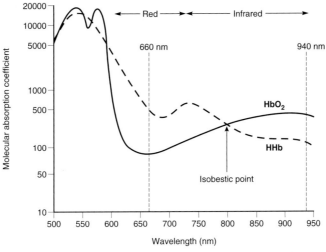

Fig. 17.27 Absorption spectra of reduced *(HHb)* and oxygenated *(HbO₂)* haemoglobin.

The absorption of radiation passing through a sample is measured. The degree of absorption of light, defined by the ratio of incident to emergent light intensities on a logarithmic scale, is proportional to the concentration of the molecules absorbing light (Beer's law) and the thickness of the absorbing layer (Lambert's law).

Oxyhaemoglobin and deoxyhaemoglobin differ at both the red and infrared portions of the absorption spectrum (Fig. 17.27). The differential absorption of two wavelengths of red and infrared light permits the calculation of the ratio of the concentrations of oxygenated and reduced haemoglobins. Additional wavelengths are added in co-oximeters for the calculation of the proportions of other species of haemoglobin, such as carboxyhaemoglobin and methaemoglobin, and the absolute absorbance is used to estimate total haemoglobin concentration from the sum of the various haemoglobins. This is important in measurements of oxyhaemoglobin for use in the calculation of oxygen content.

Commercial co-oximeters draw a small blood sample which is haemolysed before entering a cuvette. Light is filtered to produce monochromatic beams, shone through the cuvette and detected by a photocell. The absorption by the sample is the difference in the intensity of incident and transmitted light, and both must be measured. Spectrophotometers apply a double-beam technique that improves the accuracy and precision. Light from the monochromator is split into two beams, which pass through the test sample or a reference sample. Photocells generate two signals corresponding to the sample and the reference light intensities. Electronic processing compares the two signals and generates an output proportional to the difference. This greatly improves the SNR because any variation which affects both the sample

and reference beams equally is ignored and the difference remains constant.

The saturation of mixed venous blood may be measured using an oximeter incorporated into a pulmonary artery catheter. Fibreoptic cables transmit incident light of at least two wavelengths and carry reflected light from red blood cells back to a detector.

The same spectrophotometric principles used by co-oximeters in vitro on haemolysed blood samples have been applied to patients in vivo.

Pulse oximetry

Light transmitted through tissues is absorbed not only by arterial blood but also by other tissue pigments and venous blood. However, the variation in light absorption with each pulse beat results almost entirely from pulsatile arterial blood flow. Two light-emitting diodes – red (660 nm) and infrared (940 nm) – shine light through a finger or earlobe and a photocell detects the transmitted light. The output of the sensor is processed to display a pulse waveform and the arterial oxygen saturation.

The pulse oximeter progresses through the following steps.

1. The sensor first measures the ambient light and subtracts this value from all other measurements. This implies that sudden changes in ambient light levels, such as after drapes are moved, may cause transient errors.
2. A light emitting diode (LED) is turned on and off rapidly. The absorption of transmitted light is then measured, and the variations with time are recorded. The result is a waveform with a trough as blood flows into the finger (more absorption) during systole and a peak as blood

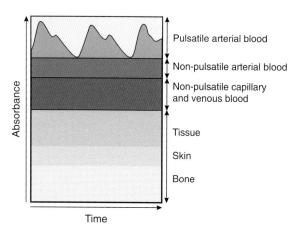

Fig. 17.28 Schematic representation of the contribution of pulsatile arterial blood, non-pulsatile blood and tissues to the absorbance of light.

Box 17.8 **Disadvantages of pulse oximetry**

Damage to skin caused by pressure from probe
Failure to detect hypoventilation
Slow response times: instrument and circulatory delay
Signal quality adversely affected by hypoperfusion
Inter-instrument variability
Failure to detect hypoxaemia in carbon monoxide poisoning

flows into the veins in diastole. The monitor requires around eight heartbeats to make a calculation and then assumes the frequency of this waveform is the heart rate. Frequent ectopic beats or atrial fibrillation may lead to a delay in calculation or unreliable results.

3. The monitor then analyses the measurements and splits the absorption into two components. The fixed or unchanging absorption is assumed to result from tissues such as skin, muscle and bone (Fig. 17.28). The varying absorption is then assumed to be caused by arterial blood moving into the tissue. In situations such as hypotension, hypovolaemia or hypothermia, pulsation may be reduced to a point at which the monitor is not able to make any calculations, and it fails to read. When a patient is on cardiac bypass the tissues are perfused, but if the flow is non-pulsatile, pulse oximeters cannot provide a reading.

4. Steps 1–3 are repeated sequentially using light of at least two different wavelengths at around 120 Hz. When the absorptions of each different wavelength are known, the proportion of oxygenated and deoxygenated haemoglobin may be calculated. The measurements are processed and a new value displayed around every 8 s. Whilst improving reliability, this averaging introduces delay. Another source of delay is circulatory, dependent on the distribution of blood from the lungs to the tissues. The response time to changes in arterial oxygenation can be prolonged, particularly if the probe is anatomically distant from the heart (e.g. the toe) or with low cardiac output or vasoconstriction.

Pulse oximeter calculations assume that the blood contains only normal haemoglobin and that no abnormal light-absorbing substances (dyes) are present. For example, if the patient has breathed carbon monoxide, the monoxy-carboxyhaemoglobin (as it has a similar absorption spectrum)

is measured as oxyhaemoglobin. The result is that the pulse oximeter reading in patients suffering from carbon monoxide poisoning is usually close to 100%, even though they have severe hypoxaemia. The use of intravascular dyes as markers may produce unpredictable results. Lastly, if the probe slips partially off the patient, some light passes directly from the LEDs to the light sensor and also through the sensor. This also causes unreliable readings.

Pulse oximeters provide a rapid, non-invasive measurement of pulse rate and an estimate of oxygen saturation. They are viewed as an essential component of safe surgery. Pulse oximeters are also used to measure oxygen saturation in patients with intermittent respiratory problems, such as postoperative patients and those with sleep apnoea. Advances in technology have resulted in several small battery-powered devices becoming available for out-of-hospital use and can even be found in personal fitness trackers. Calibration points between 80% and 100% are derived from volunteer studies, and accuracy of pulse oximeters is around ±2% greater than an oxygen saturation of 70%. Accuracy at less than 70% is not known precisely, because it is not ethical to conduct trials at these levels. It is important to note that, especially when oxygen therapy is used, normal oxygen saturation does not equate to normal ventilation. For example, in opioid overdose, hypoventilation may lead to potentially fatal hypercapnia without any decrease in oxygen saturation if the patient is breathing a high concentration of oxygen. Complications are rare. The major drawbacks and source of error of pulse oximetry are summarised in Box 17.8.

Respiratory quotient

The accurate measurement of gas volumes and concentrations of CO_2 and O_2 are key to determining the respiratory quotient (RQ). This is the ratio of carbon dioxide production to oxygen consumption and is useful in assessing patient nutritional requirements as well as in the alveolar gas equation. It is most commonly determined using indirect calorimetry, a process that determines the volume of carbon dioxide produced and the volume of oxygen consumed. The key components to the indirect calorimeter devices are measurements of gas concentrations (using infrared and paramagnetic analysers) and gas volumes (using flowmeters such as a pneumotachograph). These are used to compare inspired gases with expired gases to determine RQ.

Respiratory quotient and its related resting energy expenditure (REE) can be used to guide nutrition in the critically ill, mainly to prevent over- or underfeeding as well as to identify the correct balance of nutritional components for an individual patient. Limitations include variations in respiratory cycle, positive end-expiratory pressure and circuit leaks which contribute to inaccurate results. More importantly, there is a paucity of evidence for improved patient outcome with nutrition guided by indirect calorimetry.

The nervous system

The best monitor of cerebral function is the patient, who can report symptoms such as numbness, loss of function or pain. This is not possible during general anaesthesia, and so it is possible for patients to develop a major neurological deficit that becomes apparent only on recovery. For example, patients with traumatic brain injury may develop cerebral oedema under anaesthesia or sedation that is only detectable if monitoring (e.g. intracranial pressure measurement) is in place.

Depth of anaesthesia is difficult to monitor, and traditional signs such as heart rate, blood pressure, sweating and pupillary dilation are unreliable. Anaesthesia itself is also not well defined. Whilst accepted as a lack of perception, lack of responsiveness and inability to recall, these are poorly defined concepts and essentially unmeasurable. Monitoring depth of anaesthesia may minimise patient exposure to maintenance anaesthetic agents and so reduce side effects and improve recovery time.

Depth of anaesthesia
The isolated forearm technique

In the isolated forearm method a patient is anaesthetised and then a tourniquet is applied to the upper arm and inflated to above systolic arterial pressure. A muscle relaxant is then administered (if required as part of the appropriate anaesthetic technique). Because the tourniquet prevents the muscle relaxant passing to the arm, the forearm muscles still function and are supplied by nerves passing under the tourniquet. If awareness occurs, the patient can signal by moving the forearm. Unfortunately the technique signals only that the patient is already awake, and its duration is limited by the ischaemia caused by the tourniquet. The technique and its interpretation remain controversial as responses do not seem to be associated with explicit recall.

The electroencephalogram and evoked potentials

The EEG is a small complex signal, which is recorded usually from at least four electrodes fixed to specially prepared sites around the head. It has an amplitude of 50–200 μV and a frequency content which is classified conventionally into four categories:

- Delta waves: 0–4 Hz
- Theta waves: 4–8 Hz
- Alpha waves: 8–13 Hz
- Beta waves: 13 Hz and above

The spiking, transient depolarisation, then repolarisation, of action potentials in neurons in the brain is sufficiently asynchronous and transient to be unrecordable from the scalp or surface of the brain. The EEG is probably generated by the summation of synchronous postsynaptic potentials on the dendrites of sheets of large and symmetrically arranged pyramidal cells in cortical layers III and IV. Recording of these microvolt signals with acceptable levels of artefact and interference is difficult. Visual analysis of EEG recordings is subjective and requires training and experience.

The complexity of raw EEG signals makes its use in the operating theatre impractical. Cerebral function monitors using fewer electrodes have been developed which average the EEG signal but have been found to be unreliable in monitoring depth of anaesthesia. However, they can identify aberrant cerebral activity or seizures. Cerebral function analysing monitors (CFAMs) are useful in neurosurgery and critical care. For example, sedated and paralysed patients are unable to display classical tonic-clonic activity during generalised seizures. A CFAM enables detection of seizure activity in neurosurgical ICU patients and so sedation can be titrated against burst-suppression of the EEG. Two symmetrical pairs of EEG electrodes are placed on either side of the patient's head. The monitor then analyses the EEG amplitude and the frequency of the waveforms into delta, theta, alpha and beta waves as well as displaying wave suppression information.

Spectral analysis makes the EEG signal easier to interpret. Any complex wave may be broken down into a series of sine waves. Fast Fourier analysis determines the proportion of each frequency which contributes to the total signal. The alternative bispectral analysis determines the relationships between the phase and power of different frequencies within the original signal.

Spectral analysis has indicated that general anaesthesia produces a reduction in the mean frequency and spectral edge (frequency below which 95% of activity occurs). Increasing doses of anaesthetic drugs produce a suppressed or isoelectric EEG, but these changes are unreliable as a measure of depth of anaesthesia.

Bispectral index (BIS) monitors generate a number from 100 (awake) to 0 (deeply anaesthetised). It is important to understand that the BIS is an empirical value derived by

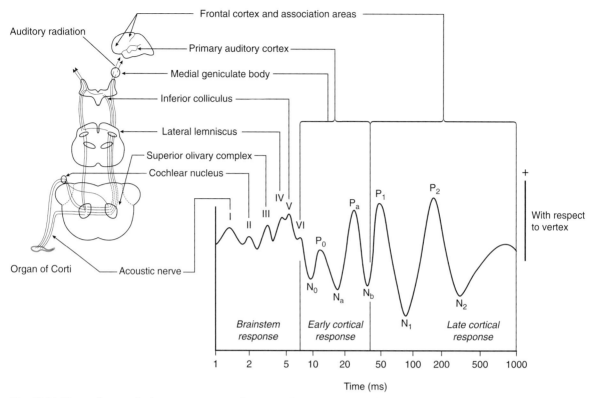

Fig. 17.29 The auditory evoked response consists of a series of waves generated from specific anatomical sites in the auditory pathway as indicated. Activity passes from the cochlea through the brainstem to the cortex.

statistical modelling of processed EEG data from individuals at various degrees of hypnosis. Four components are used – the significance of each of these varies by depth of sedation/anaesthesia: high-frequency activations (14–30 Hz); low-frequency synchronisation; presence of nearly suppressed EEG; fully suppressed (isoelectric) EEG. It uses data from the previous 15–30 s, updated at 1 s intervals. It appears to provide reliable measurements in clinical use. However, it is not clear how factors such as different anaesthetic agents, hypoxaemia or epileptic activity affect the results. For example, ketamine can cause BIS values to rise despite inducing anaesthesia, and neuromuscular blocking drugs have been associated with reductions in BIS values despite patients being awake (suggesting that EMG does contribute to BIS). Furthermore, an awake BIS value may be different at induction compared with emergence; such hysteresis for anaesthetic concentrations and depth of anaesthesia remains an area of research.

Auditory evoked potentials

Auditory evoked potential monitors measure the slowing of auditory information processing produced by anaesthetic agents. The patient wears headphones which repeatedly play soft clicks. Each click produces neuronal activity in the auditory cortex. A signal from a single click would be masked by other brain activity, so repeated clicks are used, which can be averaged to isolate the auditory signal. The activity in the auditory cortex is then displayed as the auditory evoked potential (Fig. 17.29). The time delay for some waves can then be measured and the result converted into a value from 0 to 100, reflecting depth of anaesthesia. Monitors using this principle are commercially available but are not widely used. Limitations include the slow response times, wide variability in values in conscious patients and significant overlap between anaesthetised and awake patients. It also cannot be used on some patients with impaired hearing. Equipment using either visual or somatosensory stimulation has also been developed.

Other techniques

Respiratory sinus arrhythmia is the normal variation in heart rate related to the respiratory cycle. This variability is reduced by anaesthesia and has formed the basis of a commercially available monitor. However, it has not achieved widespread use.

Monitors based on physiological measures such as frontalis muscle myography and lower oesophageal contractility have not proved reliable enough for clinical use.

Intracranial pressure

Intracranial pressure is often measured in neurointensive care units and forms the basis of neuroprotective treatment strategies in brain injuries. The principle is similar to arterial pressure monitoring: An invasive device is connected via a rigid fluid-filled column to an electromechanical transducer which enables display of the waveform on a monitor. The gold standard is a catheter inserted into the lateral ventricle. Alternatively the subdural space can be used, although this provides a less accurate monitor of ICP. More modern systems are less invasive and use either a catheter-tip miniature transducer or a microchip sensor which sits within the parenchyma of the brain. These systems do not require a fluid-filled column or an external transducer and so avoid errors of positioning. However, they cannot be recalibrated once inserted and do not necessarily reflect global ICP.

Brain oxygenation

Monitoring of brain oxygenation is mainly limited to the ICU, although it has a place in cardiac surgery. Near-infrared spectroscopy (NIRS) uses a similar principle to pulse oximetry, except it uses near-infrared light that has better depth penetration, even through bone. A series of optodes are attached to the patient's head that emit near-infrared light. This light is reflected back to sensors at set distances away. The returned signal is a complex product of cerebral oxygenation within the light path, the light-path distance and oxygenation of the intervening soft tissues (scalp). Different monitors claim to correct for this, but changes must be interpreted with caution if vasoactive agents are given as these may affect scalp blood flow more than cerebral blood flow. Near-infrared spectroscopy does not differentiate arterial and venous oxygenation, and because 70%–80% of blood in the superficial frontal cortex is venous, NIRS provides an indicator of the balance of cerebral oxygen delivery and demand.

Transcranial Doppler involves a trained operator using a Doppler probe to measure the velocity of red cells in cerebral arteries. It may detect vasospasm after subarachnoid haemorrhage but also has an important role during carotid endarterectomy to demonstrate adequacy of blood flow in the circle of Willis during contralateral carotid artery clamping.

Jugular venous oxygen saturation monitoring involves passing a catheter in retrograde fashion up the internal jugular vein into the jugular venous sinus. A saturation <55% indicates increased oxygen extraction and therefore relative ischaemia. It is a useful technique in ICU but only measures global perfusion and fails to detect small areas of ischaemia. It also does not inform the clinician as to whether a low saturation is due to inadequate oxygen supply or increased cerebral demand.

Cerebral oxygenation can also be measured directly using specialised intracerebral sensors. The Licox PMO is a combined brain tissue oxygen and brain temperature monitor which detects regional changes in oxygenation. Essentially it is a Clark polarographic electrode with a thermistor and sits within the brain parenchyma, ideally within the damaged but salvageable region of tissue (the penumbra). Assuming the monitor is sited in the correct area, it can measure regional oxygen tension accurately, although with a slight tendency to underread.

More recently, microdialysis catheters have been introduced. These comprise a catheter with a surface dialysis membrane and a perfusion system that slowly circulates dialysis fluid within the catheter. The returning fluid is analysed either remotely or continuously for cerebral metabolites such as lactate, pyruvate and other indicators of cerebral stress such as glutamate and glycerol. The lactate/pyruvate ratio is useful as a marker of cerebral ischaemia. As with intraparenchymal ICP monitors and the Licox system, the measurements are necessarily regional and dependent on accurate positioning of the catheter.

Neuromuscular junction

This is covered in Chapter 8.

Temperature

The body is considered to have an inner core temperature and an outer peripheral temperature. In reality the temperature decreases with distance down limbs and proximity to the skin. The difference between core and peripheral temperatures is related strongly to the cardiac output and degree of vasoconstriction. In practice a core–periphery difference of >2°C is suggestive of a low cardiac output state and has been used as a marker of hypovolaemia.

Commercial thermometers make use of several temperature-dependent phenomena.

Liquid expansion thermometers

Liquid expansion thermometers are simple, reliable instruments. A glass bulb is filled with a liquid (generally alcohol or mercury) and connected to an evacuated, closed capillary tube. The temperature is recorded by the position of the meniscus in the capillary tube against a calibrated scale. If the cross-sectional area of the capillary tube is constant, movement of the meniscus with changing temperature is linear. Glass thermometers are, however, fragile. A large thermal capacity results in a slow response. The instrument is handheld, awkward to read and reset and cannot be used for remote measurement or recording. Traditional mercury-in-glass thermometers are no longer used because of the risk of breakage and mercury contamination.

Chemical thermometers

Reversible chemical thermometers contain several cells filled with liquid crystals, each of slightly different composition. At a critical temperature, the optical properties change because of realignment of the molecules, causing reflection instead of absorption of the incident light. An alternative technique consists of rows of cells filled with chemical mixtures which melt at specific temperatures, releasing a dye; this single-use, disposable design prevents cross-infection but is relatively expensive.

Infrared thermometers

The amount of infrared radiation emitted by the tympanic membrane depends on its temperature, emissivity compared with a black body at the same temperature and the Stefan–Boltzmann constant. Infrared tympanic membrane thermometers based on this principle are in common clinical use. They are inserted into the external ear with the tip protected by a disposable sheath. They measure the infrared radiation produced from the eardrum and produce a digital readout in less than 3 s. Unfortunately, because of factors such as earwax and variations in the angle of insertion, results are less reliable than fixed probes and they cannot produce continuous readings. They are therefore used principally in postoperative recovery and ward areas.

Remote reading instruments

Temperature-dependent electrical properties may be incorporated into thermometers suitable for automation (e.g. targeted temperature management systems for therapeutic cooling of patients) and are also commonly used for monitoring peripheral and core temperature.

Resistance-wire thermometers

Resistance-wire thermometers are based on the principle that the resistance of metal wires increases as their temperature increases. Platinum resistance thermometers have a large temperature coefficient of resistance and are very sensitive to small changes in temperature but are fragile and slow to respond. Single-use probes which incorporate a tiny copper element have been marketed with an acceptable clinical accuracy and response time.

Thermistor thermometers

Thermistors are semiconductors made from the fused oxides of heavy metals such as cobalt, manganese and nickel. They demonstrate marked and non-linear variation in resistance with temperature, which is usually compensated for by electronic processing. Most thermistors in clinical use are negative temperature coefficient (NTC) devices – contrary to a metal wire, resistance decreases as temperature increases. Disadvantages include inconsistent variation between individual thermistors, change in resistance over time, and hysteresis during rapid heating and cooling. However, the large temperature coefficient permits the detection of small temperature changes and the tiny pinhead size results in a rapid response. They are used widely in invasive temperature monitoring (e.g. in pulmonary artery catheters).

Thermocouple thermometers

If two dissimilar metals are joined to create an electrical circuit and the junctions are at different temperatures, current flows from one metal to the other (Seebeck effect). The potential difference which is generated is a function of the temperature difference between the two junctions. All junctions made from the same metals have identical properties. The reference junction must be kept at a constant temperature or incorporate temperature compensation into the measurement. Common combinations of metals include copper–constantan or platinum–rhodium. The output is small (about 40 mV per °C temperature difference between the junctions), but this is sufficient to be sensed by a galvanometer.

Temperature probes using these properties can measure peripheral and core temperatures continuously. Peripheral temperature is measured by attaching a probe to either a finger or toe. Core temperature probes may be inserted into the nasopharynx, oesophagus or rectum, and although complications are rare, it is possible to cause mucosal trauma, bleeding and even penetration of the pharynx or rectum. When used for prolonged periods, mucosal damage is possible as a result of pressure-related ischaemia. Core temperature probes may also form part of an intravascular catheter – for example, within a PAFC. Many monitors accept two probes and automatically display the temperature difference. Care must be taken to avoid the peripheral probe being exposed to warmth from heating blankets.

Dial thermometers

Dial thermometers exploit the increase in pressure caused by the temperature-dependent expansion of a liquid or gas in an enclosed cavity. This is sensed by a Bourdon pressure gauge and recorded on a dial. Although cheap and robust, they are relatively inaccurate, slow to respond and are only suitable for large temperature changes in heated equipment (e.g. autoclaves).

Bimetallic strip thermometers

If strips of two metals with different coefficients of expansion are fastened together throughout their length, the combined strip will bend when heated. Sensitivity is improved by using a long strip which is usually bent in a spiral or coil, with one end fixed and the other connected to a recording pointer. This technique is used for temperature compensation in some anaesthetic vaporisers and in cheap mechanical thermometers for measuring air temperature.

Blood loss and transfusion

During surgery, blood loss is common, but it may be difficult to measure accurately because blood may soak into surgical drapes and swabs, find its way into suction bottles or fall onto the floor. Although it is usually impossible to measure the blood loss accurately, an attempt should be made to estimate blood loss in all cases. This is particularly important in paediatric cases, where, for example, in a 2 kg child, a blood loss of more than 20 ml equates to a major haemorrhage.

Red cell loss

Red cell loss may be estimated by weighing the swabs after use but is notoriously inaccurate. Measuring the haemoglobin concentration of a known volume of solution after all the swabs have been washed in it provides a more accurate result, but usually too late to be of immediate clinical use. Regular estimation of blood haemoglobin concentration is the only reliable method of determining the effect of blood loss.

Blood clotting

Clotting efficacy is assessed by measuring the platelet count, prothrombin time (intrinsic system), activated partial thromboplastin time (extrinsic system) and fibrinogen concentration. In addition to laboratory-based tests, several near-patient tests of coagulation are available. These are described in Chapter 14.

Near-patient testing

During long operations, or when there is a need for infusion of large volumes of fluid, it may be necessary to measure physiological variables such as pH, haemoglobin and electrolyte concentrations. Traditionally this necessitated samples being sent to a laboratory, but increasingly a variety of devices are used for near-patient analysis.

These usually comprise a small disposable cartridge containing a combination of reagents and often some electronic circuitry. A sample is placed in the cartridge, which is then inserted into a larger analyser. Serum glucose concentration may be measured by a reagent strip, which is compared with a colour chart or by insertion into a reader. These machines provide rapid results at the bedside and avoid the delays of transporting samples to the laboratory. However, the accuracy of the results produced by such devices is usually dependent on the skill of the operator, and results may be affected by poor storage of the reagent or monitor. They also usually lack the organised quality control checks used in laboratories. Results are therefore less reliable and should be confirmed by laboratory analysis where possible.

Monitoring standards

The presence of an appropriately trained and experienced anaesthetist is the most essential patient monitor. However, human error is inevitable, and there is substantial evidence that many incidents are attributable, at least in part, to error by anaesthetists.

Appropriate monitoring will not prevent all adverse incidents in the perioperative period. However, there is substantial evidence that it reduces the amount of harm to patients, not only by detecting problems as they occur but also by alerting the anaesthetist that an error has occurred. In one study the introduction of modern standards of monitoring halved the number of cardiac arrests, principally because of the reduction in arrests caused by preventable respiratory causes. In the Australian Incident Monitoring Study, 52% of incidents were detected first by a monitor, and in more than half of these cases it was the pulse oximeter or capnograph which detected the problem.

There has never been a study comparing outcomes from anaesthesia with and without monitoring, and now such a study would be unethical.

The current recommendations from the Association of Anaesthetists are shown in Box 17.9. However, not only should monitors be available, but they must also be operational, maintained and serviced correctly and staff trained in their use.

All anaesthetists must ensure that they are familiar with the equipment used in their hospital and that all equipment has been checked before use. The need for training and practice cannot be overemphasised because the increasing complexity of modern monitoring devices implies that they can behave in unexpected ways at inopportune moments.

Alarms

All electronic monitors now include alarms which sound (and illuminate) when variables are outside a preset range.

Manufacturers usually set default limits (often password protected), but temporary limits may be set by the user. Failure to reset alarm limits to appropriate values between cases is a common cause of false alarms. This may result in the anaesthetist cancelling a series of false alarms, risking a genuine alarm being inadvertently cancelled without proper acknowledgement.

Alarms alert the anaesthetist to a developing physiological change and allow it to be corrected. However, alarms may not respond to a serious problem. For example, marked hypotension in an elderly hypertensive patient may still fall within the range of a normal arterial pressure as set for the monitor. Alarms must therefore be set to appropriate levels before induction, ensuring alarms trigger for only genuine abnormalities. For example, adult alarm limits for paediatric cases would be hazardous.

Alarms are often triggered by artefacts; for example, electrical interference during diathermy often triggers ECG arrhythmia alarms. Alarms may cause unnecessary distractions when triggered for spurious reasons such as an apnoea alarm during intubation. Such alarm signals are not useful and are either recurrently ignored or given inappropriate attention.

Further, the distracting cacophony of alarms during a genuine crisis may result in the cause of the crisis being overlooked. For example, alerts to a patient's bradycardia may mask the fact that the breathing circuit had become disconnected.

Oxygen supply

The use of an oxygen analyser with an audible alarm is mandatory for all patients breathing anaesthetic gases. The sampling port must be placed such that the gas mixture delivered to the patient is monitored continuously. The analyser should provide a clearly visible readout of the concentration of oxygen in the inspired gas and sound an audible alarm if a hypoxic mixture is delivered.

Breathing systems

The principal problems are of disconnection, leak or excessive pressure. During spontaneous ventilation, the movement of a reservoir bag confirms continuing ventilation. However, a capnograph ensures that ventilation is adequate. When positive pressure ventilation is used, a measure of airway pressure and appropriate alarms are also required.

Monitors cannot detect every abnormality. For example, a capnograph attached to an airway filter in a spontaneously breathing patient will not detect disconnection of the breathing circuit. Because the patient continues to breathe room air through the filter, the capnograph trace would remain unchanged and so no alarm would be triggered.

Vapour analyser

A vapour analyser is essential whenever anaesthetic vapours are used, both to prevent accidental overdose and to prevent awareness. However, many commonly used vaporisers are not able to detect when they are empty (the TEC 6 desflurane vaporiser is one exception). A procedure may commence with an empty vaporiser, or the vaporiser may empty during a long procedure; agent monitoring mitigates this problem.

Cardiovascular

Non-invasive arterial pressure and ECG are always required as monitors of the cardiovascular system. Although these provide useful information, clinical measures such as capillary refill and urine output remain important monitors. The ECG is probably the least useful of all the routinely used monitors.

Infusion devices

Increasingly, anaesthetic drugs are being delivered by infusion devices of varying complexity. Even simple fixed-rate infusion pumps now contain occlusion (pressure) and end-of-infusion alarms.

Many infusion pumps now contain preset and/or user-defined programmes (algorithms). At their simplest these presets are designed to reduce user error by limiting doses, prompting correct drug concentrations and so on. Anaesthetists and other professionals need to be trained in their use and must understand how these devices work before using them. Serious harm continues to occur as a result of failure to program devices correctly and failure to complete the feedback control loop (e.g. blood glucose monitoring, depth of anaesthesia). Importantly, although many infusion devices display information about drug dosing and/or plasma concentration, these depend on assumptions about the patient and the absence of leaks. A serious problem is disconnection of the infusion line under surgical drapes. Factors such as size of fluid compartments or rate of drug transport may also differ from those assumed by the pump, particularly in acutely unwell patients (see also Chapter 1).

General guidelines for monitoring during anaesthesia

Box 17.10 summarises the required monitors for different components of anaesthesia. Monitors should be applied to the awake patient and readings taken to ensure that they are functioning correctly before induction of anaesthesia. If uncooperative patients make application of monitoring impossible before induction, the monitors should be applied as soon as possible after induction and the reason recorded on the anaesthetic chart.

For short procedures such as electroconvulsive therapy (ECT) or orthopaedic manipulations, the standards for induction of anaesthesia are appropriate. However, if the procedure is prolonged then the standards for maintenance of anaesthesia should be applied. A high standard of monitoring should be applied continuously until the patient has recovered fully from anaesthesia. If the recovery room is not immediately adjacent to the operating theatre or if the patient's condition is poor, equipment should be available so that these standards are applied during transfer of the patient.

Additional monitoring

The standards in Box 17.10 are the minimum acceptable levels and apply to healthy patients undergoing minor surgery. If the patient is unwell before surgery or major surgery is planned, additional monitoring should be applied. It is difficult to give strict guidelines on what conditions or

---

Box 17.10 Essential monitoring

Presence of the anaesthetist throughout anaesthesia

A. Induction and maintenance of anaesthesia

Pulse oximeter
Non-invasive blood pressure monitoring
Inspired and expired oxygen, carbon dioxide, nitrous oxide and vapour
Airway pressure
A nerve stimulator whenever a muscle relaxant is used
Temperature (pre-op) and for any procedure >30 min anaesthesia duration

B. Recovery from anaesthesia

Pulse oximeter
Non-invasive blood pressure monitor
Electrocardiograph
Capnograph if the patient has a tracheal tube or supraglottic airway device *in situ*, or is deeply sedated
Temperature

C. Additional monitoring

Some patients will require additional monitoring: e.g. intravascular pressures, cardiac output (see Box 17.11). Depth of anaesthesia monitors recommended when patients are anaesthetised with total intravenous techniques.

D. Regional techniques & sedation for operative procedures

Pulse oximeter
Non-invasive blood pressure monitoring
Electrocardiograph
End-tidal carbon dioxide monitor if the patient is sedated

Pre-op, Preoperative.
(Modified from the Association of Anaesthetists (2015).)

surgery should prompt the use of each monitor. Suggestions are given in Box 17.11.

Monitoring during transfer

It is essential that the standard of care and monitoring during transfer is as high as that applied in the operating theatre and that staff with appropriate training and experience accompany the patient.

During transfer, vibrations may make devices which rely on pressure change, such as non-invasive arterial pressure monitors, inaccurate or non-functional. Vibration may also cause connections to work loose and equipment may suffer physical damage. Movement may make an ECG trace useless for diagnosis of arrhythmias. Noise and poor lighting make the displays of many monitors difficult to read and make audible alarms inaudible. Adequate supplies must be taken for the entire journey, together with additional supplies to anticipate any unforeseen delays. This includes oxygen cylinders, batteries (the internal batteries of a monitor may have short lives) and anaesthetic drugs.

Before transfer, the patient should be in a stable physiological state. The patient should be moved onto the transport trolley and all transport monitors applied to the patient and their functions checked. All equipment should then be fastened securely and all catheters and leads taped into position. A check should be made that, from a single position, the anaesthetist is able to attend to the airway,

see all the monitors and be able to administer drugs and fluids. The process is made much easier and safer with a dedicated transport trolley so that all the equipment is fixed permanently in place. Patient transfer is discussed further in Chapter 48.

Anaesthetic recordkeeping

It is the professional responsibility of every doctor to maintain accurate records of the treatment patients receive and their response to it. The anaesthetic record forms a part of a patient's medical record. The purpose of the anaesthetic chart is to detail the anaesthetic technique, physiological changes associated with anaesthesia and surgery and any complications or problems encountered during the procedure. This information may assist other doctors if complications ensue or if anaesthesia is required in the future. Furthermore, the anaesthetic record may be a valuable source of information if any complication results in litigation; the absence of a full record makes it difficult for an anaesthetist to demonstrate, for example, that postoperative renal failure was not attributable to untreated intraoperative hypotension.

The design of anaesthetic records varies widely, but all should facilitate recording and display of all relevant data. Suggestions for the content of an anaesthetic record are shown in Box 17.12.

In addition to the data described here, the record should include details of discussions with the patient, together with any risks or benefits outlined and the management plan agreed. If the patient has any specific requests or concerns, such as a desire to avoid blood transfusion, they should also be recorded.

Automated records

Estimates are that 20% of the anaesthetist's time is taken up with documentation. Although the anaesthetic record is usually completed as the anaesthetic proceeds, there are times, such as during induction or a crisis, when it is not possible to complete the chart contemporaneously. This delay leads to inaccuracies. In addition, studies have found that anaesthetists tend to record normalised data – that is, the record tends to minimise any physiological changes which occur.

Most modern anaesthetic monitors and machines may be connected to automatic data-recording systems. These log all the monitoring data and should enable the anaesthetist to add information such as drugs used and comments on events such as the start of surgery. The data may be stored electronically for later study and printed out in a variety of

Box 17.12 **Suggested data for inclusion on anaesthetic records**

Relevant patient- and surgery-specific additional information should be included (see especially Chapters 19, 20, 30 and 44).

Many of these data will be available on other records. Duplication is discouraged, but anaesthetists must ensure relevant information is to hand when needed.

There is no single perfect anaesthesia record, and local custom and practice will dictate what information is recorded where.

General   Standards for all documentation
- Legible
- Patient identifiers (name, date of birth, unique ID)
- Name of person completing documentation
- Date, time and place

Planned surgery and date
Urgency of surgery (see Chapter 44)
- Scheduled – listed on a routine list
- Urgent – resuscitated, not on a routine list
- Emergency – not fully resuscitated
A more nuanced approach is taken in many centres reflecting the degree of urgency of urgent and emergency cases.

Preoperative   Relevant medical history
Cardiorespiratory fitness
Relevant anaesthetic history
- Personal
- Familial

Drug use
- Alcohol
- Smoking
- Herbal remedies

Current and recent medication, including hormonal contraceptives
- Time/date of last dose when appropriate
  - For example, anticoagulants, steroids, paracetamol

Drug and other allergies or intolerances
- Nature of reaction should be recorded

Airway assessment including dentition
Aspiration risk
- Reflux
- Delayed gastric emptying/full stomach

Baseline physiology
- Weight
- Height
- Blood pressure (primary care values are preferred)

Investigations
Estimation of 30-day mortality in high-risk patients
Discussion with patient (±family/friends)
- Procedures
- General risks
- Specific risks
- Benefits and alternatives
- Specific instructions
  - Medication to take/omit
  - Starvation

Outstanding issues
- Referrals
- Investigations
- Critical care bed availability

Anaesthetic plan

Induction   Time and place
All anaesthetists and role
Preinduction checks
- Anaesthesia machine, breathing circuit
- WHO

Vascular access used and placed
Monitoring
Drugs used
Airway management
- Ease or difficulty of:
  - Mask ventilation
  - Supraglottic airways
  - Laryngoscopy and intubation
- Airway devices used
- Mode (settings) of ventilation
- Throat pack – insertion *and* removal

Regional anaesthesia
- Sterile precautions
- Verification of correct site
- Patient state (awake/GA/sedation)
- Type/site of block(s)
- Equipment used
  - Needles
  - Ultrasound
  - Nerve stimulators
- Indicators of uneventful insertion
  - For example, negative aspiration
  - Absence of pain/paraesthesia
- Drug(s) administered
- Clinical efficacy

Complications and incidents

Continued

Box 17.12 **Suggested data for inclusion on anaesthetic records—cont'd**

Maintenance	Operation(s) performed
	Continuous record of physiological
	monitoring (at least every 5 min)
	• Pulse
	• Blood pressure
	• SpO_2
	• Gas monitoring
	  • FIO_2
	  • $PE'CO_2$
	  • End-tidal anaesthetic agent(s)
	• Depth of anaesthesia if used
	Temperature and warming devices used
	Monitoring used
	Drugs administered
	• Dose
	• Time
	• Route
			Fluids administered
			• Volume
			• Time
			Blood loss/urine output
			Positioning and protection
			• Limb positions
			• Eye/skin/pressure points
			• VTE precautions used
			Complications and incidents

		Postoperative	Formal handover Analgesia/antiemetics Intravenous fluids Planned discharge destination Other investigations/actions/reviews required • Blood sugar/gases/haemoglobin • Chest radiograph • Critical care review Reviews undertaken and further actions required

GA, General anaesthesia; *VTE*, venous thromboembolism

formats. They have the potential to interact with other sources of information so that patient details, laboratory results, scans and outpatient letters can all be accessed. These systems have the potential to make audits and quality control much easier to perform. The Association of Anaesthetists recommends that departments consider their procurement.

However, these systems are expensive and all monitors have numerous sources of error; although most anaesthetists tend to ignore erroneous readings, they are recorded and printed by an automated system. Printouts should therefore be checked and errors marked before being included in the patient's medical record.

References/Further reading

Al-Shaikh, B., Stacey, S., 2018. Essentials of equipment in anaesthesia, critical care and perioperative medicine, fifth ed. Elsevier.

Association of Anaesthetists, 2015. Recommendations for standards of monitoring during anaesthesia and recovery. https://www.aagbi.org/sites/default/files/Standards_of_monitoring_2015_0.pdf.

Davis, P.D., Kenny, G., 2001. Basic physics and measurement in anaesthesia, fifth ed. Butterworth-Heinemann, Oxford.

NAP5, Accidental Awareness during General Anaesthesia in the United Kingdom and Ireland. https://www.nationalauditprojects.org.uk/NAP5report?newsid=1187.

National Institute for Health and Care Excellence Guidance, 2012. Depth of anaesthesia monitors – Bispectral Index (BIS), E-Entropy and Narcotrend-Compact M. https://www.nice.org.uk/guidance/dg6.

Pinsky, M., Teboul, J.L., Vincent, J.L., 2019. European society of intensive care medicine. Hemodynamic monitoring. Springer International.

Sykes, M.K., et al., 1991. Principles of measurement and monitoring in anaesthesia and intensive care. 3rd ed. Oxford, Blackwell Scientific.

Section | 3 |

Fundamentals of anaesthesia & perioperative medicine

Chapter | **18** |

Quality and safety in anaesthesia

Iain Moppett

Quality in healthcare is hard to define. One approach is based around six goals: safety; effectiveness; patient focus; timeliness; efficiency; and equity (Table 18.1). Although errors and incidents are commonly discussed in relation to safety, the same fundamental principles apply to all aspects of healthcare quality.

Culture of quality and safety

Understanding generation of errors: systems approach

The cause of preventable deaths in healthcare systems is not usually incompetent or careless people but bad systems (Box 18.1). A safety incident should be seen in an organisational framework of latent failures – the conditions that produce error and violation – and active failures. Some active failures (such as simple mistakes, slips or lapses) have only a local context and can be explained by factors related to individual performance and/or the task at hand. Major incidents usually evolve over time and involve many factors.

Organisational factors create latent failures, which result from management decisions, organisational strategy and/or planning. Latent failures then permeate through departmental pathways to the workplace, creating conditions that allow violations and commission of errors. The errors generated in the workplace environment may be prevented by a front-end clinician (near-miss). This concept of the trajectory of error is often referred to using Reason's Swiss cheese model. There are multiple layers of defence, each containing holes: organisational, supervisory, preconditions (such as an unfamiliar team, IT failures) and specific acts (slips, lapses; see Box 18.1). When these holes line up, a hazard can lead to a failure (incident).

To facilitate a quality and safety culture, several aspects are required:
- Healthcare organisations must accept that system failure has a major role in all errors and accidents.
- Openness and transparency must be reflected in organisational policies and procedures.
- The organisation's response to an incident must be just and usually non-punitive for the individual involved.
- Mechanisms are needed that promote learning and feed this in a sustainable way into practice.

Safety behaviour and non-technical skills

In clinical practice, some personal attributes of healthcare workers naturally render them safer than other colleagues.
- *Conscientiousness*. Being sensible and meticulous, checking the information/drugs/equipment themselves, ensuring that the job is done properly and being thorough.
- *Honesty*. Accepting limitations, giving correct and complete information, accepting their own mistakes, compliance with procedures and protocols.
- *Humility*. Thanking colleagues of any grade and profession for their help and contribution, taking and seeking advice from other members of the team.
- *Self-awareness*. Knowing limitations, knowing when they are tired or preoccupied.
- *Confidence*. Knowing capabilities and being confident about them, able to speak up if necessary.

Non-technical skills are defined as 'the cognitive, social and personal resource skills that complement technical skills and contribute to safe and efficient task performance'. They are not new or mysterious skills but are essentially what the best practitioners do to achieve consistently high performance and what the rest of us do on a good day.

Table 18.1 Aims of a high-quality healthcare system

1. Safe	Prevention of injuries to patients from the care that is intended to help them.
2. Effective	Provision of services based on scientific knowledge to all who could benefit, and refraining from providing services to those not likely to benefit.
3. Patient-centred	Providing care that is respectful of and responsive to individual patient preferences, needs and values, and ensuring that patient values guide all clinical decisions.
4. Timely	Reducing waits and sometimes harmful delays for both those who receive care and those who give it.
5. Efficient	Avoiding waste, including waste of equipment, supplies, ideas and energy.
6. Equitable	Providing care that does not vary in quality because of personal characteristics such as gender, ethnicity, geographic location and socioeconomic status.

Box 18.1 **Taxonomy of error**

LATENT FAILURES are factors that exist within an organisation or process and which increase the risk of another error causing an incident. They are separated in time and often in place from the occurrence of the incident. Reason described these as organisational influences, unsafe supervision and preconditions for unsafe acts.

Organisational influences may include aspects such as training budgets and curricula and organisational safety culture.

Unsafe supervision might be reflected by a trainee anaesthetising a complex case near the limits of their competence without adequate consultant supervision.

Preconditions for unsafe acts include lack of robust checking procedures, near-identical drug ampoules and inadequate rest breaks for staff.

Active errors are unsafe acts which cause (or could cause) an incident. They may be errors of commission (doing the wrong thing) or omission (not doing the right thing). Various categories of active error are often described.

Execution failures occur when the knowledge and the intent are appropriate, but for a variety of reasons the correct actions do not ensue. These are often referred to as slips (observable actions, related to attention) and lapses (internal events, related to memory failures). They may be failures of *recognition, attention, memory* and *selection*. These are exemplified by drug errors in anaesthesia: every anaesthetist will be able to recall events where each of these failures has happened in their own practice.

Mistakes mean that the action proceeds as intended, but the wrong course has been chosen. These may be:

Rule based: Prior knowledge, intuition or a protocol is available for this situation (e.g. failed tracheal intubation) but is wrongly applied. This may be by omission, too late or by applying the wrong rule.

Knowledge based: An unfamiliar or novel situation requires the calculation of a solution based on the (usually incomplete) evidence. These require thought and are particularly prone to confirmation bias – evidence which supports the current model is sought, and contrary evidence is ignored.

Violations: These are deliberate choices to deviate from agreed practice (formal standing operating procedures (SOPs) or informal custom and practice). Again, these can be subdivided:

Routine violations: Corners are routinely cut. This may be at an individual or departmental level. 'Normalisation of deviance' may occur, where unacceptable practice becomes accepted practice over time. The risk is that practice becomes further and further away from good practice gradually, such that it is not noticed or dealt with until too late.

Self-serving violations: Breaking the rules for personal gratification.

Situational violations: Breaking the rules because (correctly) the situation demands it. There will always be circumstances when rules and procedures do not fit. A safety-conscious organisation seeks to learn from these incidents.

The underlying premises are that:

- the operating theatre is a complex environment with complicated tasks;
- many people come together to work in this environment;
- there is heightened potential for accidents and disasters in operating theatres; and
- every human has limitations.

These non-technical skills are learned and can be taught. In particular, for the operating theatre environment, the following skills are important:

- Communication, sharing of information
- Teamwork
- Situational awareness
- Anticipation and preparedness
- Decision-making

Communication and teamwork

The ideal scenario would be when all members of the team know each other, have mutual trust, are able to discuss problems and issues openly, learn from each other, are well-led and work together for a common goal. In practice this ideal is difficult to accomplish. Therefore organisations must actively explore and implement tools and training programmes that allow employees to enhance their level of communication and teamworking. Pre-list briefings are an important component of this process. They are tools to foster good communication, planning and learning for the whole operating theatre team. Debriefings are a complement to the briefing process. Good practice is reinforced, and areas of improvement are discussed constructively. Information from debriefings should be shared with other team members, and necessary actions should be completed and fed back to the team.

Situational awareness

Situational awareness refers to the ability to appraise the overall picture, to acquire relevant information quickly by scanning the whole environment and to monitor the environment continuously, in particular for any change. This term implies a broader understanding of what is going on and how events may unfold, more than just paying attention to the task. The core elements of situational awareness include:

- continuous information gathering;
- anticipation of events which may unfold; and
- processing current information to interpret the situation in view of anticipated events.

Under stress, individuals tend to develop task fixation and lose an overall perspective of the situation. Patients continue to be harmed because anaesthetists fixate on tracheal intubation at the expense of maintaining oxygenation (see Chapter 27).

Anticipation and preparedness

Anticipation is the key component of full situational awareness. It involves thinking ahead about all reasonably predictable hazards, such as 'What if there is severe bleeding?', 'What if I am unable to see the larynx?', 'What if the blood pressure drops on tourniquet release?', 'What if there is a power failure?' Having considered what can go wrong, it is useful to mentally try responses and then work out whether these responses would address the problem. These mental exercises allow the clinician to adjust or prepare the environment. The aim is to avoid the hazards and/or prepare to deal with the hazards if they were to arise in a calm, systematic manner.

Decision-making

Decisions are taken based on previous experience, knowledge, intuition and good prevailing sense at the time. Decision-making for an individual in a condition of uncertainty can be very challenging. However, the process of decision-making can be evolved and evaluated using crisis management scenarios in a simulated environment. Here there are no clinical consequences, and the evaluation can be non-threatening. Examples of training in such scenarios include rapid-sequence induction, failed tracheal intubation, unexpected severe hypotension, cardiac arrest, malignant hyperthermia and anaphylaxis. All anaesthesia departments should have working protocols to deal with crisis situations to help clinicians make logical, systematic decisions under stressful conditions (see Chapter 27). The scenarios should be practised regularly in teams, and the experience of training should be enhanced by debriefing on teamwork and individual decisions. Existing protocols will never cover all possible eventualities. Therefore decisions will still need to be made on individual choices and judgements. A culture of openness within the department should allow healthy discussion of decisions if alternative options are possible; the value of collective decision-making should be emphasised.

Measuring safety and quality

Safety culture

Safety culture is 'the product of individual and group values, attitudes, competencies and patterns of behaviour that determine the commitment to, and the style and proficiency of, an organisation's health and safety programmes'. One can also think in terms of culture being 'what happens when no-one is watching?' A positive safety culture in an organisation is characterised by its individual members respecting and trusting each other, perceiving safety to be important and having confidence that the safety interventions would be effective. *Safety climate* refers to 'surface features of safety culture from attitudes and perceptions of individuals at a given point in time', or 'measurable components of safety culture'. The two terms, *safety culture* and *safety climate,* can be differentiated by comparing the culture to an individual's personality, and climate to his or her mood.

The most common method of measuring safety culture and climate in healthcare involves using quantitative questionnaires and qualitative methods including observations, semistructured interviews and focus groups. Safety culture can be described in terms of five different levels of maturity:

1. *Pathological.* 'Who cares so long as we are not caught?'
2. *Reactive.* 'We do a lot of "safety" whenever we have an accident'.
3. *Calculative.* 'We have systems in place to manage all hazards'.
4. *Proactive.* 'We anticipate problems before they arise'.
5. *Generative.* 'Safety is how we do business around here'.

Measuring quality

A comprehensive measurement of quality would assess, and somehow measure, all the individual components of the quality matrix, such as safety, clinical effectiveness, patient experience, timeliness, efficiency and equity. Avedis Donabedian introduced a framework for assessing quality in healthcare (Table 18.2). This framework is based on three core domains – structure, processes and outcomes. These domains of measuring quality are interdependent. Good processes depend upon good structures, and they often lead to good outcomes. Consequently, assessment of only one domain (e.g. outcome – mortality) cannot assess quality or serve to improve it. It becomes useful only when this assessment is combined with finding the gaps in structure (e.g. staff shortage) or processes (e.g. non-adherence to guidelines).

Clinical outcomes: real or surrogate

In anaesthesia there is a lot of reliance on real clinical outcomes to indicate quality of care, such as incidences of epidural haematoma, nerve damage, brain damage or death. Although apparently straightforward, the use of real outcomes has limitations:

- The real outcomes may depend on many factors, including the patient's pre-existing condition, population dynamics, surgical factors and individual reactions (e.g. unknown allergies), which may not necessarily indicate quality of care *per se.*
- Direct anaesthesia-related mortality is rare and serious morbidity infrequent. Consequently, measuring anaesthesia-related mortality and morbidity are very crude measures and may not provide enough data to monitor quality on a frequent basis.

Table 18.2 Donabedian's framework for measuring quality

Domain	Description
Structure	*Setup for providing care,* including: Material resources Facilities Human resources Technology infrastructure Equipment Guidelines and implementation programmes Teaching programmes Rotas
Process	*What happens around delivery of care,* including: Patient pathway from evaluation through diagnosis to treatment Assessment before anaesthesia Optimisation of comorbidities Adherence to guidelines and teaching programmes Checklists Monitoring Incident reporting and actions Ongoing audits of different aspects of care delivery Quality improvement programmes
Outcome	*The effects of care,* including: Morbidity Mortality Patient satisfaction Other clinical outcomes as decided by the department

Adverse events and near misses are often taken as surrogate clinical outcomes. By monitoring the surrogates, a comprehensive picture can be obtained of the workflow and processes. Overall, more than 100 outcome measures have been described, so departments and individuals will make their own choices about what to measure.

Selecting a good quality indicator

No single indicator is sufficient as a quality measure in anaesthesia. Recording only major morbidity and mortality has limitations. Surrogate measures give a better picture of workflow and processes and potential problems, but they do not replace real outcomes. Characteristics of a good indicator include the following:

- Easy to define and record
- Finite frequency of occurrence so that it can be monitored regularly

• Rate of occurrence must be influenced by quality and also must indicate something important about the process

Quality improvement tools

Requirements for quality improvement

In addition to collecting all the data at an individual patient level, the challenge for a department is to analyse the data systematically, disseminate the findings as widely as possible and identify learning outcomes and areas for improvement. To improve quality, departments must develop interventions targeted at areas for improvement, implement them, and monitor progress and the impact of implementation on outcomes. Embedding a culture of incident reporting and learning is vital. Morbidity and mortality meetings and other network opportunities at which all quality issues can be aired and discussed without fear of a punitive outcome are absolutely essential for embedding quality consciousness. Barriers, facilitators and approaches in engaging staff into quality improvement are summarised in Table 18.3.

Checklists

Although they existed earlier, the modern era of the safety checklist is generally attributed to the crash of the newly designed Model 299 Boeing bomber in 1935. The cause of the crash was straightforward – the elevator lock had been left on. However, two extremely important facts emerged from the investigation. First, the pilot was extremely experienced and competent. Second, taking the elevator lock off was not an unusual requirement. The pilot would do this normally, but on this occasion, presumably because of distraction by other things, he forgot. The response of pilots was to create a process which ensured that simple things did not get missed, regardless of the situation.

The introduction of the WHO checklist as a strongly encouraged or mandated part of theatre practice has refocussed attention on the potential benefits and risks of checklists in healthcare, and particularly perioperative care. Checklists are not new in anaesthesia; various national bodies produced anaesthetic machine checklists in the 1980s and 1990s. This was in response to the emerging data that demonstrated a significant number of patient safety incidents could have been avoided by proper checking of equipment.

The term *checklist* is used for documents which may have a variety of purposes. Conceptually they can be thought of as:

• cognitive aids for crisis situations;
• checking;
• briefing; and
• planning.

Most checklists are tabulations or summaries of accepted best practice. We would hope that anaesthetists would recognise the need to undertake these actions regardless of

Table 18.3 Barriers, facilitators and approaches to engage staff in quality improvement

Barriers	Top-heavy approach Lack of involvement at the beginning Punitive actions Lack of evidence Lack of assurance Lack of control
Facilitators	Role models Peer pressure Evidence Common sense Good outcomes Enhancement of professional position Rewards
Approaches	**Science approach** Safety research Research into causes of errors Research into prevention of errors Research into systems **Educational approach** Curriculum Training Courses Cross-learning modules Faculty **Management approach** Vision Strategy Organisational change Risk management Implementation Professional leadership Networking

whether a checklist exists. Their role is, therefore, about **ensuring** that these actions take place for **every** patient, **every** time. The human memory is fallible and, regardless of professional status, cannot be **relied** upon to remember more than about seven items.

Anaesthetists are not particularly good at completing all the necessary checks. This applies to the anaesthesia machine, drug checking and WHO checklist. The reasons for this are multifactorial and relate to all aspects of safety and quality discussed in this chapter. Specific barriers to full engagement with checklist processes include the following:

• *Perceived importance.* The rate of incidents related to the items on the checklists is very low and therefore the overwhelming likelihood is that there will be nothing amiss. The anaesthetist may, therefore, choose (consciously or subconsciously) to prioritise another activity.

- *Organisational culture.* Perceptions of organisational prioritisation of efficiency over safety may encourage an individual to save time by shortening or omitting checklists. Conversely, an organisation that fails to monitor compliance with checklists or hold individuals to account when appropriate sends a message that it does not value them either.
- *Resistance to standardisation.* Anaesthetists are highly trained individuals with a large amount of professional autonomy. Checklists, by definition, standardise and consequently restrict practice and may therefore be resisted. This may manifest itself in academic arguments about the validity of evidence in favour of specific checklists.
- *Professional behaviour and stereotypes.* As a result of the three previous aspects, senior medical staff may view the checklist process as beneath them and something to be delegated to more junior staff. This may in turn promote a culture of non-importance.
- *Checklist design.* Undoubtedly some checklists are badly worded and designed. There may be too many questions, questions asked at the wrong time in the process or questions that encourage yes/no answers without true engagement.

The evolution of the Association of Anaesthetists' anaesthetic machine checklist demonstrates improvements in layout and wording to encourage full compliance.

- *Human fallibility.* However well designed the checklist process, humans make mistakes. Most commonly reported are automatic responses – answering yes when the checks have not actually been done and performing checklists by rote.

Well-designed cognitive aids assist performance in crisis periods, especially when they have been used in training or drill rehearsal. Anaesthetists are strongly encouraged to use them (see Chapter 27).

WHO checklist

The WHO checklist is a hybrid checklist. It involves elements of planning, briefing and checking (Table 18.4).

There are three phases to the checklist:

1. Sign-in: Is it safe to start anaesthesia?
2. Time-out: Is it safe to start surgery?
3. Sign-out: Has surgery been completed safely? Is it safe to hand over to the next phase of care?

Table 18.4 Examples of different purposes of checklists

Checklist	Purpose	Example	Notes
Anaesthesia machine	Checking	Check that the anaesthetic apparatus is connected to a supply of oxygen and that an adequate reserve supply of oxygen is available from a spare cylinder.	Printed cards attached to machine Long-list
Advanced life support (4 Hs and 4 Ts)	Checking	Potential causes or aggravating factors for which specific treatment exists must be sought during any cardiac arrest. For ease of memory, these are divided into two groups of four, based upon their initial letter, either H or T (see Chapter 28).	Memorisation encouraged Time-critical
WHO Checklist	Multiple/hybrid		No explicit differentiation between checking, briefing and planning
WHO Checklist	Checking	Is the anaesthesia machine and medication check complete? (Sign-in) Have the specimens been labelled (including patient name)? (Sign-out)	Refers to another process/SOP
WHO Checklist	Briefing	Are there any critical or unexpected steps you want the team to know about? (Time-out)	A 'stop–go' moment, but mainly a confirmation of adequate staff briefing
WHO Checklist	Planning	Are there any specific equipment requirements or special investigations? (Time-out)	Really a planning question May be too late to solve the problem

SOP, Standard operating procedure.

Local adaptation is encouraged, both to match local circumstances and to ensure the appropriate questions are asked. For instance, cataract surgery under local anaesthesia is ill-served by questions related to airway management but may have specific issues around preoperative biometry. There are other surgical checklists, notably the SURPASS system pioneered in the Netherlands. The basic principles are the same.

There is reasonable evidence that implementation of the WHO checklist is associated with improvement in outcomes after surgery. The degree of compliance with perioperative checklists appears to be associated with both intraoperative teamwork and postoperative outcomes. In other words, doing it well is as important as doing it at all. As with all checklists, lack of engagement, overfamiliarity and tick-boxing are significant risks from its continued use. Efficacy of the WHO checklist is enhanced by processes such as briefings and debriefings, which promote wider team communication and allow problems to be identified and addressed without the pressure of having a patient present.

Designing problems out of the system

Human error is inevitable. A key approach to minimising error is therefore to limit the possibility for human error. The example of drug errors in anaesthesia is discussed in Box 18.2.

Safety by design

The anaesthetic machine is a device designed to deliver a safe mixture of gases to a patient. Over the years, almost every method of failing to do this has happened, often with tragic consequences. It is now difficult to deliver hypoxic mixtures regardless of human interaction. Specific design features include non-interchangeable screw threads and valves on gas supplies, hypoxic guards and linkages on flowmeters, and standardised connections for breathing systems. The same approach can be taken with presetting of infusion protocols for intravenous and epidural infusions.

Organisational design

There are theoretical safety (and financial) advantages to limiting the variation in drugs and equipment available to anaesthetists. There is often scant evidence to suggest that one drug or device is better than another, but by limiting choices, individuals are more likely to be familiar with what is available and possibly less likely to confuse one for another. This approach can be seen in the rationalisation of anaesthetic drug cupboards to have the same core drugs,

---

Box 18.2 Drug errors in anaesthesia

Drug errors in anaesthesia are common. They are estimated to occur in around 1 in 300 drug administrations.

Errors can be classified at each of the steps of safe drug management:
- Diagnosis
- Prescription
- Selection
- Preparation
- Labelling
- Syringe swaps
- Administration
- Dosage
- Documentation

Reason's taxonomy of human errors can be applied to each of these steps (see Box 18.1).

No single approach can eliminate these errors. Taking the Swiss cheese analogy, every barrier to error has its own holes.

Strategies to reduce drug errors include the following:
- Protocols and policies for prescription (e.g. antiemetics, analgesics, antibiotics)
- Limiting availability of drugs (e.g. neat potassium chloride is not kept in a routine anaesthetic cupboard)
- Facilitating rapid access to drugs required in high-workload periods (e.g. resuscitation drugs, sugammadex) using 'grab boxes', preprepared syringes etc.
- Clear labelling
- Colour coding to facilitate initial drug class selection
- Deliberate drug separation within drug cupboards and the workspace (e.g. keeping local anaesthetics separate) (Fig. 18.1)
- Bar-coding and automated readout technology
- Formal reading out loud of drug labels (alone or with an independent member of the team)
- Formal training and assessment of safe drug preparation/administration practices
- Adoption of sterile cockpit principles such that drug preparation is treated as a mission-critical activity that should not be disturbed by non-essential conversation

---

laid out in the same way. 'Dangerous' drugs that are used rarely but with potentially catastrophic consequences (e.g. neat potassium chloride) are kept out of standard anaesthetic drug cupboards.

Making it easy to do the right thing

Most individuals will choose the easiest option if there are no other considerations. If the system is designed to make

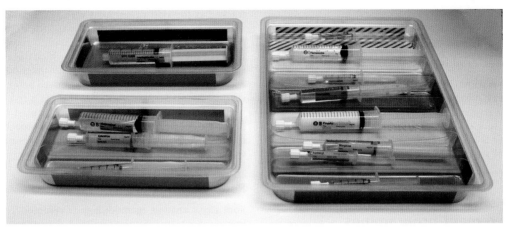

Fig. 18.1 Example of an anaesthesia drug tray system designed to aid correct drug selection through colour coding and separation of general, vasoactive and local anaesthetic drugs.

the correct option the easiest option, then safety should be enhanced. For instance, providing procedure packs with full sterile protective equipment and drapes is associated with better compliance with sterile precautions and reduction in central venous catheter–associated infections. No new equipment or policies are required, simply a redesign of the process.

Understanding workarounds

Even with these designs, individuals may deliberately circumvent the system. When this occurs, organisations and departments need to understand why this has happened. The answer will often reveal deficiencies in the current design and a lack of understanding of why processes are designed in the current way. Organisations with proactive and generative safety cultures will seek to address these rather than simply exhorting staff to follow policies and procedures.

Learning from incidents

To quote Sir Liam Donaldson, a past UK chief medical officer, 'To err is human, to cover up is unforgiveable, and to fail to learn is inexcusable'. There are several key components to learning from incidents and near misses.

Acknowledging and recording that they happen

Unfortunately there is still a common perception that responses to incidents may be punitive, which contributes to significant under-reporting. A cultural failure to recognise

the importance of incidents and near misses may result in some organisations simply not reporting incidents that have occurred. There are structural barriers to reporting in many organisations, with cumbersome paper or electronic systems.

Appropriate analysis of incidents

Large industrial companies have specific teams trained to collate, analyse and investigate incidents. Such an approach is relatively rare within healthcare. The anaesthetic profession has made significant progress in this area with prospective studies of rare events (such as the UK National Audit Projects investigating complications of neuraxial blocks, airway management, unintentional awareness and anaphylaxis); analysis of legal claims (US Closed Claims, NHS Litigation Authority database in the UK); and prospective studies of incidents (Australian Incident Monitoring Study). Many countries now have some form of national reporting system, although these are of course only as good as the data entered.

Analysis of individual incidents and aggregated data is a skill. This requires training to ensure that the correct interpretation of events is made and that any recommendations will reduce the risk of recurrence without introducing new risks.

Feedback to relevant staff

A common reason why staff choose not to fill in incident reports is that they feel nothing changes. Departments and organisations have to develop processes which allow staff

369

to receive meaningful feedback about incidents without being swamped by an overload of information.

Organisational memory

Most errors within healthcare have happened before. Sadly, healthcare has too often forgotten the lessons it learnt last time. This happens particularly when events are separated widely in time or geography. National professional organisations have a key role in ensuring that the lessons learnt previously are passed on to successive generations.

Models for implementing quality improvement programmes

Different models used in quality improvement programmes involve identifying an area for improvement, carefully defining an improvement and developing tools that can be used to measure improvement. A multidisciplinary team then considers and develops the interventions aimed at making these improvements; interventions are implemented and progress is monitored. If the intervention leads to improvements, it is then integrated into everyday practice. A clear understanding of the aims and a positive workplace quality culture are required for the success of any such programme, which requires an integrated approach at organisational, departmental and individual levels. Some of the models of quality improvement which are often used in healthcare settings are described below.

Plan-Do-Study-Act

The Institute of Healthcare Improvement has used the Plan-Do-Study-Act (PDSA) method widely for rapid cyclical improvements. At the beginning of the cycle, the nature of the problem is determined. The next stage is that of planning for a specific targeted change. The change is then implemented, and data and information are collected to study the impact. The last part of the cycle involves taking action by either implementing the change or starting the process again. The overall improvement may require many small and frequent PDSA cycles rather than one big and slow cycle. There are risks that locally developed solutions fail to consider wider organisational contexts and hence introduce new problems.

Lean production system

This system aims to minimise waste and improve efficiency by simplifying overcomplicated processes and avoiding duplications and rework. The frontline staff are involved throughout the process, and the problems are rigorously tracked as the staff experiment with potential improvements. The lean system is driven by the identification of customer (patient or staff) needs. With a focus on the needs of the customers, any activity which does not add value (waste) is then removed. Thus the value-added activities are maximised, waste is removed and efficiency savings are made. As with PDSA, there is a risk that the bigger picture may be lost. Problems caused by inappropriate partial application of lean approaches (e.g. reducing stock levels without considering resupply) are well reported.

Root cause analysis

Root cause analysis methodology is commonly used for improvements at organisational and departmental levels. The analysis is triggered by an adverse event. A retrospective systematic analysis is undertaken to tease out the underlying causal or contributory factors. The spirit of analysis is the belief that systems, rather than individual incompetence, are likely to be the root causes of most problems. With an overarching systems approach to understanding the problem in a non-punitive manner, a trained multidisciplinary team investigates the event to ask a series of questions: What happened? Why did it happen? What factors caused it? What contributed to it? What system improvements could prevent it? The team then makes recommendations for changes in system improvements. There are risks that root cause analysis focuses on a single cause when numerous interconnected contributing factors are present and that a simple (superficial) cause is identified without exploring the issues deeply enough.

Failure modes and effects analysis

The methodology and the underlying principles of failure modes and effects analysis are similar to root cause analysis. The difference is that failure modes and effects analysis is undertaken proactively. The processes and systems are observed and analysed for any potential failure by a multidisciplinary team. The team then evaluates a number of options which can mitigate potential failures and finally makes recommendations for systems improvements.

Safety II

The preceding models have all been predicated on examination of what goes wrong. However, despite all its challenges, healthcare is dominated by things going right. There is a move towards complementing the reactive (Safety I) approach with an approach that seeks to learn, systematically, from the everyday successes of individuals, teams and organisations (Safety II).

Infection prevention and control

Surgery in its current breadth and depth would be impossible without modern practices and methods to prevent, mitigate and treat infection. Hospital-associated infections affect approximately 6% of patients; most common are respiratory, urinary and surgical site infections. The incidence of surgical site infection varies by operative site, degree of contamination and the presence of foreign material (which encourages formation of antibiotic-resistant biofilms). Longer operations are associated with higher risk. Patient factors include age, comorbidities (notably diabetes, obesity and high ASA grade) and smoking.

The principles of infection management are deceptively simple – to reduce the opportunities for infective organisms to cause infection by:

- reducing microbial load (numbers);
- reducing transmission between people (healthcare staff, visitors and patients);
- reducing auto-infection;
- maintaining and enhancing natural defences (innate and acquired immunity); and
- appropriate use of antimicrobial agents.

Reducing transmission

Handwashing

The single most effective method to reduce hospital-associated infections is consistent, effective handwashing between patient contacts. The importance of handwashing was demonstrated in 1847 by Igor Semmelweis, who caused a 90% reduction in puerperal fever when handwashing was instituted (thereby reducing cross-contamination between the autopsy room and the maternity clinic). The lesson keeps having to be relearned. It matters less what the hands are washed with than that they are washed effectively. International guidance suggests the following:

- Use alcohol gel unless hands are visibly soiled as it is faster, more effective (if done properly) and better tolerated.
- Use soap and water if hands are visibly dirty, soiled with blood or other body fluids or after using the toilet.
- If outbreaks of spore-forming organisms (e.g. *Clostridium difficile*) are suspected or specific precautions are in place at patient (e.g. patients with vomiting or diarrhoeal illness) or ward level, then soap and water should be used as alcohol gels are ineffective against spores.

Effective handwashing requires attention to technique to ensure all areas are covered:

- Palm to palm
- Palm to dorsum (both hands)
- Palm to palm with fingers interlaced
- Backs of fingers to opposing palms
- Rotational rubbing of thumbs in clasped palm
- Rotational rubbing, backwards and forwards with clasped fingers of hand in palm
  The hands must be allowed to dry.

Gloves

Gloves must be worn for:

- invasive procedures;
- contact with sterile sites, non-intact skin or mucous membranes; and
- activities assessed as high risk of exposure to:
  - blood, body fluids;
  - secretions; or
  - sharp/contaminated instruments.

In practice this means almost all clinical contact by anaesthetists in the theatre suite. Gloves are **not** required for routine human contact such as shaking or holding hands or most physical examinations. Gloves are single-use items, and anaesthetists should resist the temptation to keep a single pair on for multiple episodes of care. Hands should be cleaned after removal.

Aprons

Disposable plastic aprons are single-use items intended to reduce contamination of clothing. As with many aspects of infection control, their benefit may arise from awareness of the need to keep clean rather than a strong effect of their own.

Disposal of contaminated equipment

Contaminated equipment must be disposed of as soon as is practical, in line with local policies. Disposal of high-risk waste (sharps, heavily contaminated waste) is expensive, and many hospitals now take a risk-assessed approach, where low-risk items are disposed of separately. Anaesthetic practice generates a fair amount of household waste (packaging etc.) and these should not be placed in clinical waste (and ideally recycled where appropriate).

Reusable equipment that needs to be sterile should be returned in a safe manner (covered, without sharps) to the sterile services unit. Other items should be cleaned and disinfected. The anaesthetic machine, particularly flow controls, vapourisers and ventilator switches, are well recognised as being bacterially contaminated.

Equipment sterility

Most surgically related infections probably come from the patient themselves rather than the environment. However,

371

this is a consequence of high standards of cleanliness in the operating theatre. A key component of this is keeping bacterial counts as low as possible in the surgical field. To provide acceptable equipment for use in invasive or high-risk procedures, three phases are required:

- *Cleaning*: the physical removal of foreign material (organic matter and infectious agents). This will reduce, but not eliminate, the population of viable infectious agents. Without effective cleaning, disinfection and sterilisation do not work effectively. Cleaning can be by hand in cool water and detergent (hot water risks formation of coagulated proteinaceous coatings). Increasingly, automated systems are used; some but not all items can be cleaned using ultrasonic cavitation.

- *Disinfection*: the elimination or inactivation of pathogenic organisms, but not spores. Its efficacy depends upon time and the physicochemical conditions. Disinfection can be achieved with chemicals or pasteurisation. Different chemicals have differing antimicrobial properties and potential harmful effects (equipment damage, irritation to staff). Common chemical disinfectants are detailed in Table 18.5. Disinfectants used on the body are usually known as antiseptics.

- *Sterilisation*: the killing of all infectious agents (bacteria, viruses, fungi and spores). This can be achieved with:
  - chemical agents:
    - glutaraldehyde (with long contact time >10 h);
    - ethylene oxide (used for heat and moisture sensitive equipment);
  - steam at high temperature (121 °C–134 °C); high-pressure autoclaving (up to 200 kPa) is used to decrease the time required;
  - hydrogen peroxide plasma; and
  - radiation.

Sterilisation is ineffective against the infectious agents causing prion disease. There are strict rules on reuse of surgical equipment used in high-risk procedures (brain, retina and optic nerve). New sets of instruments are required for these procedures in patients born after 1996 and should not be reused on people born before then.

Sterile precautions

Invasive procedures are usually carried out using sterile precautions or aseptic technique. In practice the procedural field is not sterile. Room air contains bacteria from the patient, the staff and the wider environment.

Skin antisepsis is usually achieved with solutions of biguanides (e.g. chlorhexidine) or iodophors (iodine-releasing compounds such as Betadine) dissolved in alcohol or water. Alcohol-containing products are more effective, but there is probably little clinical difference between products otherwise. The antiseptics must be allowed to dry to achieve their full effect. A red dye is added to chlorhexidine to aid

visibility – its use may also help prevent inadvertent injection. Chlorhexidine has been associated with neurological injury after neuraxial anaesthesia; lower concentrations and allowing time for drying are advocated to reduce this rare risk. Skin antisepsis does not sterilise the skin – viable bacteria remain in the deeper layers and hair follicles, and the skin (of patient or staff) will become recolonised relatively quickly.

Of themselves, hats and masks have never been found to reduce infection. Masks become ineffective as microbial screens very quickly when worn, and hats do not prevent skin squames from shedding. However, they are a well-accepted and cheap part of operating room rituals. The most important role of masks (and eye shields) is to prevent body fluids from contaminating the operator.

Covering the procedural field widely probably has an important role. In the past, anaesthetists commonly made do with small sterile fields for neuraxial blocks and central venous access. This risks inadvertent desterilisation of equipment or working in cramped, suboptimal positions and should be avoided. Insertion of central venous catheters using a full antiseptic technique (hat, gowns, mask, gloves and large sterile field) has been associated with lower infection rates.

Cross-infection

Cross-infection is the infection of one individual with an organism originating from another. It first requires cross-contamination followed by infection.

The main modes of cross-contamination are:
- direct physical contact;
- indirect physical contact (contamination of an intermediate inanimate object, e.g. anaesthetic machine, unsterile invasive equipment);
- airborne and droplets (coughing, sneezing, aerosols);
- faeco-oral and contamination of food and drink; and
- blood-borne.

Contamination is more likely to cause infection if natural barriers and immunity are weakened through wounds, invasive devices or comorbidity. Patients can also become infected with their own microorganisms. For example, nasally carried methicillin-resistant *Staphylococcus aureus* (MRSA) may be transferred to invasive devices by staff or patient activities.

In the hospital environment, common or high-risk cross-contaminating organisms include the following:
- *S. aureus*, *Acinetobacter baumannii* (direct/indirect)
- *Mycobacterium tuberculosis* (droplet/aerosols)
- *Clostridium difficile*, norovirus (faeco-oral via direct/indirect contact)
- Respiratory viruses such as influenza (droplets/aerosols)
- *Pseudomonas aeruginosa* (environmental (water) via direct/indirect contact e.g. neonatal unit)
- *Burkholderia cepacia* in cystic fibrosis (droplet/aerosols)

Table 18.5 Antimicrobial activity of disinfectants

Disinfectant	Mycoplasma	G+	G–	Pseudomonads	Enveloped viruses	Non-enveloped viruses	Fungal spores	Mycobacteria	Bacterial spores	Prions
Alcohols	++	++	++	++	+	–	+/–	–	+/–	–
Aldehydes	++	++	++	++	++	+	+	+	+	–
Biguanides (chlorhexidine)	++	++	++	+/–	+/–	+/–	+	–	–	–
Chlorine	++	+	+	+	+	+	+	+	+	–
Iodine	++	+	+	+	+	+/–	+	+	+	–
Oxidising agents (hydrogen peroxide, peracetic acid[a])	++	+	+	+	+	+/–	+/–	+	+	–
Phenols	++	++	++	++	+/–	+/–	+	+/–	–	–

Efficacy varies with composition and duration of application. Susceptibility of organisms to disinfectants decreases from left to right across the table.
[a]Peracetic acid has sporicidal activity.
+, Effective; ++, highly effective; –, no activity; +/–, limited efficacy; G+, gram positive; G–, gram negative.

Surveillance of infection assists in the control of cross-infection by identifying potential human, process or environmental sources. Appropriate actions to manage the underlying causes can then be taken, such as deep cleaning of rooms and wards to eliminate spores, decolonisation policies and source isolation.

Antimicrobial agents

A useful adage is that all antimicrobial agents are harmful to humans and micro-organisms; occasionally they are more harmful to the latter. Indiscriminate use of antimicrobials puts current and future patients at risk.

Antimicrobial agents can be classified by their mechanism of action (Table 18.6), their spectrum of activity (Table 18.7) and their pharmacokinetics. Effective clinical use is determined by these factors as well as patient toler-

ability (Table 18.8), effects on the patient microbiome, cost, and patterns of current and future microbial resistance.

Mechanism of action

Ideally antimicrobials would selectively affect processes and structures that exist only within the micro-organism and not in the human patient. Bacteria have a greater distinction from humans than fungi and viruses; hence efficacy and toxicity of antiviral and antifungal agents is more of a problem. For example, bacterial cell walls contain unusual D-amino acids, and the ribosomal subunits (30S and 50S) are different to human ribosomes (40S and 60S).

There are broadly five mechanisms of action (see Table 18.6):
1. Inhibition of cell wall synthesis
2. Inhibition of protein synthesis

Table 18.6 Mechanism of action of common antimicrobial agents

Mechanism of action	Specific action	Antimicrobial
Inhibition of cell wall synthesis	Inhibition of peptidoglycan cross-linkage (penicillin-binding protein)	Penicillins, cefalosporins, aztreonam, carbapenems
	Binding to terminal D-ala-D-ala to prevent polymerisation and cross-linkage	Vancomycin, teicoplanin
	Interaction with phospholipid carrier of peptidoglycan	Bacitracin
	Prevention of incorporation of D-ala	Cycloserine
	Inhibition of glycosidic bonds	Fosfomycin
Inhibition of protein synthesis	Bind to 50S ribosome subunit	Macrolides, clindamycin, chloramphenicol, linezolid
	Bind to 30S ribosome subunit	Aminoglycosides, tetracyclines
Inhibition of nucleic acid synthesis	Inhibition of nucleic acid synthesis	Flucytosine, griseofulvin
	Inhibition of topoisomerase and DNA gyrase	Quinolones
	Inhibition of mRNA synthesis	Rifampicin
	Inhibition of folate synthesis (cofactor for nucleic acid synthesis)	Sulfonamides, trimethoprim
Inhibition/interaction with fungal cell membrane sterols	Inhibition of ergosterol synthesis	Antifungal imidazoles
	Binding to membrane sterols	Amphotericin B, nystatin, polymyxins
Inhibition of other specific metabolic processes	Inhibition of mycolic acid synthesis (pro-drug, activated by mycobacterial enzyme)	Isoniazid
	Disruption of microbial DNA (pro-drug, undergoes intracellular reduction to active form in anaerobic bacteria)	Metronidazole
	Detergent-like action on gram-negative membranes	Colistin, polymyxin
	Disruption of cell membrane causing cellular depolarisation, inhibiting nucleic acid and protein synthesis	Daptomycin

Table 18.7 Spectrum of antimicrobial activities

Antibiotic	GRAM POSITIVE								GRAM NEGATIVE								
	S. aureus (MSSA)	S. aureus (MRSA)	CONS	β-haemolytic streptococci	Enterococcus faecalis	Enterococcus faecium	S. pneumoniae	C. difficile	Bacteroides fragilis	N. meningitidis	H. influenzae	Escherichia coli	E. coli (ESBL)[a]	Enterobacteriaceae[a]	Pseudomonas spp	Legionella spp	Mycoplasma spp
Penicillins																	
Benzylpenicillin	−	−	−	+	+	−	+	−	−	+	−	−	−	−	−	−	−
Amoxicillin	−	−	−	+	+	−	+	−	−	−	+/−	+/−	−	−	−	−	−
Co-amoxiclav	+	−	−	+	+	−	+	−	+	−	+	+	−	+/−	−	−	−
Flucloxacillin	+	−	+/−	−	−	−	−	−	−	−	−	−	−	−	−	−	−
Piptazobactam	+	−	−	+	+	−	+	−	+	−	+	+	−	+/−	+	−	−
Cefalosporins																	
Cefuroxime	+	−	+/−	+	−	−	+	−	−	−	+	+	−	+/−	−	−	−
Cefotaxime	+	−	−	+	−	−	+	−	−	+	+	+	−	+/−	−	−	−
Ceftriaxone	+	−	−	+	−	−	+	−	−	+	+	+	−	+/−	−	−	−
Ceftazidime	−	−	−	+	−	−	−	−	−	−	+	+	−	+/−	+	−	−
Carbapenems																	
Meropenem	+	−	−	+	+	−	−	−	+	−	+	+	+	+	+	−	−
Macrolides																	
Clarithromycin/erythromycin	+	+/−	−	+	−	−	+	−	−	−	−	−	−	−	−	+	+
Lincosamides																	
Clindamycin	+	+/−	−	+	−	−	+	−	+	−	−	−	−	−	−	−	−
Aminoglycosides																	
Gentamicin/amikacin	+	+/−	−	−	−	−	−	−	−	−	−	+	+/−	+	+	−	−
Quinolones																	
Ciprofloxacin	+	+	−	−	−	−	−	−	−	P	+	+	+/−	+	+	+	+
Levofloxacin	+	+	−	−	−	−	−	−	−	−	+	+	−	+	+	+	+
Glycopeptides																	
Vancomycin i.v.[b]/Teicoplanin[b]	+	+	+	+	+	+	+	−	−	−	−	−	−	−	−	−	−
Vancomycin p.o.	−	−	−	−	−	−	−	+	−	−	−	−	−	−	−	−	−

Continued

Table 18.7 Spectrum of antimicrobial activities—cont'd

Antibiotic	GRAM POSITIVE								GRAM NEGATIVE								
	S. aureus (MSSA)	S. aureus (MRSA)	CONS	β-haemolytic streptococci	Enterococcus faecalis	Enterococcus faecium	S. pneumoniae	C. difficile	Bacteroides fragilis	N. meningitidis	H. influenzae	Escherichia coli	E. coli (ESBL)[a]	Enterobacteriaceae[a]	Pseudomonas spp	Legionella spp	Mycoplasma spp
Lipopeptides																	
Daptomycin	+	+	+	+	+	+	+	–	+	–	–	–	–	–	–	–	–
Tetracyclines																	
Doxycycline	+	+	–	+/–	–	–	+	–	–	–	–	+	–	–	–	+	+
Tigecycline	+	+	+	+	+	+	+	–	–	–	–	+	+	+/–	–	–	–
Oxazolidinones																	
Linezolid	+	+	+	+	+	+	+	–	–	–	–	–	–	–	–	–	–
Others																	
Trimethoprim	+/–	+/–	–	–	–	–	–	–	–	+/–	+	–	+	–	–	–	–
Metronidazole	–	–	–	–	–	–	–	–	+	–	–	+	+	+/–	–	–	–
Rifampicin	+	+	+	–	–	–	–	–	–	P	–	–	–	–	–	–	–
Colistin	–	–	–	–	–	–	–	–	–	–	+	–	+	+	+/–	–	–
Fosfomycin	+	+	+	+/–	+	+	+	–	–	–		+	+	+	+	–	–

There is significant variability in resistance between and within countries, and local, contemporary data should be referred to when available. Microbiological sensitivity is not the same as clinical efficacy – penetration to the site of action is important. Some drugs are only used as combination therapy.

[a]Multiply resistant strains of *E. coli* and *Enterobacteriaceae* exist.

[b]Vanocmycin-resistant enterococci are resistant to vancomycin and/or teicoplanin (dependent on strain).

+ *(green)*, Usually sensitive; +/– *(yellow)*, variable sensitivity; – *(red)*, resistant (or inappropriate therapy); *P (blue)*, used only for prophylaxis. *CONS*, Coagulase negative Staphylococci; *ESBL*, extended spectrum β-lactamase.

3. Inhibition of nucleic acid synthesis
4. Inhibition/interaction with fungal cell membrane sterols
5. Inhibition of other specific metabolic processes

Pharmacokinetics

The metabolism and physical properties of antimicrobials affect their therapeutic efficacy and formulation.

Vancomycin is not absorbed when given orally; as a consequence it can be used orally for treatment of *C. difficile* infection without systemic effects, but conversely it is ineffective when given intravenously. Some antibiotics are concentrated in the urine or biliary tree, whilst others do not readily cross the blood–brain barrier.

Tolerability

Adverse effects of antimicrobials largely relate to non-target actions, induction or inhibition of the cytochrome P450 family of enzymes, alterations in host microbiome and idiosyncratic reactions (see Table 18.8). Alteration in the host microbiome may result in loss of competitive non-pathogenic

Table 18.8 Selected adverse reactions of antimicrobials

Drug class	Adverse effects
Penicillins/cefalosporins	Previously thought to interact with oral contraception through interference with enterohepatic circulation of steroid hormones; no longer believed to be a significant issue Rashes very common and may result in withholding of appropriate therapy because of misplaced fear of anaphylaxis
Aminoglycosides	Irreversible hearing loss caused by damage to inner ear hair cells Reversible renal tubular damage Interaction with NMBAs
Macrolides	Nausea and vomiting; hepatic cholestasis
Glycopeptides	Red man syndrome – histamine-mediated marked vasodilation, associated with rapid intravenous infusion of vancomycin; has been reported (rarely) with other drugs
Carbapenems	Seizures may be dose limiting

NMBA, Neuromuscular blocking agents.

bacteria and selection of resistant organisms. The most visible consequence of this is patients presenting with *C. difficile*–associated diarrhoea and pseudomembranous colitis after antibiotic therapy.

Resistance

Resistance to antibacterials may be:
- inherent to the organism (e.g. lack of a cell wall precluding β-lactam sensitivity);
- acquired through genetic mutation;
- acquired through phenotypic changes; or
- physical, because the location of the organism is inaccessible to the drug.

Resistance and sensitivity may not be absolute. Testing usually refers to the minimum inhibitory concentration (MIC): the lowest concentration that prevents visible growth of an organism. The minimum bactericidal concentration (MBC) is the concentration that results in cell death (inability to reculture). Clinical efficacy is in part determined by the ability to achieve MIC or MBC at the site of the organism. Organisms with high MIC can sometimes be treated by local application of antibiotics which would be toxic if systemically administered. This is used in the treatment of deep orthopaedic infection by local placement of antibiotic impregnated beads.

There are five general mechanisms that mediate resistance to antimicrobials:
- Reduction in entry (cell permeability)
  - Inability of vancomycin to penetrate outer membrane of gram-negative organisms
  - Modification of porins leading to reduced influx of imipenem

- Increase in efflux
  - Efflux pumps may be relatively drug specific (e.g. tetracyclines, macrolides) or broad spectrum, as found in multiple drug–resistant organisms
- Inactivation / destruction of the drug
  - Aminoglycoside-modifying enzymes
  - β-Lactamases (destroy β-lactams; in turn inhibited by β-lactamase inhibitors such as clavulanic acid and tazobactam)
- Changes in the target
  - Protection through competitive antagonists – quinolone resistance protein competes for DNA binding site
  - Mutations of the target site – linezolid resistance mediated by change in ribosomal binding site
  - Enzymatic alteration – macrolide resistance conferred by enzymatic methylation of the ribosomal binding site
  - Replacement of pathway – vancomycin resistance can involve new pathways that use alternatives to the D-ala-D-ala ending to which vancomycin binds

Phenotypic alterations may alter microbial sensitivity. This is most classically seen in the formation of biofilms on implanted material (central venous catheters, urinary catheters, surgical implants). When bacteria form a biofilm they become 'hidden' from the body's immune systems and antibiotics through production of an extracellular matrix. In addition, key bacterial functions (cell wall synthesis, replication) are switched off, leading to inactivity of key antibiotic targets. Biofilms are hard to treat, so technological solutions aimed at preventing their formation, such as silver or antibiotic impregnated devices, are now in clinical practice.

Genetic acquisition of resistance may occur through primary mutation of genetic material. More common is acquisition of foreign DNA through horizontal gene transfer. Horizontal gene transfer can occur through the following means:

- *Transformation.* Incorporation of naked DNA. This is relatively uncommon.
- *Transduction.* Phages (viruses) transfer DNA between bacteria, and the DNA is incorporated into the genetic material. This can occur across species.
- *Conjugation.* Plasmids can be thought of as auxiliary chromosomes, usually circles of double-stranded DNA, that can transfer between bacteria. They carry genes that are useful in specific contexts but not essential for bacterial growth and replication. Integrins are sections of genetic material found within plasmids and the chromosome that contain specific elements that facilitate transfer and integration of genetic material.

Safe use of antibiotics

Antibiotics are harmful and should only be used when benefits outweigh the risks. Within anaesthesia this is generally for prophylaxis of surgical infection or treatment of established infection in critical care.

Local antibiotic policies should be followed, because they:
- match antibiotics to the most likely infecting organism(s) based on:
  - type of surgery;
  - type of infection; and
  - local microbiological flora;
- choose antibiotics that reach MIC at the infection site;
- match antibiotics to local resistance patterns (e.g. MRSA is variably sensitive to gentamicin);
- limit spectrum and duration of therapy to an acceptable minimum by narrowing the spectrum of antibiotics as soon as infective organisms are known;
- restrict use of last line antibiotics to reduce the rate of emergence of resistance.

Prophylactic antibiotics need to be given at the appropriate time to achieve adequate tissue concentrations at the time of incision and surgery. Generally this is within 30–60 min of incision or tourniquet inflation. Due thought should be given if antibiotics with prolonged preparation (teicoplanin) or administration (vancomycin) times are required or if there is a long interval between induction of anaesthesia and start of surgery.

Immunisation

Healthcare workers have a responsibility to protect themselves and their patients from harm. Immunisations are part of this responsibility as they:
- protect staff and their families;
- protect patients from cross-infection, including those who may not respond well to immunisation or are at particular risk from cross-infection (e.g. pregnant women, immunocompromised persons, those with comorbidity);
- protect other healthcare staff; and
- reduce sickness-related absence in the healthcare workforce.

Most healthcare organisations have mandatory or strongly recommended immunisations for frontline staff. These cover the usual national programmes (such as measles, mumps, rubella, diphtheria, polio, tetanus, *Haemophilus influenzae* B, *Neisseria meningitidis* (A, C, W, Y), *Streptococcus pneumoniae*, rotavirus). In addition, frontline staff in exposure-prone roles may need selected additional vaccinations, including:
- BCG for those in contact with infectious patients;
- hepatitis B;
- varicella – depending on immune status;
- influenza – influenza mutates rapidly, and past infection and immunisation are not effective against future outbreaks. The patient population is vulnerable to infection from staff, including those with pre- or asymptomatic infection. Annual vaccination against the currently expected strains is strongly recommended.

References/Further reading

Almghairbi, D.S., Sharp, L., Griffiths, R., et al., 2018. An observational feasibility study of a new anaesthesia drug storage tray. Anaesthesia 75, 356–364.

Hollnagel, E., 2014. Safety-I and safety–II: the past and future of safety management. Ashgate Publishing, Ltd.

Merry, A.F., Webster, C.S., Hannam, J., et al., 2011. Multimodal system designed to reduce errors in recording and administration of drugs in anaesthesia: prospective randomised clinical evaluation. BMJ **343**, d5543.

Munita, J.M., Arias, C.A., 2016. Mechanisms of antibiotic resistance. Microbiol Spectr **4**.

Reason, J., 2000. Human error: models and management. BMJ **320**, 768.

Reason, J., 2005. Safety in the operating theatre–Part 2: human error and organisational failure. BMJ Qual. Saf. **14**, 56–60.

Sabir, N., Ramachandra, V., 2004. Decontamination of anaesthetic equipment. Continuing Education in Anaesthesia, Critical Care & Pain **4**, 103–106.

Chapter | **19** |

Preoperative assessment and premedication

Alexa Mannings, Damian Doyle, Jonathan Wilson

All patients scheduled to undergo surgery should be assessed in advance to ensure optimal preparation and perioperative management. This is a standard of care proposed by the Association of Anaesthetists, RCoA and similar bodies worldwide. It is one mechanism by which the standard and quality of care provided by an individual anaesthetist or an anaesthetic department may be measured. Failure to undertake this activity places the patient at increased risk of perioperative morbidity or mortality and exposes the patient to avoidable day of surgery cancellation, which is both inconvenient and distressing.

The principle aims of preoperative assessment are to assess perioperative risk, minimise that risk by producing a tailored and individualised care plan, and educate the patient about the process, choices and expectations of the surgical episode to support informed consent and active participation.

Individualising care may include alteration to the original surgical plan (e.g. arranging for laparoscopic rather than open surgery or reducing the surgical magnitude); medical and social optimisation (potentially involving specialist referral and review); specific preoperative interventions such as enhanced recovery programmes, drug commencement or cessation; and decision on the level of postoperative care required (e.g. ward, High Dependency Unit (HDU) or ICU).

Preoperative assessment is the foundation stone of the emerging discipline of perioperative medicine. Anaesthetists need to develop and maintain knowledge of surgical procedures and pathways and appreciate the necessary anaesthetic management to predict the potential issues and likely progress of an individual patient during the perioperative period. Whilst many units organise elective preoperative assessment within specialist nurse-led clinics, working to local and national guidance and protocols under the oversight of enthusiasts from the anaesthetic department, every anaesthetist needs to remain current in the

discipline, as patients requiring urgent surgery may bypass the usual processes.

The process of preoperative assessment

Who, when and where?

All patients listed for surgery should undergo preoperative assessment. The extent of the assessment process may differ depending on the urgency and magnitude of surgery and the intended anaesthetic technique.

A patient may be selected for surgical intervention after a single consultation in surgical clinic; increasingly, decisions regarding major surgery are made at multidisciplinary team meetings, particularly in cancer care, where options of neoadjuvant therapy need consideration. Currently very few multidisciplinary teams include an anaesthetist, though this may change as complex risk–benefit analysis is improved by relevant specialist input to the discussion regarding treatment options. Patients are usually assessed between surgical listing and an intended surgical date, the timing of which is often dictated by non-clinical logistics and can leave limited opportunities for optimisation. Services that are organised on a walk-in (same day as listing) basis can maximise the opportunity for optimisation and minimise journeys to the hospital for the patient.

The core of preassessment is the gathering of relevant administrative and medical information. This can be achieved by patients completing paper or electronic health questionnaires, which are then verified by appropriately trained staff. Questionnaires are particularly useful in patients who are younger or otherwise well and in those undergoing minor or intermediate surgery (e.g. cataract surgery under local anaesthesia). It is preferable that older patients, those with recognised comorbidity and those scheduled for major or complex surgery are assessed by face-to-face interview. This is generally undertaken by trained nurse practitioners with an extended skill set including physical examination and the remit to order specific investigations (both routine screening and other targeted tests). Using local and national protocols, nurse practitioners can make many of the admission arrangements, give general and surgery specific advice and information and refer patients at risk to an anaesthetist responsible for perioperative care for further management.

Hospital admission on the day of surgery is now routine practice. A comprehensive preoperative assessment document (complete with systems review, examination findings, results of screening and specific investigations and specialist instructions where necessary) allows the anaesthetist responsible to concentrate the immediate preoperative discussion on areas of particular relevance, such as discussion of the risks and benefits of regional or general anaesthesia.

History

This should cover all relevant information needed to provide safe anaesthesia and perioperative management of comorbidity (see Chapter 20). Both open and direct questioning are necessary to achieve this, and previous hospital and general practice records may require review to verify details.

Presenting condition

The operation, indication and urgency must be clearly understood. Many surgical conditions can have systemic effects that should be sought out, e.g. bowel cancer that can lead to anaemia and malnutrition.

Functional capacity

Fitness strongly influences perioperative risk and outcome, and even those patients with no comorbidities should be questioned regarding their ability to perform exercise. If limited, the reason for this should be explored, as an undiagnosed cardiorespiratory pathological condition may be present. Questioning should be wide ranging and open. Verbatim description of maximum exercise (e.g. runs 5 km twice a week) or conversion to metabolic equivalents (Table 19.1) should be clearly documented. One metabolic equivalent task (MET) is basal metabolic oxygen consumption at rest ($\sim$3.5 ml min^{-1} kg^{-1}). The inability to climb two flights of stairs ($\sim$4 METs) is associated with an increased risk of cardiac complications after major surgery. Whilst good exercise capacity is reassuring, many patients are sedentary and often do not describe activity greater than 4 METs. These patients should be considered for further fitness evaluation.

Table 19.1 Metabolic Equivalents of Task (MET)

Metabolic equivalent	Task
1.5	Bathing, sitting
2.5	Dressing, undressing, standing or sitting
3.0	Standing tasks, light effort (e.g. bartending, store clerk, filing)
3.5	Scrubbing floors, on hands and knees
4.0	Walks up two flights of stairs
4.3	Walking, 3.5 mph, brisk speed, not carrying anything
5.0	Mowing lawn, walking, power mower, moderate or vigorous effort
7.5	Carrying groceries upstairs
9.0	Moving household items upstairs, carrying boxes or furniture
10.0	Bicycling, 14–15.9 mph, racing or leisure, fast, vigorous effort

Concurrent medical history

All coexisting medical disease must be identified and the degree of severity, control and stability should be assessed by symptomatology, level of care (general practitioner or specialist) and/or recent investigations. The anaesthetic implications of comorbid conditions are discussed in detail in Chapter 20. It is essential to establish the presence and severity of cardiorespiratory disease by direct questioning regarding exertional dyspnoea, paroxysmal nocturnal dyspnoea, orthopnoea, angina, palpitations and so on.

A thorough systems enquiry should also be undertaken, with specific questioning for relevant issues that might influence perioperative management (e.g. symptoms such as indigestion and reflux within the gastrointestinal review).

Some conditions require active screening to identify sufferers or those at risk. Most pertinent are the following:
- obstructive sleep apnoea (OSA);
- frailty;
- anaemia; and
- chronic kidney disease

Obstructive sleep apnoea

Obstructive sleep apnoea is highly prevalent in the surgical population, yet often undiagnosed. Patients with OSA have a higher incidence of difficult airway management and perioperative complications, notably respiratory events, delirium and atrial fibrillation. Current recommendations are that patients be considered for continuous postoperative

Box 19.1 STOP-BANG questionnaire for obstructive sleep apnoea (OSA)

S: Do you **S**nore loudly (loud enough to be heard through closed doors or your bed partner elbows you for snoring at night)?

T: Do you often feel **T**ired, fatigued or sleepy during daytime (such as falling asleep during driving or talking to someone)?

O: Has anyone **O**bserved you stop breathing or choking or gasping during your sleep?

P: Do you have or are you being treated for high blood **P**ressure?

B: **B**MI: >35 kg m^2

A: **A**ge: >50 years

N: **N**eck circumference: >40 cm

G: Male **G**ender

    Score 0–2: Low risk of OSA
    Score 3–4: Intermediate risk of OSA
    Score 5–8: High risk of OSA
    As score increases, so does the likelihood of moderate to severe OSA.

oximetry by using a screening questionnaire progressing, if circumstances allow, to formal diagnosis by sleep studies. Although many questionnaires are in clinical use, the STOP-BANG questionnaire is currently the only tool validated in the surgical population (Box 19.1).

Frailty

Frailty is the cumulative loss of physiological reserve across body systems and is common in older people, affecting 10% of those aged older than 65 years, increasing to 25%–50% of those aged older than 85 years. It can be present with or without other comorbidities and renders patients vulnerable to adverse outcomes, even after minor health events. Measurements of the degree of frailty outperform traditional critical care illness severity scores in predicting outcome for older persons in critical care. Frailty can be described by a phenotype model (unintentional weight loss, reduced muscle strength, reduced gait speed, self-reported exhaustion and low energy expenditure) or a cumulative deficits model (symptoms such as poor hearing, low mood, tremor, comorbidity such as dementia and disability). Frailty requires active consideration to be consistently identified. Assessment methods include observation of gait speed around the clinic, timed up-and-go test and the Clinical Frailty Scale. Frailty in the older patient is also discussed in detail in Chapter 31.

Anaesthetic history

Details of previous anaesthetic episodes should be documented. Some sequelae such as sore throat, headache or postoperative nausea may not seem of great significance to the anaesthetist but may be the basis of considerable preoperative anxiety for the patient. The patient may be unaware of anaesthetic problems in the past if they were managed uneventfully, so previous anaesthetic records should be examined if available. More serious problems such as difficult tracheal intubation or other procedures (e.g. insertion of an epidural catheter) should have been documented. Operating theatre booking systems can record alerts regarding a patient, and any flagged adverse event within these systems should be explored. Other serious problems can be suggested by events such as unexpected ICU admission after previous surgery. These episodes should be explored carefully to identify contributing factors that may be re-encountered. Reviewing old notes can be vital to appreciate the course of events, as often patients and relatives can be unsure of the precipitating factors.

Family history

Several hereditary conditions can influence anaesthetic management, such as malignant hyperthermia, cholinesterase abnormalities, porphyria, some haemoglobinopathies and dystrophia myotonica (see Chapter 20). Some of these disorders have little relevance or impact in daily life. Their presence can be suggested by the report of immediate family members suffering problems with anaesthetics. Establishing the details of these problems and any referral or investigations made can guide the anaesthetic choice to a suitably safe technique. It is important to remember that a negative family history does not guarantee that there are no familial issues.

Drug history

All current medication must be carefully documented, including over-the-counter preparations. This will help inform understanding of comorbidity – both presence and severity. In addition, many drugs may interact with agents or techniques used during anaesthesia. Anaesthetists must maintain up-to-date knowledge of pharmacological advances as new drugs continue to emerge on the market.

Maintenance of the usual drug regimen, including on the morning of surgery, should be considered the norm, with some notable exceptions (Table 19.2). Consideration must also be given to possible perioperative events that influence subsequent drug administration (e.g. delayed gastric emptying, postoperative ileus) and appropriate plans made to use an alternative route or product with similar action for essential medication.

It is advised that some drugs be discontinued several weeks before surgery if feasible (e.g. oestrogen-containing oral contraceptive pill, long-acting monoamine oxidase inhibitors) because of the potential severity of perioperative complications. The pros and cons of these decisions should be considered carefully as severe consequences (unintended pregnancy, relapse of severe depression) may result.

Table 19.2 Routine medication: relevance to anaesthesia and surgery

Drug group	Comments
Cardiovascular	
Antiplatelet agents Aspirin Dipyridamole P2Y12 receptor inhibitors	Require management in perioperative period to minimise risk of serious surgical bleeding and permit neuraxial techniques. Some peripheral and superficial surgery does not require cessation. Dual antiplatelet therapy of most significance. Do not omit in patients within 6 months of cardiovascular event or stroke without specialist advice, particularly if drug-eluting coronary artery stent(s) inserted as stent thrombosis is catastrophic. Consider delay to surgery if feasible rather than disruption of therapy. Low-dose aspirin (75 mg daily) can be continued perioperatively for most surgeries. Consider reducing higher doses to low dose. Omit dipyridamole 24 h preoperatively. Some P2Y12 receptor inhibitors bind irreversibly and require longer omission for manufacture of functioning platelets – cessation for 3–5 days (ticagrelor) and 5–10 days (clopidogrel) before surgery is recommended.
Anticoagulants Warfarin Direct oral anticoagulants (DOACs) Low molecular weight heparin (LMWH)	Require management in the perioperative period to minimise risk of serious surgical bleeding and permit neuraxial techniques. Some peripheral and superficial surgery does not require cessation (e.g. hand surgery, cataracts). Indication for anticoagulation dictates management strategy. Those at higher risk of thrombotic event (e.g. metallic heart valve) require transition from long-acting oral to alternative shorter-acting agents (bridging anticoagulation). Those at lower risk (e.g. atrial fibrillation with no previous stroke) may be able to omit medication without replacement. Warfarin requires omission for 5 days preoperatively, with INR check 48 h before surgery and administration of vitamin K if inadequate reduction in effect. DOACs (e.g. rivaroxaban, apixaban) require between 2 and 4 days' omission preoperatively (according to renal function). LMWH is often the drug of choice to bridge from oral anticoagulants. Check carefully if the dose prescribed is intended to be therapeutic or prophylactic. Dosing is weight based. The last therapeutic dose of LMWH should be given 24 h before surgery. Fondaparinux requires omission for between 3 and 5 days (according to renal function).
Angiotensin-converting enzyme inhibitors	Hypotensive effects may be potentiated by anaesthetic agents. Consider omitting 24–36 h preoperatively.
Angiotensin II receptor blockers	May be associated with severe intraoperative hypotension. Omit 24 h preoperatively.
Beta-blockers	Can cause exaggerated hypotension and mask compensatory tachycardia. Acute withdrawal may result in angina, ventricular extrasystoles or precipitate myocardial infarction. Do not omit and ensure ongoing dosing throughout the perioperative period.
Calcium channel blockers Verapamil	Interacts with volatile anaesthetic agents leading to bradyarrhythmias and decreased cardiac output. Do not omit.
Diltiazem Nifedipine	Interacts with volatile anaesthetic agents to cause hypotension. Acute withdrawal may exacerbate angina. Do not omit.

Table 19.2 Routine medication: relevance to anaesthesia and surgery—cont'd

Drug group	Comments
Other antihypertensives Clonidine Guanethidine Methyldopa Reserpine	Hypotension seen with all anaesthetic agents, requiring extreme care with dosage and administration. Acute withdrawal of long-term treatment may result in a hypertensive crisis. Do not omit.
Digoxin	Toxicity enhanced by hypokalaemia and suxamethonium. Beware of bradyarrhythmias. Do not omit.
Diuretics	Preparations often taken at variable times for convenience by patients. Omission acceptable.
Central nervous system	
Anticonvulsants	Sudden withdrawal may produce rebound convulsive activity. Do not omit.
Benzodiazepines	Additive effect with many CNS-depressant drugs. Do not omit.
Monoamine oxidase inhibitors (MAOIs)	Severe hypertensive response to pressor agents as a result of inhibition of metabolism of indirectly acting sympathomimetics. Treatment of regional anaesthetic-induced hypotension may be difficult. Consider withdrawal 2–3 weeks before surgery and use of alternative medication.
Tricyclic antidepressants	Potentiation of indirectly acting sympathomimetics can precipitate hypertensive crisis. Abrupt withdrawal should be avoided because of risk of cholinergic symptoms. Do not omit.
Phenothiazines, butyrophenones	Interact with other hypotensive agents. Do not omit.
Lithium	Renal excretion with narrow therapeutic window. Consider omission 24 h before major surgery and monitoring with dose adjustment postoperatively after major surgery and those with acute kidney injury.
L-dopa	Multiple drug interactions. Ensure regular administration throughout perioperative period; note short half-life requires stringent dosing intervals. Do not omit.
Diabetic medication	
Insulin	Dose reduction required for insulins of all duration, except extended release (weekly dosing) preparations. Close monitoring required; avoid variable-rate insulin infusion where possible. Do not omit.
Oral hypoglycaemic agents	Meglitinides (e.g. repaglinide) and sulphonylureas (e.g. gliclazide) require omission because of risk of hypoglycaemia. Sodium-glucose cotransporter-2 (SGLT2) inhibitors (e.g. dapagliflozin) require omission because of risk of ketoacidosis. Acarbose, dipeptidyl peptidase-4 (DPP-4) inhibitors (e.g. sitagliptin), glucagon-like peptide-1 (GLP-1) analogues (e.g. liraglutide) and pioglitazone can be taken whilst fasting. Metformin can be taken whilst fasting (except in those with chronic kidney disease stage ≥3 or those expected to receive a dose of contrast media).

Continued

Table 19.2 Routine medication: relevance to anaesthesia and surgery—cont'd

Drug group	Comments
Immune modulation and suppression	
Oral preparations (e.g. azathioprine, leflunomide, hydroxychloroquine, methotrexate, tacrolimus)	Whilst infective risks may be increased, these drugs should be continued in the perioperative period. Methotrexate can cause leucopenia, and a full blood count should be checked preoperatively. Omit if significant leucopenia and consider omission in patients with renal impairment.
Biological disease-modifying agents (e.g. infliximab, etanercept, adalimumab, rituximab)	Continuation or omission dependent on the likelihood of relapse or loss of disease control vs. the infective risks of the procedure proposed. May require specialist advice. Cessation is variable, between 1 and 12 weeks before surgery, and restart only after wounds healed and dry.
Steroids	Potential adrenocortical suppression. Additional steroid cover may be required for the perioperative period.
Oral contraceptive pill	Increased risk of thromboembolic complications with oestrogen-containing formulations. Discuss stopping 4 weeks before elective surgery, with substitution of alternative reliable contraception. If continued, ensure adequate thromboembolic prophylaxis.
INR, international normalised ratio.	

Patients can present for surgery with an illicit drug habit. Abuse of opioids and cocaine is not uncommon, and there is significant information available about potential perioperative problems related to acute or chronic toxicity. The same is not true for the increasing number of designer drugs, nor is much published regarding anabolic steroid use and other image-enhancing drugs. Route of administration should be sought when discussing illicit drug use because of the transmission of bloodborne viruses with s.c. or i.v. injection.

There are potential interactions from herbal remedies used during the perioperative period:

- Garlic, ginseng and gingko: increased bleeding
- St John's wort: induces cytochrome P4503A4 and cytochrome 2C9
- Valerian: modulates γ-aminobutyric acid (GABA) pathways
- Traditional Chinese herbal medicines: variety of adverse effects, including hypertension and delayed emergence

The clinical importance of these interactions is not clear. Current guidance is that patients should be asked explicitly about their use and, if possible, should discontinue them 2 weeks before surgery. There is no evidence to postpone surgery purely because patients are taking herbal remedies.

History of allergy

A history of allergy to specific substances must be sought, whether drug, food or adhesives, and the exact nature of the symptoms and signs should be elicited and documented to distinguish true allergy from other predictable adverse reactions (see Chapter 26).

- Latex allergy is becoming increasingly common; it requires latex-free equipment and a theatre with a full air change to be used for surgery. Logistically this is often achieved by placing the latex-allergic patient first on the morning list.
- A small number of patients describe an allergic reaction to previous anaesthetic exposure. A careful history and examination of the relevant medical notes should clarify the details of the problem, together with the documentation of any postoperative investigations.
- Reported allergy to local anaesthetics is usually a manifestation of anxiety or a response to peak concentrations of local anaesthetic or adrenaline. There are a small number of individuals who are allergic to sulphites, which are commonly found in local anaesthetic preparations (and other drugs).

Smoking history

Long-term deleterious effects of smoking include peripheral vascular disease, coronary artery disease, many cancers and chronic obstructive pulmonary disease (COPD). There are several potential mechanisms by which cigarette smoking can contribute to an adverse perioperative outcome:

- The cardiovascular effects of smoking (tachycardia and hypertension) are caused by the action of nicotine on the sympathetic nervous system.

- Smoking causes an increase in coronary vascular resistance; cessation of smoking improves the symptoms of angina.
- Cigarette smoke contains carbon monoxide, which converts haemoglobin to carboxyhaemoglobin (COHb).
  - In heavy smokers this may result in a reduction in available oxygen by up to 25%.
  - As the half-life of COHb is short, abstinence for 12 h leads to an increase in arterial oxygen content.
- The effect of smoking on the respiratory tract leads to a sixfold increase in postoperative respiratory morbidity.

It appears sensible to advise all patients to cease cigarette smoking for at least 12 h before surgery, and if seen with sufficient lead time, be abstinent for 6 weeks to reduce bronchoconstriction and mucus secretion. The preoperative period can be considered an opportunity for health education; preoperative assessment clinics should be able to refer patients freely to smoking cessation services.

E-cigarettes are used by many smokers alongside cigarettes in an attempt to reduce consumption. These deliver an aerosol containing nicotine, propylene glycol and various flavours, without smoke, tar or carbon monoxide. There is concern regarding the wide variety of chemicals and metals found in vapour; however, it would appear advantageous to advise smokers using both cigarettes and e-cigarettes to switch entirely to e-cigarettes in the preoperative period if they are unwilling to stop smoking entirely. As nicotine is a sympathomimetic, ceasing e-cigarette smoking for some hours before surgery should be advocated.

Alcohol history

Patients may present with acute intoxication, sequelae of chronic consumption (liver disease and cirrhosis) or other non-specific features of secondary organ damage such as cardiomyopathy, pancreatitis and gastritis. Obtaining a clear history of consumption can be difficult. Where patients admit to regular daily consumption, careful questioning regarding dependence and features of risk should be undertaken. The Alcohol Use Dependence Identification Test (AUDIT) developed by the WHO for use in primary care can also be used in the preoperative assessment clinic.

Social circumstances

Suitability for day-case surgery should be established in the clinic; it is a requirement that the patient is escorted home and stays in the presence of a responsible adult in a suitable environment for the first 24 h after anaesthesia. Some patients can be identified as requiring occupational therapy or physiotherapy assessment preoperatively to allow smooth discharge planning.

Physical examination

Examination should complement the clinical history and systems enquiry, and all patients should have basic clinical observations, including recording of height and weight and an airway assessment (see Chapter 23). Detailed physical examination of a patient who is fit and well is arguably unnecessary, but it is a simple and safe method to confirm or refute the expectations of the history. Examination can provide information in case morbidity arises postoperatively e.g. foot drop after poor positioning during anaesthesia and surgery. Occasionally, occult morbidity of particular interest (e.g. aortic stenosis) can be revealed. Features of particular relevance are presented in Table 19.3.

Investigations

Before ordering investigations, these questions should be considered:

- Will this investigation yield information not already apparent from clinical assessment?
- Will the results of the investigation give additional information on diagnosis or prognosis relevant to the planned surgery?
- Will the results of the investigation alter the perioperative preparation and management of the patient and meaningfully reduce perioperative risk?

The number of routine investigations should be minimised by using stringent protocols. The UK National Institute for Health and Care Excellence (NICE) has produced

Table 19.3 Features of clinical examination particularly relevant to the anaesthetist

System	Features of interest
General	Nutritional state, fluid balance Skin and mucous membranes (anaemia, perfusion, jaundice) Temperature Evidence of frailty (slow to undress, weak grip, reduced muscle mass)
CVS	Peripheral pulse (rate, rhythm, volume) Arterial blood pressure Heart sounds Carotid bruits Dependent oedema
RS	Central or peripheral cyanosis Oxygen saturations on air, sitting and supine Respiratory rate and observation for dyspnoea Auscultation of lung fields
Airway	Specific airway assessment tests Dentition
CNS	Any dysfunction of special senses Cranial/peripheral motor and sensory nerves

comprehensive guidance on routine testing (NG45), considering both patient and surgical factors. The advice regarding routine testing presented here is based upon this (Table 19.4).

By reviewing recent investigations undertaken in the community or surgical clinic, unnecessary blood sampling and expense can be avoided, particularly where there has been no change in symptoms in a patient with chronic disease.

All tests ordered in the preassessment clinic should be reviewed and serious abnormalities acted upon promptly. This may involve direct communication with the patient, primary care specialists, waiting list coordinator and/or admitting team.

Cardiorespiratory investigations

Routine investigations should be minimised, and patients with known stable cardiorespiratory disease do not require repeated investigation where recent results are available. However, preoperative assessment often uncovers functional incapacity or unstable cardiorespiratory disease. In these situations, basic investigations should be arranged to decide the most likely pathological condition, direct onward referral and provide a baseline. The perioperative management of patients with significant cardiorespiratory disease is discussed in Chapter 20.

Plasma biomarkers

Biomarkers are biochemical substances that can be assayed from plasma samples, and abnormal concentrations may be associated with certain disease states. Concentrations of B-type natriuretic peptide (BNP), a hormone secreted by cardiac cells in response to stretching of the myocardium, are raised in patients with heart failure, resulting in increased sodium excretion and decreased systemic vascular resistance and correlate with the degree of severity of the disease. A raised BNP concentration is associated with a higher risk of adverse cardiac events and mortality after surgery, and normal concentrations are negative predictors of complications. Cardiac troponin is a marker of myocardial damage, and an elevated preoperative value confers a twofold to threefold increase in the risk of postoperative mortality in major non-cardiac surgery.

ECG

A 12-lead ECG is of greatest value in the assessment of rhythm and should be performed in patients with persistent tachycardia or an irregular pulse. However, it has a low sensitivity for the detection of pathological cardiac conditions and can appear essentially normal in the face of a wide variety of conditions, including clinically significant coronary artery disease, valvular heart disease and even the presence of an internal defibrillator. The indications for a preoperative ECG are shown in Table 19.4.

Resting transthoracic echocardiography

Echocardiography is the investigation of choice for valvular heart disease and can be required in the evaluation of patients with newly detected heart murmurs (see Table 19.4). Murmurs are common; where there is an absence of cardiac symptoms, the murmur is unlikely to represent significant valve disease. An echocardiogram should only be requested when the patient is symptomatic or has an undiagnosed heart murmur but whose function is so limited that they do not increase cardiac output (CO) sufficiently to reveal symptoms. Those with diagnosed heart murmurs or replacement valves may also require echocardiography before surgery when they have developed symptoms or if they are approaching or have exceeded a planned surveillance interval.

It is important to remember that an echocardiogram is performed at rest, at a singular point in time, and thus does not inform the anaesthetist of how the heart may respond to increased demands. Patients with severe left ventricular impairment on a recent echocardiogram can demonstrate normal oxygen delivery on subsequent functional testing. Similarly, normal left ventricular function in terms of ejection fraction on resting echocardiogram does not necessarily mean that the risk of cardiac complications is low, as a significant proportion of patients with heart failure have a preserved ejection fraction. These patients may have diastolic dysfunction and have an increased postoperative risk of adverse cardiac events.

Dobutamine stress echocardiography

Resting echocardiography is not a very useful investigation for patients with suspected ischaemic heart disease; a more commonly used test is dobutamine stress echocardiography (DSE). Stenosed coronary arteries may flow normally at rest but will produce a mismatch between flow and demand in susceptible areas of the myocardium with stress. By giving an infusion of dobutamine to increase heart rate and work and then performing an echocardiogram, regions where mismatch occurs will not contract normally. Dobutamine stress echocardiography has a low positive predictive value (25%–30%) but a high negative predictive value (95%) for perioperative cardiovascular complications after major surgery.

Pulmonary function tests

Peak expiratory flow (PEF) measurements are a useful tool to monitor asthma, and the test should be offered in clinic to those with asthma who feel that current control is suboptimal (for comparison to usual home values) and considered in those with no recent record of PEF who feel normal (to allow onward comparison).

Spirometry (forced expiratory volume in 1 s (FEV_1), forced vital capacity (FVC) and slow vital capacity (VC)) can be easily performed with small portable units. Whilst not

Table 19.4 Guidelines for preoperative investigations

Pregnancy tests	Discuss on day of surgery with women of childbearing age. Test with patient consent. Develop and adhere to local protocols for checking pregnancy status.
Urine tests	Do not routinely offer urine dipstick tests. Consider microscopy and culture of midstream urine sample where presence of UTI would influence decision to operate. Perform microscopy and culture of midstream urine sample in patients symptomatic of UTI.
Full blood count	Do not routinely offer test to any patient for minor surgery. Do not routinely offer test to ASA 1 or 2 patients for intermediate surgery. Consider in ASA 3 or 4 patients with cardiovascular or renal comorbidity if any symptoms not recently investigated, for intermediate surgery. Perform test in all patients for major or complex surgery. Various groups will also require an FBC depending on clinical presentation, including: patients with a surgical pathological condition that causes bleeding or with clinical evidence of anaemia; those undergoing treatment for anaemia without recent check of therapeutic efficacy; patients with a history of long-term immunosuppressive medication use, current neoadjuvant chemotherapy use, or taking some antiepileptic medications; those with recognised blood or bone marrow disorders; patients with a positive bleeding history or known bleeding disorder; those with alcohol dependency or anorexia nervosa; and patients who would refuse blood transfusion.
Urea, creatinine and electrolytes	Do not routinely offer test to ASA 1 or 2 patients for minor surgery. Consider in ASA 3 or 4 patients for minor surgery at risk of AKI. Do not routinely offer test to ASA 1 patients for intermediate surgery. Consider in ASA 2 patients for intermediate surgery at risk of AKI. Perform test in ASA 3 or 4 patients for intermediate surgery. Consider in ASA 1 patients for major or complex surgery at risk of AKI. Perform test in ASA 2, 3 or 4 patients for major or complex surgery. Consider in patients who have hypertension and those taking medication that can cause renal impairment (e.g. diuretics, ACE inhibitors, ARA, aminoglycoside antibiotics). Consider measuring venous bicarbonate in those with STOP-BANG score ≥ 5 (≥ 28 mmol L^{-1} is a sensitive indicator of hypoventilation with ensuing hypercarbia). Patients at risk of AKI include: those undergoing emergency surgery, particularly in the context of sepsis or hypovolaemia, or intraperitoneal surgery; patients with CKD (eGFR <60 ml min^{-1} 1.73 m^{-2}), heart failure, diabetes or liver disease; patients aged older than 65 years; and patients prescribed drugs with nephrotoxic potential in the perioperative period.
Liver function tests	Do not routinely offer. Consider before hepatobiliary surgery and in patients with liver disease, previous hepatitis, high alcohol intake, jaundice, unexplained bleeding or bruising, morbid obesity, anorexia, malnutrition or HIV.
Haemostasis	Do not routinely offer test to any patient for minor surgery. Do not routinely offer test to ASA 1 or 2 patients for intermediate or major or complex surgery. Consider in ASA 3 or 4 patients with chronic liver disease for intermediate or major surgery. Consider in patients who score positively on a structured bleeding questionnaire and those with significant malabsorption. Note: Patients taking direct acting oral anticoagulants will have abnormal coagulation tests that do not reflect the degree of anticoagulation. To assess the regression of these agents after cessation and before surgery requires specific assays such as anti-Xa; specialist haematological advice should be sought.

Continued

Table 19.4 Guidelines for preoperative investigations—cont'd

HbA1c	Do not routinely offer test to patients without a history of diabetes. Those referred for surgery with a history of diabetes should have their most recent HbA1c result included in the surgical referral. Offer HbA1c testing to patients with diabetes having surgery if they have not been tested in the previous 3 months. Consider random glucose and HbA1c testing in obese patients and other groups at high risk, particularly patients with symptoms suggestive of occult diabetes such as recurrent soft tissue infections, fatigue, polydipsia and polyuria.
Sickle-cell disease or sickle-cell trait tests	Do not routinely offer test. Consider testing in context of family history.
Chest radiograph	Do not routinely offer test. Consider only if acute symptoms of infection or failure.
Other radiographs	Consider cervical spine radiographs in selected patients where there is a possibility of vertebral instability (e.g. those with rheumatoid arthritis).
ECG	Do not routinely offer test to ASA 1 or 2 patients for minor surgery. Consider in ASA 3 or 4 patients for minor surgery if no ECG result available from prior 12 months. Do not routinely offer test to ASA 1 patients for intermediate surgery. Consider in ASA 2 patients for intermediate surgery with cardiovascular or renal comorbidity or diabetes. Perform in ASA 3 or 4 patients for intermediate surgery. Consider for ASA 1 patients for major or complex surgery aged older than 65 if no ECG result available from prior 12 months. Perform in ASA 2, 3 and 4 patients for major or complex surgery. Perform before referral for echocardiography. Perform if new stage of hypertension (stage 2/3) is diagnosed. Consider where assessment suggests or reveals conditions that can lead to cardiomyopathy (e.g. high alcohol intake, illicit steroid use, illicit cocaine use, anorexia nervosa) or if high risk for OSA.
Resting echocardiography	Do not routinely offer test. Consider if patient has a heart murmur and any cardiac symptom (e.g. breathlessness, presyncope, syncope or chest pain). Consider if patient has signs or symptoms of heart failure.
Lung function tests (spirometry and blood gas analysis)	Do not routinely offer test to any patient for minor surgery. Do not routinely offer test to ASA 1 or 2 patients for intermediate or major surgery. Consider seeking advice of senior anaesthetist for patients who are ASA 3 or 4 because of known or suspected respiratory disease for intermediate or major surgery.

ACE, Angiotensin-converting enzyme; *AKI,* acute kidney injury; *ARA,* angiotensinogen receptor antagonists; *ASA,* American Society of Anesthesiologists; *CKD,* chronic kidney disease; *eGFR,* estimated glomerular filtration rate; *FBC,* full blood count; *HbA1c,* glycated haemoglobin; *HIV,* human immunodeficiency virus; *OSA,* obstructive sleep apnoea; *UTI,* urinary tract infection.

particularly predictive for postoperative complications, values are very useful in the diagnosis of the breathless patient and as reference or monitoring in patients with progressive lung disease.

Arterial blood gas analysis is most often undertaken before thoracic surgery. It retains a place in the comprehensive assessment of the severely breathless patient or the patient with low resting oxygen saturations whilst breathing room air and can assist in appreciating the impact of OSA (see Table 19.4).

Tests of functional capacity

Rather than relying on a patient's report of function, exercise capacity can be observed or tested. The most basic assessment is simply to observe the patient moving about the clinic and undressing/dressing for examination. A stair climb can usually be easily achieved near most clinic areas and can reveal reduced cardiorespiratory function. Simple walking or stair climbing tests are useful in giving an overall impression of a patient's reserve but have limitations. Some elderly patients will have mobility problems due to osteoarthritis and may find walking difficult. These basic tests have a good negative predictive value but give little useful information about the underlying causes of impaired functional capacity in those patients who do not perform well. This is relevant as some patients will perform poorly because of an underlying disease state, most commonly cardiac impairment, whilst others will perform poorly simply through being deconditioned from lack of physical activity.

Six-minute walk test

The simplest formal evaluation is the 6-minute walk test, where patients walk on a flat 30-m course around two cones, achieving as far a distance as possible in 6 min. Stopping to rest is allowed. Full observations should be performed at the start and end of the test, and patients should wear a portable pulse oximeter throughout. It is most often used to evaluate the effect of interventions in severe chronic lung and heart conditions (e.g. COPD, pulmonary hypertension), and there is little evidence for its use in surgical patients.

Incremental shuttle walk test

The significant advantage of the incremental shuttle walk test over the 6-minute walk test is the requirement to increase power output through the test. Patients move around an oval course of 10 m marked by two cones and need to complete an increasing number of circuits with each passing minute; audible beeps and the test technician help the patient keep to time. The test ends when the patient cannot keep up with the beep or develops significant symptoms, such as angina or desaturation to less than 80%. Outcome is distance walked to the nearest 10 m; distances of more than 350–360 m in patients scheduled for oesophagogastrectomy and intra-abdominal surgery have identified those of normal risk in observational studies.

Both the incremental shuttle walk test and 6-minute walk test correlate to peak oxygen consumption ($\dot{V}O_2$) as measured by cardiopulmonary exercise testing (CPEX; see later). Hence these tests are of interest where resources are limited, and their relative simplicity can allow testing of a larger patient cohort. However, compared with CPEX, both tests fail to accurately place many patients into high- or normal-risk categories.

Cardiopulmonary exercise testing

Cardiopulmonary exercise testing has been used for more than 20 years in the preoperative evaluation of patients, particularly in major vascular and colorectal cancer surgery. The most common preoperative protocol is a ramp bicycle test. After a rest and unloaded warm-up phase, the resistance to pedalling is increased in small increments every few seconds, creating a test of steadily increasing power output to maximum. Measurements continue after the cessation of exercise for several minutes to observe recovery and resolution of any exercise-provoked abnormal response. It is an intensively monitored test, with oxygen consumption, carbon dioxide production, respiratory measurements, ECG, blood pressure and oxygen saturations all routine.

Variables used to risk assess and stratify patients include:
- anaerobic threshold (AT) – the point at which $\dot{V}O_2$ ceases to be wholly aerobic, with anaerobic metabolism added to supplement performance (Fig. 19.1);
- peak O_2 – the greatest oxygen consumption ($\dot{V}O_2$) demonstrated in that test, which may or may not genuinely reflect the true maximum oxygen consumption ($\dot{V}O_2$ max); and
- ventilatory equivalents for CO_2 ($\dot{V}_E$ [minute ventilation] / $\dot{V}CO_2$ [volume of CO_2 produced]).

These three variables relate to both short- and long-term perioperative outcomes. Anaerobic threshold generally occurs at 50%–60% of peak $\dot{V}O_2$ and is not effort dependent. This is advantageous in the very frail or elderly as the test can be curtailed deliberately or, in those who stop exercising before maximum for whatever reason, at least provide some risk assessment.

Values consistent with a high risk of postoperative morbidity and mortality are:
- AT <11 ml kg^{-1} min^{-1} (sixfold increase in mortality rates);
- Peak $\dot{V}O_2$ <15 ml kg^{-1} min^{-1}; and
- $\dot{V}_E/\dot{V}CO_2$ >34 (particularly if present in combination with a reduced AT).

Approximately 25% of patients having major surgery aged older than 55 years will have CPET measures that place them in a high-risk group. The most useful parameters are ventilatory efficiency and the ability to diagnose myocardial dysfunction from heart failure or ischaemic heart disease through an abnormal oxygen pulse ($\dot{V}O_2$/heart rate (HR)).

Ventilatory efficiency. Ventilatory efficiency is estimated from the $\dot{V}_E/\dot{V}CO_2$. This is normally between 25 and 30; an increasing ratio suggests that there is impairment of V/Q matching from either cardiac or respiratory causes. In heart failure patients $\dot{V}_E/\dot{V}CO_2$ >34 is associated with a poor prognosis, and if >44 the survival is less than 50% at 2 years. The long-term outcomes for patients having major surgery have an almost identical pattern as those with heart failure when divided into those with good or poor ventilatory efficiency, despite less than 5% of surgical patients actually having a diagnosis of heart failure.

Identification of myocardial dysfunction. Oxygen uptake per heartbeat, or $\dot{V}O_2$/HR (also known as the oxygen pulse), is a surrogate measure for stroke volume (SV) responses, knowing that oxygen consumption is the CO multiplied by the arteriovenous oxygen content difference:

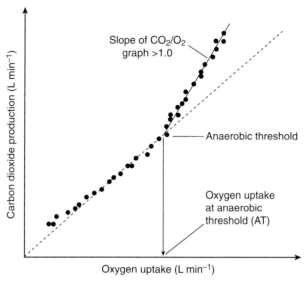

Fig. 19.1 V-slope method for estimating anaerobic threshold. Oxygen uptake increases as exercise intensity increases. During the initial aerobic phase the slope of the graph of CO_2 production versus O_2 uptake is <1. After the onset of lactate production from anaerobic pathways (the anaerobic threshold), extra CO_2 is generated by the buffering of lactate with bicarbonate, and the slope of the CO_2/O_2 graph is >1.

$$\dot{V}O_2 = CO \times (CaO_2 - CvO_2)$$

$$\text{As } CO = HR \times SV, \dot{V}O_2 = (HR \times SV) \times (CaO_2 - CvO_2)$$

Rearranging the equation:

$$\dot{V}O_2 / HR = SV \times (CaO_2 - CvO_2)$$

Oxygen pulse should increase steadily during exercise as a reflection of increases in underlying SV initially, followed by increases in oxygen extraction (Fig. 19.2A). If the slope of the graph flattens during exercise, this may reflect underlying myocardial wall motion abnormalities (Fig. 19.2B), and if the slope starts to decrease, this indicates the onset of wall motion abnormality caused by ischaemia. If the patient is symptomatic, he or she should be referred for cardiology assessment; otherwise, secondary protection with a β-blocker may be helpful. It is advisable to repeat testing after any intervention before surgery to see if the test result has improved.

Power output is measured during CPEX testing and should be linearly related to $\dot{V}O_2$, with a 1 W increase in work rate being associated with a 10 ml min^{-1} increase in $\dot{V}O_2$ a falling value can indicate heart failure (Fig. 19.3); however, care should be taken in interpretation – some patients do demonstrate a plateau in $\dot{V}O_2$ that is actually their genuine maximum oxygen consumption.

It is possible to differentiate the merely unfit or decon-ditioned patient from those with pathological limitation of oxygen delivery and consumption, which can guide

optimisation. Some patients demonstrate particular strategies or responses that can be manipulated advantageously intra- and postoperatively by the attending anaesthetist.

The stratification of patients into high- or normal-risk groups allows a more specific and honest conversation regarding the likely perioperative course, with shared decision-making where choices exist between interventions. Objective testing also allows standard-risk patients to be de-escalated from critical care environments and high-risk patients, who may not carry any diagnostic label, to access critical care postoperatively.

Much interest now lies in the possibility of exercise-based preoperative interventions to improve fitness before surgery (prehabilitation) and move patients from the high-risk to the normal-risk group. Small studies demonstrate that many patients are exercise responsive and will engage in some styles of programme; however, simply telling people to do more, rather than offering a structured and personalised intervention, is much less effective in improving fitness.

Risk assessment and optimisation

With all relevant information collated, the key questions to be answered are as follows:
- Do the anticipated benefits of surgery outweigh the combined risks of undergoing anaesthesia and surgery for this patient?

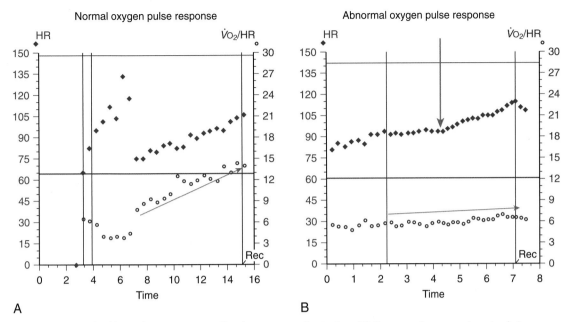

Fig. 19.2 Oxygen pulse ($\dot{V}o_2$/HR) response to cardiopulmonary exercise testing. (A) The normal response is a steady increase in oxygen pulse during exercise *(purple arrow)* as a reflection of increases in underlying stroke volume initially, followed by increases in oxygen extraction. (B) Abnormal oxygen pulse response. The slope of the oxygen pulse graph flattens during exercise *(purple arrow)* despite an increase in heart rate *(red arrow)*. This may reflect underlying myocardial wall motion abnormalities.

- Is there a specific risk that can be mitigated by planning and communication?
- Is the patient in optimum physical condition for anaesthesia and surgery? If not, how long would be required to improve comorbidity, and would this effect a significant risk reduction?

Quantifying the risk of postoperative morbidity and mortality is increasingly important to undertake shared decision-making. It must be clear that the risks quoted are for a population as no tool can predict risk for an individual; this can be challenging to convey to patients. Using both words *(common, rare, very rare)* and numbers (10% or 1 person in 10) to convey risk can help, as can using anchors such as one person in a street (around 1:100).

Prediction of non-specific adverse outcome

Across Europe the overall mortality rate within 7 days of surgery is approximately 4% over a broad range of operations and age. It is often difficult to decide if patient factors, anaesthetic technique or aspects of surgery are most influential. The incidence of deaths to which anaesthesia has made a significant contribution or has been the sole cause is very low (approximately 1 in 10,000) compared with overall short-term mortality. In large studies, common factors contributing to anaesthetic mortality include inadequate preoperative assessment of patients, inadequate supervision and monitoring in the intraoperative period and inadequate postoperative supervision and management.

Whatever the contribution from anaesthesia, the impact of postoperative complications is significant. Those who suffer postoperative complications and survive the immediate postoperative period have an increased mortality several months and even years after their operation. Some data indicate that reducing complications improves outcome, suggesting that this link is not solely identifying patients with poor reserve.

Published prospective studies evaluating risk factors for the development of morbidity tend to agree on several factors from physiological, demographic and laboratory data which can combine to indicate the likelihood of adverse outcome. These include:
- older age (>70 years);
- major, urgent or palliative surgery;
- significant organ dysfunction (as evidenced by clinical features such as jaundice or confusional state, or laboratory evidence, such as significantly deranged urea and electrolytes or anaemia); and

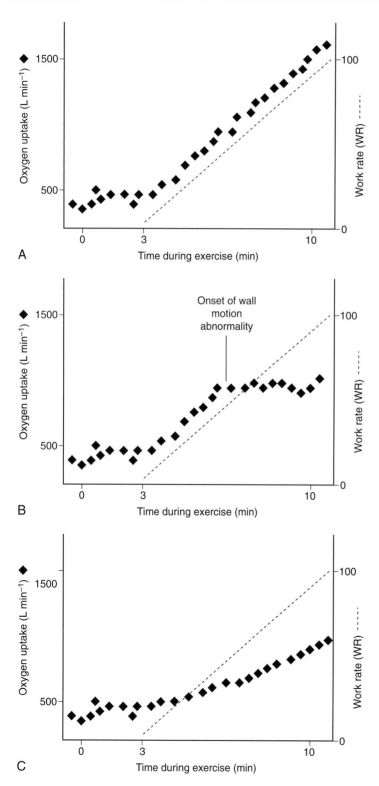

Fig. 19.3 Relationship between oxygen uptake and work rate ($\dot{V}_{O_2}$/WR). (A) Normal: for each 1 W increase in work rate intensity, oxygen uptake increases by 10 ml min^{-1}. In this example, O_2 uptake is 500 ml min^{-1} at the onset of loaded cycling and 1500 ml min^{-1} after 100 W, an increase of 10 ml min^{-1} W^{-1}. (B) Ischaemic heart disease: the $\dot{V}_{O_2}$/WR relationship starts normally, but O_2 uptake abruptly stops increasing at the critical ischaemic point as wall motion abnormalities develop. (C) Chronic heart failure: $\dot{V}_{O_2}$/WR is significantly decreased, as the myocardial pump does not respond normally to increasing exercise intensity.

Table 19.5 American Society of Anesthesiologists physical status classification system and associated mortality rates

ASA classification	Description of patient	48-h mortality (%)[a]
1	A normally healthy individual	0.001
2	A patient with mild systemic disease (without substantive functional limitations)	0.002
3	A patient with severe systemic disease that is not incapacitating (one or more moderate to severe diseases, with substantive functional limitation)	0.028
4	A patient with severe systemic disease that is a constant threat to life	0.304
5	A moribund patient who is not expected to survive 24 h with or without operation	6.232
6	A declared brain-dead patient whose organs are being removed for donor purposes	

The suffix E can be added to indicate that surgery is emergency, where delay would lead to increased risk to life or limb.
[a]Contemporary cohort of elective procedures (2009–2014).
ASA, American Society of Anesthesiologists.

- acute concurrent medical issues, particularly unstable cardiac conditions.

To better manage patients at increased risk of postoperative morbidity and mortality, clinicians should routinely undertake a risk evaluation and document the predicted risk of complications before surgery; re-evaluation after surgery is also advisable. There is reasonable evidence that clinical judgement alone is not a particularly good predictor of the need for critical care in the postoperative period; thus using a specific risk scoring tool or CPEX testing can assist in ensuring the high-risk cohort are identified (see Chapter 30).

American Society of Anesthesiologists (ASA) physical status classification

The ASA physical classification system (Table 19.5) was introduced as a simple description of the physical state of a patient, along with an indication of whether surgery is elective or emergency. It is very straightforward, requiring no investigation results, and correlates with the risks of anaesthesia and surgery in both historic and contemporary cohorts. However, the ASA classification is not a predictive risk calculator for individual patients; it is rather subjective, particularly across the crucial ASA 2/ASA 3 line, and although recent clarifications regarding obesity, smoking and alcohol intake have been made, there is still significant variation in assigned scores between anaesthetists. It serves as a useful shorthand descriptor and should be completed for all patients.

Surgical Outcome Risk Tool

The ASA physical classification system has been included in the Surgical Outcome Risk Tool (SORT), in addition to patient age (<65, 65–80, >80 years), cancer status and surgical site (thoracic, gastrointestinal or vascular), severity and urgency. This was designed to predict 30-day mortality risk for the adult UK general surgical population, using information readily available preoperatively, and has used National Confidential Enquiry into Patient Outcome and Death (NCEPOD) data to generate and validate the scoring system. It is recommended that an estimate of surgical risk in terms of mortality is written on the surgical consent form to ensure the patient understands the risks, and SORT is a straightforward way of producing this risk estimate.

Physiological and Operative Severity Score for the Enumeration of Mortality and Morbidity

The Physiological and Operative Severity Score for the Enumeration of Mortality and Morbidity (POSSUM) was first reported in 1991 to compare mortality and morbidity over a wide range of general surgical procedures. It consists of 12 physiological and six operative factors which are either readily available or predictable in the immediate preoperative period (Table 19.6). These factors are weighted according to their value, and a logistic regression formula is applied to calculate the risk of mortality or morbidity. The formula has been modified after suggestions that the original system overestimated the risk of death in low-risk patient groups

Table 19.6 Factors contributing to the POSSUM score for risk of perioperative mortality and morbidity

Physiological factors	Operative factors
Age (years)	Operative complexity
Cardiac status (heart failure)	Single *vs.* multiple procedures
Respiratory status (breathlessness, COPD)	Expected blood loss
Systolic blood pressure	Peritoneal contamination (blood, pus, bowel content)
Pulse rate	Extent of any malignant spread
ECG rhythm	Urgency of surgery
Haemoglobin concentration	
White cell count	
Serum urea concentration	
Serum sodium concentration	
Serum potassium concentration	
Glasgow Coma Scale score	

A higher score is awarded for increasing deviation from the normal value or range.
COPD, Chronic obstructive pulmonary disease; *POSSUM,* Physiological and Operative Severity Score.

(p-POSSUM); others have produced speciality-specific variants (e.g. v-POSSUM for elective vascular surgery). It should be emphasised that the POSSUM scoring system was designed to compare observed with expected death rates among populations rather than to predict mortality for an individual, and it should be applied only in this way.

American College of Surgeons National Surgical Quality Improvement Program surgical risk calculator

Built using outcome data from 2.7 million procedures undertaken in the United States and recorded in the National Surgical Quality Improvement database, the American College of Surgeons National Surgical Quality Improvement Program (ACS NSQIP) surgical risk calculator requires 20 pieces of information and usefully allows adjustment of the risk estimates where a specific concern is not addressed with routine data collection. A graphical display of the risk of any, and specific, complications, mortality and discharge to nursing facility is produced, with average risks for comparison and duration of stay estimate.

Prediction of specific adverse perioperative events
Major adverse cardiac events

Major adverse cardiac events (MACE) include myocardial infarction, pulmonary oedema, ventricular fibrillation (or other primary cardiac arrest) and complete heart block. The overall rate of symptomatic MACE is about 2%–3% in a mixed surgical population. However, between 5% and 25% of patients have increases in troponin after surgery, suggesting myocardial injury, with an increased risk of death for up to 1 year after surgery. A postoperative myocardial infarction is associated with a fivefold increase in 30-day mortality.

Initial work by Goldman and colleagues analysed preoperative risk factors associated with an adverse cardiac event after non-cardiac surgery. This topic has been re-evaluated extensively in the intervening years, with many studies agreeing broadly with Goldman's conclusions. However, conflicting opinions exist regarding identification of the most accurate predictors, probably because of the diversity of methods used in these studies, together with significant and continued advances made in the understanding and management of cardiovascular pathophysiology. The most widely used risk index is Lee's revised cardiac risk index (Table 19.7).

Patients are classified into four classes:
- (no risk factors): 35% of population, 0.4% incidence of MACE
- (one factor): 41% of population, 0.9% incidence of MACE
- (two factors): 19% of population, 6.6% incidence of MACE
- (≥ three factors): 5% of population, 11% incidence of MACE

Lee's revised cardiac risk index is simple to use but assumes all factors carry equal weight of risk, when, for example, heart failure is clearly a higher risk than ischaemic heart disease.

American and European guidance now focuses attention on those at highest risk of adverse cardiac events by the identification of patients presenting for surgery with unstable and severe cardiac disease (Table 19.8). Where these are evident, if at all possible, surgery should be delayed to permit investigation and management of these conditions.

Patients with stable cardiac disease can be considered in the context of their surgical intervention, which can be divided into low (<1%), intermediate (1%–5%) and high (>5%) risk of cardiac events in the 30 days after surgery, related to the physiological stress engendered (Table 19.9). In very general terms, those with stable cardiac disease should

Table 19.7 Lee's Revised Cardiac Risk Index

Factor	Definitions
High-risk surgical procedures	Intraperitoneal Intrathoracic Suprainguinal vascular
History of ischaemic heart disease	History of myocardial infarction History of positive exercise test Current ischaemic chest pain Use of nitrate therapy ECG with pathological Q waves
Congestive heart failure	History of congestive heart failure, pulmonary oedema or paroxysmal nocturnal dyspnoea Physical examination showing bilateral rales or S3 gallop Chest radiograph showing pulmonary vascular redistribution
Cerebrovascular disease	History of transient ischaemic attack or stroke
Insulin therapy for diabetes	
Preoperative serum creatinine >177 µmol L^{-1}	

Table 19.8 Unstable and high-risk cardiac conditions which warrant, where time allows, further investigation and multidisciplinary team decision-making as to the priority of treatment

Unstable coronary syndromes	Unstable or severe angina Recent (<3 months) myocardial infarction
Decompensated heart failure	
Significant arrhythmias	Mobitz II atrioventricular block Third-degree atrioventricular block Symptomatic ventricular arrhythmias Supraventricular arrhythmias (including atrial fibrillation) with uncontrolled ventricular rate (>100 beats min^{-1} at rest) Symptomatic bradycardia Newly recognised ventricular tachycardia
Severe valvular disease	Severe aortic stenosis (mean pressure gradient >40 mmHg, aortic valve area <1.0 cm^2, or symptomatic) Symptomatic mitral stenosis (progressive dyspnoea on exertion, exertional presyncope or heart failure)

not undergo extra assessment and intervention simply because surgery is planned. Rather, patients should be treated according to best practice for their condition. Revascularisation for coronary artery disease should only be undertaken if the patient warrants the intervention per se, not with a specific intent to diminish the perioperative risk. Those with poor functional capacity and recognised cardiac disease are most likely to warrant non-invasive cardiac investigation in the preoperative phase (e.g. biomarkers such as natriuretic peptides). Specific cardiac conditions are discussed in detail in Chapter 20.

Postoperative pulmonary complications

Postoperative pulmonary complications (PPCs) include atelectasis, infection and pneumonia, pleural effusion, pulmonary oedema, bronchospasm, aspiration pneumonitis, respiratory failure, acute lung injury and pulmonary embolus. The heterogeneity of this list demonstrates why prediction of this group of complications remains difficult. These complications in combination probably occur more often than cardiac complications, with the quoted incidence varying widely between 1% and 23%; both short- and long-term mortality are significantly elevated.

Factors classically associated with being at risk of developing PPCs include current smokers, those with pre-existing lung disease, the obese and those undergoing thoracic or abdominal surgery. Several risk prediction models have been devised to identify the high-risk cohort, but there is a lack of consensus as to the best performing tool. Two prospective multicentre tools (ARISCAT (Assess Respiratory Risk in Surgical Patients in California), which identifies multiple pulmonary complications, and PERI-SCOPE (Prospective Evaluation of a Risk Score for Postoperative Pulmonary Complications in Europe), which identifies respiratory failure; Table 19.10) are helpful in that they reveal several risk factors that can be identified in clinic and some that are optimisable. The ARISCAT scores assign points for each risk factor, with overall scores allowing risk classification for the development of PPCs:

- Low risk (<26 points): 77% of patient population, 1.6% incidence of PPC
- Intermediate risk (26–44 points): 16% of population, 13.3% incidence of PPC

Table 19.9 Approximate risk of 30-day postoperative cardiovascular death and myocardial infarction by surgical intervention, without considering patient comorbidity

Low risk (<1%)	Intermediate risk (1%–5%)	High risk (>5%)
Superficial surgery	Abdominal intraperitoneal	Aortic/major vascular
Breast	Carotid: symptomatic	Duodenopancreatic surgery
Dental	Peripheral arterial angioplasty	Liver resection, bile duct surgery
Endocrine: thyroid	Endovascular aneurysm repair	Oesophagectomy
Eye	Head and neck	Repair perforated bowel
Reconstructive	Neurological (e.g. spines)	Adrenal resection
Carotid: asymptomatic	Orthopaedic – major (e.g. joint replacement)	Total cystectomy
Gynaecology – minor	Renal transplant	Liver transplant
Orthopaedic – minor (e.g. meniscectomy)	Urology and gynaecology – major	
Urology – minor (e.g. TURP)		

TURP, Transurethral resection of the prostate.

Table 19.10 Independent variables associated with postoperative pulmonary complications from the ARISCAT and PERISCOPE risk prediction models

ARISCAT	PERISCOPE
Preoperative peripheral oxygen saturation <96%	Preoperative peripheral oxygen saturation <96%
Respiratory infection in the last month	At least one preoperative respiratory symptom
Age	Chronic liver disease
Preoperative anaemia <100 g L^{-1}	Congestive heart failure
Intrathoracic/upper abdominal surgery	Intrathoracic/upper abdominal surgery
Duration of procedure >2 h	Duration of procedure >2 h
Emergency surgery	Emergency surgery

ARISCAT, Assess Respiratory Risk in Surgical Patients in California; *PERISCOPE,* Prospective evaluation of a risk score for postoperative pulmonary complications in Europe.

The difficult airway

The preoperative identification of the potentially adverse airway allows for the appropriate equipment and personnel to be available on the day of surgery. Airway assessment is discussed in full in Chapter 23.

Venous thromboembolism

The perioperative period is a time of significant risk for the development of DVT and PE. The risk varies across the surgical population, and stratification ensures that patients receive appropriate mechanical or chemical thromboprophylaxis, whilst minimising the risk posed by unnecessary anticoagulant therapy. Patient and surgical risk factors should be balanced against an individualised bleeding risk assessment (Table 19.11).

Optimisation

In the urgent or emergency situation, optimisation is focused on adequate resuscitation and restoration of physiological, biochemical and haematological abnormalities. This is discussed in Chapter 44.

In more controlled circumstances, consideration should be given to delaying to surgery in order for concurrent comorbidities to be addressed and improved. This might entail very long delays in cases where weight loss or smoking and alcohol cessation are to be tackled. These decisions can be complex and require an understanding of what improvement can realistically be expected. The severity and reversibility of the medical disease process, risks of deterioration of the

- High risk (>44 points): 7% of population, 44.9% incidence of PPC

This is a highly sensitive and specific score, using easily obtained information. For the patient at medium or high risk, assessment by a respiratory physician may be helpful and interventions such as preoperative physiotherapy or incentive spirometry considered.

Table 19.11 Risk factors for the development of venous thromboembolism and bleeding risk evaluation

Patient factors	Surgical factors	Bleeding risk factors
Age >60 years	Orthopaedic surgery, particularly lower limb	Active bleeding
Obesity	Major abdominal, gynaecological, urological surgery	Acquired bleeding disorders (e.g. liver failure)
Active cancer or cancer treatment	Major trauma or burns (spinal cord injury)	Concurrent use of anticoagulants (e.g. warfarin)
Known thrombophilia	Longer operative times (>90 min total anaesthetic and surgical time or >60 min if pelvic/lower limb)	Lumbar puncture/epidural/spinal anaesthesia within the previous 4 h or expected within next 12 h
One or more significant medical comorbidity (e.g. heart disease, metabolic, endocrine conditions)	Anticipated significantly reduced mobility for 3 days postoperatively	Lumbar puncture/epidural/spinal anaesthesia performed within previous 4 h
Dehydration	Acute surgical admission for inflammatory condition or intra-abdominal condition	Acute stroke
Personal history or first degree relative with history of previous DVT/PE	Anticipated critical care admission	Thrombocytopenia (platelets <75 $\times 10^9$ L^{-1})
Taking hormone replacement therapy		Uncontrolled systolic hypertension (>230/120 mmHg)
Taking oral contraceptive pill		Untreated inherited bleeding disorders (e.g. haemophilia)
Varicose veins with phlebitis		
Pregnant or <6 weeks postpartum		
Indwelling venous catheter		

surgical pathological condition and patient motivation must be considered to enable a balanced plan for optimisation.

Decisions regarding optimisation often require discussion with specialists and in some instances referral. A clear time frame for optimisation should be set, with reassessment at a set interval. Options include escalated efforts, acceptance that surgery goes ahead with suboptimal gain or removal from the waiting list. A specific goal such as 'achieve a BMI <38 kg m^{-2}, is preferable to generic advice to 'lose weight'; this also makes the reassessment of the patient more straightforward. Delay for optimisation requires discussion with the surgical team and clear communication to the clerical and administrative staff.

It is common to find patients incompletely compliant with regular prescription therapy, and optimisation can be as straightforward as reinforcing the importance of compliance in the weeks preoperatively e.g. to use steroid inhalers for asthma regularly.

Recent acute respiratory tract infection is commonly seen in the preoperative assessment clinic. If significant infection (pyrexia, clinical signs on examination, productive cough) is identified, where possible, elective, non-urgent surgery should be rescheduled for 6 weeks after resolution to reduce the risk of respiratory complications.

Examples of shorter-term optimisation strategies include the following:

- preoperative venesection to reduce haematocrit in significant polycythaemia (days before surgery);
- treatment of asymptomatic atrial fibrillation with rapid ventricular rate with β-blockers (titrated over 2–4 weeks);
- treatment of iron deficiency anaemia with i.v. iron (expectation of some improvement of haemoglobin at 1 week after first dose, maximal gain seen at 4 weeks); and
- intensive escalation of insulin therapy where diabetic control is suboptimal (i.e. HbA1c >75 mmol mol^{-1}) over 6–8 weeks

Stage 3 or 4 hypertension (i.e. >180/110 mmHg) should be referred back to primary care for blood pressure control as per Association of Anaesthetists guidelines (see Chapter 20).

Preparation for elective surgery

Providing information to the patient and obtaining consent

Much of the administration and process of care information can be given to patients in the preoperative assessment clinic by nurse practitioners, who can also signpost patients to reliable sources of information regarding the risks and benefits of types of anaesthesia, such as the RCoA and NHS Choices for UK patients.

Consent for anaesthesia is a vital part of preoperative preparation and is a process, not an event. It is discussed more fully in Chapter 21.

Generic preparation of the patient

All patients should receive clear advice regarding the practical arrangements of admission (where and when to arrive to the hospital, what to bring with them), including expectation of duration of stay or same-day discharge.

Preoperative fasting instructions should be given well in advance and reiterated when booking arrangements are confirmed, with cessation of intake of solids 6 h before intended anaesthesia start, and encouragement to maintain clear fluid intake up to 2 h before anaesthesia. All patients should receive tailored advice regarding medication (see Table 19.2). Those patients enrolled in an enhanced recovery protocol should adhere to this (see Chapter 35).

Specific preparation of the patient

Certain comorbidities can require additional preoperative preparation. Examples include:
- admission in the immediate preoperative phase for blood product administration;
- i.v. hydration for those at particularly high risk of renal impairment or significant hypercalcaemia; and
- management of bridging anticoagulation in the high-risk patients.

These requirements should be decided by the preoperative assessment clinic, having sought specific specialist advice and clearly documented and communicated this to all relevant members of the surgical team. The requirements for specific medical conditions are discussed in Chapter 20.

Communication of anticipated perioperative care needs

Patients requiring booking to extended recovery, HDU or ICU can be identified in clinic. Similarly, care requirements such as wheelchair transfer for the patient with poor mobility or bariatric equipment for the morbidly obese patient can be highlighted to theatres and ward areas.

Premedication and other prophylactic measures

Premedication refers to the administration of drugs in the two-hour period before induction of anaesthesia. Note that many regularly prescribed medications should have been taken at the usual time, and if the patient has omitted a drug, many can be given in the hours before surgery. The objectives of premedication are to:
- allay anxiety and fear;
- reduce secretions;
- reduce the volume and increase the pH of gastric contents;
- reduce PONV; and
- provide pre-emptive analgesia

Relief from anxiety

Surgical patients have a high incidence of anxiety, which in addition to its undesirable psychological effects has been associated with reduced patient satisfaction and an increased risk of PONV and acute postoperative pain. Relief from anxiety is accomplished most effectively by non-pharmacological means: establishing a rapport at the preoperative visit; providing a clear explanation of the process and events; seeking to address specific fears with honest advice; empathy; reassurance; and basic psychotherapeutic and relaxation techniques.

In selected patients it may be appropriate to offer anxiolytic medication such as benzodiazepines or α_2-agonists (see Chapter 4).

Reduction in secretions

Historically, premedication with an anticholinergic agent was common, as older agents, particularly ether, stimulated the production of secretions from pharyngeal and bronchial glands. This problem occurs rarely with modern anaesthetic agents, and anticholinergic premedication is seldom used, except in awake fibreoptic intubation (when excessive salivation can create extra difficulty) or occasionally before using ketamine.

Reduction in gastric volume and elevation of gastric pH

In patients at risk of vomiting or regurgitation (e.g. emergency patients with a full stomach, elective patients with hiatus hernia, obstetric patients), it may be desirable to promote gastric emptying and elevate the pH of residual gastric contents. Gastric emptying may be enhanced by the administration of metoclopramide, which also possesses some antiemetic properties, whereas elevation of the pH of gastric contents may be produced by administration of sodium citrate or H_2-receptor antagonists.

PONV prophylaxis

Nausea and vomiting are common sequelae of anaesthesia. Antiemetics (see Chapter 7) may be given as an oral premedication, particularly in day-case surgery (see Chapter 34). Acupuncture at the wrist PC6 point is also effective and should be sited before surgery.

Pre-emptive analgesia

The preoperative administration of oral analgesia (e.g. paracetamol or NSAIDs) is effective and economical. This is often embedded into care pathways in day-case and paediatric units. Care must be taken to ensure that a second dose is not delivered intraoperatively. Premedication with opioids is now rarely used in elective surgery, but it is common for trauma and emergency patients to have received opioids before arriving to theatre.

Other prophylactic measures
Steroid supplementation

Steroid supplementation is discussed in Chapter 20.

Chapter | **20** |

Intercurrent disease and anaesthesia

Damian Doyle, Alexa Mannings

The number of surgical procedures carried out in patients previously considered unfit for surgery is increasing. A growing proportion have significant coexisting medical conditions, are older and may have a limited physiological reserve. These factors influence the conduct of anaesthesia and surgery and must be considered when assessing and managing an individual patient.

Intercurrent disease and drug therapy may affect anaesthesia and surgery in a number of ways.

- The effects of anaesthesia
- The choice of anaesthetic technique
- The choice of surgical procedure or technique
- Normal compensatory responses to anaesthesia or surgery
- The investigations required, preoperative preparation and timing of surgery
- Postoperative management and resources (e.g. availability of ICU beds)
- The course of the disease may be modified by anaesthesia and surgery

In severe cases the patient's condition may preclude a successful outcome from the proposed anaesthesia and surgery.

Cardiovascular disease

Ischaemic heart disease

The presence of coronary, cerebral or peripheral vascular disease defines a group of patients at increased risk of perioperative cardiac complications. These are described as major adverse cardiac events (MACE) and are estimated to complicate between 1.4% and 3.9% of surgeries. They include myocardial ischaemia, myocardial infarction (MI), arrhythmias, cardiac failure and death from myocardial causes.

Preoperative assessment

The preoperative assessment of patients with ischaemic heart disease (IHD) should follow a stepwise approach.

Clinical features

A detailed history and examination should identify recent or previous MI, unstable angina, significant arrhythmias or valvular heart disease. Diabetes, stroke, renal insufficiency and pulmonary disease are significant related comorbidities. The presence of one or more of the following active conditions is considered to make a patient at high risk for MACE:

- acute coronary syndrome (ACS), unstable angina or recent MI;
- decompensated heart failure;
- significant arrhythmias; and/or
- severe valvular disease (aortic stenosis with a gradient >40 mmHg/valve area <1.0 cm^2 or symptomatic mitral stenosis)

The presence of these active conditions requires urgent management and may result in delay to non-urgent surgery.

Functional capacity

A simple assessment of physiological reserve can be made by quantifying a patient's metabolic equivalents (METs) (see Chapter 19). If a patient has no major cardiac risk factors and can achieve more than 4 METs of activity without significant cardiorespiratory symptoms, then the perioperative risk of an adverse cardiac event is low. A more detailed assessment of reserve can be made through the use of cardiopulmonary exercise (CPEX) testing. It may be possible to improve cardiorespiratory reserve before surgery in some patients (see Chapter 30).

Extent of surgery

The extent of surgery determines the level of physiological stress which the patient will experience. Examples of high-risk (cardiac morbidity >5%), intermediate-risk (cardiac morbidity 1%–5%) and low-risk (cardiac morbidity <1%) procedures are shown in Table 20.1.

Cardiac risk stratification

The revised cardiac risk index (RCRI) can be used to identify several risk factors in patients undergoing non-cardiac surgery. It includes six predictors of risk:

1. High-risk surgery
2. History of IHD
3. Biventricular cardiac failure
4. Cerebrovascular disease
5. Preoperative treatment with insulin
6. Renal impairment (serum creatinine >177 μmol L^{-1})

Table 20.1 Surgical risk estimate according to type of surgery or intervention

High risk (reported cardiac risk >5%)	Vascular: aortic aneurysm repair (elective and ruptured); lower limb amputation. Thoracic: lung resection; oesophagectomy; gastric surgery. General surgery: emergency laparotomy; open bowel resection; open hepatic/pancreatic resection.
Intermediate (reported cardiac risk 1%–5%)	Vascular: endovascular aneurysm repair; lower limb vascular bypass surgery. General surgery: open cholecystectomy; laparoscopic hepatic/splenic/colorectal resection.
Low risk: (reported cardiac risk <1%)	Gynaecology: hysterectomy; hysteroscopy. Orthopaedic: arthroscopy; hip/knee arthroplasty. Urological: transurethral resection of prostate. General surgery: hernia; laparoscopic/open appendicectomy; laparoscopic cholecystectomy; rectal surgery.

(Adapted from Glance, L. G., Lustik, S. J., Hannan, E. L., et al. (2012) The surgical mortality probability model: derivation and validation of a simple risk prediction rule for noncardiac surgery. *Annals of Surgery.* 255, 696–702.)

The presence of two risk factors has been equated to a risk of MACE approaching 7% and three risk factors, 11%.

The American College of Surgeons National Surgical Quality Improvement Program (ACS NSQIP) surgical risk calculator (available as an Internet-based calculator) has been developed to provide surgery-specific risk calculation. Up to 21 patient variables are used to calculate the risk of 10 outcomes, including MACE and death.

Management

Having made the assessment, subsequent management may be outlined as shown in Fig. 20.1.

- If the patient requires *emergency* non-cardiac surgery, they should proceed to surgery without any further cardiac testing.
- If the surgery is *elective, but the patient has evidence of ACS*, surgery should be deferred. The patient should undergo further cardiac assessment. Once optimised, the patient's perioperative risk should be reassessed.
- In patients scheduled for *elective surgery without any evidence of ACS*, a risk assessment of MACE should be made based on surgery type, RCRI or NSQIP tools.
- Those patients with a risk of MACE estimated to be < 1% should proceed to surgery. No further testing is required in this group of patients.
- The management of patients with a risk of MACE ≥ 1% depends on their functional capacity. In the group of patients with an unknown or poor functional capacity (<4 METs), consideration should be given to non-invasive cardiac testing. Cardiac testing, however, should only be undertaken if results are going to change anaesthetic or surgical management; those patients with a good functional capacity (≥ 4 METs) should proceed to surgery.

Investigations

Recent guidelines from the UK National Institute for Health and Care Excellence (NICE) have reviewed the tests recommended before elective surgery, and these are discussed in detail in Chapter 19.

Management of pre-existing cardiovascular disease

Ischaemic heart disease. Medical therapy should be reviewed and optimised if symptoms are poorly controlled. The American College of Cardiology recommends at least a 60-day interval between an ACS event and elective non-cardiac surgery.

Previous coronary bypass graft surgery. Few data are available to clarify the interval required before undertaking non-cardiac surgery after coronary artery bypass grafts (CABGs). Asymptomatic patients may constitute a low-risk group at 6 weeks postoperatively, although studies have

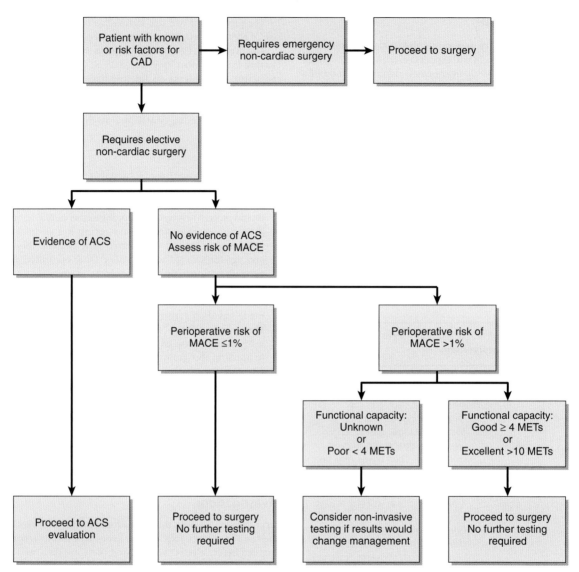

Fig. 20.1 Stepwise approach to perioperative cardiac assessment for coronary artery disease. *ACS,* Acute coronary syndrome; *CAD,* coronary artery disease; *MACE,* major adverse cardiac event; *METS,* metabolic equivalent of task. (Adapted from Fleisher, L. A., Fleischmann, K. E., & Auerbach, A. D., et al. (2014) 2014 ACC/AHA guideline on perioperative cardiovascular evaluation and management of patients undergoing noncardiac surgery: Executive summary. *Journal of the American College of Cardiology.* 64, 2373–2405.)

found an increased risk associated with the presence of a low ejection fraction < 45% or a right ventricular systolic pressure > 40 mmHg. In those patients a delay of at least 3 months is advised.

Previous percutaneous coronary intervention. Percutaneous coronary intervention (PCI) has become a standard and increasingly common intervention in patients suffering from ACS. Fewer than 10% of patients undergo angioplasty alone; the remaining patients have an intracoronary stent inserted to maintain coronary artery patency. The major risk with coronary stents is restenosis by thrombus formation or re-endothelialisation resulting in an MI, which may be associated with a mortality of up to 50%. Bare metal stents (BMS) are only used in up to 15% of cases. The remainder are drug-eluting stents (DES), which have a lower restenosis rate. A cytotoxic agent is released by the DES to limit the risk of endothelialisation. In both types of stents, dual antiplatelet therapy (DAPT) with aspirin and a P2Y12 inhibitor (e.g. clopidogrel; see Chapter 14) is recommended to reduce stent thrombosis. Current guidelines recommend DAPT after PCI for a minimum of 1 month in patients with BMS and 6 months with DES. If DAPT is tolerated without risk of bleeding, it may be reasonable for it to be continued beyond 12 months. This is an important clinical problem as it is estimated that as many as 5%–10% of patients with coronary stents may present for surgery within 1 year of stent implantation.

Guidelines now recommend elective non-cardiac surgery should be delayed 14 days after balloon angioplasty and 30 days after BMS implantation. In patients with DES the highest risk of stent thrombosis persists for the 3 months postimplantation, and surgery should initially be deferred if

possible. With newer second-generation–type DES, the risk of stent thrombus falls at 6 months. At that point DAPT can be discontinued to allow surgery. Between 3 and 6 months it is a balance of risk, considering urgency of surgery, risk of bleeding if DAPT is continued perioperatively and risk of thrombus if it is discontinued. Low-dose aspirin should be continued perioperatively provided surgical bleeding risk allows and P2Y12 inhibitors should be restarted postoperatively. More recently an alternative type of polymer-free stent has been introduced (e.g. BioFreedom). This type of stent is claimed to have a restenosis risk similar to that of DES, with the advantage of requiring DAPT for only 1 month. This may represent a significant advantage in those patients who are at high risk of bleeding if prescribed long-term DAPT. Appropriate management will require discussion with the patient, surgeon and cardiologists (Fig. 20.2).

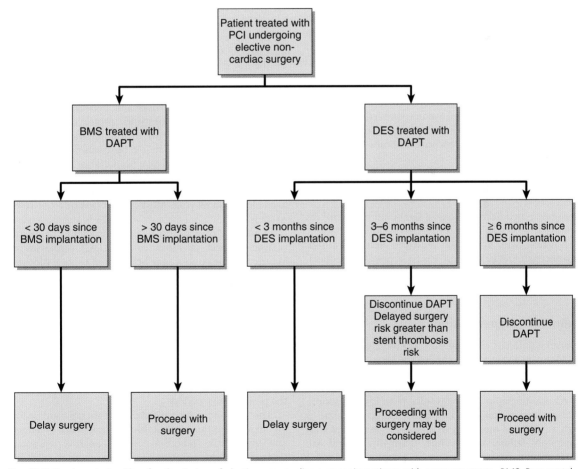

Fig. 20.2 Treatment algorithm for the timing of elective non-cardiac surgery in patients with coronary stents. *BMS,* Bare metal stent; *DAPT,* dual antiplatelet therapy; *DES,* drug-eluting stent; *PCI,* percutaneous coronary intervention. (Reprinted with permission. *Circulation.* 2016; 134, e123–e155. ©2016 American Heart Association, Inc.)

Hypertension

Raised arterial pressure is one of the major preventable causes of morbidity and mortality in the general population. It is a major risk factor for ischaemic and haemorrhagic stroke, MI, heart failure, chronic kidney disease (CKD) and premature death. British Hypertension Society guidelines recommend starting antihypertensive therapy for sustained pressures greater than 140/90 mmHg. However, in the perioperative setting there is little evidence that patients with stage 2 hypertension (<180/110 mmHg) and no evidence of end-organ damage have an increased risk of cardiovascular complications. Isolated hypertension below this level is classified as a low risk factor. If hypertension is identified preoperatively the risks of anaesthesia and surgery are dependent on the presence and severity of end-organ damage.

Current UK recommendations are that a patient with a recorded blood pressure measurement less than 160/100 mmHg in the preceding 12 months should proceed to surgery. In those patients without a recording in the preceding 12 months, a blood pressure of less than 180/110 mmHg at the time of preassessment is acceptable to proceed with surgery. For non-urgent surgery, patients with severe hypertension (i.e. >180/110 mmHg) should be referred back to primary care for blood pressure control. Patients with hypertension, both controlled and uncontrolled, have a more labile haemodynamic profile intraoperatively. The perioperative management of antihypertensive medication is discussed in Chapter 19.

Heart failure

Decompensated heart failure is a significant risk factor for perioperative MACE. Patients may have systolic or diastolic dysfunction, with or without preserved ejection fraction. Treatment should be optimised as far as possible preoperatively and investigation of underlying coronary artery disease undertaken as appropriate.

Pulmonary hypertension

A mean pulmonary artery pressure >25 mmHg is diagnostic of pulmonary hypertension. This may be idiopathic in nature or secondary to left-sided heart disease, lung disease or chronic thromboembolic disease. Diagnosis is confirmed by echocardiography and right-sided heart catheterisation. Perioperative mortality in non-cardiac surgery may be as high as 18% and morbidity of up to 42%, associated with respiratory failure, heart failure, dysrhythmias and MI. Intraoperative management can be complex, requiring a balance of maintaining right ventricular output and avoiding excessive afterload. Senior experienced management is essential.

Cerebrovascular disease

A history of previous ischaemic stroke is a recognised risk factor for MACE as measured by the RCRI. There may be up to a fivefold increase in risk of 30-day mortality and MACE regardless of timing between stroke and surgery. This risk is highest in those patients suffering a stroke less than 3 months before surgery and appears to stabilise after 9 months. The type of surgery does not seem to affect the risk of cerebrovascular event.

Treatment and additional interventions

β-blockers. Established β-blocker therapy should be maintained throughout the perioperative period either orally or i.v. if necessary. Sudden preoperative cessation may be associated with rebound effects such as angina, MI, arrhythmias and hypertension. Intraoperative bradycardia usually responds to i.v. atropine or glycopyrronium bromide. There is evidence to support starting perioperative β-blocker therapy for patients at high cardiac risk. It should, however, be initiated days to weeks before elective surgery and not started on the day of surgery. This practice may reduce non-fatal MI but with an increased risk of postoperative stroke, hypotension and death. Thus patients must be carefully counselled regarding the risks and benefits of initiating perioperative β-blockers for cardiac protection.

Arrhythmias. Preoperative arrhythmias should be treated before surgery. The patient should be screened for predisposing factors such as IHD, valvular heart disease and electrolyte and endocrine abnormalities.

Atrial fibrillation (AF) affects up to 5% of the population aged older than 69 years. Most cases of new-onset AF revert to sinus rhythm spontaneously within 24 h. Haemodynamically unstable or symptomatic patients should be offered pharmacological or direct current (DC) cardioversion. Ventricular rate control may be required using β-blockers, calcium channel blockers or digoxin, with a target ventricular rate before surgery of less than 90 beats min^{-1}. Sustained AF is associated with a risk of thromboembolic events, including stroke. This risk can be calculated by the use of the CHA$_2$DS$_2$-VASc scoring system. Depending on the score, patients will require long-term anticoagulation with either warfarin or direct oral anticoagulants (DOACs). These drugs may need to be discontinued perioperatively as described earlier. Antiarrhythmic therapy should continue throughout the perioperative period.

The indications for antiarrhythmic therapy and pacing are identical to those applicable in the absence of surgery and anaesthesia. Indications for preoperative temporary pacing include:

- bradyarrhythmia unresponsive to atropine if associated with syncope, hypotension or ventricular arrhythmias;
- risk of asystole;

- complete heart block;
- second-degree heart block (Mobitz type II);
- first-degree heart block associated with bifascicular block; and
- sick sinus syndrome.

Angiotensin-converting enzyme inhibitors (ACEIs) and angiotensin II receptor antagonists. Angiotensin-converting enzyme inhibitors (ACEIs) and angiotensin II receptor antagonists have disease-modifying effects in patients with vascular disease, heart failure and diabetes, with a long-term reduction in cardiac morbidity and mortality. Their continued use preoperatively may be associated with intraoperative hypotension.

Antiplatelet agents. Aspirin is an irreversible cyclo-oxygenase (COX) inhibitor, blocking the synthesis of thromboxane A_2. The antiplatelet effect lasts for the life span of a platelet (7–10 days). P2Y12 receptors are adenosine diphosphate (ADP) receptors expressed on the surface of thrombocytes, which can be blocked chemically, resulting in reduced platelet aggregation. Currently clopidogrel, prasugrel and ticagrelor are in use as P2Y12 receptor antagonists. Patients may be on DAPT, either aspirin combined with a P2Y12 receptor antagonist or a combination of clopidogrel and ticagrelor if intolerant of aspirin. Management of antiplatelet drugs in the perioperative period is a balance of bleeding risk if continued and risk of cardiovascular complications (stent thrombosis, stroke) if discontinued (see Chapter 19 and Fig. 20.2).

Anticoagulants. Warfarin and the newer DOACs are widely used as oral anticoagulants in patients at risk of thrombosis. As with DAPT, management of these during the perioperative period is a balance of risk of thrombosis and risk of bleeding (see Chapter 19).

Statins. Statins reduce morbidity and mortality in patients with vascular disease even in the presence of a normal cholesterol concentration. This is thought to result from stabilisation of atheromatous plaques. There is some evidence in patients undergoing high-risk vascular surgery that initiating statin therapy may reduce cardiovascular complications. Treatment should continue perioperatively in those patients on long-term statins.

General anaesthetic principles in patients with cardiovascular disease

Having ensured that management of the patient's cardiovascular disease is optimised (see Chapters 19 & 30), anaesthesia should comprise a balanced technique aimed at maintaining cardiovascular stability. A variety of options may be suitable, including general or regional anaesthesia or a combination of both. Tachycardia should be avoided and an adequate arterial pressure maintained; there should not be a sustained reduction in arterial pressure of >20% of the patient's normal blood pressure. Coronary perfusion and myocardial oxygen delivery are thus maintained without increasing myocardial work and oxygen requirements.

The level of intraoperative monitoring should be dictated by risk assessment. The following should be considered in addition to standard monitoring:

- *Five-lead ECG.* The usual ECG configuration for anaesthetic monitoring is standard limb lead II. Whilst this is useful for identifying arrhythmias, myocardial ischaemia occurs most commonly in the left ventricle and is detected more sensitively with a CM5 configuration.
- *Direct arterial pressure recording.*
- *CVP monitoring* (with or without central venous oxygen saturations).
- *Oesophageal Doppler or transoesophageal echocardiography (TOE).* These provide a measurement of cardiac function, output and intravascular filling.
- *Minimally invasive cardiac output monitors.* These are devices that derive cardiac output and other variables from the arterial pressure waveform using internal algorithms. Some (FloTrac or LiDCO (Lithium Dilution Cardiac Output) devices) use a standard arterial catheter, whereas others (PiCCO (Pulse Index Continuous Cardiac Output)) require a dedicated thermistor-tipped catheter in a proximal (femoral or axillary) artery.

For patients identified as high-risk, specific consideration should be given to reducing the surgical stress response (see Chapter 13). Measures to achieve this are dictated by the patient and operative factors. These include:

- *Use of neuraxial blockade.* This has been associated with reduced risk of perioperative myocardial ischaemia and infarction. However, this must be balanced against the accompanying sympathetic block and associated hypotension, which may be pronounced, particularly with a high spinal block. Early judicious use of vasopressors, coupled with maintenance of intravascular volume, should limit this problem. However, neuraxial blockade, particularly spinal block, is relatively contraindicated if there is severely limited cardiovascular reserve and if maintenance of adequate arterial pressure is critical, such as in severe aortic stenosis.
- *Effective perioperative analgesia.* This is essential because pain is a potent stimulator of the stress response, and uncontrolled sympathetic activation increases myocardial work and oxygen demand, predisposing to myocardial ischaemia or infarction.
- *Maintaining oxygenation, normocapnia and electrolyte balance at all times.*
- *Close attention to fluid balance.* This begins preoperatively when fluid depletion secondary to factors such as excessive fasting times and bowel preparation should be corrected. As far as possible, euvolaemia should be maintained. Intravascular volume depletion is known to compromise organ perfusion and oxygen delivery, but

Table 20.2 Generic pacemaker codes

Letter 1	Letter 2	Letter 3	Letter 4	Letter 5
Pacing chamber	Sensing chamber	Response to sensing	Programmability	Multisite pacing
O = None A = Atrium V = Ventricle D = Dual (atrium and ventricle)	O = None A = Atrium V = Ventricle D = Dual (atrium and ventricle)	O = None I = Inhibited T = Triggered D = Dual (inhibited and triggered)	O = None R = Rate modulation	O = None A = Atrium V = Ventricle D = Dual (atrium and ventricle)

there is increasing evidence that postoperative recovery is also compromised by excessive volume and sodium loading in the immediate perioperative period.

- *Monitoring haemoglobin concentrations.* Patients at high risk from cardiovascular disease do not tolerate anaemia. The optimal concentration of haemoglobin is the subject of much discussion but is probably around 100 g L^{-1}.
- *Active patient warming to avoid hypothermia.* Hypothermia activates the stress response, predisposes to arrhythmias and increases oxygen consumption postoperatively as a result of shivering.

Before embarking on anaesthesia and surgery, the patient's management and destination postoperatively should be planned; for example, would benefit be derived from a period of mechanical ventilation or continued close monitoring in HDU/ICU? Good communication between all the relevant clinicians, including anaesthesia, critical care, surgical and cardiology teams, is important.

Anaesthetic agents

Volatile anaesthetic agents may have cardioprotective effects through both pre- and postischaemic conditioning. Propofol is also likely to be cardioprotective via free radical scavenging and an antioxidant effect. There is conflicting evidence in cardiac surgery to support either a volatile- or propofol-based type of anaesthetic; trials in non-cardiac surgery indicate no difference in cardiovascular outcomes. High-dose opiates are thought to be cardioprotective. Remifentanil is widely used for its potent analgesic effect and fast offset.

Cardiac implantable electronic devices

The number of patients presenting for surgery with cardiac implantable electronic devices (CIEDs) is increasing. They fall into three categories.

1. Implantable loop recorders: leadless and have a diagnostic function only.
2. Permanent pacemakers (PPMs): inserted for symptomatic bradycardia, caused by atrioventricular (AV) block and

for sick sinus syndrome. Biventricular PPMs are indicated for patients with moderate to severe cardiac failure.

3. Implantable cardioverter-defibrillators (ICDs): sense and analyse myocardial electrical activity and are capable of pacing and shock therapy when necessary.

Pacemakers are classified by a series of five letters relating to their various functions (Table 20.2).

Specific issues in anaesthetic management

- The indication(s) for pacemaker insertion, its history and mode of action noted and any evidence of malfunction should be sought. Patients should carry a pacemaker patient identification card. The underlying rhythm and rate should be determined and the consequences in case of pacemaker malfunction failure known to determine the need for backup support. Guidelines vary, but it is generally acceptable for a PPM to have been checked within 12 months and an ICD within 6 months.
- Before surgery the cardiology department or pacemaker clinic should be liaised with. Loop recorders require no intervention. If a patient is pacemaker dependent, the device will require reprogramming to a fixed pacing mode. All ICDs will require tachycardia therapies switching off.
- Standard perioperative monitoring should be used. An appropriate ECG lead should be used to demonstrate any pacing spikes.
- Hypoxia, hypercapnia, acidaemia and electrolyte abnormalities (potassium and magnesium) should be avoided as they may precipitate arrhythmias or interfere with pacemaker capture.
- Central venous catheters may dislodge pacing leads, particularly if the pacemaker has only recently been inserted. Consideration should be given to use of the femoral vein for central venous access and to alternative monitors of cardiac output.
- Equipment should be immediately available for external defibrillation or temporary pacing as required. Defibrillator/pacing pads should be sited before surgery. Anteroposterior pad positioning is preferred.

- Magnetic resonance imaging is contraindicated in the presence of older CIEDs; some newer cardiac-conditional devices are now being inserted.
- Electromechanical interference (EMI): Although modern pacemakers and ICDs are designed with a high tolerance to EMI, a variety of effects may still occur such as pacemaker inhibition, induction of fixed rate pacing, software reset or triggering of shocks with an ICD. The potential sources of EMI include:
  - *Diathermy.* Should be avoided wherever possible. Bipolar is safer than monopolar. If monopolar is required, cables and pads should be kept away from the CIED implant site. Short bursts and cutting rather than coagulation current should be used.
  - *Radiofrequency ablation.* Defibrillator function of ICDs should be disabled.
  - *Electroconvulsive therapy (ECT).* The short electrical stimulus (1–2 s) with ECT is unlikely to be significant. Subsequent seizure activity may cause oversensing. Pacemakers should be converted to asynchronous mode; ICDs should be disabled.

Most PPMs will revert to an asynchronous (fixed-rate) mode when a magnet is held over the generator. For ICDs, placing a magnet over the device will switch off the anti-tachycardia therapy but will have no effect on the pacing mode. The use of magnets to adjust CIED function should only be done with expert supervision.

All CIEDs should be routinely checked postoperatively either before discharge or via an early appointment at the pacemaker clinic.

Valvular heart disease

In both aortic and mitral stenosis, there is a low fixed cardiac output, which leaves no reserve to compensate for changes in heart rate or vascular resistance. Regurgitant lesions are usually better tolerated. As with IHD, specific intervention such as valve replacement or valvuloplasty is indicated before non-cardiac surgery only if the valvular lesion merits intervention in its own right. Clearly, in an emergency situation, this is not an option.

General principles

- The patient's functional reserve is a good indicator of the severity of a valve lesion.
- Routine antibiotic prophylaxis is no longer recommended for all patients with valvular heart disease.
- Patients with valvular heart disease may be receiving anticoagulants; adhering to local bridging protocols is necessary.
- No specific anaesthetic technique is preferred for valvular heart disease. The aim is to maintain cardiovascular stability. In severe disease this is often best achieved

using a general anaesthetic technique with opioids and controlled ventilation.
- Invasive monitoring is often required in these patients.

Aortic stenosis

Isolated aortic stenosis is associated most commonly with calcification, often on a congenitally bicuspid valve. In rheumatic heart disease, aortic stenosis occurs rarely in the absence of mitral disease and is combined usually with regurgitation. The diagnosis is suggested by the findings of an ejection systolic murmur, low pulse pressure and clinical and ECG evidence of left ventricular hypertrophy. It is important to distinguish between aortic stenosis and the murmur of aortic sclerosis found in some older patients. Clinical signs provide a guide: a slow-rising, low-volume pulse with reduced pulse pressure; reduced intensity of the second heart sound; and the presence of a click are suggestive of stenosis, as is evidence of left ventricular hypertrophy on ECG. However, echocardiography with Doppler flow monitoring is essential for confirmation and assessment of severity. The American Heart Association classification of aortic stenosis is shown in Table 20.3. The heart size on chest radiograph is normal until late in the disease, whereas symptoms of angina, exertional syncope and left ventricular failure indicate advanced disease. Untreated severe symptomatic stenosis has a 50% 1-year survival rate.

Perioperative mortality is increased in patients with aortic stenosis. Left ventricular systolic function is usually good, but the hypertrophied ventricle has reduced compliance. Tachycardia and arrhythmias that compromise ventricular filling are poorly tolerated and should be avoided. In aortic stenosis, up to 40% of ventricular filling results from atrial systole; therefore, maintenance of sinus rhythm is important. Tachycardia also reduces the duration of coronary perfusion,

Table 20.3 American Heart Association classification of severity of aortic stenosis based on echocardiographic measurements

	Mild	Moderate	Severe
Aortic valve area (cm²)	2.5–1.5	1.5–1.0	< 1.0
Mean pressure gradient across aortic valve (mmHg)	25–15	40–25	> 40
Velocity across aortic valve (m s⁻¹)	< 3.0	3.0–4.0	< 4.0

compromising blood supply to the hypertrophied ventricle, particularly if there is concomitant coronary artery disease. The resulting myocardial ischaemia causes further cardio-vascular deterioration, which may be catastrophic. Excessive bradycardia also compromises cardiac output. Adequate venous return must be maintained to ensure ventricular filling, and hypotension, which compromises coronary flow, must be avoided.

Mitral stenosis

Mitral stenosis is usually a manifestation of rheumatic heart disease. Characteristic features include AF, arterial embolism, pulmonary oedema (may be acute and precipitated by AF), pulmonary hypertension and right-sided heart failure. Patients with mitral stenosis who present for surgery are often receiving digoxin, diuretics and anticoagulants. Preoperative control of ventricular rate, treatment of pulmonary oedema and management of anticoagulant therapy (see Chapter 19) are necessary. During anaesthesia, control of heart rate is important. Tachycardia reduces diastolic ventricular filling and thus cardiac output, whereas bradycardia also results in decreased cardiac output because stroke output is limited. As with aortic stenosis, drugs which produce vasodilatation and neuroaxial block may cause severe hypotension. As a result of pre-existing pulmonary hypertension, patients are particularly vulnerable to hypoxaemia. Both hypoxaemia and acidaemia are potent pulmonary vasoconstrictors and may produce acute right ventricular failure. Thus opioid analgesics should be prescribed cautiously and airway obstruction avoided.

Aortic regurgitation

Acute aortic regurgitation (e.g. resulting from infective endocarditis) causes rapid left ventricular failure and may require emergency valve replacement, even in the presence of unresolved infection. Chronic aortic regurgitation is asymptomatic for many years. Left ventricular dilatation occurs, with eventual left ventricular failure. Patients with mild or moderate aortic regurgitation without left ventricular failure or major ventricular dilatation tolerate anaesthesia well. A slightly increased heart rate of approximately 100 beats min^{-1} is desirable because this reduces left ventricular dilatation. Bradycardia causes ventricular distension and should be avoided. Vasodilator therapy increases net forward flow by decreasing afterload and is useful in severe aortic regurgitation; isoflurane anaesthesia may be beneficial. Vasopressors should be avoided.

Mitral regurgitation

Leaflet mitral regurgitation usually results from infective endocarditis, rheumatic fever or mitral valve prolapse.

Chordal or papillary muscle mitral regurgitation is more commonly secondary to ischaemia or MI. If occurring acutely, pulmonary oedema results and urgent valve replacement is required. Left ventricular failure with ventricular dilatation may cause functional mitral regurgitation. Chronic mitral regurgitation is commonly associated with mitral stenosis. In pure mitral regurgitation, left atrial dilatation occurs with a minimal increase in atrial pressure. The degree of regurgitation may be limited by reducing the volume of the left ventricle and the impedance to left ventricular ejection. Thus inotropic agents and vasodilators may be useful, whereas vasopressors should be avoided. A slight increase in heart rate is desirable unless there is concomitant stenosis.

Mitral valve prolapse

Mitral valve prolapse is most common in young women and may be an incidental finding in up to 5% of patients. It is associated with atypical chest pains, palpitations and embolic phenomena. Patients may be taking antiarrhythmic agents which need to be continued perioperatively.

Infective endocarditis

This is caused predominantly by the viridans group of streptococci, occasionally by gram-negative organisms or enterococci, and also by staphylococci, especially after cardiac surgery or in i.v. drug abusers. *Coxiella burnetii* also accounts for some cases. Patients with rheumatic or congenital heart disease, including asymptomatic lesions (e.g. bicuspid aortic valve), are at higher risk.

Hypertrophic cardiomyopathy

Hypertrophic cardiomyopathy (HOCM) is a genetic cardiac disorder affecting 1 in 500 adults. There is a variable degree of ventricular muscle hypertrophy affecting mainly the interventricular septum. Patients may remain asymptomatic, or they may suffer dyspnoea, angina and syncope as a result of muscle hypertrophy and subsequent left ventricular outflow obstruction. Hypertrophic cardiomyopathy is also a cause of sudden cardiac death caused by arrhythmias. Diagnosis is confirmed by echocardiography. Anaesthetic issues include the following:

- Acute changes in volume status cause severe haemo-dynamic consequences, and hypovolaemia should be avoided.
- Outflow obstruction is exacerbated by catecholamines so inotropic agents should be avoided.
- Patients are usually receiving a β-blocker, which should be continued perioperatively.
- Patients with previous malignant ventricular arrhythmias are likely to have an ICD *in situ*.

Respiratory disease

Successful anaesthetic management of the patient with respiratory disease depends on accurate assessment of the nature and extent of functional impairment and an appreciation of the effects of surgery and anaesthesia on pulmonary function.

Assessment

History

Of the six cardinal symptoms of respiratory disease (cough, sputum, haemoptysis, dyspnoea, wheeze and chest pain), dyspnoea provides the best indication of functional impairment. Specific questioning is required to elicit the extent to which activity is limited by dyspnoea. Dyspnoea at rest or on minor exertion clearly indicates severe disease. A cough productive of purulent sputum indicates active infection. Chronic copious sputum production may indicate bronchiectasis. A history of heavy smoking or occupational exposure to dust may suggest pulmonary pathology.

A detailed drug history is important. Long-term steroid therapy ($\geq$ prednisolone 5 mg day^{-1} or equivalent (Table 20.4)) within 3 months of the date of surgery necessitates augmented cover for the perioperative period (see later; Table 20.9); adverse effects include hypokalaemia and hyperglycaemia. Bronchodilators should be continued during the perioperative period. Patients with cor pulmonale may be receiving digoxin and diuretics.

Examination

A full physical examination is required, with emphasis on detecting signs of airway obstruction, increased work of breathing, active infection which may be treated preoperatively, and

Table 20.4 Equivalent doses of glucocorticoids

Glucocorticoid	Dose (mg)
Betamethasone	3
Cortisone acetate	100
Dexamethasone	3
Hydrocortisone	80
Methylprednisolone	16
Prednisolone	20
Triamcinolone	16

evidence of right-sided heart failure. The presence of obesity, cyanosis or dyspnoea should be noted. In addition, a simple forced expiratory manoeuvre may reveal prolonged expiration, and a simple test of exercise tolerance may be useful, such as a supervised walk test (see Chapter 19). Measurement of oxygen saturation provides a quick and useful indication of oxygenation; SpO_2 greater than 95% on air excludes significant hypoxaemia and, by inference, hypercapnia.

Investigations

These are discussed in Chapter 19.

Effects of anaesthesia and surgery

The effects of anaesthesia alone on respiratory function are generally minor and short lived but may tip the balance towards respiratory failure in patients with severe disease. These effects include:

- mucosal irritation by anaesthetic agents;
- ciliary paralysis;
- introduction of infection by aspiration or tracheal intubation; and
- respiratory depression by neuromuscular blocking agents (NMBAs), opioid analgesics or volatile anaesthetic agents.

In addition, anaesthesia is associated with a decrease in functional residual capacity (FRC), especially in older and obese patients. This leads to closure of basal airways and shunting of blood through inadequately ventilated areas of lung, an effect which is magnified by inhibition of the hypoxic pulmonary vasoconstrictor reflex. After recovery from anaesthesia, residual concentrations of anaesthetic agents and the presence of opioids inhibit the hyperventilatory responses to both hypercapnia and hypoxaemia so that, without close monitoring with pulse oximetry and appropriate blood gas analysis, serious hypoxaemia and hypercapnia may occur. After thoracic and upper abdominal surgery, the decrease in FRC is more profound and persists for 5–10 days, with a parallel increase in alveolar–arterial oxygen tension difference. Complications, including atelectasis and pneumonia, occur in approximately 20% of these patients. The effects of surgery are dependent on its type and magnitude. Clearly, patients with pre-existing respiratory disease are at much greater risk after upper abdominal and thoracic surgery than after limb, head and neck or lower abdominal surgery.

The use of appropriate regional anaesthetic techniques, where possible, confers several advantages in patients with respiratory disease both intra- and postoperatively, including:

- avoidance of tracheal intubation and controlled ventilation;
- reduced or absent requirement for respiratory depressant agents such as volatile anaesthetic agents and opioids;

- effective analgesia, allowing the patient to undergo chest physiotherapy and take deep breaths thereby maintaining FRC. This may potentially reduce hypoxaemia.

Obstructive pulmonary disease

Obstructive pulmonary disease includes both chronic obstructive pulmonary disease (COPD) and bronchial asthma. Patients with bronchiectasis and cystic fibrosis may also demonstrate marked airways obstruction and justify a similar management approach.

Chronic obstructive pulmonary disease

Chronic obstructive pulmonary disease is characterised by the presence of productive cough for at least 3 months in two successive years. Airways obstruction is caused by bronchoconstriction which has minimal or no reversibility, bronchial oedema and hypersecretion of mucus. In the postoperative period, pulmonary atelectasis and pneumonia result if sputum is not cleared. Severe disease may be accompanied by the signs and symptoms of right-sided heart failure.

Asthma

Asthma is characterised by airway inflammation and hyper-responsiveness causing reversible airway obstruction resulting in episodic wheeze, chest tightness, cough and breathlessness. It is estimated that just over 5 million people in the UK are treated for asthma. Management of asthma follows a stepwise approach dependent on the frequency and severity of symptoms and attacks (e.g. British Thoracic Society and Scottish Intercollegiate Guidelines Network guidelines):

- Short-acting β_2-agonists (salbutamol) are the first-line treatment.
- Regular or frequent attacks will require the use of inhaled corticosteroids (e.g. beclomethasone) as preventative therapy.
- Patients who are not adequately controlled with low-dose inhaled steroids will require additional therapies such as long-acting β_2-agonists (e.g. salmeterol), leukotriene-receptor agonists (e.g. montelukast) or a long-acting antimuscaric agent (e.g. tiotropium). Further treatments options include the use of oral theophyllines.

Preoperative management

The current state of the patient's disease is assessed by:

- history – frequency and severity of attacks, factors provoking attacks, recent episodes of infection, drug history;
- examination – presence or absence of wheeze, prolonged expiratory phase, overdistension, evidence of infection (cough, sputum, temperature, raised white cell count);
- pulmonary function tests – peak expiratory flow rate (PEFR) or forced expiratory volume in 1 s (FEV_1)/forced vital capacity (FVC) before and after inhalation of bronchodilator; and
- blood gas analysis, including changes in $PaCO_2$ to varying inspired oxygen concentrations.

Treatment of airways obstruction

Elective surgery should not be undertaken unless or until airways obstruction is well controlled. Existing bronchodilator therapy should be continued perioperatively. Patients prescribed long-term inhaled or systemic steroid therapy who are suboptimally controlled may require a course of augmented steroid therapy to cover the anaesthetic and postoperative periods (see Table 20.9). The steroid dose should be gradually reduced postoperatively, titrated against the severity of the asthma.

Treatment of active infection

Sputum for culture and sensitivities should be obtained to allow an appropriate choice of antibiotic. Chest physiotherapy and humidification of inspired gases aid expectoration. Elective surgery should be deferred whenever possible for a period of at least 4–6 weeks after lower respiratory tract infection.

Treatment of cardiac failure

Biventricular failure resulting from concurrent IHD and cor pulmonale often complicates COPD. Diuretics are indicated, and nitrates or digoxin may have a role.

Weight reduction

Weight reduction should be encouraged before elective surgery in obese patients with respiratory disease.

Smoking

Patients should be strongly encouraged to stop smoking for at least 6 weeks before elective surgery.

Anaesthesia

The anaesthetic technique in obstructive airways disease should be guided by the nature of the surgery and also the severity of the disease.

An approach with minimal intervention

Spontaneous ventilation with the option of local or regional anaesthesia is indicated for minor body surface operations. The use of a supraglottic airway (SAD) avoids tracheal intubation with its attendant risk of provoking bronchoconstriction, and if undue respiratory depression occurs, ventilation may be readily assisted. Volatile anaesthetic agents, being bronchodilators, are well tolerated in patients with asthma. Nerve plexus blocks and low subarachnoid or epidural anaesthesia enable limb, lower abdominal or pelvic surgery in patients with severe respiratory impairment. Sedation should be administered carefully to avoid respiratory compromise.

Elective mechanical ventilation

A decision may be made to undertake intermittent positive-pressure ventilation (IPPV) during anaesthesia and for a variable period after operation, at least until elimination of NMBAs and anaesthetic agents has occurred. This also permits optimal provision of analgesia without fear of opioid-induced depression of ventilation. Care should be taken with ventilator settings. A sufficiently long expiratory phase should be allowed to enable lung deflation and prevent gas trapping, and the inspiratory time should be adequate to avoid unduly high inflation pressures, with the attendant risk of pneumothorax.

Regional anaesthesia

A combined general/epidural anaesthetic technique is often useful for major abdominal or thoracic surgery, as there is good evidence of a reduction in postoperative pulmonary complications with effective epidural analgesia. This approach may avoid a need for postoperative IPPV in some patients or may be usefully combined with non-invasive ventilation (NIV).

Anaesthetic agents

Drugs that are associated with histamine release, such as atracurium and morphine, are perhaps best avoided, whereas rocuronium and fentanyl are preferred; β-blockers should also be avoided. If bronchospasm occurs during anaesthesia, it may result from easily remedied causes such as light anaesthesia or tracheal tube irritation, and these should be corrected. If bronchospasm persists, first-line treatment is the use of salbutamol, either 6–8 puffs of a metered dose inhaler down the tracheal tube or nebulised salbutamol 2.5–5 mg administered into the anaesthetic breathing circuit. If this is not immediately beneficial, salbutamol 125–250 µg or aminophylline 5 mg kg^{-1} should be administered by slow i.v. injection over at least 20 min, under ECG monitoring. The aminophylline dose should be modified if the patient is receiving oral theophylline. Thereafter, an infusion of aminophylline (up to 0.5 mg kg^{-1} h^{-1}) or salbutamol (5 µg min^{-1}) should be started. Hydrocortisone 200 mg i.v. should be given simultaneously, although it has no immediate effect. Other therapies include magnesium 50 mg kg^{-1} over 20 min to a maximum of 2 g or ketamine 10–20 mg boluses.

Postoperative care

Patients with severe disease or those undergoing major surgery should be nursed in an HDU or ICU setting. Elective NIV is increasingly used in high-risk patients, reducing the need for tracheal intubation. Modalities used include CPAP or non-invasive positive-pressure ventilation (NIPPV). High-flow nasal oxygenation (HFNO) provides some a low concentration of CPAP (approximately 3 cmH$_2$O) and is being used increasingly after tracheal extubation. This avoids the need for a tight-fitting mask or CPAP hood and is often better tolerated by patients. Patients who are likely to benefit or require NIV should be identified early in the surgical pathway. This facilitates careful anaesthetic management, familiarisation by the patient with equipment used and early implementation (including use in PACU if appropriate). Effective analgesia, either via epidural or regional techniques, is crucial in minimising postoperative respiratory complications.

Analgesia

Simple non-opioid analgesics and/or local and regional techniques should be used where possible. Non-steroidal anti-inflammatory drugs (NSAIDs), such as diclofenac or ibuprofen, are useful in reducing opioid requirements after major surgery. However, NSAIDs may aggravate bronchospasm in around 10% of people with asthma as a result of increased leukotriene production. These agents should not be given to patients with a history of aspirin hypersensitivity. Opioid analgesics are best administered, where necessary, in small i.v. doses under direct supervision or using patient-controlled analgesia. Physiotherapy, bronchodilators and antibiotics should be continued postoperatively.

Obstructive sleep apnoea

Obstructive sleep apnoea (OSA) is characterised by periods of complete or partial airway obstruction accompanied by oxygen desaturation and sympathetic activation. The condition may affect up to 5% of middle-aged individuals. Night-time sleep disturbance is associated with daytime somnolence. Long-term complications include hypertension, IHD, pulmonary hypertension and heart failure. Perioperatively, patients with OSA have a higher incidence of airway management difficulties, and postoperatively, they can be particularly sensitive to the sedative effects of anaesthetics and analgesics. Patients at risk may be identified using the STOP-BANG questionnaire (see Chapter 19, Box 19.1), with a score > 5 strongly suggestive of OSA. Diagnosis is confirmed by formal sleep studies, and the severity of OSA is graded by the apnoea–hypopnoea index (AHI) – that is, the number of events per hour of sleep. Treatment and symptom management are through weight loss and the use of CPAP. Patients with known OSA treated with CPAP should be encouraged to bring their machine with them to hospital to be used postoperatively. Patients with a high STOP-BANG score should be referred for sleep studies before elective surgery. Opioid use should be kept to a minimum and regional or local anaesthetic techniques used wherever possible. Patients with significant OSA are usually nursed in HDU during the initial postoperative period.

Bronchiectasis

The patient should receive intensive physiotherapy with postural drainage for several days before surgery. Appropriate antibiotics, based on sputum culture, should be prescribed. Severe disease localised in one lung should be isolated during anaesthesia using a double-lumen tracheal tube.

Restrictive lung disease

Restrictive lung disease includes a wide range of conditions which affect the lung and chest wall. Lung diseases include sarcoidosis and fibrosing alveolitis, and lesions of the chest wall include kyphoscoliosis and ankylosing spondylitis. Pulmonary function tests reveal a decrease in both FEV_1 and FVC, with a normal FEV_1/FVC ratio and decreased FRC and total lung capacity (TLC). Small airways closure occurs during tidal ventilation, with resultant shunting and hypoxaemia. Lung or chest wall compliance is decreased; thus the work of breathing is increased, and the ability to cough and clear secretions is impaired. There is an increased risk of postoperative pulmonary infection.

Anaesthesia causes little additional decrease in lung volumes and is tolerated well, provided that hypoxaemia is avoided. However, inadequate basal ventilation and retention of secretions may occur postoperatively, partly as a result of pain, opioid analgesics and residual effects of anaesthetic agents. High concentrations of oxygen may be used without risk of respiratory depression. A short period of mechanical ventilation may be necessary in patients with severe disease to allow adequate analgesia and clearing of secretions. Non-invasive ventilation may avert the need for prolonged tracheal intubation and IPPV. Effective epidural analgesia may help to reduce postoperative respiratory complications.

Bronchial carcinoma

Patients with bronchial carcinoma often suffer from coexisting COPD. In addition, there may be infection and collapse of the lung distal to the tumour. Patients with bronchial carcinoma may have myasthenic syndrome, whereas oat-cell tumours may secrete a variety of hormones, among the most common being adrenocorticotrophic hormone (ACTH), (producing Cushing's syndrome) and antidiuretic hormone (ADH) (producing dilutional hyponatraemia, the syndrome of inappropriate ADH secretion).

Tuberculosis

Tuberculosis should be considered in patients with persistent pulmonary infection, especially if associated with haemoptysis or weight loss. It is becoming more common in the UK. If active disease is present, all anaesthetic equipment should be changed after use to avoid cross-infection.

Haematological disorders

Anaemia

Anaemia occurs as a result of decreased red cell production or increased loss caused by bleeding or destruction. A number of congenital or acquired conditions can result in anaemia (Table 20.5). Anaemia is defined as a haemoglobin less than 130 g L^{-1} (men) or 120 g L^{-1} (women), but the level of anaemia at which physiological dysfunction occurs in everyday life or under the stress of surgery, is unclear.

Symptoms associated with anaemia include dyspnoea, angina, vertigo, syncope, palpitations and limited exercise tolerance. These symptoms may be better tolerated in younger patients or in those in whom the onset is more gradual. Anaemia detected in the preoperative period should ideally be investigated and treated before major surgery in all patients where >500 ml blood loss or ≥10% probability of red cell transfusion is expected. This is true of even relatively mild anaemia because patients with a low haemoglobin concentration at the outset are at higher risk of transfusion-related problems (see Chapter 14, Table 14.6).

Anaemia is classically subdivided into three diagnostic categories:
- *Microcytic, hypochromic* anaemia (mean cell volume (MCV) <78 fl and mean cell haemoglobin (MCH) <27 pg). Common causes include iron deficiency anaemia, chronic blood loss, anaemia of chronic disease, thalassaemia or sideroblastic anaemia.
- *Macrocytic* anaemia (MCV >100 fl). Common causes include vitamin B12 or folate deficiency/malabsorption, alcoholism, liver disease, myelodysplasia and hypothyroidism. If the reticulocyte count is high (>2.5%), acute blood loss or haemolytic anaemia may be considered.
- *Normocytic normochromic* anaemia (normal MCV and MCH). Common causes include anaemia of chronic disease, aplastic anaemia, haematological malignancy and bone marrow invasion or fibrosis. If the reticulocyte count is high, this may also represent acute blood loss or haemolysis.

Haemoglobinopathies

Haemoglobinopathies, which include sickle-cell disease and thalassaemia, may be associated with systemic complications. In the case of sickle-cell disease these complications may be triggered or exacerbated by anaesthetic techniques.

Table 20.5 Causes of anaemia

Decreased Production	
Bone marrow failure	Aplastic anaemia Chemotherapy or bone marrow transplant conditioning Marrow infiltration or destruction • Non-haematological cancers (e.g. breast, lung, kidney or thyroid cancers) • Lymphoma • Myelofibrosis • Myeloma • Tuberculosis
Decreased erythropoiesis	Alcoholism Chronic disease Hypothyroidism Infection Renal failure Sideroblastic anaemia Thalassaemia
Nutritional deficiencies	Iron Folic acid Vitamin B12 Vitamin C Note: Nutritional deficiencies may be caused or exacerbated by a number of conditions, including: • Alcoholism • Drugs (e.g. methotrexate) • Impaired absorption (e.g. Crohn's disease, pernicious anaemia, tropical sprue, Whipple's disease) • Inherited disorders (e.g. homocystinuria)
Increased Loss	
Bleeding	Acute haemorrhage Chronic bleeding (e.g. haematuria or occult GI blood loss)
Haemolysis or sequestration	Acquired haemolytic disease • Heart valve defects/mechanical heart valves • Immune-mediated haemolysis (e.g. drug-related haemolysis, incompatible blood transfusion) • Malaria • Microangiopathic haemolytic anaemia (MAHA)* • Paroxysmal nocturnal haematuria Inherited red cell disorders • G6PD deficiency • Pyruvate kinase deficiency • Sickle-cell disease • Spherocytosis • Thalassaemia
Artefactual	
	Hypervolaemic haemodilution Laboratory error

*Causes of MAHA include vasculitis, disseminated intravascular coagulation (DIC), HELLP syndrome (Haemolysis, Elevated Liver enzymes, Low Platelets) and thrombotic thrombocytopaenic purpura/haemolytic uraemic syndrome (TTP/HUS).
G6PD, Glucose-6-phosphate dehydrogenase.

Sickle-cell disease

Sickle-cell disease is a genetic variation in the synthesis of haemoglobin which occurs most commonly in people with African or Mediterranean heritage. It involves a valine substitution for glutamine in the β-globin chain to make sickle haemoglobin (HbS), and because it is an autosomal recessive condition, individuals can either have HbA and HbS present (HbAS; sickle-cell trait), or just HbS (HbSS; sickle-cell anaemia). HbS becomes less soluble when deoxygenated and aggregates, causing the red cell to deform into the classic sickle shape, which can lodge in the microcirculation, becoming sequestrated and causing areas of ischaemia. Sickling is probably not the only cause of the pathology of sickle-cell disease. HbS is unstable as well as insoluble, resulting in cell breakdown, and oxidative/ endothelial damage. Surgical stress may, therefore, trigger vaso-occlusion through an inflammatory rather than sickling process. Sickle cell trait is relatively protected from this effect because approximately 70% of red cells contain HbA, whereas up to 95% of red cells contain HbS in sickle-cell anaemia. HbS can be detected in a laboratory blood sample. However, it is extremely unlikely for adults to have unknown sickle-cell disease (as opposed to sickle-cell trait), particularly if they are not anaemic.

As well as potentially being chronically anaemic, patients with sickle-cell disease are more likely to have preoperative renal or splenic disease (in which case splenectomy prophylaxis may be required, even in the absence of a surgical splenectomy). They are also more likely to have suffered from lung or cardiovascular disease, which may include previous cerebral infarctions or increased cardiac output at rest. Because of recurrent painful sickle cell crisis episodes these patients suffer, they are often not opioid naïve, which may present challenges in perioperative pain management.

During anaesthesia, and during the postoperative period, HbS is prone to sickling in the presence of hypoxaemia, dehydration, acidaemia or mild hypothermia. In patients with HbS, sickling may occur even at high oxygen saturations and become progressively worse such that all red cells will be sickled at approximately 50% saturation. If sickling causes lung ischaemia, further hypoxaemia may develop. Patients with sickle-cell trait are less susceptible to ischaemic complications, but this does depend on the proportion of HbS present, and there are case reports of thrombotic complications in this patient group. There is some evidence to suggest that patients with sickle-cell trait are at increased risk of venous thromboembolism and pregnancy-related complications. In patients with sickle-cell disease, haematology input is required, and advice should be sought preoperatively, as an elective transfusion to lower the proportion of HbS may be indicated.

Intraoperative anaesthetic techniques should avoid hypoxaemia and acidaemia, and this may involve general or regional anaesthesia. If general anaesthesia is required, IPPV may be preferable as a means of optimising oxygenation and avoiding respiratory acidosis (or potentially providing a respiratory alkalosis in high-risk patients). Intravenous fluids (including in the preoperative period) and active warming of the patient are likely to be required to avoid dehydration and hypothermia. Vasopressors and limb tourniquets should be used with due consideration to risks and benefits. Intraoperative cell salvage is not currently recommended. Continuation of monitoring and support with oxygen and i.v. fluids are likely to be required into the postoperative period, and the presence of a postoperative fever should alert clinicians to the possibility of an ischaemic crisis.

There are no specific guidelines as to which analgesic regimens should be used, although the presence of renal disease may be a relative contraindication to NSAIDs. Anaesthetists may also be called upon to provide analgesia, including patient-controlled morphine, to patients suffering from a non-surgical sickle-cell crisis. These are often extremely painful.

Thalassaemia

Thalassaemia is an abnormality of globin synthesis which occurs in patients of Mediterranean, Middle Eastern or Asian descent. There are two common forms, α and β, and both forms are inherited in a recessive pattern and can thus be present in minor or major forms. The minor forms have few clinical implications except in states of increased haemodynamic stress such as pregnancy, when anaemia may occur. In the major forms, haemolytic anaemia occurs, which is often managed with regular blood transfusions to prevent anaemia and bony deformation caused by bone marrow hyperplasia. In untreated individuals, marrow hyperplasia can result in craniofacial abnormalities, which may directly affect anaesthetic techniques such as laryngoscopy. Iron overload can also occur, resulting in cardiac hypertrophy, pulmonary hypertension and liver disease; detailed cardiac history and preoperative assessment are required. In rare cases the splenomegaly or folate deficiency associated with thalassaemia has resulted in thrombocytopenia or neutropenia being present, and this should be excluded preoperatively.

Various drugs are relatively contraindicated in thalassaemia because they may trigger haemolysis; these include prilocaine, nitroprusside, penicillin, aspirin and vitamin K. Advice should be sought before administering such agents.

Neutropenia

Neutropenia creates a significantly immunocompromised state, leaving patients at increased risk of infections, including those infections usually considered unusual or atypical. A white cell count less than 1×10^9 L^{-1} is considered significant and often requires prophylactic medications against fungal, viral or *Pneumocystis jirovecii* infections.

The most common causes of neutropenia are haematological malignancies and their treatments, as well as chemotherapy for other malignancies. When neutropenic patients require surgery, the benefits must be weighed against the increased risk of postoperative infections. Strict asepsis is essential when dealing with neutropenic patients, and it should be noted that they are at increased risk of ventilator-associated pneumonia, urinary catheter infections and infections associated with i.v. cannulation, particularly CVCs. If possible, these interventions should be avoided or limited to as short a time as possible. Various antimicrobial regimens are recommended in patients with neutropaenic sepsis, which include broad-spectrum agents with antipseudomonal and antifungal cover. Most hospitals have their own policies for management of suspected neutropaenic sepsis.

Gastrointestinal disease

Gastrointestinal disease presents several problems for the anaesthetist including:
• Malnutrition
• Fluid and electrolyte depletion
• Gastro-oesophageal reflux

Malnutrition cannot usually be corrected fully before surgery, but fluid and electrolyte depletion and anaemia may be remedied and appropriate measures taken to minimise the risk of regurgitation and aspiration.

Malnutrition

Malnutrition may be caused by decreased nutritional intake (including eating disorders), malabsorption or gut losses. Patients are at increased risk of perioperative morbidity and mortality, with infections, poor wound healing and thromboembolic complications being prominent. If patients are undergoing major surgery, consideration should be given to commencing preoperative nutritional support with enteral or total parenteral nutrition (TPN) before surgery. Vitamin supplementation is essential.

Fluid and electrolyte depletion

Fluid and electrolyte depletion may result from decreased fluid intake caused by dysphagia, vomiting or diarrhoea. Significant fluid depletion may also be caused by preoperative bowel preparation with hypertonic solutions, and fluid may be given i.v. before surgery to maintain hydration.

Clinical assessment of volume depletion (poor perfusion, decreased tissue turgor, postural hypotension) should be supplemented by measurement of serum urea and electrolyte concentrations and fluid and electrolyte deficits replaced. Patients with intestinal obstruction may have extreme fluid and electrolyte depletion, with a consequent risk of cardiovascular collapse if vigorous fluid resuscitation is not provided before induction of anaesthesia. These patients require invasive cardiovascular monitoring throughout the perioperative period.

Gastrointestinal reflux

Patients at risk of GI reflux include those with symptoms such as heartburn and regurgitation, and those with proven hiatus hernia. Patients with intestinal obstruction or ileus secondary to peritonitis from any cause and those presenting with vomiting may have a full stomach and be at risk for regurgitation. Another factor associated with reflux is raised intra-abdominal pressure, with obesity, pregnancy and the lithotomy position being particular risk factors.

The risk of aspiration of gastric acid and subsequent pneumonitis is reduced by administration of an H_2-receptor antagonist (e.g. ranitidine) or a proton pump inhibitor (e.g. omeprazole) on the night before and morning of surgery. Sodium citrate 30 ml 5 min before induction neutralises residual gastric acid. A prokinetic (e.g. metoclopramide) is sometimes given to promote gastric emptying.

In patients with intestinal obstruction, emptying the stomach before induction of anaesthesia using a large-bore nasogastric tube may be attempted. However, this may precipitate vomiting, and even if apparently effective, an empty stomach cannot be assumed. Prevention of regurgitation and aspiration of gastric contents is based on early securing of the airway using rapid-sequence induction of anaesthesia with cricoid force (see Chapter 23).

Liver disease

Causes of chronic liver disease include sustained excessive alcohol intake, hepatitis B and C, and fatty liver disease. The prevalence of cirrhosis is increasing in the UK. The presence of cirrhosis is associated with an increase in postoperative complications and mortality. Anaesthesia and surgery may adversely affect liver function, whereas pre-existing liver disease may affect the conduct of anaesthesia.

Preoperative assessment

Preoperative assessment should be directed to the degree of liver dysfunction and complications of liver disease. Clinical features of liver disease include jaundice, ascites, oedema and impaired conscious level (encephalopathy). Preoperative investigations should include full blood count, coagulation screen, serum urea and electrolytes, bilirubin, alkaline phosphatase and transaminases, protein, albumin and blood sugar concentrations. Hypoglycaemia and hyperlactaemia indicate hepatic metabolic dysfunction and a prolonged international normalised ratio (INR) suggests impaired synthetic function.

Two risk assessment tools are available to estimate the perioperative risk of patients with liver disease. The Child–Turcotte–Pugh (CTP) score is predominately used for prognostication in cirrhosis and considers five variables: pro-thrombin time (PT); albumin; bilirubin; degree of ascites; and encephalopathy. Patients may be classified as class A, B or C, with increasing associated mortality. The model for end-stage liver disease (MELD) score is used to prioritise patients awaiting liver transplantation and may have greater accuracy in estimating postoperative risk. The variables included are requirement for haemodialysis, creatinine, bilirubin, INR and sodium.

Particular problems relevant to the anaesthetist are discussed below.

Cardiovascular function

Patients with liver disease tend to be vasodilated and hypotensive. This may be aggravated by loss of fluid from the circulation as a result of hypoalbuminaemia and low oncotic pressure. Hypotension can also be caused by alcoholic cardiomyopathy.

Respiratory function

There may be respiratory compromise caused by diaphragmatic splinting secondary to ascites and/or pleural effusions. In severe disease, intrapulmonary shunting may cause disproportionate hypoxaemia.

Acid–base and fluid balance

Many patients are overloaded with salt and water. Hypoal-buminaemia results in oedema and ascites and predisposes to pulmonary oedema. Secondary hyperaldosteronism produces sodium retention (even though the plasma sodium concentration may be low) and hypokalaemia. Diuretic therapy, often including spironolactone, may also affect the serum potassium concentration. In hepatic failure a combined respiratory and metabolic alkalosis may occur, which shifts the oxygen dissociation curve to the left, potentially impairing tissue oxygenation.

Hepatorenal syndrome

Hepatorenal syndrome is defined as acute renal failure developing in patients with pre-existing chronic liver failure. Jaundiced patients are at risk of developing postoperative renal failure. This may be precipitated by hypovolaemia.

Prevention involves adequate preoperative hydration, with i.v. fluids for at least 12 h before surgery and close monitoring of urine output intra- and postoperatively. Intravenous 100 ml mannitol 20% may be given pre- and postoperatively if the hourly urine output decreases to less than 50 ml, though there is limited evidence for its efficacy. Close cardiovascular monitoring is essential, and measurement of cardiac output should be considered.

Bleeding problems

Production of clotting factors II, VII, IX and X is reduced because of decreased vitamin K absorption. Production of factor V and fibrinogen is also reduced. Thrombocytopenia occurs if portal hypertension is present. Gastrointestinal haemorrhage from gastro-oesophageal varices may cause major management problems. Preoperatively, vitamin K and fresh frozen plasma (FFP) may be required to correct coagulation abnormalities. Cryoprecipitate may also be required in the presence of a prolonged PT. Desmopressin (DDAVP) and tranexamic acid may also be useful. Close liaison with the haematology service is essential, and local protocols should be in place for the management of major haemorrhage.

Infection

Impairment of the filtering function of the liver's Kupffer cells leads to a higher incidence of endotoxaemia and infection. Bacterial peritonitis is a potential problem in patients with ascites.

Drug metabolism

Significant impairment of liver function will affect protein binding as a result of decreased synthesis. Drug metabolism, detoxification and excretion are likely to be affected, resulting in prolonged drug half-lives. Propofol is safe to use, but sensitivity to its sedative and cardiorespiratory effects may be increased. Suxamethonium may have a prolonged duration of action because of reduced plasma cholinesterase activity. Atracurium is commonly used as its metabolism is not dependent on hepatic function. The metabolism and elimination of morphine and fentanyl can be variable. Remifentanil is useful as it is metabolised by plasma and tissue esterases. Of the volatile anaesthetic agents, desflurane is least metabolised, with minimal effects on hepatic blood flow (see Chapter 3).

Hepatic failure

The management of hepatic failure is beyond the scope of this chapter. The main issues are recognition, assessment, initial resuscitation and transfer to a specialist centre.

Conduct of anaesthesia

Anaesthesia with tracheal intubation and IPPV is commonly required to enable procedures to control GI bleeding, such as endoscopy with injection or banding of oesophageal varices, to be undertaken safely. Controlled ventilation to a normal $PaCO_2$ is important, as hypocapnia is associated with decreased hepatic blood flow. Hypoxaemia should be avoided throughout the perioperative period.

The liver is particularly vulnerable to hypoxia, hypovolaemia and hypotension. During anaesthesia, cardiovascular stability should be maintained as far as possible. Blood loss should be replaced promptly and overall euvolaemia maintained. In the adequately volume-expanded patient, hypotension may be reversed by infusion of noradrenaline. However, in the unstable patient, expert help should be sought, and monitoring should include measurement of cardiac output. In the presence of oesophageal varices, oesophageal Doppler monitoring is contraindicated, and other cardiac output monitors should be used.

Drugs that depress cardiac output or arterial pressure, including volatile anaesthetic agents and β-blockers, should be used with caution to avoid reductions in hepatic blood flow. The neuromuscular blocking agents (NMBAs) of choice are those with cardiovascular stability and a short duration of action; atracurium may be preferable because its elimination is independent of hepatic and renal function. Opioids should be administered with caution unless ventilatory support is planned postoperatively. Short-acting agents such as remifentanil should be infused intraoperatively, and fentanyl PCA may be suitable for postoperative analgesia. NSAIDs should be avoided.

Renal disease

Renal dysfunction has important implications for anaesthesia, and a full assessment is required before even minor surgical procedures are contemplated (see Chapter 19).

The major causes of CKD are diabetes, hypertension, intrinsic kidney disease (e.g. glomerulonephritis, polycystic kidney disease) and obstructive uropathy. Chronic kidney disease is currently classified according to estimated glomerular filtration rate (eGFR) (Table 20.6). Increasing severity of CKD is associated with increased mortality and morbidity. In part, this relates to the associated comorbidities.

It should be noted that, although eGFR can be a useful estimate of renal function, it requires a steady-state creatinine concentration for calculation and is inaccurate in acute renal failur; it should not be used in the acutely ill or unstable patient. It is also inaccurate where muscle mass or creatinine intake are at extremes, such as in cachectic patients or those on a vegetarian diet. In this context the term *chronic* means two or more creatinine concentrations measured at least 90 days apart.

Preoperative assessment

Preoperative assessment should be directed to several specific problems that require correction before anaesthesia.

Fluid balance

In acute kidney injury, fluid overload may develop suddenly and is uncompensated. In chronic renal failure, overload may be controlled with diuretic therapy or dialysis. Pulmonary oedema and hypertension may result from fluid overload and must be treated before induction of anaesthesia. This may require fluid removal using dialysis or haemofiltration. In patients with nephrotic syndrome, hypoalbuminaemia results in oedema and ascites. Circulating blood volume in these patients is often decreased, and care should be taken at induction of anaesthesia to avoid hypotension. Invasive monitoring and measurement of cardiac output should be considered in these patients.

Sodium

Sodium retention occurs in renal failure and, through increased secretion of ADH, is associated with water

Table 20.6 Kidney Disease: Improving Global Outcomes (KDIGO) categories of chronic kidney disease		
Stage	**Description of function**	**GFR (ml min^{-1} 1.73 m^{-2})**
1	Normal, but other renal damage (e.g. haematuria, proteinuria) present	>90
2	Mildly decreased (compared with young adult)	60–89
3a	Mild to moderately decreased	45–59
3b	Moderate to severely decreased	30–44
4	Severely decreased	15–29
5	Kidney failure	<15
GFR, Glomerular filtration rate.		

retention, oedema and hypertension. Hyponatraemia is also common in renal disease. It is the result either of sodium losses through the kidney/GI tract (e.g. diuretic therapy, vomiting or diarrhoea) or secondary to water overload causing dilutional hyponatraemia. The renal tubules may have a reduced ability to conserve sodium, such as in pyelonephritis, analgesic nephropathy or recovering acute renal failure.

Potassium

Hyperkalaemia occurs typically in renal failure, often in association with metabolic acidaemia, and causes delayed myocardial conduction; if this is untreated, it may lead to cardiac arrest due to asystole or ventricular fibrillation.

Hyperkalaemia should be treated promptly when the serum potassium concentration exceeds 6 mmol L^{-1} or when ECG changes are evident (peaked T-waves, increased P-R interval, prolonged QRS, conduction blocks and ultimately a sinusoidal waveform). Treatment is as follows:

- Calcium salts (e.g. 10–20 ml calcium gluconate 10% over 5 min or 5–10 ml calcium chloride 10% over 10 min). These do not lower plasma potassium concentrations but stabilise cardiac membranes.
- 50 ml glucose 50% with 5–15 units of soluble insulin followed by an infusion of 20% glucose with insulin (depending on blood sugar estimation). This drives potassium back into cells.
- Nebulised salbutamol 2.5–5 mg repeated regularly. This drives potassium back into cells.
- Sodium bicarbonate 1.4% to improve the metabolic acidaemia if pH is less than 7.2. The use of bicarbonate is controversial, and its use may be associated with risk of sodium and fluid overload.
- Ion exchange resin (e.g. calcium polystyrene sulphonate p.o. or p.r.). This provides longer-term control in chronic renal failure.
- Haemodialysis or haemofiltration. The former is more effective in lowering serum potassium concentration rapidly, but haemofiltration may be more familiar for emergency use on ICU.

Calcium

Retention of phosphate and vitamin D depletion (1,25-dihydroxycholecalciferol) in chronic renal failure lead to hyperparathyroidism. The development of a parathyroid adenoma leads to hypercalcaemia (tertiary hyperparathyroidism).

Cardiovascular effects

Hypertension may occur for several reasons:

- Raised plasma renin concentration secondary to decreased perfusion of the juxtaglomerular apparatus results in hypertension through increased secretion of angiotensin and aldosterone.

- Fluid retention results in increased circulating blood volume.

Both pulmonary and peripheral oedema may occur from a combination of fluid overload, hypertensive cardiac disease and hypoproteinaemia. Heart failure should be treated preoperatively. Uraemia may cause pericarditis and haemorrhagic pericardial effusion, which may reduce cardiac output and require aspiration, although this is now a rare event.

Neurological effects

Severe uraemia causes drowsiness and eventually coma. Electrolyte disturbances and rapid fluid shifts, such as during dialysis, may also affect level of consciousness by causing cerebral oedema. Sedative drugs, including opioids, should be used with care in these patients. Morphine may be a problem because renally excreted metabolites, in particular morphine-6-glucuronide, accumulate. A combined motor and sensory peripheral neuropathy may also occur.

Haematological effects

Anaemia is common in patients with CKD because of:

- reduced renal erythropoietin secretion;
- bone marrow suppression secondary to uraemia;
- increased GI blood loss;
- impaired iron absorption; and
- reduced red blood cell lifespan (especially if on haemodialysis).

Patients are usually well compensated, with an increased cardiac output, so preoperative blood transfusion is unnecessary. Increasingly, patients are treated with long-term erythropoietin. There is often a bleeding tendency, in part caused by platelet dysfunction. Conventional tests of coagulation are normal, but bleeding time is prolonged and correlates with the degree of bleeding tendency. Platelet dysfunction may be improved with DDAVP 0.3 µg kg^{-1} i.v./s.c.

Other

Patients with CKD are often undernourished and tend to be vulnerable to infection. Patients who have received a renal transplant and are immunosuppressed are particularly vulnerable to opportunistic pathogens, such as *Pneumocystis jirovecii*.

Drug treatment

Drug treatment is important for several reasons:

- Patients are often receiving concurrent medication for attendant problems (e.g. hypertension).
- Many drugs are renally excreted, and doses may require modification and plasma concentrations monitoring (e.g. aminoglycosides, digoxin).
- Some drugs have active metabolites which are renally excreted (e.g. morphine, midazolam) and require careful titration or the use of alternative agents (e.g. fentanyl).

- Some drugs adversely affect renal function even in normal dosage:
  - NSAIDs and cyclo-oxygenase-2 inhibitors inhibit vasodilator prostaglandin production in the kidney and thus reduce glomerular blood flow and sodium excretion. This may be critical in septic or shocked patients, those with pre-existing renal dysfunction or those undergoing surgery associated with major blood loss. Their use should be avoided in such high-risk patients.
  - ACEIs dilate the postglomerular arterioles in the kidney and thus reduce glomerular filtration pressure; this may precipitate renal failure in hypotensive patients. Patients receiving these agents should be monitored carefully, and fluid should be replaced adequately to avoid hypotension. It may be prudent to omit the immediate preanaesthetic dose in the high-risk patient. Angiotensin-converting enzyme inhibitors may also cause hyperkalaemia, particularly in patients with renal dysfunction.

Anaesthesia

- Minor procedures, such as the establishment of vascular access for dialysis, may be carried out satisfactorily under regional anaesthesia.
- Patients receiving long-term dialysis for CKD may require dialysis before surgery to correct fluid overload, acid-base disturbances and hyperkalaemia. Ideally there should be some delay before surgery to allow correction of anticoagulation.
- The i.v. cannula for induction and fluid infusion should be sited in the contralateral limb from the arteriovenous shunt or fistula in patients undergoing dialysis, and care should be taken to protect the fistula during the operation.
- Careful monitoring of arterial pressure and ECG is required. Intravenous fluid administration should be cautious, and cardiac output monitoring may be helpful.
- Excessive sodium administration and potassium-containing solutions should be avoided in renal failure.
- If the patient is anaemic preoperatively, intraoperative blood loss should be replaced promptly.
- Suxamethonium should be avoided in hyperkalaemic patients in view of its effect of releasing potassium from muscle cells. An increase of up to 0.6 mmol L^{-1} may be expected with normal dosage.
- Drugs excreted primarily via the kidneys should be used with caution in renal failure. In anaesthetic practice the principal drugs involved are the NMBAs. Atracurium, elimination of which is independent of kidney and liver function and which has minimal cardiovascular effects, is the drug of choice. All other NMBAs depend to some extent on renal elimination and should be avoided, particularly in repeated doses.

- Many drugs, including morphine, are conjugated in the liver before excretion in the urine. Depending on the activity of the conjugated metabolite, these drugs may have adverse effects after repeated doses. Morphine-6-glucuronide, an active metabolite of morphine, accumulates in renal failure and may result in prolongation of clinical effects after administration of morphine.
- Modern volatile anaesthetic agents avoid metabolism to fluoride ions to any great extent and are free of any deleterious effects on renal function.

Perioperative acute kidney injury

Perioperative acute kidney injury (AKI) is recognised as a leading cause of morbidity and mortality, with increased risk of sepsis, anaemia, coagulopathy and need for mechanical ventilation. The classification criteria of AKI are based on increases in creatinine and reductions in urine output (see Chapter 11, Table 11.4).

Preoperative risk factors include:
- chronic hypertension;
- poor diabetic control;
- obesity; and
- use of nephrotoxic drugs.

Intraoperative risk factors include:
- emergency and major vascular surgery;
- sepsis;
- hypovolemia;
- hypotension (MAP <55 mmHg); and
- direct renal injury.

Raised intra-abdominal pressure (>12 mmHg) may be significant during laparoscopic surgery but can also occur in the postoperative phase as a result of ascites, blood, oedematous bowel and intra-abdominal sepsis.

High-risk patients should be identified and optimised preoperatively. Perioperatively the aim is to ensure kidney perfusion by targeting a MAP > 60–65 mmHg and by maintaining intravascular volume. Balanced crystalloid solutions are preferred. Diuretics or dopamine have no role in the prevention of AKI. The use of vasopressors in preventing AKI is not entirely clear. They have the potential to maintaining MAP whilst causing renal vasoconstriction at the same time. Evidence does not support the use of one vasopressor agent over another.

Diabetes mellitus

Diabetes mellitus (DM) is common, affecting 6%–7% of the general population and up to 30% of hospital inpatients. Studies have found that presence of diabetes in surgical patients is associated with a 50% increase in mortality and a 100% increase in the incidence of surgical infections, MI and AKI. The reasons for this increase in morbidity and mortality are multifactorial:

- Complications of diabetes:
  - IHD
  - Autonomic neuropathy
  - Diabetic ketoacidosis (DKA)/metabolic consequences
  - Chronic kidney disease
- Hyperglycaemia leading to increased risk of infective complications and impaired healing (including anastomotic failure)
- Hypoglycaemia, the clinical signs of which may be masked completely by anaesthesia

There are two main types of diabetes: type 1, an autoimmune condition with pancreatic β-cell destruction; and type 2, caused by a complex interplay of genetic and environmental factors resulting in defective insulin secretion and insulin resistance. Approximately 10% of people with diabetes have type 1 and 90% type 2. Both groups suffer from hyperglycaemia. However, the complete lack of insulin in the former group allows unrestrained glycogenolysis, gluconeogenesis and protein and fat catabolism with subsequent production of keto acids if insulin treatment is interrupted. These effects are limited by residual insulin production in people with type 2 diabetes. However, additional significant stress such as major surgery or sepsis may be sufficient to precipitate ketoacidosis in this group too.

Complications of diabetes mellitus

Cardiovascular

Ischaemic heart disease, cerebrovascular disease and peripheral vascular disease are common in diabetic patients, and there is an increased risk of perioperative MI. There may be significant IHD in the absence of warning symptoms, and as discussed earlier, patients with diabetes often require further cardiovascular investigation before major surgery.

Renal disease

Microvascular damage produces glomerulosclerosis with proteinuria, oedema and eventually chronic renal failure.

Ocular problems

Cataracts, exudative or proliferative retinopathy, vitreous haemorrhage and retinal detachment may occur. In the long term, good blood glucose control has been found to reduce the frequency of such complications.

Infection

Diabetic patients are prone to infection and an increased risk of septicaemia, abscess formation and wound infection. Infection is associated with increased insulin requirements, which return to normal on its eradication.

Neuropathy

Chronic sensory peripheral neuropathies are common; mononeuropathies and acute motor neuropathies (amyotrophy) are associated with poor control of blood glucose. Loss of sensation together with peripheral vascular disease may lead to ulceration after trivial trauma. Consequently, care in positioning patients in the operating theatre is important. Local anaesthetic nerve or plexus blocks should be used with caution in patients with an acute neuropathy, as neurological deficits may be attributed to the local anaesthetic solution.

Autonomic neuropathy

Autonomic neuropathy may cause postoperative urinary retention or vasomotor instability (e.g. postural hypotension or hypotension during anaesthesia). Spinal or epidural anaesthesia may be associated with significant hypotension; preoperative intravascular volume status should be assessed and fluids given to achieve euvolaemia before performing a block. Precise cardiovascular monitoring, use of vasopressors and careful anaesthetic management are essential.

Measuring glycaemic control

Capillary blood glucose (CBG) samples are used to measure immediate control. In the UK the units used are mmol L^{-1}. Hyperglycaemia is defined as a concentration > 6.0 mmol L^{-1}. Glycated haemoglobin (HbA1c) is a measure of long-term glycaemic control, reflecting the level of exposure of haemoglobin to plasma glucose in the preceding 3–4 months. Glycated haemoglobin is now expressed as mmol mol^{-1}. An HbA1c concentration > 48 mmol mol^{-1} on repeated testing is diagnostic of diabetes.

Treatment regimens

Some form of insulin therapy is required in all people with type 1 diabetes. Those with type 2 diabetes may be managed by dietary control alone or with non-insulin glucose-lowering drugs. Poorly controlled type 2 diabetes may require the addition of insulin.

Non-insulin glucose-lowering drugs

There are currently eight different classes of non-insulin glucose-lowering drugs. Some (sulphonylureas, meglitinides and to some extent thiazolidinediones) act to lower glucose concentrations and may cause hypoglycaemia. The remainder act to prevent glucose concentrations increasing.

1. Sulphonylureas (e.g. glibenclamide and gliclazide) are insulin secretagogues relying on adequate β-cell function in the pancreas. With a long half-life and partial renal

excretion, they should be avoided in the elderly and patients with inspired renal function.

2. Meglitinides (e.g. nateglinide) are short-acting insulin secretagogues, similar to sulphonylureas. They are rarely used because of frequent dosing requirements.

3. Intestinal α-glucosidase inhibitors (e.g. acarbose) inhibit monosaccharide absorption in the gut. Their use is limited by GI adverse effects.

4. Sodium-glucose transporter 2 inhibitors (e.g. canagliflozin) prevent glucose reabsorption from the proximal convoluted tubule of the kidney.

5. Biguanides (e.g. metformin) are recommended by most guidelines as first-line treatment for type 2 diabetes. They act by a combination of decreasing gluconeogenesis, increasing insulin sensitivity and reducing intestinal absorption of glucose. Metformin may be associated with the development of lactic acidosis, though this is rare. Dosage should be reviewed in patients with reduced renal function. Previous guidelines advised discontinuing metformin up to 48 h before surgery. Current guidelines support its continued use in patients with short fasting times and who are at low risk of AKI.

6. Thiazolidinediones (e.g. pioglitazone) increase cellular sensitivity to naturally released insulin. Their use is reducing because of the associated risks of heart failure, bladder cancer and bone fracture.

7. Glucagon-like peptide-1 (GLP-1) analogues (e.g. dulaglutide) act to mimic the effect of incretin hormones such as GLP-1. Incretin hormones are released by the upper GI tract in response to glucose in the gut lumen increasing glucose-dependent insulin secretion, reducing glucagon secretion and reducing gastric emptying. They can be given as a weekly s.c. injection.

8. Dipeptidyl peptidase-4 (DPP-4) inhibitors (e.g. alogliptin and linagliptin) act by inhibiting the enzyme DPP-4 responsible for the inactivation of GLP-1.

Insulins

Many formulations of insulin are available with a wide variety of pharmacokinetic profiles. Although some patients continue to use animal-derived insulin preparations, the majority of patients use a genetically-engineered human insulin produced by recombinant DNA technology. Insulins in current use can be classified by:

- Pharmakokinetic profile: speed of onset and duration of action (e.g. NovoRapid, 10-min onset, or Levemir, 24-h duration of action);
- Insulin type: human analogue, bovine or porcine; or
- Formulation: single type or mixture, also described as biphasic (e.g. NovoMix).

Further classification may be used when considering the type of insulin administration regime:

- Once daily: used in patients with type 2 diabetes to supplement their oral medication.

- Twice daily: a biphasic formulation injected at breakfast and evening meal, commonly used in both type 1 and type 2 diabetes.
- Basal bolus: typically a long-acting insulin given at night with a rapid-acting insulin given three times a day with meals.
- Continuous s.c. insulin infusion (CSII): a pump delivers an hourly basal rate of a very rapid insulin analogue. The rate can be adjusted in response to oral intake or CBG concentrations.

Perioperative management

For elective surgery, the aim should be for same-day admission, minimal fasting period, normoglycaemia (CBG 6–10 mmol L^{-1}) and minimal change to the patient's normal routine. For both type 1 and type 2 diabetic patients undergoing surgery who are stable and expected to miss one meal only, glycaemic control can be achieved by simple manipulation of their usual medications (Tables 20.7 and 20.8).

In patients with longer expected fasting times or whose diabetic control is labile an insulin infusion is required. The term *variable-rate intravenous insulin infusion (VRIII)* is now used to replace the previously used term *sliding scale*. There is increasing recognition of the iatrogenic complications associated with the incorrect management of a VRIII in the perioperative period. These include significant hypoglycaemia, hyperglycaemia, hyponatraemia and hypokalaemia. Development of ketosis is also a risk if there is significant delay in setting up a VRIII in a fasted patient or delayed administration of s.c. insulin on discontinuation.

National guidelines have been published in the UK with the aim of standardising and improving the care and outcomes of diabetic patients in the perioperative period. Most hospitals have local guidelines which reflect these national guidelines, including the appropriate use of VRIIIs. These guidelines should be followed wherever possible, with support of the local diabetic team whenever required.

Key points of these recommendations include the following:

- Comorbidities should be recognised and optimised before admission.
- Glycaemic control is optimised before surgery, aiming for an HbA1c < 69 mmol mol^{-1}.
- Day-of-surgery admission should be the default position. Diabetes-specific preadmission should be avoided. Diabetic patients should be prioritised on the operating list.
- Patients with a short starvation period (one missed meal) should be managed by modification of their usual diabetes medication. A VRIII should be avoided wherever possible.

421

Table 20.7 Guidelines for the perioperative adjustment of oral hypogylcaemic agents (short starvation period, no more than one missed meal)

Drug Type	Day before admission	DAY OF SURGERY a.m. Surgery	DAY OF SURGERY p.m. Surgery	Whilst a VRIII is used
Meglitinides	Take as normal	Omit a.m. dose	Give a.m. dose if eating	Stop until eating and drinking normally
Sulphonylureas		Omit a.m. dose	Omit	
SGLT2 inhibitors		Halve a.m. dose, evening meal dose unchanged		
Acarbose		Omit a.m. dose if fasting	Give a.m. dose if eating	
DPP-4 inhibitors		Take as normal	Take as normal	
GLP-1 analogues				Take as normal
Metformin				Stop until eating and drinking normally
Pioglitazone				

DPP-IV, Dipeptidyl peptidase-4; GLP-1, glucagon-like peptide-1; SGLT2, sodium-glucose contransporter-2; VRIII, variable-rate intravenous insulin infusion.
(Adapted from Association of Anaesthetists of Great Britain and Ireland. (2015) Perioperative management of the surgical patient with diabetes 2015. *Anaesthesia.* 70, 1427–1440.)

Table 20.8 Guidelines for the perioperative adjustment of insulin (short starvation period, no more than one missed meal)

Insulin Regime	Day before admission	Day of surgery	Whilst a VRIII is used
Once daily			
p.m. Injection	Reduce dose by 20%	CBG o/a	Continue at 80% of usual dose
a.m. Injection		Reduce dose by 20%, CBG o/a	
Twice daily			
Biphasic or ultra long-acting Short-acting	No dose change	Halve a.m. dose, CBG o/a, Evening meal dose unchanged Give half of usual a.m. insulin as intermediate acting, CBG o/a, evening meal dose unchanged	Stop until eating and drinking normally
Three to five injections daily			
	No dose change	**Morning surgery** *Basal & bolus regimen:* Omit a.m. and lunch time short acting insulin, Keep basal unchanged *Premixed morning insulin:* Halve a.m. dose, Omit lunchtime dose CBG o/a	• Afternoon surgery Give usual a.m. dose Omit lunchtime dose CBG o/a	Stop until eating and drinking normally

CBG o/a, Capillary blood glucose on admission; VRIII, variable-rate intravenous insulin infusion.
(Adapted from Association of Anaesthetists of Great Britain and Ireland. (2015) Perioperative management of the surgical patient with diabetes 2015. *Anaesthesia.* 70, 1427–1440.)

- Capillary blood glucose should be measured and recorded at least hourly during the surgical procedure.
- The target blood glucose during the perioperative period should be 6–10 mmol L^{-1} (maximum 12 mmol L^{-1}).
- VRIIIs are preferred in patients who will miss more than one meal, patients with type 1 diabetes who have not received background insulin, patients with poorly controlled diabetes (HbA1c >69 mmol mol^{-1}) and most diabetic patients requiring emergency surgery.
- Use of 5% dextrose in 0.45% sodium chloride with either 0.15% or 0.3% potassium chloride (as appropriate) as the substrate fluid of choice if VRIII is required.
- Whenever a VRIII is administered, patients should also receive a long-acting insulin analogue. The dose should equate to 80% of their normal insulin dose. This reduces the risk of ketosis on discontinuation of the VRIII.
- Avoid unnecessary use of VRIII, but never stop an insulin infusion in someone with type 1 diabetes unless s.c. insulin has been given.

Concurrent drug therapy

Thiazide diuretics, adrenergic agents (e.g. salbutamol) and corticosteroids tend to increase blood glucose concentration. β-blockers tend to potentiate hypoglycaemia and may mask its clinical signs. Blood glucose concentration should be monitored if any of these drugs is administered and insulin dosage altered accordingly. Some drugs, including phenylbutazone, displace sulphonylureas from protein-binding sites and potentiate their hypoglycaemic effect. Dexamethasone, used as an antiemetic, may cause hyperglycaemia and should be used with caution in diabetic patients. Preoperative carbohydrate loading given as part of an enhanced recovery protocol should be avoided unless a VRIII is expected to be used.

Emergency surgery and diabetic ketoacidosis

Physiological stressors such as pain and sepsis contribute to hyperglycaemia and increased insulin requirements. Emergency patients may also be subjected to erratic and prolonged starvation periods. A VRIII will therefore be required in the majority of diabetic patients undergoing emergency surgery. Dextrose 5% with saline 0.45% should be used for fluid maintenance. Ideally patients should arrive in the operating theatre with a CBG of 6.0–10.0 mmol L^{-1}, having been adequately resuscitated and without any evidence of DKA.

Diabetic ketoacidosis can occur in people with both type 1 and type 2 diabetes. The diagnosis is based on the presence of ketosis (ketonaemia >3.0 mmol L^{-1} or ketonuria >2+ on urine testing sticks), CBG greater than 11.0 mmol L^{-1} and

acidaemia (bicarbonate <15 mmol L^{-1}, venous pH <7.3). The most common causes are infection (which may require surgical intervention), missed insulin treatment or as a first presentation of diabetes. Management of a patient with DKA will require fluid replacement and insulin administration: 0.9% saline with added potassium is used, initially 1000 ml given at 1000 ml h^{-1}, 2000 ml given at 500 ml h^{-1}, reducing to 250 ml h^{-1} thereafter. While the patient remains ketotic, a fixed-rate insulin infusion (FRIII) is used rather than a VRIII, initially started at a rate of 0.1 unit kg^{-1} h^{-1}. Capillary blood glucose concentrations are regarded as a poor marker for the resolution of DKA. Use of an FRIII rather than a VRIII is usually associated with a faster resolution of DKA. The FRIII should be continued until pH > 7.3, bicarbonate > 15.0 mmol L^{-1} and blood ketone concentration > 0.6 mmol L^{-1}. Surgery on a patient with DKA is associated with significant mortality and should only be undertaken with involvement of senior surgeons, anaesthetists, diabetologists and intensivists.

Other endocrine disorders

Pituitary disease

The clinical features of pituitary disease depend on the local effects of the lesion and its effects on the secretion of pituitary hormones. Local effects include headache and visual field disturbances. The effects on hormone secretion depend on the cells involved in the pathological process.

Acromegaly

Acromegaly is caused by increased secretion of growth hormone from eosinophil cell tumours of the anterior pituitary gland. If this occurs before fusion of the epiphyses, gigantism results. Problems for the anaesthetist include the following:

- Upper airway obstruction may result from an enlarged mandible, tongue and epiglottis; thickened pharyngeal mucosa; and laryngeal narrowing. Maintenance of a clear airway and tracheal intubation may be difficult, and postoperative care of the airway must be meticulous. Obstructive sleep apnoea is common.
- Cardiac enlargement, hypertension and biventricular cardiac failure occur commonly and require preoperative treatment.
- Growth hormone increases blood sugar concentration, and hyperglycaemia should be controlled perioperatively.
- Thyroid and adrenal function may be impaired because of decreased release of thyroid-stimulating hormone (TSH) and ACTH.

Treatment involves hypophysectomy, which requires steroid cover perioperatively (see later).

Cushing's disease

Cushing's disease results from basophil adenomas, which secrete ACTH (see later).

Hypopituitarism

Causes of hypopituitarism include chromophobe adenoma, tumours of surrounding tissues (e.g. craniopharyngioma), skull fractures, infarction after postpartum haemorrhage and infection. Clinical features include loss of axillary and pubic hair, amenorrhoea, features of hypothyroidism and adrenal insufficiency, including hypotension, but with a striking pallor, in contrast to the pigmentation of Addison's disease. The fluid and electrolyte disturbances are not as marked as in primary adrenal failure because of intact aldosterone production but may be unmasked by surgery, trauma or infection. Anaesthesia in these patients requires steroid cover (see later), cautious administration of induction agent and volatile anaesthetic agents, and careful cardiovascular monitoring.

Diabetes insipidus

Diabetes insipidus is caused by disease or damage affecting the hypothalamic posterior pituitary axis. Common causes are pituitary tumour, craniopharyngioma, basal skull fracture and infection; it also may occur as a result of pituitary surgery. In 10% of cases, diabetes insipidus is renal in origin. Dehydration with hypernatraemia follows excretion of large volumes of dilute urine. Patients require fluid replacement and treatment with DDAVP.

Thyroid disease

Goitre

Thyroid swelling may result from iodine deficiency (simple goitre), autoimmune (Hashimoto's) thyroiditis, adenoma, carcinoma or thyrotoxicosis. Nodules of the thyroid gland may be 'hot' (secreting thyroxine) or 'cold'. The goitre may occasionally cause respiratory or superior vena caval obstruction. The anaesthetic implications of this are discussed in Chapter 37.

Thyrotoxicosis

Thyrotoxicosis is characterised by excitability, tremor, tachycardia, arrhythmias (commonly atrial fibrillation), weight loss, heat intolerance and exophthalmos. Diagnosis is confirmed by measurement of total serum thyroxine, tri-iodothyronine (T_3) and TSH concentrations. Elective surgery should not be carried out in hyperthyroid patients; they should first be rendered euthyroid with carbimazole or radioactive iodine (see Chapter 37). However, urgent surgery and elective subtotal thyroidectomy may be carried out safely in hyperthyroid patients using β-blockade alone or in combination with potassium iodide to control thyrotoxic symptoms and signs. Emergency surgery carries a significant risk of thyrotoxic crisis. Control is best achieved in these circumstances by i.v. potassium iodide and a nonselective β-blocker (e.g. propranolol). If patients are unable to absorb oral medication, an i.v. infusion is indicated; for propranolol the daily i.v. dose is approximately 10% of the p.o. dose.

Hypothyroidism

Hypothyroidism may result from primary thyroid failure, Hashimoto's thyroiditis, as a consequence of thyroid surgery or secondary to pituitary failure. The diagnosis is suggested by tiredness, cold intolerance, loss of appetite, dry skin and hair loss. It may be confirmed by the finding of a low serum thyroxine concentration associated, in primary thyroid failure, with a raised serum TSH concentration.

Cardiac output is decreased, with little myocardial reserve, and hypothermia may be present. Treatment is with thyroxine, which should be started at a dose of 50–100 μg daily, and titrated to clinical and biochemical response. Rapid correction of hypothyroidism may be achieved using i.v. T_3, but this is inadvisable in older patients and those with IHD (which is common in hypothyroidism) as the sudden increase in myocardial oxygen demand may provoke ischaemia or infarction. Electrocardiographic monitoring is advisable during treatment. Elective surgery should be avoided in hypothyroid patients, but if emergency surgery is necessary, close cardiovascular, ECG and blood gas monitoring is essential. Basal metabolic rate is decreased, resulting in slower drug distribution and metabolism; all anaesthetic agents must, therefore, be administered in reduced doses.

Disease of the adrenal cortex

Clinical symptoms are associated with increased or decreased secretion of cortisol or aldosterone.

Phaeochromocytoma

Phaeochromocytoma is discussed in Chapter 39.

Hypersecretion of cortisol

Most commonly caused by pituitary adenomas which secrete ACTH and thus cause bilateral adrenocortical hyperplasia (Cushing's disease). In 20%–30% of patients an adrenocortical adenoma or carcinoma is present (Cushing's syndrome). Rarely, an oat-cell carcinoma of bronchus, secreting ACTH, is the cause. Prolonged corticosteroid therapy and ACTH cause similar clinical features, including obesity, hypertension, proximal myopathy and diabetes mellitus. Biochemically there is a metabolic alkalosis with hypokalaemia. Depending on the cause, treatment may involve hypophysectomy or adrenalectomy.

Anaesthetic management of these patients involves preoperative treatment of hypertension and biventricular cardiac failure, and correction of hypokalaemia. Adrenal surgery is now commonly laparoscopic, often with the patient in the prone position. Intraoperative management is directed towards careful monitoring of arterial pressure and maintenance of cardiovascular stability, with careful choice and administration of anaesthetic agents and NMBAs. Postoperative steroid therapy is required for hypophysectomy and adrenalectomy (see later). Fludrocortisone 0.05–0.3 mg day^{-1} is required after bilateral adrenalectomy.

Primary hypersecretion of aldosterone (Conn's syndrome)

Conn's syndrome is caused by an adenoma of the zona glomerulosa of the adrenal cortex and presents with hypertension, hypernatraemia, hypokalaemia and oliguria. Anaesthetic management involves preoperative treatment of hypertension, administration of spironolactone and potassium replacement; meticulous intra- and postoperative monitoring of arterial pressure is essential.

Adrenocortical insufficiency

Primary adrenocortical insufficiency (Addison's disease) most commonly occurs due to autoimmune destruction of the adrenal glands. Other causes include tuberculosis, HIV infection, amyloid, metastatic carcinoma or haemorrhage into the adrenal glands (e.g. as a result of meningococcal septicaemia). Secondary hypoadrenalism is caused by anterior pituitary disease; aldosterone secretion is maintained and fluid and electrolyte disturbances are less marked. Hypoadrenalism after prolonged corticosteroid therapy is similar to secondary hypoadrenalism. Clinical features include weakness, weight loss, hyperpigmentation, hypotension, vomiting, diarrhoea and volume depletion. Hypoglycaemia, hyponatraemia, hyperkalaemia and metabolic acidaemia are characteristic but late biochemical findings. The stress of infection, trauma or surgery provokes profound hypotension. Diagnosis is made by measurement of plasma cortisol concentration and the response to ACTH stimulation.

All surgical procedures in these patients must be covered by increased steroid administration (see later). Patients with acute adrenal insufficiency require urgent fluid and sodium replacement with invasive monitoring, glucose infusion to combat hypoglycaemia and hydrocortisone 200 mg 24 h^{-1} by continuous infusion, or 100 mg i.m. every 6 h. Patients should be cared for in HDU/ICU. Antibiotics are advisable

to cover the possibility that infection has provoked the crisis. In cases of primary adrenal failure, mineralocorticoid replacement with fludrocortisone is required.

Steroid cover for anaesthesia and surgery

Replacement therapy in cases of primary adrenocortical failure and hypopituitarism is given as oral hydrocortisone 20 mg in the morning and 10 mg in the evening. Fludrocortisone 0.05–0.1 mg daily is given additionally to replace aldosterone in primary adrenocortical failure. Equivalent doses of other steroid preparations are shown in Table 20.4. Prednisolone and prednisone have less mineralocorticoid effect, and betamethasone and dexamethasone have none. Requirements increase after infection, trauma or surgery.

Indications for perioperative steroid supplements include:
- patients with pituitary adrenal insufficiency, receiving steroid replacement therapy;
- patients undergoing pituitary or adrenal surgery (unless underlying Cushing's disease);
- patients receiving ≥ 5 mg prednisolone or equivalent per day for 4 weeks or longer;
- patients no longer receiving systemic steroid therapy but who received steroids within the 3 months before surgery; and
- patients on high-dose inhaled steroids, greater than 2 mg beclomethasone or 1 mg fluticasone.

Supplementation is usually with i.v. hydrocortisone at induction of anaesthesia, with ongoing dosing for some days after surgery, depending on the magnitude of surgery (Table 20.9). Continued administration is vital; where oral absorption appears unreliable, i.v./i.m. dosing should be continued. High doses of hydrocortisone (e.g. 100 mg) given i.v. often exceed the capacity of cortisol-binding globulin, which is necessary for cellular delivery; i.m. delivery may, therefore, be superior.

Neurological disease

General considerations

Neurological disease embraces a wide range of differing conditions, the effects of which may influence the conduct of perioperative care in a number of ways:
- Depressed level of consciousness may compromise airway protection and result in depressed respiratory drive.
- Peripheral neuromuscular disease may lead to impaired ventilatory function and reduced ability to clear secretions.
- Autonomic dysfunction may result in blood pressure instability, cardiac arrhythmias and dysfunction of GI motility.

Table 20.9 Intra- and postoperative steroid cover for adults at risk of adrenal suppression (prednisolone equivalent ≥ 5 mg for ≥ 4 weeks)

	Intraoperative	Postoperative
Major surgery (including caesarean section)	Hydrocortisone 100 mg i.v. at induction, followed by continuous infusion of hydrocortisone 200 mg per 24 h^{-1}. Dexamethasone 6-8 mg i.v., if used, will suffice for 24 h	Hydrocortisone 100 mg 24 h^{-1} by i.v. infusion while nil by mouth. Resume usual p.o. steroid dose if recovery is uncomplicated. If not, double regular p.o. dose for 48 h., then return to regular dose.
Intermediate/body surface surgery	As for major surgery	Double regular p.o. dose for 48 h, then return to regular dose.
Bowel procedures requiring laxatives/enemas	Continue normal steroid dose. Switch to equivalent i.v. dose if unable to take p.o.	
Labour and vaginal delivery	Hydrocortisone 100 mg i.v. at onset of labour, followed by immediate initiation of a continuous infusion of hydrocortisone 200 mg 24 h^{-1} Alternatively, hydrocortisone 100 mg i.m. followed by 50 mg every 6 h i.m.	

Adapted from: Management of glucocorticoids for patients with adrenal insufficiency during the peri-operative period Association of Anaesthetists, Royal College of Physicians and Society for Endocrinology UK.

- Significant adverse effects can occur with specific drug treatments, and there are several important drug interactions which need to be recognised.

Assessment

In addition to standard history and examination, a detailed drug history should be obtained. Many patients with neurological disease (e.g. epilepsy, parkinsonism, myasthenia gravis) should have their medication continued up to the time of surgery and reinstated as soon as possible thereafter. Respiratory function should be assessed using pulmonary function tests, including vital capacity and measurement of arterial blood gas tensions. Erect and supine arterial pressure should be measured when appropriate and a 12-lead ECG performed to assess QT interval and possible heart block.

Respiratory impairment

Inadequate ventilatory function may result from:
- reduced central drive (e.g. because of an impaired conscious level);
- motor neuropathy (e.g. Guillain–Barré syndrome, motor neuron disease);
- neuromuscular dysfunction (e.g. myasthenia gravis);
- muscle weakness (e.g. muscular dystrophies); or
- rigidity (e.g. Parkinson's disease).

These patients are sensitive to anaesthetic agents, opioids and NMBAs. If intraoperative mechanical ventilation is undertaken, a period of elective postoperative ventilation may be needed until full recovery from the effects of anaesthesia has occurred. If appropriate, procedures may be carried out under a regional anaesthetic technique. Bulbar muscle involvement may lead to inadequate protection of the airway such that regurgitation and aspiration can occur. Any pulmonary infection should be treated preoperatively and, in the elective situation, this may necessitate postponing surgery.

Altered innervation of muscle and hyperkalaemia

Suxamethonium may cause life-threatening hyperkalaemia in some neurological conditions. An altered ratio of intracellular to extracellular potassium tends to produce sensitivity to non-depolarising, and resistance to depolarising, NMBAs. If there is widespread denervation of muscle with lower motor neuron damage, such as in Guillain–Barré syndrome, disorganisation of the motor end-plate occurs, resulting in hypersensitivity to acetylcholine and suxamethonium, with increased permeability of muscle cells to potassium. A similar potassium efflux occurs in the presence of direct muscle damage, widespread burns involving muscle, upper motor neuron lesions, spinal cord lesions with paraplegia and tetanus. In upper motor neuron and spinal cord lesions, the reason for this shift is less clear. Patients undergoing mechanical ventilation in ICU who are suffering from sepsis and multiple organ failure may develop a critical illness polyneuropathy, with a similar hyperkalaemic response to suxamethonium. The resulting increase in serum potassium concentration after suxamethonium may be 3 mmol L^{-1} (compared with 0.6 mmol L^{-1} in other patients) and may occur from 24 h after acute muscle denervation or damage.

Autonomic disturbances

Autonomic disturbances may occur as part of a polyneuropathy (e.g. diabetes mellitus, Guillain–Barré syndrome and porphyria) or from central nervous system involvement (e.g. in parkinsonism). Sympathetic stimulation, such as tracheal intubation or after administration of catecholamines, may produce severe hypertension and arrhythmias. More commonly, blood loss, head-up posture or neuraxial regional blocks may be associated with severe hypotension. Cardiac arrhythmias may also occur.

Raised intracranial pressure

Elective surgery should be postponed if raised intracranial pressure is suspected, until investigation by CT scan and treatment have been undertaken. This is discussed fully in Chapter 40.

Epilepsy

Epilepsy may be caused by birth injury, hypoglycaemia, hypocalcaemia, drug overdose or withdrawal, fever, head injury, cerebrovascular disease or cerebral tumour; however, in most patients with epilepsy, no identifiable cause is found. Epilepsy developing after the age of 20 years usually indicates organic brain disease. Patients with refractory epilepsy may also present for surgical treatment, e.g. implantation of intracranial electrodes, vagal nerve stimulators or resection of the epileptic focus.

Patients should receive their maintenance anticonvulsant therapy throughout the perioperative period. The effects of i.v. anaesthetic agents are complex in epilepsy, being proconvulsant at low concentrations and anticonvulsant at high concentrations. Propofol was previously avoided but is now used widely. The inhalational anaesthetic agents are safe to use. Alfentanil is a potent enhancer of epileptiform activity and should be used with caution. Other opioids are regarded as safe to use. Local anaesthetic agents may cause convulsions at lower than normal concentrations, and the safe maximum dose should be reduced. All NMBAs are safe to use; laudanosine, a metabolite of atracurium, has been associated with seizures in animals only. Dopamine antagonists used as antiemetics (prochlorperazine, metoclopramide and droperidol) may cause extrapyramidal effects and dystonic reactions. Their use should be avoided. Postoperatively, i.v. or p.r. formulations of antiepileptic therapies are available.

Status epilepticus

Management of status epilepticus is aimed at cessation of the fits while maintaining tissue oxygenation. Initial treatment should be lorazepam 0.1 mg kg^{-1}, repeated after 10–20 min. Second-line treatment is with i.v. phenytoin 15–18 mg kg^{-1} given at 50 mg per min or i.v. levetiracetam 30 mg kg^{-1} (to maximum of 3 g). If seizures remain refractory, a general anaesthetic is administered, with airway control, ventilation and transfer to ICU.

Parkinson's disease

The clinical signs of resting tremor, muscle rigidity and bradykinesia characterise Parkinson's disease. This illness affects more than 100,000 people in the UK, with a prevalence of approximately 1% in those aged older than 65. It is caused by cell death in areas of the basal ganglia, with loss of dopaminergic neurons. Similar symptoms and signs occur with loss of dopaminergic function secondary to drugs such as antipsychotic agents and after encephalitis in some patients. Patients commonly present for urological, ophthalmic or orthopaedic surgery. There are various considerations for the anaesthetist.

Respiratory

The airway may be difficult because of fixed flexion of the neck. Upper airway muscle dysfunction may lead to aspiration. Excessive salivation may necessitate administration of a preoperative antisialagogue. An obstructive ventilatory pattern is present in around 35% of patients, and muscle rigidity and tremor may also impair ventilation.

Cardiovascular

Postural hypotension may be present, and there is an increased risk of cardiac arrhythmias. Autonomic failure may cause or exacerbate these problems.

Gastrointestinal

There is an increased risk of gastro-oesophageal reflux.

Medications

Medications may have cardiovascular adverse effects, and there are several potential interactions with antiemetics, analgesics and vasoactive drugs (Table 20.10).

Anaesthetic management

- Medication should be continued up to the time of surgery and be reinstated as soon as possible thereafter.
- A technique which avoids pulmonary aspiration should be used when appropriate. Regional techniques offer several advantages such as the avoidance of opioid drugs and less effect on respiratory function. Isoflurane and sevoflurane are the inhalational agents of choice, although hypotension may be a problem, particularly in the presence of autonomic neuropathy and when bromocriptine or selegiline have been administered.
- In the patient requiring general anaesthesia, nasogastric L-dopa can be administered during prolonged operations.

427

Table 20.10 Potential drug interactions in patients with Parkinson's disease

Drug	Effect
Contraindicated	
Phenothiazines (e.g. prochlorperazine) Butyrophenones (e.g. droperidol) Benzamides (e.g. metoclopramide) Antipsychotics (e.g. haloperidol)	All are dopamine antagonists causing exacerbation of parkinsonian symptoms
Caution	
Centrally acting anticholinergics (e.g. atropine)	May precipitate central anticholinergic syndrome
Direct-acting sympathomimetics if taking MAOBI	Exaggerated vasoconstrictor effects
Adrenaline if taking COMTi	Exaggerated sympathomimetic response
Fentanyl, alfentanil	Large doses may cause muscle rigidity

COMTi, Catechol-*O*-methyltransferase inhibitors; *MAOBI,* monoamine oxidase-B inhibitor.
(Reproduced from Chambers DJ, Sebastian J, and Ahern DJ (2017) Parkinson's disease. *British Journal of Anaesthesia Education.* 17(4), 145–149.)

If the enteral route is not possible, parenteral apomorphine can be used. This should be preceded by administration of domperidone for 72 h.

- Transdermal rotigotine, a dopamine agonist, may be used as an alternative.
- Parkinsonian patients have an increased risk of postoperative confusion and hallucinations and may exhibit abnormal neurological signs such as decerebrate posturing, upgoing plantars and hyperreflexia after general anaesthesia.

Multiple sclerosis

A deterioration in symptoms of multiple sclerosis (MS) tends to occur after surgery, but no specific anaesthetic technique has been implicated. Postoperative relapses are related to the incidence of infection and pyrexia. For most patients with MS there is no evidence of a greater risk of complications associated with general or regional anaesthesia. Anaesthetic management does not need to be altered in women with MS during labour and delivery.

Peripheral neuropathies

Peripheral neuropathies may exhibit axonal dying back degeneration or segmental demyelination. They are classified by anatomical distribution, the most common being a symmetrical peripheral polyneuropathy. Motor, sensory and autonomic fibres are involved. Causes include:
- metabolic disorders (e.g. diabetes, porphyria);
- nutritional deficiency;
- toxicity (e.g. heavy metals, drugs);
- collagen disease;
- carcinoma;
- infection;
- inflammation; and
- critical illness polyneuropathy.

Problems for the anaesthetist include the effects of autonomic neuropathy, respiratory impairment and bulbar involvement.

Motor neuron disease

Motor neuron disease is characterised by slow-onset and progressive deterioration in motor function. Several patterns of motor loss occur, with both upper and lower motor neuron loss. Problems for the anaesthetist include sensitivity to all anaesthetic agents and NMBAs, respiratory inadequacy and laryngeal incompetence. Regional techniques may be useful. Prolonged mechanical ventilation should generally be avoided, but NIV has a definite role in palliation of dyspnoea.

Spinal cord lesions with paraplegia

Assessment of ventilatory function is important, as impaired cough and poor inspiration may indicate a need for postoperative controlled ventilation. In cervical spine lesions, patients are dependent on the diaphragm for breathing. In the acute situation the loss of intercostal muscle function, to which patients may take some time to adjust, coupled with general anaesthesia may lead to postoperative respiratory failure, necessitating controlled ventilation. Regional anaesthetic techniques may be useful in these patients, reducing the autonomic reflexes stimulated by surgery and avoiding compromise of ventilatory function. Release of potassium from muscle cells by suxamethonium precludes its use within 6–12 months of cord injury.

Myasthenia gravis

Myasthenia gravis usually presents in young adults and is characterised by episodes of increased muscle fatigue caused by decreased numbers of acetylcholine receptors at the neuromuscular junction. Treatment comprises an anticholinesterase (e.g. pyridostigmine 60 mg every 6 h or neostigmine 15 mg every 6 h) with a vagolytic agent (atropine or propantheline) to block the muscarinic adverse effects. Steroid therapy is useful in some cases, and thymectomy may benefit many patients. Anticholinesterase therapy should be continued throughout the perioperative period.

The principal anaesthetic problems concern adequacy of ventilation, ability to cough and clear secretions and the increased secretions resulting from anticholinesterase therapy. If there is evidence of respiratory infection, surgery should be postponed. Serum potassium concentration should be kept within the normal range because hypokalaemia potentiates myasthenia. Local and regional anaesthesia, including subarachnoid or epidural block, may be suitable alternatives to general anaesthesia, although the maximum dose of local anaesthetic agents should be reduced because of their neuromuscular blocking action. All myasthenic conditions are extremely sensitive to the effects of NMBAs. Intraoperative management of NMBAs can be difficult in terms of dose, duration and reversal. Awake fibreoptic intubation should be considered. The use of rocuronium and sugammadex may be beneficial. Suxamethonium has a variable effect in myasthenia and is best avoided. The use of a peripheral nerve stimulator to monitor neuromuscular block is essential.

Factors associated with the need for postoperative ventilation include coexisting respiratory diseases, previous myaesthenic crisis, FVC < 2.1 L and existing bulbar symptoms. Frequent chest physiotherapy and tracheal suction are required. Steroid cover is given if appropriate. If extreme muscle weakness occurs, neostigmine 1–2 mg and atropine 0.6–1.2 mg may be given i.v.. Care must be taken to titrate the doses of anticholinesterase or a cholinergic crisis may occur, characterised by a depolarising neuromuscular block, with sweating, salivation and pupillary constriction. An infusion of neostigmine is required if resumption of oral intake is delayed after surgery; 0.5 mg i.v. is equivalent to 15 mg neostigmine or 60 mg pyridostigmine orally and should be combined with an anticholinergic agent.

A myasthenic state may also be associated with carcinoma, thyrotoxicosis, Cushing's syndrome, hypokalaemia and hypocalcaemia. In these patients, non-depolarising NMBAs should be avoided or used in reduced dosage.

Dystrophia myotonica

Dystrophia myotonica is a disease of autosomal dominant inheritance characterised by muscle weakness and muscle contraction persisting after the termination of voluntary effort. Other features may include frontal baldness, cataract, sternomastoid wasting, gonadal atrophy and thyroid adenoma. Problems which affect anaesthetic management include the following:

- *Respiratory muscle weakness.* Respiratory function should be assessed fully before operation. Respiratory depressant drugs should be used with care; there is sensitivity also to non-depolarising NMBAs. Planned mechanical ventilation may be required after surgery. Postoperative care of the airway must be meticulous, and pulmonary infections are common.
- *Cardiovascular effects.* There may be cardiomyopathy and conduction defects, including complete heart block. Patients may have a cardiac pacemaker *in situ*. Arrhythmias are common, particularly during anaesthesia, and may result in cardiac failure. Echocardiographic assessment may be required preoperatively.
- *Muscle spasm.* This may be provoked by administration of depolarising NMBAs or anticholinesterases; suxamethonium and neostigmine should be avoided. The spasm is not abolished by non-depolarising NMBAs.
- *Gastrointestinal.* Oesophageal dysmotility may predispose to regurgitation and aspiration.

Psychiatric disease

There are several considerations in the anaesthetic management of patients with psychiatric disease:

- Psychiatric patients are often depressed, with little understanding of, or interest in, anaesthesia.
- Patients are receiving a variety of medications with potential for serious drug interactions with anaesthetic agents.
- Patients may have associated pathological conditions as a result of drug and/or alcohol abuse.
- Repeated anaesthetics are required for ECT (see Chapter 46).

Drug interactions in psychiatric disorders

Antidepressants

Antidepressant drugs include selective serotonin reuptake inhibitors (SSRIs), serotonin and noradrenaline reuptake inhibitors (SNRIs), tricyclic antidepressants (TCAs) and monoamine oxidase inhibitors (MAOIs). They all act by increasing brain concentrations of serotonin and noradrenaline. Serotonin syndrome, hyperreflexia, agitation and hyperthermia can occur in patients taking SSRIs when given fentanyl or tramadol. SSRIs can also inhibit the cytochrome P450 enzyme system, affecting the metabolism of several drugs. TCAs and MAOIs are now used less often in current practice. Both TCAs and MAOIs can have a profound pressor effect in response to sympathomimetic agents. MAOIs are usually discontinued 2 weeks before surgery.

Antipsychotics

Most antipsychotics act by blocking the action of dopamine. Newer antipsychotics have an additional serotonin effect.

429

They may have extrapyramidal side effects. Neuroleptic malignant syndrome is a rare adverse effect of their use and shares many of the signs and symptoms of malignant hyperpyrexia.

Mood stabilisers

Mood stabilisers are drugs used in the management of bipolar disorders for the treatment and prevention of mania. They include lithium, carbamazepine and sodium valproate. Lithium has a range of adverse effects, including interference with ADH, arrhythmias, GI disturbance and tremor. Its use may prolong the effect of NMBAs, and it is usually discontinued 24–48 h before surgery. Carbamazepine is an enzyme inducer and may reduce the effectiveness of many drugs. Sodium valproate may interfere with platelet function.

Connective tissue disorders

Connective tissue disorders are multisystem diseases which can present with a variety of problems relevant to anaesthesia and surgery and which show a wide degree of overlap.

Rheumatoid arthritis

Rheumatoid arthritis is by far the most common connective tissue disorder; it is a multisystem disease with several implications for anaesthesia which must be considered at the time of preoperative assessment.

Airway

The arthritic process may involve the temporomandibular joints, rendering laryngoscopy and tracheal intubation difficult. The cervical spine may be fixed or subluxed (and potentially be unstable, especially when the patient is anaesthetised). Cervical spine flexion/extension radiographs are required before surgery. Cricoarytenoid involvement should be suspected if hoarseness or stridor is present.

Respiratory system

Costochondral involvement causes a restrictive defect, with reduced vital capacity. Pulmonary involvement with interstitial fibrosis produces ventilation/perfusion abnormalities, a diffusion defect and thus hypoxaemia.

Cardiovascular system

Endocardial and myocardial involvement may occur. Coronary arteritis, conduction defects and peripheral arteritis are other, uncommon, features. Immobility caused by arthritis may make assessment of cardiorespiratory function difficult.

Anaemia

A chronic anaemia, hypo- or normochromic, but refractory to iron therapy, occurs. Treatment with NSAIDs may cause GI blood loss. Preoperative transfusion to a haemoglobin concentration of approximately 100 g L^{-1} is advisable before major surgery.

Renal function

Renal impairment, or nephrotic syndrome, may occur as a result of amyloidosis or drug treatment. NSAIDs should be used with caution in the perioperative period.

Drug therapy

In addition to standard analgesics, disease modifying anti-rheumatic drugs (DMARDs) may be prescribed. These include methotrexate, sulfasalazine, cyclophosphamide and the newer biological agents, many of which have an antitumour necrosis factor action. Methotrexate may cause liver and hepatic dysfunction. Most DMARDs are discontinued before surgery because of increased infection risk. Many patients are also receiving long-term steroid therapy and require augmented steroid cover for the perioperative period (see Table 20.9).

Conduct of anaesthesia

Specific anaesthetic considerations include:
- consideration of general versus regional anaesthesia;
- how to secure and maintain the patient's airway if a general anaesthetic is required;
- vascular access;
- steroid replacement where indicated;
- positioning for surgery; and
- analgesia for a group of patients who may have significant preoperative pain and may be on regular opioids and other analgesics.

Particular care should be taken with venepuncture and insertion of i.v. cannulae because of atrophy of skin and subcutaneous tissues and fragility of veins. Careful positioning of the patient on the operating table is required because these patients may have multiple joint involvement. Padding may be required to prevent pressure sores.

The anaesthetist should be prepared for a difficult tracheal intubation. If tracheal intubation is essential, awake fibreoptic intubation is often the technique of choice. When tracheal intubation is not essential, a SAD is often satisfactory, but a backup plan should be made in case of difficulties.

Alternatively the use of regional anaesthesia may negate the need for complex airway management.

Other connective tissue diseases

Implications for the anaesthetist regarding patients with other connective tissue disorders are similar to those associated with rheumatoid arthritis. However, some specific features may be more prominent, such as vasculitis (including cerebral vasculitis), glomerulonephritis, pulmonary fibrosis or peri- or myocarditis. Steroid and immunosuppressive therapy are other potential problems.

- *Scleroderma (systemic sclerosis)*. This disorder is associated with restricted mouth opening, lower oesophageal involvement with increased risk of regurgitation, pulmonary involvement, renal failure, steroid therapy and peripheral vascular disease.
- *Systemic lupus erythematosus (SLE)*. Anaemia and renal and respiratory involvement may be severe. Cardiac involvement may include mitral valve disease. Cerebral vasculitis may occur. Steroid therapy is usual.
- *Ankylosing spondylitis*. The rigid spine makes tracheal intubation difficult, and spinal and epidural anaesthesia may be technically impossible. Awake fibreoptic intubation is often required for airway control and may be difficult. Costovertebral joint involvement restricts chest expansion. Postoperative ventilatory support may be required.

Human immunodeficiency virus

Statistics in 2016 suggest about 90,000 people are living with HIV in the UK. With early diagnosis and effective treatment, individuals with HIV can expect a near normal life expectancy. It is estimated that more than 30% of people accessing HIV specialist care are aged 50 years or older. Current treatment of HIV is described as highly active antiretroviral therapy (HAART) and typically involves a combination of three different antiviral medications. A patient's HIV status and response to treatment can be assessed by measurement of his or her HIV viral load and CD4 lymphocyte cell count. A high HIV count indicates a high risk of infective transmission, whereas a low CD4 count means immune system dysfunction in the patient. Patient compliance with an effective HAART regime should result in an undetectable HIV viral load.

Preoperative evaluation and intraoperative management of the HIV-infected patient is similar to that of the general population. Universal precautions should be followed at all times. Patients with HIV are at risk of liver dysfunction as an adverse effect of HAART therapy or infection with hepatitis B or C. There may be risk of increased bleeding as a result of coagulopathy or thrombocytopenia. There is an increased prevalence of renal dysfunction from HIV-associated nephropathy (HIVAN). Cardiac issues can occur with advanced HIV disease, with a higher incidence of coronary artery disease and conduction defects. Respiratory complications can occur as a result of an increased risk of bacterial pneumonia and a high prevalence of smoking in HIV-infected patients. Rates of alcohol, substance abuse and methicillin-resistant *Staphylococcus aureus* (MRSA) are also higher in this group of patients.

In the event of significant exposure to infected body fluids, postexposure prophylaxis (PEP) should be given. The local occupational health department or infectious diseases unit should be contacted for advice urgently, because treatment should ideally commence within 1–2 h. Postexposure prophylaxis regimes may involve up to four antiviral agents taken for 4 weeks.

Myeloma

Myeloma is a neoplastic condition that affects plasma cells and has several features of significance to the anaesthetist.

- Widespread skeletal destruction occurs, and careful handling of the patient on the operating table is essential. Pathological fractures are common.
- Bone pain may be severe and often requires large doses of analgesics.
- Hypercalcaemia occurs as a result of bone destruction and may precipitate renal failure.
- Chronic renal failure may also result from direct nephrotoxicity.
- Anaemia is almost invariable, and preoperative blood transfusion is often necessary.
- Thrombocytopenia is common during cytotoxic therapy.
- Patients are susceptible to infection, especially during chemotherapy.
- Increased plasma immunoglobulin concentrations may increase blood viscosity, predisposing to arterial and venous thrombosis. Drug binding may be affected.
- Neurological manifestations include spinal cord and nerve root compression.

Porphyria

The porphyrias are an inherited group of disorders of haem biosynthesis. Deficiencies in the intermediary enzymes in the haem pathway result in an accumulation of 5-aminolaevulinic acid (ALA) and elevated concentrations of porphobilinogen (PBG). Porphyrias are classified as acute or non-acute. The acute porphyrias have the potential to

431

precipitate acute neurovisceral crises. Clinical features include the following:

- GI: Abdominal pain and tenderness, vomiting, constipation and occasionally diarrhoea may occur.
- CNS: Motor and sensory peripheral neuropathy is common. It may involve bulbar and respiratory muscles. Epileptic fits and psychological disturbance may occur.
- CVS: Hypertension and tachycardia often occur during the attacks. Hypotension has also been reported.
- Fever and leucocytosis occur in 25%–30% of patients.

Precipitating factors are commonly seen in the surgical patient, namely: fasting; dehydration; infection; stress (physical or emotional); and smoking. Numerous drugs can also precipitate porphyria, many of which are commonly used perioperatively (Table 20.11). Diagnosis is made by checking PBG concentrations in fresh urine: normal values effectively exclude acute porphyria. Treatment consists of supportive measures, removal of the precipitating agent and administration of haem arginate 3 mg kg^{-1} i.v. (to a maximum of 250 mg) once daily for 4 days.

Table 20.11 Safety of drugs commonly used in anaesthesia for patients with acute porphyrias

Class of drug	Safe	Unsafe	Undetermined
Intravenous anaesthetic agents	Propofol (bolus)	Thiopental	Propofol (infusions) Etomidate
Inhalational anaesthetic agents	Isoflurane Desflurane Nitrous oxide	Sevoflurane	
Local anaesthetic agents	Bupivacaine Prilocaine Lidocaine		Levobupivacaine Ropivacaine
Neuromuscular blocking drugs	Suxamethonium Atracurium Rocuronium Pancuronium Neostigmine		
Analgesics	Fentanyl Alfentanil Remifentanil Morphine Tramadol Diamorphine Codeine phosphate Celecoxib Aspirin Paracetamol	Oxycodone Diclofenac	Pentazocine Mefenamic acid
Sedatives	Lorazepam Temazepam Midazolam		
Antibiotics	Gentamicin Co-amoxiclav Penicillins, cephalosporins Vancomycin Teicoplanin Meropenem	Rifampicin Erythromycin	

Table 20.11 Safety of drugs commonly used in anaesthesia for patients with acute porphyrias—cont'd

Class of drug	Safe	Unsafe	Undetermined
Cardiovascular drugs	Adrenaline, noradrenaline Atropine Glycopyrronium bromide β-blockers Magnesium Adenosine	Ephedrine	Vasopressin Metaraminol
Miscellaneous	Syntocinon Carbaprost Ondansetron Tranexamic acid		Dexamethasone Hydrocortisone

An up-to-date list of drugs considered safe in acute porphyria is available at www.wmic.wales.nhs.uk/specialist-services/drugs-in-porphyria/.

References/Further reading

Association of Anaesthetists of Great Britain and Ireland, 2016. The measurement of adult blood pressure and management of hypertension before elective surgery 2016. Anaesthesia 71, 326–337.

Dhatariya, K., Levy, N., et al., 2016. Joint British Diabetes Societies for inpatient care. Management of adults with diabetes undergoing surgery and elective procedures: improving standards.

Fleisher, L.A., Fleischmann, K.E., Auerbach, A.D., et al., 2014. 2014 ACC/AHA guideline on the perioperative cardiovascular evaluation and management of patients undergoing noncardiac surgery: executive summary. J. Am. Coll. Cardiol. 64, 2373–2405.

Levine, G.N., Bates, E.R., et al., 2016. ACC/AHA guideline focused update on duration of dual antiplatelet therapy in patients with coronary artery disease. Circulation 134, e123–e155.

The National Confidential Enquiry into Patient Outcome and Death, 2018. Highs and Lows, London.

Chapter 21

Consent and information for patients

David Bogod, Kate McCombe

Whenever we seek consent from a patient before medical examination, investigation or treatment, we demonstrate our respect for the ethical principles of autonomy and the patient's right to self-determination. Consent is always **given** or withheld by the patient; it is not something done **to** a patient, and anaesthetists, along with other healthcare professionals, should avoid using phrases such as *consenting the patient*. Seeking consent is a process, not an event, and it must not be reduced to getting the patient to sign a piece of paper merely to protect us from litigation. In the simplest of terms, when patients offer us their consent, they give us permission to make physical contact with them in the manner we have explained to them. Without this permission, we may find ourselves accused of battery or assault, no matter how well intentioned our actions.

Capacity

A patient must have the *capacity* to consent to medical intervention. In what is often referred to as the 'four-step assessment of capacity', capable patients can **understand**, in broad terms, the nature of the proposed intervention; **retain** this information for long enough to **weigh** it in the balance; and use it to make a decision. Finally, they can **communicate** their decision.

In the UK, all patients older than age 16, including those with mental illness, are assumed to have capacity to consent to their treatment unless serious doubt exists to the contrary. Capacity is not an all-or-nothing state, and so a patient's ability to make a choice may depend on how complex the factors involved in that decision are. Capacity may also

fluctuate, and where possible, doctors should defer making treatment decisions if they anticipate the return of the patient's ability to decide.

Voluntariness

Consent should be given voluntarily – that is, without coercion. The anaesthetist should take appropriate steps to satisfy himself or herself that, however well meaning, the patient is not being coerced by other people or by the situation. In normal practice this involves nothing more than straightforward discussion with the patient.

In our increasingly multicultural society, it is not uncommon to find that language barriers prevent us from communicating easily with our patients. The Association of Anaesthetists advises that, in these situations, we should not rely on the patient's family members or friends to translate as we cannot be certain of the quality or accuracy of information relayed. Instead we should use independent professional translators provided by the hospital or translation telephone services.

The law does permit doctors to offer their advice as to the best course of action, but they must not pressure the patient to accept their advice.

Types of consent

For most patients the consent process begins when they first present to their primary care provider. At every subsequent interventional step, they give consent, however informally, before proceeding. A patient with capacity has the absolute right to accept or refuse medical intervention and so, if the patient refuses, we *may not* proceed. This remains the case even if we believe that the treatment is in their best interests and their refusal is irrational and may result in dire consequences, including death. Disagreeing with one's doctors is not diagnostic of a lack of capacity. Although patients have the right to *refuse* treatment, they cannot *insist* on receiving treatment which the medical team does not consider to be in their best interests.

Written consent is not a legal requirement for all medical interventions; much of what we do in our clinical practice is permitted with the patient's *implied* or *verbal* consent. For example, if a doctor asks to check the patient's pulse and the patient holds out a wrist, or asks to insert a cannula and the patient says yes, then the doctor may reasonably continue.

The Association of Anaesthetists is of the view that a signed consent form is not necessary for anaesthetic procedures performed to facilitate another treatment because a signed form 'does nothing to validate or invalidate the consent. The anaesthetic can be considered a component of another treatment or part of a larger and interrelated process (e.g. epidural pain relief for childbirth), rather than a treatment in itself. The Association of Anaesthetists advises, however, that, 'whether consent is verbal or written, [we] should document the patient's agreement to the proposed intervention and the discussion that lead to that agreement, including the patient's questions and the responses given'. Discussions can be recorded on the anaesthetic chart, a preprinted consent form or in the patient's medical notes. When the anaesthetic intervention is the primary procedure, for example, therapeutic injections for chronic pain, hospitals may insist on formal, written consent, and anaesthetists should follow the guidelines of the institution in which they work.

The General Medical Council (GMC) advises that written consent should be sought if:

1. the investigation or treatment is complex or involves significant risks;
2. there may be significant consequences for the patient's employment or social or personal life;
3. providing clinical care is not the primary purpose of the investigation or treatment; or
4. the treatment is part of a research programme or is an innovative treatment designed specifically for their benefit.

Although written consent is usually facilitated by preprinted consent forms for operative procedures, it is important to appreciate that these forms do not make the consent any more 'valid'. Written consent provides a useful record of the process but does not, in itself, add to the quality of that consent. It is the two-way sharing of information that renders consent valid, not simply a signed piece of paper.

Information

We must give patients sufficient information to ensure that their consent is 'informed' or 'valid' (Table 21.1). If patients can demonstrate that their decision to proceed would have been altered by different information, then they may successfully sue in negligence.

The ruling of the Supreme Court in the case of *Montgomery vs. Lanarkshire Health Board* clarified the legal standard we must reach when disclosing information to ensure that our patients are able to give valid consent. The Court ruled that patients must be warned of 'all material risks' inherent in the proposed treatment or procedure. To allow them genuine choice, they must also be counselled about alternative treatments, including the option for no treatment at. The Court defined a risk as 'material' if 'a reasonable person in the patient's position would be likely to attach significance to the risk, or the doctor should reasonably be aware that the particular patient would be likely to attach significance to it'.

This means that consent must be tailored to the individual, and each patient must be warned of all risks he or she might find significant, no matter how unlikely they are to materialise. This demands that we know our patients well enough to understand what each might find uniquely significant. In the same ruling the Court goes on to caution against bombarding patients with information and technical details for fear of omitting material risks, because this may promote confusion rather than autonomy.

These standards might seem incredibly stringent, but in fact this Supreme Court ruling has done nothing more than bring the law into line with the long-standing guidance on consent issued by the GMC and Association of Anaesthetists. We may feel it is impossible to counsel the patient adequately within the time constraints of the system; however, the Court says that lack of time will provide no defence for inadequate provision of information. If doctors are not allowed sufficient time for these essential discussions, then they must raise this issue with their employing Trust.

There are only three situations where it is acceptable, in law, *not* to provide patients with information about diagnosis or risks of treatment:

1. When the patient has expressed a repeated wish not to be told about his or her treatment. In this situation the doctor should explore and revisit this request in a sensitive manner before acquiescing.
2. Where disclosure of information will cause harm to the patient; this must be harm beyond merely causing distress, such as exacerbating the risk of suicide.
3. In cases of necessity where a patient needs lifesaving treatment and cannot give consent because of temporary incapacity, such as after a head injury.

The judges in the Montgomery ruling warned that these exceptions must not be abused.

Table 21.1 Broad summary of information appropriate for patients during the consent process

Common components of anaesthetic technique	Fasting Administration and effects of premedication Transfer from ward to anaesthetic room Cannula insertion Non-invasive monitoring Induction of general and/or local anaesthetic Discomfort/awareness of the procedure/surroundings, if awake/sedated Transfer to recovery area Return to ward Postoperative analgesia/antiemetics/fluids Techniques of a sensitive nature (e.g. insertion of an analgesic suppository) Alternative techniques where appropriate, including if one technique fails (e.g. general anaesthesia for Caesarean section as an alternative to regional anaesthesia or if the latter is inadequate)
Specific aspects related to procedure or condition	Invasive monitoring and associated risks Recovery in a critical care environment Sedation Tracheal intubation/tracheostomy
Common/significant adverse effects	Nausea and vomiting Sore throat Damage to teeth/lips Cognitive dysfunction Numbness/weakness/return of pain after local anaesthetic techniques Suxamethonium pains Postdural puncture headache
Serious adverse effects	Nerve/eye damage Awareness during anaesthesia Death

Methods and timing of information provision

Patients not only need to be given information but also need time to reflect before coming to a decision. We should not be presenting patients with new information immediately before surgery as they will not have sufficient time for assimilation or reflection; one could argue that these circumstances are coercive and will invalidate the consent. In its guidance the Association of Anaesthetists stipulates categorically that taking consent 'immediately before the induction of anaesthesia, for example in the anaesthetic room, is not acceptable…other than in exceptional circumstances'.

Information about anaesthesia should be provided in advance of the day of surgery, and there are numerous ways of conveying that information to the patients aside from the traditional face-to-face consultation. Written information, which can be sent to the patient ahead of time, provides an opportunity to give more extensive information; the patient can read and discuss this at their leisure. Shared decision-making aids are also becoming more prevalent across all specialties. These tools help patients to weigh the pros and cons of proposed treatment and usefully quantify risk.

Producing good quality, user-friendly information, regardless of the medium, is a time-consuming and skilled process that requires consultation with patients, colleagues and experts. There is plenty of high-quality information available from national bodies such as the Royal College of Anaesthetists, Obstetric Anaesthetists' Association, Royal College of Surgeons' Patient Liaison Group and other surgical specialty associations. Patients can be directed to these and other trusted websites, and information leaflets can be downloaded to save individual departments both time and expense.

Communicating risk

Humans are not very good at judging risk. A variety of factors influence people's acceptance and interpretation of risk; for example, self-inflicted risk is generally better accepted than externally imposed risk. There is also a tendency to overestimate rare but serious risks while underestimating common, less serious ones. People everywhere are subject to the optimism bias – that is, the belief that the risk is real but is unlikely to befall them.

Patients prefer to be given numerical estimates of risk, whereas doctors prefer to provide less precise qualitative estimates. In truth, neither is more accurate, and the risk to the individual patient is not usually known with any precision. Verbal likelihood scales are therefore most commonly used, but these bring with them the problem of interpretation; *never* and *always* are straightforward, but *common, rare* and *unusual* are subjective terms. To provide more personal context, the population scale is sometimes used, comparing the risk with the number of people on a street, village, town, and so on.

How we frame risk changes its perception, and so a 90% success rate is generally better received than a 10% chance of failure. Relative risks and benefits may have a greater influence on an individual than is necessarily warranted. The absolute risk of dying due to anaesthesia-related complications is very small, regardless of technique; however, the relative risk (e.g. regional versus general anaesthesia for caesarean section) may be quite large. Risk assessment is discussed further in Chapters 19 and 30.

The Mental Capacity Act and incapacity

The vast majority of patients will have capacity to make their own decisions. However, a number of patients may be unable to give valid consent, either temporarily or permanently. In England and Wales, the Mental Capacity Act 2005 provides a legal framework governing the treatment of patients who lack capacity to consent to their care. Similar legislation exists in other countries.

Doctors must do everything practicable to maximise the capacity of their patients. People's lack of capacity cannot be assumed solely because they have taken drugs, alcohol or premedication, nor because they have learning difficulties or mental illness or they seem to be making 'the wrong' choices. In particular, the inability to communicate verbally does not imply a lack of capacity.

Best interests

Section 5 of the Mental Capacity Act dictates that decisions made on behalf of incapable patients must be in their best interests and that we must choose the least restrictive of the possible therapeutic options. When making these decisions, the term *best interests* refers to more than just the patient's *medical* interests. A best interests decision must take into account *all* of the patient's interests: physical, emotional, cultural and spiritual. Family members and, where appropriate, others close to the patient should be consulted when making best interest decisions.

The concept of best interests has been criticised as being unknowable and unachievable. However, the phrase emphasises the ethical importance of placing patients at the centre of decisions made about them.

Decisions by proxy

In the UK, no one can give consent on behalf of an incapable adult unless they have been legally invested with this authority (see later). Simply being the patient's next-of-kin *does not* bestow any powers to make treatment decisions.

a. **Lasting power of attorney**

If the patient anticipates his or her own loss of capacity, for example, because of advancing dementia, the patient may appoint a proxy decision maker with lasting power of attorney (LPA) for health and welfare. These individuals have the right to give or withhold consent to treatment on behalf of the patient. They may not, however, refuse lifesaving treatment unless specific provision is made for this in the legal documentation.

b. **Court-appointed deputies**

The Court may appoint a 'deputy' to act on behalf of the incapacitated patient. A court-appointed deputy can never refuse lifesaving treatment considered to be in the patient's best interests.

c. **The medical team**

In the vast majority of situations, there is no designated LPA or court-appointed deputy, and the responsibility of making best interests decisions falls to the medical team caring for the patient.

d. **Independent mental capacity advocates (IMCA)**

If an incapacitated patient needs to undergo serious medical treatment (i.e. where the merits of treatment are finely balanced or serious consequences may arise) but there are no family or friends to consult, or disagreement exists between parties, then an IMCA should be appointed. These independent professionals act as the patient's advocate in best interest decision-making.

e. **Advance decisions**

Before losing capacity, a patient may make an advance decision (often known as an 'advance directive' or 'living will') forbidding specific treatments or interventions in predefined situations, such as refusal of tracheal intubation and ventilation if suffering severe pneumonia. Many Jehovah's Witnesses carry advance decisions refusing treatment with blood or blood products.

Advance decisions do not have to be written to be valid unless they are concerned with refusal of lifesaving treatment. In this case the advance decision must be in writing, signed and witnessed and must clearly state that it applies even when life is at risk. Valid advance decisions must be honoured by the medical team, even if they do not believe them to be the best interests of the patient. If doubt exists as to the validity of an advance decision

437

in an emergency situation, doctors should err on the side of preserving life.

Restraint and deprivation of liberty

The Mental Capacity Act permits the restraint of patients who lack capacity to facilitate treatment in their best interests so long as the restraint is **necessary** and **proportional** to the harm that we are trying to prevent. Restraint may be physical or chemical, and the anaesthetist is often called upon to administer the latter. We must keep in mind that if restraint is prolonged or complete, then it may evolve into a deprivation of the patient's liberty. A deprivation of liberty occurs when a patient is subject to constant supervision and control and is not free to leave. Whether or not the patient attempts to leave is irrelevant because depriving the patient of his or her liberty without the correct legal authorisation contravenes Article 5 of the European Convention of Human Rights (ECHR), the right to liberty and security of person, and is against the law. When it proves necessary to deprive a patient of his or her liberty to protect the patient from harm, a legal process called the Deprivation of Liberty Safeguards is triggered. Trusts must submit a formal application to their local authority, who may grant permission after independent review of the case. At the time of writing, this legislation is undergoing government review and is likely to change.

The Deprivation of Liberty Safeguards and intensive care

Thankfully the Court of Appeal has ruled that patients treated in the ICU fall outside Article 5 of the ECHR because it is their underlying illness that prevents them from leaving the hospital, rather than medical intervention. Hence, the procedural safeguards are not triggered and these patients *do not* need deprivation of liberty authorisation.

Consent in special circumstances

Emergency

Most emergency patients have capacity, and the same considerations about consent and information apply. However, the urgency of a situation does not preclude the requirement to ensure understanding and to clearly document any discussions held. For patients who lack capacity (e.g. loss of consciousness as a result of head injury), the stipulations of the MCA (or similar) apply and the doctor must act in the patient's best interests in the least restrictive way possible.

Children

The laws around paediatric consent can seem confusing. In legal terms a **minor** is someone younger than age 18 years.

When patients are aged younger than 16 years, consent to treatment must be given on their behalf by the adult with parental responsibility. Patients *older than* age 16 years are assumed to have capacity, as per the Mental Capacity Act, but, rather confusingly, reaching the age of capacity does not confer adult status. This results in a period between the ages of 16 and 18 years (when patients are often referred to as **'young people'**) when the minor's refusal of treatment can still be overruled by his or her parents or by the Court.

A minor aged younger than 16 years may be assessed as having capacity, and such children are often referred to as being 'Gillick competent'. This term originates from the case *Gillick vs. West Norfolk and Wisbech* in which Lord Scarman ruled that the parents' right to consent for their child terminates when the child has reached sufficient maturity to understand what is proposed. In spite of this clear legal principle it is sensible to gain consent to treatment from the responsible adult as well as from a Gillick-competent child.

Minors who have tried to refuse lifesaving treatment in the UK have, without exception, had their wishes overruled by the Court, which has considered them lacking in capacity to make such significant decisions. Even when the minor's arguments to the contrary are rational and considered, the Court seems to have no appetite for watching a child dying as a result of withheld treatment. In practice, minors may give their consent to treatment but may not refuse lifesaving treatment thought to be in their best interests.

The GMC advises caution before accepting a minor's refusal of treatment, which the court might over-rule. It says, 'In the UK the law on parents overriding young people's competent refusal is complex. You should seek legal advice if you think treatment is in the best interests of a competent young person who refuses'.

Obstetrics

The pregnant woman retains absolute autonomy over her body and has exactly the same rights to give or withhold consent as any other person. Association of Anaesthetists guidance states that 'Drugs, fatigue, pain or anxiety may compromise the capacity of the adult parturient, but do not necessarily lead to incapacity unless the degree of compromise is severe.' The fetus has no legal rights until it is born, and its interests should only be considered as an extension of its mother's best interests.

Epidural analgesia

Labour is not the time to burden women with new information, and so every attempt should be make to inform them in the antenatal period about options for pain relief. Once labour has started, women may not wish to hear (and almost certainly will not retain) a long list of potential complications. However, the anaesthetist has a responsibility to provide information about the material risks of the procedure. This **must** be documented at the time because there is good evidence that the mother's recollection of the discussion may not be complete, even the next day.

A woman who has decided against epidural analgesia in her birth plan retains the right, and capacity, to change her mind during labour, and the anaesthetist should act upon her request in the usual way.

In the rare situation that a woman loses capacity during labour, Association of Anaesthetists guidance advises that we use an existing birth plan as an advance decision, and therefore in this situation we should accept any documented refusal of therapy.

Caesarean delivery

Situations requiring urgent delivery of the baby are not uncommon in obstetrics. When these arise, we must tailor the consent process to facilitate timely delivery, which can reasonably be assumed to be in the mother's best interests. Consent in this setting can be written, verbal or implied, and subsequent documentation should reflect that delivery was time-critical and that the chosen technique was performed in the mother's best interests.

In rare circumstances a woman may refuse Caesarean delivery even when the obstetric team believes it will lead to the death of the fetus. If the woman has capacity, this remains her right, no matter how distressing it may be for all involved. If there is doubt as to her capacity, and it is likely that her capacity *will* be questioned in this situation because the decision to refuse is so unusual, then the team *must* refer the case to the Court of Protection, where the judge will make the ultimate decision with regards to the woman's capacity and whether forced Caesarean section is in her best interests. There is always an emergency out of hours judge available, and decisions can usually be made within the hour. A recent case where a Trust was severely criticised acts as a useful reminder that courts should be given as much time as possible to make these difficult decisions and that doctors should, therefore, try to anticipate issues relating to capacity and refusal early in pregnancy, rather than leaving them to the last minute.

Teaching and learning

Patients want to be cared for by experts, but we all have to learn, and every expert was once a novice. The conundrum of how to provide optimal care to each individual patient whilst allowing doctors to practise and develop new skills may seem insoluble. However, setting the problem in a less individualistic context makes it less difficult:

- Patients are part of a wider society, and they benefit from the altruism of those who went before; therefore society *and* the individual benefit from the ongoing development of its medical staff.
- Outcomes are often better when trainees are involved because their work is scrutinised – corners will not be cut and standards are maintained or elevated.
- Teaching others and being questioned by them ensures that experts keep their own skills up to date.

The Association of Anaesthetists advises that the harms inherent in skill acquisition should be minimised where possible; for example, students should practice on manikins or using simulation before moving to closely supervised practice with patients.

When teaching airway skills, for example, to medical students or paramedics, the risk–benefit analysis must always be borne in mind. Specific consent should be sought from the patient to allow the involvement of these less skilled and non-medically qualified individuals. Studies show that the majority of patients understand the need for teaching and training and are happy to be involved when asked. Patients always have the right to know who is doing what to them, regardless of the influence of anaesthesia.

Summary

Consent is a process, and patients have a fundamental right to give or withhold their consent for anaesthesia. Anaesthetists must respect this fact and help patients make decisions about their management by providing high-quality information in a timely manner. They must ensure that all material risks have been discussed and that the patient understands, in broad terms, the nature of the proposed treatment. When patients lack capacity, decisions must be made in their best interests.

References/Further reading

Association of Anaesthetists of Great Britain and Ireland, 2017. Information and consent for anaesthesia 2017. AAGBI, London.

https://www.aagbi.org/sites/default/files/AAGBI_Consent_for_anaesthesia_2017_0.pdf. (Accessed 30 July 2017).

Ferreira v Coroner of Inner South London, 2017. EWCA Civ 31. http://www.mentalhealthlaw.co.uk/R_(Ferreira)_v_HM_Senior_Coroner

_for_Inner_South_London_(2017)_EWCA_Civ_31,_(2017)_MHLO_2. (Accessed 20 October 2017).

General Medical Council, 2008. Consent: patients and doctors making decisions together. GMC, London. http://www.gmc-uk.org/GMC_Consent_0513_Revised.pdf_52115235.pdf. (Accessed 30 July 2017).

Gillick v West Norfolk and Wisbech Area Health Authority, 1985. 3 All ER 402. (1). http://www.hrcr.org/safrica/childrens_rights/Gillick_WestNorfolk.htm (Accessed 20 October 2017).

Montgomery v Lanarkshire Health Board, 2015. UKSC 11. https://www.supremecourt.uk/decided-cases/docs/UKSC_2013_0136_Judgment.pdf. (Accessed 20 October 2017).

Re CA (Natural Delivery or Caesarean Section), 2016. EWCOP 51. http://www.bailii.org/ew/cases/EWCOP/2016/51.html. (Accessed 20 October 2017).

Chapter | **22** |

The practical conduct of anaesthesia

David Kirkbride

The conduct of anaesthesia is planned after obtaining details of the surgical procedure and medical condition of the patient. All patients should be visited preoperatively for anaesthetic assessment, including review of the results of relevant investigations. This is also an important opportunity to form a rapport, gain patients' trust and answer any questions about their anaesthetic and postoperative pain relief. Preoperative assessment and selection of appropriate premedication are discussed in Chapter 19.

Preparation for anaesthesia

Before commencing anaesthesia and surgery, the anaesthetist must be satisfied that there is functioning equipment, the correct monitoring is attached and set up, the trained assistant is present and the WHO patient safety checklist has been completed (see Chapter 18).

Equipment checks

Anaesthetic equipment should be up-to-date and maintained regularly and the instruction manuals available and accessible. An equipment check must be performed before an operating theatre session begins, because a common cause of problems is the use of a machine that has not been checked properly and which malfunctions. An adequate check of anaesthetic apparatus is an integral part of good practice; failure to check the anaesthetic equipment properly may amount to malpractice.

Operating theatre staff usually carry out checks when setting up an operating theatre for use or after apparatus has been serviced or repaired, but the ultimate responsibility for ensuring that the apparatus is safe for its intended use rests with the anaesthetist. Sophisticated tests may have been performed after major servicing, but key control settings may have been altered, and it is essential that the anaesthetist checks that the equipment is in proper working order and ready for clinical use. The final check is the sole responsibility of the anaesthetist who is to use the machine; it cannot be delegated to any other person. There is no justification for proceeding with an anaesthetic when faults have been identified in the equipment. If there is no record of an adequate preoperative check of equipment and a problem occurs as a result of equipment failure, it is very difficult to defend an allegation of negligence.

At its most basic, the function of an anaesthetic machine is to enable the anaesthetist to administer oxygen under pressure without leaks. If all else fails, this allows the anaesthetist to maintain cerebral oxygenation. Anaesthetic apparatus should be checked before the start of each operating session in a logical sequence, as recommended on the Association of Anaesthetists checklist (Table 22.1). Further checks should be undertaken between cases (Box 22.1). The primary intention of the anaesthetic machine check is to ensure that it is safe to use and will deliver gases under pressure without leaks. These checklists are available as laminated cards intended to be attached to all anaesthetic machines in the UK and Ireland.

In most industries in which complex equipment is used, full training is provided for users. It is not acceptable for anaesthetists to assume that they intuitively understand an anaesthetic machine they have not used before. Those new to the specialty require detailed instruction and training in the use of anaesthetic equipment, but even experienced anaesthetists need tuition in the use of new equipment.

Alternative means of ventilation

The early use of an alternative means of ventilation, namely a self-inflating bag that does not rely on a source of oxygen to function, may be lifesaving. A self-inflating bag must be immediately available in any location where anaesthesia

Table 22.1 Association of Anaesthetists guidelines for the checking of anaesthetic equipment

Checks at the start of every operating session Do not use this equipment unless you have been trained	
Check self-inflating bag available	
Perform manufacturer's (automatic) machine check	
Power supply	• Plugged in • Switched on • Backup battery charged
Gas supplies and suction	• Gas and vacuum pipelines – tug test • Cylinders filled and turned off • Flowmeters working (if applicable) • Hypoxic guard working • Oxygen flush working • Suction clean and working
Breathing system	• Whole system patent and leak-free using two-bag test • Vaporisers – fitted correctly, filled, leak-free, plugged in (if necessary) • Soda lime – colour checked • Alternative systems (e.g. Bain, T-piece) – checked • Correct gas outlet selected
Ventilator	• Working and configured correctly
Scavenging	• Working and configured correctly
Monitors	• Working and configured correctly • Alarms limits and volume set
Airway equipment	• Full range required working, with spares
RECORD THIS CHECK IN THE PATIENT RECORD	
Don't forget!	• Self-inflating bag • Common gas outlet • Difficult airway equipment • Resuscitation equipment • TIVA and/or other infusion equipment

TIVA, Total intravenous anaesthesia.
(Adapted from Association of Anaesthetists of Great Britain and Ireland. (2012) Checking anaesthetic equipment 2012. *Anaesthesia*. 67(6), 660–668.)

might be given. An alternative source of oxygen should also be readily available.

Perform manufacturer's machine check

Modern anaesthesia workstations may perform many of the following checks automatically during start-up. Anaesthetists must know which are included and ensure that the automated check has been performed.

Power supply

The anaesthetic workstation and relevant ancillary equipment must be connected to the mains electrical supply (where appropriate) and switched on. The anaesthetic workstation should be connected directly to the mains electrical supply and only correctly rated equipment connected to its electrical outlets. Multisocket extension leads must not be plugged into the anaesthetic machine outlets or used to connect the anaesthetic machine to the mains supply. Hospitals should have backup generators, and many operating theatres have

Box 22.1 **Association of Anaesthetists guidelines for checking anaesthetic equipment between cases**

Breathing system

- Whole system patent and leak-free using two-bag test (see Box 22.2)
- Vaporisers – fitted correctly, filled, leak-free, plugged in (if necessary)
- Alternative systems (e.g. Bain, T-piece) – checked
- Correct gas outlet selected

Ventilator

- Working and configured correctly

Airway equipment

- Full range required working, with spares

Suction

- Clean and working

(Adapted with permission from Association of Anaesthetists of Great Britain and Ireland. (2012) Checking anaesthetic equipment 2012. *Anaesthesia.* 67(6), 660–668.)

their own backup system. Backup batteries for anaesthetic machines and other equipment should be charged.

Gas supplies and suction

The gas supply master switch (if one is fitted) should be switched on. On some workstations it is necessary to disconnect the oxygen pipeline to check the correct function of the oxygen failure alarm, although on machines with a gas supply master switch, the alarm may be operated by turning the master switch off. Repeated disconnection of gas hoses may lead to premature failure of the Schrader socket and probe, and current guidelines recommend that the regular check of equipment includes a tug test to confirm correct insertion of each pipeline into the appropriate socket (see later). It is also recommended that the oxygen failure alarm is checked once a week by disconnecting the oxygen pipeline with the oxygen flowmeter turned on; the alarm must sound for at least 7 s. Oxygen failure warning devices are also linked to a gas shut-off device. Anaesthetists must be aware of both the tone of the alarm and which gases will continue to flow on the anaesthetic machine.

Suction

The suction apparatus should be checked to ensure that it is clean and functioning, all connections are secure and an adequate negative pressure is generated.

Medical gas supplies

The gases that are being supplied by pipeline should be identified, confirming with a tug test that each pipeline is correctly inserted into the appropriate gas supply terminal. Only gentle force is required; excessive force during a tug test may damage the pipeline or gas supply terminal. It is essential to check that the anaesthetic machine is connected to a supply of oxygen and that an adequate reserve supply of oxygen is available from a spare cylinder. It is also necessary to check that adequate supplies of any other gases intended for use are available and connected.

All cylinders should be seated securely and turned off after checking their contents. Carbon dioxide cylinders should not be present on the anaesthetic machine. If a blanking plug is supplied, it should be fitted to any empty cylinder yoke.

All pressure gauges for pipelines connected to the anaesthetic machine should indicate a pressure of 400–500 kPa.

If flowmeters are present, their function should be checked, ensuring that each control valve operates smoothly and the bobbin moves freely throughout its range without sticking. If nitrous oxide is to be used, the hypoxic-guard device should be tested by first turning on the nitrous oxide flow and ensuring that at least 25% oxygen also flows. The oxygen flow should then be turned off to check that the nitrous oxide flow also stops. The oxygen flow should then be turned back on, the nitrous oxide flow should be turned off, and a check made that the oxygen analyser display approaches 100%. All flow control valves should then be turned off; machines fitted with a gas supply master switch will continue to deliver a basal flow of oxygen.

The emergency oxygen bypass control should be operated to ensure that flow occurs from the gas outlet without a significant decrease in the pipeline supply pressure. It is important to ensure that the emergency oxygen bypass control ceases to operate when released; there is a risk of awareness if it continues to operate.

Breathing system and vaporisers

All breathing systems which are to be used must be checked and a two-bag test performed before use (Box 22.2). Breathing systems should be inspected visually for correct configuration and assembly. All connections within the system and to the anaesthetic machine should be checked to ensure that they are secured by push and twist. It should be ensured that there are no leaks or obstructions in the reservoir bags or breathing system. A pressure leak test (between 20 and 60 cmH$_2$O) should be performed on the breathing system by occluding the patient end and compressing the reservoir bag.

Manual leak testing of vaporisers (see later) was previously recommended. It should only be performed on basic Boyle

Box 22.2 **Association of Anaesthetists two-bag test**

A two-bag test should be performed after the breathing system, vaporisers and ventilator have been checked individually.
1. Attach the patient end of the breathing system (including angle piece and filter) to a test lung or bag.
2. Set the fresh gas flow rate to 5 L min^{-1} and ventilate manually. Check that the whole breathing system is patent and that the unidirectional valves are moving. Check the function of the adjustable pressure-limiting (APL) valve by squeezing both bags.
3. Turn on the ventilator to ventilate the test lung. Turn off the fresh gas flow or reduce to a minimum. Open and close each vaporiser in turn. There should be no loss of volume in the system.

(Adapted with permission from Association of Anaesthetists of Great Britain and Ireland. (2012) Checking anaesthetic equipment 2012. *Anaesthesia.* 67(6), 660–668.)

machines because it may be harmful to modern anaesthetic workstations. Manufacturer's recommendations should be reviewed before performing a manual test.

The anaesthetist should check that the vaporisers for the required volatile anaesthetic agents are fitted correctly to the anaesthetic machine, any locking mechanism is fully engaged and the control knobs rotate fully through the full ranges. Vaporisers should be adequately filled but not overfilled, and the filling port must be tightly closed. Tilting vaporisers can result in delivery of dangerously high concentrations of vapour, and therefore they must always be kept upright. All vaporisers must be turned off after they have been checked.

It may be necessary to change a vaporiser during use, although this should be avoided if at all possible. If a change is necessary, repeat the leak test because failure to do so is a common cause of critical incidents. Some anaesthetic workstations automatically test the integrity of vaporisers.

It is only necessary to remove a vaporiser from a machine to refill it if the manufacturer recommends this.

Manual leak test of vaporiser

With the vaporiser turned off, a flow rate of oxygen of 5 L min^{-1} should be set, and the common gas outlet should be temporarily occluded. There should be no leak from any part of the vaporiser, and the flowmeter bobbin (if present) should dip. If more than one vaporiser is present, turn each one on in turn and repeat this test. After the tests, ensure that the vaporisers and flowmeters are turned off.

Carbon dioxide absorber

The contents and connections should be checked to ensure that there is an adequate supply of CO_2 absorbent and that it is of an appropriate colour.

Alternative breathing systems

If a coaxial system is in use, an occlusion test should be performed on the inner tube and a check should be made that the adjustable pressure-limiting (APL) valve, where fitted, can be fully opened and closed.

Correct gas outlet

Special care must be exercised if the anaesthetic machine incorporates an auxiliary common gas outlet (ACGO). Incidents of patient harm have resulted from misconnection of a breathing system to an ACGO or incorrect selection of the ACGO.

Breathing systems

Whenever a breathing system is changed, either during a case or a list, its integrity and correct configuration must be confirmed. This is particularly important for paediatric cases, when breathing systems may be changed frequently during an operating list.

Ventilator

It is important to check that the ventilator is configured correctly and the ventilator tubing is attached securely. The controls should be set according to the intended use of the ventilator, and the system should be checked to ensure that adequate pressure is generated during the inspiratory phase. Ventilator alarms should be checked to ensure that they are working and correctly configured. The pressure relief valve should be checked to ensure that it functions correctly at the set pressure.

Scavenging

The anaesthetic gas scavenging system should be checked to ensure that it is switched on and functioning and that the tubing is attached to the appropriate exhaust port of the breathing system, ventilator or anaesthetic workstation.

Airway equipment

Airway equipment includes bacterial filters, catheter mounts, connectors, face masks, tracheal tubes and supraglottic airways (SADs). These should all be available in the appropriate sizes for patients on the operating list and **must** be checked for patency.

A new, single-use bacterial filter and angle piece or catheter mount must be used for each patient. It is important that these are checked for patency and flow, both visually and by ensuring that gas flows through the whole assembly when connected to the breathing system. This check must occur whenever new airway equipment is provided and is a standard part of the WHO checklist for every patient.

Appropriate laryngoscopes must be available and checked to ensure that they function reliably. Equipment for the management of the anticipated or unexpected difficult airway must be available and checked regularly in accordance with departmental policies. The anaesthetist and anaesthetic assistant should both be aware of the location of the nearest difficult airway trolley.

Single-use devices

Any part of the breathing system, ancillary equipment or other apparatus that is designated 'single-use' must be used for one patient only and not reused. Packaging should not be removed until the point of use, for infection control, identification and safety purposes.

Ancillary and resuscitation equipment

The patient's trolley, bed or operating table must be capable of being placed rapidly into a head-down position; as with all equipment, the anaesthetist must be familiar with the operating mechanism before anaesthesia starts. A resuscitation trolley and defibrillator must be available in all locations where anaesthesia is given and checked regularly in accordance with local policies. Equipment and drugs for rarely encountered emergencies, such as malignant hyperthermia and local anaesthetic toxicity, must be available and checked regularly in accordance with local policies. The location of these must be clearly signed.

Machine failure

In the event of failure, some modern anaesthetic workstations may default to little or no flow of oxygen with no vapour. The anaesthetist must know the default setting for the machine in use. Alternative means of oxygenation, ventilation and anaesthesia must be available.

'Shared responsibility' equipment

As a member of the theatre team, the anaesthetist has shared responsibility for the safe use of other equipment (e.g. diathermy, intermittent compression stockings, warming devices, cell salvage and tourniquets) and should have received appropriate training. Involvement with this equipment, especially troubleshooting problems which arise intraoperatively, must not be allowed to distract anaesthetists from their primary role.

Monitoring the patient during anaesthesia

During anaesthesia the patient's physiological state and adequacy of anaesthesia need continual assessment. Whilst the primary 'monitor' is the anaesthetist, additional monitoring devices are attached to the patient to supplement this clinical observation throughout the anaesthetic (see Chapter 17). The following are considered to be the minimum additional monitoring modalities for the safe provision of anaesthesia:

- pulse oximetry
- blood pressure; measurement (indirect or direct);
- ECG;
- measurement of inspired and expired oxygen, carbon dioxide (capnography), nitrous oxide and volatile anaesthetic agent values;
- continuous airway pressure measurement;
- peripheral nerve stimulator assessment of neuromuscular blockade (if used); and
- temperature for any procedure longer than 30 min duration.

Depending on patient and surgical factors, additional monitoring may be required, such as to measure intravascular pressures, cardiac output and biochemical and haematological variables. The use of additional monitoring is at the discretion of the anaesthetist but should be discussed with the team to ensure availability and readiness.

All monitoring devices must be calibrated periodically according to manufacturer's recommendations and checked before each case to ensure that they are functioning and that appropriate parameters and alarms have been set. This includes the cycling times of automatic non-invasive blood pressure monitors. Gas sampling tubing must be properly attached and checked to ensure it is free from obstruction or kinks.

Recording and audit

A clear note must be made in the patient's anaesthetic record that the anaesthetic machine check has been performed, appropriate monitoring is in place and functional, and the integrity, patency and safety of the whole breathing system has been assured. A logbook should also be kept with each anaesthetic machine to record the daily presession check and weekly check of the oxygen failure alarm. Modern anaesthesia workstations may record electronic self-tests internally. Such records should be retained for an appropriate time.

445

Patient safety checklists

Before patients arrive in the anaesthetic room or theatre, the WHO team brief should take place (see Chapter 18).

Trained ancillary staff

Skilled and dedicated help is required to be available to the anaesthetist at all times. In the majority of hospitals in the UK, this is provided by operating department practitioners (ODPs), who undergo a two-year diploma training programme in recognised institutions and once qualified are required to register with the Health and Care Professions Council (HCPC). Nationally there is a move towards a degree course in operating department practice. In some hospitals, anaesthetic nurses perform essentially the same functions as an ODP. It is important to differentiate between anaesthetic nurses and the nurse anaesthetists who are trained to deliver anaesthesia in some countries.

Roles of the ODP/anaesthetic nurse include:

- preparation and preliminary checking of equipment. It should be stressed that this does not absolve the anaesthetist from the responsibility of checking the equipment fully before an operating list is started;
- alleviation of anxiety by reassurance and communication with the patient while awaiting anaesthesia;
- checking the correct identity of the patient and participating in the WHO checklist procedures, preparation of intravenous infusions and cardiovascular monitoring transducers and so on;
- assistance during anaesthesia, particularly during tracheal induction, when special manoeuvres such as cricoid pressure may be required, and after transfer to the operating theatre to assist in re-establishment of monitoring;
- assistance in positioning the patient for local or regional blocks;
- assistance in obtaining drugs or equipment if complications arise during anaesthesia; and
- assistance in the immediate postoperative period before the patient is transferred to the recovery room.

The ODP or anaesthetic nurse should never be left alone with an anaesthetised patient unless a dire emergency requires the anaesthetist's presence elsewhere.

Physicians' assistants (anaesthesia)

Physicians' assistants (anaesthesia) (PA(A)s) are fully trained professionals who have completed a specific postgraduate diploma. They work under the direction and supervision of a consultant anaesthetist at all times, often in a 2:1 model where one consultant supervises two theatres with a trainee and a PA(A) or two PA(A)s. They are allowed to provide anaesthesia without an anaesthetist present, but overall responsibility for the care of the patient remains with the supervising consultant anaesthetist. Their role is to improve theatre utilisation through reductions in theatre downtime, assisting with preoperative assessment and regional anaesthesia. Availability of a PA(A) does not negate the requirement for a trained assistant to be available throughout the case.

For every case, the supervising consultant anaesthetist must:

- be present in the theatre suite, must be easily contactable and must be available to attend within 2 min of being requested to attend by the PA(A);
- be present in the anaesthetic room/operating theatre during induction of anaesthesia;
- regularly review the intraoperative anaesthetic management;
- be present during emergence from anaesthesia until the patient has been handed over safely to the recovery room staff; and
- remain in the theatre suite until control of airway reflexes has returned and airway devices have been removed or the ongoing care of the patient has been handed on to other appropriately qualified staff (e.g. in ICU).

Induction of anaesthesia

Anaesthesia is usually induced using an inhalational or i.v. technique. Whichever technique is chosen, appropriate personal and protective equipment (PPE) should be used (see Chapter 18).

Inhalational induction

The most common indications for inhalational induction of anaesthesia are:

- paediatric anaesthesia in young children;
- upper airway obstruction, e.g. epiglottitis;
- lower airway obstruction with foreign body;
- bronchopleural fistula or empyema; and
- inability to achieve i.v. access for intravenous induction.

The proposed procedure should be explained to the patient before starting. A technique using a cupped hand around the fresh gas delivery tube may be preferred for young children; otherwise a face-mask is used. The mask or hand is introduced *gradually* to the face from the side; the use of a transparent perfumed mask can render the procedure less unpleasant. While talking to the patient and encouraging normal breathing, the anaesthetist adjusts the mixture of the fresh gas flow and observes the patient's reactions. Initially either nitrous oxide 70% in oxygen or 100% oxygen is used, and anaesthesia is deepened by the gradual introduction of increments of a volatile agent. Sevoflurane is typically used and can be increased up to an inspired concentration of 8%. Maintenance concentrations of isoflurane (1%–2%) or sevoflurane (2%–3%) are used when anaesthesia has been established. A single-breath technique of inhalational induction has been advocated for patients who are able to cooperate. One vital capacity breath from a prefilled 4-L reservoir bag containing a high concentration of volatile agent (e.g. sevoflurane 8%) in oxygen (or nitrous oxide 50% in oxygen) results in smooth induction of anaesthesia within 20–30 s.

If spontaneous ventilation is to be maintained during the procedure, airway patency is ensured by use of an oropharyngeal airway, SAD or tracheal tube once anaesthesia has been established.

Complications and difficulties

Complications and difficulties can include the following:
- slower induction of anaesthesia;
- problems particularly during stage 2 of anaesthesia (see later), when stimulation of the pharynx or larynx may result in laryngeal spasm;
- airway obstruction or bronchospasm; and
- environmental pollution.

Signs of anaesthesia

Guedel's classic signs of anaesthesia are those seen in patients premedicated with morphine and atropine and breathing ether in air. The clinical signs associated with anaesthesia produced by other inhalational agents follow a similar course, but the divisions between the stages and planes are less precise (Fig. 22.1).

Stage 1: analgesia. This is the stage attained when using nitrous oxide 50% in oxygen, as used in the technique of relative analgesia.

Stage 2: excitement. This is seen with inhalational induction but is passed rapidly during i.v. induction. Respiration is erratic, breath-holding may occur, laryngeal and pharyngeal reflexes are active and stimulation of pharynx or larynx (e.g. by insertion of an oropharyngeal airway or SAD) may produce laryngeal spasm. The eyelash reflex

STAGE	RESPIRATION	PUPILS	EYES	RESPIRATORY
1 Analgesia	Regular Small volume	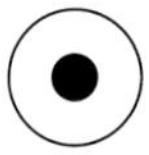		
2 Excitement	Irregular	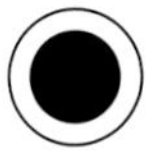	Eyelash reflex absent	
3 Anaesthesia Plane I	Regular Large volume	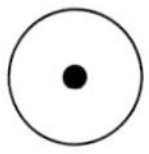	Eyelid reflex absent Conjunctival reflex depressed	Pharyngeal and vomiting reflexes depressed
Plane II	Regular Large volume	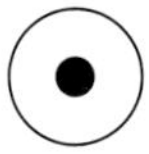	Corneal reflex depressed	
Plane III	Regular Becoming diaphragmatic Small volume	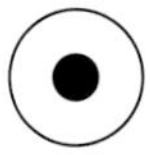		Laryngeal reflex depressed
Plane IV	Irregular Diaphragmatic Small volume	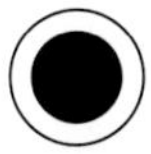		Carinal reflex depressed
4 Overdose	Apnoea	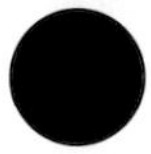		

Fig. 22.1 Stages of anaesthesia. (Modified from Guedel.)

(used as a sign of unconsciousness with i.v. induction) is abolished in stage 2, but the eyelid reflex (resistance to elevation of eyelid) remains present.

Stage 3: surgical anaesthesia. This deepens through four planes (in practice, three: light, medium, deep) with increasing concentration of anaesthetic drug. Respiration assumes a rhythmic pattern, and the thoracic component diminishes with depth of anaesthesia. Respiratory reflexes become suppressed, but the carinal reflex is abolished only at plane IV (therefore, a tracheal tube which is too long may produce carinal stimulation at an otherwise adequate depth of anaesthesia). The pupils are central and gradually enlarge with depth of anaesthesia. Lacrimation is active in light planes but absent in planes III and IV – a useful sign in a patient not premedicated with an anticholinergic.

Stage 4: impending respiratory and circulatory failure. Brainstem reflexes are depressed by the high anaesthetic concentration. Pupils are enlarged and unreactive. The patient should not be permitted to reach this stage. Withdrawal of the anaesthetic agents and administration of 100% oxygen lightens anaesthesia.

Observation of other reflexes provides a guide to depth of anaesthesia.
- Swallowing occurs in plane I of stage 3.
- Gag reflex is abolished in plane III of stage 3.
- Stretching of the anal sphincter produces reflex laryngospasm even at plane III of stage 3.

Intravenous induction

Induction of anaesthesia with an i.v. agent is suitable for most routine purposes and avoids many of the complications associated with the inhalational technique. It is the most appropriate method for rapid induction of the patient undergoing emergency surgery, in whom there is a risk of regurgitation of gastric contents.

All drugs that may be required at induction should be prepared beforehand and a cannula inserted into a suitable vein. If an existing i.v. cannula is to be used, its function must be checked. Cannulae with a top injection port are useful; large-bore cannulae (i.e. 14G/16G) are necessary for the rapid administration of fluids or blood. A vein in the forearm or on the back of the hand is preferable; veins in the antecubital fossa should be avoided because of the risks of intra-arterial injection and problems with elbow flexion. After selection of a suitable vein and skin preparation with 2% chlorhexidine in alcohol, s.c. local anaesthetic can be used for wide-bore cannula insertion. Alternatively, local anaesthetic cream (EMLA or Ametop) can be applied preoperatively (see Chapter 5). Transparent cannulae dressings are preferred to allow regular inspection of the skin entry site.

Preoxygenation of the lungs may begin, using a close-fitting face-mask and 100% oxygen delivered by a suitable breathing system for 3–5 min. Alternatively, three to four vital capacity breaths may be used. Preoxygenation before routine elective induction of anaesthesia minimises the risk of transient hypoxaemia before establishment of effective lung ventilation (see Chapter 23).

Intravenous induction agents are discussed in detail in Chapter 4. The induction dose varies with the patient's weight, age, state of nutrition, circulatory status, premedication and any concurrent medication. A small test dose is commonly administered, and its effects are observed. Slow injection is recommended in the older patient and in those with a slow circulation time (e.g. shock, hypovolaemia, cardiovascular disease) while the effects of the drug on the cardiovascular and respiratory systems are assessed.

A rapid-sequence induction technique is indicated for patients undergoing emergency surgery and for those with potential for vomiting or regurgitation (see Chapter 23).

Complications and difficulties

Complications and difficulties can include the following:
- *Respiratory depression.* Slow injection of an induction agent can reduce the extent of respiratory depression. Respiratory adequacy must be assessed carefully, and the anaesthetist should be ready to assist ventilation of the lungs if necessary.
- *Cardiovascular depression.* This is likely to occur particularly in the older, hypovolaemic or untreated hypertensive patient. Reducing the dose and speed of injection is essential in these patients. Infusion of i.v. fluid (e.g. 500 ml colloid or crystalloid solution) is usually successful in restoring arterial pressure, but other agents (e.g. ephedrine 3–12 mg i.v.) may be required.
- *Histamine release.* Thiopental in particular may cause release of histamine with subsequent formation of typical wheals. Severe reactions may occur to individual agents, and appropriate drugs and fluids should be available in the anaesthetic room for treatment. Guidelines for emergency management of anaphylaxis are discussed in Chapter 27.
- *Inadvertent intra-arterial injection* (see Chapter 27).
- *Regurgitation and vomiting* (see Chapter 27).

Maintenance of anaesthesia

Anaesthesia may be continued using inhalational agents, i.v. anaesthetic agents or i.v. opioids either alone or in combination. Tracheal intubation, with or without neuromuscular blockade may be used. Regional anaesthesia may be used to supplement any of these techniques to achieve the components of the familiar anaesthetic triad of hypnosis, neuromuscular blockade and analgesia.

Inhalational anaesthesia with spontaneous ventilation

Indications

This is an appropriate form of maintenance for superficial body surgery, minor procedures which produce little reflex or painful stimulation and operations for which profound neuromuscular blockade is not required.

Conduct

After induction of anaesthesia, a mixture of nitrous oxide or air in oxygen supplemented with a volatile anaesthetic agent is used, with the patient breathing spontaneously. The patient's response is assessed by observation of ventilation, circulation and heart rate/rhythm. Typically the volatile anaesthetic agent is used with an inspired concentration equivalent to 1 MAC (minimum alveolar concentration) (see Chapter 3).

Maintenance of the airway is one of the most important of the anaesthetist's tasks. Inhalational anaesthetic agents may be delivered via a face-mask SAD or tracheal tube. The use of these devices is discussed in detail in Chapter 23.

Tracheal intubation may be performed under local anaesthesia (using topical spray, e.g. lidocaine) or under general anaesthesia (either i.v. or inhalational, with or without the use of neuromuscular blockade). The usual approach is to provide general anaesthesia and neuromuscular blockade to perform laryngoscopy and direct vision tracheal intubation, and then to maintain anaesthesia via the tracheal tube with spontaneous or controlled ventilation.

Inhalational technique for tracheal intubation

Adequate depth of anaesthesia is necessary to depress the laryngeal reflexes and provide a degree of relaxation of the laryngeal and pharyngeal muscles. Sevoflurane 8% provides rapid attainment of the necessary depth, which can be judged from the pattern of respiration with predominance of diaphragmatic breathing (a useful sign in children is the dissociation of the thoracic and abdominal excursion). The mask is removed and laryngoscopy and tracheal intubation performed. The anaesthetic circuit is then connected to the tracheal tube and anaesthesia maintained at a depth appropriate for surgery.

Anaesthesia using neuromuscular blocking agents

Indications

The use of a neuromuscular blocking agent (NMBA) provides muscle paralysis, permitting lighter anaesthesia with less risk of cardiovascular depression. Thus, the technique is appropriate for: major abdominal, intraperitoneal, thoracic or intracranial operations; prolonged operations in which spontaneous ventilation would lead to respiratory depression; and operations in a position in which ventilation is impaired mechanically.

Conduct

After i.v. or inhalational induction of anaesthesia, an intubating dose of an NMBA is administered. The choice of NMBA depends upon operative indications and/or the patient's clinical condition (see Chapter 8). Assisted ventilation is maintained via the face-mask until neuromuscular blockade is adequate as measured by train-of-four monitoring; laryngoscopy and tracheal intubation are then performed. Inhalational anaesthesia may be continued with manual ventilation until the effects of the NMBA have ceased, whereupon spontaneous ventilation is resumed. Otherwise controlled ventilation is commenced, first manually by compression of the reservoir bag and then by a mechanical ventilator delivering the appropriate tidal and minute volumes. Anaesthesia and analgesia are provided by nitrous oxide/oxygen or air/oxygen, together with a volatile inhalational agent and i.v. analgesic. The inspired and end-expired concentrations of volatile anaesthetic agents should be monitored. Analgesia may also be supplemented by analgesic premedication or by use of regional or local anaesthetic techniques (see Chapter 25).

Adequacy of anaesthesia

Autonomic reflex activity with lacrimation, sweating, tachycardia, hypertension or reflex movement in response to surgery indicate inadequate depth of anaesthesia or insufficient analgesia. Accidental awareness under general anaesthesia is discussed in Chapter 26.

Adequacy of neuromuscular blockade

Clinical signs of return of muscle tone include retraction of the wound edges during abdominal operations and abdominal muscle, diaphragmatic or facial movement. An increase in airway pressure (with a time- or volume-cycled ventilator) may also indicate a return of muscle tone. Quantitative estimation of neuromuscular block should be obtained with a peripheral nerve stimulator and train-of-four monitoring. Increments (e.g. 20%–35% of the original dose) of NMBA may be given to maintain neuromuscular blockade; alternatively, an i.v. infusion may be a more convenient method of administration.

Reversal of neuromuscular blockade

At the end of surgery the degree of neuromuscular block should be reassessed and residual neuromuscular blockade

449

antagonised (see Chapter 8). Resumption of spontaneous ventilation should occur if normocapnic ventilation has been used and ensured by monitoring the end-tidal CO_2.

Total intravenous anaesthesia

Total intravenous anaesthesia (TIVA) techniques for induction and maintenance of anaesthesia without inhaled hypnotic agents are widely used. Some indications for TIVA are shown in Box 22.3. The pharmacokinetic and pharmacodynamic profiles of agents such as propofol and remifentanil (fast onset and offset times) permit rapid titration of drug dose to the required effect in individual patients (see Chapter 1). Target-controlled infusion (TCI) devices use pharmacological models to enable the theoretical drug concentration in the plasma and brain of propofol and remifentanil to be controlled continuously and administered without the need for complex calculation by the anaesthetist. This is discussed in detail in Chapter 4. Processed EEG monitoring (e.g. bispectral index) is recommended during TIVA to help prevent awareness, particularly when NMBAs are used.

Practical aspects of TIVA

The use of TIVA requires a secure and reliable i.v. cannula which ideally is accessible for inspection throughout the case. Observation for disconnection, leakage or extravasation of the i.v. anaesthetic agents should occur regularly. A dedicated two- or three-way TIVA set should always be used, including antisiphon valves on drug administration lines,

---

a non-return valve on the i.v. fluid line and minimal dead space distal to the point of agent and i.v. fluid mixing. Only Leur-Lock syringes should be used to help prevent disconnection from giving sets. Dedicated TCI pumps which are regularly serviced are required. Checks to ensure that a secure mains connection and an operational battery backup exist should be completed. Care must be taken to ensure accurate patient data are entered and the program applies to the drug contained in the syringe actually attached to it. Alarm settings for low and high pressures should also be set. The Association of Anaesthetists have produced detailed guidelines relating to TIVA use (Nimmo et al., 2018).

Patient positioning for surgery

After induction of anaesthesia, the patient is placed on the operating table in a position appropriate for the proposed surgery. When positioning the patient, the anaesthetist should take into account surgical access, patient safety, anaesthetic technique, monitoring and position of i.v. cannulae, etc. Some commonly used positions are shown in Figs 22.2–22.9. Each may have adverse effects in terms of skeletal, neurological, ventilatory and circulatory effects.

Positioning for newer, specialised surgical techniques such as robotic surgery may present challenges because of the prolonged duration of the procedures (e.g. 'extreme' Trendelenburg position). Movement or slippage of the patient may also result in injury from the robotic arms. Complications of positioning during anaesthesia are discussed in more detail in Chapter 26.

- *Supine.* Carries the risk of aortocaval compression during pregnancy (see Chapter 43) or in patients with a large abdominal mass.
- *Trendelenburg (head down).* May produce upward pressure on the diaphragm because of the weight of the abdominal contents. Damage to the brachial plexus may occur as a result of pressure from shoulder supports, especially if the arms are abducted.
- *Lithotomy and Lloyd-Davies.* Differ in the degree of hip and knee flexion, but both may result in nerve damage on the medial or lateral side of the leg from pressure exerted by the stirrups, which must be well padded. Care must be taken to elevate both legs simultaneously so that pelvic asymmetry and resultant backache are avoided. The sacrum should be supported and not allowed to slip off the end of the operating table.
- *Lateral.* May result in asymmetrical lung ventilation. Care is required with arm position and i.v. infusions. The pelvis and shoulders must be supported to prevent the patient from rolling either backwards (with a risk of falling from the table) or forwards into the recovery position.

Box 22.3 Indications for total intravenous anaesthesia (TIVA)

Malignant hyperthermia risk
History of severe PONV
Anaesthesia in non-theatre environments
Day-case surgery
Avoidance of neuromuscular blockade
    Myasthenia gravis
    Myotonic dystrophy
    Surgery requiring neurophysiological monitoring (e.g. spinal surgery)
Transfer of anaesthetised patients between locations (e.g. theatre and ICU)
Upper airway/thoracic surgery undertaken without a tracheal tube (e.g. rigid bronchoscopy)
Patient choice

PONV, Postoperative nausea and vomiting.

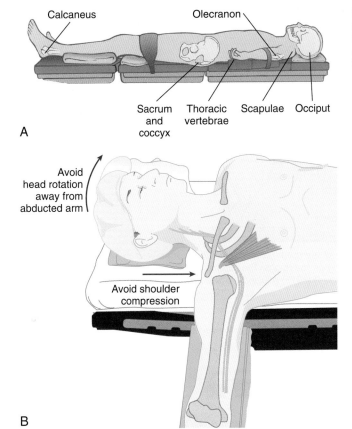

Calcaneus   Olecranon

Sacrum   Thoracic   Scapulae   Occiput
and   vertebrae
coccyx

A

Avoid
head rotation
away from
abducted arm

Avoid shoulder
compression

B

Fig. 22.2 (A) Supine position with potential pressure areas. Care must be taken to avoid (B) traction injury to the brachial plexus. (From Rothrock, J. (2015) *Alexander's care of the patient in surgery*. 15th ed. St. Louis, MO, Mosby.)

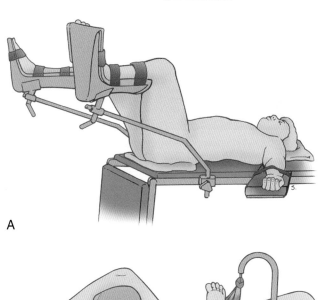

A

B   C

Fig. 22.3 Lithotomy position using (A) boot-type, (B) knee crutch and (C) candy cane stirrups. (From Rothrock, J. (2015) *Alexander's care of the patient in surgery*. 15th ed. St. Louis, MO, Mosby.)

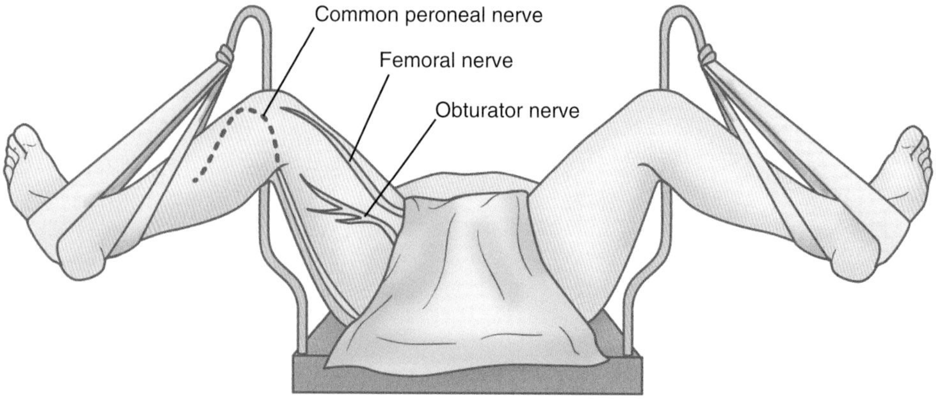

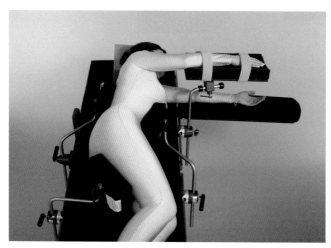

Fig. 22.4 Lower limb nerves at risk of damage when stirrups are used. Femoral and obturator nerves can be stretched by overextension of the hips or surgical team members leaning on the thighs. The common peroneal nerve can be compressed if the lateral knee rests against the stirrup bar. (From Rothrock, J. (2015) *Alexander's care of the patient in surgery.* 15th ed. St. Louis, MO, Mosby.)

Fig. 22.5 Lateral position with three lateral braces (abdomen, lower back and upper posterior thigh) and arm supports. (From Rothrock, J. (2015) *Alexander's care of the patient in surgery.* 15th ed. St. Louis, MO, Mosby.)

- *Sitting or beach-chair.* Requires careful attention to the support of the head. In addition, venous pooling and resultant cardiovascular instability may occur. During craniotomy, venous air embolism is possible (see Chapter 40).
- *Prone.* The most common specialised position; its safe management requires manual handling teamwork and specialist equipment. Equipment such as the Jackson table sandwich the patient, allowing careful positioning before mechanical turning (see Fig. 22.6A). Other options include foam or gel head and face supports and tabletop body supports such as the Montreal mattress and Wilson frame (see Fig. 22.6B). Prone positioning under general anaesthesia requires a number of physiological and practical issues to be considered:
  - Cardiovascular
    Decreased venous return can be caused by abdominal compression or venous pooling in the legs.
    Dislodgement and/or inaccessibility of i.v. cannula after turning is not uncommon.
  - Respiratory:
    Functional residual capacity is often increased in the prone position, which may improve lung compliance.
    Abdominal compression can cause increased ventilatory pressures.

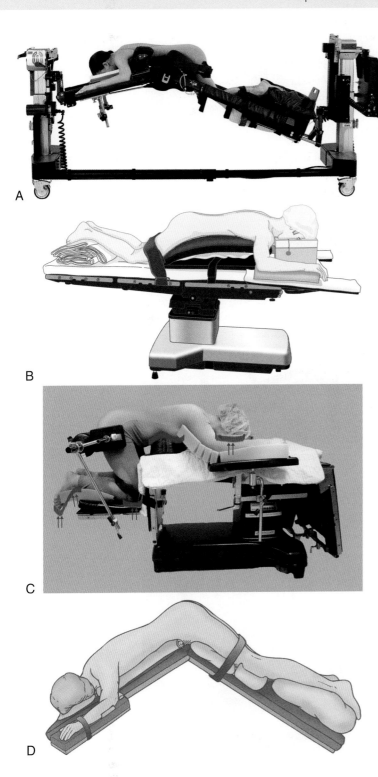

Fig. 22.6 Prone positioning on (A) Jackson table and (B) Wilson frame. Variations of the prone position include the (C) knee-chest (pressure areas at risk are highlighted in red) and (D) jack-knife positions. (From Rothrock, J. (2015) *Alexander's care of the patient in surgery*. 15th ed. St. Louis, MO, Mosby.)

A

B

C

D

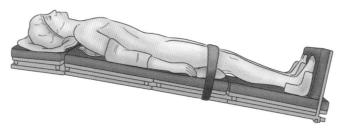

Fig. 22.7 Reverse Trendelenburg position with shoulder roll *in situ*. (From Rothrock, J. (2015) *Alexander's care of the patient in surgery.* 15th ed. St. Louis, MO, Mosby.)

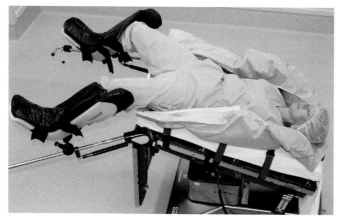

Fig. 22.8 Steep Trendelenburg position often used in robotic-assisted surgery. The model is supported in vacuum beanbag device. (From Rothrock, J. (2015) *Alexander's care of the patient in surgery.* 15th ed. St. Louis, MO, Mosby.)

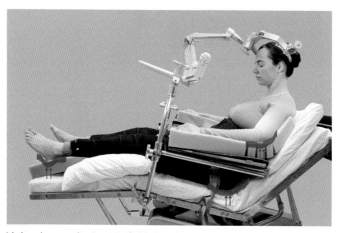

Fig. 22.9 Sitting position with head secured using Mayfield pins. (From Rothrock, J. (2015) *Alexander's care of the patient in surgery.* 15th ed. St. Louis, MO, Mosby.)

There is a reduced risk of pulmonary aspiration. The tracheal tube may potentially be dislodged.

- Nerve injury:
  Blindness secondary to retinal artery occlusion or retinal vein thrombosis has been described.
  Traction injuries to the brachial plexus are possible with extensive abduction of the arms in the forward position.

To prevent this, support must be provided beneath the shoulders and iliac crests. Excessive extension of the shoulders should be avoided. The face, and particularly the eyes, must be protected from external pressure or trauma. The tracheal tube must be secured firmly in place as it is almost impossible to reinsert it with the patient in this position.

Emergence and recovery

After surgery has ended and the WHO sign-out checklist is completed, anaesthetic agents are withdrawn and oxygen 100% is delivered. Patients whose trachea has been intubated should be extubated before transfer to recovery areas unless postoperative mechanical ventilation in ICU is planned.

Conduct of tracheal extubation/ SAD removal

Tracheal extubation/SAD removal is discussed in Chapter 23.

Recovery

After removal of the tracheal tube or SAD, the patient's airway is supported until respiratory reflexes are intact. The patient is then ready for transfer from the operating table to a bed or trolley. Supplemental oxygen is delivered by face-mask during transport, and further patient recovery takes place in a recovery area of theatre or in the recovery ward (see Chapter 29).

References/Further reading

Association of Anaesthetists of Great Britain and Ireland, 2015. Recommendations for standards of monitoring during anaesthesia and recovery 2015. AAGBI, London.

Association of Anaesthetists of Great Britain and Ireland, 2012. Checklist for anaesthetic equipment 2012. Anaesthesia 66, 662–663.

Difficult Airway Society UK, 2011. DAS Extubation Guidelines. https:// www.das.uk.com/content/ das-extubation-guidelines.

Nimmo, A.F., Absalom, A.R., Bagshaw, O., Biswas, A., Cook, T.M., Costello, A., et al., 2018. Guidelines for the safe practice of total intravenous anaesthesia (TIVA) Joint Guidelines from the Association of Anaesthetists and the Society for Intravenous Anaesthesia. Anaesthesia https://doi. org/10.1111/anae.14428.

Royal College of Anaesthetists, 2016. Scope of practice for a PA(A) on qualification. (2016 revision). https:// www.rcoa.ac.uk/document-store/scope -of-practice-paa-qualification.

WHO Surgical Safety Checklist. http:// www.who.int/patientsafety/ safesurgery/checklist/en/.

Chapter | **23** |

Airway management

Tim Cook

This chapter is divided into four parts:

1. Airway equipment
2. Routine airway management
3. Emergency airway management
4. Difficult airway management

It does not cover airway management in paediatric, obstetric or emergency anaesthesia. These are covered in Chapters 33, 43 and 44, respectively.

Section 1

Anaesthetic airway equipment

Anaesthetists must have a sound understanding and firm knowledge of the functioning of all anaesthetic equipment in common use. It is essential that anaesthetists check that all equipment is functioning correctly before they proceed to anaesthetise a patient (see Chapter 22). It is not possible to describe the whole range of anaesthetic airway equipment here; rather an overview is provided with specific detail described where relevant later in the chapter.

Face-masks

Face-masks are designed to fit the face so that no leak of gas occurs, but without applying excessive pressure to the skin. An appropriate size of face-mask must be used to ensure a proper fit. Most modern masks consist of a hard plastic cone with a soft deformable gas-filled cuff to place against the face. Traditional rubber masks have been replaced by transparent single-use devices (Fig. 23.1). These are preferred by patients and enable the anaesthetist to observe the airway for vomitus or secretions during use.

Oropharyngeal and nasopharyngeal airways

The Guedel oropharyngeal airway (Fig. 23.2) consists of a rigid plastic flattened tube that is straight in its proximal section and curved distally. It is designed to be placed into the mouth to reverse the effects of gravity on the tongue (which falls back and can occlude the oral cavity and posterior pharynx) after induction of anaesthesia and thus maintain a patent airway. Size can be estimated from laying the airway on the cheek and it should be approximately the distance from the angle of the mandible to the midline of the lips.

The nasopharyngeal airway is a small plastic tube (6.0–7.0 mm ID) designed to be placed through the nose so the tip lies in the upper pharynx (Fig. 23.3). It is designed to lift the soft palate off the pharyngeal wall and so eliminate this mode of airway obstruction. The proximal end of the airway has a flange to prevent loss of the device into the nose. Complications include bleeding (common) and submucosal passage (very uncommon).

Connectors and catheter mounts

The anaesthetic circuit is constructed from plastic tubes joined together by connectors. The distal end of the anaesthetic circuit is a plastic connector of 22-mm external diameter. Between the distal end of the anaesthetic circuit and the proximal end of the airway device sits the catheter mount with a 22-mm connector at the proximal end and a 15-mm connector distally. These push fit connectors must be actively pushed and twisted to connect reliably; failure to do this is a common cause of circuit disconnection. The catheter mount may be straight or angled, fixed length or concertinaed and may serve additional functions (e.g. including a self-sealing diaphragm at the angled end to facilitate endoscopic inspection through the airway device). The catheter mount enables positioning of the anaesthetic circuit such that there is no excessive traction on the airway device that may lead

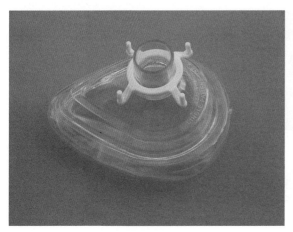

Fig. 23.1 Face mask.

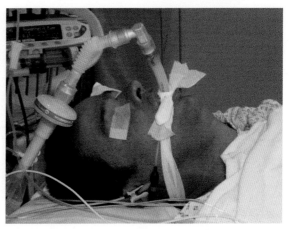

Fig. 23.4 Classic laryngeal mask airway (LMA) in place with attached catheter mount and heat and moisture exchange filter (HMEF).

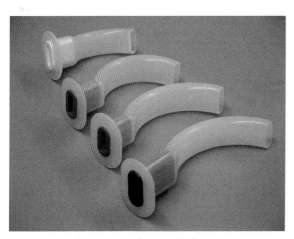

Fig. 23.2 Oropharyngeal airways.

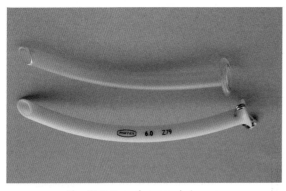

Fig. 23.3 Nasopharyngeal airways.

to displacement. Proximal to the catheter mount a heat and moisture exchange filter (HMEF) is usually placed (Fig. 23.4). This helps maintain airway gases temperature and humidity and isolates the anaesthetic circuit from the patent so that it may be used for multiple patients.

Supraglottic airway devices

Supraglottic airway devices (SADs) are the mainstay of airway management during low-risk, elective anaesthesia. There are numerous devices that generally consist of a proximal tube ('stem') that runs from the anaesthetic circuit through the mouth, and a 'head' or 'mask' that forms a seal with the larynx (or rarely with just the pharynx above). In most designs this mask portion is cuffed, but some are cuffless and rely on their shape to create a seal.

There are several classifications of SADs, none of them entirely satisfactory. The most widely used divides SADs into first- and second-generation devices. First-generation devices are simple SADs (tube and mask) without specific design features to reduce the risk of aspiration. These include the classic laryngeal mask airway (cLMA), flexible LMA (fLMA) and equivalent single-use devices. Second-generation SADs have design features that aim to reduce the risk of aspiration. These often have a drain tube running parallel to the stem of the SAD that exists at the tip of the device and therefore sits at the top of the oesophagus when correctly placed. They often also have an integral bite block and create a better seal with the airway than first-generation SADs (though neither are part of the second-generation definition). Second-generation SADs include the i-gel, ProSeal LMA (PLMA) and LMA Supreme (SLMA). The 2015 Difficult Airway Society (DAS)

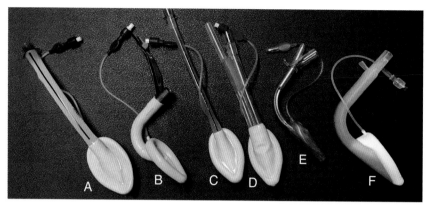

Fig. 23.5 Supraglottic airway devices. Left to right, the devices are (A) classic laryngeal mask airway (LMA); (B) Intubating LMA; (C) Flexible LMA; (D) ProSeal LMA; (E) LMA Supreme; (F) LMA Protector.

guidelines for difficult tracheal intubation recommend a second-generation SAD for airway rescue after failed tracheal intubation. Their provision and training in their use therefore needs to be widespread. The classification does not include the term third-generation SAD, though some manufacturers erroneously use this for marketing.

Supraglottic airway devices are generally made of silicone (most reusable devices) or polyvinyl chloride (PVC) (most single-use devices). Polyvinyl chloride is generally somewhat more rigid than silicone, and as a result the airway seal is often less good and the risk of airway trauma higher.

First-generation SADs
Classic LMA

The cLMA is the forerunner of many modern SADs and consists of a silicone tube with an elliptical distal mask, which has a cuff, inflated through a pilot tube (Fig. 23.5A). The cuff, which resembles a miniature face mask, is designed to seal around the posterior perimeter of the larynx. In the middle of the bowl two soft bars run longitudinally to prevent the epiglottis entering the airway tube and occluding the airway. When correctly positioned, the bowl of the cLMA surrounds the laryngeal inlet and epiglottis, and the cuff of the mask extends from the base of the tongue to the upper oesophagus. Seven sizes are routinely available, enabling use in all patients from neonates to large adults (Table 23.1).

The cLMA (in common with most other SADs) is reusable up to 40 times. There are numerous single-use devices based on the cLMA, collectively referred to as laryngeal masks. Performance of laryngeal masks may be similar to the cLMA, but in many cases this is unproven, and some devices perform less well.

Flexible LMA

The fLMA (Fig. 23.5C) differs from the cLMA only in the fact that it has a flexible, wire-reinforced airway tube. The

Table 23.1 Laryngeal mask airway (LMA) sizes

Mask size	Patient weight (kg)	Cuff volume (ml)
1	<5	2–5
1.5	5–10	5–7
2	10–20	7–10
2.5	20–30	12–14
3	>30	15–20
4	n/a	25–30
5	n/a	35–40

tube is longer and narrower compared with the cLMA, which modestly increases airway resistance. The flexible tube means that once the mask is placed the tube can be moved (carefully) without displacing the mask, and this makes it suitable for many head and neck surgeries including (in skilled hands) shared-airway work. However, the flexible stem means placement requires scrupulous attention to detail and good technique. Poor technique can lead to axial rotation of the stem so the mask portion faces sideways or backwards. Because of the wire in the tube, the fLMA is unsuitable for use in MRI suites.

Second-generation SADs
ProSeal LMA

The PLMA is a reusable device with a drain tube, posterior inflatable cuff, reinforced airway tube, integral bite block and no epiglottic bars (Fig. 23.5D). Like all laryngeal masks, the distal end must sit in the oesophageal inlet to ensure best performance. The dual tubes of the PLMA and the high seal pressures achieved within the airway (30–40 cmH$_2$O) and the upper oesophagus (>60 cmH$_2$O) mean the tubes create a 'functional separation of the respiratory and gastrointestinal tracts' (i.e. airway tube in continuity with the larynx, drain tube in continuity with the oesophagus). The drain tube vents gases leaking into the oesophagus and fluid if regurgitation occurs, and it facilitates insertion of an orogastric tube. The PLMA can be inserted in an identical way to the cLMA or mounted on an introducer to be inserted in a similar way to the intubating LMA (ILMA) (see later). It can also be inserted by passing a bougie (straight end first) into the oesophagus and then railroading the PLMA into place over the drain tube. With its improved airway and oesophageal seal, the performance of the PLMA is arguably equal or superior to all other SADs, with insertion difficulty (overcome by good technique) perhaps its only drawback.

LMA Supreme and LMA Protector

The SLMA (Fig. 23.5E) has features of the PLMA (drain tube), ILMA (rigid curved stem) and single-use SADs (PVC construction). Its airway seal is intermediate between the cLMA and PLMA at 24–28 cmH$_2$O. Because of its rigid construction and PVC cuff it is slightly more traumatic to the airway than the reusable devices. The drain tube runs centrally in the stem with two small airway tubes running laterally. This arrangement means the airway tubes are small and this makes the SLMA poorly suited as a tracheal intubation conduit (see difficult airway management section).

Recently the LMA Protector (Fig. 23.5F), which is similar in design to the SLMA but is made of silicone, has been introduced; its role in clinical practice is yet to be established.

Other cuffed second-generation SADs include the Ambu Aura-Gain and Guardian CPV.

i-gel

The i-gel is a single-use SAD with a non-inflatable mask made of a soft thermoplastic elastomer (Fig. 23.6). The mask is a preformed soft mould which fits into the per-ilaryngeal structures. It has a narrow-bore drain tube, short

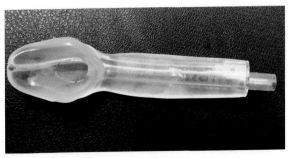

Fig. 23.6 i-gel supraglottic airway device.

wide-bore airway tube and integral bite block. The mask portion is shorter than other laryngeal masks, and it therefore sits less deeply, and seals less well, in the upper oesophagus. It has now been used for many millions of anaesthetics and has a good efficacy and safety record. Sore throats and dysphagia may occur less commonly after i-gel use than with other SADs. It is well suited to guided tracheal intubation during difficult airway management, and because it is extremely simple to insert, it has become widely used for airway management during cardiac arrest.

Baska mask

The Baska mask is a silicone device with two large drain tubes and a central airway tube. The mask is reduced to a thin soft head that creates a seal around the airway during positive pressure by becoming partly inflated. The drain tubes open onto the posterior of the mask and serves dual functions as sump for secretions and drain tubes.

Intubating LMA

The ILMA is a specialised LMA designed to facilitate tracheal intubation (Figs 23.5B and 23.7). It is described in the section on Difficult Airway Management later in this chapter.

Laryngeal tubes

These devices are formed of a slim tube with two cuffs, one distal and one approximately 7–10 cm proximal to the tip. Between the cuffs lies an airway orifice. Reusable and single use variations exist and also versions with a standard drain tube or an expanded one (for use in upper gastrointestinal endoscopy). These devices are easy to insert, but prone to rotate leading to obstruction. In a small number of counties they are popular for use during resuscitation or anaesthesia.

Laryngoscopes

There are many designs of laryngoscope, and only the main devices are described here. Traditional laryngoscopes comprise a handle attached to a metal blade with a light usually halfway along its length. The blade is designed to enable displacement of tissues and illumination of the airway so that a tracheal tube may be passed under direct vision into the larynx (direct laryngoscopy) (Fig. 23.8). This requires almost perfect alignment of the oral, pharyngeal and laryngeal axes (Fig. 23.9), which may require significant force and is often difficult.

Over the last decade, cameras have become incorporated into laryngoscope blades (videolaryngoscopes), enabling

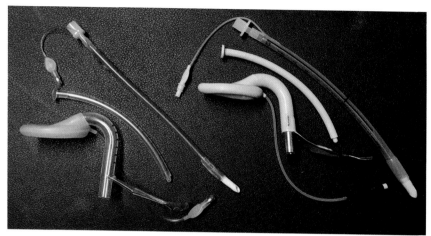

Fig. 23.7 Intubating laryngeal mask airway (ILMA) – single use version on the left and reusable version on the right.

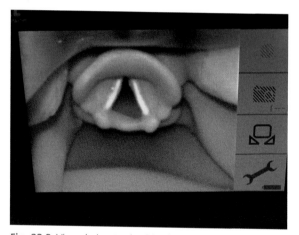

Fig. 23.8 View during tracheal intubation of a manikin, with the tip of the laryngoscope in the vallecular.

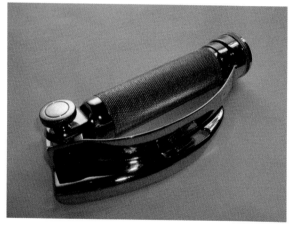

Fig. 23.10 Macintosh laryngoscope.

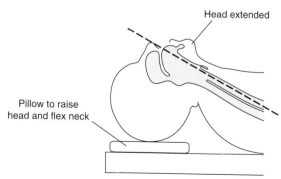

Fig. 23.9 Head position for laryngoscopy with alignment of oral, pharyngeal and laryngeal axes.

display of an image from the blade onto an incorporated or separate screen. Depending on the design of the videolaryngoscope, the need for tissue displacement and alignment may be reduced or eliminated completely. The technique is called indirect laryngoscopy or, more usefully, videolaryngoscopy.

Macintosh laryngoscope

The most commonly used adult laryngoscope blade is the Macintosh blade (Fig. 23.10), which is manufactured in several sizes. Similar to other laryngoscopes, the handle contains batteries, and clicking the blade into place (90 degrees to the handle) turns the light on. Older laryngoscopes had bulbs in the blade, but these have largely been replaced by a light on the handle that is transmitted along the blade via cold fibreoptics.

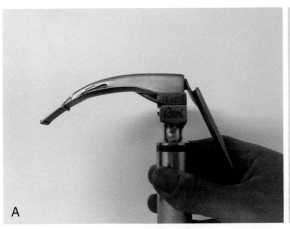 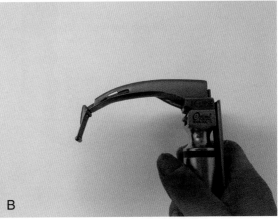

A   B

Fig. 23.11 (A) McCoy laryngoscope; (B) flexion of the hinged distal portion of the blade.

Specialised blades

Straight blade

There are various designs of straight, or nearly straight, bladed laryngoscopes (e.g. Henderson, Miller, Magill and Wisconsin). Although each have their advocates and have an important role in paediatric practice (see Chapter 33), their use is infrequent in adult practice in the UK.

McCoy (levering) laryngoscope

The blade of the McCoy laryngoscope (Fig. 23.11) is hinged in its distal portion and can be flexed by squeezing a lever on the handle. This moves the fulcrum of laryngoscopy from the teeth to the end of the blade. When deployed, the tip lifts the epiglottis and often improves laryngeal view by one Cormack-Lehane grade (see Airway Assessment section). However, the device is somewhat cumbersome and has largely been replaced by videolaryngoscopes.

Videolaryngoscopes

Videolaryngoscopes use high-resolution electronic video cameras incorporated in a laryngoscope blade. The image is relayed to a dedicated video display which may be on the laryngoscope handle or separately. Videolaryngoscopy enables the anaesthetist to 'see around the corner' and effectively gain a view from the blade. This converts the very narrow angle view obtained with direct laryngoscopy ($\approx$15 degrees) into a wider angle view ($\approx$60 degrees) (Fig. 23.12). An exception to this electronic design is the Airtraq (Fig. 23.13), which projects its light and image through a series of prisms.

There are three main designs of videolaryngoscopes:

- Bladed
  - Macintosh-shaped blade, such as C-MAC (Fig. 23.14), GlideScope Titanium, McGRATH MAC (may be used for both direct and videolaryngoscopy)
  - Hyperangulated blade, such as C-MAC D blade, GlideScope original (Fig. 23.15)
- Conduited, such as Airtraq, Pentax AWS
- Optical stylets, such as Bonfils, Shikani optical stylet, C-MAC VS videostylet.

Optical stylets are metal rods with an internal fibreoptic or video system which enables the user to view the image from the distal end directly from the viewing port or on a remote screen (Fig. 23.16). Most stylets are rigid with a fixed angle (e.g. Bonfils, Levitan). The Shikani stylet is semimalleable and the SensaScope has a flexible fibreoptic tip which allows some manipulation. Optical stylets are placed within the lumen of the tracheal tube and then directed into the larynx before the tracheal tube is advanced into the airway. The main advantage of stylets is that they require minimal mouth opening (as little as 1 cm) and can be advanced with negligible tissue disruption. Their main disadvantage is the inability to manipulate and displace airway structures in the manner that a bladed instrument can. Bladed videolaryngoscopes are increasingly popular, with optical stylet use restricted to expert local use.

The potential advantages of videolaryngoscopy compared with direct laryngoscopy include:

- ability to 'see round corners';
  improved view at laryngoscopy (especially when there is difficulty)
- reduced head and neck movement to achieve a view of the larynx, which is important in patients with potentially unstable cervical spines;

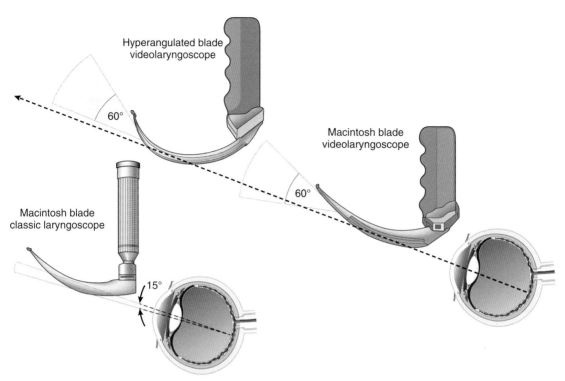

Hyperangulated blade
videolaryngoscope

60°

Macintosh blade
videolaryngoscope

60°

Macintosh blade
classic laryngoscope

15°

Fig. 23.12 Videolaryngoscopy angle *versus* direct laryngoscopy view.

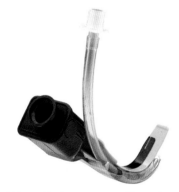

Fig. 23.13 Airtraq videolaryngoscope. (Reproduced from
http://www.airtraq.com/downloads/#downloadstitle2.
© Prodol Meditec.)

- improved ease of tracheal intubation and reduced failed intubation;
- reduced tissue distortion and haemodynamic responses to laryngoscopy;
- reduced airway trauma;
- reduced postoperative hoarseness;

- ability to display the image on a remote screen, which permits:
  - improved supervision by trainers of tracheal intubation performed by trainees;
  - an assistant to observe what the intubator sees (e.g. guiding cricoid force);
  - improved skill acquisition of direct laryngoscopy by trainees;
  - recording for medical notes and medicolegal reasons; and
  - recording of an objective image or video for presentation, teaching or research purposes.

These benefits are particularly apparent to those experienced with videolaryngoscopy.

When laryngoscopy is easy, use of a hyperangulated or conduited, but not a Macintosh-type videolaryngoscope may overcomplicate tracheal intubation and, therefore, slow it down and increase the number of attempts.

Use of a hyperangulated blade prevents direct laryngoscopy as the blade is too curved to enable direct vision of its distal end. To overcome this problem, many manufacturers advise the use of a rigid or semirigid stylet to pre-form the shape of the tracheal tube before insertion. There is a risk of damage to other tissues in the airway as the tracheal tube/stylet assembly is introduced (blindly). This is minimised if the tip of the

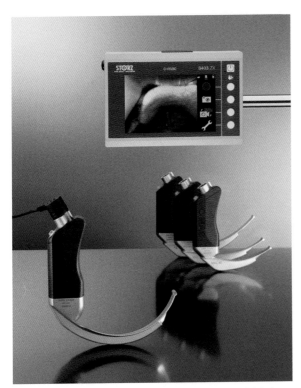

Fig. 23.14 C-MAC videolaryngoscope with Macintosh blades in the background and hyperangulated 'D-blade' in the foreground. (Reproduced from https://www.karlstorz.com/gb/en/anesthesiology-and-emergency-medicine.htm. © Karl Storz.)

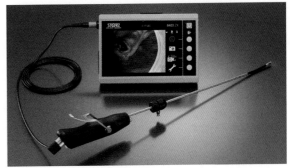

Fig. 23.16 C-MAC VS video stylet. (© Copyright KARL STORZ SE & Co. KG, Germany.)

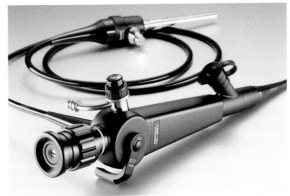

Fig. 23.17 Flexible endoscope. (Reproduced from https://www.pentaxmedical.com/pentax/en/106/1/Fiber-Naso-Pharyngo-Laryngoscopes. © Pentax Medical.)

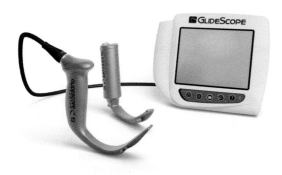

Fig. 23.15 GlideScope videolaryngoscope – Macintosh blades in the background and hyperangulated blade in the foreground. (Reproduced from https://verathon.com/glidescope-titanium-reusable/. © Verathon Inc.)

tracheal tube is advanced for as long as possible under direct vision and then along the blade of the videolaryngoscope.

The 2015 DAS guidelines for difficult tracheal intubation state that 'videolaryngoscopy should be rapidly available (in any location where tracheal intubation is performed) and that all anaesthetists should be trained and expert in the use of videolaryngoscopy'. This makes it a mainstream technique that should be taught during routine anaesthetic care. As videolaryngoscopy becomes more widely available, there is a strong argument for initially selecting a device with a Macintosh type blade (suitable for direct or videolaryngoscopy), reserving a specialised (i.e. hyperangulated, conduited or stylet) device only for when there is difficulty.

Flexible intubating laryngoscope and bronchoscope

The term 'fibreoptic scope' or 'fibrescope' (Fig. 23.17) describes a flexible fibreoptic endoscope suitable for introduction into the airway via the nose or mouth to guide tracheal

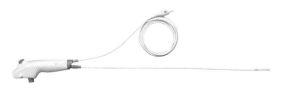

Fig. 23.18 Ambu aScope. (Reproduced from https://www.ambu.com/products/flexible-endoscopes/bronchoscopes/product/ambu-ascope-4-large. © Ambu A/S.)

intubation. Traditionally fibrescopes contain tiny fibres (20 μm glass fibres) in bundles that either transmitted an external light to the tip of the device to illuminate the subject or transmitted an image from the tip of the device to the eyepiece, or a connected screen. The fibres transmitting light (light guide) are arranged in a random fashion but those returning the image (image guide) are precisely located relative to each other to ensure integrity of the transmitted image. The flexible fibrescope consists of a long flexible cord, the distal tip of which is manipulated by controllers operated the proximal end. Various working channels are incorporated in the cord, their size varying with device diameter and function; this enables suction, instrumentation and drug or oxygen administration. Proximally there are directional controls and an eyepiece. The light source may be externally mains- or battery-powered. The eyepiece consists of the viewing lens and dioptre adjustment ring. A camera can be attached to the eyepiece either to take photographs or to transmit the pictures to a monitor.

The term 'fibrescope' is increasingly redundant as many modern devices (flexible videoscopes) no longer contain fibreoptic bundles but rather a distal electronic camera that captures a high-definition video image and transmits it electronically to a screen. This is a rapidly developing technology. Disposable flexible videoscopes (e.g. the aScope Fig. 23.18) are now available.

The size of flexible fibrescopes varies from 1.8–6.4 mm to fit inside tracheal tubes of 3.0–7.0 mm ID. Most intubating videoscopes are ≈3–5 mm diameter.

Tracheal tubes

Most tracheal tubes are constructed of plastic or silicone. The rigidity of the plastic used and the angle of the distal bevel of the tube varies considerably and can have an impact on airway trauma during tracheal intubation. Plastic tubes are almost entirely single use and are presented in a sterile pack. Cuffed tubes have a distal cuff to seal with the airway, and this is inflated via a pilot balloon with a self-sealing valve (Fig. 23.19). The internal diameter is marked on the side in millimetres and the distance from the tip of the tube

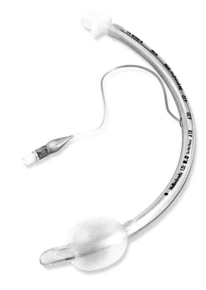

Fig. 23.19 Standard cuffed tracheal tube showing tube markings, pilot balloon and radio-opaque marking line. (Reproduced from http://www.medtronic.com/covidien/en-us/products/intubation/shiley-cuffed-basic-endotracheal-tubes.html. © Medtronic.)

is marked along its length in centimetres. The tube also has a radio-opaque line running along its length. This enables the position of the tube to be determined on a chest radiograph. Many tracheal tubes (but not all) have a depth indicator distally indicating where the tube should lie against the larynx. Silicone rubber is used in some tracheal tubes. These are softer than plastic tubes and some can be sterilised and reused but are more expensive than plastic tubes.

Tracheal tube size

Choice of size of tracheal tube is a matter for debate. Where the patient's lungs are ventilated there is little to be gained from using a large tracheal tube, and a smaller tube (e.g. 6.0–6.5 mm ID for women, 6.5–7.0 mm ID for men) may make tracheal intubation less traumatic, especially where there is an awkward view at laryngoscopy. If the patient will breathe spontaneously whilst the trachea is intubated (e.g. planned postoperative ICU admission), a larger tracheal tube (e.g. 7.0–7.5 mm ID for women, 8.0–8.5 mm ID for men) may lead to less airway resistance and improved access for passage of suction catheters.

Plain and cuffed tracheal tubes

Uncuffed tracheal tubes are generally only used in children (see Chapter 33). In adults, as the larynx is the narrowest part of the airway, a cuff is necessary to seal with the trachea (as inserting a tube large enough to seal with the larynx would cause trauma). Use of a cuffed tube facilitates positive pressure ventilation and (largely) protects the airway from soiling with secretions, regurgitated gastric contents, blood, pus and so on.

Cuff design, volume and pressure

Tracheal tube cuffs are generally described as low-volume/high-pressure or high-volume/low-pressure. A tracheal tube with a low-volume cuff needs almost complete inflation (high pressure) to create a seal within the trachea, whereas a large-volume cuff needs only partial inflation (low pressure). Most tracheal tube cuffs are now high-volume/low-pressure as, although not all pressure within the cuff is transmitted to the tracheal mucosa, these have a reduced likelihood of mucosal ischaemia. The volume of air inserted into the cuff need only be enough to create a seal and leak-free ventilation. For prolonged periods of tracheal intubation, manometry may be used to ensure the cuff pressure remains less than 30 cmH$_2$O. Some tracheal tubes now incorporate a pilot tube on which the pilot balloon is replaced by an integrated 'traffic light' pressure indicator to assist in maintaining safe pressures. If nitrous oxide is used, this can diffuse into the cuff as inspired concentration rises (and out as it falls), and cuff pressure should be checked 20 min after any increase in fractional concentration of nitrous oxide. Alternatively, the cuff volume may be inflated with fluid to avoid this problem.

High-volume/low-pressure plastic cuffs are incompletely inflated, and as a result small folds occur longitudinally, leading to microchannels which may enable fluid to bypass the cuff. Silicone cuffs (e.g. on ILMA tracheal tubes) inflate without microchannels and are generally low-volume/high-pressure (reusable ILMA tracheal tubes) or intermediate-volume/intermediate-pressure (single-use ILMA tracheal tubes). Herniation of an overinflated cuff may occlude the distal end of the tracheal tube and cause partial or total airway obstruction, but this is extremely rare.

Tube shape

A curved tracheal tube is used in most settings. Preformed tubes in shapes which either fit the pharyngeal contour or move the proximal end of the tracheal tube away from the mouth are used particularly for head and neck surgery (see Chapter 37). The preformed shape means bronchial intubation is more common, especially if the head is extended.

Specialised tracheal tubes

A flexible tube made of softer plastic or silicone and reinforced with an internal spiral of nylon or wire may be

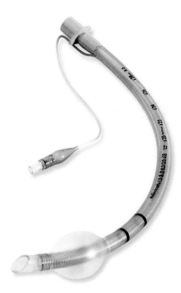

Fig. 23.20 Reinforced ('armoured') flexible tracheal tube. (Reproduced from http://www.medtronic.com/covidien/en-us/products/intubation/shiley-oral-nasal-endotracheal-tube-reinforced.html. © Medtronic.)

useful if there is a danger of the tube kinking during surgery, such as during head and neck surgery or prone positioning (Fig. 23.20). Flexible tubes are often straight and are more awkward to place at laryngoscopy, so use of a bougie or stylet is recommended. The internal spiral means they cannot be cut and care needs to be taken to avoid bronchial intubation.

The tip of many tracheal tubes is a rigid lateral bevel, and when used to railroad over a bougie, stylet or fibrescope, this can catch on the glottic tissues and cause hold-up and trauma. The ILMA tracheal tube is a wire-reinforced straight tube with a soft silicone bullet tip. The tip is designed to deviate when it hits tissue and to wrap around a fibrescope (Fig. 23.21A). This makes for atraumatic, smooth insertion when used for fibreoptic intubation. The Parker and GlideRite tracheal tubes (Fig. 23.21B and C), which have anterior-posterior bevels and softer tips, may also be useful when railroading.

Other specialised tubes include laser, micolaryngeal, double-lumen and laryngectomy tracheal tubes. These are discussed in Chapters 37 and 41.

Cricothyroidotomy devices

Cricothyroidotomy is the creation of an opening in the cricothyroid membrane to gain access to the airway either as an elective procedure in an anticipated difficult airway

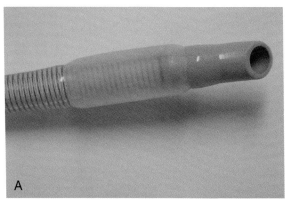

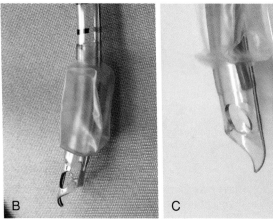

Fig. 23.21 (A) Intubating LMA (ILMA), (B) Parker and (C) GlideRite tracheal tube tips.

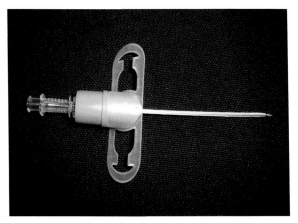

Fig. 23.22 Ravussin cricothyroidotomy cannula.

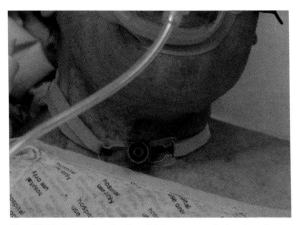

Fig. 23.23 Ravussin cricothyroidotomy cannula in place (but not being used for ventilation).

or as an emergency to rescue a lost airway (e.g. in the 'cannot intubate, cannot oxygenate' (CICO) situation).

Cricothyroidotomy can be carried out using a:

- small cannula (≤ 2-mm ID);
- large-bore cannula (≥ 4.0-mm ID); or
- tracheal tube (5–6 mm ID).

If a small cannula is used (cannula over needle technique), there is a risk of failure to insert, kinking or device failure. A specifically designed device, such as the Ravussin cannula (Figs 23.22 and 23.23), is recommended over the use of a standard i.v. cannula to ensure it is long enough, to reduce kinking and to improve ventilation. After insertion, ventilation needs to be provided by a high-pressure source (e.g. gas cylinder or wall oxygen) during which there is a risk of barotrauma. Devices such as the VBM Manujet III (Chapter 16, Fig. 16.37) and Rapid-O_2 insufflation device assist ventilation in these settings and are preferred to ad hoc equipment. Technical failure and complications of ventilation are much more common in an emergency. The Ventrain device (Fig. 23.24) facilitates ventilation through a

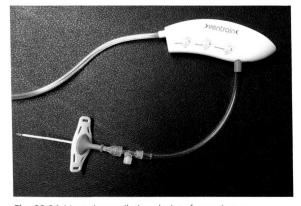

Fig. 23.24 Ventrain ventilation device, for expiratory ventilatory assist, with attached cannula.

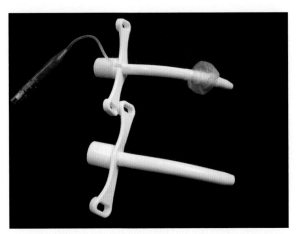

Fig. 23.25 Cook Melker cricothyroidotomy devices (5-mm cuffed and 6-mm uncuffed) which are inserted using a Seldinger technique.

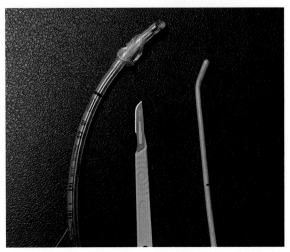

Fig. 23.26 Equipment for scalpel-bougie criciothyroidotomy.

narrow-bore cricothyroidotomy device (or a narrow tracheal tube) by providing high-flow gas for inspiration and using the Bernoulli principle to provide active expiration. Using this manual device, normal minute ventilation can be achieved through a 2-mm ID cannula.

Large-bore cannulae are inserted either with a cannula-over-needle technique (e.g. VBM Quicktrach) or with a Seldinger technique (e.g. Cook Melker cuffed and uncuffed devices, Fig. 23.25). They provide a tracheal tube through which an adult can breathe spontaneously (≥ 4.5-mm ID). The cannula-over-needle designs may be too short to reach the trachea in obese patients. The Portex cricothyroidotomy kit is designed for emergency use and has a spring-loaded Veress needle with a blunt stylet to aid insertion of a 6.0-mm ID tracheal tube. The Portex Minitrach II is a wire-guided kit which provides a 4-mm ID uncuffed airway designed for tracheal suction and specifically not for use in an emergency situation.

Insertion of a tracheal tube via the cricothyroid membrane can be achieved with a scalpel and bougie (Fig. 23.26). It is a versatile and quick technique and is described later in the chapter. It is currently the technique recommended in the DAS guidelines for both non-obese and obese patients. Unfamiliarity and bleeding are the main concerns with this technique.

Other apparatus

Bougie

If the larynx cannot be seen adequately during laryngoscopy, or if the tracheal tube cannot be manoeuvred into the

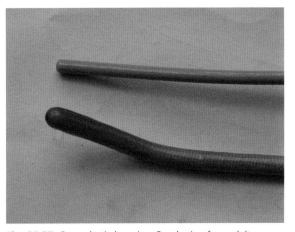

Fig. 23.27 Gum elastic bougies. Coude tip of an adult bougie (front) and straight tip of a paediatric bougie (rear).

laryngeal inlet, a bougie (diameter ≈5 mm, length ≈70 cm; Fig. 23.27) may facilitate this. The lubricated bougie is inserted into the trachea to act as a guide for the tracheal tube. The bougie's tip is bent distally (Coude tip) to aid insertion into the glottis. The bougie should never be inserted beyond the carina (maximum insertion distance 25 cm). The tracheal tube should be rotated as it is advanced over the bougie so that the bevel does not become lodged against the aryepiglottic fold or the vocal cord. Single-use disposable bougies are now available, but they may be rigid (increasing risk of trauma), have poor memory (i.e. they unfurl too rapidly after curling) or lack the Coude tip. They have not been shown to be better than the reusable Eschmann (gum elastic) in practice.

Stylet

An (often malleable) metal stylet may be used to adjust the degree of curvature of a tracheal tube as an aid to its insertion (Fig. 23.28). The stylet must not protrude from the distal end of the tube, in order to prevent trauma. Stylets have traditionally been used much more in North America, with the bougie more commonly used in the UK; recently this has changed as stylets are particularly suited to aiding

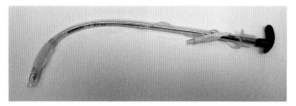

Fig. 23.28 Preformed stylet for use with the hyperangulated GlideScope blade.

tracheal intubation with hyperangulated videolaryngoscope blades. Stylets for use with videolaryngoscopes may be device specific and may be rigid or malleable. The Parker Flex-It stylet is a single-use plastic stylet that can be used to increase the curvature of the tracheal tube and so facilitate tracheal intubation (Fig. 23.29).

Aintree intubating catheter

The Aintree Intubation Catheter (AIC) is a 56-cm hollow catheter designed to facilitate tracheal intubation via a SAD (Fig. 23.30). It is supplied with special (Rapi-Fit) adapters that connect to either a 15-mm connector for use with conventional anaesthetic circuits or a Luer-Lok for use with a high-pressure oxygen source (Fig. 23.31). Although the connectors enable oxygenation via the AIC, this is rarely necessary or effective and risks barotrauma if a high-pressure source is used. The catheter has a 4.8-mm ID, which enables it to be preloaded over a videoscope. A standard 7.0-mm ID tube (or a 6.5-mm ID ILMA tube) fits over the AIC.

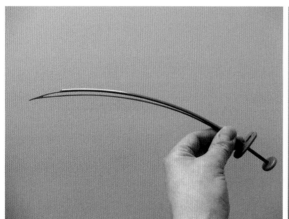

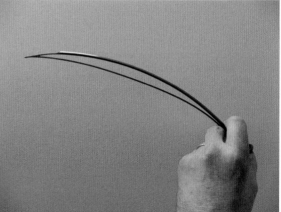

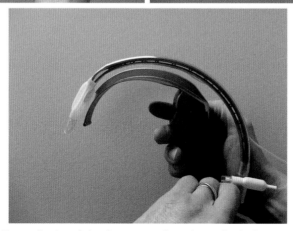

Fig. 23.29 Parker Flex-It stylet. The application of thumb pressure allows the tracheal tube curvature to be continuously varied during tracheal intubation enabling the tracheal tube to follow the curvature of the airway.

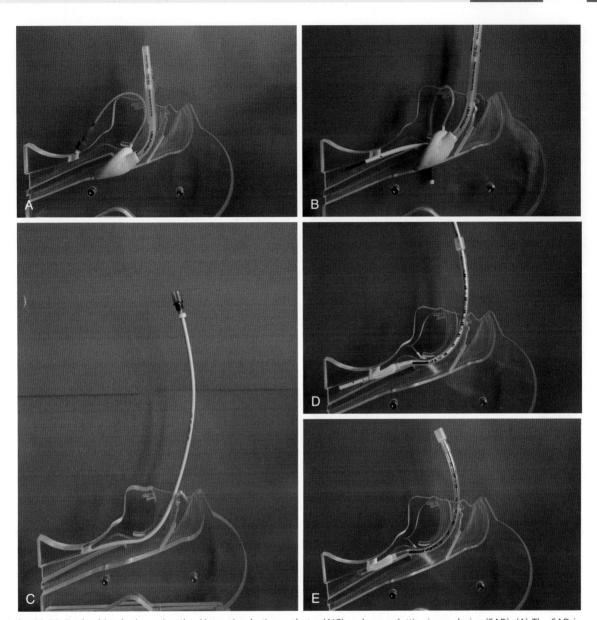

Fig. 23.30 Tracheal intubation using the Aintree intubation catheter (AIC) and supraglottic airway device (SAD). (A) The SAD is inserted; (B) the AIC is passed into the trachea through the SAD under fibrescope guidance; (C) the SAD and fibrescope are removed, leaving the AIC in place; (D) a tracheal tube is then railroaded over the AIC; (E) the AIC is then removed, leaving the tracheal tube in place.

Airway exchange catheters

Airway exchange catheters (AECs) are long (45–140 cm), narrow (external diameter 2.67–6.33 mm) catheters that are used to exchange one tracheal tube for another. The AEC is inserted through the tracheal tube, which is then removed and a new tracheal tube railroaded into place. Like

the AIC, AECs may be hollow and be provided with adaptors enabling administration of oxygen, including from a high-pressure source. Airway exchange catheters have been associated with barotrauma, which may be serious or even fatal, and this is best avoided by: (a) never inserting the tip of the AEC beyond the carina (approximately 25 cm); and (b) not using the AEC for oxygen administration, but only

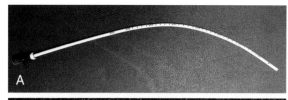

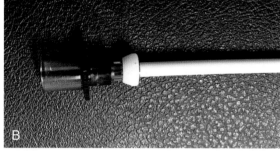

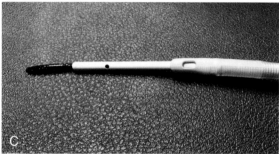

Fig. 23.31 Aintree intubating catheter (A) with 15-mm connector attached (B) magnified view of 15-mm connector and (C) with fibrescope within and with intubating laryngeal mask airway (ILMA) tracheal tube mounted.

for tracheal tube exchange. Some AECs have soft tips, but it is not known if this reduces complications.

Airway exchange catheters may also be used to facilitate high-risk tracheal extubation. In this setting either the AEC or a firm wire (over which the AEC can be railroaded) is left in the trachea after tracheal extubation until the airway is stable. The AEC should be fixed in place to avoid displacement or inward migration. Oxygen should be delivered by alternative routes.

Section 2

Routine airway management

Whether anaesthesia is induced by i.v. or gaseous induction, once consciousness is lost, the airway must be maintained.

Preoxygenation

At the core of safe anaesthesia and airway management is maintenance of oxygenation. After induction of anaesthesia, apnoea is common, and a degree of atelectasis (worsened by supine position, obesity, abdominal distension, etc.) means that hypoxia will occur rapidly if this is not prevented by administration of oxygen via a patent airway. The time until critical hypoxia occurs (the safe apnoea time) is dramatically prolonged by *preoxygenation* (administering oxygen to replace the nitrogen in the lungs with oxygen – also termed denitrogenation) and by *per-oxygenation* (administering oxygen after loss of consciousness).

Safe apnoea time can be prolonged by:
- sitting the patient upright;
- preoxygenation: administering 100% oxygen for 3–5 min via a closely fitting face-mask during tidal ventilation;
- per-oxygenation:
  - oxygen delivered by standard nasal cannulae at up to 15 L min^{-1};
  - oxygen delivered via a buccal or pharyngeal cannula or tube;
  - high-flow humidified nasal oxygen (HFNO) at 60–70 L min^{-1};
- mask ventilation after induction of anaesthesia; and
- CPAP.

Importantly, each of these techniques relies entirely on a patent airway to transmit oxygen from the upper airway to the alveoli.

Use of the face-mask

Face-mask ventilation is part of most anaesthetics but is now rarely used throughout surgery, having been replaced by the use of a SAD. In most settings the patient will be breathing spontaneously via a face-mask and anaesthetic circuit until the point of loss of consciousness; the airway must then be maintained and ventilation of the lungs assisted manually.

If the patient is breathing spontaneously, the anaesthetist need only maintain a clear airway. Soft tissue indrawing in the suprasternal and supraclavicular areas is evidence of upper airway obstruction, as is noisy ventilation or inspiratory stridor. Capnography should be used to confirm the airway is clear and ventilation adequate.

Face-mask ventilation is a core anaesthetic skill, but its difficulty should not be underestimated: honing the skill requires training and practice. The patient's head and neck should be maintained with the lower cervical spine flexed and the upper cervical spine extended (variously termed 'sniffing the morning air', 'first sip of beer' or 'flextension') (Fig. 23.32). Face-mask ventilation requires the combination of:
- establishing a seal between the mask and the face;
- maintaining a clear upper airway; and
- ventilation of the lungs.

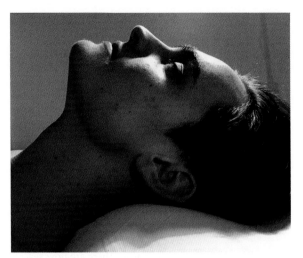

Fig. 23.32 Patient position for airway management: 'Sniffing the morning air' or 'flextension'.

Using a C-grip, the thumb and first finger are used to hold the mask, pushing downwards, while the remaining three fingers pull the chin and jaw (with fingers holding the bony elements of the mandible) and soft tissues up into the mask and also maintain head and neck positions. Manual ventilation is performed with the anaesthetist's other hand (Fig. 23.33). Where there is difficulty (novice anaesthetist, wrong face-mask size, obese or hirsute patient) it may be necessary to use two people (one maintaining position and face-mask seal and one manually ventilating) (Fig. 23.34) or three people (two maintaining the airway and seal and one manually ventilating) (Fig. 23.35). Patients for whom obtaining an adequate mask seal is often problematic include those who are edentulous bearded and/or require high ventilation pressures, such as the morbidly obese.

If there is airway obstruction, an oropharyngeal, nasopharyngeal airway or SAD may be of benefit. A nasopharyngeal airway is tolerated at the lightest plane of anaesthesia followed by an oropharyngeal airway and then a SAD. Insertion at an inadequate depth of anaesthesia can precipitate coughing, breath holding, retching, vomiting or laryngospasm.

Use of a SAD

A SAD is the mainstay of routine anaesthetic airway management and is used for airway maintenance in approximately 60% of general anaesthetics.

Indications
- To provide a clear airway without the need for the anaesthetist's hands to support a face-mask
- To maintain an airway when tracheal intubation is not required
- To rescue the airway after failed face-mask ventilation or tracheal intubation
- After airway rescue, to facilitate tracheal intubation using the SAD as a conduit

Contraindications
- A patient with a full stomach or with any condition leading to delayed gastric emptying
- A patient in whom the risk of regurgitation of gastric contents into the oesophagus is increased (e.g. hiatus hernia)
- Where surgical access (e.g. to the pharynx) is impeded by the cuff of the SAD

All these contraindications are relative and require clinical judgement in their interpretation. Suitable cases for SAD anaesthesia will depend on many factors, including the planned surgery, the experience and skills of the anaesthetist and surgeon and the device chosen. However, avoiding SAD use when aspiration risk is high is a fundamental principle of safe care.

Conduct of SAD insertion
Most evidence around SAD insertion comes from studies with the cLMA, with other devices much less well studied. An appropriate depth of anaesthesia is required for successful insertion. Agents that specifically improve insertions for SAD insertion include propofol (compared with other intravenous anaesthetic agents), a rapid-onset opioid such as fentanyl or alfentanil, lidocaine up to 1.5 mg kg^{-1} and nitrous oxide. Neuromuscular blockade is not necessary.

The appropriate size of SAD is chosen according to the weight or sex of the patient (see Table 23.1). In general, choosing a larger size is most effective (typically size 4 for a female patient and size 5 for a male patient). The lubricated mask is inserted fully deflated, with the patient's head and neck in the sniffing position (lower neck flexed and upper neck extended, flextension) (see Fig. 23.32). The tongue and epiglottis should be avoided during insertion by pushing the device (with a finger placed at the junction of the stem and mask) upwards and backwards. The tip passes along the hard palate, soft palate, and posterior pharyngeal wall and into the upper oesophagus, where the tip of the mask is stopped by the horizontal fibres of the cricopharyngeus muscle (the upper oesophageal sphincter). The cuff is then inflated to a pressure that does not exceed 60 cmH$_2$O, measured with a manometer. The device is very effective in maintaining a patent airway in spontaneously breathing patients and in many patients during positive pressure ventilation. The cLMA is not suitable for patients who are at risk of regurgitation of gastric contents. The airway seal of the cLMA rarely exceeds 20 cmH$_2$O, so positive pressure ventilation in patients who need higher airway pressures (obese patients,

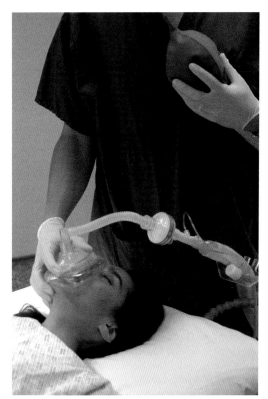

Fig. 23.33 Face-mask ventilation. Note the C-grip of the fingers over the mask and the three fingers supporting the airway.

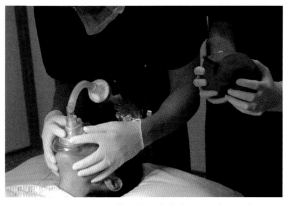

Fig. 23.34 Two-person (four-handed) face-mask ventilation.

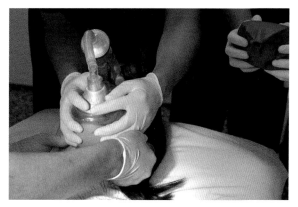

Fig. 23.35 Three-person (six-handed) face-mask ventilation.

poorly compliant lungs, certain patient positions) is likely to lead to leakage of gas from the airway. A poorly positioned airway also leads to gas leak during controlled ventilation and reduces safety. Leaking gases increasingly enter the stomach as airway pressure rises and increase the risk of gastric distension and regurgitation. There are now several SADs that are better suited to use if controlled ventilation is required.

After placement, adequacy of seal and ventilation must be checked by gentle manual ventilation of the lungs. The breathing system is attached via a catheter mount to the 22-mm proximal connector. The SAD is secured in place with tape or a tie. Anaesthesia may continue with either spontaneous or controlled ventilation according to patient needs and status.

Tracheal intubation

Tracheal intubation is used in approximately 40% of general anaesthetics, including the majority of higher-risk cases and emergencies.

Indications (many are relative)
- Protection of the airway when there is a risk of aspiration of gastric contents (e.g. most emergency surgery)
- Thoracic or abdominal procedures
- Airway maintenance in unusual or prolonged positions (e.g. prone or sitting)
- Operations on the head and neck (e.g. ENT, dental surgery)
- Protection of the respiratory tract (e.g. from blood during upper respiratory tract or oral surgery)
- To facilitate suction of the respiratory tract

Contraindications
There are few contraindications.

Preparation
Before starting, the anaesthetist must check the availability and function of the necessary equipment. The anaesthetist should have a dedicated, trained, experienced assistant. Laryngoscopes of the correct size are chosen, and their

function checked. The patency of the tracheal tube should be checked and the integrity of the cuff ensured.

Anaesthesia for tracheal intubation

In most circumstances tracheal intubation is facilitated by general anaesthesia with neuromuscular blockade, as this produces optimal conditions.

Alternatives include the following:
- Awake placement of a tracheal tube after topical or regional anaesthesia
  - Guided by a flexible videoscope
  - Guided by videolaryngoscopy
- General anaesthesia without neuromuscular blockade
  - Deep inhalational or i.v. anaesthesia
  - Supplementation with high-dose opioids (especially remifentanil)

Laryngoscopy

- The patient is placed in position with the lower cervical spine flexed and the upper cervical spine flexed – this best aligns the axes of mouth, pharynx and trachea (see Figs 23.9 & 23.32).
- The laryngoscope is held in the left hand and inserted into the right side of mouth with the lips parted and jaw open. Care is needed throughout to avoid contact with the upper incisor teeth.
- The blade is passed along the right side of the tongue, gently controlling and moving the tissues to the left. As the blade advances, it is returned to the midline and into the vallecula (the point where the base of the tongue meets the base of the epiglottis) (see Fig. 23.8).
- The tip of the blade is pulled upwards (along the axis of the handle), and the tip of the blade is pushed into the vallecula, which stretches the hyoepiglottic ligament to make the epiglottis hinge forwards.
- As the laryngoscope is pulled upwards, the aim is to create a direct line of sight from upper incisors to the larynx. There is a danger of using the incisor teeth as a fulcrum to lever the tip of the blade upwards, and this must not be done.
- In about 90% of cases a good view of the larynx is achieved, and the tracheal tube can be inserted directly.
- The supraglottic area and cords can be sprayed with local anaesthetic (lidocaine 4%) to reduce the stress response to tracheal intubation and to improve tracheal tube tolerance.
- The tracheal tube is passed from the right side of the mouth and between the vocal cords into the trachea until the cuff is below the vocal cords.
- If there is a partial view of the cords this may be improved by an assistant larynx pressing on the anterior neck to reverse the forces applied by the intubator (*b*ackwards *u*pwards *r*ightwards *p*ressure – BURP) or the intubator

manipulating the larynx with their right hand (*o*ptimal *ex*ternal *l*aryngeal *p*ressure – OELM).
- In approximately 6% of patients a poor view of the larynx is obtained, and additional tools or techniques are needed (see later).
- The tube is inserted so the cuff lies 1–2 cm below the vocal cords and the distance at the teeth or lips recored (usually 18–23 cm).
- The tube is then connected to the anaesthetic circuit with a catheter mount and HMEF between tracheal tube and circuit.
- The tracheal tube cuff is inflated until there is no gas leak during gentle ventilation of the patient's lungs.
- Correct insertion and ventilation of the lungs is confirmed by waveform capnography (see Chapter 17).
- Clinical signs (inspection to see both sides of the chest rising equally and auscultation in each axilla for equal breath sounds) assist in confirming the tracheal tube tip is above the carina and both lungs are ventilated.
- If there is unilateral air entry, the tracheal tube should be withdrawn slowly and carefully until air entry is equal in both lungs. If there is uncertainty over correct intubation, oesophageal placement should be assumed and actively excluded. If doubt remains, remove the tracheal tube and reintubate or secure the airway by other means.
- Where there is minor difficulty in passing the tracheal tube (which may occur despite a good view of the cords) tracheal intubation may be facilitated by use of a bougie or stylet.
- Once placed, the tracheal tube should be tied or taped securely. The choice and technique of tracheal tube fixation varies according to the clinical setting, but the anaesthetist should ensure it is adequately secured for the duration of surgery.

Nasal intubation

Nasal intubation may be used for some dental, otorhinolaryngology, maxillofacial, plastics and neurosurgical operations, though the fLMA has replaced many indications for minor surgery. To avoid trauma, a small tracheal tube is used (e.g. 6.0–6.5 mm ID), and a soft plastic or silicone tube is preferred. Either nostril may be used, though the left-facing bevel of the tube means the right may be preferable. The tracheal tube is passed posteriorly along the floor of the nose and advanced gently into the pharynx, avoiding excessive force. Once the tube passes into the pharynx, laryngoscopy facilitates tracheal intubation either by manipulation of the proximal end of the tube or by grasping the distal tip with Magill's intubating forceps to pass it between the cords.

When surgery may lead to blood, pus or debris soiling the pharynx, a throat pack can be placed to manage this. The pack can be made with moist gauze or preformed foam packs may be used. Failure to remove a pharyngeal pack is a serious cause of morbidity, and it is mandatory that the presence of a pack is clearly documented and that it is removed at the end of surgery (see Chapter 18). The responsibility for removing the pack lies with the person who inserted it.

Difficult tracheal intubation

The incidence of difficult tracheal intubation varies widely with clinical setting, patient groups and intubator skill. However, a poor view of the larynx (requiring use of a bougie or another adjunct) occurs in approximately 6% of tracheal intubation attempts. Poor technique of laryngoscopy is the most common cause. Difficulty with tracheal intubation is a significant cause of anaesthetic morbidity and mortality (see Chapter 26). Sequelae range from the minor (dental trauma, mucosal injury, minor hypoxaemia) to severe (major airway trauma, severe hypoxaemia, aspiration, death).

Aetiology

Box 23.1 shows the common causes of difficult tracheal intubation. The single most important cause is an inexperienced or inadequately prepared anaesthetist.

During traditional laryngoscopy the anaesthetist must achieve a direct line of sight from the upper incisors to the laryngeal inlet (see Fig. 23.9). This requires:
- flexion of the lower cervical spine;
- extension of the upper cervical spine;
- mouth opening; and
- displacement of the soft tissues behind the mandible and in the upper anterior neck.

The cause of difficult laryngoscopy is much easier to understand armed with these concepts. Any anatomical variation that impedes these movements will likely make laryngoscopy more difficult:
- Reduced lower cervical flexion (e.g. ankylosing spondylosis)
- Reduced upper cervical extension (e.g. atlanto-occipital disease or arthritis)
- Reduced mouth opening (e.g. mandibular abscess, temporomandibular joint disease)
- Increased volume of soft tissues (e.g. obesity, acromegaly, Down's syndrome)
- Decreased deformability of tissues (e.g. base of tongue tumours, dental abscesses, previous radiotherapy or burns)
- Reduced mandibular space (e.g. Treacher Collins and similar syndromes)

Conditions that alter the appearance (e.g. tumour), position (e.g. goitre) or structure (e.g. papillomata, strictures) of the larynx also impede both laryngoscopy and tracheal intubation.

In clinical practice the cause of difficult laryngoscopy is often multifactorial (e.g. a patient with morbid obesity,

pregnancy and rheumatoid arthritis). Tracheal intubation is made particularly difficult when there is also time pressure, when preoxygenation has either been omitted or is not feasible.

Obesity merits its own mention: it is likely to be the most common cause of airway difficulty. Laryngoscopy is not notably more difficult, but compared with the non-obese, preoxygenation is less effective, face-mask ventilation is often more difficult, desaturation is notably more rapid, re-oxygenation may be slower and all rescue techniques are more likely to fail (see Chapter 32).

Airway assessment

Traditionally airway assessment has focussed on identifying patients in whom direct laryngoscopy and tracheal intubation will be difficult. As modern airway management is more varied, it is important to consider all aspects of airway care, including difficult face-mask ventilation, SAD placement and other rescue techniques. It is logical to first assess ease of the intended airway maintenance technique and focus on planned backup techniques if there are concerns.

Airway assessment should be focussed around patient oxygenation, and a patient with a relatively easy airway but at high risk of hypoxia (e.g. obesity, sepsis, pregnancy) after induction of anaesthesia may be a far greater challenge than a patient with a moderately difficult airway but no problems with oxygenation.

Important aspects of airway assessment include the following:
1. ease of face-mask ventilation;
2. ease of laryngoscopy and tracheal intubation;
3. ease of SAD insertion;
4. overall ease of oxygenation;
5. where there are any concerns about 1-4, assess for ease of front of neck airway (FONA);
6. assess risk of regurgitation and aspiration.

Patients who have indicators of increased risk need careful planning. They should be discussed with senior staff, and alternative techniques should be considered (e.g. regional anaesthesia, establishing the airway while the patient is awake). General anaesthesia should only be undertaken with clear plans for management of the airway if the primary technique fails.

Problems occur quite commonly:
- Difficult face-mask ventilation: use approximate symbol (wavy equals sign) 1 in 20 cases
- Impossible face-mask ventilation: use approximate symbol (wavy equals sign) 1 in 1500 cases
- Difficult laryngoscopy (unable to view larynx): up to 5%
- Impossible tracheal intubation: 1 in 2000 electively, but as many as 1 in 200 emergencies
- Failed rescue techniques: use approximate symbol (wavy equals sign) 1 in 10–20 cases

Box 23.1 **Common causes of difficult tracheal intubation**

Anaesthetist

Inadequate preoperative assessment
Inadequate equipment preparation
Inexperience
Poor technique

Equipment

Wrong choice
Malfunction
Unavailability
No trained assistant

Patient

Congenital		Syndromes such as Down's, Pierre Robin, Treacher Collins, Marfan's, Klippel–Feil
		Mucopolysaccharidoses
		Achondroplasia
		Cystic hygroma
		Encephalocoele
Acquired	Reduced neck movement	Rheumatoid/osteoarthritis
		Ankylosing spondylitis
		Cervical fracture/instability/fusion
	Reduced jaw movement	Trismus (abscess/infection, fracture, tetanus)
		Fibrosis (post-infection/radiotherapy/trauma)
		Rheumatoid arthritis, ankylosing spondylitis
		Tumours
		Jaw wiring
	Airway	Oedema (abscess/infection, trauma, angio-oedema, burns)
		Compression (goitre, surgical haemorrhage)
		Scarring (radiotherapy, infection, burns)
		Tumours/polyps
		Foreign body
		Nerve palsy
		Morbid obesity
		Acromegaly
	Others	Pregnancy
		Rapid sequence induction

Importantly, failures cluster together; a patient whose trachea is difficult to intubate is considerably more likely to fail mask ventilation and SAD placement.

Simple bedside tests are used routinely to detect signs of airway difficulty. Complex tests are rarely required. The tests used are imperfect, with a low specificity and positive predictive value. As a result, there are a large number of false positives, and only approximately 1 in 20–30 patients identified as high risk proves to be so. False negatives are also a problem as approximately 6% of patients with no features to predict airway difficulty present with difficult tracheal intubation. Sensitivity is also low, so the tests miss many difficult patients; more than 90% of cases of difficult laryngoscopy and more than 90% of cases of combined difficult face-mask ventilation and laryngoscopy are not predicted by bedside tests. Despite these stark statistics it is beholden on all anaesthetists to assess all patients to identify where risk factors are identifiable. Combining multiple tests increases the specificity (i.e. reduces false positives) but decreases sensitivity (i.e. leads to missing even more truly difficult cases).

Defining difficulty

- *Difficult face-mask ventilation* occurs when mask ventilation cannot be maintained by a single operator with simple adjuncts.
- *Difficult SAD insertion* occurs when either the SAD cannot be inserted without multiple attempts or, after insertion, effective ventilation of the lungs is not possible.
- *Difficult laryngoscopy* is variously defined but in practice occurs when the laryngeal inlet cannot be seen.
  - Cormack and Lehane described a grading of laryngeal view (Fig. 23.36), which correlates only moderately with measures of difficulty with tracheal intubation.
  - The Cook classification (Fig. 23.37) of laryngeal view appears to expand the scale but can be functionally divided into 'easy', 'restricted' and 'difficult': Difficulty

with tracheal intubation is likely if the glottis cannot be seen and insertion of a bougie is not possible (i.e. grades 3b and 4).

- *Difficult tracheal intubation* may be caused by difficult laryngoscopy or difficulty passing the tracheal tube despite a good view of the larynx, requiring multiple attempts, multiple operators or adjuncts.
- *Difficult oxygenation* occurs when hypoxia (SpO_2 <92%) occurs despite routine preoxygenation and efforts at airway maintenance after induction.

History

Many conditions described above and listed in Box 23.1 may be identified. The history should include full exploration of the surgical condition as this may affect airway management (e.g. quinsy, temporomandibular joint arthroscopy, cervical surgery, facial burns, laryngeal surgery). Risk factors for reduced functional respiratory reserve and cervical spine instability should also be identified.

The most important aspect of the airway history is identifying problems during previous anaesthetics (e.g. a history of difficulty, dental damage or severe sore throat). A previous problem with airway management is arguably the

single strongest predictor of future difficulty. Many conditions worsen with age. Anaesthetic records should be consulted whenever possible, and the patient may carry an airway alert.

A history of obstructive sleep apnoea (OSA) is very important to identify (see Chapter 19). In most patients with OSA this is undiagnosed preoperatively, and it is commonly missed. Obstructive sleep apnoea increases difficulty with many aspects of airway management but especially increases risk of airway obstruction and rapid hypoxia.

Examination

- The patient's facies, airway and respiration should all be examined.
- Poor dentition is important to identify and document (including warning the patient) as loose or rotten teeth may impede airway management and may be displaced during airway management.
- Facial hair interferes with face-mask ventilation, and a beard may mask adverse anatomical features.
- Anatomical features associated with difficulty are shown in Box 23.2. Difficulty can also arise from obesity and large breasts.
- Examination should identify and assess the impact of abscesses, tumours, radiotherapy burns or other scars.
- Mobility of the cervical spine and temporomandibular joint and mouth opening should all be assessed.
- If there is a plan for nasal tracheal intubation, it is important to confirm patency of the nasal passages.
- If difficulty is anticipated with any aspect of airway management or oxygenation, the location and ease of access to the cricothyroid membrane should be identified.

Preoperative airway assessment is summarised in Box 23.3 and described in detail later.

Predictors of difficult face-mask ventilation

Difficult face-mask ventilation is predicted by:
- BMI > 26 kg m^{-2};
- history of snoring;
- age > 55 years;

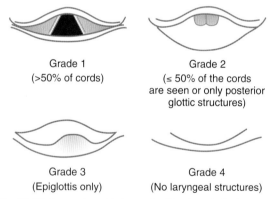

Grade 1 (>50% of cords)

Grade 2 (≤ 50% of the cords are seen or only posterior glottic structures)

Grade 3 (Epiglottis only)

Grade 4 (No laryngeal structures)

Fig. 23.36 Cormack and Lehane classification of glottic visualisation at direct laryngoscopy.

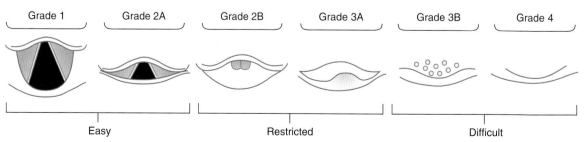

Grade 1 Grade 2A Grade 2B Grade 3A Grade 3B Grade 4

Easy Restricted Difficult

Fig. 23.37 Cook's modified classification of laryngeal view. *1-4* refer to Cormack and Lehane classification. 'Easy' views require no adjuncts, 'restricted' views need a bougie, and 'difficult' views require advanced techniques. In grade 3a the epiglottis can be lifted from the pharyngeal wall, whereas in grade 3b it cannot.

- presence of a beard; and
- absence of teeth.

Multiple features increase likelihood of difficulty (≥ 2 has a 70% sensitivity and specificity). Patients with facial abnormalities preventing a face-mask seal, an underslung jaw or OSA also present significant difficulty.

Predictors of difficult SAD insertion or failure

Predictors of difficult SAD are poorly defined and have only been defined for the Unique LMA. Predictors include:

- male sex;
- raised BMI;
- poor dentition; and
- rotation of the operating table after induction of anaesthesia.

Limited mouth opening also interferes with SAD placement (difficult if < 2.5 cm, impossible if < 2.0 cm) as do any intraoral or pharyngeal masses (e.g. swollen tongue, lingual tonsil).

Specific tests to predict risk of difficult laryngoscopy

Most risk prediction tests identify a likely problem with gaining a direct line of sight from upper teeth to larynx. It

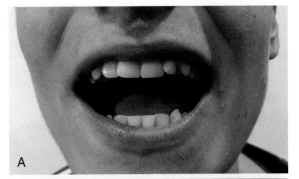
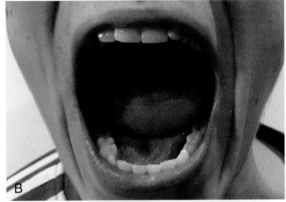
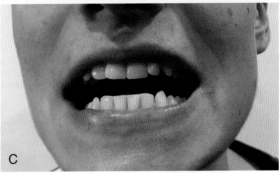

Fig. 23.38 Interincisor gap assessment: (A) normal; (B) large; (C) markedly reduced.

is normal to assess, as a minimum, mouth opening and upper cervical spine movement. Where features indicate an increased risk of difficulty with the chosen airway technique, further assessment should be undertaken.

Mouth opening – interincisor gap

Measure the distance between the incisors (or alveolar margins) with the mouth fully open (Fig. 23.38). This distance is affected by upper cervical spine and temporomandibular joint mobility. A gap < 3 cm increases likelihood of difficult tracheal intubation.

Mallampati test

Mallampati described three classes, and Samsoon and Young added a fourth. The patient should be asked to open the mouth as wide as possible and protrude the tongue as far as possible; the view of the posterior pharyngeal wall should then be examined (Fig. 23.39). This should be done with the anaesthetist opposite the patient but can be done standing, sitting or lying.

- Class 1: faucial pillars (palatoglossal and palatopharyngeal folds), soft palate and uvula visible.
- Class 2: faucial pillars and soft palate visible; uvula masked by base of tongue.
- Class 3: only soft palate visible.
- Class 4: soft palate not visible.

Class 3–4 views (i.e. when the posterior pharyngeal wall cannot be seen) are associated with increased risk of difficult laryngoscopy and face-mask ventilation. A positive test has a positive predicted value of only 3%–5% and sensitivity of 50%.

Flexion/extension of the upper cervical spine

The range of movement of the upper cervical spine normally exceeds 90 degrees and, when reduced, the risk of difficult laryngoscopy is increased (Fig. 23.40). The patient's lower cervical spine should be immobilised manually, then the patient asked to fully flex and then extend the head, with a pen placed on the vertex to observe the arc of movement.

Alternatively the patient can be asked to sit straight. One finger should then be placed on the patient's occipital prominence and another on the patient's chin. The patient should then fully extend the neck.

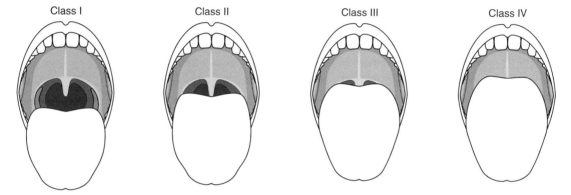

Fig. 23.39 Classification of the pharyngeal view when performing the Mallampati test. The patient must fully extend the tongue during maximal mouth opening. Class I: pharyngeal pillars, soft palate, uvula visible. Class II: only soft palate, uvula visible. Class III: only soft palate visible. Class IV: soft palate not visible. Note that the posterior pharyngeal wall is visible in class 1 and 2 but is not visible in class 3 and 4.

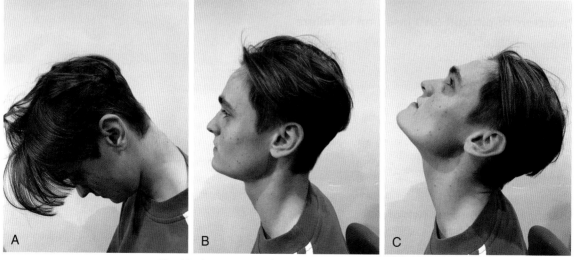

Fig. 23.40 Assessment of upper cervical spine extension.

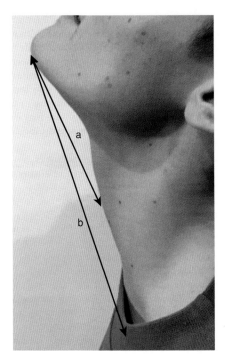

Fig. 23.41 Assessment of (A) thyromental and (B) sternomental distances.

- Class 1 (normal): the chin rises above the occiput.
- Class 2 (moderate limitation): both fingers are at the same level.
- Class 3 (severe limitation): the chin remains lower than the occiput.

Thyromental distance (Patil test)

With the patient's head and neck fully extended and the mouth closed, a measurement should be taken from the tip of the thyroid cartilage to the mentum (tip of the mandible) (Fig. 23.41A).

- > 7.0 cm is normal.
- < 6.0 cm has a 75% sensitivity for detecting difficult laryngoscopy.
- < 5.5 cm means a difficult laryngoscopy is very likely.

Sternomental distance (Savva test)

The Savva test is conducted as earlier but measurement is taken from the upper border of the manubrium to the tip of the mandible (Fig. 23.41B). A distance < 12.5 cm predicts difficult laryngoscopy.

Protrusion of the mandible (prognathism)

To identify prognathism, the patient should be asked to move the lower jaw in front of the upper jaw.

- Class A (normal): the lower incisors lie anterior to the upper incisors.

- Class B (abnormal): lower incisors reach the upper incisors.
- Class C (very abnormal): lower incisors do not reach the upper incisors.

Combined tests

Combining tests increases the positive predictive value and specificity at the cost of sensitivity.

Combining thyromental distance and Mallampati tests (< 7 cm and class 3–4) increases specificity (97%) but reduces sensitivity (81%).

The Wilson score combines five factors (weight, upper cervical spine mobility, jaw protrusion, buck teeth, receding mandible) each rated 0–2 (normal to abnormal). A score > 3 identifies 75% of patients with difficult laryngoscopy.

Advanced testing

Where increased risk is identified, further tests may be indicated. These include:

- ultrasound of the airway to identify the cricothyroid membrane and measure the depth of the tongue base.
- nasendoscopy to directly image the airway with the patient awake; this is an underused technique.
- CT/MRI scanning. This has particular value in cases of airway obstruction. It is important to note that the patient lies flat during the scan (this affects gravitational effects) and in severe obstruction may be unsafe. With modern technology it is possible to create a three-dimensional (3D) image of the patient's airway, and this can even be 3D printed to enable airway planning of the most complex cases. Although plain radiographs or CT scanning may be of value with acute cervical pathological conditions (e.g. trauma to identify fractures), this imaging has less value in some chronic conditions such as rheumatoid arthritis where anatomical abnormality correlates poorly with mobility and stability.

Predicting difficulty with FONA

Features include:

- obesity;
- goitre or other anterior neck mass;
- deviated trachea;
- fixed neck flexion;
- previous radiotherapy; and
- surgical collar or external fixator (remove!).

Predicting difficulty securing the airway awake

The most important predictor of difficulty with awake techniques is lack of patient co-operation. Secretions and bleeding make flexible fibrescopic techniques difficult. Airway obstruction makes an awake technique increasingly difficult and requires a skilled and experienced operator for safe management.

Assessing risk of regurgitation and aspiration

Assessing the risk of regurgitation and aspiration is an essential part of preoperative history taking (see Chapter 19). The degree of risk determines to a great degree what technique can be safely chosen.

Conduct of anaesthesia

Conduction of anaesthesia is discussed in detail in Chapter 22. Issues specific to the airway include the following.

Preparation

Premedication is rarely indicated specifically for airway management reasons, though an antisialagogue (e.g. Glycopyrronium bromide 0.2 mg) reduces airway secretions and may be of value before awake techniques. Sedative premedication is contraindicated in patients with significant airway obstruction. A trained, briefed assistant is essential, and the availability of an experienced anaesthetist and a special difficult airway trolley is necessary.

General anaesthesia

Unless tracheal intubation is essential for airway protection or surgical access, a SAD-based technique is a safe option. Spontaneous or controlled ventilation may be indicated and, importantly, controlled ventilation does not require neuromuscular blockade provided an appropriate SAD is well placed and depth of anaesthesia adequate. If tracheal intubation is indicated, the appropriate anaesthetic technique depends on the anticipated degree of difficulty, presence of airway obstruction and risk of regurgitation and aspiration.

Preoxygenation should be performed routinely before general anaesthesia. The technique used for preoxygenation will depend on the setting, but a technique suitable for almost all circumstances is:

- a minimum of 3 min of tidal ventilation (or until the end-tidal oxygen is > 85%);
- via the anaesthetic circuit;
- FiO_2 1.0; and
- via a patent airway.

Delivering oxygen throughout attempts at establishing an airway is a neglected technique. It is rational to do this for all patients who are at risk of hypoxia or in whom difficult airway management may occur. Techniques include:

- nasal oxygen (5–15 L min^{-1}) via nasal cannulae;
- buccal oxygen delivered via a Ring-Adair-Elwyn (RAE) tracheal tube hooked around the angle of the mouth;

- high-flow humidified nasal oxygen (50–70 L min^{-1}) delivered via specifically designed nasal cannulae. This technique provides a degree of PEEP and carbon dioxide clearance and, when used in the apnoeic patient, has been termed THRIVE (transnasal humidified rapid-insufflation ventilatory exchange). The technique prolongs safe apnoea time in most patients but may not be as effective in the obese and critically ill. The bulky nasal cannulae may need to be removed to re-establish an airway seal during face-mask ventilation.

Before attempting any airway manoeuvres:

1. care should be taken to position the airway correctly (flextension);
2. depth of anaesthesia should be adequate for the technique; and
3. if a neuromuscular blocking agent (NMBA) is used, this should be given time to work fully.

The safest anaesthetic technique may usually be chosen from the following clinical examples:

1. *Patients with little anticipated difficulty and no airway obstruction.* General anaesthesia, with choice of airway and neuromuscular blockade according to anaesthetic and surgical indications. If difficulty is encountered, the patient is woken up and the procedure replanned.
2. *Patients with an increased risk of regurgitation and aspiration (e.g. full stomach, intra-abdominal pathological condition, pregnancy).* Regional anaesthesia may be preferable. An RSI (see later) is appropriate. If there is also a high degree of anticipated difficulty, an awake technique is recommended (see later).
3. *Patients with significant risk of difficulty and no airway obstruction.* The choice of technique is controversial and the best technique unproven. A senior anaesthetist is required. Optimal techniques include regional anaesthesia to avoid general anaesthesia or securing the airway awake. If general anaesthesia is chosen, this may be i.v. or gaseous induction.
4. *Patients with airway obstruction (e.g. burns, infection, trauma).* These patients usually require general anaesthesia to secure and maintain the airway. Securing the airway awake is often preferable but in severe cases may be impractical. Advanced techniques are often needed.
5. *Extreme clinical situations of severe difficulty and airway obstruction.* Tracheostomy performed under local anaesthesia may be the safest technique, but this also is fraught with difficulty.

When there is an intention to provide neuromuscular blockade (whether for tracheal intubation or surgical reasons), traditional teaching is that this should not be done until the ability to perform face-mask ventilation has been confirmed. There is now clear evidence that, in the vast majority of patients, neuromuscular blockade either improves the ease of face-mask ventilation or has no impact. The one caveat is that this has not been confirmed in patients with pre-existing airway pathological conditions or airway obstruction (see difficult airway management section).

Awake tracheal intubation and induction of anaesthesia while maintaining spontaneous ventilation

Awake tracheal intubation and induction while maintaining spontaneous ventilation are discussed in the difficult airway management section.

Complications of airway management

Complications may be mechanical, respiratory or cardiovascular and may occur early or late. Complications are notably more common with tracheal intubation but may also occur with SADs and face-mask ventilation. Multiple instrumentation of the airway increases the risk of complications. This is discussed further in Chapter 26.

Airway removal at the end of surgery

Before removing any airway, the patient should have recovered full ventilatory capacity. This should be actively assessed by observation of the patient's respiratory pattern and rate, augmented by examination of capnography and spirometry. Where an NMBA has been used, neuromuscular monitoring should be used routinely to assess any residual paralysis and to confirm full reversal before airway removal (see Chapter 8).

Supraglottic airway device removal

A SAD should usually be left in place until the patient has recovered full ventilatory capacity and regained consciousness. At the point of return of consciousness, airway reflexes are also recovering and patients will normally protect their own airway. It is not necessary for patients to be turned on their side, and lying semirecumbent is optimal.

The SAD should not be removed simply when spontaneous respiration resumes or when the patient starts swallowing. A better measure of return of consciousness is response to voice, making spontaneous movements towards the SAD or following commands. Suction should be used to clear the oropharynx of secretions, the patient should be asked to open the mouth and the SAD should be removed. The need to deflate the device cuff varies with SAD, but for LMAs, retaining some air in the cuff and deflating as the device is removed will assist in clearing secretions. After removing the SAD, oxygen should be administered by mask or nasal cannulae and respiration should be monitored.

If a SAD is removed while the patient is unconscious, airway obstruction is a significant risk. Coughing and laryngospasm may occur during SAD removal but are much less common than during removal of a tracheal tube. Because SADs are well tolerated during light anaesthesia and complications of removal are infrequent, it is reasonable to delegate SAD removal to an appropriately trained nurse in an appropriately monitored recovery environment, though expert anaesthetic assistance must remain immediately available (see Chapter 29).

Tracheal tube removal (extubation)

Tracheal extubation can be done with the patient supine or sitting up, provided the airway is kept patent and there is no risk of regurgitation. In patients at risk of regurgitation and potential aspiration, the lateral position is preferred unless the patient is fully awake. The tracheal tube may be removed with the patient unconscious (deep tracheal extubation) or awake. Deep tracheal extubation is a higher-risk procedure and should be reserved for very low-risk patients; airway obstruction, breath holding, respiratory inadequacy and laryngospasm may all occur. Awake tracheal extubation is generally preferred unless the stimulus will have a negative impact on the patient's physiology. When awake tracheal extubation is planned, it is prudent to inform patients preoperatively that they may be aware of the presence and then removal of the tracheal tube on awakening. To avoid complications of tracheal extubation, or to facilitate safe deep tracheal extubation, the tracheal tube may be exchanged for a SAD (placed behind the tracheal tube before removing the tracheal tube – Bailey's manoeuvre) or an AEC may be placed in the trachea (via the tracheal tube) before it is removed; these are advanced techniques.

Routine tracheal extubation can be conducted as follows:
- Before lightening anaesthesia, clear secretions from the mouth and pharynx (with a Yankeur sucker, ideally under direct vision, avoiding trauma to the pharyngeal mucosa, uvula or epiglottis) and, if indicated, from the trachea (using a soft sterile suction catheter with an external diameter less than half the tracheal tube ID).
- Administer 100% oxygen to create an oxygen reservoir in the lungs in case airway problems occur after tracheal extubation.
- Insert an oropharyngeal airway.
- When ready for tracheal extubation, deflate the tracheal tube cuff fully and remove the tracheal tube during patient inspiration. Positive pressure may be applied by squeezing the bag as the cuff is removed.
- After tracheal extubation, administer 100% oxygen by mask.

- Assess the patient's ability to maintain and protect the airway and ensure ventilatory sufficiency.
- Remove monitoring only after tracheal extubation is complete and the airway is stable.

Because complications and difficulty at the time of tracheal extubation are common, it is normal for this to take place in the operating theatre, under the direct supervision of the anaesthetist.

Complications of tracheal extubation

Laryngeal spasm (laryngospasm), bronchospasm or coughing

Laryngospasm, bronchospasm and coughing are all more likely in those with an irritable airway (smokers, patients with asthma, patients with current or recent respiratory tract infection), children and when tracheal extubation occurs in the stage between deep anaesthesia and full wakefulness. Clearance of secretions before tracheal extubation reduces the risk.

Airway obstruction

Airway obstruction is more likely when the airway is removed before return of consciousness.

Regurgitation/aspiration

Aspiration and regurgitation are increased in all patients at high risk and by airway removal in the light plane of anaesthesia before full wakefulness. If a nasogastric tube is present, this should be suctioned before airway removal.

All these complications are more common during tracheal extubation than when removing a SAD. The management of these complications are discussed in Chapter 27.

Airway management during emergency anaesthesia

The conduct of anaesthesia in the emergency setting is discussed in Chapter 44. Two important issues relating to airway management and emergency surgery are: (1) risk of regurgitation; and (2) RSI.

Airway assessment should be performed as normal where this is feasible. During emergency anaesthesia there is an increased risk of regurgitation, and there should be a lower threshold for tracheal intubation, including use of RSI. Rapid sequence induction is associated with an increased likelihood of airway difficulty (approximately 10-fold higher than in elective surgery). Increased difficulty may arise from the patient's usual anatomy, surgical pathological condition, limited time available to secure the airway when RSI is used and risk of poorly applied cricoid force making laryngoscopy

difficult. If preoperative assessment indicates a high risk of difficulty in tracheal intubation, an awake technique may be necessary.

All patients should be assessed for risk of regurgitation (and therefore risk of aspiration) before anaesthesia, but this is particularly important before emergency anaesthesia.

A SAD may be appropriate for airway maintenance during emergency surgery, but only when the risk of aspiration is judged to be very low. In this setting it is logical to select a second-generation device. More commonly, a tracheal tube is selected, and where there is any significant risk of aspiration and general anaesthesia is planned, RSI should be routine practice.

Anaesthesia for the patient at increased risk of regurgitation/aspiration

The anaesthetic management of a patient at increased risk of aspiration may be described in five phases: preparation; induction; maintenance; emergence; and postoperative management.

Preparation

The risk of aspiration must be weighed against the risk of delaying an urgent procedure; however, in the setting of an acute surgical condition, such delay will often not decrease this risk. Three manoeuvres may reduce risk:

- A nasogastric tube may be inserted to decompress the stomach and to provide a low-pressure vent for regurgitated fluid. Aspiration through the nasogastric tube may be useful if gastric contents are liquid (as in bowel obstruction) but is less effective when contents are solid. Cricoid force is still effective with a nasogastric tube in place.
- Liquid oral antacids (e.g. 30 ml sodium citrate 0.3 M) may be used to raise the pH of gastric contents immediately before induction. Particulate antacids should not be used, as they may be very damaging to the airway if aspirated.
- H_2-receptor antagonists raise gastric pH and may reduce the chance of chemical pulmonary injury occurring in the event of aspiration. These need to be given at least 2 h before anaesthesia. Proton pump inhibitors have the same effect but need to be used at least 12 h before anaesthesia and so have little role in the emergency setting. Although this is standard practice in obstetric anaesthesia, few anaesthetists employ these measures for emergency general surgery.

Increasingly, preoperative gastric ultrasound is being proposed as a method for determining whether the stomach is empty. It is not yet standard practice but has acceptable sensitivity and specificity for determining whether there is a clinically significant volume within the antrum of the stomach.

Induction

Rapid sequence induction is the technique used most often for the patient with a full stomach. The aim of RSI is to minimise the time between loss of consciousness and tracheal intubation, during which the patient is at greatest risk of aspiration of gastric contents. At its most basic RSI involves:

- preoxygenation;
- administration of a predefined dose of i.v. hypnotic agent;
- administration of an intubating dose of rapid-onset NMBA immediately after the induction dose;
- application of cricoid force as consciousness is lost and until the airway is secured; and
- laryngoscopy and tracheal intubation.

Much of the technique of RSI is controversial and open to academic debate. The decision to employ the RSI technique balances the risk of losing control of the airway against the risk of aspiration. A careful airway assessment is, therefore, mandatory. If difficult laryngoscopy or tracheal intubation is anticipated, performing surgery under local anaesthesia or securing the airway with an awake technique should be actively explored. In all cases, consider the airway strategy that will be employed where tracheal intubation proves difficult or fails. For RSI to be consistently safe and successful it should be performed with meticulous attention to detail and careful preparation is necessary.

Preparation

- The patient should be informed of the planned technique, and particularly about cricoid force and awake tracheal extubation.
- The patient *must* be on a tipping trolley or table, preferably with an adjustable headpiece so that the degree of neck extension/flexion may be altered quickly.
- To reduce the risk of difficult airway management, the patient's head should be positioned with the neck flexed on the shoulders and the head extended on the neck (flextension, or sniffing position) (Fig. 23.32).
- Sitting the patient up or tilting the whole table 20–30 degrees head-up may improve oxygenation and reduce risk of aspiration, but the table should be positioned so the intubator is comfortable during laryngoscopy.
- The anaesthetist *must* be aided by at least one skilled assistant to perform cricoid force, assist in turning the patient, obtain smaller tracheal tubes, supply a bougie or stylet and so on.
- High-volume suction apparatus *must* be functioning and the suction catheter should be within easy reach of the anaesthetist's right hand (commonly placed under the patient's pillow).

- An i.v. cannula should be sited and connected to running fluid to confirm its patency.

Full monitoring should be applied; if a processed EEG monitor is to be used, this can be applied before induction. Before inducing anaesthesia, the patient's lungs should be preoxygenated with 100% oxygen. The patient should breathe 100% O_2 for 3–5 min or until the end-tidal oxygen concentration is 85% or greater. In extreme emergencies this process can be quickened by asking the patient to make four to eight vital capacity breaths, though to be effective this requires a 2 L reservoir bag and the oxygen flush on continuously.

The use of nasal oxygen, either via standard nasal cannulae (2 L min^{-1} increasing to 15 L min^{-1} after loss of consciousness) or high-flow nasal cannulae (50–70 L min^{-1}), should be considered where there is a risk of hypoxia after induction of anaesthesia.

Cricoid force

Cricoid force (also called cricoid pressure) involves pushing the cricoid cartilage backwards against the vertebral column during and after loss of consciousness. The cricoid is a complete ring, and with appropriate force it occludes the hypopharynx (just above the oesophagus), thereby preventing regurgitant matter reaching the larynx and causing pulmonary aspiration.

Cricoid force is an important part of RSI but if done poorly can be either ineffective or an active hindrance to airway management; it should therefore only be performed by someone who is appropriately trained. It is important that the assistant can identify the cricoid cartilage, as compression of the thyroid cartilage distorts laryngeal anatomy and interferes with laryngoscopy. The cricoid cartilage is below the hyoid bone and the thyroid notch (the Adam's apple); it is often at the same level as the second skin crease of the neck and is also generally at the mid-point of the neck. Ultrasound can also be used to identify the cricoid cartilage.

The assistant may practise the force required by either pressing down on weighing scales or compressing an air-filled syringe; for most syringes, compressing a closed 20-ml syringe from 20 ml to 12 ml or a 50-ml syringe from 50 ml to 32 ml requires approximately 30 N (3 kg) force. To perform cricoid force, the thumb and forefinger press the cricoid cartilage firmly in a posterior direction and the middle finger stabilises these fingers on the trachea (Fig. 23.42). The force applied should be 10 N (1 kg) as the patient loses consciousness, increasing to 30 N (3 kg) with loss of consciousness. A force less than 20 N (2 kg) is ineffective and more than 40 N (4 kg) leads to airway distortion, tracheal intubation difficulty and airway obstruction during rescue mask ventilation.

In cases of trauma, cricoid force can still be applied. The cervical spine should be immobilised with manual inline stabilisation and the anterior part of any neck collar removed (as a minimum).

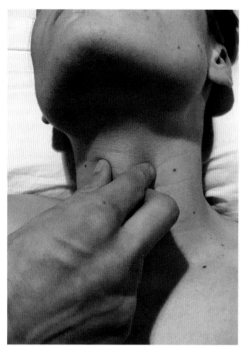

Fig. 23.42 Cricoid force position.

Induction

- With the assistant in position, a precalculated dose of i.v. anaesthetic induction agent is administered.
- This is followed immediately by the administration of a rapid-acting NMBA (suxamethonium 1.5 mg kg^{-1} or rocuronium 0.9 mg kg^{-1}) without waiting to assess the effect of the induction agent.
- Cricoid force is applied.
- Manual ventilation of the patient's lungs whilst waiting for neuromuscular blockade may be performed if there is a risk of hypoxia.
- As soon as the fasciculations have stopped (suxamethonium) or after 45–60 s (rocuronium), laryngoscopy is performed and the trachea intubated.
- Cricoid force is maintained until the cuff of the tracheal tube has been inflated and correct placement of the tracheal tube has been confirmed by capnography and auscultation of both lungs.
- In the very rare situation of active vomiting at the point of induction, cricoid force should be released to avoid risk of oesophageal rupture.
- If laryngoscopy is difficult, cricoid force may be partly released or removed altogether to see if this improves the laryngeal view. Use of a videolaryngoscope during RSI enables the assistant to observe the effect of cricoid force on the airway and laryngeal view and adjust it accordingly.

- After successful tracheal intubation, the lungs are gently ventilated, noting that excessive increases in intrathoracic pressure may worsen hypotension. One of the main disadvantages of RSI is the risk of haemodynamic instability if the dose of induction agent is excessive (hypotension, circulatory collapse) or inadequate (hypertension, tachycardia).
- Although thiopental is historically regarded as the i.v. induction agent of choice for RSI, propofol and ketamine (for high-risk patients) are now generally favoured. Whatever drug is chosen a significantly reduced dose should be used in the older, frail or hypovolaemic patient.

There are many modifications to the RSI technique, and adding an opioid is common. If this is done, a rapid-onset opioid should be selected (e.g. alfentanil or fentanyl) and should be given in a modest dose immediately before the induction agent. An opioid may enable a smaller dose of hypnotic agent to be used and result in a smoother induction.

The choice of NMBA between suxamethonium and rocuronium is debated. The most important characteristic of each drug for RSI is rapid onset. Suxamethonium is the classic NMBA for RSI and provides slightly better tracheal intubating conditions than rocuronium if thiopental is used and no opioids are administered. If propofol is used and an opioid is also administered, the conditions are similar for either agent.

Failed intubation during RSI

Failed intubation during RSI is 5–10 times more common than during elective surgery. This may be because of the clinical setting, the impact of cricoid force or because of limited time available before failed intubation is declared. It is essential that a plan for the management of difficult or failed intubation is established and communicated to all members of the intubation team before undertaking RSI. The default plan should be to wake the patient, where this is feasible. It is often taught, incorrectly, that the short-acting nature of suxamethonium enables rapid wake up when tracheal intubation fails during RSI; in many settings suxamethonium lasts at least 10 min and outlasts the duration of induction agents. Therefore severe hypoxia (and awareness) will occur if the airway is not managed actively.

Maintenance

A nasogastric tube may be passed and the stomach contents aspirated if this has not been done preoperatively.

Reversal and emergence

Once surgery is complete and if the patient is stable enough for tracheal extubation, conduct is broadly similar to that described earlier; however, the nasogastric tube should be suctioned and left on free drainage. Because the risk of aspiration of gastric contents is as great on recovery as at induction, tracheal extubation should only be performed when the patient is awake and responds to commands. It is prudent to warn the patient about awake extubation before a planned RSI. Complications of tracheal extubation are increased during emergency surgery and the anaesthetist and assistant should be prepared to manage laryngospasm, breath holding, bronchospasm and vomiting. Where the risk of aspiration remains high, tracheal extubation may be performed in the lateral position, although this makes subsequent airway management difficult if complications occur. The alternative is sitting up at an angle greater than 45 degrees.

Management of the difficult airway

This important topic can be divided into anticipated and unanticipated difficult airway management. Although both situations may require similar techniques, the approach, urgency and risk of adverse outcomes differ considerably between the two settings.

Difficulties arise most commonly at the start or end of anaesthesia, with the former more common. Difficulty at the end of anaesthesia involves either airway obstruction or aspiration; when the problem is airway obstruction, difficulty may be categorised in the same manner as difficulty after induction.

Difficult airway management may involve any of the four main categories of airway management:
- face-mask ventilation;
- SAD placement and ventilation;
- tracheal intubation; and
- emergency front of neck airway (eFONA), including surgical techniques and cannula cricothyroidotomy.

Airway management is usually routine and straightforward, but each of these techniques may fail. Anaesthetists are used to high levels of success at what they do, and routine airway management does not usually fail. Airway management failure rates vary depending on definitions used, operator experience and the group of patients examined; for example, difficult laryngoscopy (and hence difficult tracheal intubation) occurs in about 6% of unselected patients, but in selected groups, such as those presenting for cervical spine surgery, this may be as high as 20%. About 25% of major airway emergencies occur in the ICU or emergency department, and it is necessary to ensure that the same response to airway difficulty can be provided in these locations as in the operating theatre. In the emergency department, tracheal intubation may be difficult in 1 in 12, fail as often as 1 in 50, and an eFONA has been reported to be needed as often as 1 in 200 tracheal intubation attempts. Although it is important not to dismiss complications arising during uncomplicated airway management, the vast majority of complications occur during difficult airway management.

Before managing the difficult airway

Preparedness

The key to safe management of the difficult airway is *preparedness*.

Organisational preparedness

Guidelines
Organisational preparedness requires that those events which might reasonably be anticipated to occur can be managed appropriately in the organisation. This in turn requires guidelines (or policies) and equipment. As a minimum, the guidelines should cover the following:
- management of unanticipated difficult tracheal intubation;
- management of unanticipated CICO;
- triggers and mechanisms for getting assistance when airway difficulty is anticipated or unexpectedly encountered; and
- information to provide to a patient after a difficult airway event.

Guidelines will also ideally include unexpected failed face-mask ventilation and unexpected failed insertion of a SAD. Guidelines might also address the indications for awake tracheal intubation and management of tracheal extubation of the difficult airway. These guidelines need not be created by every institution, and there is much to be said for nationally accepted or published guidelines being adopted as local policy (e.g. DAS guidelines in the UK). There are several advantages to widespread adoption of this approach; for example, practice becomes based on available evidence, and clinicians who move between hospitals will be immediately familiar with emergency protocols.

Equipment
Logic dictates that the equipment needed to satisfy institutional preparedness is that which is needed for all the guidelines to be carried out in their entirety. This equipment should be procured, stored, maintained and checked appropriately to ensure that it is readily available whenever and wherever it is required. Difficult airway equipment (perhaps better described as advanced airway equipment) is usually maintained in an airway trolley. It is advisable for all airway trolleys in an organisation to have the same content and layout; this includes areas such as ICU and emergency department. Organising the airway trolley so that the layout of the equipment matches the flow of the airway guideline may improve compliance with the guideline and patient care; an example based on the DAS guideline is shown in Fig. 23.43.

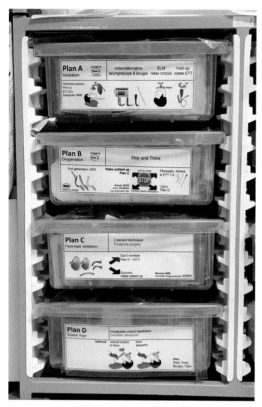

Fig. 23.43 Advanced airway equipment trolley encompassing the Difficult Airway Society difficult tracheal intubation flow chart.

Communication and training

Guidelines are of limited value if they are not understood, accepted and practised by the relevant staff. Many hospitals have access to training in advanced airway management. Training should involve the use of local guidelines and locally available equipment to ensure relevance. Where possible, those individuals who work together in teams should be trained together so that the chances of the team working well in an emergency are enhanced. The team need not be limited to the anaesthetist and anaesthetic assistant, and some training (rather like a trauma team) allocates specific roles to surgeons, scrub nurses and other anaesthetists who attend to help in an airway crisis. Although there is no evidence that such an approach improves outcome in real airway emergencies, it probably enables an organised, systematic approach and has the value of enabling a team leader to oversee the management of the crisis, perhaps avoiding task fixation and promoting situation awareness. Task fixation is the tendency to, having started a task (e.g. tracheal intubation), persevere with attempts to complete that task, even when it is not in the patient's interest (e.g. repeated attempts risking airway trauma and progression

to CICO). Situation awareness should enable the anaesthetist (or someone else in the team) to realise that the task is failing and that another technique or approach is necessary, or perhaps that priorities have changed (e.g. from tracheal intubation to oxygenation and waking the patient).

Personal preparedness

Individual anaesthetists have a clear responsibility to be prepared to manage the difficult airway. At different stages of training and expertise the responsibilities will differ. The elements of individual preparedness are education, training and patient assessment and planning.

Through appropriate education, individual anaesthetists should ensure that they have the appropriate knowledge and skills to deal with anticipated and unanticipated airway difficulties and emergencies which they may reasonably expect to encounter. It is also important that the less experienced know the limitations of their expertise and when to call for assistance. To the trained anaesthetist, management of the difficult airway should become a part of routine practice.

Assessment and planning a strategy

Although it is accepted that not all cases of airway difficulty can be anticipated (perhaps 50% are unanticipated), many can be. Airway assessment is discussed in detail earlier in this chapter. Assessment is a pointless ritual unless the chosen technique is adjusted as necessary according to the findings. The chosen strategy should be consistent with the findings at assessment.

When difficulty with one technique is identified, particular attention is required in assessment of other techniques, first because that rescue technique is more likely to be required, and second because in patients in whom one technique fails there is an increased likelihood that other techniques will also fail. Multiple airway problems tend to coexist in the same patient.

The importance of assessment and planning is underlined by the fact that several large studies examining major airway complications have identified failure to assess, failure to alter technique in the light of findings and failure to have backup plans as causes of poor outcomes.

A strategy is a logical sequential series of plans that aim to achieve oxygenation, ventilation and avoidance of aspiration and which are appropriate to the patient's specific features and condition. Airway management should not rely on the success of 'plan A' and should be based on a clear strategy that is communicated to all. An aphorism that may encapsulate this is 'in order to succeed, it is necessary to plan for failure'. Guidelines are, in essence, a strategy for unexpected difficulty. The strategy should usefully identify a 'place of safety'; this is a preplanned rescue plan when problems arise. For example, if insertion of a SAD is known to be successful, this may be the place of safety, but alternatively the safest option may be to awaken the patient.

Management of the unanticipated difficult airway

The ASA and DAS guidelines and the Vortex approach

The introduction of difficult airway guidelines in the United States led to a reduction in death and brain damage medicolegal claims (and therefore probably critical incidents) related to airway management, most notably at the time of induction of anaesthesia. Many European countries have also developed their own guidelines. Although all these claim to be evidence based, the paucity of robust evidence means that most guidelines differ significantly from each other, often reflecting local preferences. The UK guidelines were published by DAS in 2004 and revised in 2015. Although these guidelines are intended for the unanticipated difficult tracheal intubation, many of the principles can be applied to anticipated difficulty. Both the ASA and DAS guidelines emphasise the most important principles in airway management:

- To have devised a plan for airway management in the eventuality of it proving difficult and a backup plan(s) which has been prepared for and practised.
- That priority must be given to ensuring oxygenation and preventing iatrogenic trauma to the airway at all times. The 2015 DAS guidelines (Figs 23.44 and 23.45) are didactic and present a single recommended pathway arranged in plans A–D, with only minor modifications between the patient undergoing routine tracheal intubation or RSI. They do not prescribe any advanced techniques but recommend simple procedures using equipment that should be familiar to all anaesthetists in training. They also strongly emphasise the need for regular practice of the recommended techniques using simulators and manikins where appropriate. The DAS has also produced guidelines for difficult airway management in obstetrics, paediatrics, critical illness and for managing tracheal extubation.

Difficult face-mask ventilation

The first problem encountered in any difficult airway situation is often difficulty with face-mask ventilation. This is a vital step because it represents the basic and least invasive way of ensuring oxygenation of the patient. For face-mask ventilation to occur, a sealed and patent airway from face mask to the lower airway is required. Difficulty can be diagnosed when there is inadequate chest movement despite high airway pressures (in the case of obstruction) or very low airway pressures (because of a leak during inspiration). Capnography and spirometry, both of which are available on most modern anaesthetic machines, can help to identify poor ventilation before hypoxaemia occurs. Difficulties with face-mask ventilation can be due to:

- failure to maintain a patent upper airway (by far the most common problem);
- laryngeal obstruction (either laryngospasm or pathological condition); or
- obstruction below the larynx, in the trachea, bronchi or in patients with reduced pulmonary compliance.

If there are problems with maintaining patency of the airway, the following simple measures should be employed:
- Correct positioning of head and neck
- Jaw-thrust
- Chin-lift
- Insertion of an appropriately sized oropharyngeal airway
- Consideration of a nasopharyngeal airway
- A two-person ventilation technique
- A three-person ventilation technique

In an alternative technique, one or two people maintain the airway and the reservoir bag is squeezed by a foot, or mechanical ventilation is employed. If ventilation is still not possible and the depth of anaesthesia is adequate, an appropriate SAD should be inserted. Adequate depth of anaesthesia and neuromuscular blockade should be ensured where appropriate.

Difficult SAD insertion and ventilation

Difficult SAD insertion is a neglected topic, perhaps because it is commonly considered that if a SAD cannot be used effectively, then face-mask ventilation or tracheal intubation can be used. However, it is not uncommon for a major airway problem to have started because of failed SAD use, and rescue ventilation with a SAD is at the core of airway rescue techniques.

When the routine insertion technique does not work for an LMA-type device, the following may be helpful:
- Ensure the device is appropriately lubricated.
- Ensure the cuff is carefully and fully deflated so its shape is not distorted.
- Ensure adequate depth of anaesthesia.
- NMBAs are not routinely required.
- Ensure the assistant is performing jaw-thrust correctly.
- Consider a modified insertion technique: insert the device turned 90 degrees until it reaches the soft palate. At this point rotate the device into the correct position and advance into the hypopharynx.
- Ensure the cuff is neither over- nor underinflated; inflate to 60 cmH$_2$O, measured with a manometer.
- A ProSeal LMA may be inserted over a bougie to improve success where there is difficulty. The bougie is carefully inserted into the oesophagus straight end first (under direct vision); the proximal tip of the bougie is lubricated and passed into the distal end of the drain tube of the ProSeal; the ProSeal is then railroaded over the bougie while the assistant performs jaw-thrust; the bougie is removed and the cuff inflated. A similar technique using

a gastric tube or bougie inserted via the mouth into the oesophagus and used as a guide may be suitable for other SADs with a drain tube.

Management of unanticipated difficult tracheal intubation

Every anaesthetist should have a strategy prepared for dealing with problems with tracheal intubation, including plans for the more serious situation of CICO. The DAS algorithm is a suitable approach and is shown in Figs 23.44 and 23.45. This,

or another equally valid strategy, should be familiar to all anaesthetists who are practising without direct supervision.

General principles of management are as follows:
- Administer high-flow 100% oxygen at all times.
- Limit attempts at instrumenting the airway. Each failed attempt risks airway injury, making CICO more likely. Repeating a technique that has just failed is illogical. Change something.
- Transition through the steps of the algorithm at the key failure points without delay.
- Communicate each step of failure/transition to all members of the team in clear non-technical language so all members understand evolving priorities.

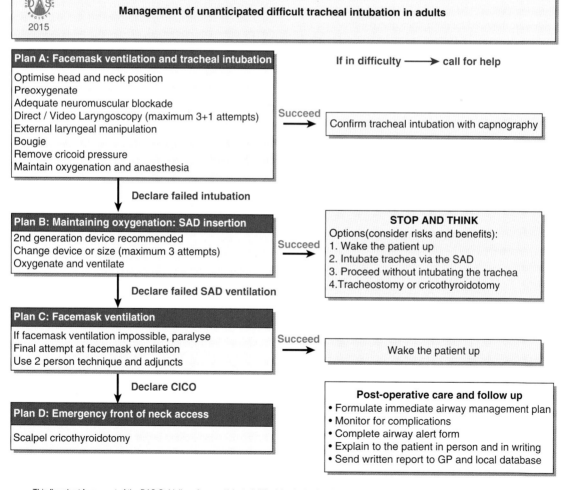

Fig. 23.44 Difficult Airway Society (DAS) guideline for management of unexpected difficult tracheal intubation. *CICO,* 'can't intubate, can't oxygenate'; *GP,* general practitioner; *SAD,* supraglottic airway devices.

Failed intubation, failed oxygenation in the paralysed, anaesthetised patient

2015

CALL FOR HELP

Continue 100% O$_2$
Declare CICO

Plan D: Emergency front of neck access

Continue to give oxygen via upper airway
Ensure neuromuscular blockade
Position patient to extend neck

Scalpel cricothyroidotomy

Equipment: 1. Scalpel (number 10 blade)
2. Bougie
3. Tube (cuffed 6.0mm ID)

Laryngeal handshake to identify cricothyroid membrane

Palpable cricothyroid membrane
Transverse stab incision through cricothyroid membrane
Turn blade through 90° (sharp edge caudally)
Slide coude tip of bougie along blade into trachea
Railroad lubricated 6.0mm cuffed tracheal tube into trachea
Ventilate, inflate cuff and confirm position with capnography
Secure tube

Impalpable cricothyroid membrane
Make an 8-10cm vertical skin incision, caudad to cephalad
Use blunt dissection with fingers of both hands to separate tissues
Identify and stabilise the larynx
Proceed with technique for palpable cricothyroid membrane as above

---

Post-operative care and follow up
- Postpone surgery unless immediately life threatening
- Urgent surgical review of cricothyroidotomy site
- Document and follow up as in main flow chart

Fig. 23.45 Difficult Airway Society (DAS) guidance plan D: scalpel cricothyroidotomy. *CICO*, 'can't intubate, can't oxygenate'.

- Where aspiration is a high risk, make attempts to prevent this where possible.

Management is in four parts (plans A–D), which should be approached in sequence in the event of deteriorating oxygenation and increasing difficulty with ventilation.

Plan A: Primary tracheal intubation attempt

Plan A involves the first and best attempts at tracheal intubation. It requires good preoxygenation, optimal positioning and anaesthesia, appropriate neuromuscular blockade and the correct laryngoscope blade. Use of external laryngeal manipulation and a high-quality bougie are also appropriate. Attempts at tracheal intubation must be limited to no more than three (preferably fewer), as multiple attempts at laryngoscopy are associated with dramatically increased risk of airway trauma, failed rescue techniques, CICO and mortality. A fourth attempt is deemed appropriate only if a more experienced anaesthetist arrives and adequate face-mask ventilation can be maintained.

After one failed attempt at laryngoscopy, help should be summoned, but do not send away the primary assistant. The difficult airway trolley should also be called for.

There is no necessity to use the same laryngoscope blade for all attempts at tracheal intubation. The most recent guidelines advocate using a videolaryngoscope if initial attempts at fail.

Videolaryngoscopy has a major role to play in reducing and managing difficult tracheal intubation. Its use has largely superseded that of other specialised blades (e.g. McCoy levering laryngoscope or straight-bladed laryngoscopes such as the Miller or Henderson designs). Videolaryngoscopy should no longer be considered an advanced or optional technique but should be viewed as a fundamental part of all anaesthetists' armamentarium. All anaesthetists should be trained and expert in the use of any videolaryngoscope they intend to use to manage a difficult tracheal intubation.

When tracheal intubation fails, this should be declared aloud – so all around are aware – and the priority transitions to plan B.

Plan B: Maintaining oxygenation and SAD insertion

A SAD is inserted to enable ventilation and oxygenation. Success rates for airway rescue are reported to be as high as 95% for the cLMA and are likely to be equally high or higher with second-generation devices. The DAS 2015 guidelines recommend that a second-generation SAD is used. Patients who require airway rescue are often obese, male, scheduled to undergo emergency surgery and likely to have received an NMBA either before or during the airway emergency. Many are at a significantly increased risk of regurgitation and aspiration of gastric fluid because of obesity, urgency of surgery and possible gastric inflation during attempts to ventilate by face-mask. These are not the type of patients whom most anaesthetists would choose to manage with a standard laryngeal mask. In this circumstance the require-ments for a SAD to rescue the airway are:

- speedy and reliable insertion;
- reliable ventilation (even if lung compliance is low);
- early detection of regurgitation and increased protection against aspiration;
- ability to empty the stomach; and
- suitable as a conduit for subsequent fibreoptic–guided tracheal intubation.

There is, therefore, a good argument for choosing a second-generation SAD with a high airway seal for airway rescue. Suitable devices include the ProSeal LMA (probably inserted over a bougie to increase success) and i-gel. The SLMA and Laryngeal Tube Suction II enable airway rescue but are less suited as conduits for tracheal intubation.

If this succeeds (i.e. it achieves adequate ventilation and oxygenation as judged by capnography and oximetry and

supported by clinical signs), the team should stop and consider the next step.

Options are to:
- wake the patient;
- attempt to intubate the trachea via the SAD (discussed later);
- continue without tracheal intubation;
- perform cricothyroidotomy or tracheostomy.

Waking the patient should be the default option. Surgery should then be postponed or the airway established using an awake technique. If neuromuscular blockade has been established, this must be allowed to wear off or be reversed; sugammadex may have an important role if rocuronium (or vecuronium) has been used to induce neuromuscular blockade but will not reverse CICO which has an anatomical or mechanical cause. However, waking the patient is not practical in many emergencies, most commonly because the airway is incompletely rescued. Less commonly, the urgency of the surgery demands that it must proceed and the airway must be secured come what may.

If SAD insertion is difficult or initially unsuccessful, subsequent attempts should consider repositioning, use of a different size or type of device or a different operator. Multiple attempts at SAD insertion also risk airway trauma and should be limited to three attempts.

If SAD insertion and ventilation fails, the situation is critical. The failure should be declared aloud and the priority transitions to plan C.

Tracheal intubation via a SAD

If the decision is to intubate via the SAD, fibreoptic guidance is recommended. Second-generation SADs are recommended because they perform better than first-generation devices and are likely to be safer; the ILMA is an alternative. All anaesthetists should be expert with the device they may need to use in this circumstance.

Blind tracheal intubation via any standard SAD is extremely unlikely to be successful (< 20% success rate) and cannot be recommended. The use of a fibrescope through a SAD has a high success rate, is a relatively low-skill pro-cedure and may be practised both in manikins and in patients in a non-emergency setting, with appropriate consent.

The AIC is a useful adjunct to fibreoptic intubation. It is slid over the fibrescope, and fibreoptic tracheal intubation is then performed via the SAD. The procedure is described in Fig. 23.31.

Tracheal intubation via an ILMA

The ILMA is also an option for management of plan B. Although it is not a second-generation SAD, it has a well-established role in management of difficult tracheal intuba-tion. The ILMA has a mask end which is similar to a cLMA but the grille is replaced by an 'epiglottic elevating bar', which is a firm piece of silicone anchored at one end only.

The stem of the ILMA is both shorter and wider than other LMAs and is rigid, with a handle attached on the concave side (see Fig. 23.7); the stem passes through an angle of approximately 110 degrees. The ILMA is supplied with a specifically designed ILMA tracheal tube which is straight, reinforced and has a soft bullet-shaped tip (Fig. 23.21A). The ILMA is supplied in three sizes for patients of 30–100 kg, and each accommodates all sizes of ILMA tracheal tube from 6.0–8.0 mm ID. The ILMA can be used for blind or fibreoptic–guided tracheal intubation; the success rate of the blind technique is approximately 75%, rising to close to 100% with a fibreoptic–guided technique. The fibre-optic–guided technique is the technique advocated in the DAS guidelines. The ILMA is supported by robust evidence of performance but has also been implicated in fatalities during difficult airway management. The use of the ILMA is technically demanding, and a clear understanding of the steps required and of potential pitfalls is required before using it in clinical practice. Training and practice is therefore essential.

Plan C: Final attempt at face-mask ventilation

If tracheal intubation and SAD insertion have both failed, then ventilation should be attempted again using a face-mask if this succeeds the patient should be woken up where this is feasible. If this fails (or if it succeeds but waking is not feasible), the team should transition to performing eFONA.

Management of unanticipated difficult intubation during RSI

Failed intubation during RSI is 5–10 times more common than during elective surgery. The default plan should be to wake the patient, where this is feasible. It is often taught, incorrectly, that the short-acting nature of suxamethonium enables rapid waking when tracheal intubation fails during RSI. In many settings suxamethonium lasts at least 10 min and outlasts the duration of induction agents. Therefore severe hypoxia will occur if the airway is not actively managed.

The principal goals in the guidelines for unanticipated difficult intubation during RSI are the same as in non-RSI settings (i.e. maintain oxygenation, avoid trauma, avoid aspiration). Minor differences include the following:
- The patient is always fully preoxygenated, which may create more time before oxygen desaturation, but often the patient's general condition hastens desaturation.
- There should be a lower threshold for starting high-flow nasal oxygen before induction to prolong safe apnoea time.
- Cricoid force is in place, and this may interfere with laryngoscopy, making tracheal intubation difficulty more likely.

- There should be a low threshold for using videolaryngoscopy as this will improve the view of the larynx, decrease the risk of failed tracheal intubation and help the assistant in optimising cricoid force.
- Cricoid force should be reduced or removed if it is impeding laryngoscopy; this should be done with sucker in hand so that regurgitated material can be removed promptly.
- If rocuronium is used as part of the RSI technique, sugammadex may be used to reverse it, although this can only be achieved in a timely fashion if the drug is immediately available *before* induction starts.

Plan D: Management of 'cannot intubate, cannot oxygenate' (CICO)

Although CICO can arise unexpectedly during routine anaesthesia, it is more common when multiple attempts at laryngoscopy/tracheal intubation have changed a 'cannot intubate, can ventilate' situation into CICO. All organisations should have a guideline, and all individuals a plan, for the management of CICO; the DAS guideline is one option (see Fig. 23.45). This includes the following:
- Call for help if this has not already been done or it has not yet arrived.
- Call for and open the eFONA equipment.
- Administer an NMBA if not already done this may facilitate face-mask ventilation or SAD insertion and may also improve conditions for establishing eFONA.
- Insert a second-generation SAD, as this may rescue the airway even at this point.
- *If the situation is not resolved, declare a 'cannot intubate, cannot oxygenate' situation and proceed directly to establishing eFONA.*

It is not necessary to wait for hypoxia before transitioning to eFONA. At this point the situation is critical and will result in hypoxic-ischaemic brain injury, cardiac arrest or death unless an airway is secured within 3–5 min. There have been numerous studies which illustrate that many cases of eFONA are performed too late to prevent brain injury or death. Harm caused by delay in recognising and managing CICO is dramatically more common than harm caused by complications of eFONA techniques.

CICO and obesity

It is notable that obesity is an important factor when considering CICO. Obesity is a risk factor for all aspects of airway difficulty, and when this occurs, profound hypoxia can result in as little as 60 s, even after full preoxygenation. Therefore, many patients who develop CICO may be obese. eFONA is technically more challenging on the obese patient as the cricothyroid membrane is often impalpable and soft tissues interfere with access.

Emergency front of neck airway

When managing a CICO situation, eFONA should be performed via the cricothyroid membrane. This is readily identifiable in most patients and is relatively avascular. As the trachea descends lower, it lies deeper in the neck and bleeding risk is increased, especially where the thyroid gland lies over it. Concerns about long-term injury as a result of cricothyroid rather than tracheal access are overstated and of negligible consequence in the emergency setting.

There are three options:

- Scalpel (surgical) cricothyroidotomy
- Narrow-bore cannula with high-pressure source ventilation
- Wide-bore cannula

The best technique is controversial, with competing evidence bases and opinions. The 2015 DAS guidelines recommend scalpel cricothyroidotomy as the default technique (see Fig. 23.45). This is because it is relatively simple and quick, uses limited specialist equipment, is readily adapted for the obese patient and results in a wide-bore airway which avoids complications of ventilation after the airway is secured. The DAS guidelines support use of other techniques only in the setting of a fully trained and experienced department.

Scalpel cricothyroidotomy

There are four steps:

1. The neck is fully extended and the cricothyroid membrane is identified.
2. A horizontal stab incision is made in the neck over the cricothyroid membrane with a wide round-ended (e.g. number 10 or 20) scalpel blade extending deep into the membrane. The scalpel is rotated to face vertically with the sharp side caudad and slightly pushed away to create space.
3. A bougie is inserted alongside the scalpel blade and into the trachea 8–10 cm.
4. A 5.5–6.0 mm ID tracheal tube (or tracheostomy tube) is inserted.

Identifying the cricothyroid membrane may be difficult. In a slim patient it can be palpated just below the thyroid prominence (Adam's apple), and it is generally right in the middle of the neck. The membrane, or the midline, may be identified with ultrasound and marked, and although this is useful if difficulty is anticipated, there is rarely time for this when CICO occurs. The 'laryngeal handshake' (Fig. 23.46) has been described in which the trachea and hyoid bone are grasped – this helps identify the relations of the hyoid (upper most), thyroid lamina (lower) and trachea (lowest). The larynx can then be held between thumb and middle finger and the index finger used to palpate the cricothyroid membrane. The main advantage is likely to be avoiding mistaking the hyoid bone for the thyroid. In an

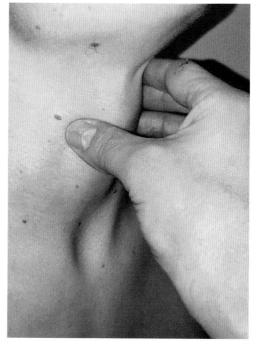

Fig. 23.46 Laryngeal handshake to identify cricothyroid membrane.

obese patient these landmarks may all be impalpable. Where the cricothyroid membrane cannot be reliably identified, the scalpel technique is modified:

1. Make a large longitudinal (up to 10 cm long) incision through the skin, starting above the manubrium.
2. Use blunt dissection to dissect down to the trachea and identify the cricothyroid membrane.
3. Proceed as for the slim neck.

Other scalpel cricothyroidotomy techniques are described that include use of tracheostomy dilators or a cricoid hook. The important feature is to ensure that, once the cricothyroid membrane has been entered, something stays in it, keeping the tract open at all times.

Bleeding is the most common complication of scalpel cricothyroidotomy and should be anticipated. Various simulation studies suggest that a scalpel technique can be performed as rapidly as a Seldinger cannula technique, although these are typically performed in bloodless fields.

Narrow-bore cannula with high-pressure source ventilation

A narrow-bore cannula (most are approximately 2 mm ID) is usually inserted as a cannula-over-needle technique through the cricothyroid membrane. Once inserted, ventilation is based on two important principles:

1. a high driving pressure is required to inflate the lungs because of the enormous resistance to flow through the cannula; and

2. expiration must take place though the patient's upper airway.

Complications of ventilation, especially barotrauma, are more problematic than complications of device insertion. It is appropriate to use specifically designed devices which sit against the neck correctly and are less likely to kink. These are described in the equipment section of this chapter.

Although the narrow-bore technique has the appeal of simplicity, it is prone to failure. In a recent study of major complications of airway management, more than 60% of emergency cannula cricothyroidotomies inserted by anaesthetists failed. The causes were numerous and included use of inappropriate equipment, misuse of appropriate devices, device failure, poor technique and inappropriate ventilation via a correctly placed narrow-bore device. Complications of this technique are especially high in the emergency setting.

Wide-bore cannula (≥ 4-mm ID)

Wide-bore cannulae may be cannula-over-needle devices (e.g. QuickTrach) or those requiring a Seldinger insertion technique (e.g. Cook Melker cricothyroidotomy devices; see Fig. 23.25). Cannula-over-needle devices require a large sharp needle, which risks significant tissue trauma if misplaced, and such devices may be too short to reach the trachea in patients with an obese neck. Seldinger-type devices take somewhat longer to insert, but the technique is familiar to anaesthetists.

Ventilation and expiration via cricothyroidotomy devices

Wide-bore cannula and scalpel cricothyroidotomy
Wide-bore cannulae are defined as those with an internal diameter ≥ 4 mm because this is the minimum calibre through which an adult can spontaneously exhale with adequate speed to maintain a normal minute volume. After the device has been inserted, ventilation can be achieved with a low-pressure gas source (e.g. a standard anaesthetic machine). Large-bore cannulae without a cuff require that the upper airway is obstructed during inspiration to avoid the ventilating gas being vented via the upper airway. This may be achieved by actively obstructing the upper airway (e.g. a SAD is inserted and the proximal end obstructed) or, preferably, by the use of a cuffed cannula. Spontaneous ventilation via a wide-bore cannula is also possible.

Narrow-bore cannula
When ventilating through a narrow-bore cannula, a high-pressure source is needed to overcome the resistance of the cannula. However, the pressure changes in the trachea during this type of ventilation are similar to those during conventional ventilation. The technique should not be confused with jet ventilation or oscillation; what is achieved is high-pressure source conventional ventilation. Appropriate sources of the high pressure for such ventilation are either wall oxygen or an oxygen cylinder (both deliver approximately 400 kPa). If wall oxygen is used, the flow rate should be set at more than 15 L min⁻¹. When using an anaesthetic machine, pressure regulators and blow-off valves reduce the pressure available; an attached anaesthetic breathing system with a conventional anaesthetic reservoir bag limits pressure to 6 kPa, which is inadequate for ventilation through a narrow cannula. If the anaesthetic flush is deployed continuously, a pressure of 30–60 kPa can be achieved, and this may be just sufficient to ventilate the lungs. Maximum flow rates from an anaesthetic machine are 15 L min⁻¹ via a flowmeter and 30–60 L min⁻¹ when the oxygen flush button is depressed. An anaesthetic machine cannot provide a reliably high-pressure source unless a connection is made to a high-pressure source outlet at the back of the machine (usually a mini Schroeder connector; Fig. 23.47), which can then be used to drive an injector or similar device.

An oxygen injector such as a Sanders or Manujet injector can deliver a high-pressure source ranging from 50–400 kPa at a flow of up to 1 L s⁻¹. Because such high pressures and flows are needed to ventilate through a narrow-bore cannula, there is a high risk of severe barotrauma, particularly if the device is displaced (e.g. surgical emphysema, pneumothorax, pneumomediastinum), inspiration is prolonged or inspiration occurs before expiration is complete. In CICO situations, the upper airway is sufficiently patent during expiration to allow exhalation in up to 90% of patients. Whenever ventilating through a narrow-bore cannula, it is essential to ensure that expiration is complete (e.g. with a hand on the chest)

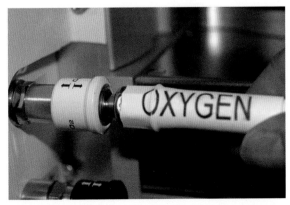

Fig. 23.47 Mini Shroeder valve, a source of high-pressure oxygen on the anaesthetic machine.

before administering the next inspiration. The Rapid-O2 and Enk oxygen flow modulator devices are alternative methods for providing inspiration via a narrow bore cannula (with lower risk of barotrauma).

The Ventrain device (Fig. 23.24) uses a driving gas that bypasses a narrow airway cannula during the expiratory phase and, by entraining gas from the cannula to achieve assisted exhalation, can achieve normal minute ventilation.

To summarise, this is a complex and often confused topic. There are three methods of achieving oxygenation and ventilation via a cricothyroidotomy:

1. Scalpel techniques enable insertion of a large tube into the trachea and conventional (low-pressure) ventilation.
2. Large cannula techniques enable ventilation with lower pressures but require either a tracheal cuff or the upper airway to be obstructed to prevent loss of driving gas through the upper airway. Entrainment is minimal or non-existent.
3. Small cannula techniques require a high-pressure gas source to overcome device resistance and rely on a patent upper airway for exhalation. Expiration must be confirmed before subsequent breaths are administered.

The Vortex approach

The Vortex approach to airway management has recently been proposed as a model for crisis airway management (Fig. 23.48). The approach describes two areas: a 'green zone' of airway safety; and a 'vortex' of spiralling failure. The vortex may be entered when any chosen airway device (face-mask ventilation, SAD or tracheal intubation) fails. Once in the vortex, successful airway management returns the patient to the safe green zone. While in the vortex, each of the modalities of airway rescue (face-mask ventilation, SAD insertion, tracheal intubation) may be attempted a

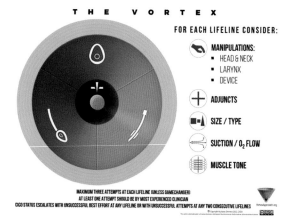

Fig. 23.48 The Vortex approach. (With permission of Dr Nick Chrimes.)

maximum of three times, in any order. If an optimal attempt with any device is made and fails, further attempts with that device are not indicated. If there is clinical deterioration during rescue attempts, the guideline directs transitioning to eFONA. Importantly, if each of the (up to) three attempts with each device have been exhausted, transition to eFONA is also indicated, even if oxygenation is maintained. The approach aims to (1) better reflect the variety of clinical situations leading to development of airway difficulty; (2) better represent real-life responses to airway difficulty; and (3) actively promote avoidance of excessive attempts at airway instrumentation and early transitioning to eFONA.

This approach has much appeal and creates the possibility of increasing unity between the currently numerous and disparate national guidelines.

Management of the predicted difficult airway

The main difference between management of the unanticipated and the predicted difficult airway is that the latter enables the anaesthetic team to plan and prepare more thoroughly and to fit a strategy to the specific needs of the patient rather than following a guideline designed to fit all situations. Because of the limitations of airway assessment, many patients with a predicted difficult airway will not prove to be difficult, but this is not a reason to ignore a history of difficulty or preoperative findings. Many airway disasters are preceded by anaesthetists ignoring the history or signs of difficulty and then getting into avoidable trouble.

When airway management is predicted to be difficult, the strategy can be based around achieving the:
- right plan (strategy);
- right place;
- right time;
- right person.

The *right plan* has been discussed earlier in the chapter in the section describing strategy. In patients with a predicted difficult airway, careful assessment is vital to determine which specific routes of access and techniques are likely to be problematic or successful so that a logical individualised strategy can be constructed. The plan will usually include tracheal intubation.

Ensuring the *right place* may require that the patient is transferred to a location where appropriate monitoring, equipment and skills are available to manage the airway safely. However, transfer of a patient with a critical airway is fraught with danger, and an assessment of specific risks should be made, including a plan for management of deterioration during transfer. In the operating theatre setting, patients in whom airway difficulty is anticipated should usually be managed in the operating theatre rather than the anaesthetic room for reasons of space, visibility, monitoring, communication and teamwork.

The *right time* implies patients with anticipated difficulty should be managed at the time that is safest for the patient. Urgent and emergency patients must be managed with appropriate promptness, but patients undergoing elective procedures should be managed with enough time for assessment, collecting all necessary information (e.g. retrieving notes and scans as necessary) and gathering the equipment and personnel needed for optimal management.

The *right person* may not be the anaesthetist to whom the patient presents. The right person may also not be one individual but a number of individuals with the skills to carry out specialised parts of the airway strategy. If possible, the right personnel should be present from the start of airway management. Most airway difficulties provide ample opportunity for teaching, and these opportunities should be seized.

Although the detail may differ, the principles of managing the patient with predicted airway difficulty are no different to managing unanticipated problems.

Training, teamwork and human factors

Human factors associated with airway management complications include:
- misuse of equipment through lack of knowledge or training;
- task fixation;
- poor situation awareness;
- communication problems;
- lack of leadership;
- poor teamworking; and
- failure to follow guidelines and, in particular, to transition through the phases of the guidelines appropriately.

Before approaching the difficult airway

Several questions can usefully be considered before approaching any anticipated difficult airway. These questions are based on the preamble to the American Society of Anesthesiologists difficult airway algorithm.
- Will delivery of oxygen be difficult?
- Will face-mask ventilation be difficult?
- Will SAD placement be difficult?
- Will tracheal intubation be difficult?
- Will direct access to the trachea (i.e. eFONA) be difficult?
- Will there be problems with patient consent or co-operation?
  Consider the relative merits of:
- securing the airway with the patient awake or anaesthetised;

- making the initial approach to tracheal intubation direct or indirect; and
- maintaining spontaneous ventilation or ablating it during airway management.

The ASA also recommends actively pursuing opportunities to deliver supplemental oxygen throughout the process of difficult airway management.

Securing the airway awake

When airway difficulty is anticipated, the point at which the anaesthetist risks loss of control is likely to be when general anaesthesia is induced. At this point, respiratory drive is diminished or obliterated, airway reflexes are largely ablated, and the loss of muscle tone of the airway means that the risk of airway obstruction increases dramatically. If general anaesthesia is induced, the time from stopping administration of drugs to patient waking is often up to 10 min, which is more than sufficient to cause profound hypoxaemia, hypoxic tissue injury or even death.

Securing the airway awake should be considered actively whenever significant difficulty in tracheal intubation is predicted. The argument for this increases when face-mask ventilation is predicted to be difficult, when rescue techniques such as eFONA are predicted to be difficult and when there is a high risk of aspiration. The main contraindications to awake techniques are lack of patient co-operation or refusal. Reassurance and appropriate (very light) sedation and anxiolysis may enable many patients to accept awake techniques. If there is critical airway obstruction, great care is needed as topical anaesthesia of the airway or even light sedation may lead to total airway obstruction.

Although awake fibreoptic intubation (AFOI) is generally considered the standard mode of awake tracheal intubation, there are several methods reported. These include:
- awake fibreoptic intubation via oral or nasal routes;
- awake direct laryngoscopy (standard laryngoscope);
- awake videolaryngoscopy;
- awake tracheal intubation via an ILMA;
- awake tracheal intubation via another SAD; and
- awake FONA.

Although not all anaesthetists currently have the skills and experience to perform AFOI, such skills must be available in every anaesthetic department at all times and should be deployed whenever indicated.

Administration of NMBAs in the patient with a difficult airway

When general anaesthesia is administered, NMBAs can be friend or foe during difficult airway management. It is notable that neuromuscular blockade is not usually necessary for face-mask ventilation or SAD insertion but does facilitate tracheal intubation and probably insertion of eFONA.

When face-mask ventilation is problematic, administration of an NMBA usually makes ventilation easier. This has led some to promote the use of neuromuscular blockade when face-mask ventilation is difficult in patients with a difficult airway. However, it is important to note that the evidence of easier ventilation is derived from patients who are not particularly difficult in the first place. In contrast, there is no robust evidence that neuromuscular blockade makes ventilation *reliably* easy when dealing with patients with abnormal anatomy or an anticipated difficult airway. There is also a lack of evidence that neuromuscular blockade reliably converts CICO to a situation in which ventilation is possible. A disadvantage of inducing neuromuscular blockade in this situation is that it commits the anaesthetist to securing the airway promptly and may remove the option of waking the patient. Patients who are difficult or impossible to ventilate using a face-mask are also at increased risk of failed tracheal intubation. Thus, administration of an NMBA may be reasonable when difficult face-mask ventilation occurs and waking the patient is not desirable, but the anaesthetist must be prepared to manage a critical airway if it does not improve the situation. In contrast, when both face-mask ventilation and tracheal intubation have failed, if waking the patient is not possible, there is little to be lost and much to be gained by administering an NMBA. If successful, it will avoid an unnecessary eFONA and may save the patient's life.

Selecting an appropriate size of tracheal tube

In the circumstance of difficult airway management, there is a strong argument for using a smaller tracheal tube. A smaller tracheal tube:
- passes though some narrow lumens through which a larger tracheal tube will not pass;
- passes through a narrow lumen with greater ease and with less risk of trauma to the airway; and
- is easier to railroad over a bougie or AEC with less risk of hold-up during insertion.

Spontaneous ventilation is rarely required for prolonged periods after tracheal intubation. Selection of a tracheal tube of 6.0–6.5 mm ID may make airway management easier, and use of tracheal tubes larger than 7.0 mm ID is rarely indicated.

Oxygenation for predicted difficult airways

Because time is available when difficulty is predicted, this provides an opportunity which must be taken to optimise oxygenation before and during airway management. Pre-oxygenation should be thorough; 100% oxygen should be delivered via any device that enables it during difficult airway management (e.g. nasal cannulae, high-flow nasal oxygen, or buccal oxygen) to prolong safe apnoea time.

Planning a strategy and 'place of safety' planning

Before starting airway management, the airway strategy should be established, agreed and communicated to all present to ensure a shared mental model within the team. It is useful to identify transition points in the strategy: points at which the plan should change. A place of safety plan should also be made. That is the default plan for the situation when there is increasing difficulty; in most cases the place of safety involves waking the patient, as it is the safest option. The airway can subsequently be secured awake.

Fibreoptic intubation

Fibreoptic intubation may be performed by the nasal or oral route but requires special equipment, skill and time. There are three phases to fibreoptic intubation:
1. Topicalisation of the airway
2. Fibreoptic endoscopy
3. Railroading the tracheal tube
   The procedure may fail at each stage.

Topicalisation of the airway

Before topicalising the airway, secretions may be decreased with glycopyrronium bromide 0.1–0.2 mg and nasal co-phenylcaine. Anxiolysis or sedation, if appropriate, may be achieved with low doses of sedative drugs, amongst which propofol, remifentanil or dexmedetomidine are commonly used. Topical anaesthesia is achieved by spraying the nasal and oropharyngeal mucosa and/or gargling viscous preparations. Nebulised lidocaine may be used, and atomising devices improve mucosal coverage. Typically, lidocaine preparations of 2%–4% are used to progressively anaesthetise the nasal or oral route. Although specific nerve blocks (sphenopalatine, glossopharyngeal, superior laryngeal) may be performed, a spray-as-you-go technique is also effective and widely used. Injection of 2–3 ml lidocaine 2% through the cricothyroid membrane induces coughing and anaesthetises the tracheal and laryngeal mucosa. Total lidocaine dose should not exceed 8 mg kg^{-1}.

Fibreoptic endoscopy

Before performing the endoscopy:
- Explain to the patient what will happen and keep communicating throughout the procedure.
- Apply routine monitoring.
- Optimise patient positioning, usually sitting up at least 45 degrees.

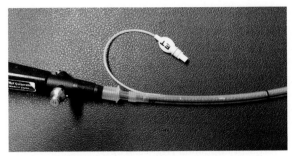

Fig. 23.49 Fibrescope with tracheal tube loaded for awake fibreoptic tracheal intubation.

- Optimise patient sedation – if it is used, the patient must be co-operative and able to follow commands.
- Perform airway suction to clear any secretions and assess quality of topical anaesthesia. Take care to avoid trauma and bleeding which interferes with endoscopy.
- Administer oxygen, either by nasal cannulae or using a Hudson-type face mask with hole cut into it to enable the fibrescope access.
- Set up the fibrescope screen so the best view is achieved.
- Place an appropriate tracheal tube over the fibrescope for subsequent railroading and secure it close to the handle of the fibrescope (Fig. 23.49). A small tracheal tube with a tip that hugs the fibrescope is best as this avoids a large gap between fibrescope and tracheal tube that risks nasal trauma and catching at the glottis; an ILMA (6.0 mm ID) or Parker tip tracheal tube is suitable. Rigid and large tracheal tubes with sharp bevels should be avoided.

Endoscopy can then be undertaken.

- For nasal tracheal intubation, the fibrescope is inserted into the nose and gently moved forward below the inferior turbinate, at all times seeking to keep the fibrescope tip away from the mucosa.
- The fibrescope is advanced to the back of the nose, deflected caudad, advanced into the nasopharynx and thence towards the hypopharynx where the epiglottis and then the vocal cords should be visible.
- Additional topical anaesthesia can be applied via an epidural catheter inserted through the fibrescope channel and dribbled onto the mucosa. This is particularly useful at the vocal cords to improve anaesthesia without causing coughing.
- Where there is difficulty passing the endoscope or identifying a clear passage, it may be helpful to ask the patient to take a deep breath, stick the jaw forward or tongue out or phonate (e.g. ask the patient to say "eeeeeee").
- As the larynx is entered, the patient should be informed not to talk. The fibrescope is then advanced into the

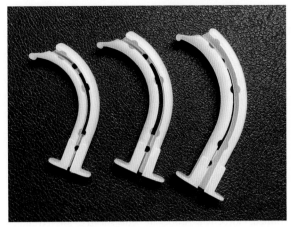

Fig. 23.50 Berman intubation guides.

trachea to just above the carina and this position maintained while the tracheal tube is railroaded.

- If an oral route is chosen, endoscopy may be improved by use of a fibreoptic guide (e.g. Ovassapian or Berman airway; Fig. 23.50). These are curved conduits similar to an oropharyngeal airway that are split to enable removal after endoscopy is complete. Although useful, sizing is important and they can interfere with endoscopy or cause gagging if they are the wrong size.

Railroading the tracheal tube

- The position of the fibrescope is maintained while the lubricated tracheal tube is passed through the nose or mouth and into the larynx and trachea. The patient should be warned this may be briefly uncomfortable.
- If the correct tracheal tube is chosen, there should be no hold-up. If there is hold-up, the tracheal tube should be gently advanced while rotating it; minimal force should be used to avoid trauma or displacement of the fibrescope from the trachea.
- Once the tracheal tube is in place, the fibrescope should be withdrawn while watching the screen so the position of the tracheal tube within the trachea can be confirmed.
- The tracheal tube is then connected to the breathing circuit and correct placement reconfirmed with capnography.
- The tracheal tube cuff is then inflated, and anaesthesia can be induced. Some advocate inducing anaesthesia before cuff inflation because of concerns about discomfort; provided topical anaesthesia is good, cuff inflation is well tolerated and minimises the risk of aspiration or tracheal tube displacement.

At the end of surgery, it is useful to remember that the tracheal tube will be tolerated to very light planes of anaesthesia because of the topical anaesthesia, and this may delay waking. Unless the airway problem has been resolved by surgery, tracheal extubation should be treated as high risk (see later). The patient will also not reliably protect the airway from aspiration, even when awake, while topical anaesthesia of the larynx continues to be effective. The patient should remain starved until topical anaesthesia has resolved.

Conventional laryngoscopy or videolaryngoscopy

Conventional laryngoscopy or videolaryngoscopy may also be performed in awake patients. After topically anaesthetising the oropharynx, larynx and trachea, laryngoscopy is performed. Videolaryngoscopes are better suited to this technique as they require less force to be applied to the tissues, and if a hyperangulated device is used there may be minimal displacement of tissues and negligible force applied.

Awake SAD placement

Careful topicalisation is applied and an appropriate SAD is inserted with minimal force. It may be sensible to use one size smaller SAD than normal. This technique requires excellent topical anaesthesia and a motivated patient. Once adequate positioning of the SAD is confirmed, it may be used as a conduit for tracheal intubation (see earlier). Only in rare circumstances would it be logical to then proceed with general anaesthesia with just the SAD in place, as this lacks a backup plan.

Awake FONA

A narrow-bore cannula (e.g. Ravussin cannula; see Fig. 23.22) may be placed in the cricothyroid membrane relatively simply. This may be useful if the planned anaesthetic technique is transtracheal high-pressure source ventilation. It may also be useful if there are concerns that the airway may be lost during attempts to secure the airway from above. Placing the cannula before inducing anaesthesia then means a rescue technique is readily available if problems occur. The insertion technique is as follows:

- The cricothyroid membrane is located (Fig. 23.51A); ultrasound may be appropriate if there is time and appropriate expertise.
- Local anaesthesia is applied to the skin and through the cricothyroid membrane.
- The cannula is attached to a 5-ml syringe partially filled with saline.
- The syringe and needle are advanced perpendicular to the skin while gently aspirating the syringe (Fig. 23.51B). On entering the trachea, a clear inrush of air to the syringe will be seen as bubbles (Fig. 23.51C).

- The needle should be directed to face 45 degrees caudad and the cannula advanced over the needle into the trachea (Fig. 23.51D). Care should be taken during insertion not to advance the cannula too far, as this will lead to damage to the posterior wall of the trachea, risking oesophageal injury and mediastinitis.
- Correct positioning is then confirmed again with the syringe and with capnography.
- High-pressure source ventilation (see earlier) is required, with careful monitoring of expiration before each subsequent inspiration (Fig. 23.51E).

A wide-bore cricothyroid cannula or surgical tracheostomy may also be performed awake. When this is done in the context of airway obstruction, particularly as an emergency, it is far from a simple procedure. The patient may be hypoxic, distressed and agitated. Surgical tracheostomy may take a considerable time, and perhaps the hardest part of the anaesthetic technique is resisting the temptation to give sedation or anaesthesia.

Tubeless techniques

In some settings the airway may be shared completely with the surgeon. The surgeon establishes an airway with a straight rigid bronchoscope (placed into the trachea) or laryngoscope (placed above the vocal cords). A narrow tube within the endoscope enables the anaesthetist to administer high-pressure source ventilation (Fig. 23.52) either manually or via a high-frequency jet ventilator or oscillator. This mandates the use of total intravenous anaesthesia (TIVA), and neuromuscular blockade must be maintained to (1) prevent glottic closure or coughing during high-pressure ventilation with subsequent risk of barotrauma; and (2) prevent patient movement and injury during surgery.

An alternative is placement of a very fine tracheal tube of only a few millimetres' diameter (e.g. Hunsaker tube) through the larynx and into the upper airway (transglottic ventilation). A plastic cage at the end of the tube keeps the tube tip off the tracheal wall, and ventilation is again with a high-pressure source.

In each of these modes of ventilation significant amounts of air are entrained during ventilation.

Induction of anaesthesia while maintaining spontaneous ventilation

Inhalational induction is now rarely used as a technique for difficult airway management. The idea behind inhalational induction for the difficult airway while maintaining spontaneous breathing was that if the airway obstructs, the delivery of volatile agent is reduced, anaesthesia will lighten and the patient will awaken. In practice there are numerous problems with the technique:

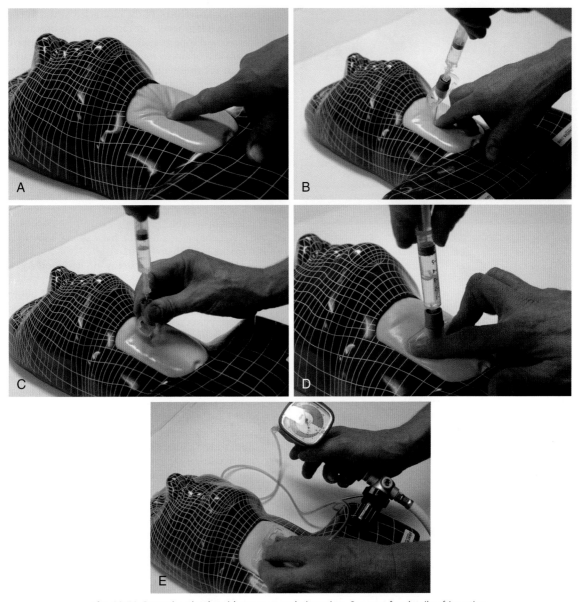

Fig. 23.51 Ravussin cricothyroidotomy cannula insertion. See text for details of insertion.

- It is extremely slow in cases of airway obstruction.
- Breath holding and coughing are very common.
- It is difficult to reliably assess when depth of anaesthesia is adequate for airway instrumentation.
- There is often a temptation to accelerate the technique with i.v. agents or manual ventilation, which subverts the technique entirely.

- In practice the airway can easily be lost during this technique, without guarantee that the patient will wake promptly.

Inhalational technique

Traditionally an antisialagogue is administered. Depth of anaesthesia is slowly increased while the patient breathes

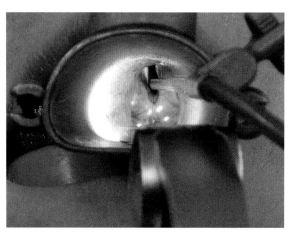

Fig. 23.52 High-pressure source ventilation via a surgical laryngoscope.

spontaneously. Sevoflurane is the volatile of choice and may be administered in 100% oxygen or with nitrous oxide. Once adequate depth of anaesthesia is achieved, laryngoscopy and tracheal intubation are performed.

Intravenous technique

The goals of maintaining spontaneous ventilation during induction can also be achieved with a slow, incremental TIVA technique. The main advantage of this technique is that the airway reflexes are ablated (rather than stimulated with an inhalational technique) and this may enable assessment of ease of ventilation at very light depths of anaesthesia. Clearly the patient will not awaken if problems occur unless anaesthesia is stopped.

Management of the obstructed airway

The management of the obstructed airway represents a very dangerous, although uncommon, situation. Obstruction may occur from the pharynx to any point distally and may be due to many causes, including infection or trauma, but the most common cause is malignancy. The patient may present late or occasionally be referred incorrectly to the ICU team with a diagnosis of worsening asthma or chronic obstructive pulmonary disease, having failed to respond to treatment and perhaps *in extremis*. To manage these patients safely and achieve a successful outcome requires careful preparation, planning and good communication between anaesthetists, otolaryngology specialists, the operating theatre team and, in some situations, cardiothoracic surgeons.

Optimal management of the obstructed airway is controversial, but it is generally the case that airway obstruction becomes worse during anaesthesia because of supine positioning and loss of airway tone and reflexes. All approaches may lead to life-threatening complications (e.g. complete obstruction after induction of anaesthesia, haemorrhage or swelling in the airway). Involvement of anaesthetists and surgeons with appropriate experience is essential, and backup plans should be established and communicated to all.

Precise management depends on the level and cause of the obstruction, the urgency for intervention and several other factors. Assessment should determine the following factors:

- What is the level of the obstruction?
- What is the degree of obstruction?
- Is it fixed or variable?
- What is its cause (e.g. tumour, haematoma, infection)?
- Is it friable or likely to bleed?
- Has there been previous airway or neck surgery, or radiotherapy?
- Can the patient's airway be improved? If time allows, nebulised adrenaline or steroids may improve the airway for short periods. Heliox may be beneficial before anaesthesia in critical cases.
- Is there any important comorbidity?
- What is the surgical plan and preferred route for anaesthetic access? These patients illustrate the complexity of a shared airway, and there is no point in planning an anaesthetic approach which is not compatible with an agreed surgical plan.
- What is the urgency of the intervention? It is important to differentiate patients in whom anaesthesia is planned to achieve surgery to improve the airway from those in whom anaesthesia is necessary to secure the airway in order to preserve life.

Important features of the history and clinical examination are noisy breathing, waking up in the middle of the night fighting for breath (having a panic attack) and/or having to sleep in an upright position. These features enable the anaesthetist to determine the patient's best breathing position to be used during induction of anaesthesia. If a patient cannot tolerate lying flat when awake, that position is likely to be dangerous after induction of anaesthesia. Stridor (inspiratory noise) is a concerning sign as it represents significant upper airway narrowing; however, it is not always present, and patients with chronic obstruction may present with a very narrow airway and no stridor. Expiratory noise (wheeze) may indicate a lower level of obstruction.

Other than in the most urgent cases, or if the patient's condition makes it impossible, full investigation is warranted. This usually involves CT or MRI, nasendoscopy and lung function tests. Imaging is performed supine and is a static image; it does not necessarily reflect the airway in the sitting position or the dynamic nature of the obstruction. It is also important to note the date of any imaging; lesions may progress rapidly.

Nasendoscopy is underused by anaesthetists and, although discussion of the surgical findings may be useful, it is often sensible for the anaesthetist to perform awake nasendoscopy, even when a fibreoptic approach is not planned. Lung function tests, including flow-volume loops, may help in assessing the extent of physiological compromise and the level of the obstruction. If these tests are not possible, a walk test may be of value because it enables the accompanying anaesthetist to assess exercise tolerance and respiratory pattern and may elicit signs such as noisy breathing, which add information not acquired at the bedside.

Patients with an obstructed airway can be considered according to the level of obstruction.

Upper airway obstruction

In patients with upper airway obstruction, the cause is usually malignancy, trauma or infection affecting the larynx and other supraglottic structures such as the tonsils and tongue. The management depends on whether or not it is judged that tracheal intubation from above the vocal cords is going to be possible. Usually an informed decision can be made after nasendoscopy and imaging. If it is clear that tracheal intubation will not be possible, the safest approach is to perform a tracheostomy under local anaesthesia. Lesions of the base of the tongue and floor of the mouth often interfere with laryngoscopy, particularly if there has been previous surgery or radiotherapy. Where there is doubt, awake fibreoptic (or perhaps videolaryngoscopic) tracheal intubation is a safe method for trying to secure the airway.

Laryngeal lesions may interfere with all forms of tracheal intubation. Awake fibreoptic or videolaryngoscopic intubation may be options, but surgical technique may require unrestricted access to the larynx. Supraglottic (from above), transglottic (via a narrow 2–3 mm catheter placed through the cords) or transtracheal (via a catheter placed in the trachea) ventilation may all be options or necessities, and each requires attention and good communication between the anaesthetist and surgeon. Whichever method is chosen, a clear plan for airway management and back-up (including whether waking the patient is an option) is needed, with all relevant equipment and personnel present. A senior ear, nose and throat surgeon should be in the operating theatre and prepared to carry out immediate surgical cricothyroidotomy (or tracheostomy) if the airway is lost.

Mid-tracheal obstruction

A mid-tracheal obstruction presents an entirely different problem and is often caused by a retrosternal thyroid mass, although malignancies and infections also may be the cause (Fig. 23.53). In the presence of a thyroid mass, the onset

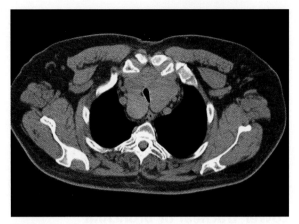

Fig. 23.53 A thyroid mass partially obstructing the mid trachea.

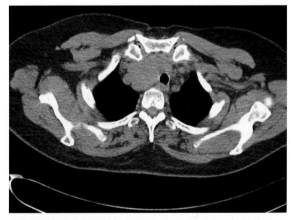

Fig. 23.54 A thyroid mass displacing but not narrowing the retrosternal trachea.

of airway compromise is usually slow and further radiological assessment is possible. A CT scan is vital to show the level and extent of the obstruction. Lesions below the larynx do not interfere with laryngoscopy (although the larynx and trachea may be displaced; Fig. 23.54) or the ability to use a face mask or SAD, but they may interfere with ventilation after induction of anaesthesia and the ability to insert a tracheal tube.

There are several key issues which must be clarified before anaesthesia.

- How wide is the tracheal lumen and what size of tracheal tube may be used? Remember it is the *external* diameter of the tracheal tube that is important here.
- Is there space below the obstruction and above the carina to accommodate the end of the tracheal tube and the cuff?
- Is the tracheal wall itself invaded? If so, there is a risk of collapse after any external mass has been removed.

501

- Would an eFONA be possible and would a standard tracheostomy tube be long enough to bypass the obstruction?
- Will surgery make the airway better or worse?

If laryngoscopy is predicted to be straightforward, there is no tracheal invasion and there is a clear distance below the obstruction and above the carina, a standard anaesthetic induction technique followed by administration of an NMBA can be considered. Otherwise, the safest way of securing the airway is likely to be awake fibreoptic intubation, although the problem of obstructing the airway while the obstruction is passed ('cork in a bottle') remains and may be distressing to the patient. A rapid tracheostomy would not be possible in this situation, so plan B is the use of a rigid bronchoscope by a skilled operator.

Lower tracheal or bronchial obstruction

Bronchial obstruction is a very difficult clinical problem, and life-threatening complications may occur. The cause is usually a malignant mediastinal mass, and obstruction of the superior vena cava often coexists. Sudden and total obstruction to ventilation can occur at any time, particularly if the patient becomes apnoeic or an NMBA is used. Sub-atmospheric intrapleural pressure during inspiration may contribute to holding the airways open; if lost, the pressure from any mass external to the airway can cause airway collapse and complete obstruction. A tissue diagnosis should be obtained under local anaesthesia if possible, and an emergency course of chemotherapy and/or radiotherapy should be considered; stenting or laser resection may be surgical options. Management is complex, and if possible, the patient should be transferred to a cardiothoracic centre where rapid induction of anaesthesia and skilled rigid bronchoscopy may be the technique of choice. Extracorporeal oxygenation may be required.

Tracheal extubation and recovery

Airway problems during emergence and in the recovery room account for approximately one third of major airway complications of anaesthesia. Most involve airway obstruction after tracheal extubation, some with secondary aspiration of fluid into the lungs. At the time of tracheal extubation, there is a change from a controlled situation, with airway protection, suppressed airway reflexes and the ability to deliver 100% oxygen, to one of absent airway protection, partial recovery of airway reflexes and an ability to reliably deliver only much lower oxygen concentrations. Airway obstruction which occurs during emergence and recovery needs to be rapidly recognised and resolved to prevent hypoxaemia and post-obstructive pulmonary oedema, which considerably worsens the situation.

Factors which increase the risk of problems at the time of extubation/emergence and recovery include:
- patients who had problems at induction or tracheal intubation;
- blood in the airway from surgical or anaesthetic causes;
- patients who may have airway oedema from anaesthetic or surgical interventions;
- obese patients, particularly those with OSA; and
- intraoral or airway surgery (risks both oedema and aspiration of blood).

Management of at-risk tracheal extubation requires recognition of the potential problems, planning, preparation, preoxygenation and, sometimes, special procedures. Communication with the operating theatre team is important because there is a natural tendency for the surgical and nursing team members to relax and attend to other tasks at the end of surgery.

Planning involves creating a strategy for tracheal extubation (plan A and backup plans), communicating this to assistants and colleagues and ensuring that the right equipment is immediately available and that personnel with the necessary skills are present. This may require having the difficult airway trolley present, summoning senior anaesthetic assistance or that the surgeon assists in the event that an eFONA is required. Planning also includes making a clear decision as to whether the airway will be removed with the patient 'deep' or awake.

Preoxygenation is part of preparation but is separated for emphasis; it is the single most important preparatory step before tracheal extubation.

Preparation involves optimising the patient for tracheal extubation. This includes (but is not limited to) ensuring full reversal of neuromuscular blockade (train of four ratio >0.9), adequate offset of anaesthetic and opioid medication, pharyngeal and bronchial suction as necessary and emptying the stomach if there is a risk of aspiration. Dexamethasone may be administered to minimise airway swelling, although its effect is delayed and its administration does not influence the immediate consequences of tracheal extubation. Direct inspection of the airway may be necessary to assess oedema and is specifically indicated when there has been blood in the airway to ensure that there is no risk of aspiration. A leak test may be performed in which the tracheal tube cuff is deflated and positive pressure applied while listening for an audible leak around the trachea. The test assesses only laryngeal swelling and is very dependent on the size of tracheal tube used and the pressure applied, so its efficacy in predicting safe extubation is limited.

Special procedures are non-routine actions at tracheal extubation performed to improve the safety of extubation and to facilitate reintubation if that is necessary. Examples include:
- insertion of a cricothyroid needle or AEC before tracheal extubation;

- exchange of the tracheal tube for a SAD immediately before (Bailey's manoeuvre) or after tracheal extubation; and
- tracheal extubation followed immediately by CPAP or high-flow nasal oxygen.

If it is considered that there is very high risk of airway compromise at tracheal extubation, an elective tracheostomy may be appropriate. Alternatively, tracheal extubation may be delayed and the patient transferred to ICU.

Guidelines on the management of tracheal extubation

In 2012, DAS published the first national guidance on extubation of adult patients (Fig. 23.55). This guidance divides tracheal extubation into four phases: plan, prepare, perform and postextubation care. It recommends that an early assessment is made to determine whether extubation

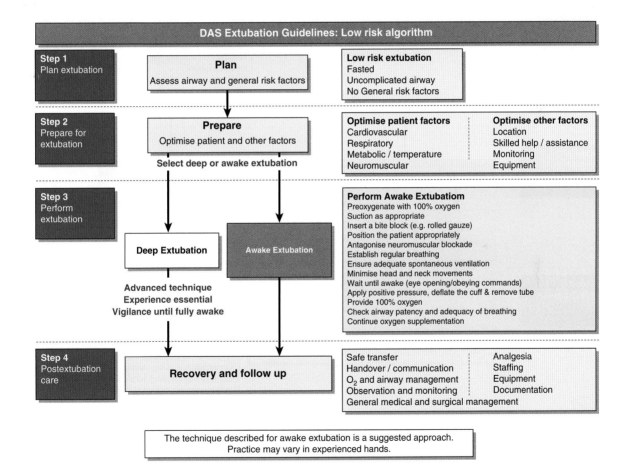

Fig. 23.55 Difficult Airway Society (DAS) tracheal extubation guidelines. (A) low-risk and (B) high-risk cases. *HDU,* High dependency unit.

Continued

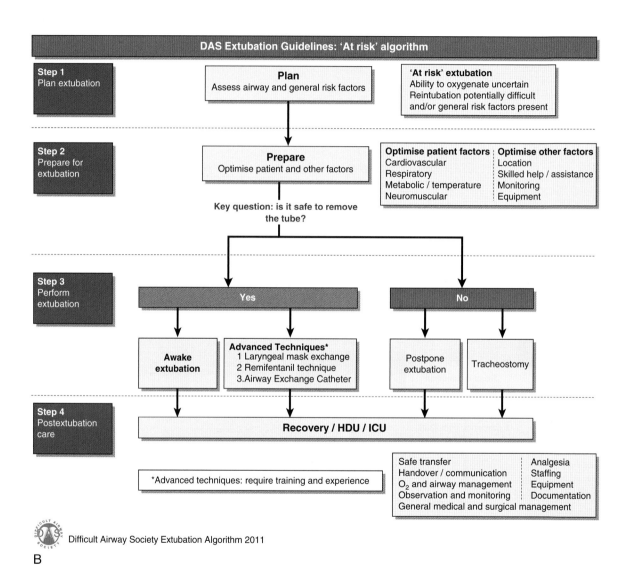

DAS Extubation Guidelines: 'At risk' algorithm

Step 1
Plan extubation

Plan
Assess airway and general risk factors

'At risk' extubation
Ability to oxygenate uncertain
Reintubation potentially difficult
and/or general risk factors present

Step 2
Prepare for
extubation

Prepare
Optimise patient and other factors

Optimise patient factors	Optimise other factors
Cardiovascular	Location
Respiratory	Skilled help / assistance
Metabolic / temperature	Monitoring
Neuromuscular	Equipment

Key question: is it safe to remove
the tube?

Step 3
Perform
extubation

Yes

No

**Awake
extubation**

Advanced Techniques*
1 Laryngeal mask exchange
2 Remifentanil technique
3. Airway Exchange Catheter

Postpone
extubation

Tracheostomy

Step 4
Postextubation
care

Recovery / HDU / ICU

*Advanced techniques: require training and experience

Safe transfer	Analgesia
Handover / communication	Staffing
O_2 and airway management	Equipment
Observation and monitoring	Documentation
General medical and surgical management	

Difficult Airway Society Extubation Algorithm 2011

B

Fig. 23.55, cont'd

is low risk (fasted, uncomplicated airway, no other risk factors) or high risk (all others). After taking the precautions described earlier, low-risk tracheal extubation can usually be managed awake or 'deep' according to the anaesthetist's preference and judgement, though the default method is awake. For patients requiring high-risk tracheal extubation, a number of options are offered:

* Awake tracheal extubation
* Advanced techniques as described earlier
* Delayed tracheal extubation
* Tracheostomy

Deep tracheal extubation in the high-risk setting is not advocated.

The difficult airway in other locations

A difficult airway is encountered most commonly in the operating theatre suite around the time of surgery, but most deaths from airway management difficulty occur elsewhere. At least a quarter of major airway events occur outside theatres, with ICU and emergency department being particularly important areas. When such events occur in these sites, the risk of injury is increased compared with the risk in the operating theatre environment. The reasons for this are complicated.

Patients in ICU are critically ill, with markedly reduced physiological reserve. Approximately 8% have a difficult airway. Most have pre-existing respiratory compromise and increased intrapulmonary shunt and, therefore, tolerate airway obstruction or apnoea very poorly. Initial tracheal intubation may be performed as an extreme emergency, and enabling the patient to wake if difficulty occurs is often not an option. Although intubation in ICU is accepted to be very high risk, a large proportion of critical airway events in this setting occur at a time well after tracheal intubation. Dislodgement of tracheal tubes and particularly tracheostomies, followed by airway difficulty, especially in the obese, is a notable cause of morbidity and mortality. The airway is often oedematous for a considerable period after prolonged tracheal intubation, and reintubation may be more difficult. The management of displaced tracheostomies is discussed in Chapter 37.

In the emergency department, patients often have reduced physiological reserve as a result of the pathophysiological problem that led to admission. Trauma is a specific condition in the emergency department which often increases the difficulty of airway management. The combination of an at-risk cervical spine requiring immobilisation of the neck, blood in the airway and multiple trauma with pulmonary injury and hypovolaemia is a major challenge.

There are also extrinsic factors which may lead to an increased likelihood of difficulty and to poor management of the difficult airway outside the operating theatre suite.

* Hazardous environment: an environment not designed for airway management and where this is sometimes not considered a main priority
* Failure to recognise and plan for patients with a known or predictably difficult airway
* A more limited range of equipment for management of the difficult airway than in theatres
* Less skilled intubators, if not from an anaesthetic background
* Lack of experienced and skilled assistance
* Absence of guidelines for management of routine airway problems (tracheostomy or tracheal tube displacement or failed RSI)
* Lack of routine use of capnography

Although some of these factors are unavoidable, many are not. All staff who manage the airway in ICU emergency department and in remote hospital locations should recognise that both patient factors and extrinsic factors interact to increase the likelihood of difficult airway management. Preparation for such difficulty is vital.

After difficult airway management

Although there is often considerable focus on securing a safe airway in patients with a predicted or known difficult airway, it is equally important to establish a strategy for future management if there is a need for further anaesthesia.

When the patient has recovered fully and before discharge from hospital, the senior anaesthetist involved should inform the patient of the relevant facts and the ways in which the difficulties experienced may affect future airway management. It is probably appropriate that any patient whose airway is *likely to prove difficult to manage during RSI by a junior anaesthetist* is given written information to that effect. The anaesthetic record should contain a clear record of the problem, what was done, what did and did not work, and a judgement as to the likely problems and solutions in the future. This information should be given to the patient, sent to the patient's general practitioner and filed in the hospital records. An example of a pro forma is shown in Fig. 23.56. The general practitioner should be asked to include the information in any future referrals. It may be appropriate for the patient to wear a medical alert bracelet.

Royal United Hospital, Bath

AIRWAY ALERT

Tel ....

Name	
Date of birth Hospital number	
Home address Telephone	
GP address Tel	

To the patient:
Please keep this letter safe and show it to your doctor if you are admitted to hospital.
Please show this letter to the anaesthetic doctor if you need an operation.
This letter explains the difficulties that were found during your recent anaesthetic, and the information may be useful to doctors treating you in the future.

To the GP:
Please copy this letter with any future referral.
READ CODE SP2y3 / ICD-10, T88.4 / SNOMED CT 718447001 Difficult intubation (finding)

Summary of Airway Management

Date of operation:

Type of operation:

		Reasons/comments
Difficult mask ventilation?	**YES/NO**	
Difficult SAD insertion	**YES/NO**	
Difficult direct laryngoscopy?	**YES/NO**	
Difficult videolaryngoscopy	**YES/NO**	
Difficult tracheal intubation?	**YES/NO**	
Laryngoscopy grade	1 / 2a / 2b / 3a /3b / 4	
Extubation		
Further investigation		

Equipment used:

Other information:

Is awake intubation necessary in the future?

Follow up care (tick when completed)

Copies of letter
YES/NO One copy to patient
YES/NO One copy to GP
YES/NO One copy in case notes
YES/NO One copy in anaesthetic department

YES/NO Spoken to patient
YES/NO Anaesthetic chart complete
YES/NO Information on front of case notes
YES/NO Medic Alert or Difficult Airway
          Society referral (Specify)

Name of anaesthetist:
Grade: Consultant   Date:

If you require further information please contact the Hospital.

Fig. 23.56 Airway alert. *GP,* General practitioner; *SAD,* supraglottic airway devices.

Chapter | 24 |

Pain

Lesley Colvin, Lorraine Harrington

The experience of pain is much more complex than nociception, where there is a reflex response to a noxious stimulus. The total pain experience is influenced by several factors, as outlined in the biopsychosocial model of pain (Fig. 24.1). Successful pain management depends on addressing all these aspects. Neuroimaging studies of pain reveal that multiple areas in the brain are activated in acute and chronic pain, the 'pain neuromatrix'. The International Association for the Study of Pain defines pain as *'an unpleasant sensory and emotional experience associated with actual or potential tissue damage, or described in such terms'*.

This definition highlights the subjective nature of the pain experience that can pose challenges in assessment and management; two individuals can suffer the same potential tissue damage, yet the experience of pain can be totally different, modulated by social and cultural factors. This effect of an individual's emotions can have a huge impact on their perception of pain. For example, the analgesic requirements for a straightforward elective Caesarean section are significantly less than for an elective uterine myomectomy, despite the operations being very similar in terms of surgical technique, approach and trauma.

Optimal management of both acute and chronic pain is important to allow early mobilisation after surgery or injury, reduce morbidity, and minimise long-term impact on function and quality of life. Pain management concerns postoperative, acute and chronic pain and cancer-related symptom control in children and adults. The RCoA and the Faculty of Pain Medicine (UK) have developed a comprehensive training curriculum to cover all these areas, with the majority of acute and chronic pain services being led by anaesthetists.

Acute pain

Acute pain is associated with body tissue injury and is thought to have evolved as a protective mechanism to prevent or minimise further tissue damage. Placing a hand in a fire causes pain, and the individual instinctively removes his or her hand. Once the hand is removed, the pain diminishes and further tissue damage is reduced. As the healing process begins and completes, the pain subsides and disappears. Acute pain should resolve within 6 weeks of the tissue injury repairing itself.

Organisation and objectives of the acute pain service

The Association of Anaesthetists have published guidelines that state: 'All hospitals performing major surgery should have a multidisciplinary acute pain team with an anaesthetist in overall charge and a senior nurse running the day-to-day basis'. The role of the acute pain service is aimed at improving analgesia, maintaining safety and education. In addition, in the long term, improvements may also be seen in morbidity and mortality and, potentially, duration of hospital stay. In broad terms these teams have the following functions:
- assessment of pain;
- standardisation of orders of analgesic preparations and monitoring of patients;
- education of nurses, doctors and staff allied to medicine who deal with patients who deal in acute pain;

507

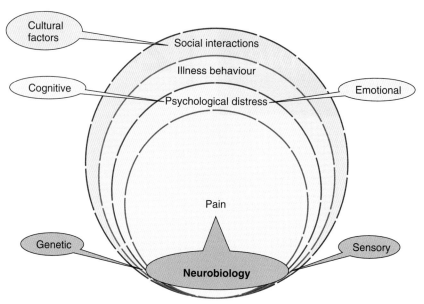

Fig. 24.1 An illustration of pain as biopsychosocial phenomenon.

- provision and monitoring of new or specialist analgesic methods;
- advice to staff on managing acute pain;
- constant evaluation of analgesic regimens (e.g. efficacy, adverse effects and safety);
- audit and quality improvement projects; and
- adherence to national standards

The teams are usually multidisciplinary but managed by senior nursing staff trained in pain management. Team members are often trained to manage and administer drugs via epidural systems or other local anaesthetic pumps; many have postgraduate qualifications in pain and are able to prescribe analgesia. Guidance and assistance, which are both practical and educational, are provided by a consultant anaesthetist trained in pain management. Trainee anaesthetists often form part of the pain team, either as part of their on-call or for modular pain training. Assistance at ward level is provided by a system of link nurses who have a special interest in pain management.

Pain teams now deal with a wide variety of pain problems, both surgical and medical. The move away from managing exclusively postoperative patients has undoubtedly improved pain control in all areas within the hospital. This is particularly true in medical wards, where, historically, pain was often left unmanaged. The acute pain team often reviews preoperatively those patients who have been identified as potentially having difficult to manage pain after surgery. This could be because of pre-existing chronic pain conditions or concomitant opioid use.

In patients with underlying chronic pain states, it should be anticipated that the patient will have a greater postoperative pain experience than normally expected. It is important this is discussed, consent obtained and an appropriate individualised analgesic regimen designed. In patients who are already regularly taking opioid medication, either appropriately as prescribed by their primary care provider (e.g. slow-release morphine or oxycodone formulations, fentanyl patches, methadone) or those sourcing opioids illegally (e.g. heroin), standard-dose opioid prescriptions will often leave the patient's pain unmanaged. Several issues need consideration:

1. Tolerance may have developed, and consequently a higher dose of opioid will be required to produce a similar level of analgesia, with a higher risk of adverse effects. The use of a regional anaesthetic technique and/or opioid-sparing analgesics should be considered, as these help reduce the overall opioid requirement.
2. The patient may have developed dependence, meaning withdrawal effects will occur if they do not receive an approximately equivalent opioid dose. This is particularly important to consider when a regional technique is used. Whilst the patient may be pain-free from surgery, they will still require opioid to prevent any withdrawal symptoms and provide analgesia for additional pain conditions. Symptoms of withdrawal may be relatively non-specific but can include anxiety, sweating, GI disturbance, myalgia and increased pain.
3. Opioid-induced hyperalgesia (OIH), where there is a paradoxical increase in pain as the dose is increased,

may occur. There are specific mechanisms by which this may occur, including activation of *N*-methyl-D-aspartate (NMDA) receptors.

There is greater awareness of the potential for some patients to have difficult manage pain after surgery, or indeed develop chronic postoperative pain. Such patients should be referred to the acute pain team for discussion of analgesic strategies. This allows a full assessment and individualised planning, with postoperative monitoring as appropriate. Discussions with surgeons may be beneficial in choosing the most appropriate surgical technique.

Pain measurement tools

Although pain is subjective, it is important to have validated scoring tools to assess the severity of a patient's pain and their response to analgesia. This guides ongoing analgesic therapy, quality improvement work and research. In addition, the importance of pain as a vital sign is well recognised and it is now routinely incorporated into scoring systems, such as the modified early warning score (MEWS). Often a sudden worsening in pain can suggest a serious underlying pathological condition, which may not be overtly obvious from other vital signs. For example, necrotising fasciitis, compartment syndrome or anastomotic leak can often be suspected from acutely worsening pain scores.

In the assessment of acute pain, unidimensional, straightforward self-reporting tools are more practical than the complex multidimensional time-consuming tools used in chronic pain or research (Table 24.1). The four main types of pain rating scales are as follows:

1. *Verbal rating scales.* Tend to be short, easy to administer and understand (e.g. mild, moderate or severe) but less accurate than other methods.
2. *Visual analogue scale (VAS).* Composed of an unmarked line 10 cm long. It is anchored with no pain at 0 and the worst pain imaginable at 100 on the right. Patients mark on the line where they think their pain lies, and this can subsequently be measured to give their actual pain rating. Traditionally the VAS has been recorded using pencil and paper, but electronic VAS recording is now available.
3. *Numerical rating scale (NRS).* Typically 11-point scoring systems, with 0 meaning no pain and 10 meaning the worst pain imaginable. Advantages of NRS systems are that the patient can compare with earlier delivered scores and scores can be transferred easily onto patient vital signs observation chart.
4. *Pictorial rating systems.* Devised for use in children. These are age-appropriate charts which allow children to select face images to describe their pain. These include the Faces Pain Score (FPS) and its revised version (FPS-R),

Table 24.1 Pain assessment tools with examples of suitable patient groups

Neonatal infant pain scale (NIPS)	Infants up to 1 year old
CRIES Pain Scale	Infants up to 1 year old
Wong-Baker FACES Pain Rating Scale	Children aged >3 years
Pain Assessment in Advanced Dementia (PAINAD)	Adults with dementia
Abbey pain scale	Adults with dementia
Assessment of discomfort in dementia protocol (ADD)	Adults with dementia
Critical-Care Pain Observation Tool (CPOT)	Sedated patients in the ICU
Behavioural Pain Scale	Sedated patients in the ICU

ICU, Intensive care unit.

Wong-Baker FACES Pain Rating Scale (Fig. 24.2) and the OUCHER scale. The FLACC (face, legs, activity, cry, consolability) Scale is used to assess pain in babies and younger children.

Other tools have been devised and validated for use in other groups of patients in whom traditional scoring tools would be difficult or inaccurate (see Table 24.1).

It is important to measure pain scores on movement as well as pain scores at rest and adjust analgesia appropriately. Effective relief of pain on movement is required for patients to deep breathe, cough and mobilise, reducing the risk of postoperative cardiorespiratory complications and facilitating earlier hospital discharge.

Irrespective of what tool is used, the information provided by the scoring tool must be used to guide analgesic therapy. Clearly if a high pain score is recorded, additional analgesia needs to be provided and the pain score reassessed in addition to recognising and managing any associated adverse effects.

Analgesic ladder

In 1986 the World Health Organization (WHO) devised the cancer analgesic ladder to assist with pain management in patients suffering from cancer. This has been adapted to provide a framework for providing symptomatic relief from

509

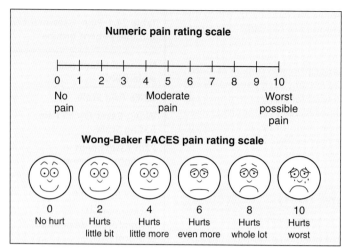

Fig. 24.2 Diagram showing numerical pain rating scale and Wong-Baker FACES Pain Rating Scale. (From Wong-Baker FACES Foundation. (2016) Wong-Baker FACES® Pain Rating Scale. Available from: http://www.wongbakerfaces.org/ (Accessed with permission 21 January 2018). Originally published in *Whaley & Wong's Nursing Care of Infants and Children.* © Elsevier Inc.)

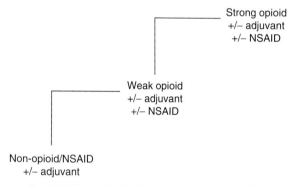

Fig. 24.3 World Health Organization analgesic ladder.

pain from multiple sources (Fig. 24.3). Whilst initially designed so that patients would be moved up each step if analgesia at that step of the ladder was insufficient, there is now a greater realisation that it may be more appropriate to start at a midpoint or higher, with adjuvants used as indicated by the pain type.

Analgesic strategy

When planning analgesia for the acute postoperative period, a multimodal strategy will deliver the best quality of analgesia with a minimum of adverse effects. This includes the appropriate regional or local anaesthetic technique in addition to choice of analgesic drugs. Regional anaesthesia (see

Chapter 25) has played a major role in delivering optimum perioperative anaesthesia and analgesia over extended periods of time. Options include epidural, intrathecal (spinal) or individual nerve/plexus blockade.

Epidural analgesia can provide excellent pain relief not just for labour but also for patients undergoing thoracic, abdominal, pelvic and orthopaedic surgery. Relatively small volumes of local anaesthetic delivered directly to the epidural space can effectively block pain transmission to groups of nerves and thus facilitate comfort and analgesia. Epidural infusion of small doses of opioid, clonidine or ketamine can enhance the epidural block achieved and reduce the local anaesthetic dose required. In addition to blocking pain transmission along A and C fibres (see Chapter 6), effective epidural analgesia also blocks the sympathetic chain with a consequent reduction in the surgical stress response (see Chapter 13). This has been demonstrated to reduce postoperative complications including ileus, thrombosis and pulmonary complications. Epidural analgesia is not, however, without risk. The 3rd National Audit Project (NAP3) report quantified the small, but potentially significant risk, associated with regional anaesthesia. This, coupled with a changing pattern leaning towards minimally invasive surgery, is leading towards a general reduction in the use of perioperative epidural analgesia.

Intrathecal injections of local anaesthetic are primarily used for surgical anaesthesia. However, the addition of long-acting intrathecal opiates (e.g. diamorphine 0.3–0.5 mg) is common in many surgical specialties, providing up to 24 h of good quality analgesia.

Local anaesthetic applied around a nerve plexus or individual nerves can effectively block pain transmission and thus postoperative pain (see Chapter 5). With the increasing use of ultrasound techniques, the risk of neuronal damage from nerve blocks is diminishing. The accuracy in placement of the local anaesthetic solution is increased with the use of ultrasound, theoretically improving the quality of the block provided. The duration of the block depends on the specific local anaesthetic solution placed, and an analgesic plan needs to be considered for when the block wanes or in the event of block failure.

Opioids

Opioids (see Chapter 6) form the backbone of most postoperative analgesic regimens. However, the increasing use of NSAIDs, paracetamol, local anaesthetics and adjuvants can reduce opioid requirements and potential opioid-related adverse effects.

Patient-controlled analgesia

For major surgery requiring opioid delivery postoperatively, patient-controlled analgesia (PCA) can be an effective technique. The key to this is that the patients themselves determine the rate of i.v. administration of the drug, thereby providing feedback control. That is, if a patient self-administers significant amounts of opioid and becomes sedated, he or she will stop pressing the delivery device; opioid delivery will cease until the sedation level decreases and further opioid can be self-administered.

Patient-controlled analgesia equipment (see Chapter 16) comprises an accurate source of infusion via an i.v. cannula and controlled by a patient–machine interface device. Safety features are incorporated to limit the preset dose, number of doses that may be administered and lockout period between doses. Morphine is the drug most commonly used with PCA. For opioid-naïve patients, the demand dose is usually 1–2 mg with a lockout period of 5–10 min. Fentanyl (10–20 µg) and oxycodone (1–2 mg) may also be used. The PCA pump may also be set with a background infusion rate. This can be particularly useful in patients who would normally take opioids before surgery or to allow high doses to be infused. There is, however, a slightly higher risk of overdose, as patients will continue to receive the opioid even when their conscious level may be impaired, thus negating the benefits of the feedback loop.

Intravenous PCA is a standard method of providing postoperative analgesia in hospitals worldwide. It provides superior pain relief compared to conventional intermittent subcutaneous (s.c.) or intramuscular (i.m.) administration of opioids. It is generally considered a safe technique, which can be managed by nursing staff on a general ward. The effective and safe use of PCA requires frequent monitoring of the patient. PCA charts are required to be completed by nursing staff hourly, with the patient's observations, including respiratory rate, sedation score, oxygen saturations, heart rate and blood pressure, recorded. In addition, most PCA pumps have inbuilt computers that allow staff to check the dose of opioid infused and number of requests for analgesia by the patient. These are valuable tools for assessing the adequacy of analgesia.

Many hospitals have standard protocols for setting up PCAs and use prediluted drug concentrations to minimise the risk of handling error. The use of PCA prevents any delay in the delivery of opioid. This potential delay is caused by the requirement to have a nurse, or in some situations, two nurses, collect the drug from the drug cupboard and perform the necessary checks before administering it to the patient. The immediate i.v. delivery of the drug minimises unnecessary delay in the patient receiving analgesia and allows for a predictable dose delivery independent of other physiological or pharmacokinetic considerations (see Chapter 1). After the insertion of the initial i.v. cannula, repeated injections are not required for further doses of analgesia, as occurs with i.m. analgesic regimens.

In patients unable to use PCA (because of impaired physical or cognitive function) or who do not require moderate doses of opioid, alternative routes of delivery are available.

Subcutaneous

A small-gauge s.c. cannula can be inserted relatively painlessly in patients who are likely to require the delivery of regular or as required opioid analgesia. After the initial insertion, repeated doses can be delivered to a patient without the need for further injections. The cannula can be left *in situ* for 2–3 days provided there is no evidence of infection. This can be particularly useful in older patients, children or adults with learning difficulties.

Intramuscular

Whilst i.m. injections were previously favoured as a route for opioid delivery, their use is now largely limited to situations where no other route is available. Intramuscular injection is painful and disliked by patients. Drug absorption is variable, particularly in patients with hypothermia, hypovolaemia, hypotension or excessive adipose tissue; this may result in the formation of a depot of opioid, which may be absorbed later and add to already adequate plasma concentrations of the drug, resulting in toxicity. In addition, there is an inevitable delay between the request for analgesia and subsequent administration while controlled drugs are checked and prepared.

Transdermal

Transdermal opioids are rarely used for acute postoperative analgesia. This is largely because of the delay in time from patch application to steady-state plasma drug concentrations being reached and variable drug absorption in the perioperative period (see Chapter 1). Fentanyl patches, however, are often used in step-down plans from epidural analgesia if there is uncertainty regarding gastric absorption, such as postoperative ileus or after GI surgery.

Oral

Oral opioids undergo extensive metabolism in the gut wall and liver (first-pass metabolism; see Chapter 1) and therefore bioavailability is low. However, if this is accounted for when dose prescribing, and there is no concern regarding gastric absorption, oral opioids can provide excellent postoperative analgesia without the need for i.v./s.c. cannulae or i.m. injections. In addition to the standard immediate-release opioid preparations, there is a selection of long-acting strong opioids that provide analgesia for up to 12 h; sustained-release preparations of morphine or oxycodone are typically prescribed. Similarly, oral preparations can be used to replace parenteral opioids when gastric absorption resumes and a predictable dose can be estimated. Oral preparations have the advantage that patients can be discharged home from hospital with these formulations, reducing the duration of hospital admission and potential for infection or thrombo-embolic complications. Importantly, as with all opioid prescriptions, a limited supply should be provided, with a clear end date to minimise the risk of dependency or drugs becoming abused within the community. Oral transmucosal fentanyl has been prepared as a palatable solid matrix (presented as a lollipop). The time of onset of pain relief is in the order of 9 min, and both transmucosal (buccal) and gastric routes contribute to the absorption of the fentanyl. These, along with effervescent fentanyl tablets, are only licensed for use in cancer pain and are therefore rarely used outside these settings.

Non-opioid adjuncts

Non-steroidal anti-inflammatory drugs

Non-steroidal anti-inflammatory drugs (NSAIDs; see Chapter 6) can provide excellent analgesia in the acute postoperative period. These drugs counteract inflammation and swelling caused by the trauma of surgery. They are particularly helpful in managing the nociceptive pain associated with orthopaedic surgery. Although some parenteral preparations of NSAIDs are available (e.g. diclofenac, parecoxib), these often require specific preparation and dilution, with dose titration over time. Consequently, these drugs are typically delivered intraoperatively. An alternative to the parental route of administration is to deliver the drug per rectum (p.r.); diclofenac and ibuprofen are available as suppositories. These are often inserted perioperatively and can deliver up to 12 h of analgesia as the suppository is absorbed slowly. NSAIDs have several potential adverse effects and therefore should be used with caution, especially in older patients (see Chapter 6).

NMDA receptor antagonists

Ketamine is an NMDA receptor antagonist (see Chapter 4) that has analgesic properties in subanaesthetic doses. Administration of low-dose ketamine can reduce postoperative opioid requirements and enhance the quality of analgesia produced, being particularly efficacious where there is a strong neuropathic component to the pain. Ketamine is useful when:

- the nature of the surgery results in high analgesic requirements;
- patients have a pre-existing opioid tolerance; or
- high dose-opioid use should be avoided because of the risk of respiratory complications.

Adverse effects, such as tachycardia, hypertension, agitation and hallucinations, are dose related and can be quite unpleasant. Ketamine can be given as an i.v. infusion (e.g. 5–15 mg h^{-1}) or bolus (0.2–0.3 mg kg^{-1}); however, care must be taken as the latter is more likely to precipitate adverse effects.

α_2-Agonists

Clonidine and dexmedetomidine are examples of commonly used α_2-agonists. When given perioperatively i.v. (clonidine 1–2 µg kg^{-1}, dexmedetomidine loading dose 0.5 µg kg^{-1} followed by an infusion of 0.1–0.4 µg kg^{-1} h^{-1}), there is an associated decrease in pain score intensity, opioid consumption and postoperative nausea and vomiting. Dose-related adverse effects include hypotension and bradycardia.

Lidocaine

When given perioperatively, i.v. lidocaine has anti-inflammatory, antihyperalgesic and analgesic properties. In colorectal surgery, an i.v. lidocaine infusion has been found to decrease postoperative pain, reduce the time for gut function to return to normal and reduce duration of stay. Lidocaine infusions typically consist of a 1.5–2 mg kg^{-1} bolus at the start of surgery with an i.v. infusion (1.33–3 mg kg^{-1}) continued for up to 24 h postoperatively. As yet, there is no consensus as to the optimal infusion regimen in terms of dose or duration. Disappointingly, the beneficial effects found in colorectal patients have not been replicated in other surgical settings. There is no absolute definition of the drug doses required to cause toxicity or the level of monitoring required postoperatively. Whilst many patients require admission to a high-dependency unit to facilitate monitoring for potential cardiac complications after major surgery, a greater pressure on bed availability has led some units to deliver lidocaine infusions to patients on the ward.

Gabapentinoids

The gabapentinoids, gabapentin and pregabalin, are licensed for the management of chronic neuropathic pain, epilepsy and anxiety but over the last 10 years have also been used as adjuncts in acute pain management. They are particularly useful in patients who have a neuropathic component of postoperative pain or acute neuropathic pain.

The use of gabapentin preoperatively has been found to improve functional recovery, with earlier mobilisation and pulmonary function postoperatively. This is presumed to be due to the opioid-sparing effects of gabapentin and consequent reduction in opioid adverse effects. The optimal perioperative dose is uncertain, but doses of 300–600 mg are commonly used. The main adverse effects are sedation, dizziness and nausea, particularly when the drug is administered for the first time preoperatively. Pregabalin has a worse adverse effect profile, with visual disturbance, sedation, somnolence and nausea all reported despite a variation in doses (225–600 mg). Consequently there is no absolute consensus on the use of the gabapentinoids perioperatively,

and the risk of harm needs careful consideration, particularly in the older or frail patient population.

Inhalational analgesics

Entonox and methoxyflurane are discussed in Chapters 3 and 44, respectively.

Rescue analgesia

The key to prescribing rescue analgesia is to assess the patient and determine why the current analgesia regimen has been ineffective (Table 24.2).

The implementation of the WHO analgesic ladder (see Fig. 24.3) is an effective means of stepping up the analgesia provided. However, it is not always appropriate to begin at the bottom. For example, if a patient who has undergone major abdominal surgery wakes in pain (because the patient has not pressed the PCA whilst asleep), a bolus dose of opioid may be required to allow the patient to become comfortable again. Conversely, a patient receiving regular paracetamol and ibuprofen after minor surgery may only require an oral weak opioid to achieve better analgesia. Hence the important steps are to:

- assess the patient using an appropriate pain scoring tool (see Table 24.1);
- calculate what analgesia has been given and where this is on the analgesic ladder;
- consider stepping up to the next level or increasing the drug dose at the current level; and

---

Table 24.2 Management of inadequate pain control

Potential reason for ineffective analgesia	Suggested management
Patient not receiving prescribed analgesia	Address underlying cause, such as lack of trained nurses; route of prescription or drug not available; fault with PCA.
Impaired patient communication about pain	Explain to patient importance of regular maintenance analgesia and inform nursing staff of alternative scoring tools (e.g. for dementia, children, etc.; see Table 24.1).
Insufficient analgesia prescribed	Increase doses prescribed, both regular and as required.
Pre-existing opioid tolerance	Increase opioid prescription doses; consider adding non-opioid adjunct.
Neuropathic component to pain	Consider non-opioid adjunct, such as ketamine, gabapentin (see Table 24.7).
New pathophysiology contributing to pain	Ensure surgical/medical review in parallel with managing analgesia.
PCA, Patient-controlled analgesia.	

- reassess the patient after analgesic delivery to ensure an appropriate response has been achieved.

Acute preoperative pain

Managing acute pain before surgery is as important as treating postoperative pain. The same basic formula should be applied, beginning with pain assessment and then commencing a multimodal strategy derived from the WHO analgesic ladder. It is also important to consider any possible psychological upset related to the illness and that abnormal physiology may persist despite adequate analgesia. Acute physiological changes (e.g. acute kidney injury, hypovolaemia) affect the pharmacokinetics and pharmacodynamics of analgesic agents, and dose reduction may be necessary. Frequent reassessment is required to ensure adequate analgesia without significant adverse effects.

The route of drug administration should be considered. Gastrointestinal absorption is unpredictable in the presence of an abdominal pathological condition or severe pain. The enteral route may be best avoided as inadequate absorption of analgesics will result in persistent pain. In patients with sepsis, where skin blood flow is variable, s.c. injections are best avoided; in addition to the potential for initial underdosing, as peripheral perfusion improves, rapid absorption of the subcutaneous drug depot may cause dangerous adverse effects (e.g. delayed respiratory depression with s.c. morphine). The same considerations apply to transdermal opioid patches. If a patient presents with an opioid patch *in situ*, it is best to remove the patch and substitute with a more controlled method of opioid delivery, such as PCA with background infusion.

The role for regional anaesthesia in acute preoperative pain is small but may be invaluable in some circumstances. In vulnerable older patients, proximal femoral fractures are associated with significant morbidity and mortality, which may partly relate to opioids prescribed for pain. Regional techniques, such as femoral nerve or fascia iliaca blocks (see Chapter 25), are simple to perform, can be done in the emergency department and reduce opioid requirements. In patients with a high opioid requirement, such as intravenous drug abusers, opioid-tolerant patients or patients with major trauma, adequate analgesia may be impossible to achieve with opioids alone because the high doses needed carry a significant risk of respiratory depression. Such patients may also benefit from regional techniques if applicable. If regional anaesthesia is not appropriate (e.g. because of the site of trauma or risk of bleeding), small doses of i.v. ketamine ($0.2-0.3$ mg kg^{-1}) may be useful. Ketamine has the advantage of working synergistically with opioids to enhance the quality of analgesia without the potential for adverse effects such as hypotension or impairment in respiratory function. Care should also be taken when managing a patient who has received significant amounts of opioid and then has his or her painful stimulus removed (e.g. joint relocation or performance of regional technique). These patients may subsequently develop respiratory depression or impaired consciousness, especially if multiple agents have been used.

Paediatric pain

Managing pain in children in the acute postoperative period should follow the same basic principles as for adults – that is, a multimodal technique with regional anaesthesia, if applicable, and regular assessment. There are, however, a few additional specific considerations in children.

Most drug doses are calculated according to patient weight. Consequently, meticulous attention needs to be paid when calculating doses of all drugs to avoid overdose and inadvertent adverse effects. This is especially true in neonates and premature babies, in whom enzyme handling systems may not have fully matured, resulting in longer drug metabolism or excretion times. Examples of typical analgesic drug doses are shown in Table 24.3.

The use of codeine is now restricted to children aged >12 years with acute moderate pain because of the unpredictable metabolism of codeine and potential for morphine toxicity. In addition, a risk of serious or life-threatening adverse reactions to codeine was identified in children with obstructive sleep apnoea after tonsillectomy or adenoidectomy. Consequently, codeine is now contraindicated in all children aged <18 years who have obstructive sleep apnoea.

With considered the use of regional techniques, adequate analgesia for most paediatric day surgery can be provided using paracetamol, NSAIDs and a local anaesthetic block (e.g. caudal). Local anaesthetic techniques are discussed in detail in Chapters 25 and 33.

If simple analgesia and use of a regional technique is either insufficient or inappropriate, an opioid should be used. Ideally this will be prescribed orally, in an appropriate

Table 24.3 Analgesic doses for paediatric patients

Drug	Dose
Paracetamol	15 mg kg^{-1} every 6 h (if < 50 kg; max 60 mg kg^{-1} per 24 h)
Ibuprofen	5–10 mg kg^{-1} every 6 h (if > 5 kg weight; max 2.4 g per 24 h)
Diclofenac	1 mg kg^{-1} every 8 h (if > 6 months of age)
Morphine (i.v.)	0.1–0.2 mg kg^{-1}
Fentanyl	1–2 µg kg^{-1}

dose according to body weight. Older children may understand and be able to use a PCA, but younger children, neonates or children with learning difficulties may require a background opioid infusion with appropriate monitoring or nurse-controlled analgesia (NCA). A variety of PCA handsets more suited to children are available.

Pain in pregnancy

Pregnant patients need special consideration when prescribing an appropriate analgesic regimen for non-labour pain. Some drugs cross the placenta (see Chapter 43) and thus could potentially harm the fetus. For example, NSAID use (except aspirin) in the first trimester is associated with an increased risk of miscarriage and fetal malformations, and use in the third trimester is associated with premature closure of the foetal ductus arteriosus. Other drugs, such as opioids, are generally considered safe if used in the short term. Long-term use, however, is associated with neonatal abstinence syndrome. Whilst no drug is without risk, a balanced approach needs to be taken, with consideration of the individual risk/benefit ratio in each case.

The use of antineuropathic pain medication during pregnancy is difficult. There are minimal published data on the safety or efficacy of these drugs in pregnancy. An increased risk of miscarriage and fetal anomalies has been reported, particularly with the gabapentinoids, in patients inadvertently becoming pregnant whilst taking them. Hence, these agents are not routinely prescribed in pregnant patients; a full risk/benefit analysis should be considered and discussed with the patient before their use.

Sickle-cell crisis

Patients with sickle-cell disease can present in crisis, where sickling of the haemoglobin leads to vaso-occlusion and subsequent tissue hypoxia and necrosis. These attacks can vary in severity and duration, with the worst requiring i.v. opioid and several nights' hospitalisation. As with all pain conditions, patients should be assessed and their pain managed as per the WHO analgesic ladder, commencing on the most appropriate step. Patients with sickle-cell disease are rarely opioid naïve, and thus potentially higher doses of opioid may be required.

Patients with burns

The tissue damage caused by burns can be extensive, and patients can suffer severe pain from both the injury and

during treatments (e.g. dressing changes). Partial thickness burns cause more pain than deep burns because nervous tissue is preserved. Patients with burns often require high-dose opioids to manage their pain. In addition, neuropathic pain is a common phenomenon, and ketamine or a gabapentinoid is commonly used.

Acute to chronic pain

Unrelieved acute pain may lead to chronic pain, with a variety of factors that may increase an individual's risk of developing persistent pain. These may include:
- type of surgery;
- younger age;
- female sex;
- preoperative pain;
- severe pain in the immediate postoperative period;
- high doses of opioids postoperatively;
- psychological factors (e.g. anxiety, catastrophising); and
- pre-existing vulnerability (e.g. genetic factors, reduced descending noxious inhibitory control (DNIC))

The management of acute and chronic pain overlaps in many areas. Pain is increasingly viewed as a continuum rather than two separate entities, with subsequent merging of management techniques and staff.

Chronic pain

Recent advances in the understanding of the fundamental mechanisms involved in the transmission and modulation of noxious impulses have significantly extended the range of assessment tools and treatments that clinicians can offer to patients with pain (see Chapter 6). With increasing awareness of the complexity of the pain experience there has been recognition that a multidisciplinary approach involving anaesthetists/pain specialists, psychologists, physiotherapists, occupational therapists and nurse specialists is the preferred management model. Pain management clinics are available in most hospitals in the United Kingdom, with variation in the services offered locally. Some offer specialist clinics for specific conditions (e.g. pelvic pain clinic, paediatric pain clinic) or treatments (e.g. spinal cord stimulators).

Current health trends are focusing on the delivery of pain management services in primary care and the community. Early involvement of the patient as an active participant in treatment and including self-management strategies as part of the management plan should help minimise long-term disability.

Epidemiology

Understanding the epidemiology of chronic pain is important, as it allows us to identify modifiable risk factors and to develop maximally effective healthcare systems to address the problem. Around 18% of people will suffer from chronic pain at some point during their life, with 10%–15% having moderate to severely disabling pain. Chronic pain is the presenting complaint in at least 22% of primary care consultations and is estimated to account for 4.6 million primary care visits per year. Patients with persistent pain consult primary care services five times more often than those without. Many patients with persistent pain have significant functional, social and financial consequences, with a major impact on their quality of life. Mood and sleep disturbances, sickness absence and job loss are common.

The incidence of chronic pain increases with age, with around 40% of older adults affected. There is also an association with social deprivation, mental health problems and female sex. Genetic factors are still poorly understood, although there are multiple genes associated with chronic pain, and there is a possibility that some individuals may be more vulnerable to developing chronic pain.

Assessment of chronic pain

Patients present with pain as a result of many different pathological processes. Some examples of chronic pain conditions are shown in Box 24.1, with some definitions of relevant clinical terms shown in Table 24.4. The first step in successful pain management is proper assessment. To address all the issues, a full biopsychosocial assessment is required (see Fig. 24.1). Although chronic pain has been accepted as a chronic long-term condition, it is important to ensure that all appropriate tests and investigations have been carried out to exclude any treatable causes. It is essential to not just determine pain intensity but also to assess other aspects of chronic pain and its impact. The Initiative on Methods, Measurement and Pain Assessment in Clinical Trials (IMMPACT) has recommended that clinical trials assessing new analgesics do more than just measure changes in pain intensity. A number of core domains have been suggested that are also applicable in the routine clinical setting (Table 24.5).

Pain history

The key elements of a pain history should be ascertained using a structured interview to address the domains outlined in Table 24.5. The interview should include assessment of the pain, effect of pain on the patient's mood and the impact of the pain on quality of life and functioning. Many patients

---

Box 24.1 **Common conditions associated with chronic pain**

Malignant causes

Primary tumour(s) or metastases

Non-malignant causes

Musculoskeletal
- Back pain
- Osteoarthritis
- Rheumatoid arthritis
- Osteoporotic fracture

Neuropathic
- Trigeminal neuralgia
- Post-herpetic neuralgia
- Brachial plexus avulsion
- Radicular pain of spinal origin
- Peripheral neuropathy
- Complex regional pain syndrome (CRPS)

Visceral
- Urogenital pain
- Pancreatitis

Postoperative
- Phantom pain
- Stump pain
- Scar pain
- Post-laminectomy pain

Ischaemic
- Peripheral vascular disease
- Raynaud's phenomenon/disease
- Intractable angina

Cancer treatment related
- Surgery
- Chemotherapy
- Radiotherapy

Headaches

---

with pain become physically deconditioned, and their mood can deteriorate. The assessment can be recorded using tools such as the Brief Pain Inventory, which can be useful for monitoring changes in pain over time and with treatment. Key elements in a pain history include the following:
- Mode of onset
- Location and radiation (a pain diagram can be helpful)
- Frequency
- Precipitating, aggravating and relieving factors
- Pain intensity using a scale (see Table 24.1)
- Pain quality, to determine a possible somatic or neuropathic cause (e.g. burning, shooting; several validated screening tools, e.g. the Leeds Assessment of Neuropathic Symptoms and Signs (LANSS), are available)
- Current and previous treatments (analgesics and others; prescribed medication often does not reflect actual medication as compliance can be variable)

Table 24.4 Definitions of pain and related terms

Term	Definition
Pain	An unpleasant sensory and emotional experience associated with actual or potential tissue damage or described in terms of such damage
Acute pain	Pain associated with acute injury (including surgery) or disease
Chronic or persistent pain	Pain that either occurs in disease processes in which healing does not take place or persists beyond the expected time of healing[a]
Allodynia	When a normally non-painful stimulus is perceived as painful; may be mechanical (e.g. light touch) or thermal (e.g. pain from touching cool or warm surfaces)
Hyperalgesia	Increased or exaggerated pain from a painful stimulus
Pain management programme	Usually a group-based multidisciplinary programme for patients with persistent pain and disability using cognitive behavioural principles

[a]Arbitrarily 3 months, although for persistent postoperative pain some definitions use 2 months as a cut-off point.

Table 24.5 Suggested core domains for assessment in chronic pain

Domain	Areas to assess
Pain	Location, intensity, character
Physical function	Include activities of daily living and social functioning
Mood/emotional function	Anxiety, depression and distress
Sleep	Duration and quality
Quality of life	Can use a standardised tool (e.g. EQ-5D)
Relations with others	Family, friends, social support
Effect of any treatments	Efficacy and adverse effects should both be assessed; global improvement

Adapted from Dworkin RH, Turk DC, Farrar JT, Haythornthwaite JA, Jensen MP, Katz NP, Kerns RD, Stucki G, Allen RR, Bellamy N, Carr DB. Core outcome measures for chronic pain clinical trials: IMMPACT recommendations. *Pain*. 2005 Jan 1;113(1):9–19.

- Concurrent conditions and medical history (including history of mental health issues and drug and alcohol misuse)
- Basic psychological assessment (including mood, coping skills, pain beliefs and self-reported disabilities); if required, a full psychological evaluation should be performed by a psychiatrist or by a clinical psychologist with expertise in pain management
- Impact on different aspects of life (sleep, work, activity, family life, etc.)
- Family and social history
- Patient's own ideas as to causation and expectations of treatment

Many patients, especially older patients and those with malignancy, have more than one site of pain, and separate histories should be taken for each complaint because their causes may differ. Particular care and skill are needed when taking a pain history from children and older patients.

Physical examination

A physical examination relevant to the pain complaint should be performed and may include a full musculoskeletal or neurological assessment. Signs implicating involvement of the sympathetic nervous system, including vasomotor, sudomotor and trophic changes, should be considered. Physiotherapy assessment may be part of the initial screening interview.

Investigations

Additional laboratory, radiological and electrophysiological tests may be needed for full evaluation. It is important to ensure that all relevant tests and investigations have been carried out, particularly in those patients who have seen many different healthcare professionals, or where factors may have affected their ability to attend for requested investigations (e.g. substance misuse population). It is important, however, to avoid overinvestigation, and investigations should only be carried out if they are likely to change management.

Explanation

Chronic pain is a complex phenomenon and often multifactorial in aetiology. The diagnosis, where possible, is based on history, examination and results of any investigations. Classification of the pain aids treatment decisions in some cases, but many pains are of mixed aetiology. The pain complaint and results of any investigations should be discussed with the patient. This may involve an explanation that there is no obvious structural explanation for the pain, impressing upon the patient that this is a reflection of our currently inadequate methods for imaging pain and does not imply that the pain is imagined. A patient-led problem list should be formulated and patient expectations for treatment should be explored and, if necessary, rationalised. The limitations of the medical model of disease for some chronic pain complaints should be explained.

Chronic pain syndromes

Chronic pain syndromes can adversely affect the patient in various ways, including depressed mood, fatigue, reduced activity and libido, excessive use of drugs and alcohol, dependent behaviour and disability out of proportion to impairment. It does not respond to the medical model of care and is best managed with a multidisciplinary approach.

Classification of pain

Pain may be classified according to its cause. This can be useful where there are specific treatment options. However, the assessment and impact of chronic pain are often not specific to cause. The Scottish Intercollegiate Guidelines Network (SIGN) guidance on the management of chronic pain (see Further Reading) gives an evidence-based approach to assessment and management.

Nociceptive pain

Nociceptive pain results from tissue damage causing continuous nociceptor stimulation. It may be either somatic or visceral in origin.

Somatic pain
Somatic pain results from activation of nociceptors in cutaneous and deep tissues, such as skin, muscle and subcutaneous soft tissue. Typically it is well localised and described as aching, throbbing or gnawing. Somatic pain is usually sensitive to opioids.

Visceral pain
Visceral pain arises from internal organs. It is characteristically vague in distribution and quality and is often described as deep, dull or dragging. It may be associated with nausea, vomiting and alterations in blood pressure and heart rate. Stimuli such as crushing or burning, which are painful in somatic structures, often evoke no pain in visceral organs. Mechanisms of visceral pain include abnormal distension or contraction of smooth muscle, stretching of the capsule of

solid organs, hypoxaemia necrosis or irritation of viscera by algesic substances. Visceral pain is often referred to cutaneous sites distant from the visceral lesion. One example of this is shoulder pain resulting from diaphragmatic irritation. Hyperalgesia (increased response to a stimulus which is normally painful) can occur in visceral pain. There are three types:

1. *Visceral hyperalgesia*: increased sensitivity in the painful organ. Pain threshold is lowered in some patients with functional GI disease and patients complain of abdominal pain in response to normally innocuous stimuli of the gut.
2. *Referred hyperalgesia*: from viscera, in which hypersensitivity is localised in the muscles and often associated with a state of sustained contraction. For example, patients with urinary colic typically display hypersensitivity in the muscles of the lumbar region.
3. *Visceroviseral hyperalgesia*: pain in one visceral organ can be enhanced by pain in another visceral organ. Women with repeated urinary stones who were also dysmenorrhoeic manifested a higher number of episodes of renal colic than non-dysmenorrhoeic women.

Neuropathic pain

Neuropathic pain is defined as 'pain arising as a direct consequence of a lesion or disease affecting the somatosensory system'. It is characteristically dysaesthetic in nature and so patients complain of unpleasant abnormal sensations. There may be marked allodynia (a normally non-painful stimulus, such as light touch, evokes pain), and pain can be described as shooting or burning and may occur in areas of numbness. Neuropathic pain may develop immediately after nerve injury or after a variable interval. It is often persistent and can be relatively resistant to opioids.

There are many causes of neuropathic pain. Lesions in the peripheral nervous system include peripheral nerve injuries, peripheral neuropathies, HIV infection, some drugs and tumour infiltration. Central neuropathic pain is associated with lesions of the central nervous system, such as infarction, trauma and demyelination, and is very resistant to treatment.

Complex regional pain syndrome

Complex regional pain syndrome (CRPS) was previously known as sympathetically-maintained pain because of the postulated involvement of sympathetic nerves or circulating catecholamines. It is considered a form of neuropathic pain. Sympathetic nerve blocks may provide at least temporary reduction of pain, but current thinking is that this does not imply a mechanism for the pain. It is classified into two types, although this distinction does not influence treatment:

Type 1 CPRS. A minor injury, including mild soft tissue trauma or a fracture, precedes the onset of symptoms, without any overt nerve lesion (Fig. 24.4).
Type II CPRS. Develops after injury to a peripheral nerve.

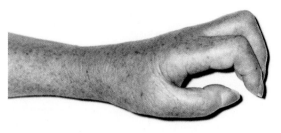

Fig. 24.4 Complex regional pain syndrome (CPRS) type I after Colles' fracture.

Pain is the prominent feature in CPRS. It is characteristically spontaneous and burning in nature and associated with allodynia (abnormal sensitivity of the skin) and hyperalgesia. Autonomic changes may lead to swelling, abnormal sweating and changes in skin blood flow. Atrophy of the skin, nails and muscles can occur, and localised osteoporosis may be demonstrated on a radiograph or bone scan. Movement of the limb is usually restricted as a result of the pain, and contractures may result. Treatment is directed at providing adequate analgesia to encourage active physiotherapy and improvement of function, with some evidence for graded motor imagery and spinal neuromodulation being helpful.

Management of chronic pain

Total relief of persistent pain is rarely possible; it is therefore important that patients are given information on strategies to reduce the impact of the pain on their everyday life. These self-management strategies should include advice about the importance of remaining active, increasing fitness levels, planning and pacing all activities and avoiding overactivity/ underactivity cycles. Self-management booklets and online resources, such as the Pain Toolkit (www.paintoolkit.org), can be given to patients.

A management plan should be formulated jointly with the patient after discussion of appropriate treatments, the potential benefits and adverse effects of those options and the option of deciding against treatment. Several methods of treatment may be used in the same patient, either concomitantly or sequentially. Some of the management options available are shown in Fig. 24.5, with most effective management often requiring a multidisciplinary approach using a range of individualised strategies.

Physical therapies

There is good evidence for the effectiveness of increasing physical activity in improving outcomes from chronic pain.

There is no clear evidence of what type of exercise is best (e.g. land- or water-based activities). It is likely that this is down to individual circumstances and preference. The marked fear/avoidance of activity that can accompany established chronic pain needs to be addressed to allow an increase in activity levels. Activities can range from very basic household activities to more formal supervised exercise programmes. Advice alone is insufficient to increase activity levels, with additional intervention and support needed for many chronic pain patients.

Psychological therapies

Pain is not merely a sensation of tissue damage, but a complex interaction of biochemical, behavioural, cognitive and emotional factors. Unless all these factors are addressed effectively, long-term management is unlikely to be successful. There is good evidence for the use of cognitive behavioural therapy (CBT) and related approaches to allow patients to self-manage their chronic pain and improve their quality of life and coping strategies. A cognitive and behavioural approach investigates how thoughts (often negative) and behaviours (often maladaptive) reinforce the chronic pain state. Other psychological approaches using relaxation, mindfulness and acceptance and commitment therapy (ACT) can also be used. A clinical psychologist is an important member of the pain management team.

Pain management programme

A pain management programme is a psychologically based rehabilitative treatment for patients with chronic pain in which physical therapies and psychological techniques are delivered by a multidisciplinary team to maximise function and quality of life. It is usually delivered in a group format, either as a daily intensive programme or spaced out over a number of weeks. Key clinical staff include a doctor, clinical psychologist, physiotherapist and occupational therapist, all of whom should be trained in pain management. Information and education about the nature of pain and its management, medication review and advice, psychological assessment and intervention, physical reconditioning, advice on posture and graded return to the activities of daily living are components of pain management programmes. There is good evidence of efficacy, although there is a drop-off in treatment effect over time.

Pharmacological therapies

Many patients in pain are prescribed analgesic drugs. The pharmacology of most of these agents is discussed elsewhere (see Chapter 6) and only aspects of particular relevance to their use in chronic pain are mentioned here.

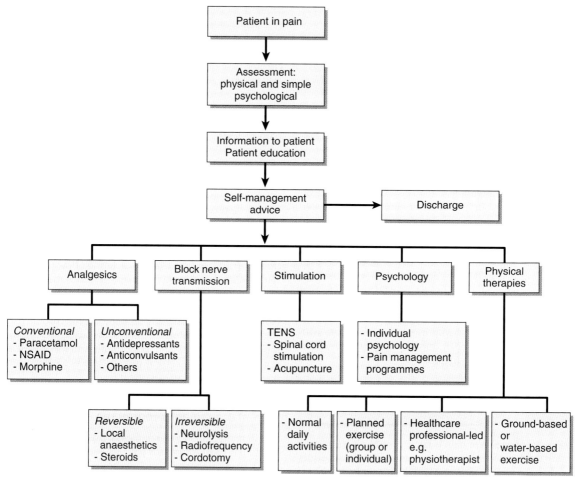

Fig. 24.5 Management pathway for patient in pain. *TENS*, Transcutaneous electrical nerve stimulator. (Adapted from Moore, A., Edwards, J., Barden, J., & McQuay, H. (2003) *Bandolier's little book of pain*, Oxford, Oxford University Press.)

Cancer pain

Approximately 75% of patients with advanced cancer develop significant pain before death. Most cancer pain responds to pharmacological measures, and successful treatment is based on simple principles that have been promoted by the World Health Organization. As with chronic pain, a full biopsychosocial assessment is needed. Many patients will have more than one site and/or type of pain, with each needing full assessment. If possible, medication is given orally unless intractable nausea and vomiting occur or there is a physical impediment to swallowing.

Analgesic drugs should be taken regularly and according to the analgesic ladder (see Fig. 24.3). The first step is a non-opioid, such as paracetamol, or an NSAID. If this is

inadequate, a weak opioid such as codeine is added. The third step is substitution of the weak opioid with a strong opioid. Inadequate pain control at one level requires progression to a drug on the next level rather than to an alternative of similar efficacy. There is some debate as to the role of step 2 of the analgesic ladder, with an alternative approach being to add in a strong opioid (at an appropriate dose) much earlier to optimise symptom control. Adjuvant analgesics, such as tricyclic/serotonin-noradrenaline reuptake inhibitor (SNRI) antidepressants or anticonvulsants, may be used at any stage.

Using these strategies, pain may be controlled successfully in about 90% of patients with cancer pain without resorting to other interventions. In the remaining 10%, some form of anaesthetic intervention may be indicated. Other treatments also need to be discussed with the oncology team, such as palliative radiotherapy for bone pain or chemotherapy to reduce disease progression. Communication among palliative medicine, oncology and pain specialists is important to ensure treatment is delivered as and when needed.

Non-cancer pain

Paracetamol. Paracetamol (4 g daily) is a better analgesic than placebo, but probably not as effective as NSAIDs. However, in the older patient, paracetamol may be useful because of its low adverse effect profile. Dose reduction should be considered in frail patients (e.g. 500 mg qds)

NSAIDs. NSAIDs possess analgesic and anti-inflammatory actions and are used widely in the management of mild to moderate pain. They are effective analgesics for pain from osteoarthritis, rheumatoid arthritis and dysmenorrhoea. NSAIDs are not without adverse effects, including an increased incidence of GI tract ulceration, adverse effects on renal function and increased thrombotic risk. This has resulted in the European Medicines Agency stating that NSAIDs should be used in the lowest effective dose for the shortest possible duration.

Opioid analgesics. These are covered in detail in Chapter 6. Weak opioid drugs, such as dihydrocodeine, may be useful for moderate pain, although they may be less useful in the longer term. As with all opioids, they may be taken in excess, and often with only little benefit, by the patient with chronic non-malignant pain.

The use of strong opioids in non-malignant pain is controversial, with limited evidence of long-term benefit and accumulating evidence of harm, including increased mortality, misuse, dependence, hyperalgesia, endocrine dysfunction, GI problems, increased fracture risk and increased risk of cardiovascular events. The RCoA and SIGN have published useful guidance for clinicians and patients on the clinical use of opioids (see Further Reading). When opioids are used, long-acting preparations may be more useful for chronic pain than immediate-release preparations.

Morphine is the strong opioid used most commonly. Immediate-release oral morphine, either in liquid or tablet form, can be given as often as necessary in increasing dosage until pain is controlled. When the required daily dose has been established, it is usual to convert to sustained-release morphine tablets, which need to be taken only once or twice daily. If breakthrough dosing is needed, for example, in cancer pain, the dose of morphine necessary to treat breakthrough cancer pain is one-sixth of the total daily morphine requirement. For example, if the patient is taking morphine 120 mg b.d., the breakthrough dose is (120 + 120) / 6 = 40 mg; this can be prescribed as required every 4 h.

Physical dependence normally occurs, and patients should be warned not to stop opioids precipitously. Nausea and vomiting may occur when treatment with morphine is started, and an antiemetic should be prescribed for the first week; this can then often be stopped. Sedation and cognitive impairment may occur as the dose is increased, but these usually resolve. There is no tolerance to the constipating effect of morphine, and laxatives need to be taken regularly. A phenomenon of OIH has been described, in which the patient suffers increasing pain, often of a widespread nature. The treatment of OIH involves decreasing the dose of opioid, switching to another opioid or the use of centrally acting analgesics such as ketamine.

Continuous subcutaneous administration of opioids is an alternative method of administration if oral medication cannot be taken, although this is rarely appropriate for non-cancer pain. A small, portable battery-operated syringe driver is usually used. Because of its greater solubility, diamorphine is the drug of choice in the UK for this route of administration. A conversion ratio of 3 mg oral morphine to 1 mg s.c. diamorphine is used.

Opioids may also be administered via the epidural or intrathecal routes for patients whose pain is controlled effectively by oral opioids but who suffer intolerable adverse effects (e.g. drowsiness or vomiting) or whose pain cannot be controlled by the use of oral or systemic opioids. These routes can be used for chronic pain, although there is limited evidence of long-term benefits. Much smaller doses of drug are required when given intrathecally, and thus adverse effects are minimised. The daily dose of morphine via the epidural route is 1/10 of the daily oral dose, and the intrathecal dose is 1/10 of the epidural dose. Adverse effects, such as respiratory depression, itching and urinary retention, which cause such concern in the opioid-naïve patient are rare in cancer patients who have been chronically exposed to systemic opioids.

Adjuvant analgesics. Adjuvant analgesics are drugs which may have primary indications for conditions other than pain but have an analgesic effect in certain situations. A recent comprehensive systematic review and meta-analysis outlines a suggested evidence-based approach to the treatment for neuropathic pain, where adjuvant agents are most commonly used (Table 24.6).

Anticonvulsants. Anticonvulsants are primarily used in the treatment of neuropathic pain. The precise mechanism of action varies among different agents. For example, it is thought that carbamazepine blocks activity-dependent sodium channels and gabapentin and pregabalin act on the $\alpha_2\delta$ subunit of the calcium channel. Therefore, if one anticonvulsant at maximum dosage is ineffective, then it is worthwhile trying another. Gabapentin, pregabalin, carbamazepine, oxcarbazepine, lamotrigine and phenytoin can be used for neuropathic pain and trigeminal neuralgia. Sedation, ataxia and weight gain are common adverse effects of these drugs and may limit dose escalation, especially in older patients.

521

Table 24.6 Evidence-based pharmacological treatment for neuropathic pain

Recommendation	Treatment	Daily dose
First line	Gabapentin Pregabalin SNRIs (e.g. duloxetine) TCA (e.g. amitriptyline)	1200–3600 mg in three divided doses 300–600 mg in two divided doses 60–120 mg 25–150 mg in two divided doses
Second line	Capsaicin 8% patches Lidocaine patches Tramadol	30–60 min treatment every 3 months Once a day for up to 12 h 200–400 mg in divided doses
Third line	Strong opioids	Individual titration

SNRIs, Serotonin-noradrenaline reuptake inhibitors; *TCAs*, tricyclic antidepressants.
(Adapted from Finnerup, N. B., Attal, N., Haroutounian, S., et al. (2015) Pharmacotherapy for neuropathic pain in adults: a systematic review and meta-analysis. *Lancet Neurology*. 14, 162–173.)

Tricyclic and SNRI antidepressants. Tricyclic and SNRI antidepressants have a role in the management of pain, independent of their effect on mood. Tricyclic drugs and SNRIs are postulated to act as analgesics by reducing the reuptake of the amine neurotransmitters noradrenaline and serotonin into the presynaptic terminal, increasing the concentration and duration of action of these substances at the synapse and thereby enhancing activity in the descending inhibitory pain pathway. Tricyclics also block sodium channels and suppress ectopic neuroma discharge. Amitriptyline is the most common tricyclic drug prescribed as an analgesic, and the normal starting dose is 10–25 mg at night. Adverse effects include sedation (which can be beneficial), constipation and a dry mouth. Other tricyclic drugs used as analgesics include imipramine and nortriptyline. Selective serotonin reuptake inhibitors (SSRIs), such as fluoxetine, appear to be relatively ineffective analgesics.

Antiarrhythmic drugs. Sodium channel blockers may be used to reduce pain caused by nerve damage. Intravenous lidocaine (bolus of 1–2 mg kg^{-1}, followed by infusion of 0.5–3 mg kg^{-1} h^{-1}) can be used to reduce neuropathic pain, although there is a limited evidence base. Although oral mexiletine does block sodium channels and has been used for neuropathic pain, evidence would recommend against its use because of inefficacy and adverse effects.

Ketamine. Ketamine (see Chapter 4) has been used successfully as an analgesic via intravenous, subcutaneous and oral routes. Psychometric adverse effects may be a problem.

Capsaicin. Capsaicin is an alkaloid derived from chillies which acts at the transient receptor potential vanilloid receptor (TRPV1), which is also activated by noxious heat stimuli. It is used topically either as a cream (0.025%–0.075%)

applied up to four times per day or as a single application of a high-dose 8% plaster that can be repeated after 12 weeks. It selectively denervates C fibres expressing the TRPV1 receptor. The cream can be used for osteoarthritis, with limited evidence for neuropathic pain, whereas the patch is licensed for neuropathic pain.

Cannabinoids. Animal studies suggest that cannabinoids reduce hyperalgesia and allodynia in neuropathic, inflammatory and cancer pain. Human trials have also reported modest benefit in neuropathic pain. Cannabinoids act on CB_1 receptors, which are located in the brain, and CB_2 receptors found peripherally. Current clinical evidence is limited, with international guidelines giving a weak recommendation against use of cannabinoids. Further research is needed to identify which cannabinoids may produce analgesia without psychotropic adverse effects.

Interventional pain therapies. Therapeutic interventional therapies in the management of chronic and malignant pain have been performed for many years and include various types of nerve block and minimally invasive surgical procedures. There has been discussion and controversy regarding effectiveness, but significant progress has been made over the last two decades in establishing some evidence base for their use. Such techniques are often included as part of the multidisciplinary management of chronic pain.

For chronic pain management, a nerve block often comprises an injection of a local anaesthetic combined with steroid, although the optimal dose and type of steroid has not been established and it is not licensed for some blocks around a peripheral or central sensory nerve, sympathetic plexus or trigger point. The use of neurolytic agents is predominantly restricted to cancer pain management. Correct use of interventional procedures in the treatment

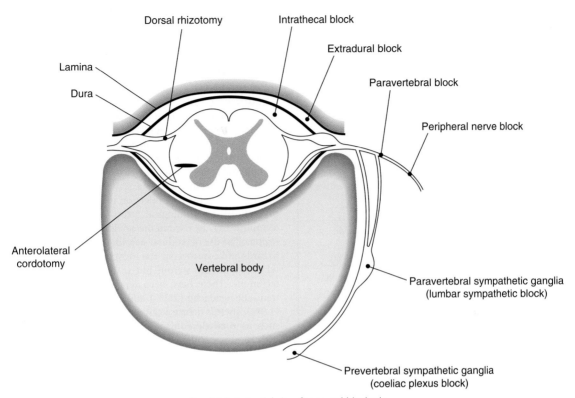

Fig. 24.6 Potential sites for neural blockade.

of chronic pain requires an experienced practitioner with a thorough knowledge of anatomy and an understanding of pain syndromes. Interventions should be undertaken in appropriate locations, usually ambulatory surgery theatre suites, by clinicians who are fully acquainted with the techniques involved and who are competent to manage the complications that may arise. The use of radiological imaging and contrast media, ultrasound guidance or peripheral nerve stimulation is strongly advocated to confirm accurate needle placement. Potential sites for neural blockade are shown in Fig. 24.6, and indications for neural blockade are listed in Table 24.7. For a full description of the techniques of neural blockade, the reader should consult more detailed texts (see Further Reading).

Local anaesthetics. Local anaesthetics block sodium channels (see Chapter 5) and may be used for both diagnostic and therapeutic injections. They have been injected into muscle trigger points for the relief of myofascial pain, and it has been shown that prolonged relief of pain may result from local anaesthetic blocks to peripheral nerves.

Botulinum toxin. Botulinum toxin has been used for the treatment of temporomandibular dysfunction, migraine and vulvodynia.

Neurolytic techniques. Neural destruction can be produced by chemical or thermal means. In general, the use of neurolytic techniques has diminished in the last two decades. There are many reasons for this, including the improved use of analgesic drugs, recognition that the effect of neuroablative procedures is often transient, the development of neurostimulatory techniques and appreciation of the cognitive and behavioural elements of pain. The clinical indications for neurolytic techniques are now limited to patients with cancer pain and a few selected non-cancer conditions. Careful thought with regard to the potential benefits and risks of the procedure, appropriate patient selection and fully informed consent are essential.

The most common neurolytic agents used are phenol and ethyl alcohol. Phenol acts by coagulating proteins and destroys all types of nerves, both motor and sensory. The most common indication is for lumbar sympathetic block for peripheral vascular disease. Large systemic doses cause convulsions followed by central nervous system depression and cardiovascular collapse. Alcohol is the neurolytic agent of choice for coeliac plexus block in patients with intractable abdominal pain from pancreatic cancer, when the large

Table 24.7 Indications for neural blockade

Nerve block	Indications
Trigger point injections	Myofascial pain, scar pain
Somatic nerve block	Nerve root pain, scar pain
Trigeminal nerve block and branches	Trigeminal neuralgia
Stellate ganglion block	SMP, CRPS
Coeliac plexus block	Intra-abdominal malignancy, especially pancreatic
Superior hypogastric plexus block	Malignant pelvic pain
Lumbar sympathetic block	Ischaemic rest pain, SMP, CRPS, phantom and stump pain
Epidural steroids/root canal injections	Nerve root pain, benign or malignant
Lumbar and cervical medial branch blocks	Back pain, whiplash cervical pain
Intrathecal neurolytics	Malignant pain
Percutaneous cervical cordotomy	Unilateral somatic malignant pain, short life expectancy

CRPS, Complex regional pain syndrome; SMP, sympathetically maintained pain.

volume required prohibits the use of phenol. It produces a higher incidence of neuritis than phenol and is not used for other blocks.

Radiofrequency lesioning. Radiofrequency is indicated for patients in whom non-invasive treatments have failed. A destructive heat lesion is produced by a radiofrequency current generated by a lesion generator. The radiofrequency electrode comprises an insulated needle with a small exposed tip. A high-frequency alternating current flows from the electrode tip to the tissues, producing ionic agitation and a heating effect in tissue adjacent to the tip of the probe. The magnitude of this heating effect is monitored by a thermistor in the electrode tip. Damage to nerve fibres sufficient to block conduction occurs at temperatures above 45°C, although in practice most lesions are made with a probe tip temperature of 60°C–80°C. An integral nerve stimulator is used to ensure accurate positioning of the probe. Whereas the spread of neurolytic solutions is unpredictable, radiofrequency lesions are more precise. Lower-temperature lesions are now being used in an attempt to produce analgesia without nerve destruction in pulsed radiofrequency lesioning. Radiofrequency lesions of the trigeminal nerve may be used

to treat trigeminal neuralgia in the older patient whose pain is uncontrolled by anticonvulsant drugs and who is unsuitable for microvascular decompression. Radiofrequency lesions of spinal nerves (most commonly the medial branch of the dorsal ramus supplying facet joints) are used in some spinal conditions.

Corticosteroids. Corticosteroids have been found to block transmission in normal unmyelinated C fibres and to suppress ectopic neural discharges in experimental neuromas. They are sometimes added to local anaesthetics in nerve blocks and for injection into painful scars.

Epidural steroids have been used for more than 50 years for nerve root pain. Either a standard epidural injection or a targeted nerve root injection may be used, depending on indication; radiological screening is important. This technique may be used in the cervical, thoracic and lumbar regions. The use of epidural steroids is not without potential hazards and controversy. The most common adverse effects relate not to the steroid but to technical aspects of the technique. There have been reports of dural tap (2.5%), transient headache (2.3%) and transient increase in pain (1.9%). There is debate around the use of particulate steroids, such as methylprednisolone acetate and triamcinolone, with non-particulate steroids, such as dexamethasone, a potentially safer option because of the risk of harmful effects if injected inadvertently into the subarachnoid or subdural spaces.

Medial branch block of the dorsal ramus (lumbar and cervical facet nerve blocks). Chronic back and neck pain are common complaints in pain management clinics, and lumbar and cervical facet joints may be causative. Injections of local anaesthetic and steroid into both lumbar and cervical facet medial branch nerves are performed commonly, although there is controversy about long-term benefit. Radiofrequency lesions of the facet nerves have been reported to give long-term relief in appropriately selected patients.

Sympathetic nerve blocks. Visceral nociceptive afferents travel in the sympathetic nervous system to the spinal cord. Visceral pain tends to be less opioid-sensitive than somatic pain. Percutaneous sympathetic blocks may, therefore, be useful in the management of severe cancer-related visceral pain which is poorly controlled with opioids or controlled only with intolerable adverse effects.

Percutaneous coeliac plexus block using 50% alcohol is one of the most commonly used and effective blocks performed for cancer pain. It is used for pain resulting from upper GI neoplasms, in particular carcinoma of the pancreas. Radiological screening, either X-ray imaging or CT, is mandatory, although this does not ensure absence of complications. Hypotension, especially postural hypotension, should be anticipated and managed appropriately. Serious complications are rare but include paraplegia. The superior hypogastric plexus innervates the pelvic viscera. Superior hypogastric

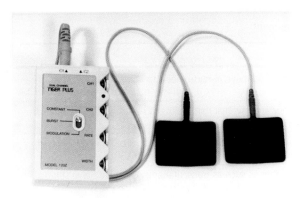

Fig. 24.7 Transcutaneous electrical nerve stimulator (TENS).

plexus block with phenol has been used for pelvic pain from cervical, prostatic, colonic, rectal, bladder, uterine and ovarian malignancy and for rectal tenesmus.

Chemical lumbar sympathectomy using phenol is performed for inoperable ischaemic leg pain. Radiological screening using contrast medium is necessary to ensure correct positioning of the needle. The most common complication is genitofemoral neuralgia (4%–15%).

Stellate ganglion and lumbar sympathetic block with local anaesthetic is sometimes helpful in the treatment of sympathetically mediated pain, CRPS types I and II, amputation stump and phantom pain.

Transcutaneous electrical nerve stimulation. Transcutaneous electrical nerve stimulation (TENS) is based on the gate control theory of pain. It is thought that large-diameter primary afferents exert a specific inhibitory effect on dorsal horn nociceptive neurons and that stimulation of these fibres alleviates pain. Conventional TENS produces high-frequency, low-intensity stimulation which relieves pain in the area in which it produces paraesthesia. Stimulation variables of TENS may be altered to produce low-frequency acupuncture-like TENS, which unlike conventional TENS produces analgesia that is antagonised by naloxone. A small battery-powered unit is used to apply the electrical stimulus to the skin via electrodes (Fig. 24.7). These are placed over the painful area, on either side of it or over nerves supplying the region, and stimulation is applied at an intensity which the patient finds comfortable. Adverse effects are minimal, with allergy to the electrodes being the most common problem encountered. The presence of a pacemaker is the main contraindication. TENS is used for a variety of musculoskeletal pains and has been advocated recently for refractory angina. Tolerance to TENS does occur sometimes; it may be possible to overcome this by changing stimulation variables.

Spinal cord stimulation. The National Institute for Health and Care Excellence (NICE) has produced guidance recommending spinal cord stimulation as a treatment option for adults with severe chronic neuropathic pain. Electrical stimulation may be applied to the spinal cord via electrodes implanted surgically or positioned percutaneously in the epidural space under radiological guidance. To be effective, the stimulating electrode must be positioned to produce artificial paraesthesia in the distribution of the pain. It is usual practice for the patient to undergo a period of trial stimulation. Patients showing substantial improvement in pain relief and other outcome measures may be considered for permanent implantation of a battery-driven stimulus generator.

Acupuncture. According to Chinese philosophy, *chi*, the life force, circulates around the body in pathways termed meridians. Injury and illness can block the flow of *chi*, causing pain and disease. Acupuncture is believed to release these blocks and balance the energy of the patient. Traditionally, acupuncture points are stimulated by the insertion of fine needles, which are then rotated manually or stimulated by heat (moxibustion) or electrically. Acupuncture is widely used for treating chronic pain, and yet there is little evidence that it is effective in the long term.

Costs of pain management services

There is little information on the costs of pain management services. A detailed study of the costs incurred by users of specialty pain clinic services in Canada found that users incurred less direct healthcare costs than non-users with similar conditions. Similar results were reported by a small study of NHS pain clinic attendees. This found that the pain clinic covered its costs by reducing consumption elsewhere and by reducing GP consultations and private treatments.

Advances in knowledge of pain pathophysiology and new methods of brain imaging, such as functional MRI and positron emission tomography scanning, and increasingly close co-operation between scientists and clinicians have led to a better understanding of mechanisms sustaining chronic pain and an increase in therapeutic options. In addition, the increasing acceptance by the medical profession and the general public of the importance of psychological factors in chronic pain has opened up new treatment opportunities. There is evidence of the effectiveness of many of the treatments used in the management of chronic pain, but further work is needed on those interventions for which information is lacking and in identifying which patients may benefit most from specific treatments. It is clear, however, that a multidisciplinary approach is most likely to be successful. Key components of this are outlined in Table 24.8.

Table 24.8 Key components in multidisciplinary pain management

Treatment approach	Comments
Physical therapy	Good evidence base of efficacy and minimal harm; need to address barriers such as fear avoidance
Psychological therapy	Good evidence base of efficacy and minimal harm; aims to reduce distress and teach psychological techniques for long-term self-management
Pharmacological therapy	Good evidence base of variable efficacy; adverse effects of agents; limited long-term studies in some areas; complete pain relief unusual
Stimulation techniques	Ranges from simple, low-risk options such as transcutaneous electrical nerve stimulation (TENS) to more invasive techniques such as spinal cord stimulation (SCS)
Injection therapy	Range of techniques, very limited evidence base; includes nerve root injections, radiofrequency lesioning (e.g. facet joint injections)

References/Further reading

Faculty of Pain Medicine. Clinical use of opioids. https://www.rcoa.ac.uk/faculty-of-pain-medicine/opioids-aware/clinical-use-of-opioids.

Faculty of Pain Medicine. Opioids Aware: A resource for patients and healthcare professionals to support prescribing of opioid medicines for pain. https://www.rcoa.ac.uk/faculty-of-pain-medicine/opioids-aware.

Finnerup, N.B., Attal, N., Haroutounian, S., et al., 2015. Pharmacotherapy for neuropathic pain in adults: a systematic review and meta-analysis. Lancet Neurol. 14, 162–173.

Moore, R.A., Straube, S., Wiffen, P.J., Derry, S., McQuay, H.J., 2009. Pregabalin for acute and chronic pain in adults. Cochrane Database Syst. Rev. (3), Art. No.: CD007076, doi:10.1002/14651858.CD007076.pub2.

Scottish Intercollegiate Guidelines Network 2013. Management of chronic pain. http://www.ckp.scot.nhs.uk/Published/PathwayViewer.aspx?id=608.

SIGN Guideline Development Group (Chair L Colvin), 2013. SIGN 136: Management of chronic pain. http://sign.ac.uk/guidelines/fulltext/136/contents.html -71.

The Association of Anaesthetics of Great Britain and Ireland, 2010. The anaesthesia team. AAGBI, London. https://www.aagbi.org/sites/default/files/anaesthesia_team_2010_0.pdf.

Wiffen, P.J., Derry, S., Bell, R.F., et al., 2017. Gabapentin for chronic neuropathic pain in adults. Cochrane Database Stst. Rev. (6), Art. No.: CD007938, doi:10.1002/14651858.CD007938.pub4.

Wong-Baker FACES pain rating scale. http://www.wongbakerfaces.org/.

Chapter | **25** |

Regional anaesthetic techniques

David Hewson, Jonathan Hardman

Regional anaesthetic techniques are used for both operative anaesthesia and postoperative analgesia. They are becoming more popular as a result of advances in drugs and equipment and improved techniques of anatomical localisation, particularly ultrasonic location. In addition, there is a greater appreciation of the need to improve postoperative pain control using techniques that not only reduce pain but also have the ability to abolish it and potentially improve outcome. This chapter outlines the basic principles of patient management in regional anaesthesia and the methods used in the performance of a variety of common neuraxial and peripheral nerve blocks. Regional anaesthetic techniques for obstetrics, ophthalmological and dental surgery, and airway instrumentation and tracheal intubation are described in other chapters.

Features of regional anaesthesia

Regional anaesthesia may be used alone or in combination with sedation or general anaesthesia, depending on individual circumstances. Neuraxial regional anaesthetic procedures include spinal, epidural or combined spinal-epidural techniques. *Peripheral nerve blockade* refers to any technique using local anaesthetic drugs to prevent transmission of nerve impulses along the course of one or more peripheral nerves.

Advantages of regional techniques include the following:

1. *Avoidance of the adverse effects of general anaesthesia.* These may range from relatively minor complaints such as postoperative nausea and vomiting or sore throat to major issues such as airway complications, aspiration pneumonitis, postoperative respiratory impairment, myocardial infarction or accidental awareness. In addition, the management of many patients with significant medical comorbidity, such as diabetes, obesity or pulmonary disease, can be improved or simplified by the use of regional anaesthesia. In older patients, postoperative cognitive dysfunction may be limited by reducing or avoiding psychoactive drugs associated with general anaesthesia and maintaining contact with their surroundings.

2. *Postoperative analgesia.* Regional anaesthetic techniques can be used to provide effective, prolonged postoperative analgesia whilst avoiding the systemic effects of other analgesic drugs, especially opioids. Analgesia can be provided using: long-acting local anaesthetics; continuous catheter techniques, either neuraxial or peripheral; or pharmacological adjuncts, either systemic or perineural. A common adjunct is dexamethasone, which usefully prolongs the analgesic duration of peripheral nerve blockade when given i.v. or when added to local anaesthetic and delivered perineurally as part of the peripheral nerve block itself (Chong et al 2017). If a long-acting local anaesthetic is used to provide prolonged postoperative analgesia, it is important that the nursing staff and the patient are aware of the risk of tissue damage to any blocked area, whether from direct trauma or indirect pressure from poor positioning or prolonged immobility. Simple techniques such as supporting the arm in a sling after brachial plexus block may help prevent injury and encourage earlier mobilisation.

3. *Preservation of consciousness during surgery.* The ability to assess neurological status continuously may be an advantage in patients with a head injury or diabetes or those undergoing carotid endarterectomy. Patient positioning may be safer and more comfortable and damage to pressure areas or joints avoided if the patient is awake. Airway and neck manipulation can be avoided; this may be especially important in a patient with severe rheumatoid arthritis or an unstable cervical spine.

4. *Sympathetic blockade and attenuation of the stress response to surgery.*

5. *Improved gastrointestinal motility and reduced nausea and vomiting.* This can allow earlier feeding and more rapid mobilisation and discharge.

There are now several studies suggesting that the net effect of these features may lead to a reduction in the incidence of major postoperative pulmonary complications, though claims of other pathophysiological benefits remain unproven. Some patients may be unhappy at the prospect of being awake during surgery. In this situation, the combination of a regional anaesthetic technique with target-controlled i.v. sedation or general anaesthesia may be valuable. Similarly, this combination works well for prolonged surgery, where patient positioning may be compromised by generalised discomfort or where surgery at several sites is necessary.

Complications of regional anaesthetic techniques

The incidence of complications may be minimised by ensuring adequate supervision and training in regional anaesthetic techniques and by exercising care in the performance of all blocks. Many anaesthetists recommend performing blocks in the awake (or lightly sedated) patient. This offers several advantages:

- it encourages careful, meticulous practice;
- it provides the anaesthetist with information on block onset and efficacy; and
- it alerts the anaesthetist to early complications such as inadvertent i.v. injection, signifying possible local anaesthetic toxicity, or intraneural injection, signifying possible nerve damage.

Sufficient expertise and equipment must always be available to deal with potential complications. Regional anaesthesia carries a small risk of injury to either the central or peripheral nervous systems (see Chapter 26). Anaesthetists should be familiar with the emergency management of total spinal anaesthesia, local anaesthetic toxicity and anaphylaxis because these are recognised complications of regional anaesthesia (see Chapter 27).

Patient assessment and selection

Careful preoperative evaluation is as important before a regional anaesthetic as it is before general anaesthesia and the same principles apply (see Chapter 19). It is inappropriate to proceed with surgery under local or regional anaesthesia for the sake of convenience in the poorly prepared patient.

- *Consent.* The preoperative visit should be used to establish rapport with the patient. A clear description of the proposed anaesthetic technique should be given in simple terms. Patients require an explanation of the reasons for selecting a particular regional technique, its advantages, material risks and alternatives. Consent should be an individualised process, considering the particular circumstances of the specific patient in question (see Chapter 21). There should be no attempt at coercion to accept a particular technique. An explanation that nerve blockade by local anaesthetic abolishes pain sensation but may preserve some sensation of touch, pressure and proprioception is often helpful.
- *Practical considerations and absolute contraindications.* Potential problems related to the intended block should be anticipated. Anatomical deformities or pain affecting patient positioning may render some blocks impractical. Contraindications to regional anaesthesia are discussed later.
- *Abnormalities of coagulation.* Anticoagulant therapy and bleeding diatheses are not automatic contraindications to the use of regional anaesthesia. The decision to perform neuraxial anaesthesia and the timing of catheter removal in a patient receiving antithrombotic therapy should be made on an individual basis, weighing the small but definite risk of vertebral canal or perineural haematoma against the benefits of regional blockade for a specific patient. The patient's coagulation status should be optimised at the time of needle or catheter placement and indwelling catheters should not be removed in the presence of therapeutic anticoagulation because this seems to increase the risk of haematoma significantly. Importantly, neuraxial techniques and peripheral nerve blocks at sites which are not externally compressible (e.g. the lumbar plexus) carry a higher risk of uncontrolled haemorrhage than those at easily compressible sites (e.g. the axilla). Close monitoring is vital to allow early evaluation of neurological dysfunction and allow prompt intervention where necessary.
- Anaesthetists must be familiar with all new classes of novel anticoagulant drugs because these are increasingly used. Tests of coagulation, including platelet count and function, prothrombin time and activated partial prothrombin time, are a useful adjunct to the decision-making process; however, the concept that particular test results alone can be applied to categorise a block as 'safe' or 'unsafe' is misleading and unhelpful. Guidelines for the use of neuraxial blockade in the presence of anticoagulants are shown in Table 25.1.
- *Pharmacological therapy.* The use of NSAIDs is not a contraindication to neuraxial or peripheral nerve block unless combined with other anticoagulant agents.
- *Cardiovascular comorbidity.* Sympathetic blockade with consequent vasodilatation may lead to profound hypotension, and this can be particularly dangerous in patients with significant aortic or mitral stenosis. Careful consideration

Table 25.1 Association of Anaesthetists recommendations for the performance of neuraxial procedures (spinal anaesthesia, epidural catheter insertion or removal, combined spinal-epidural techniques) in patients with normal renal function in association with drugs used to modify coagulation (Association of Anaesthetists 2013)

Drug	Acceptable time after drug dose for neuraxial block performance	Administration of drug while neuraxial catheter *in situ*	Acceptable time after neuraxial block performance or catheter removal for next drug dose
NSAIDs	No additional precautions	No additional precautions	No additional precautions
Aspirin	No additional precautions	No additional precautions	No additional precautions
Clopidogrel or prasugrel	7 days	Not recommended	6 h
Dipyridamole	No additional precautions	No additional precautions	6 h
Unfractionated heparin (i.v. treatment)	4 h or normal APTTr	Caution	4 h
LMWH (s.c. prophylactic dose)	12 h	Caution	4 h
LMWH (s.c. treatment dose)	24 h	Not recommended	4–24 h
Fondaparinux (prophylactic dose)	36–42 h (consider anti-Xa levels)	Not recommended	6–12 h
Fondaparinux (treatment dose)	Avoid (consider anti-Xa levels)	Not recommended	12 h
Warfarin	INR ≤ 1.4	Not recommended	After catheter removal
Rivaroxaban (prophylactic dose)	18 h	Not recommended	6 h
Rivaroxaban (treatment dose)	48 h	Not recommended	6 h
Dabigatran (prophylactic or treatment dose)	48 h (provided CrCl > 80 ml min^{-1})	Not recommended	6 h
Apixaban (prophylactic dose)	24–48 h	Not recommended	6 h
Thrombolytics (alteplase, reteplase, streptokinase)	10 days	Not recommended	10 days

APTTr, Activated partial thromboplastin time ratio; *CrCl*, creatinine clearance; *INR*, international normalised ratio; *LMWH*, low-molecular-weight heparin.

of the best way to maintain systemic vascular resistance during anaesthesia should be taken in such patients. Significant hypovolaemia must be corrected before contemplating spinal or epidural anaesthesia.

- *Neurological comorbidity.* There is no evidence that neuromuscular disorders or multiple sclerosis are adversely affected by regional anaesthetic techniques, but most anaesthetists use regional anaesthesia in such patients only if there are obvious benefits to be gained; any perioperative deterioration in the neurological condition may be associated by the patient with the regional anaesthetic procedure. Raised intracranial pressure is a contraindication to central neuraxial blockade, but peripheral techniques may be considered.

Selection of technique

Local anaesthetic drugs may be administered by:
1. single dose; and/or
2. continuous infusion or repeated intermittent bolus administration via an indwelling catheter.

It is essential that the technique selected is tailored to, and sufficient for, the planned surgery. The anaesthetist's primary objective is to ensure adequate intraoperative anaesthesia and/ or postoperative analgesia. The duration of surgery, its site (which may be multiple, e.g. the need to obtain bone graft from the iliac crest) and the likelihood of a change of procedure in mid-operation should all be considered. The problem of multiple sites of surgery can be met using one block that covers both sites or by more than one regional anaesthetic procedure where indicated. The duration of anaesthesia may be tailored to the anticipated duration of surgery by selection of an appropriate local anaesthetic agent or may require the use of a technique that allows further administration of drug through an indwelling catheter. If regional anaesthesia has been selected primarily to provide analgesia during and after surgery under general anaesthesia, a more peripheral technique that provides more selective sensory blockade with less motor impairment may be more appropriate.

Premedication

Premedication before performance of regional anaesthesia is very rarely required. Patient anxiety regarding being awake for block performance or surgery itself, is often very amenable to simple explanation and reassurance. It is helpful to enquire about specific patient concerns, such as being able to see or hear the procedure, because these are often easily addressed. A small dose of i.v. benzodiazepine is useful in some patients to achieve anxiolysis when performing a block. Nerve blocks can themselves sometimes be considered a form a premedication, such as a femoral nerve block performed to alleviate the pain of proximal femoral fracture before definitive surgical fixation. Patients undergoing regional anaesthesia should be fasted preoperatively in the same manner as if they were undergoing general anaesthesia.

Timing

A well-organised operating list will not be delayed by delivery of regional anaesthesia, which when conducted appropriately can improve theatre suite efficiency. It is essential that sufficient time is allowed to perform the block without undue haste on the part of the anaesthetic team. The risk of inadvertent wrong-sided nerve block is increased if time pressure and other distractions are allowed to impinge, even subconsciously, on the concentration of the anaesthetic team.

Regional block equipment

Needles

The use of very fine spinal needles (25–27G) reduces the incidence of postdural puncture headache (PDPH), as does the use of pencil-point Whitacre and Sprotte needles (Fig. 25.1). The 27G Whitacre needles appear to be associated with the lowest incidence of PDPH, but confident and successful use of these needles requires greater expertise than is needed for the use of larger needles.

For peripheral blocks, short-bevelled needles allow greater tactile appreciation of fascial planes and may reduce the

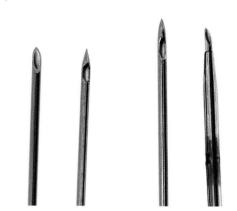

Fig. 25.1 Left to right: Quincke, Whitacre, Sprotte and Spinocath spinal needles.

likelihood of nerve damage because they displace nerves rather than penetrate them. A variety of insulated needles are available for plexus and peripheral nerve blockade using a nerve stimulator. Needle visibility during ultrasound guidance may be improved by using echogenic needles that have 'corner stone' reflectors positioned at the distal end of the cannula shaft. For peripheral nerve blocks, syringes are usually connected to the block needle via flexible tubing. This allows the anaesthetist to hold the needle steady while aspiration tests are performed and syringes are changed, as required. The system must be primed to prevent air embolism and to avoid ultrasound image artefacts.

Catheters

Continuous administration of local anaesthetic drugs has been made possible by the development of high-quality perineural catheters, which may be left in position for several days. Careful fixation is essential to maintain the position of the catheter in the postoperative period. Skin adhesive glues are useful in this regard because they provide excellent fixation and minimise leakage of local anaesthetic from the catheter puncture site. Catheters should be labelled clearly to prevent inadvertent injection of i.v. medication.

Non-Luer connection systems for regional anaesthesia

The accidental connection of an intravenous infusion line or syringe to an epidural, intrathecal or perineural needle or catheter (or vice versa) can result in fatal harm. The Luer connector has been in use for more than 100 years and has become the most common small-bore medical connection system. The ubiquity of the Luer system poses an intrinsic risk of inadvertent wrong-route administration of medication. International standard ISO 80369 applies a dedicated non-Luer connector (neuraxial connectors or NRFit) for epidural, intrathecal and perineural devices that cannot connect to intravenous Luer connectors, with the aim of reducing the risk of wrong-route drug administration. This represents a major change to the equipment of hospitals and is expected to take several years to implement fully.

Nerve stimulators

Few anaesthetists continue to use the historical technique of deliberately eliciting paraesthesia to confirm perineural needle tip position when performing a peripheral nerve block. Some anaesthetists use a peripheral nerve stimulator (Fig. 25.2), but an increasing number now use ultrasound guidance to identify needle tip placement. If using peripheral nerve stimulation, it is important to explain to the patient the sensation elicited by electrical stimulation; this usually causes very little discomfort, unless the contracting muscle crosses a fracture site, when duration of stimulation should be kept to the absolute minimum necessary to confirm needle position.

Stimulators that deliver a constant current and give a digital display of the current used are readily available. One lead is attached to an electrode on the patient's skin, and the other lead to the needle. After skin puncture, the stimulator is set to a frequency of 1–2 Hz and an initial current of 1–2 mA. Most stimulators have a visual display to confirm a complete circuit when the needle touches the patient. If this fails, connections should be checked or the electrode replaced. Failure to confirm a complete circuit could result in unwanted paraesthesia or nerve injury from repeated needling.

As the nerve is approached, motor nerve fibre stimulation causes muscle contraction in the appropriate distribution. The muscle contraction sought from nerve stimulation is often different from contractions resulting from direct contact of the needle tip with muscle tissue that overlies the target nerve. The current is reduced until visible muscle contraction is still present at a current of (optimally) 0.5 mA; reducing the current still further, the twitch should be seen to disappear when current is very low (e.g. 0.2 mA). A gentle aspiration test is then performed and 1–2 ml local anaesthetic solution slowly injected. Muscle contraction should cease immediately because of nerve displacement. If it does not, and an insulated needle is being used, the tip may have moved beyond the nerve or be placed intravascularly. In this circumstance gentle aspiration should be repeated, the needle withdrawn slightly and the procedure repeated. Severe pain on injection suggests intraneural injection, in which case the needle should be withdrawn and repositioned. When the needle tip has been correctly positioned, the remainder of the anaesthetic solution should be injected slowly with occasional test aspirations.

Ultrasound

A variety of high-quality ultrasound machines are now readily available and these have contributed greatly to advances in regional anaesthetic techniques. All ultrasound machines consist of a display, keyboard or touchscreen menu with transducer controls, computer processing unit and transducer. Many are also equipped with disk storage facilities or printers to allow a record to be made of procedures. The principles of ultrasound are discussed in Chapters 15 and 17. Production of a clear target image and safe needle guidance requires sound cross-sectional anatomical knowledge along with excellent technical skills.

The most common transducers used for ultrasound-guided regional anaesthesia are the linear or curved array probes. Linear high-frequency probes (8–12 MHz) are used to produce superficial images of high resolution, such as would be required for interscalene or axillary brachial plexus block. Curved array low-frequency probes (4–7 MHz) provide improved penetration to visualise deeper structures but with reduced resolution. Using the curved array probe for deeper blocks will provide a broader field of view for appreciation of surrounding anatomical structures and landmarks, such as during performance of a subgluteal sciatic block. The view obtained by a chosen transducer can be optimised by altering the screen depth, the gain (screen brightness) and, on some machines, the adjustable focusing of the beam. Most ultrasound machines allow the operator to select anatomical structures of interest from a preset menu (e.g. 'nerve' or 'vascular'), and this alters these variables automatically to improve image quality. The operator can manipulate the transducer position on the patient by a combination of

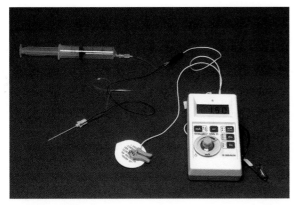

Fig. 25.2 Nerve stimulator and insulated stimulating needle attached to syringe.

Box 25.1 **Potential advantages of ultrasound-guided nerve blockade**

Visualisation of target structure
Visualisation of surrounding anatomical structures
Accuracy of needle placement
Visualisation of local anaesthetic spread in real time
Compensation for anatomical variation
Avoidance of intraneural or i.v. injection
Variety of approaches (not landmark dependent)
Rapid block onset
Reduced local anaesthetic dosage
Reduced procedure-related pain
Reduced complications

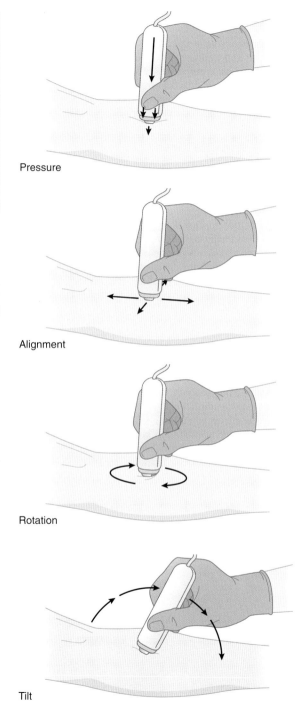

Pressure

Alignment

Rotation

Tilt

Fig. 25.3 PART (Pressure, Alignment, Rotation, Tilt) manipulation of an ultrasound transducer to optimise image quality.

pressure, alignment, rotation and tilt (Fig. 25.3). The search for an optimal screen image is made easier if each of these movements are applied systematically, rather than changing them concurrently.

Most nerves exhibit a 'honeycomb' appearance on scanning – a combination of nerve fascicles and connective tissue, which varies in appearance depending on the individual nerve, its location and the angle of incidence of the probe. More proximal nerve roots, such as with interscalene imaging, tend to appear hypoechoic or dark as a result of reduced amounts of connective tissue compared with the axilla and peripherally.

There is increasing evidence that ultrasound offers several advantages over traditional landmark or nerve stimulator nerve localisation techniques (Box 25.1).

Monitoring

Monitoring equipment should be appropriate to the anaesthetic technique and surgical procedure, with a minimum of three-lead ECG, NIBP and pulse oximetry for all blocks.

Asepsis

As a minimum for all peripheral nerve blocks, operators should wash their hands, wear gloves and draw up and store local anaesthetic syringes in a clean manner. Skin over the scanning and injection site should be prepared with a solution of chlorhexidine 0.5% in alcohol, which should be allowed to dry. Ultrasound probes should be covered with a sterile sheath. Sterile conductivity gel should be used to facilitate ultrasound wave penetration. All major blocks, such as neuraxial blocks or blocks siting a perineural catheter, should be performed under strict aseptic technique with sterile gloves, gown, hat, mask and drapes.

Inadvertent wrong-sided block

Inadvertent wrong-sided peripheral nerve blockade is an avoidable anaesthetic complication. Such events are uncommon but can have serious consequences. These include complications from the unnecessary block such as nerve injury and local anaesthetic toxicity, delayed hospital discharge, patient anxiety and distress and the risk of wrong-sided surgery if the error is not identified promptly (Royal College of Anaesthetists 2017).

A 'stop before you block' moment, undertaken as part of every peripheral nerve block, is a strong preventative measure to avert wrong-sided blocks. Many hospitals have adopted the World Health Organization (WHO) surgical safety checklist, including a 'sign in' before anaesthesia is commenced, where the surgical site marking is confirmed against the written consent form. This is not a substitute for a correctly performed 'stop before you block' moment, which should occur before every peripheral nerve block *immediately* before needle insertion and requires the anaesthetist and anaesthetic practitioner to reconfirm:

- patient identity and consent form;
- the side of the block; and
- the surgical site marking.

Circumstances that require particular vigilance include the following:

- *Peripheral nerve blocks performed as a sole procedure rather than in conjunction with a surgical procedure, such as a femoral nerve block the day before the operative management of a proximal femoral fracture.* In these circumstances an operative marking may not have been made and a full WHO surgical safety checklist process is recommended, including relevant written procedural consent for the block and block site marking.
- *Moving or turning patients between 'sign in' and performance of the nerve block.* This can result in the block site 'moving' in relation to the anaesthetist and equipment in the room. Certain blocks often necessitate repositioning of patients (e.g. popliteal blocks), and additional care is required to use the 'stop before you block' appropriately.
- *Delays and distractions before and during performance of the peripheral nerve block.* Certain time-critical and important distractions cannot be avoided by the anaesthetist and anaesthetic assistant, and these will occasionally occur at key moments in the performance of a block. Vigilance is required by the anaesthetist to be aware of these distractors and if any disruption to the usual 'stop before you block' procedure occurs, the entire procedure should be discontinued and re-started at a more appropriate time.
- *Covering of preoperative surgical marking with blankets, dressings or drapes.*
- *Presence of an ultrasound machine in the anaesthetic room for purposes other than performance of the block (e.g. for venous access).* The use of an ultrasound machine in the anaesthetic room for this indication should alert the anaesthetist to the high risk of the wrong-sided block because of the potential unconscious selection of block side based on the presence of an ultrasound machine on one side or other of the patient.
- *Presence of negative external and internal influences on anaesthetist's performance.* Time pressure, hunger, thirst, fatigue, background noise and emotional distraction can all increase the risk of wrong-sided block. If these are present and may affect task performance, the anaesthetist should always respond and address these demands before undertaking a peripheral nerve block.

Supplementary techniques

A local anaesthetic may be the only drug administered to the patient, or it may form part of a balanced anaesthetic technique. During surgery, patients may be awake, or sedated by i.v. or inhalational means. Intermittent boluses of midazolam or target-controlled infusions of propofol are commonly used to provide intraoperative sedation. General anaesthesia may be used as a planned part of the procedure. A combination of regional and general anaesthesia may be useful to obtain advantages from both, particularly for prolonged procedures or where positioning is difficult because of trauma or arthritis.

When a surgical tourniquet is used, the chosen block must extend to the tourniquet site unless the procedure is brief. Discomfort from prolonged immobility on a hard table may be relieved by the administration of analgesia during surgery. This type of discomfort is usually not relieved by sedative drugs, which may result in the patient becoming agitated, confused and uncooperative.

Aftercare

At the end of surgery, clear postoperative instructions should be given to both patients and healthcare professionals taking over their care. This may include general advice about analgesia management when a block wears off and care of the insensate limb. It may also include a reiteration of the preoperative advice about block-specific adverse effects, such as Horner's syndrome after interscalene brachial plexus blockade.

Continuous perineural infusion of local anaesthetics

Continuous infusion techniques are suitable for use only by experienced anaesthetists but are increasingly used in both inpatient and ambulatory settings. When used correctly, administration by infusion is safer than repeated large bolus injections of drug, but regular observations are essential and nursing staff must have an adequate level of knowledge to appreciate possible complications. A clear pathway of escalation must exist to allow patients or nursing staff to bring to the attention of an anaesthetist any concerns regarding the continuous infusion.

A variety of needles, catheters, local anaesthetic mixtures and infusion devices are commercially available. Infusions of local anaesthetic can be delivered by fixed-rate infusion alone or in combination with patient-bolus demands. Syringe drivers or elastomeric infusion devices containing low-concentration ropivacaine or levobupivacaine are commonly used to deliver local anaesthetic via perineural catheters.

Block failure

When confronted with the apparent failure of a neuraxial or peripheral nerve block to produce the desired analgesic or anaesthetic effect, the anaesthetist must take a calm, step-wise approach to identify the precise problem and remedy this accordingly. In the circumstances of a block sited preoperatively this is always best done before the patient is prepared and positioned for surgery. Clear communication with the patient regarding sensory expectations is mandatory, and this should have been undertaken as part of the consent process. To determine whether particular myotomes or dermatomes are inadequately anaesthetised, a focused examination of the motor and sensory systems is required (Fig. 25.4). This requires excellent communication between clinician and patient to avoid ambiguity, and a senior anaesthetist may be required at this point. Inadequate sensory blockade in some dermatomes may sometimes be remedied by repeat nerve block, but this should be performed by an experienced practitioner and with the total dose of local anaesthetic in mind. Inadequacy of regional blockade to achieve anaesthesia to the site of surgery should not be managed by increasing doses of sedation, although i.v. analgesics such as fentanyl can be a useful adjunct in awake surgery. Occasionally, conversion to general anaesthesia is required.

Intravenous regional anaesthesia

Intravenous regional anaesthesia (IVRA) is being used less commonly by anaesthetists, who often prefer to block the brachial plexus, but it is still used by emergency department staff as a simple, safe and effective block for trauma patients. Deaths from IVRA have resulted from incorrect selection of drug and dosage, incorrect technique and the performance of the block by personnel unable to treat systemic local anaesthetic toxicity. Bupivacaine was inappropriately chosen in many of these cases and is now contraindicated for IVRA.

Indications

Intravenous regional anaesthesia is suitable for short procedures when postoperative pain is not marked, such as manipulation of Colles' fracture or carpal tunnel decompression. Recovery is rapid, and the technique is appropriate for day-case surgery.

Method

Intravenous regional anaesthesia involves isolating an exsanguinated limb from the general circulation by means of an arterial tourniquet and then injecting local anaesthetic solution intravenously. Analgesia and weakness occur rapidly and result predominantly from local anaesthetic action on peripheral nerve endings.

An orthopaedic tourniquet of the correct size is applied over padding on the upper arm. All connections must lock, and the pressure gauge should be calibrated regularly. An i.v. cannula is sited in the contralateral arm in case administration of emergency drugs is required. An i.v. cannula is inserted into a vein of the limb to be anaesthetised. A vein on the dorsum of the hand is preferred because injection into more proximal veins reduces the quality of the block and increases the risk of toxicity. Exsanguination by means of an Esmarch bandage improves the quality of the block and increases the safety of the technique by reducing the venous pressure developed during injection. In patients with a painful lesion (e.g. Colles' fracture), elevation combined with brachial artery compression is adequate. The tourniquet should be inflated to a pressure 100 mmHg above systolic arterial pressure.

In an adult, 40 ml prilocaine 0.5% is injected over 2 min ensuring that the tourniquet remains inflated. Analgesia should be achieved within 10 min, but it is important to inform the patient that the feeling of touch is often retained. The anaesthetist must be ready to deal with toxicity or tourniquet pain throughout the surgical procedure. The tourniquet should not be released until at least 20 min after injection, even if surgery is completed. This delay allows for diffusion of drug into the tissues so that plasma concentrations do not reach toxic levels after release of the tourniquet. The technique of repeated reinflation and deflation of the cuff during release has little effect on plasma concentrations and is not advised.

Tourniquet pain

Tourniquet pain may be troublesome if the cuff remains inflated for longer than 30–40 min. It is sometimes alleviated by inflating a separate tourniquet below the first on an area already rendered analgesic by the block; the first cuff is then deflated. Failing this, general anaesthesia is preferable to administration of large and often ineffective doses of opioids and sedatives.

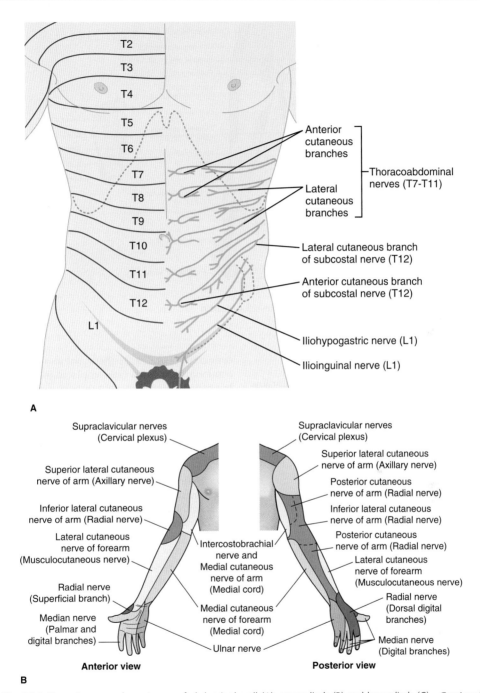

Fig. 25.4 Dermatomes and myotomes of abdominal wall (A), upper limb (B) and lower limb (C). *Continued*

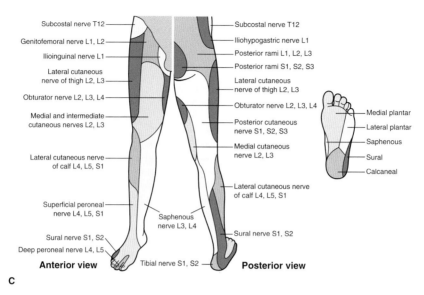

Fig. 25.4, cont'd

Choice of drug

The agent of choice for this procedure is isobaric prilocaine 0.5%. It has an impressive safety record with no major reactions reported after its use, although minor adverse effects such as transient light-headedness after release of the tourniquet are not uncommon. Prilocaine has distinct pharmacokinetic advantages for IVRA and does not cause methaemoglobinaemia in the doses used.

Lower limb

Intravenous regional anaesthesia of the foot may be produced using the same dose of prilocaine and a calf tourniquet positioned carefully at least 10 cm below the tibial tuberosity to avoid compression of the common peroneal nerve on the fibular neck.

Central nerve blocks

Spinal anaesthesia usually refers to intrathecal administration of local anaesthetic and is also known by the term *subarachnoid block*. The technique of spinal anaesthesia is basically that of lumbar puncture, but knowledge of factors which affect the extent and duration of anaesthesia, and experience in patient management are essential. Epidural block may be performed in the sacral (caudal block), lumbar, thoracic or cervical regions, although lumbar block is used most

commonly. Local anaesthetic solution is injected most commonly through a catheter placed in the epidural space but may be injected straight through a needle after the tip position has been confirmed.

Contraindications to central nerve blocks

Most contraindications are *relative,* but the following are best generally regarded as *absolute* contraindications to neuraxial blockade:
- uncorrected abnormality of coagulation;
- significant hypovolaemia;
- infection at the injection site;
- systemic sepsis manifested by pyrexia or rising inflammatory markers despite resuscitation and antibiotic therapy;
- severe stenotic valvular heart disease (particularly aortic stenosis) or obstructive cardiomyopathy;
- raised intracranial pressure;
- patient refusal; and
- allergy to local anaesthetic medication

Anatomy of the epidural and subarachnoid space

The epidural space is the space between the periosteal lining of the vertebral canal and spinal dura mater. It contains spinal nerve roots, lymphatics, blood vessels and a variable

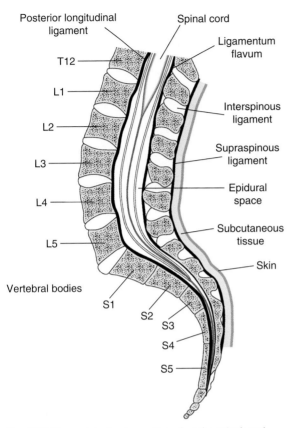

Posterior longitudinal ligament

Spinal cord

Ligamentum flavum

T12

L1

L2

Interspinous ligament

Supraspinous ligament

L3

Epidural space

L4

Subcutaneous tissue

L5

Skin

Vertebral bodies

S1

S2

S3

S4

S5

Fig. 25.5 The vertebral column. Note that the spinal cord ends at the level of L1 or L2 and that the dural sac extends to the level of the S2 vertebra.

amount of fat (Figs 25.5 and 25.6). Its boundaries are as follows:

- *Superiorly* – foramen magnum, where the dural layers fuse with the periosteum of the cranium; hence, local anaesthetic solution placed in the epidural space cannot extend higher than this
- *Inferiorly* – sacrococcygeal membrane
- *Anteriorly* – posterior longitudinal ligament
- *Posteriorly* – ligamentum flavum and vertebral laminae
- *Laterally* – pedicles of the vertebrae and intervertebral foramina

In the normal adult the spinal cord begins at the foramen magnum and ends at the level of L1 or L2 (though it may end lower); here it becomes the cauda equina. The subarachnoid space extends further than the cord, to the level of S2. Below this level, the dura blends with the periosteum of the coccyx. Between the dura and arachnoid is the subdural space, within which the local anaesthetic solution may spread extensively.

The volume of the vertebral canal is finite. An increase in volume of contents of one compartment reduces the compliance of the other compartments and increases the pressures throughout.

Spinal anaesthesia

Indications

Blockade is produced more consistently and with a lower dose of drug by the spinal route than by epidural injection. Duration of analgesia is usually limited to 2–4 h depending on surgical site and may be prolonged by use of intrathecal opioids such as diamorphine, fentanyl or morphine. These drugs carry a minimal risk of serious adverse effects such as respiratory depression, but nausea, pruritus or urinary retention are not uncommon.

Spinal anaesthesia is most suited to surgery below the umbilicus and in this situation the patient may remain awake. Surgery above the umbilicus using spinal block is less appropriate and would usually necessitate addition of a general anaesthetic to abolish the unpleasant sensations from visceral manipulation resulting from afferent impulses transmitted by the vagus nerve.

Types of surgery

- *Urology.* Spinal block is commonly employed for urological procedures such as transurethral prostatectomy, but it should be remembered that a block to T10 is required for surgery involving bladder distension. Perineal and penile operations may also be carried out using a low 'saddle block', peripheral blockade or caudal anaesthesia.
- *Gynaecology.* Minor procedures may be performed reliably with a block to T10. Pelvic floor surgery and vaginal hysterectomy may also be carried out readily with spinal anaesthesia extending to T6, but for procedures requiring laparoscopic assistance, general anaesthesia is necessary.
- *Obstetrics.* Spinal anaesthesia is considered the technique of choice for the clear majority of elective caesarean sections and a large proportion of emergency ones. The technique is discussed in detail in Chapter 43.
- *Orthopaedics.* Spinal anaesthesia is suitable for virtually every type of lower limb surgery and these are discussed in more detail in Chapter 36.

Performance of spinal anaesthesia
Preparation

Full monitoring must be applied and wide-bore i.v. access secured. A full sterile technique must be used (mask, gown, hat, gloves, sterile drapes, antiseptic skin preparation). The

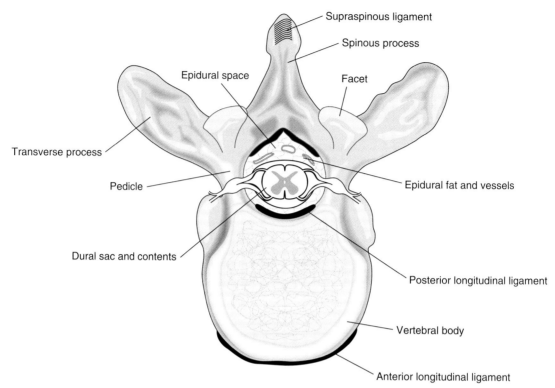

Fig. 25.6 Anatomical relations of the epidural space.

skin should be cleaned with 0.5% solution chlorhexidine in alcohol, which should be allowed to evaporate fully (to prevent wicking of the potentially neurotoxic solution into the needle when it touches the skin).

Spinal blockade may be performed with the patient sitting or in the lateral decubitus position (Table 25.2, Fig. 25.7). If it is anticipated that the procedure may be technically difficult, the midline is usually more discernible with the patient in the sitting position, but the risk of hypotension in the sedated patient or after development of the block may be increased.

Technique of spinal blockade in the lateral position

For the right-handed anaesthetist, the patient is positioned on the operating table in the left lateral position. The patient's back should lie along the edge of the table. A curled position, with knees drawn to the body and chin on chest, opens the spaces between the lumbar spinous processes. An assistant stands in front of the patient to assist with positioning and to provide reassurance.

Landmark techniques, an example of which is described next, are most commonly used to achieve spinal blockade; however, ultrasound can be used to assist in the placement of spinal (and epidural) needles and is of particular utility in obese patients or those with abnormal vertebral anatomy.

A line (Tuffier's line or the intercristal line) between the iliac crests approximates to the fourth lumbar vertebral body, and spinal injection should be performed at the L3/4 or L4/5 space (see Fig. 25.7). All drugs should be drawn into non-Luer connection syringes directly from sterile ampoules using a filter needle to prevent the injection of glass particles into the intrathecal space. A selection of non-Luer connection spinal needles (22–27G) should be available.

The skin and subcutaneous tissues are infiltrated with local anaesthetic using a narrow-gauge needle. Most fine-gauge spinal needles come with a 19G introducer needle to assist in the guidance of the flexible spinal needle to the intrathecal space. This introducer needle, or the spinal needle itself, is inserted in the midline, midway between two spinous processes. In the well-positioned patient, the needle is directed at right angles to the skin, toward the naval. Passage through the interspinous ligament and ligamentum flavum

Table 25.2 Techniques of spinal anaesthesia

Type of block	Upper level of analgesia	Position during lumbar puncture	Volume of solution
Saddle block	S1	Sitting 5 min	1 ml hyperbaric solution
Low thoracic	T10–12	Sitting/lateral decubitus	2–3 ml hyperbaric solution
Mid thoracic	T4–6	Lateral decubitus/sitting (immediately supine)	3–4 ml hyperbaric solution
Unilateral: A unilateral block, or at least a differential block between limbs, may be achieved by the slow injection of small volumes (1–1.5 ml) of hyperbaric solution in the lateral position. This position then must be maintained for at least 15 min to minimise spread. On return to the supine position there may still be some contralateral spread, and the necessity for smaller volumes and dosage may increase block failure rate.			

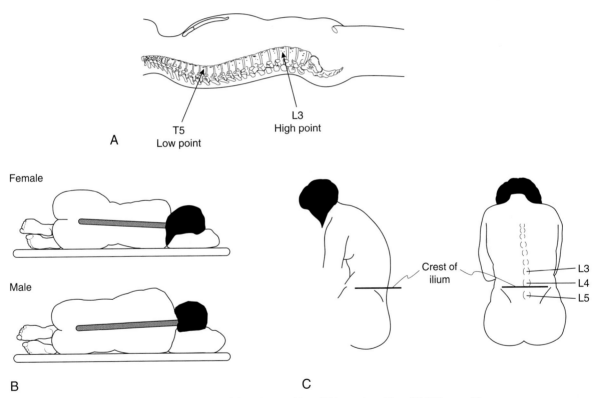

Fig. 25.7 Spinal curvature. (A) Supine position. (B) Lateral position. (C) Sitting position.

into the spinal canal is appreciated easily with a 22G needle (Fig. 25.8A), but these needles are now rarely used because of the high incidence of PDPH. With some practice, these structures can be discerned with a 25G or 27G pencil-point needle, and a click may be felt immediately after the needle tip passes beyond the ligamentum flavum and punctures the arachnoid mater. When the needle tip has breached the ligamentum flavum and epidural space to enter the intrathecal space, the stilette is withdrawn from the needle and the hub observed for CSF flow. A gentle aspiration test can be performed if free flow of CSF is not observed or the needle carefully rotated through 90 degrees.

The most common reasons for difficulty accessing the intrathecal space are incorrect patient positioning, failure

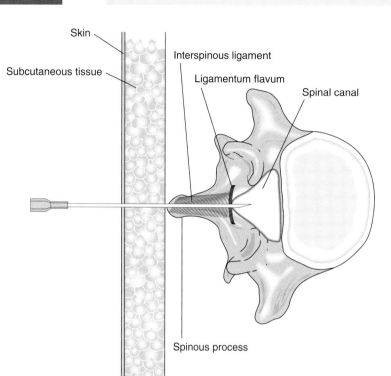

Skin

Subcutaneous tissue

Interspinous ligament

Ligamentum flavum

Spinal canal

Spinous process

A

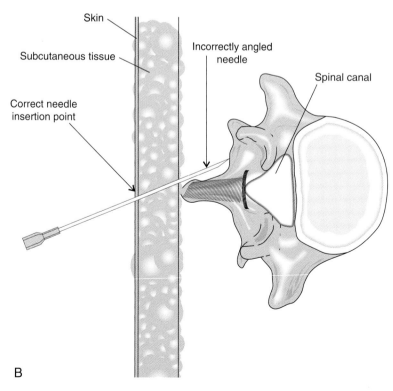

Skin

Subcutaneous tissue

Correct needle
insertion point

Incorrectly angled
needle

Spinal canal

B

Fig. 25.8 Midline approach for spinal anaesthesia. (A) Correctly angled. (B) Incorrectly angled.

to insert the needle in the midline and directing the needle laterally (Fig. 25.8B). This last fault is seen most easily from one side and is usually apparent to onlookers but not to the anaesthetist, who looks only along the line of the needle.

When CSF is obtained, the non-Luer connection syringe containing the injectate should be carefully attached to the spinal needle, taking care not to displace the tip. Gentle aspiration, with eddies of CSF seen in the local anaesthetic solution, confirms the needle tip position and the solution is injected slowly (although some have recommended rapid injection to obtain effective blocks using small volumes of injectate). Further aspiration towards the end of injection confirms that the needle tip has remained in the correct place. Needle and introducer are withdrawn together and the patient then repositioned to facilitate the desired spread of the block.

Factors affecting spread

The most important factor which affects the height of block in spinal anaesthesia (Table 25.3) is the baricity of the solution, which may be made hyperbaric (i.e. denser than CSF) by the addition of glucose. The specific gravity of CSF is 1.004. The addition of glucose 5% or 6% to a local anaesthetic produces a solution with specific gravity of 1.024 or greater. A patient who assumes the sitting position for 5 min after injection of 1 ml hyperbaric solution develops a saddle block which affects the sacral roots only. Conversely, a patient placed supine immediately after injection of 2–3 ml develops a block to around T4–8. Slightly larger volumes are advisable to ensure spread above the lumbar curvature (see Fig. 25.7), and the spread of local anaesthetic may be encouraged above the lumbar lordosis by raising the patient's knees, flattening the lumbar spine.

Factors affecting duration

The duration of anaesthesia depends on the drug used and the dose injected. Vasoconstrictors added to the local anaesthetic solution significantly increase the duration of action of tetracaine, which is widely used in the United States, but this is not so for other agents.

Agents

Only preservative-free agents should be used for spinal blockade. Local anaesthetics currently licensed in the UK for intrathecal injection include hyperbaric bupivacaine, plain levobupivacaine, hyperbaric prilocaine and chloro-procaine. Hyperbaric bupivacaine 0.5% is more predictable for abdominal procedures and consistently produces a block to the umbilicus (and usually to T5) in supine patients. As with all hyperbaric solutions, hypotension is encountered

Table 25.3 Factors influencing spread of hyperbaric spinal solutions

Factor	Effect
Position of patient	Sitting position produces perineal block only, provided that small volumes are used.
Spinal curvature	With standard volumes (2–3 ml) the block often spreads to T4. With small volumes (1 ml) the block may affect only the perineum even when the patient is placed supine immediately.
Dose of drug	Within the range of volumes usually employed increasing the dose of drug increases the duration of anaesthesia rather than the height of the block.
Interspace	Minor factor affecting height of block.
Obesity	Minor factor affecting height of block. Obese patients tend to develop higher blocks.
Speed of injection	Rapid injection makes the height of block more variable.
Barbotage	No longer used. Makes the height of block more variable.

more often because of higher concentrations of sympathetic blockade. Volumes of 1.5–3.0 ml are used and a duration of 2–3 h is usually ensured. Hyperbaric prilocaine 2% has a duration of action of 90–120 min and is useful in day-case surgery. A volume of 1.5–3.0 ml can be used for surgical procedures anticipated to last up to 60 min, allowing mobilisation around 3 h after injection. The relatively slow onset and tendency to a patchy block can be improved by the addition of an opiate (e.g. fentanyl 20 μg) to the injectate.

Almost all opioids have been tried by the spinal and epidural route with success, but diamorphine or fentanyl are the most common additives in the UK. These drugs are highly lipophilic (the octanol/water partition coefficient of fentanyl is 860 and of diamorphine is 280), so partition across the dura is rapid, propensity for cephalic spread is restricted and systemic absorption is limited in duration. In comparison, hydrophilic opioids such as morphine (octanol/water partition coefficient of 1.4) slowly diffuse across the dura, have prolonged high cerebrospinal fluid concentrations and therefore have an increased risk of late-onset respiratory depression. Clonidine combined with local anaesthetic has also been used successfully.

Continuous spinal anaesthesia

Spinal blockade can be produced incrementally or the duration prolonged by using an indwelling spinal catheter. It may be performed using either a small catheter passed through an 18G or 19G Tuohy needle or using a purpose-made catheter-over-wire kit such as the Spinocath. It can also be used after the inadvertent puncture of the dura by a 16G Tuohy needle during attempted epidural catheter insertion for labour analgesia. Perioperative spinal catheter techniques fell out of favour in the early 1990s after reports of cauda equina syndrome occurring in association with the use of 28G and 32G microcatheters and large doses of hyperbaric lidocaine 5%. It is postulated that the problem arose through pooling of high concentrations of lidocaine around the sacral nerve roots because of a slow injection rate, leading to permanent neurological damage.

The technique is relatively uncommon in current anaesthetic practice, has an attendant risk of inadvertent wrong-route medication administration and comes with the potential for misidentification of the spinal catheter for an epidural catheter and subsequent catastrophic delivery of epidural doses of local anaesthetic into the intrathecal space. As a consequence, continuous spinal anaesthesia should be limited to more experienced practitioners in specific circumstances.

Physiological effects of spinal blockade

CNS

Local anaesthetic solution injected into the CSF spreads away from the site of injection, and the concentration of the solution decreases as mixing occurs. A differential blockade of fibres occurs because small fibres are blocked by weaker concentrations of local anaesthetic solution. Sympathetic B-fibres are blocked to a level approximately two segments higher than the upper segmental level of sensory blockade. Motor blockade may be several segments caudal to the upper level of sensory block. A sensory level to T3 with spinal blockade may be associated with total blockade of the T1–L2 sympathetic outflow.

RS

Low spinal blockade has no effect on the respiratory system, and the technique is an important part of the anaesthetist's armamentarium for patients with severe respiratory disease.

Spinal anaesthesia with motor blockade extending to the thoracic level causes loss of intercostal muscle activity. This has little effect on tidal volume (because of diaphragmatic compensation), but there is a marked decrease in vital capacity resulting from a significant decrease in expiratory reserve volume. The patient may experience dyspnoea and difficulty in maximal inspiration or coughing effectively. A thoracic block may lead to a reduction in cardiac output and increased ventilation/perfusion imbalance, resulting in a decrease in PaO_2. Awake patients with a high spinal block should always be given oxygen-enriched air to breathe. Blocks which reach the roots of the phrenic nerves (C3–5) will cause apnoea.

CVS

The cardiovascular effects are proportional to the height of the block and result from denervation of the sympathetic outflow (T1–L2). This produces dilatation of resistance and capacitance vessels and results in hypotension. In awake patients, vasoconstriction above the height of the block may compensate almost completely for these changes, thereby maintaining arterial pressure, but general anaesthetic agents may reduce this compensatory response, with consequent profound hypotension.

Hypotension is exacerbated by:
- the use of head-up patient positioning;
- hypovolaemia – pre-existing or induced by surgery;
- administration of sedatives, opioids or induction agents; and
- positive pressure ventilation.

Both the incidence and degree of hypotension are reduced by limiting the height of the block and by keeping it below the level of sympathetic supply to the heart (T1–4). Changes in position (e.g. turning the patient from the supine to the prone position) may result in a sudden increase in the height of block, with consequent extension of sympathetic blockade. This may occur even after 15–20 min.

It is common practice to attempt to minimise hypotension during spinal or epidural anaesthesia by preloading the patient with 500–1000 ml crystalloid solution i.v. before or during the performance of the block. These volumes are usually ineffective even in the short term, may risk causing pulmonary oedema in susceptible individuals either during the procedure or when the block wears off, and may lead to postoperative urinary retention. Appropriate fluid should be given to replace blood and fluid losses and prevent dehydration. Severe or unwanted hypotension may be treated by i.v. fluids or drugs. Hypotension is associated commonly with bradycardia, and ephedrine 5–6 mg i.v. is an appropriate treatment. Atropine may be useful, but sympathomimetic drugs with vasoconstrictor effects are usually more effective than vagolytics.

Bradycardia may occur as a result of the following:
- Neurogenic factors, particularly in awake patients (i.e. vasovagal syndrome)
- Paradoxical Bezold–Jarisch reflex; decreased venous return and heightened sympathetic tone leads to forceful contraction of a near empty left ventricle, with consequent parasympathetically mediated arterial vasodilatation and bradycardia
- Block of the cardiac sympathetic fibres (T1–4)

Spinal anaesthesia has no direct effect on the liver or kidneys, but reductions in hepatic and renal blood flow occur in the presence of hypotension and reduced cardiac output associated with high spinal blocks.

GI

The vagus nerve supplies parasympathetic fibres to the whole of the gut as far as the transverse colon. Spinal blockade causes sympathetic denervation (proportional to height of block), and unopposed parasympathetic action leads to a constricted gut with increased peristaltic activity. Nausea, retching or vomiting may occur in the awake patient and are often the first symptoms of impending or established hypotension. If nausea occurs, the anaesthetist must assess arterial pressure and heart rate immediately and take appropriate measures.

GU

Urinary retention may follow the use of central neuraxial blocks. It is important to avoid overhydration, as bladder distension may require catheterisation. Spinal anaesthesia does not automatically warrant the insertion of a urinary catheter. If the patient has other risk factors for urinary retention (e.g. prostatic hypertrophy), catheterisation is often performed. The risks of urinary tract infection and delayed mobility associated with catheterisation should be balanced against the risk of urinary retention when undertaking spinal anaesthesia.

Epidural block

Indications

Epidural blockade may be used for procedures from the neck downwards, and the duration of anaesthesia and analgesia can be tailored to meet the needs of surgery and postoperative pain relief by using a catheter system. The duration of analgesia may be prolonged as necessary by means of an indwelling catheter and use of intermittent boluses, continuous infusion or a combination of the two. Bupivacaine, levobupivacaine or ropivacaine are the drugs of choice when continuous techniques are used. The pharmacology of these agents is discussed in Chapter 5.

Performance of epidural block

Equipment

Epidural anaesthesia is usually performed using a Tuohy needle (Fig. 25.9). The needle is marked at 1-cm intervals and has a Huber point which allows a catheter to be directed along the long axis of the epidural space. Disposable catheters

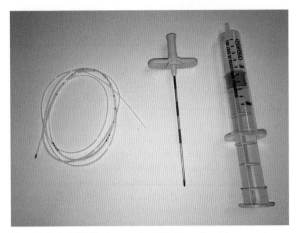

Fig. 25.9 A 16G Tuohy needle with loss of resistance syringe and catheter.

are available with a single end hole or with a sealed tip and three side holes distally.

Preparation
This is identical to the preparation for spinal block.

Technique

Epidural block may be performed at any level of the vertebral column to provide segmental analgesia over an area that can be predetermined with reasonable accuracy. Initial experience should be gained in the lumbar region before progressing to sites above the termination of the spinal cord.

The pressure in the epidural space is, at rest, slightly positive, but negative pressures are induced by sudden release of pressure when the Tuohy enters the space, having previously tented the ligamentum flavum onto the space during its passage through the ligament. Older methods of identifying the epidural space (e.g. Odom's indicator, Macintosh's balloon, hanging drop) relied on detection of this negative pressure in the epidural space; however, these techniques have been superseded by methods which depend on loss of resistance to injection of air or saline as the tip of the needle penetrates the ligamentum flavum and enters the epidural space.

A midline lumbar approach is described here, using a continuous technique with loss of resistance to saline, because this method carries the lowest risk of inadvertent dural puncture.

The patient is positioned as for spinal blockade and the vertebral level is identified from the iliac crests. The skin and subcutaneous tissues of the chosen interspace are infiltrated with local anaesthetic solution in the midline.

The Tuohy needle (16G or 18G) is introduced through the skin, subcutaneous tissue and supraspinous ligament. When inserted into the interspinous ligament or ligamentum flavum, the unsupported needle remains firm and steady, as it is held in these tissues. The stilette is withdrawn from the Tuohy and a 10 ml low-resistance syringe filled with saline attached. Steadying the dorsum of the non-dominant hand on the patient's back, the hand that holds the needle serves as a brake against sudden forward movement of the Tuohy. The needle tip is advanced by pressure on the plunger of the syringe by the dominant hand (Fig. 25.10). When the needle penetrates the ligamentum flavum, there is a sudden loss of resistance to pressure on the plunger, and the non-dominant hand serves to prevent further needle advancement. A continuous technique of forward pressure on the syringe plunger, resisted by slight opposing pressure by the non-dominant hand on the needle, is a good way to reduce the chance of inadvertent dural puncture and is practical in the forgiving lumbar ligaments of parturients. When performed correctly, the wings of the Tuohy needle should not be used to advance the needle tip, because all forward movement arises from the pressure applied to the syringe plunger, although the wings can be used to assist the non-dominant hand in its gentle resistive efforts. In young adults undergoing lumbar epidural insertion, if pressure on the plunger fails to advance the needle tip, it is most likely that the needle is not within the ligamentum flavum and should be redirected. Such a reliable continuous epidural technique may not be possible in the thoracic region, especially in older patients, who have more variation in the consistency of their ligaments and whose epidural space is less accessible via a midline approach. Thoracic epidural insertion, therefore, should only be practised by anaesthetists who have first gained competency in the lumbar region.

Single-dose technique

A syringe containing local anaesthetic can be connected to the Tuohy needle, and after aspiration, a test dose is administered to detect intravascular or intrathecal placement. After an appropriate pause, the remainder of the solution is injected at a rate not exceeding 10 ml min^{-1} while verbal contact is maintained with the patient. Such techniques are usually used in chronic pain management.

Catheter insertion

When the Tuohy needle tip is in the epidural space a note should be made of its depth using the markings on the needle. An epidural catheter, with graduated markings from its tip, can then be inserted though the needle. The catheter should pass freely into the epidural space, resistance to threading indicating the space identified with loss of resistance may not be epidural. If the catheter does not thread easily, the needle and catheter should be withdrawn together and the space found again by a second pass with the Tuohy needle. Withdrawing the catheter alone risks shearing off a piece of the catheter on the edge of the Huber point.

When a sufficient length of catheter is in the epidural space (e.g. 5 cm), the needle is carefully removed over the catheter and the catheter then withdrawn to leave 4–5 cm in the epidural space. After ensuring that there is no flow of blood or CSF down the catheter under the influence

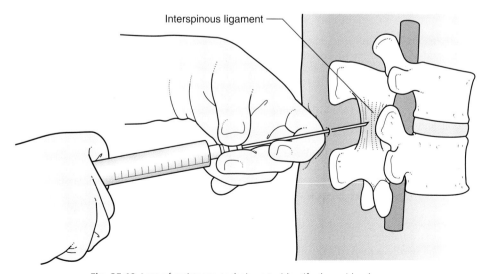

Interspinous ligament

Fig. 25.10 Loss of resistance technique to identify the epidural space.

of gravity, the hub is attached and an aspiration test performed; if blood is obtained, the catheter should be withdrawn 0.5–1.0 cm and reaspirated; if blood continues to be aspirated, a second insertion at another vertebral space should be performed. Aspiration of CSF can be confirmed using a test for glucose (saline and local anaesthetics will reliably test negative), and a decision should be made about whether to use the catheter as a continuous spinal technique or remove the catheter and reinsert at an adjacent interspace.

If neither blood nor CSF are aspirated, a filter is connected and a test dose of local anaesthetic, usually 3–5 ml bupivacaine 0.25%, is given to check for intrathecal spread. When using a test dose, motor function should be tested by asking the patient to raise the whole leg and not merely to wiggle the toes; movement of the toes may not be abolished for 20 min after intrathecal injection, if at all. Profound motor block to the lower limbs should alert the anaesthetist to the possibility of intrathecal injection. If the test dose is satisfactory, the catheter is fixed to the patient's back and a loading dose administered to establish blockade. A variety of fixing techniques can be used alone or in combination, including adhesive dressings, skin glues, locking devices and subcutaneous tunnelling.

Factors affecting spread

Epidural spread varies widely among individuals and the initial injection site will govern the distribution. The most important determinant of spread appears to be the total mass of drug injected, with the same mass of drug given in different concentrations and volumes producing similar spread of sensory blockade. Higher concentrations of drug will tend to increase the intensity of block, including motor block. Posture has a minimal effect on spread; in the lateral position, the dependent side will usually have block levels 1–3 segments higher; a supine position with head-down tilt will result in higher sensory block levels. Patients who are pregnant, obese or older than 60 years have an increased likelihood of a high block with any given dose of local anaesthetic.

Factors affecting onset

Onset time may be reduced by increasing the concentration of the local anaesthetic, using local anaesthetic associated with quicker onset of action (e.g. lidocaine), the addition of adrenaline 1 : 200,000 or alkalinisation of the solution with sodium bicarbonate.

Factors affecting duration

The choice of local anaesthetic agent has a major effect on the duration of anaesthesia. The concentration of the drug

also has an effect; higher concentrations of levobupivacaine produce a more prolonged block. To some extent this is a reflection of increased dose, which is known to increase the duration of anaesthesia.

Agents

- Lidocaine is used in concentrations of 1%–2% with or without adrenaline 1 : 200,000. Without adrenaline, the duration of action is approximately 1 h; a duration of approximately 1.0–2.5 h may be expected when solutions containing adrenaline are used, depending on surgical site.
- Bupivacaine is available in concentrations of 0.25% and 0.5%. Levobupivacaine is the pure S-isomer of bupivacaine and is less cardiotoxic than the racemic mixture but appears equipotent in terms of sensory and motor blockade. Levobupivacaine is available as 0.25%, 0.5% and 0.75% solutions. A block lasting more than 4 h may be achieved with a 0.75% solution.
- Ropivacaine is a long-acting agent that is less cardiotoxic than bupivacaine and produces less dense motor block for a similar degree of sensory blockade. It is usually regarded as being less potent than bupivacaine and slightly higher concentrations/doses are usually employed. It has a more rapid onset of action than bupivacaine or levobupivacaine.
- A variety of opioids can be given via an epidural catheter, either as boluses or as part of a low-concentration local anaesthetic solution. Boalused opioids such as fentanyl can usefully increase the density of a sensory block but are associated with pruritus in a proportion of patients.

Combined spinal-epidural anaesthesia

Combined spinal-epidural anaesthesia (CSE) is a useful technique in clinical situations benefiting from the rapid onset of spinal anaesthesia as well as the ability to prolong the sensory block using local anaesthetics delivered through an epidural catheter. The technique is most often applied in obstetrics to assist with caesarean delivery where operative duration is expected to be longer than usual, or in non-obstetric circumstances where spinal anaesthesia is an ideal choice but may not provide sufficient anaesthetic time for surgery to be completed. The use of CSE as part of an analgesic strategy during labour is dealt with in Chapter 43. Broadly there are two techniques for siting a CSE. Either the spinal and epidural components can be performed as two separate needle passes as described in their respective sections earlier and performed one after the other, or a needle-through-needle technique can be employed.

In a needle-through-needle technique the epidural space is identified using a Tuohy needle, and a long spinal needle passed through the Tuohy into the intrathecal space to allow careful intrathecal injection of local anaesthetic. The spinal needle is withdrawn and an epidural catheter then passed through the Tuohy and sited in the epidural space as described earlier. Caution must be exercised in the testing and loading of such epidural catheters because a concomitant spinal block is an integral part of the CSE technique. The catheters are most usefully tested once the initial spinal block has begun to recede, which will allow differentiation of a safe epidural catheter from an inadvertent intrathecal one.

Caudal anaesthesia

Caudal block involves injection of local anaesthetic into the epidural space through the sacral hiatus (covered by skin and sacrococcygeal membrane) into the sacral canal. This contains the sacral and coccygeal nerve roots in addition to the cauda equina, filum terminale, epidural fat and epidural veins.

Injection of very large volumes of local anaesthetic to obtain anaesthesia of lumbar and thoracic roots, although described, is seldom practised because of an unacceptable incidence of adverse effects and failure to achieve a sufficiently high block. With appropriate volumes, caudal blockade does not cause sympathetic blockade and has a low risk of dural puncture, although it does usually result in a degree of motor block to the lower limbs. The technique is used more often in children than adults, usually as a single-shot block, although it is possible to site caudal catheters.

Indications

In conjunction with general anaesthesia, caudal anaesthesia provides good intra- and postoperative analgesia. Caudal anaesthesia is suitable for perineal operations, such as haemorrhoidectomy, although in practice a low spinal block is usually preferred. It is often used in paediatric practice for postoperative analgesia after orchidopexy, inguinal hernia and hypospadias repairs.

Method

Caudal blockade may be performed with the patient in the prone position, but the left lateral position is usually easier in anaesthetised children. Palpation down the sacral spine leads to the depression of the sacral hiatus at S5, flanked by the sacral cornua, between which the needle is inserted. After thorough skin disinfection, and using a sterile technique, a non-ported cannula is introduced through skin and sacrococcygeal ligament in a *cephalad* direction at 45 degrees to the skin (Fig. 25.11). When the membrane is

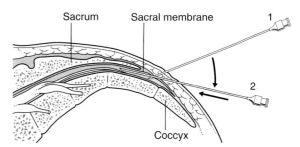
Fig. 25.11 Needle position for caudal anaesthesia.

penetrated, a small loss of resistance is felt and the cannula advanced over the needle, which is then withdrawn. After observing for CSF or blood, injection may be performed after careful and repeated aspiration. It must be remembered that the dura may extend to S3 and so intrathecal injection is a risk.

The Armitage regimen provides a useful guide to the dosing of 0.25% bupivacaine for the purposes of caudal injection in children:

- Lumbosacral block ~ L1 (e.g. circumcision) 0.5 ml kg^{-1}
- Thoracolumbar block ~ T10 (e.g. inguinal hernia) 1 ml kg^{-1}
- Midthoracic block ~ T6 (e.g. umbilical hernia) 1.25 ml kg^{-1}

Care must be taken to not exceed the maximum recommended dose of bupivacaine (2 mg kg^{-1}) with these volumes.

Physiological effects of epidural block

The physiological effects of epidural blockade are similar to those after spinal block but develop more slowly. Additional effects may occur as a result of the much larger doses of anaesthetic, as there may be appreciable systemic absorption of local anaesthetic (and of adrenaline if an adrenaline-containing solution is used).

Complications of central nerve blocks

Immediate
Possible immediate complications of spinal or epidural block include as hypotension, bradycardia, total spinal blockade, anaphylaxis and local anaesthetic toxicity. These are discussed in Chapter 27.

Late
Complications of spinal or epidural block that predominantly manifest in the postoperative period include PDPH (see Chapter 43), labyrinthine disturbances, cranial nerve palsy, meningitis, spinal cord or nerve root trauma and vertebral canal haematoma (see Chapter 26).

Peripheral blocks

This section will provide an outline of the commonest peripheral nerve blocks undertaken in perioperative practice. For the inexperienced anaesthetist, further reading and supervised learning should be undertaken before these blocks are performed under direct supervision (Ellis and Lawson, 2004; and Grant and Auyong, 2016).

Head and neck blocks

Blocks used in ophthalmic surgery are discussed in Chapter 38 and anaesthetic techniques for awake fibreoptic intubation in Chapter 23.

Stellate ganglion block

- Stellate ganglion block is usually performed in the context of chronic pain syndromes or vascular insufficiency of the upper limb.
- The stellate ganglion is a fusion of the inferior cervical ganglion and first thoracic ganglion and is present in approximately 80% of the population. It is located at the level of C7, anterior to the neck of the first rib in close approximation to the vertebral foramina, carotid sheath, dome of the pleura, vertebral artery, oesophagus and trachea.
- These anatomical relations mean the block should only be performed by experienced practitioners, who will look for ipsilateral Horner's syndrome to indicate successful blockade of the ganglion.
- The complications of the block arise mostly from needle damage or local anaesthetic spread to the aforementioned structures.

Cervical plexus blocks

- The single-injection ultrasound-guided intermediate cervical plexus block is replacing separate superficial and deep cervical plexus blocks for carrying out awake carotid endarterectomy in many hospitals.
- The cervical plexus is formed from branches of the C1–4 nerve roots. The plexus, which may not be visible as individual nerves when performing this block, lies deep to sternocleidomastoid between the superficial and deep cervical fasciae.
- Injection using an in-plane needling technique of 10–20 ml local anaesthetic between these fascial layers and around the carotid sheath (Fig. 25.12) will provide effective anaesthesia for carotid surgery.
- The phrenic nerve will, to some extent, always be blocked by this technique, so bilateral blocks of the cervical plexus are not appropriate.

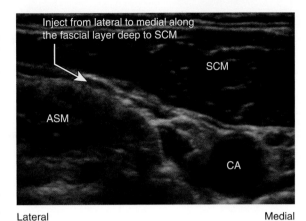

Inject from lateral to medial along the fascial layer deep to SCM

SCM

ASM

CA

Lateral   Medial

Fig. 25.12 Ultrasound anatomy relevant to the intermediate cervical plexus block. *ASM*, Anterior scalene muscle; *CA*, carotid artery; *SCM*, sternocleidomastoid muscle.

- Modifications of this technique can usefully block the skin of the anterolateral neck to assist in cervical lymph node biopsy or insertion of a CVC into the internal jugular vein.

Upper limb blocks

The upper limb is well suited to local anaesthetic techniques and these remain among the most useful and commonly practised peripheral regional techniques (Neal et al 2009). Interscalene block is the most useful approach for shoulder surgery, whilst supraclavicular, infraclavicular and axillary blocks can all be used for elbow, forearm and hand surgery. These techniques are commonly used as the sole anaesthetic for surgery but can be combined with general anaesthesia in suitable patients. Analgesic supplementation can be provided by blockade of individual peripheral nerves, typically the radial, median and ulnar, although anatomical variation in the dermatomal supply of these nerves and their subdivisions means they cannot provide reliable surgical anaesthesia without recourse to the more proximal blocks listed earlier.

Anatomy of the brachial plexus

- The nerve supply of the upper limb is derived from the brachial plexus, formed from the anterior primary rami of the fifth to eighth cervical and first thoracic nerves.
- The roots of the plexus divide repeatedly and recombine to form trunks, divisions, cords and terminal branches (Fig. 25.13).
- The roots emerge from the intervertebral foramina to lie between the anterior and middle scalene muscles invested

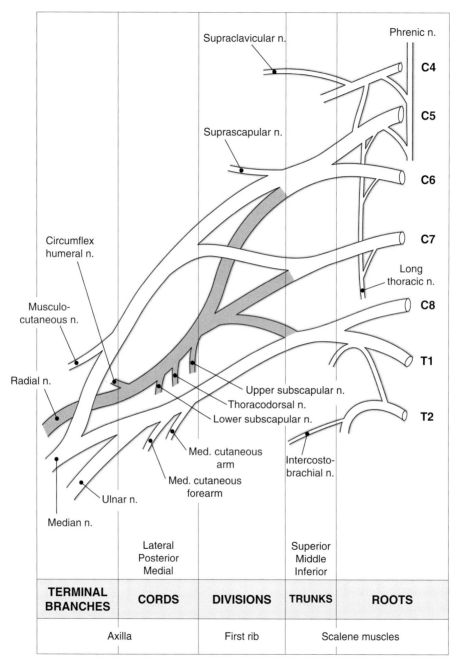

Fig. 25.13 Formation of the brachial plexus.

in a sheath derived from the prevertebral fascia. The roots combine into three trunks above the first rib.

- Each trunk separates into anterior and posterior divisions; anterior divisions supply the flexor structures of the arm and posterior divisions the extensor structures.

- The divisions recombine into three cords, which surround the second part of the axillary artery behind pectoralis minor.
- The cords divide into the terminal branches.

The cutaneous and deep nerve supplies of the upper limb are depicted in Fig. 25.14. The only parts of the

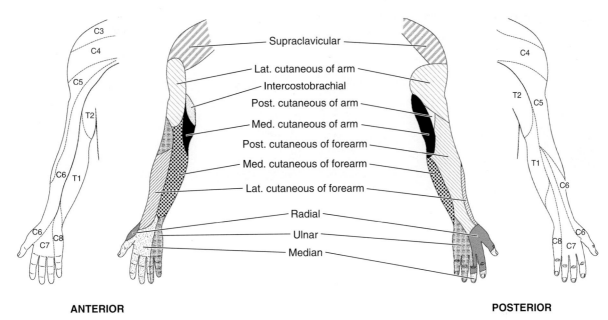

Fig. 25.14 Innervation of the upper limb: outer, dermatomal innervation of the skin; inner, cutaneous nerve supply to the upper limb.

cutaneous nerve supply of the upper limb not derived from the brachial plexus are the upper medial part of the arm, supplied by the intercostobrachial nerve (T2), and skin over the superior aspect of the shoulder, supplied by the supraclavicular branches of the superficial cervical plexus.

Interscalene block

- Interscalene is the most proximal approach to the brachial plexus and the only approach which reliably blocks the plexus above C5.
- Interscalene injection usually extends to block the cervical plexus roots C3 and C4 and is suitable for shoulder and upper arm surgery.
- Block of the C8 and T1 roots may prove difficult and makes the technique unsuitable for hand surgery.
- Complications are similar to those for supraclavicular block, but phrenic nerve blockade occurs almost universally. Ultrasound guidance, targeting the C5 and C6 nerve roots (Fig. 25.15) allows much smaller volumes of local anaesthetic (as little as 5–10 ml) to be used for postoperative analgesia, reducing the degree of phrenic paresis.
- Pneumothorax, vertebral artery puncture, and direct intrathecal injection also may occur. Seizures may result from injection into the vertebral artery with as little as 1–2 ml local anaesthetic.

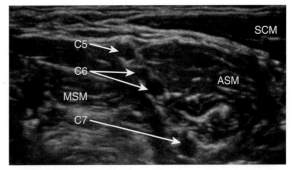

Fig. 25.15 Ultrasound anatomy relevant to the interscalene brachial plexus block. *ASM,* Anterior scalene muscle; *MSM,* middle scalene muscle; *SCM,* sternocleidomastoid muscle. The C5, C6 and C7 nerve roots can be seen lying within the interscalene groove. Note the bifid C6 nerve root.

Supraclavicular block

- This approach provides perhaps the best overall efficacy of complete arm block from a single injection as the trunks/divisions of the brachial plexus are closely related at this point.
- The key to successful and safe approaches is accurate visualisation of the plexus, subclavian artery, pleura and

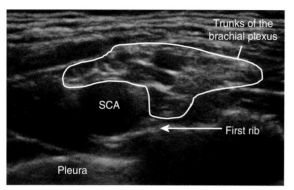

Anteriomedial   Posteriolateral

Fig. 25.16 Ultrasound anatomy relevant to the supraclavicular brachial plexus block. *SCA,* Subclavian artery.

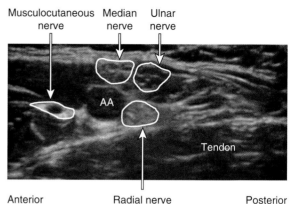

Anterior   Radial nerve   Posterior

Fig. 25.17 Ultrasound anatomy relevant to the axillary brachial plexus block. *AA,* Axillary artery; *Tendon,* conjoined tendon of teres major and latissimus dorsi. Note that multiple axillary veins have been compressed by transducer pressure.

first rib (Fig. 25.16). The needle is introduced in-plane, in a posterolateral to anteromedial direction, and should be visualised continuously to prevent inadvertent pleural puncture.

- The chief advantage of the supraclavicular block is that it can provide reliable anaesthesia to the entire arm extending from shoulder to fingertip. Unlike the axillary block, it does not require arm abduction for access to the plexus, which can sometimes be difficult in elderly patients.
- Pneumothorax is a well-described complication of supraclavicular block; the risk is small (<0.5%) in experienced hands. The identification of the first rib overlying the pleura produces a 'backstop' preventing breach by the needle into the pleural cavity.
- Phrenic nerve paralysis occurs in around one-third of patients but is usually asymptomatic.
- Sympathetic block is relatively common and results in Horner's syndrome.

Infraclavicular block

- Historically, an infraclavicular approach is less popular than the other approaches because of the variety and imprecision of landmark approaches, high vascular puncture rate and variable efficacy; however, this technique has been increasingly used since the advent of ultrasound guidance.
- Most techniques are described either below the clavicular mid-point (vertical infraclavicular block) or a more lateral approach caudal and medial to the coracoid process. The latter approach is more popular with ultrasound guidance (lateral sagittal infraclavicular block) and blocks the three cords of the plexus as they surround the second part of the axillary artery deep to pectoralis minor muscle.

- The block can be performed with the arm at the side and may be useful when access for axillary block is prevented by limitation of shoulder abduction.
- For optimal ultrasound images and ease of needle placement in the limited space below the clavicle, a small curved array probe is used. This probe not only shows the important vascular structures with which the nerves are intimately related, but with experience also demonstrates the three neural cords and the local anaesthetic spread around them.
- The approach is useful for elbow, forearm and hand surgery and is particularly useful if a catheter is placed for postoperative use, because of greater ease of secure fixation below the clavicle.
- Blockade of the phrenic nerve is unlikely with the lateral approach.

Axillary block

- An axillary block represents perhaps the safest approach to the brachial plexus. It is useful for elbow, forearm and hand surgery and is generally safe for day-case surgery.
- The most common orientation of nerves around the axillary artery is shown in Fig. 25.17. Ultrasound visualisation allows both the detection of anatomical variation and optimisation of local anaesthetic spread around these structures.
- The patient lies supine with the arm abducted to no more than 90 degrees and the elbow bent to 90 degrees. The plexus of most individuals can be visualised using a linear 10 MHz probe set to a depth of 3 cm. An anatomical survey is carried out to demonstrate the positions of the nerves:
  - *Musculocutaneous.* Generally seen lying between biceps and coracobrachialis muscles lateral to the artery.

- *Median.* Usually located adjacent to the artery in the 12 o'clock position.
- *Ulnar.* Often seen in the corresponding 2 o'clock position, a small distance from the artery, and often just below the axillary vein.
- *Radial.* Most difficult to visualise; tends to lie beneath the ulnar nerve in the 5 o'clock position.
- After local anaesthetic infiltration of the overlying tissues, the block needle is introduced either in-plane or out of plane and further local anaesthetic is then distributed around the individual nerves.
- Access is occasionally problematic if arm abduction and external rotation are limited by either shoulder trauma or arthritis.
- This approach rarely blocks the axillary nerve unless large volumes are used. If blockade of this nerve is required, a more proximal approach to the plexus should be considered.
- Puncture of the axillary artery is rarely a problem because the vessel is largely compressible at this point. Inadvertent venous injection is a possibility because venous anatomy is variable and there are often multiple veins in the axilla. Injection of local anaesthetic that does not visibly displace tissues should raise the possibility of inadvertent venous injection.
- Nerve damage occurs rarely and is more likely to result from malposition of the anaesthetised limb or failure to recognise a compartment syndrome postoperatively.

Median, radial and ulnar nerve blocks

Median, radial and ulnar nerves can be blocked individually to supplement postoperative analgesia after forearm or hand surgery. This is usually done in conjunction with a more proximal brachial plexus block because the complex and overlapping cutaneous innervation of the arm and hand is not easily amenable to surgical anaesthesia after only selective distal nerve blockade. Each nerve can be blocked using in-plane ultrasound guidance with 2–5 ml local anaesthetic.

Radial

The radial nerve can be viewed travelling posterior to anterior as it emerges from the spinal groove at the level of the mid-humerus (Fig. 25.18A). It is often accompanied by the profunda brachii artery, which can be identified using colour Doppler, before splitting into superficial and deep interosseous branches.

Median

The median nerve is readily accessible in the antecubital fossa as an oval hyperechoic structure medial to the brachial artery and deep to the pronator teres muscle (Fig. 25.18B). It can be traced down the forearm to the wrist between superficial and deep flexor muscles.

Ulnar

The ulnar nerve is best identified with the arm abducted and elbow flexed to allow ultrasound visualisation of the cubital tunnel. Distal scanning reveals the flexor carpi ulnaris muscle and tendon together with the triangular hyperechoic ulnar nerve (Fig. 25.18C). More distal scanning will show the ulnar artery becoming superficial to join the nerve as they travel down the forearm. The ulnar nerve can be blocked at this level, taking care that it has fully emerged from the non-expansible cubital tunnel and that the ulnar artery is identified and is away from the needle tip.

Truncal blocks

Fascial plane blocks of the trunk can provide opioid-sparing analgesia for a wide variety of abdominal, breast and thoracic surgical procedures. Ultrasound visualisation of individual nerves is usually not possible with these blocks, so a practical understanding of the sonographic muscular anatomy is required to ensure adequate volumes of local anaesthetic are deposited in the correct tissue layer. The analgesic area may be extended using multiple injections or by spread of a larger single bolus. Perineural catheters can be sited to prolong the duration of action of many of these blocks; however, a multiorifice catheter is recommended to ensure adequate deposition of local anaesthetic.

Thoracic paravertebral block

- Paravertebral blocks, unilateral or bilateral, with or without catheter insertion, and at single or multiple thoracic levels, can provide analgesia for thoracic, axillary, breast, gallbladder and renal surgery.
- The triangular paravertebral space is in continuity medially with the epidural space and contains the segmental spinal nerves, rami communicantes and sympathetic chain. The space is bounded medially by vertebral bodies and discs; posteriorly by transverse processes, heads of ribs and superior costotransverse ligaments; and anterolaterally by parietal pleura. The thoracic paravertebral space is continuous from T1 to T12.
- A number of landmark and ultrasound-guided approaches to the block are described or the block can be performed by the surgeon under direct vision during thoracic surgery.
- Because the paravertebral space is in direct apposition with the pleural and epidural spaces, only experienced regional anaesthetists should undertake this block.

Pectoral blocks (PECS I and PECS II) and serratus plane block

- The lateral branches of the second to sixth thoracic intercostal nerves provide cutaneous innervation to most of the chest wall and breast.

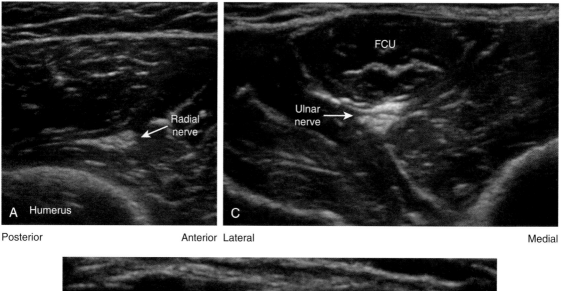

Posterior Anterior Lateral Medial

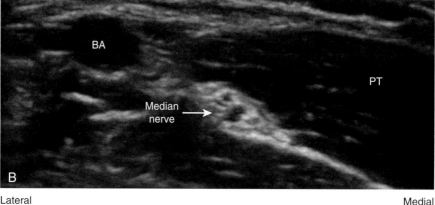

Lateral Medial

Fig. 25.18 Ultrasound anatomy relevant to the major nerves of the arm. (A) Radial nerve. (B) Median nerve. (C) Ulnar nerve. *BA*, Brachial artery; *FCU*, flexor carpi ulnaris; *PT*, pronator teres.

- Deeper tissue innervation is supplied by a complex combination of the medial and lateral pectoral nerves, which lie between pectoralis major and pectoralis minor along with the thoracoacromial artery, long thoracic nerve and thoracodorsal nerve, which lies between the latissimus dorsi and serratus anterior in the posterior-lateral chest wall.
- With the patient in the supine position with arm abducted, local anaesthetic can be deposited using an in-plane needling technique between the pectoralis major and minor muscles (PECS I) at the level of the fourth rib to block the medial and lateral pectoral nerves.
- Inserting the needle deeper to lie between pectoralis minor and serratus anterior and injecting local anaesthetic in this plane (PECS II) will block the lateral branches of the second to sixth intercostal nerves. Sliding the transducer caudad to the fifth rib and towards the posterior axillary line will bring the latissimus dorsi muscle into view, overlying serratus anterior. Deposition of local anaesthetic between these muscles (serratus plane) will block the thoracodorsal nerve.
- These blocks can provide analgesia for a variety of breast and chest wall procedures; however, the complex innervation of this region, simplified earlier, means they rarely provide adequate anaesthesia for surgery.

Ilioinguinal and iliohypogastric block

- The main nerves which supply the groin are the subcostal (T12), iliohypogastric (L1) and ilioinguinal (L1).

- Ilioinguinal and iliohypogastric blocks are usually used for postoperative analgesia after inguinal hernia surgery. When supplemented by surgical infiltration of local anaesthetic, surgery performed solely under local anaesthesia is possible.
- The traditional 'blind' approach relying on fascial clicks to identify muscle aponeuroses has largely been superseded by an ultrasound-guided approach that allows accurate deposition of anaesthetic close to the anterior superior iliac spine in the fascial layer between internal oblique and transversus abdominis to block the ilioinguinal and iliohypogastric nerves.

Transversus abdominis plane block

- A transversus abdominis plane (TAP) block provides analgesia of the anterior and lateral abdominal wall below the umbilicus by blocking the T6–L1 segmental nerves as they lie within the fascial plane between the transversus abdominis and internal oblique muscles.
- It is suitable as part of a postoperative analgesic strategy after unilateral lower abdominal surgery such as hernia repair and appendicectomy or performed bilaterally for procedures such as abdominal hysterectomy or subumbilical laparotomy. The block does not provide relief of visceral pain.
- Injection is made using an in-plane ultrasound technique to place at least 0.3 ml kg^{-1} local anaesthetic in the plane between internal oblique and transversus abdominis (Fig. 25.19). This usually takes place between the iliac crest and rib margin, with the aim of achieving spread of local anaesthetic as far posterior in this plane as possible.
- Higher 'subcostal' TAP blocks have been described, with the aim of achieving more cephalad dermatomal analgesia. Dilution of local anaesthetic to obtain adequate volumes for injection and safe total doses may be required, and care is required to identify and avoid breeching the underlying peritoneum.

Rectus sheath block

- Rectus sheath block is useful for midline abdominal incisions and is readily amenable to perineural catheter placement to provide analgesia for several days.
- The aim is to block the anterior cutaneous branches of the lower five intercostal nerves and subcostal nerve as they lie in the plane between rectus abdominis muscle and transversalis fascia.
- This can be achieved using an in-plane ultrasound technique to both sides of the rectus abdominis muscle. Like many truncal blocks, large volumes of dilute local anaesthetic are required to obtain analgesic effect, in this case typically 0.3 ml kg^{-1} to each side.

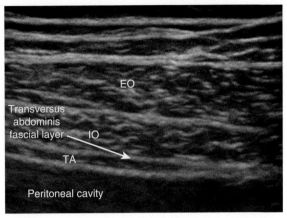

Anterior Posterior

Fig. 25.19 Ultrasound anatomy relevant to the transversus abdominis plane block. *EO*, External oblique muscle; *IO*, internal oblique muscle; *TA*, transversus abdominis muscle.

Lower limb blocks

Lower limb blocks are most useful in the following circumstances:

1. combined with spinal or general anaesthesia to provide postoperative analgesia;
2. as part of a multimodal analgesic regime after trauma to the lower limb;
3. as a sole anaesthetic technique for day-case lower limb surgery; and
4. in circumstances where severe medical comorbidity renders general or neuraxial anaesthesia unsafe but surgery may be lifesaving (e.g. amputations)

Sciatic nerve block

Sciatic block may be used alone for procedures in the foot (e.g. hallux valgus operations) or combined with femoral or saphenous nerve block for surgery that involves the anterior thigh, knee, or medial calf and foot (Enneking et al 2005).

Anatomy

- The sciatic nerve (L4–S3) arises from the sacral plexus and passes through the great sciatic foramen midway between the greater femoral trochanter and ischial tuberosity in a fascial plane between the superficial gluteus maximus muscle and deep quadratus femoris.
- The nerve descends in the posterior thigh to the popliteal fossa, where it divides into the tibial and common peroneal nerves.
- The posterior cutaneous nerve of the thigh (S1–3) may run with the sciatic nerve or separate from it proximally;

this nerve supplies the skin of the posterior thigh and upper calf.

- The tibial and common peroneal nerves, together with the saphenous nerve derived from the femoral nerve, supply all structures below the knee.

Method

There are many approaches to the sciatic nerve, most based on traditional landmark techniques. With ultrasound guidance the nerve is best visualised where it is most superficial: either subgluteal or in the popliteal fossa.

- *Subgluteal approach.* The patient lies lateral or prone. A linear or curvilinear transducer is placed distal to the buttock crease, and the hyperechoic and highly anisotropic triangular sciatic nerve is seen between the superficial muscles semitendinosus (medially) and biceps femoris (laterally) and deep adductor magnus muscle. It is not unusual to require a 150-mm insulated needle to reach the sciatic nerve at this level. The subgluteal approach may not block the posterior cutaneous nerve of the thigh, and so if blockade of this nerve is required, a parasacral approach may be needed.
- *Popliteal fossa.* Access to the nerve at this level is easiest with the patient lateral or prone and with the leg slightly flexed at the knee. Scanning the popliteal fossa will identify the popliteal artery, usually deep to the popliteal vein. More superficial, lying between biceps femoris laterally and semimembranosus and semitendinosus medially, will be the common peroneal nerve laterally and tibial nerve medially (Fig. 25.20). Tilting the transducer will often improve visualisation of the anisotropic nerve tissue. Scanning the nerves proximally will reveal the point at which they unite to form the sciatic nerve. The block can be performed at whichever level best identifies the nerves, often just distal to the bifurcation. A mesoneurium sheath encloses the nerves, and needle placement within this sheath but outside the epineurium will provide a rapid onset and dense block.

Femoral nerve block and fascia iliaca block

Femoral nerve and fascia iliaca blocks provide effective analgesia after hip fracture. These blocks are often performed to assist in preoperative lateral positioning for spinal anaesthesia and, when combined with sciatic and obturator nerve blocks, can provide anaesthesia to virtually the entire lower limb.

Anatomy

- The femoral nerve (L2–4) arises from the lumbar plexus and runs between psoas and iliacus muscles to enter the thigh beneath the inguinal ligament, 1–2 cm lateral to the femoral artery and underneath the hyperechoic fascia iliacus.
- Branches of the anterior division include the intermediate and medial cutaneous nerves of the thigh.

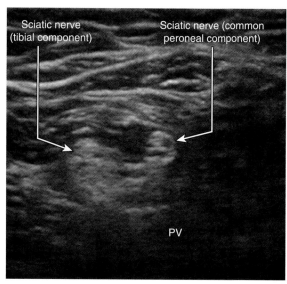

Fig. 25.20 Terminal branches of the sciatic nerve identified at level of the popliteal fossa. *PV,* Popliteal vein.

- The posterior division supplies the quadriceps muscle and the hip and knee joints. It terminates as the saphenous nerve, which supplies the skin of the medial side of the calf as far as the medial malleolus and sometimes the medial side of the dorsum of the foot.
- The lateral femoral cutaneous nerve and obturator nerve also arise from the lumbar plexus.

Method

- The patient lies supine and the femoral artery is identified proximal to its division into superficial femoral and profunda femoris arteries. Ultrasound guidance, either in-plane or out of plane, can be used to locate the nerve below the fascia lata and fascia iliaca and on top of the iliacus muscle (Fig. 25.21).
- The term *fascia iliaca block* describes an attempt to inject local anaesthetic in the plane between the fascia iliaca and iliacus muscle in sufficiently high volumes to block the major components of the lumbar plexus (femoral, lateral femoral cutaneous and obturator nerves) with one injection.
- Using this block, identification of the individual nerves is not required, because proximal spread of local anaesthetic will theoretically block all three components of the lumbar plexus.

Adductor canal block

- The dense motor block to quadriceps provided by femoral nerve blockade is unhelpful in encouraging

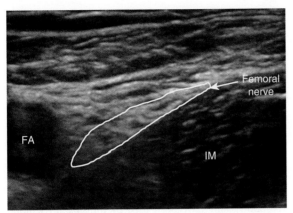

Medial   Lateral

Fig. 25.21 Ultrasound anatomy relevant to the femoral nerve block. *FA*, Femoral artery; *IM*, iliacus muscle.

early active mobilisation of the knee joint after primary arthroplasty. Consequently, femoral nerve block has fallen out of favour in many centres and has been replaced by high-volume infiltration of local anaesthetic by the surgeon or by a selective block of the saphenous nerve (the largest sensory branch of the femoral nerve) in the adductor canal.

- This can be undertaken in the mid-thigh at the adductor hiatus, where the nerve lies in close lateral proximity to the superficial femoral artery.
- The adductor canal at this level is bounded by vastus medialis anterolaterally and adductor longus and magnus muscles posteromedially, with the roof of the canal formed by the sartorius muscle.
- The saphenous nerve itself lies deep to the vastoadductor membrane, a layer of fascia connecting the muscle groups. For an effective block, local anaesthetic must be deposited deep to this fascial layer.
- Although the canal also contains the nerve to vastus medialis and branches of the obturator nerve, local anaesthetic delivered at this level is largely motor sparing, while providing effective analgesia to the knee joint.

Ankle block

Ankle block can be used in awake or anaesthetised patients to provide anaesthesia and analgesia to the entire foot. Selective nerve blockade under ultrasound guidance is readily possible for more focused perioperative analgesia.

Anatomy

Five nerves supply the foot:
- The tibial nerve enters the foot posterior to the medial malleolus, dividing into medial and lateral plantar nerves

and supplies the medial foot and great toe, deep structures within the foot and the medial plantar surface.
- The common peroneal nerve divides into deep and superficial branches; the deep peroneal nerve supplies the web space between first and second toes, and the superficial branch supplies the dorsum of the foot.
- The saphenous nerve supplies a variable area of skin on the medial side of the dorsum of the foot, occasionally reaching as far as the first metatarsophalangeal joint.
- The sural nerve is a branch of the tibial nerve; it runs posterior to the lateral malleolus and supplies skin over the lateral side of the foot and fifth toe.

Method

- Each nerve can be blocked with 2–5 ml local anaesthetic.
- Often a combination of in-plane or out-of-plane needle approaches is needed, depending on the accessibility of the nerves and patient habitus. The bony contours of the ankle mean a 25-mm linear array transducer often obtains a more complete probe–tissue interface than larger transducers.
- To block the tibial nerve, the posterior tibial artery is identified using ultrasound behind the medial malleolus. The hyperechoic tibial nerve lies posterior to the artery, superficial to the flexor hallucis longus muscle (Fig. 25.22A).
- The deep peroneal nerve can usually be identified anterior to the ankle joint line in close proximity to the anterior tibial artery and anterior tibial veins. The nerve is typically lateral to the vessels but can lie superficial or medial to them (Fig. 25.22B).
- A superficial peroneal nerve block can be performed by scanning proximally from the lateral malleolus. As the fibula becomes deeper, the extensor digitorum longus muscle becomes larger anteriorly and the peroneus brevis muscle becomes larger posteriorly. The superficial point of intersection of these muscles contains the superficial peroneal nerve (Fig. 25.22C).
- For distal saphenous and sural nerve blocks, a venous tourniquet is useful to distend the great and short saphenous veins. Ultrasound identification of the great saphenous vein in front of the medial malleolus and the short saphenous vein behind the lateral malleolus allows accurate perivenous deposition of local anaesthetic to block the saphenous and sural nerves respectively (Fig. 25.22D & E).

Continuous peripheral nerve block

Continuous peripheral nerve blocks are growing in popularity for both upper and lower limbs, as a method of prolonging postoperative analgesia and facilitating rehabilitation without the adverse effects associated with opioids and epidural analgesia. Postoperative care is simplified and may usually be carried out in a general ward environment.

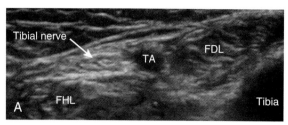

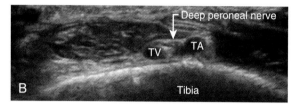

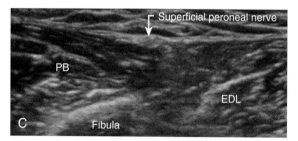

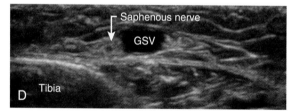

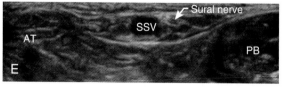

Fig. 25.22 Nerves supplying the ankle and foot. (A) Tibial nerve. (B) Deep peroneal nerve. (C) Superficial peroneal nerve. (D) Saphenous nerve. (E) Sural nerve. *AT,* Achilles tendon; *EDL,* extensor digitorum longus; *FDL,* flexor digitorum longus; *FHL,* flexor hallucis longus; *GSV,* great saphenous vein; *PB,* peroneus brevis; *TA,* tibial artery; *TV,* tibial vein; *SSV,* short saphenous vein.

The anaesthetist should be proficient in single-shot peripheral blocks – brachial plexus, femoral, lumbar plexus and sciatic – before advancing to catheter techniques. Some of the most popular techniques include continuous femoral infusion after total knee arthroplasty, sciatic infusion after below-knee amputation, interscalene infusion after major shoulder surgery and infraclavicular infusions for elbow replacement or arthrolysis. Equipment has improved greatly in recent years, and insulated Tuohy needles and facet-tipped needles are available to assist catheter placement.

Local anaesthetic agents, usually levobupivacaine or ropivacaine, are most commonly used in concentrations of 0.10%–0.25%, although much lower concentrations of levobupivacaine have been used by infusion for femoral nerve blockade after total knee arthroplasty in an attempt to minimise motor blockade and promote earlier and safer ambulation. Alternatively, local anaesthetic top-ups can be administered by intermittent bolus either by appropriately trained staff or as part of a patient-controlled system with or without a background infusion.

Periarticular techniques

Periarticular and intra-articular wound infiltration techniques, particularly after knee arthroplasty surgery, are becoming increasingly popular as part of a multimodal analgesic strategy aimed at minimising adverse effects of parenteral opioids, improving analgesia and promoting early ambulation by avoiding significant motor block. Although at an early stage of development, it appears to be cheap, simple and safe and has been suggested to improve early outcomes and reduce hospital stay. The technique for knee arthroplasty surgery involves infiltrating the entire surgical site with 100–120 ml dilute local anaesthetic solution (e.g. ropivacaine 0.1%). An intra-articular catheter can be sited for subsequent top-ups.

Special situations

Paediatric regional anaesthesia

Most nerve blocks used in adult practice are suitable for use in children. Many of these are used for postoperative analgesia and are performed after induction of general anaesthesia. Ultrasound guidance has become very useful for peripheral blockade because of the variation in depth and position of nerves and to help avoid intraneural injection in the anaesthetised child.

The disposition of local anaesthetic agents in children differs from that in adults. In children younger than 1 year, and particularly in the neonate, very high plasma concentrations of local anaesthetic may ensue after standard doses based on weight. In children older than 1 year, plasma concentrations are consistently lower than would be expected from adult data.

Topical anaesthesia

This may be achieved with either EMLA (eutectic mixture of local anaesthetic – prilocaine 2.5% and lidocaine 2.5%) or tetracaine 4% (e.g. Ametop) cream, held in place with an occlusive dressing. Both provide anaesthesia of intact skin, which is particularly useful before venepuncture in children. EMLA cream must remain in contact with the skin for at least 1 h to be effective and may be left in place for up to 5 h. Tetracaine is generally effective within 30–45 min, after which time the cream and occlusive dressing should be removed and the site marked.

References/Further reading

Association of Anaesthetists of Great Britain and Ireland, 2013. Obstetric Anaesthetists' association and regional anaesthesia UK. Regional anaesthesia and patients with abnormalities of coagulation. Anaesthesia 68, 966–972.

Chong, M.A., Berbenetz, N.M., Lin, C., 2017. Perineural versus intravenous dexamethasone as an adjuvant for peripheral nerve blocks: a systematic review and meta-analysis. Reg. Anesth. Pain Med. 42, 319–326.

Ellis, H., Lawson, A., 2004. Anatomy for anaesthetists, ninth ed. Wiley-Blackwell, Oxford.

Enneking, K.F., Chan, V., Greger, J., Hadžic, A., Lang, S.A., Horlocker, T.T., 2005. Lowe extremity peripheral nerve blockade: essentials of our current understanding. Reg. Anesth. Pain Med. 30, 4–35.

Grant, S.A., Auyong, D.B., 2016 2nd edition. Ultrasound guided regional anesthesia. Oxford University Press, Oxford.

Neal, J.M., Gerancher, J.C., Hebl, J.R., Ilfeld, B.M., McCartney, C.J., Franco, C.D., et al., 2009. Upper extremity regional anesthesia: essentials of our current understanding. Reg. Anesth. Pain Med. 34, 134.

Royal College of Anaesthetists, (2017). Wrong Site Block. Available at: https://www.rcoa.ac.uk/standards-of-clinical-practice/wrong-site-block.

Chapter | 26 |

Complications arising from anaesthesia

David Hewson, Jonathan Hardman

Complications are undesirable events arising from anaesthesia. They occur in approximately 10% of anaesthetics. Only the minority of these complications cause lasting harm to the patient. Death complicates five anaesthetics per million given in the UK (0.0005%). Every complication has the *potential* to cause lasting harm to the patient. Therefore deviations from the norm must be recognised, and managed promptly and appropriately.

Certain complications of anaesthesia manifest as emergencies during the intraoperative phase of surgery, such as arrhythmias, hypotension, adverse drug effects and inadequate ventilation of the lungs. These are commonly termed 'critical incidents' because without rapid correction they lead directly to anaesthetic mortality preventable intraoperative cardiac arrest or permanent organ injury. Such intraoperative events are described in detail in Chapter 27. The focus of this chapter is on complications that occur as a result of anaesthesia but which manifest in the postoperative period.

Causes of complications

Human error

Human error is a common contributor to anaesthetic complications, often in association with inadequate monitoring, equipment malfunction and organisational failure. Human error is commonly associated with insufficient training, fatigue, inadequate experience and poor preparation of the patient, environment or equipment. These circumstances are generally avoidable and should be preventable by good organisation. When complications do occur, effective monitoring and vigilance allow for a greater period for action before the complication grows in severity. During this 'window', when the complication is apparent but has not

yet damaged the patient, the anaesthetist must act with precision. This may be facilitated through the use of action plans or drills that have been rehearsed previously.

Communication failure

Failure of communication is often implicated in the generation of complications in the perioperative period. Poor working relationships, varying levels of training amongst staff and challenging working conditions make such failure more likely. Team training and simulation-based training are effective in reducing the incidence of this type of error.

Equipment failure

Equipment failure may result in significant risk to the patient. In particular, failures of breathing systems, airway devices and gas supplies have resulted in several deaths in recent years. In addition, malfunction of mechanical infusion pumps and infusion pressurising devices have also been responsible for patient morbidity and mortality. Meticulous checking of equipment before use is mandatory (see Chapter 22).

Coexisting disease

Some complications stem from the deterioration of the patient's medical condition, which may have existed before the anaesthetist's involvement. Although such deterioration may be coincidental, it must be recognised that anaesthesia and surgery often introduce altered conditions into a patient's finely balanced combination of pathological condition and compensatory physiological characteristics. This may be sufficient to cause instability in the patient's condition and result in sudden worsening of an apparently stable condition.

Typical examples include diabetes mellitus, ischaemic heart disease, hypertension and asthma.

Inevitable complications

There is a subgroup of complications that may be classed as inevitable. Despite excellent surgical and anaesthetic practice, the patient may still experience a complication that brings morbidity or even death. Although we must, at all times, make stringent efforts to save our patients from harm, it is also important to recognise that it is not always appropriate to assign causation of a complication to the healthcare provider.

Avoidance of complications

The most effective steps in preventing harm from complications are implemented before the complication occurs. Thorough preparation will prevent most complications. Such preparation includes:

- preoperative assessment, investigation and counselling of the patient;
- preoperative checking of equipment and the assurance of backup equipment;
- availability of an appropriately trained assistant;
- preoperative consultation with more experienced personnel, where necessary, regarding the most appropriate anaesthetic technique; and
- use of appropriate monitoring techniques.

Experience

Complications occur more commonly in inexperienced (or incautious) hands. Clearly, finite resources exist, and suitably experienced personnel cannot always be allocated to appropriate patients and procedures. It is the individual anaesthetist's responsibility to ensure that he or she has adequate training for the task presented. If the anaesthetist does not have the necessary experience, then senior assistance must be sought.

Redundant systems

The use of redundant systems helps prevent complications; the availability of at least two working laryngoscopes illustrates this. Should one system fail, another may be put in its place. Other examples include the insertion of two or more intravenous cannulae if significant blood loss is expected and monitoring of expired volatile agent concentration in addition to depth of anaesthesia monitors to minimise the risk of awareness.

Monitoring

The Association of Anaesthetists has produced guidelines stipulating the acceptable minimum level of intraoperative monitoring (see Chapter 22).

Modern monitoring systems have automatically activated alarms, and the anaesthetist selects the values at which these alarms sound. The default values are not always the optimal choices. Consideration should be given to the values at which the anaesthetist gains useful insight into the patient's deviation from the healthy *status quo*, without generating unnecessary visual and auditory pollution that may detract from the anaesthetist's concentration and reduce the effectiveness of the monitor. In general, alarms should sound before the value in question reaches a potentially damaging level but should not sound at values that would be considered within the patient's expected range. Clearly this is different for each patient, whose coexisting disease, age, anaesthesia and surgical procedure may vary greatly. The repeated sounding of an alarm should not trigger reflex silencing of the alarm but should cause the anaesthetist to consider whether treatment of the patient is required or whether the alarm limit should be altered.

Management of complications

Generic management

The majority of complications that result in serious harm to the patient compromise the delivery of oxygen to tissues. Organs that are damaged most rapidly by a deficiency in oxygen supply include the brain and heart. The liver and the kidneys are less fragile but are potentially at risk from even short interruptions in oxygen supply. Cessation of perfusion results in more rapid damage to an organ than hypoxaemia while perfusion is maintained. Treatment must be provided rapidly when organ perfusion is threatened or when arterial oxygenation is impaired. The management of virtually any significant complication should include the provision of a high inspired oxygen fraction and the assurance of an adequate cardiac output.

In general, complications should be dealt with through a sequence of:

1. continual vigilance and monitoring;
2. recognition of the evolution of a problem;
3. creation of a list of differential diagnoses;
4. choice of a *working diagnosis*, which is either the most *likely* or the most *dangerous* possibility;
5. treatment of the *working diagnosis*;
6. assessment of the response of the problem to the treatment administered;
7. refinement of the list of differential diagnoses, especially if the response has not been as expected;

8. confirmation or elimination of the choice of *working diagnosis*; if the response to treatment has been unexpected, then replacement with a more *likely* working diagnosis is indicated; and
9. return to step 5 and repeat until the problem is resolved.

The evolving problem

The early recognition of an evolving problem allows the anaesthetist time to manage the complication before it damages the patient. Appropriate selection of monitoring alarm limits and the anaesthetist's vigilance will allow more time for pre-emptive treatment to be provided to reduce the impact of the complication.

The first response to an emerging complication should be to minimise the potential harm to the patient. Such harm may be produced by the anaesthetist's treatment or by a pathological source. It is important to ensure that an abnormal reading from a monitor is not an artefact. Inaccurate information may be displayed if, for example, a pulse oximeter probe is poorly positioned or if an ECG electrode becomes displaced, and the anaesthetist should ensure, through rapid clinical assessment of the patient, that the values shown on the monitor screen are consistent with the patient's clinical appearance and the context. For example, a sudden SpO_2 reading of 70% when the values have been greater than 96% throughout the procedure should prompt a rapid examination of the patient; if the patient is not cyanosed and ventilation appears to continue uninterrupted, then the position of the pulse oximeter probe should be checked, particularly if the plethysmograph trace is poor.

In most situations in which complications become apparent, the diagnosis is simple and treatment may progress in a linear fashion. Such linear treatment of complications is detailed later in this chapter. However, the causes of some complications, such as hypoxaemia, are not always immediately clear, and several potential causes may exist. Where the differential diagnoses relating to a problem appear equally likely, the anaesthetist should treat the problem that threatens the most harm to the patient. During the management of problems during anaesthesia the anaesthetist must constantly be reconsidering the list of differential diagnoses, rearranging them mentally in order of likelihood and treating the most likely and most dangerous possibilities first.

Record keeping

Record keeping, while useful in preventing complications, is also important *during* complications. Trends in a patient's physiological data may become apparent only when charted, and new differential diagnoses may be generated through examination of the recorded data. Accurate record keeping also allows safer sharing of care

between anaesthetists, facilitating handover of care during long operations and allowing better teamwork in complex cases in which two anaesthetists are required. Review of critical incidents and complications is vitally important in preventing future repetitions of the incident and in providing continuing education to individual practitioners and departments of anaesthesia. Thorough record keeping is vital in allowing informed review of these cases. Finally, some complications result in harm to the patient, and it is very important for the practitioner and patient that detailed records are available for later review. In a minority of such cases, legal action may result, and detailed, legible records are vital in defending the actions of the staff and in providing an adequate explanation to the patient (and possibly to the court) of what happened in the operating theatre.

Medicolegal aspects of complications

A minority of complications result in a formal complaint, but litigation by patients who feel that they have been wronged by the healthcare system is becoming increasingly common. Defensive practice is consequently becoming widespread. Such practice aims to reduce the potential culpability of the anaesthetist should complications arise. In some situations this may lead to overinvestigation of patients and even to the provision of care that is not necessarily optimal for the patient. The culture of blame in which we now practise mandates that anaesthetists must protect themselves as well as their patients. Meticulous record keeping, preoperative information and consent and frank discussion of risks with the patient are vital.

Complaints by patients should be dealt with promptly and professionally. The complaint and the anaesthetist's response must be recorded clearly in the patient's records. The anaesthetist should express regret and sympathy that the complication has occurred and explain why. A frank discussion of the difficulties that occurred during anaesthetic administration may provide the patient with sufficient information. If human error has occurred, then the anaesthetist should apologise and reassure the patient that further information will be provided when it becomes available. If the anaesthetist is a trainee, then it is sensible to enlist the assistance of a consultant to attend discussions with the patient. The clinical director should be informed of all discussions with the patient. It may be prudent that the clinical director accompanies the anaesthetist during their dealings with the patient. The results and content of all such discussions must be recorded in the patient's medical records.

Any complaint that goes further than an informal conversation should be referred to the hospital's complaints department, and the anaesthetist's defence organisation should be informed, who will provide advice on subsequent action. It must be emphasised that throughout this often distressing process, meticulous and professional record keeping may make the difference between exoneration and condemnation, irrespective of the true source of fault.

Common complications

The presentation, causes and management of the most common and serious complications arising from anaesthesia are described next.

Pulmonary complications

Postoperative pulmonary complications (PPCs) occur in 10% of patients undergoing non-thoracic surgery. Many respiratory complications can be prevented, or their severity mitigated, with adequate preoperative patient assessment, careful selection of anaesthetic technique and suitable postoperative monitoring and respiratory rehabilitation (Rock and Rich, 2003). Risk factors for the development of PPCs are shown in Box 26.1 (Canet et al., 2010) (see also Chapter 19). A carefully selected regional anaesthetic technique is likely to decrease the risk of respiratory complications in individual patients compared with general anaesthesia.

The most common postoperative respiratory complications are atelectasis, pneumonia and pulmonary thromboembolism.

Atelectasis

The reduction in functional residual capacity and tendency for hypoventilation which occur during general anaesthesia

---

Box 26.1 **Risk factors for the development of postoperative pulmonary complications**

1. Age
2. Low preoperative oxygenation saturation
3. Respiratory infection in the month preceding surgery
4. Preoperative anaemia (haemoglobin concentration <100 gL^{-1})
5. Upper abdominal or thoracic surgery
6. Duration of surgery >2 h
7. Emergency surgery

From the Assess Respiratory Risk In Surgical Patients in Catalonia (ARISCAT) system.

---

make alveolar collapse, or atelectasis, common. Atelectasis causes impairment of gas exchange and increases the risk of postoperative pneumonia. The most common presentation is a gradual downward drift in arterial oxygen saturation or a gradual increase in peak inspiratory pressure during mechanical ventilation.

Risk factors for its development include:
- pre-existing lung disease;
- prolonged anaesthesia or spontaneous ventilation;
- increased intra-abdominal pressure;
- high inspired oxygen fraction;
- head-down positioning;
- extended exposure of the open airway to atmospheric pressure; and
- prolonged apnoea during anaesthesia (e.g. while awaiting the onset of spontaneous ventilation).

Atelectasis may be reduced by the use of:
- mechanical ventilation during lengthy operations;
- head-up positioning where possible;
- PEEP during mechanical ventilation; or
- CPAP or pressure-support during spontaneous ventilation.

If intraoperative atelectasis is suspected, gentle hyperinflation of the lungs usually reinflates the collapsed alveoli and results in an increase in arterial oxygen saturation. Inflation for 20–30 s at an inspiratory pressure up to 40 cmH$_2$O is often required. Such a recruitment manoeuvre is probably best performed using a mechanical ventilator and may usefully be achieved by adding substantial PEEP (e.g. 20–30 cmH$_2$O) for 20–30 s. Prevention of recollapse is best achieved by adding and/or increasing PEEP.

If atelectasis becomes established during anaesthesia, then the patient is at increased risk of pulmonary dysfunction postoperatively. In this situation the provision of good analgesia (to encourage coughing and mobilisation), use of the sitting position and physiotherapy (including incentive spirometry and deep breathing exercises) may reduce postoperative morbidity.

Pneumonia

Pneumonia is the third most common postoperative infection, after urinary tract and wound infection, with an incidence of 2%–20%. It is suggested by new cough, purulent sputum or dyspnoea, often more than 48 h after surgery. There may be systemic evidence of sepsis (tachycardia, pyrexia, hypotension) and hypoxaemia; these indicate severe infection. Chest radiography is likely to show new infiltrate(s), consolidation or effusion. Isolation of responsible organisms is possible from blood or sputum cultures but should not delay the commencement of antibiotic therapy to target likely community- and hospital-acquired organisms. Perioperative atelectasis and the aspiration of bacterially colonised subglottic secretions are thought to be responsible for pneumonia in many cases. Aspiration of gastric contents (see Chapter 27) resulting in a chemical pneumonitis predisposes the damaged lung parenchyma to subsequent bacterial infection. The prognosis for patients with postoperative pneumonia is poor, with 30-day mortality ten times higher than patients without pneumonia, and an overall mortality of approximately 10%.

Pulmonary venous thromboembolism

Embolisation of thrombus occurs usually from the deep veins of the legs or pelvis. Venous emboli usually become lodged in the lung, where they impair gas exchange and cause a local inflammatory reaction. Risk factors include the following:

- active cancer or cancer treatment;
- age >60 years;
- critical care admission;
- known thrombophilia;
- BMI >30 kg m^{-2};
- one or more significant medical comorbidities (e.g. heart or respiratory disease, acute infections, inflammatory conditions);
- personal history or first–degree relative with a history of venous thromboembolism (VTE);
- use of hormone replacement therapy/oestrogen contraceptive therapy; and
- varicose veins with phlebitis.

Venous stasis caused by venous compression, hypovolaemia, hypotension, hypothermia or the use of tourniquets also increase the risk of VTE. Pulmonary embolism (PE) may present with tachycardia, hypoxaemia, arrhythmia, hypotension and/or cardiovascular collapse. This is rare during anaesthesia and more common in the postoperative period.

The risk of postoperative VTE can be reduced by two types of intervention.

1. Mechanical
   a. Graduated compression stockings
   b. Intermittent pneumatic compressive devices
   c. Vena caval filters
2. Pharmacological
   a. Low molecular weight heparin
   b. Unfractionated heparin
   c. Vitamin K antagonists (e.g. warfarin)
   d. Newer direct oral anticoagulants (e.g. rivaroxaban).

The provision of good analgesia to facilitate early mobilisation and adequate hydration to optimise blood viscosity are also important to prevent PE. A high clinical index of suspicion and a low threshold for investigation and presumptive treatment are needed to allow effective management of PE in postoperative patients because the signs and symptoms of the condition overlap with many other respiratory and cardiovascular disease processes.

Cardiovascular complications

The most common causes of cardiac morbidity and mortality after anaesthesia are hypotension, myocardial ischaemia and arrhythmia, all of which can lead to cardiac failure. Together these account for a third of postoperative deaths.

Risk factors include:

- age;
- pre-existing cardiovascular, renal or metabolic disease;
- recent stroke or myocardial ischaemia; and
- intraoperative haemorrhage, hypotension, tachycardia or hypothermia.

The revised cardiac risk index is one model for the prediction of cardiovascular complications in patients undergoing non-cardiac surgery (see Chapter 19).

Hypotension

There is no agreed definition of intraoperative hypotension, although ≥20% reduction in MAP from the patient's usual resting value is commonly used. Hypotension may impair perfusion and consequently oxygen supply to vital organs. During anaesthesia, myocardial and cerebral metabolic rates are reduced, and intraoperative hypotension is less likely to cause permanent damage to these organs than would be the case in the conscious state. However, pathological processes (e.g. atherosclerosis) commonly compromise the arterial supply to organs, and hypotension during anaesthesia occasionally results in critical loss of flow to vital organs. Left ventricular coronary artery flow occurs predominantly in diastole, and diastolic arterial pressure is particularly important in determining myocardial viability in patients with ischaemic heart disease.

Hypotension is caused by decreases in cardiac output, heart rate and/or systemic vascular resistance. Most anaesthetic agents cause vasodilatation and have a mildly negative inotropic effect; moderate hypotension is very common during and immediately after anaesthesia. Spinal and epidural anaesthesia commonly result in hypotension through sympathetic pharmacodenervation. Concurrent hypovolaemia caused by preoperative fluid restriction, in combination with haemorrhage and/or concurrent antihypertensive drugs, may result in further decreases in MAP. The causes of perioperative hypovolaemia are listed in Box 26.2.

A MAP ≤55 mmHg is potentially harmful, even in healthy individuals, and should not be allowed to persist; in patients with significant comorbidities, persistent hypotension (even if less severe) may be detrimental. The patients most at risk from the effects of hypotension are, unfortunately, often the patients most likely to develop it because of concurrent medications, poor myocardial reserve and atherosclerosis. Older or hypertensive patients should, therefore, be observed carefully for the development of hypotension, and it should be treated promptly.

Box 26.2 Causes of hypovolaemia and fluid loss

Preoperative

Haemorrhage
  Trauma
  Obstetrics
  Gastrointestinal
  Major vessel rupture (e.g. aortic aneurysm)
Gastrointestinal
  Vomiting
  Obstruction
  Fistulae
  Diarrhoea
Other
  Fasting
  Diuretics
  Fever
  Burns

Intraoperative

Haemorrhage
Insensible loss
Sweating
Expired water vapour
Third-space loss
Prolonged procedures/extensive surgery
Drainage of stomach, bowel, or ascites

Treatment principles for hypotension in the perioperative period are to:

- seek an underlying cause (Table 26.1);
- optimise preload with i.v. fluid or blood resuscitation;
- provide systemic vasoconstriction (usually with α-adrenergic agonists, e.g. metaraminol); and
- increase myocardial contractility (using agents with some β-adrenergic effects, e.g. ephedrine).

Myocardial ischaemia and infarction

The myocardium has the largest oxygen consumption per tissue mass of almost all the organs; the oxygen extraction ratio is 70%–80%, compared with an average of 25% for other tissues (see Chapter 9). Increased oxygen consumption must be matched by an increase in coronary blood flow. Ischaemia results when oxygen demand exceeds supply. Even very brief reductions in supply result in ischaemia, which may lead rapidly to infarction and permanent loss of muscle function in the affected area.

Perioperative myocardial ischaemia may manifest in the awake patient with chest pain, dyspnoea, nausea, arrhythmia, hypotension or pulmonary oedema. It is diagnosed by ECG ST-segment changes (typically depression), elevated cardiac biomarkers (usually troponin) and/or echocardiography to detect abnormal myocardial wall motion (Somasundaram and Ball, 2013).

Increased myocardial work during the perioperative period (e.g. tachycardia and increased afterload secondary to inadequate analgesia) may precipitate further myocardial ischaemia or infarction in susceptible patients. The therapeutic management of myocardial ischaemia depends on the underlying pathological process: acute coronary syndrome with plaque rupture (also known as type 1 perioperative myocardial infarction), or prolonged oxygen supply–demand imbalance without plaque rupture (type 2 perioperative myocardial infarction); these conditions are discussed in Chapter 29. Although the risk of infarction in the general surgical population is low, the overall mortality rate is 4%–25%.

Arrhythmias

Bradyarrhythmias

Bradycardia is defined as a heart rate less than 60 beats min^{-1}. Heart rate very commonly decreases during anaesthesia because afferent input and sympathetic tone are reduced and because many anaesthetic agents and opioids have parasympathomimetic actions (see Table 26.1). Anaesthesia-induced bradycardia often leads to an escape rhythm, with a wandering suprajunctional pacemaker. Atrioventricular heart block may result in bradycardia and reduced cardiac output. Treatment is seldom necessary but minor degrees of atrioventricular block may progress to complete heart block, in which atrial impulses do not reach the ventricles. In this situation, bradycardia is usually severe and the atria no longer assist in filling the ventricles before ventricular systole. Cardiac output may fall to life-threateningly low levels, and immediate treatment is necessary. The emergency management of bradycardia is described in Chapters 28 and 29.

Tachyarrhythmias

Tachycardia is defined as a heart rate greater than 100 beats min^{-1}. Tachycardia is a normal sign of increased sympathetic nervous system activity. Perioperative tachyarrhythmias are not infrequent, and common causes are listed in Box 26.3. Tachycardia reduces diastolic coronary perfusion and simultaneously increases myocardial work. This may precipitate myocardial ischaemia in patients with coronary artery or hypertensive heart disease.

Extracellular potassium concentration has a profound effect on myocardial electrical activity. Hypokalaemia increases ventricular irritability and the risks of ventricular ectopics, tachycardia and fibrillation. This effect is potentiated in patients with ischaemic heart disease and in those receiving digoxin. Hyperventilation alters acid–base balance, with acute transmembrane redistribution of potassium. Serum potassium concentration decreases by approximately 1 mmol L^{-1}

Table 26.1 Causes of intraoperative hypotension (MAP ≈ (stroke volume × heart rate) × systemic vascular resistance)

Decreased stroke volume	Decreased heart rate	Decreased systemic vascular resistance
Reduced preload Hypovolaemia 　See Box 26.2 Obstruction 　PE 　Aortocaval compression (surgical, gravid uterus, tumour) 　Pericardial effusion/tamponade Raised intrathoracic pressure 　Mechanical ventilation, PEEP 　Pneumothorax Raised intra-abdominal pressure 　Pneumoperitoneum Head-up positioning **Reduced myocardial contractility** Drugs 　Most anaesthetic agents 　β-blockers 　Calcium channel antagonists Acidaemia Ischaemia/infarction Arrhythmias Pericardial tamponade	Cardiovascular causes 　Normal variant in athletic patient 　Myocardial ischaemia 　Sick-sinus syndrome 　Vasovagal syncope Non-cardiovascular causes 　Hypothermia 　Hypothyroidism 　Raised intracranial pressure Surgical 　Increased vagal tone (traction on eye, cervix, anus, peritoneum) 　Direct cardiac stimulation (chest surgery, CVC guidewire) Drugs 　Suxamethonium (especially with repeat dosing) 　Opioids (particularly remifentanil, alfentanil, fentanyl) 　Propofol 　Neostigmine 　β-blockers 　Calcium channel antagonists 　Digoxin	Drugs 　Relative or absolute overdose (most anaesthetic agents, antihypertensives) 　Direct histamine release (morphine, atracurium) 　Neuraxial blockade (local anaesthetics) 　Hypersensitivity reactions Sepsis

Box 26.3 Causes of perioperative tachycardia

Cardiorespiratory

Hypoxaemia
Hypotension
Hypo-/hypercapnia
Myocardial ischaemia

Metabolic

Infection
Hypovolaemia
Hyperthermia
Hyperthyroidism
Anaemia
Hypo-/hyperkalaemia
Hypomagnesaemia
Malignant hyperthermia

Physical

Painful surgical stimulus
Airway manipulation

Drugs

Vagolytics (e.g. atropine, pancuronium)
Sympathomimetics (e.g. adrenaline, ephedrine)
Ketamine
Alcohol ingestion

for every 2.5-kPa reduction in $PaCO_2$. Electrolyte disorders are discussed further in Chapter 12. The classification and management of atrial and ventricular arrhythmias are described in Chapter 28.

Neurological complications
Accidental awareness during general anaesthesia

Recall of intraoperative events occurs in 0.03%–0.3% of patients who have undergone general anaesthesia. Such recall may be spontaneous or may be provoked by postoperative events or questioning. Accidental awareness during general anaesthesia (AAGA) may be a very distressing event for a patient, particularly if it is accompanied by awareness of the painful nature of an operation or the presence of paralysis. However, most recalled events are not painful, and 80%–90% of patients recalling intraoperative events have not experienced pain. Awareness may have psychological sequelae including insomnia, depression and post-traumatic stress disorder (PTSD) with distressing flashbacks.

The risk of AAGA correlates with depth of anaesthesia. Light anaesthesia, particularly in conjunction with neuromuscular blockade, is associated with the highest risk of awareness. Awareness often is associated with poor anaesthetic technique. Errors include the omission or late commencement of volatile anaesthetic agent, inadequate dosing or failure to recognise the signs of awareness. Underdosing of anaesthetic agent may occur during hypotensive episodes, when anaesthetic is withheld to maintain arterial pressure. Breathing system malfunctions, misconnections and disconnections have also been associated with awareness.

Traditionally described signs of awareness and distress, such as sweating and signs of sympathetic activation (e.g. sweating, tachycardia, hypertension, tear formation), are not always present, and when present, they are not specific. Non-paralysed patients experiencing noxious stimulation may move or grimace. Depth of anaesthesia may be assessed through clinical examination, monitoring of the patient's end-tidal volatile anaesthetic agent concentration or using specialised monitoring equipment. Such equipment includes processed EEG such as the bispectral index and auditory evoked potential monitoring systems (see Chapter 17). If the end-tidal concentrations of inhaled anaesthetic agents summate to a total of greater than 0.7 (age-adjusted) minimum alveolar concentrarion (MAC), then it is unlikely that a patient will experience intraoperative awareness.

Risk factors for AAGA identified by the UK 5th National Anaesthetic Audit Project (NAP5) were as follows:

- Drug factors
  - Neuromuscular blockade
  - Use of thiopental
  - Rapid-sequence induction
  - TIVA techniques
- Patient factors
  - Female sex
  - Early middle age adults
  - Obesity
  - Previous episodes of awareness
  - Protracted or difficult airway management
- Surgical factors
  - Obstetric, cardiac, thoracic and neurosurgery
- Organisational factors
  - Emergencies
  - Out-of-hours operating
  - Inexperienced anaesthetists

The use of intravenous drugs for maintenance of anaesthesia (e.g. propofol) is associated with an increased risk of awareness compared with the use of inhaled anaesthetic agents. This is a result of the lack of real-time monitoring of plasma–brain drug concentrations, the necessary estimation of plasma–brain drug concentrations using a population-based model and the risk of unrecognised interruption of delivery (e.g. cannula disconnection). Many cases of awareness during TIVA occur when fixed-rate infusions of propofol are used or when drugs are manually administered as boluses. This is typically outside the operating theatre, often in an emergency setting (e.g. during transfer from the emergency department). The use of target-controlled infusions of intravenous anaesthetic is associated with a reduced risk of AAGA and is recommended by the Association of Anaesthetists guidelines (Nimmo et al., 2018).

If the anaesthetist suspects that a patient may be experiencing awareness, anaesthesia should be deepened immediately. If the arterial pressure is low despite an inadequate dose of anaesthetic agent, then arterial pressure should be supported through the use of i.v. fluids, modification of ventilatory pattern or i.v. administration of a vasopressor, and anaesthesia deepened appropriately. Consideration should be given to the use of an i.v. benzodiazepine (e.g. midazolam) because further recall is made unlikely through the anterograde amnesic effect.

If a patient complains in the postoperative period of intraoperative awareness, the anaesthetist should be informed and should visit the patient. The anaesthetist should establish the timing of the episode and try to distinguish between dreaming and awareness. If there is genuine awareness and a clear anaesthetic error, then a prompt apology and explanation should be provided. All details should be recorded in the case notes. The situation may be exacerbated if staff refuse to believe the patient. It is essential to offer follow-up counselling for the patient and to inform the patient's general practitioner. See the medicolegal aspects of complications section earlier for further detail of dealing with subsequent formal complaints.

Awareness occasionally occurs despite apparently excellent practice and in the absence of equipment malfunction. Successful defence against litigation requires that the anaesthetist has made thorough records. It is advisable that the anaesthetist always record the timing (absolute and relative to surgery) and dose of anaesthetic agents (inhaled or intravenous).

Stroke

Transient disruptions of CNS perfusion and oxygenation are common during anaesthesia. However, prolonged a reduction in oxygenation of the CNS may result in ischaemia or infarction. Ischaemic injury varies from minimal focal dysfunction to stroke or death. The mechanism is related usually to hypoxaemia or hypotension. The risk of ischaemic brain damage related to hypotension is increased in patients with atherosclerosis, and, in particular, cerebrovascular disease. A history of previous transient ischaemic attacks or stroke makes CNS injury much more likely during and after anaesthesia. Rarely, intracerebral haemorrhage may occur during anaesthesia, with consequent local cerebral tissue compression and ischaemic injury. Although the risk is increased if arterial pressure has been very high, there have been reports of intracerebral haemorrhage during anaesthesia without episodes of hypertension. It is likely that previously undetected vascular abnormalities were present in these cases.

Extreme rotation, flexion or extension of the neck or back may cause cerebral ischaemia because of vertebrobasilar insufficiency in susceptible patients. Ischaemic spinal cord injury may also occur during major vascular and spinal surgery, when the local arterial supply may be compromised. Hypoxaemia and hypotension should not be allowed to persist, particularly in patients at risk of ischaemic CNS injury. Severe hypocapnia should be avoided because of its potential for global cerebral vasoconstriction. Deep anaesthesia results in a greatly lowered cerebral metabolic rate (with all agents except ketamine), and this confers some protection against the effects of cerebral ischaemia.

Nerve injury

Nerve injury is a rare event that may occur at the time of either general or regional anaesthesia. Some cases of nerve injury can be ascribed to anaesthesia itself, but in many cases surgical factors (e.g. spinal nerve root damage as a result of incorrect pedicle screw placement or surgical retraction causing nerve stretch) are responsible.

Injury to the spinal cord or nerve roots

Injury to the spinal cord or its nerve roots occurs after a range of insults: compression; stretch; hypoperfusion; direct trauma; exposure to neurotoxic material; or combinations of these factors. Risk factors include:
* spinal canal deformity (see later);
* coagulation disorders;
* abnormal vascular supply; and
* immunosuppression.

Spinal canal stenosis is a common spinal canal deformity and can result from arthritic change, ankylosing spondylitis, Paget's disease or acromegaly. Pre-existing stenosis may contribute to spinal cord injury because the narrower canal cross-sectional area in such patients renders them more at risk of nerve compression. Underlying neurological conditions such as multiple sclerosis are not absolute contraindications to neuraxial anaesthesia, but this decision should be made on a case-by-case basis given the individual clinical circumstances.

Spinal cord ischaemia and infarction. Perioperative spinal cord ischaemia and infarction caused by hypoperfusion, thrombus or embolus can occur during any regional or general anaesthetic technique but is most often associated with surgery to the aorta, spine or heart. Risk factors include:
* atherosclerosis;
* cardiovascular disease;
* diabetes mellitus; and
* smoking history.

The clinical presentation of spinal cord infarction is variable, but the classical anterior spinal artery syndrome of paraplegia and loss of pain and temperature sense, but with intact proprioception, is the most common presentation. Such patients will need early neurological review and urgent MRI to detect ischaemic change and exclude differential diagnoses. Neuroprotective measures to reduce ongoing ischaemic damage to the cord should be instituted. These include blood pressure manipulation to prevent arterial hypotension, CSF drainage and initiation of anticoagulation in selected patients.

Spinal cord injury after neuraxial anaesthesia. Spinal cord injury after spinal or epidural blockade is very rare but can result in devastating, and often permanent, sequelae. Injury may occur as a result of direct needle trauma, vertebral canal haematoma, infection or chemical damage. The management of postdural puncture headache is described in Chapter 43.

Direct needle trauma. Direct trauma to the nerve roots of the cauda equina or the spinal cord itself is possible during spinal, epidural or caudal insertion. Needling at vertebral levels cephalad to the termination of the spinal cord (usually L2) during spinal techniques risks direct neural injury and should never be performed. Despite accurate vertebral level selection, needle trauma to neural tissue may occur. This can be due to lateral deviation of the needle towards spinal roots, usually causing paraesthesia. Paraesthesia during needling or injection should always alert the operator to potential neural injury and should prompt withdrawal of the needle; verbal confirmation should be sought from the patient that the paraesthesia has resolved and a careful redirection made before advancing the needle. A similarly cautious approach should be followed if paraesthesia is elicited during intrathecal injection of local anaesthetic. Fortunately, temporary paraesthesia, when managed with these steps, is rarely associated with permanent neurological damage.

Vertebral canal haematoma. Vertebral canal haematoma (VCH) is an accumulation of blood in either the subdural or epidural space that mechanically compresses the spinal cord or roots. Vertebral canal haematoma is a common complication of epidural catheter placement, but the majority of haematomata are asymptomatic, resolve spontaneously and are apparent only on spinal imaging. A large haematoma may cause permanent nerve injury, and importantly, neurological outcome from symptomatic haematoma is dependent on prompt diagnosis and management. National guidelines exist to inform anaesthetists of the impact of anticoagulants on neuraxial procedures (see Chapter 25).

Vertebral canal haematoma may cause pain at the site of haematoma, motor or sensory impairment, and altered bowel or bladder function. In 75% of cases this presentation will progress rapidly within a 24-h period. After neuraxial anaesthesia, any motor or sensory block that is unexpectedly prolonged outside the expected distribution or that reappears after initial block resolution should alert staff to the possibility of VCH. In the circumstances of an epidural infusion with unexpectedly dense motor block, the infusion should be stopped immediately and reassessment of neurology made every 30 min for no more than 4 h (before further investigations are undertaken). Low concentrations of local anaesthetic (e.g. 0.1% or 0.125% levobupivacaine) cause minimal weakness and numbness, and there should be a high level of suspicion of VCH if these signs arise in this context. In the event that motor power does not improve, the patient should undergo immediate MRI to confirm the diagnosis. If indicated, decompressive spinal surgery should be undertaken within 6–8 h of symptom onset.

Infection. Infection leading to spinal cord injury after neuraxial procedures may take the form of spinal epidural abscess or meningitis. The incidence of epidural abscess after neuraxial techniques is very low; the 3rd RCoA National Audit Project (NAP3) reported 20 new cases after the performance of an estimated 707,455 neuraxial blocks. Epidural abscesses typically present insidiously in the days to weeks after neuraxial blockade with:

- progressive back pain;
- localised tenderness;
- radicular pain;
- malaise;
- fever;
- sensory and motor deficit; or
- bowel and bladder dysfunction.

Management involves resuscitation like any other septic patient and the patient should be commenced on systemic antibiotics (after blood cultures) covering gram-positive cocci and gram-negative bacilli as soon as possible; *Staphylococcus* is the most commonly implicated organism. Urgent MRI is needed, and surgical drainage of the abscess and decompression of the spine or cauda equina may be necessary.

Meningitis after neuraxial blockade presents with headache, backache, meningism, fever and lethargy. It can easily be confused with postdural puncture headache, but the absence of a strong postural element to the headache and the presence of rising inflammatory and infectious markers should alert the clinician to the possibility of meningitis and the need to perform urgent diagnostic lumbar puncture. Respiratory tract commensals, such as the *Streptococcus viridans* group, are the responsible bacteria in the majority of cases, reinforcing the message that the wearing of a face mask is a vital component of neuraxial aseptic technique.

Epidural abscess and postdural puncture meningitis together carry an estimated 15% mortality, but speedy diagnosis and treatment reduce this significantly.

Chemical damage. Adhesive arachnoiditis is characterised by inflammation of the meninges, fibrous collagen band proliferation, reduced blood and CSF flow and permanent damage to neural tissues. The condition is often complicated by syringomyelia and has a bleak neurological prognosis, often resulting in paraplegia, with few treatment options. In response to concern about the role of chlorhexidine in triggering adhesive arachnoiditis, alcoholic chlorhexidine 0.5% solution is preferred to 2% solution for skin asepsis before central neuraxial blockade. The physical and temporal isolation of chlorhexidine solution from any equipment that will be used as part of the neuraxial technique is also recommended, as is the drying of the alcoholic solution before needle insertion, to optimise the antimicrobial action and to prevent wicking into the needle.

Injury to peripheral nerves

Injury to the peripheral nervous system can occur after general or regional anaesthesia, as a consequence of surgical trauma (the commonest cause), incorrect patient positioning or peripheral nerve blockade. Peripheral nerve injury of any cause occurs after approximately 0.1% of anaesthetics.

Nerve injury related to patient position. Peripheral nerve injury caused by incorrect patient positioning is an avoidable complication of anaesthesia. It can occur in patients undergoing sedation or regional or general anaesthesia and most commonly affects the ulnar nerve, brachial plexus or common peroneal nerve. The usual mechanism of injury to superficial nerves is ischaemia from compression of the vasa vasorum by surgical retractors, leg stirrups or contact with other equipment. Nerve injury may occur as part of a compartment syndrome after ischaemia from poor positioning, particularly when the legs are placed in Lloyd-Davies supports and the patient is positioned head-down. Ischaemic injury is more likely to occur during periods of poor peripheral perfusion associated with hypotension or hypothermia. Nerves may also be injured by traction (e.g. the brachial plexus during excessive shoulder abduction). Safe positioning for surgery requires careful planning, communication and compromise between surgical, anaesthetic and nursing staff. The anaesthetist must be vigilant during initial positioning for surgery and during the course of the operation, when deliberate or accidental movement and repositioning of the patient may lead to injury. The long duration of some surgical procedures undertaken in high-risk positions (e.g. laparoscopic or robot-assisted surgery in the lithotomy position) makes it prudent to set limits on the amount of time patients can be maintained in any potentially injurious position. When these limits are reached patients should be placed for at least 10 min in a neutral (respite) position before being repositioned for continuing surgery. It is difficult to prescribe safe durations because patients, positions and other circumstances vary. In general, though, it is widely held that a respite should be provided a minimum of every 4 h during at-risk positioning.

Although many injuries recover within several months, all patients with a peripheral nerve injury must be referred to a neurologist for assessment and continuing care.

Nerve injury after peripheral nerve blockade. There is a small risk of damage to nerves in association with any peripheral nerve block. Postoperative neurological symptoms suggestive of nerve injury after peripheral nerve blockade occur in approximately 2.2%, 0.8% and 0.2% of patients at 3, 6 and 12 months, respectively (Neal et al., 2015). Avoidance of direct intraneural damage by needle trauma is a prerequisite to safe regional anaesthesia. Paraesthesia or pain in the sensory distribution of a nerve are indicative of needle–nerve contact and should prompt immediate needle withdrawal. Pain commencing during the injection of local anaesthetic should cause immediate cessation of injection and withdrawal of the needle. The following potentially modifiable anaesthetic factors may influence the likelihood of nerve injury after peripheral nerve blockade.

Method of nerve and needle localisation. To date, no nerve localisation technique during needle placement (i.e. ultrasound guidance, nerve stimulation, elicited paraesthesia) has been found to be superior in terms of reducing the risk of nerve injury after peripheral nerve blockade in clinical trials; however, ultrasound guidance is now the clinical gold-standard technique for nerve and needle identification.

Block timing in relation to general anaesthesia. The main concern with performing peripheral nerve blockade in patients under general anaesthesia or deep sedation is that patients cannot communicate pain or paraesthesia during the block's performance. For this reason many anaesthetists choose routinely to perform blocks in conscious patients. In certain circumstances (e.g. paediatric practice, patients with movement disorders or developmental delay) the risk of unintended patient movement or inability of the patient to communicate paraesthesia even when awake means that performing blocks under general anaesthesia or deep sedation is preferable.

Needle design. Specialised block needles have a short bevel angle (i.e. blunted), which is designed to produce less direct nerve trauma than long (sharp) bevels because the nerve fascicle tends to be pushed away on needle contact, rather than being impaled.

Injection pressure. High injection pressure (>170 kPa) may indicate intraneural needle tip placement and should prompt immediate cessation of injection; in the absence of pain, this might simply indicate that the needle tip is against connective tissue, but if pain is present, then the needle should be withdrawn immediately. In-line manometer devices are available to monitor injection pressures. Very high injection pressures can be easily, and inadvertently, generated with small volume syringes. It is pragmatic, and therefore sensible, to use large-volume syringes (i.e.

preferably ≥ 20 ml) for peripheral nerve blockade because these make the requirement for greater force of injection more obvious.

Drug complications

Complications of drug administration during anaesthesia can be divided into adverse drug reactions and medication administration errors. Adverse drug reactions are commonly divided into type A and type B reactions. Medication administration errors in anaesthesia usually involve incorrect drug selection, inappropriate dosing, wrong route administration or incorrect drug preparation. The emergency management of perioperative critical incidents arising from drug administration, including anaphylaxis, local anaesthetic toxicity and malignant hyperpyrexia, is discussed in Chapter 27.

Adverse drug reactions

Type A reactions

These reactions are predictable from the known pharmacological properties of a drug, are dose-dependent and make up more than 80% of adverse drug reactions. Mild type A adverse drug reactions are often referred to as 'adverse effects'. Examples of reactions include gastritis associated with the perioperative use of NSAIDs and diarrhoea with antibiotics. More severe type A reactions include bleeding after anticoagulation with warfarin.

Type B reactions

These consist of fewer than 20% of adverse drug reactions and are unexpected, unpredictable and not a likely consequence of the known pharmacological properties of the drug. They are subdivided into immunological or idiosyncratic reactions.

Immunological drug reactions. Susceptible patients may display an enhanced immunological reaction to a trigger, which may be a drug but is sometimes an environmental agent. These hypersensitivity reactions may be anaphylactic or anaphylactoid.

Anaphylactic reaction. Anaphylaxis is an immunoglobulin E (IgE)–mediated reaction to an antigen. Antibodies bind to mast cells, which degranulate, releasing the chemical mediators of anaphylaxis. These include histamine, prostaglandins, platelet-activating factor (PAF) and leukotrienes. The signs produced by the actions of these mediators of anaphylaxis include:

- urticaria;
- cutaneous flushing;
- bronchospasm;
- hypotension;
- arrhythmia; and
- cardiac arrest.

Reactions are more common in women and in patients with a history of allergy, atopy or previous exposure to anaesthetic agents. More than 90% of reactions occur immediately after induction of anaesthesia. There is a clinical spectrum of severity from mild urticaria to immediate cardiac arrest. Coughing, skin erythema, difficulty with ventilation and loss of a palpable pulse are common early signs. Reactions often involve a single, major physiological system (e.g. bradycardia and profound hypotension without bronchospasm). This may make diagnosis confusing, but **every instance of bronchospasm, unexpected hypotension, arrhythmia or urticaria should be considered to be anaphylaxis until proven otherwise.** Erythema of the skin may be short-lived or absent because cyanosis from poor tissue perfusion and hypoxaemia may occur rapidly and be profound. The conscious patient may experience a sense of impending doom, dyspnoea, dizziness, palpitations and nausea.

Anaphylaxis has been reported in patients without apparent previous exposure to the specific antigen, probably because of immunological cross-reactivity. This is true particularly of reactions to neuromuscular blocking agents (NMBAs) as cosmetics and some foods contain similar structural groups. The incidence of anaphylaxis varies according to the antigen involved.

Intravenous drugs

- Of the i.v. drugs, reactions are most commonly to NMBAs (1 in 5000 to 1 in 10,000). Suxamethonium is the most immunogenic, although reactions to all non-depolarising NMBAs have also been reported. Most reactions are IgE-mediated. There is significant cross-reactivity between NMBAs and other drugs which contain a quaternary ammonium group. Pancuronium appears to be the least likely to cause anaphylaxis.
- Reactions to i.v. induction agents are far less common (1 in 15,000 to 1 in 50,000).
- Antibiotics are often implicated in allergic reactions. Penicillins are most often to blame, and there is cross-reactivity with cephalosporin antibiotics in 10% of penicillin-allergic patients.

Local anaesthetics

- Anaphylaxis to local anaesthetics is very rare. Reactions are more likely to be the result of dose-related toxicity, sensitivity to the effects of added vasoconstrictor or a reaction to preservatives such as paraben, sulphites and benzoates.
- Amide local anaesthetic agents are less allergenic than esters.

Latex

- Latex is emerging as one of the more important causes of anaphylaxis during anaesthesia and surgery. Reactions usually begin 30–60 min after exposure and may be very severe. Previous frequent exposure to latex (e.g. spina bifida) is a strong risk factor for latex allergy. There is often a history of intolerance to some foods, including banana and avocado.
- Many medical devices contain latex (e.g. arterial pressure cuffs, surgical gloves), and it is important that all such products are eliminated from the care of latex-susceptible patients.

Others

- Anaphylaxis also occurs in response to radiocontrast media, blood products, colloid solutions, protamine, streptokinase, aprotinin, atropine, bone cement and opioids.

Anaphylactoid reaction. These reactions are not IgE-mediated although the clinical presentation is identical to anaphylaxis. The precise immunological mechanism is not always evident, although many reactions involve complement, kinin and coagulation pathway activation.

Non-immunological histamine release. This is caused by the direct action of a drug on mast cells. The clinical response depends on both the drug dose and rate of delivery but is usually benign and confined to the skin. Anaesthetic drugs which release histamine directly include d-tubocurarine, atracurium, doxacurium, mivacurium (all of similar chemical derivation), morphine and meperidine. Clinical evidence of histamine release, usually cutaneous, occurs in up to 30% of patients during anaesthesia. However, some very serious reactions have been reported in association with administration of atracurium and mivacurium.

Anaesthesia in patients with known significant allergy. Unless the patient is allergic to local anaesthetics, regional anaesthesia should be used if possible. If the patient requires general anaesthesia, the preoperative use of corticosteroids and histamine H_1- and H_2-receptor antagonists can be considered as prophylaxis. The anaesthetic technique chosen should avoid exposure to implicated agents. Drugs should be chosen that have a low potential for hypersensitivity and direct histamine release. Typically, safe drugs include volatile agents, etomidate, fentanyl, pancuronium and benzodiazepines. All drugs should be given slowly in diluted form, and resuscitation facilities must be immediately available.

Idiosyncratic drug reactions. An idiosyncratic drug reaction is a qualitatively abnormal and harmful drug effect which occurs in a small number of individuals and is precipitated usually by small drug doses. There is often an associated genetic defect, and the reaction may be severe or even fatal. Suxamethonium sensitivity, malignant hyperthermia and acute intermittent porphyria are important examples of drug idiosyncrasy in anaesthetic practice.

Acute intermittent porphyria. Acute intermittent porphyria (AIP) is a rare but serious metabolic disorder caused by an inherited deficiency of an enzyme required for haem synthesis. Porphyrin precursors accumulate and cause acute neuropathy, abdominal pain (mimicking an acute abdomen), delirium and death. These precursors are produced in the liver by δ-amino laevulinic acid synthetase, and this enzyme may be induced by barbiturates, amongst other drugs. If an at-risk patient is identified, porphyrinogenic drugs (including barbiturates) must be avoided. Drugs considered safe include:

- propofol;
- midazolam;
- suxamethonium;
- vecuronium;
- nitrous oxide;
- morphine;
- fentanyl;
- neostigmine; and
  - atropine.

Physical complications

Direct physical injury is a common event in the perioperative period. Most of these injuries are preventable. Tracheal intubation and poor patient positioning are commonly to blame. Nerve, dental and ophthalmic injuries are common causes of litigation. Thermal and electrical injuries are less common, but are potentially disastrous.

Cutaneous and muscular injury

Skin is easily damaged by poor and/or prolonged positioning, use of highly adhesive tape and incautious movement of the patient. Older patients and those who have been treated with steroids for a prolonged period may have fragile skin, and this must be protected. These patients tend to heal very slowly, and an apparently minor skin injury may produce many months of suffering postoperatively. Pressure sores that originate during the intraoperative period are increasingly recognised. Muscle injury is produced most commonly by poor positioning, but tourniquets may also cause direct muscle damage.

Injury during airway management

Dental damage is the most commonly reported anaesthetic injury and is usually sustained during laryngoscopy. Damage to teeth is much more likely if laryngoscopy is difficult, or the laryngoscopist is inexperienced. Most dental injuries result from a rotational force applied to the laryngoscope during attempts to lever the tip of the laryngoscope blade upwards, using the upper incisors as a fulcrum. The correct, and much safer, practice is to apply a force upwards and away from the anaesthetist without any leverage on the incisors. Injuries vary from chipped teeth to complete avulsion. The upper incisors are most commonly involved. Dental injury has also been reported during tracheal extubation, either by pulling the tracheal tube while the patient is biting it, or by using an oropharyngeal airway as a bite-block.

Supraglottic airway (SAD) removal has also caused many dental injuries, and forceful traction should not be applied while the patient is biting on the shaft. Removal of tracheal tubes and SADs is usually most safely accomplished in the conscious patient, and such a scenario is best achieved by preventing stimulation while the patient eliminates or redistributes anaesthetic agent.

Preoperative assessment and documentation of dentition are essential. All patients should be warned of the possibility of dental injury. If a tooth is accidentally avulsed, it should be replaced in its socket with minimal interference and a dental surgeon consulted at the earliest opportunity.

Mucosal damage is common during airway management, and mucosal abrasion may be very painful postoperatively. Overinflation of the cuff of a tracheal tube in the larynx or trachea may produce local ischaemia, with consequent scarring and stenosis; cuff pressure should be checked regularly, particularly during prolonged surgery, and when nitrous oxide is used. Other reported injuries include dislocated arytenoid cartilages (tracheal intubation), recurrent laryngeal nerve damage (laryngoscopy and SAD use), uvular ischaemia (oropharyngeal airway), epistaxis and nasal turbinate fracture (nasal tracheal intubation).

Ophthalmic injury

Retinal ischaemic injury may follow prolonged pressure on the globe or orbit from equipment or prone positioning; permanent blindness may result. Prolonged hypotension, especially in the head-down position, can result in ischaemic optic nerve injury. The differentiation of venous, arterial, retinal and optic nerve injury is beyond the scope of this chapter, but in all cases, ophthalmological opinion should be sought urgently in the context of perioperative visual loss.

Corneal abrasions are associated with inadequate eye protection, especially during transfer or use of the prone position. The use of adhesive tape to close the eyelids is also a risk factor, and incautious removal of such eye protection can itself lead to corneal injury. Lubricated dressings such as sterile paraffin gauze may be a preferable method of securing the eyelids. Corneal injury may occur after removal of airway devices and ocular protection; sleepy and disorientated patients may rub their eyes, or an oxygen mask may rub the cornea. Care should be taken to minimise such possibilities.

Thermal and electrical injury

The high-density electrical current of surgical diathermy is a potential source of injury. If the return current path is interrupted by incorrect application of the diathermy pad, then ECG electrodes or other points of contact between skin and metal may provide an alternative electrical path, producing serious burns. Failure of thermostatic control on warming devices is also a source of potential thermal injury. Warming devices should always be used in accordance with the manufacturer's guidelines. In particular, hot air hoses used to inflate convective warming blankets must never be used alone to blow hot air under the patient's blankets, as serious thermal injury may result. Ignition of alcohol-based surgical preparation solutions is possible, especially if they are not allowed to evaporate fully and if diathermy is used. Airway fires have occurred during laser surgery to the larynx; it is advisable to use a low inspired oxygen fraction and omit nitrous oxide in this situation. Fires should be extinguished immediately, and the area should be soaked in cool saline or covered with saline-soaked swabs. If the burned area is significant, the opinion of a burns surgeon should be sought.

Vascular injury and tourniquets

Arterial catheters may produce significant arterial injury, resulting in ischaemia and, potentially, loss of the distal limb. Arterial tourniquets reduce surgical bleeding but also rob the distal tissue of its perfusion. An absolute maximum duration of 2 h should be observed, and inflation pressures should be high enough to just occlude arterial flow. Typically a pressure of 200–250 mmHg is adequate for the upper limb and 250–300 mmHg for the lower limb. Vascular occlusion (e.g. during tourniquet use, aortic cross-clamping) risks distal ischaemia and infarction. Assurance of an adequate arterial pressure and oxygen saturation is important in facilitating distal oxygenation via collateral flow. Parts distal to an arterial occlusion should not be warmed because this increases local metabolic rate and accelerates the onset of ischaemia.

References/Further reading

Canet, J., Gallart, L., Gomar, C., et al., 2010. Prediction of postoperative pulmonary complications in a population-based surgical cohort. Anesthesiology 113, 1338–1350.

Neal, J.M., Barrington, M.J., Brull, R., et al., 2015. The second ASRA practice advisory on neurologic complications associated with regional anesthesia and pain medicine: executive summary 2015. Reg. Anesth. Pain Med. 40, 401–430.

Nimmo, A.F., Absalom, A.R., Bagshaw, O., Biswas, A., Cook, T.M., Costello, A., et al., 2018. Guidelines for the safe practice of total intravenous anaesthesia (TIVA) Joint Guidelines from the Association of Anaesthetists and the Society for Intravenous Anaesthesia. Anaesthesia. doi: 10.1111/anae.14428.

Rock, P., Rich, P.B., 2003. Postoperative pulmonary complications. Curr. Opin. Anesthesiol. 16, 123–131.

Somasundaram, K., Ball, J., 2013. Medical emergencies: atrial fibrillation and myocardial infarction. Anaesthesia 68, 84–101.

Chapter | 27 |

Management of critical incidents

Mark Barley

Emergencies in anaesthesia and critical care are often time-critical events requiring rapid intervention to prevent patient harm. There is added complexity interpreting and managing the dynamic interaction of surgical events (physiological stimulus, haemorrhage or mechanics of surgery), patient comorbidities, physiological changes associated with anaesthesia and myriad potential problems with anaesthetic equipment, ventilators and gas and electrical supplies.

Successful management of critical incidents requires well-developed non-technical skills (see Chapter 18) including situational awareness, communication, teamwork and decision-making skills. Obtaining assistance early in the incident can facilitate diagnosis and decision making. Delegating practical tasks to an assistant expedites treatment while allowing the team leader to maintain situational awareness, a calm sense of control and clear lines of communication.

Critical incidents in anaesthesia are managed differently to those encountered in other branches of medicine. The traditional pattern of history, examination, investigation, diagnosis and treatment in series is too slow for conditions which are rapidly life threatening. The anaesthetist must be prepared to simultaneously diagnose and treat the most likely problems whilst examining and investigating for rarer conditions. After any intervention, it is vital to take a moment to think 'How do I expect this patient to respond to this treatment?' and assess the response. It can be detrimental to continue down a treatment algorithm without objective evidence of clinical improvement; an open mind may help prevent both task and diagnostic fixation.

It is useful to apply a consistent, basic approach to any potential critical incident to rapidly rule in or rule out a problem or diagnosis, as this will:
- increase the chance of identifying the underlying problem;
- reduce the risk of task fixation;
- reduce the risk of cognitive overload and allow thinking time; and
- facilitate good communication and teamwork.

This chapter presents a series of critical incidents with management guidelines along with a range of differential diagnoses, conditions to rapidly rule in and rule out, and top tips to optimise patient outcome. The management of failed tracheal intubation (see Chapter 23), 'can't intubate, can't ventilate' situations (see Chapter 23) and cardiac arrest and cardiac arrhythmias (see Chapter 28) are discussed elsewhere.

Unexpected fall in Spo_2 with or without cyanosis
A fall in Spo_2 >5%, an absolute Spo_2 <90% or Pao_2 <8kPa

Rule out: *breathing circuit disconnection or displacement; failure of oxygen supply; endobronchial intubation; bronchospasm; anaphylaxis; circuit or airway obstruction; hypotension/hypoperfusion; probe displacement.*

Alert team; pause surgery if possible.

❶ Increase oxygen delivery
- Increase FGF, give 100% O_2. Confirm measured FIO_2 approaches 100%.
- Confirm breathing circuit connections and that circle valves move freely.
- Verify ventilator bellows or reservoir bag moving and APL valve set correctly.

❷ Airway
- Confirm airway device position and listen for added noise (stridor, spasm, wheeze).
- Confirm end-tidal CO_2 waveform and shape.
- Check airway device is patent (breath sounds, pass a suction catheter).
- **Use self-inflating bag to isolate patient from machine – if high pressure resolves, assume machine problem and REPLACE.**
- If high airway pressure persists, reconnect to anaesthetic machine.
- Consider changing airway device, or tracheal intubation if SAD *in situ*.

❸ Breathing
- Assess airway pressure with reservoir bag and APL valve.
- Check chest expansion and symmetry.
- Confirm equal bilateral air entry and normal breath sounds.
- Consider neuromuscular blockade if ventilator asynchrony.
- Consider and exclude differential diagnoses *(box right)*.

❹ Circulation
- Recheck blood pressure and ensure patient has a perfusing rhythm.

❺ Anaesthesia
- Confirm and maintain adequate depth of anaesthesia and neuromuscular blockade.

Differential diagnoses

Airway
Displaced airway device/oesophageal intubation
Laryngospasm
Endobronchial intubation
Foreign body (circuit or airway)

Breathing
Diaphragmatic splinting (e.g. pneumoperitoneum/position)
Pneumothorax
Bronchospasm
Anaphylaxis
Aspiration
Pulmonary oedema
Unrecognised underlying lung disease

Circulation
Low cardiac output state (e.g. haemorrhage, MI, tamponade, PE)
Vasodilatation (e.g. sepsis)

Anaesthetic
Inappropriately low FIO_2 delivery
Oxygen supply failure
Inadequate minute ventilation
Poor pulse oximeter placement (e.g. contact with skin, peripheral vascular disease, arteriovenous fistula)
Increased metabolic oxygen demand (e.g. MH, sepsis)

Top Tips

- Treat low Spo_2 as hypoxaemia until proven otherwise.
- Exclude anaphylaxis (bronchospasm, cardiovascular collapse).
- An *absolute* inability to ventilate the patient's lungs is rarely physiological – immediately rule out a mechanical obstruction in the circuit / airway device with a self-inflating bag connected **directly** to the tracheal tube/SAD 15-mm connector.

If hypoxia not resolving, **call for help,** stop surgery.
Consider: CXR (tracheal tube position, lung fields), ABG, bronchoscopy, ECG.

ABG, arterial blood gas; *APL,* adjustable pressure limiting; *CXR,* chest radiograph; *ECG,* electrocardiogram; *FGF,* fresh gas flow; *FIO₂,* fraction of inspired oxygen; *MH,* malignant hyperthermia; *MI,* myocardial infarction; *PE,* pulmonary embolism; *SAD,* supraglottic airway device.

Unexpected increase in peak airway pressure
Peak airway pressure >40 cmH$_2$O or rise > 5 cmH$_2$O

Rule out: *kinked, obstructed or endobronchial tracheal tube; anaphylaxis; laryngospasm; bronchospasm; pneumothorax; excessive intra-abdominal pressure; foreign body.*

Alert team; pause surgery if possible.
Level operating table.

❶ **Increase oxygen delivery**
- Increase FGF, give 100% O$_2$. Confirm measured FIO_2 approaches 100%.
- Rule out surgical cause.
- Confirm breathing circuit connections and that circle valves move freely.
- Verify ventilator bellows or reservoir bag moving and APL valve set correctly.
- Manual ventilation with reservoir bag to confirm high pressure.

❷ **Airway**
- Check airway device position and listen for added noise (stridor, spasm, wheeze).
- Confirm end-tidal CO$_2$ waveform and shape.
- Check airway device is patent (breath sounds, pass a suction catheter).
- **Use self-inflating bag to isolate patient from machine – if high pressure resolves, assume machine problem and REPLACE.**
- If high airway pressure persists, reconnect to anaesthetic machine.
- Consider changing airway device, or tracheal intubation if SAD *in situ*.

❸ **Breathing**
- Check chest expansion and symmetry.
- Confirm equal bilateral air entry and normal breath sounds.
- Consider and exclude differential diagnoses.

❹ **Circulation**
- Recheck blood pressure and ensure patient has a perfusing rhythm.
- Hypotension may be secondary to high intrathoracic pressure.

❺ **Anaesthesia**
- Confirm and maintain adequate depth of anaesthesia and neuromuscular blockade.

Differential diagnoses

Airway
Kinked, displaced or endobronchial tube
Foreign body in circle, airway device or trachea
Glottic obstruction: laryngospasm or foreign body

Breathing
Bronchospasm or anaphylaxis
Raised intra-abdominal pressure or diaphragmatic splinting – obesity, pneumoperitoneum, Trendelenburg position
Reduced lung compliance (e.g. aspiration of gastric contents, atelectasis, pneumothorax)

Anaesthetic
APL or one-way flow valves in circle stuck
Oxygen flush stuck ON
Unintentionally high PEEP
Ventilator pressure or volumes set inappropriately high
Inadequate depth of anaesthesia or paralysis
Opioid-induced chest wall rigidity

Top Tips
- Pneumoperitoneum, retraction and head-down positioning all increase peak airway pressure.
- Reduce or release pneumoperitoneum (aim for IAP <15 mmHg.
- Position changes (lithotomy, head down) cause tracheal tube position to change – beware endobronchial intubation and bronchospasm.

If high airway pressures are not resolving, **call for help**, stop surgery, and release any pneumoperitoneum.
Consider: CXR (tube position, lung fields), ABG, bronchoscopy.

ABG, arterial blood gas; *APL,* adjustable pressure limiting; *CXR,* chest radiograph; *FGF,* fresh gas flow; FIO_2, fraction of inspired oxygen; *IAP,* intra-abdominal pressure; *PEEP,* positive end-expiratory pressure; *SAD,* supraglottic airway device.

Progressive fall in minute volume during spontaneous respiration or IPPV
Manifesting an unexpected decrease in minute/tidal volume with increase in end-tidal CO_2 and decrease in SpO_2

Rule out: *displaced airway device; laryngospasm; drug effect (opioids, NMBA); foreign body; bronchospasm; arrhythmia; anaphylaxis; cardiac arrest.*

Alert team; pause surgery if possible.

❶ **Increase oxygen delivery**
- Increase FGF, give 100% O_2. Confirm measured FIO_2 approaches 100%.
- Confirm breathing circuit connections and that circle valves move freely.
- Verify ventilator bellows or reservoir bag moving and APL valve set correctly.

❷ **Airway**
- Check airway device position and listen for added noise (stridor, spasm, wheeze).
- Confirm end-tidal CO_2 waveform and shape.
- Check airway device is patent (breath sounds, pass a suction catheter).
- Consider changing airway device, or tracheal intubation if SAD *in situ.*

❸ **Breathing**
- Check chest expansion and symmetry.
- Confirm equal bilateral air entry and normal breath sounds.
- Check tidal volume and feel lung compliance during manual ventilation with reservoir bag.
- Check APL valve position – exclude excess PEEP.
- Ensure mode and ventilator settings are appropriate if controlled ventilation used.
- Consider and exclude differential diagnoses.

❹ **Circulation**
- Recheck blood pressure and ensure patient has a perfusing rhythm.

❺ **Anaesthesia**
- Double-check drug administration; exclude accidental opioid or NMBA administration with spontaneous respiration.
- Ensure appropriate depth of anaesthesia.

Differential diagnoses

Airway
Displaced airway device
Laryngospasm/obstruction (stridor)
Foreign body, aspiration

Breathing
Aspiration
Bronchospasm
Pneumothorax
Anaphylaxis
Diaphragmatic splinting, pneumoperitoneum

Cardiovascular
Cardiovascular collapse (e.g. anaphylaxis, massive PE)
Arrhythmia, early cardiac arrest

Neurological
Elevated ICP, brainstem coning

Anaesthetic
Drugs: Opioids/NMBA administration
Incorrect mode or ventilator settings
Ventilator or gas supply failure

Top Tips
- Rule out an airway problem before moving on to other systems.
- Ventilator or circuit problems can be excluded with a self-inflating bag connected directly to the airway device 15-mm connector.
- Return operating table to neutral and patient to a reverse Trendelenburg position to optimise lung compliance.
- Drug errors/effect (opioid/NMBA) reduce MV.
- Cardiovascular collapse will lead to a fall in end-tidal CO_2, minute volume and tidal volume.

If ventilation not improving, **call for help.** Stop surgery.
Consider: CXR (tube position, lung fields), ABG, bronchoscopy, ECG, use of alternate means of ventilation.

ABG, arterial blood gas; *APL*, adjustable pressure limiting; *CXR*, chest radiograph; *ECG*, electrocardiogram; *FGF*, fresh gas flow; *FIO$_2$*, fraction of inspired oxygen; *ICP*, intracranial pressure; *NMBA*, neuromuscular blocking agent; *PE*, pulmonary embolism; *PEEP*, positive end-expiratory pressure; *SAD*, supraglottic airway device.

Fall in end-tidal CO_2

Rule out: *cardiac arrest; anaphylaxis; major haemorrhage; bronchospasm; laryngospasm; airway device displacement or obstruction; iatrogenic mechanical hyperventilation.*

Alert team; pause surgery if possible.

❶ **Increase oxygen delivery**
- Increase FGF, give 100% O_2. Confirm measured FIO_2 approaches 100%.
- **If no capnograph trace, check cardiac output.**
- Commence CPR if no cardiac output detected.
- Confirm breathing circuit and gas analysis/CO_2 connections and power supply.

❷ **Airway**
- Check airway device position and listen for added noise (stridor, spasm, wheeze).
- Confirm end-tidal CO_2 waveform and shape.
- Check airway device is patent (breath sounds, pass a suction catheter or bronchoscope).
- If any doubt, change airway device, or tracheal intubation if SAD *in situ.*

❸ **Breathing**
- Exclude bronchospasm and endobronchial intubation by auscultation.
- Check tidal volume and respiratory rate and feel lung compliance during manual ventilation with reservoir bag.
- Ensure mode and ventilator settings are appropriate if controlled ventilation used.

❹ **Circulation**
- Recheck blood pressure and ensure patient has a perfusing rhythm.
- Exclude major haemorrhage.
- Treat hypotension with fluids and/or drugs.
- Treat severe hypotension *without* haemorrhage as anaphylaxis until ruled out.
- Auscultate precordium for the mill wheel murmur of an air embolus. If audible, flood surgical field, position head down and summon help.
- Cross-check end-tidal CO_2 with $PaCO_2$ via ABG.

❺ **Anaesthesia**
- Optimise analgesia and depth of anaesthesia.
- Check ventilator settings.
- Treat hypothermia (if applicable).

Differential diagnoses

Airway
Airway device displacement
Airway or circuit obstruction
Laryngospasm

Breathing
Bronchospasm/anaphylaxis
Hyperventilation (spontaneous or controlled)
Endobronchial intubation

Circulation
Cardiovascular collapse (e.g. anaphylaxis, cardiac arrest, PE, air embolus)
Major haemorrhage
Arrhythmia and hypoperfusion

Neurological
Brainstem infarction or haemorrhage

Anaesthetic
Hyperventilation (e.g. pain, inadequate depth of anaesthesia, ventilator settings)
Gas analyser failure (e.g. obstructed line, moisture trap full, electrical failure)

Top Tips

- Accidental tracheal tube displacement, disconnection and extubation can occur under the drapes.
- A falling end-tidal CO_2 can be a marker of **cardiovascular collapse** – rule out anaphylaxis, PE and cardiac arrest.
- Hyperventilation can easily occur after release of a pneumoperitoneum.
- A frail elderly patient with little muscle mass is easily hyperventilated on pressure-controlled ventilator modes.
- Inadequate depth of anaesthesia or analgesia will cause hyperventilation.
- A low end-tidal CO_2 will compromise cerebral perfusion by temporary vasoconstriction.

If end-tidal CO_2 fails to improve, **call for help.** Stop surgery. Recheck peripheral pulses to exclude a cardiac cause. Consider: tracheal intubation, CXR, ABG, change of capnography and tubing if potentially faulty.

ABG, arterial blood gas; *CXR,* chest radiograph; *FGF,* fresh gas flow; *FIO_2,* fraction of inspired oxygen; *$PaCO_2$,* partial pressure of carbon dioxide in arterial blood; *PE,* pulmonary embolism; *SAD,* supraglottic airway device.

Rise in end-tidal CO_2

$Paco_2$ >6.5 kPa or presence of CO_2 in inspired gas

Rule out: *malignant hyperpyrexia; hypoventilation; soda lime exhaustion; bronchospasm; sepsis; thyroid storm; increased CO_2 delivery from pneumoperitoneum or endoscopic procedure.*

Alert team; pause surgery if possible.

❶ **Increase oxygen delivery**
- Ensure no CO_2 detected in inspired gas.
- Increase FGF and refresh soda lime if exhausted.
- Confirm breathing circuit connections and valves are functioning correctly.

❷ **Airway**
- Check airway device position and listen for added noise (stridor, spasm, wheeze).
- Confirm end-tidal CO_2 waveform and shape.
- Check airway device is not obstructed (breath sounds, pass a suction catheter or bronchoscope).
- If any doubt, change airway device, or tracheal intubation if SAD *in situ*.

❸ **Breathing**
- Auscultate to exclude bronchospasm.
- Check tidal volume and respiratory rate and feel lung compliance during manual ventilation with reservoir bag.
- Increase minute volume or switch to assisted ventilation if breathing spontaneously.
- Check ventilator settings.

❹ **Circulation**
- Cross-check end-tidal CO_2 with $Paco_2$ via ABG.
- If MH suspected, acid–base status, K^+ and CK should be measured.

❺ **Anaesthesia**
- Insert temperature probe.
- Refer to MH protocol if suspected.
- Rule out respiratory depression from opioids, accidental NMBA administration or excessive anaesthesia if spontaneously breathing.
- Release pneumoperitoneum or apply suction via endoscope to remove CO_2.

Differential diagnoses

Airway
Reduced tidal volume as a result of FGF leak from airway device
Partial airway obstruction

Breathing
Rebreathing CO_2
Hypoventilation

Cardiovascular
Malignant hyperthermia (hypercapnia, increased O_2 demand, tachycardia)
Thyroid storm (hyperthermia, hypercapnia, tachycardia, hypertension)
Neuroleptic malignant syndrome
Serotonin syndrome

Anaesthetic
CO_2 absorption exhausted or faulty
Inadequate FGF
Increased dead space and rebreathing *(inner from coaxial Bain circuit disconnected or stuck expiratory circle valve)*
Hypoventilation

Surgical
CO_2 delivery from pneumoperitoneum or endoscopic techniques

Top Tips
- Hypercapnia is a function of increased production (e.g. MH or other hypermetabolic condition) or external CO_2 (surgical insufflation) with inadequate elimination (ventilation).
- Modest hypercapnia (end-tidal CO_2 <8 kPa) is common with spontaneous ventilation anaesthetic techniques.
- Hypercapnia will increase ICP, heart rate and blood pressure.
- Significant hypercapnia causes dysrhythmias.

If end-tidal CO_2 fails to improve, **call for help.** Pause surgery. Exclude MH – if in doubt, start treatment. Consider: CXR, ABG, urinary catheter (MH, thyroid storm). Change CO_2 absorber and circuit.

ABG, arterial blood gas; *CK*, creatinine kinase; *CXR*, chest radiograph; *FGF*, fresh gas flow; *ICP*, intracranial pressure; *MH*, malignant hyperthermia; *NMBA*, neuromuscular blocking agent; *$Paco_2$*, partial pressure of carbon dioxide in arterial blood; *SAD*, supraglottic airway device.

Rise in inspired CO_2
Presence of any CO_2 in fresh gas flow

Rule out: *exhausted or faulty CO_2 absorber; very low fresh gas flow; circle unidirectional valve stuck open; faulty gas analyser; exogenous CO_2 (CO_2 cylinder on old anaesthetic machine).*

❶ Increase oxygen delivery
- Increase FGF to ≥ 10 L min^{-1}.

❷ Breathing
- Confirm breathing circuit and capnography connections.
- Visualise unidirectional circle valves move correctly. Replace machine if faulty.
- Check tidal volume, respiratory rate and feel lung compliance during manual ventilation with reservoir bag.
- Refresh CO_2 absorber.
- Check end-tidal CO_2 waveform falling to zero following these interventions.

❸ Anaesthetic
- Ensure no CO_2 cylinder on machine.
- Recalibrate gas analyser if zero calibration error suspected.
- Check for moisture contamination of gas analyser and replace analyser and tubing if water identified.
- If cause of increased $F_{I}CO_2$ cannot be identified, change machine – maintain anaesthesia with intravenous agents and ventilate with self-inflating bag during this process.

Differential diagnoses

Breathing
Inadequate FGF
Exhausted or faulty CO_2 absorption
Channelling of exhaled gases through CO_2 absorber
Faulty unidirectional flow valves causing rebreathing

Anaesthetic
Zero calibration error on gas analyser.
Moisture contamination in gas analyser.
Exogenous CO_2 – old anaesthetic machine.

Top Tips

- Exhaustion of soda lime is the commonest cause; be sure you know the colour changes of your locally used absorber. Some change from white to purple, others from purple to white!
- A high $F_{I}CO_2$ will contribute to a high end-tidal CO_2, increasing ICP and heart rate and producing respiratory acidosis.

If $F_{I}CO_2$ fails to improve, **call for help.** Pause surgery.
Consider: changing CO_2 absorption, circuit and anaesthetic machine.

FGF, fresh gas flow; $F_{I}CO_2$, fraction of inspired carbon dioxide; *ICP,* intracranial pressure.

Unexpected hypotension
Fall in systolic blood pressure > 20% of baseline value

Rule out: *anaphylaxis; cardiac arrest; myocardial ischaemia or arrhythmia; pneumothorax; high spinal or epidural block; drug error; haemorrhage or hypovolaemia; vagal response; gas, fat or pulmonary embolism*

Alert team; pause surgery if possible.

❶ Increase oxygen delivery

- Increase FGF, give 100% O_2. Confirm measured FiO_2 approaches 100%.
- Confirm breathing circuit connections and that circle valves move freely.
- Verify ventilator bellows or reservoir bag moving and APL valve set correctly.

❷ Airway

- Check airway device position and listen for added noise (stridor, spasm, wheeze).
- Confirm end-tidal CO_2 waveform and shape.
- Check airway device is not obstructed (breath sounds, pass a suction catheter).
- Palpate tracheal position (tension pneumothorax).

❸ Breathing

- Confirm equal bilateral air entry and normal breath sounds to exclude pneumothorax.
- Check tidal volume and respiratory rate and feel lung compliance during manual ventilation with reservoir bag.
- Check mean airway pressure and PEEP and exclude raised intrathoracic pressure as a cause.

❹ Circulation

- Recheck blood pressure, heart rate and perfusion.
- ***In the absence of catastrophic haemorrhage, treat severe hypotension as anaphylaxis.***
- Treat bradycardia with anticholinergic agent.
- Consider vasopressor use and head-down position.
- Administer fluid bolus (250 ml) if sinus tachycardia.
- Manage non-sinus tachycardia as per ALS protocols (see Chapter 28).
- Confirm blood loss with surgical and scrub team. Weigh swabs and check suction bottles, drapes and the floor for occult blood.
- Request a surgical 'pack and pause' to allow correction of hypovolaemia if haemorrhage confirmed.
- Release any pneumoperitoneum or bowel dilatation from endoscopy to increase venous return.
- Consider and exclude differential diagnoses.

❺ Anaesthesia

- Exclude excessive depth of anaesthesia.
- Rule out potential drug error; discard and replace partially used syringes.

Differential diagnoses

Airway
Profound hypoxaemia

Breathing
Tension pneumothorax
Raised intrathoracic pressure

Circulation
Anaphylaxis
Hypovolaemia
Reduced venous return (e.g. pneumoperitoneum or aortocaval compression)
Gas, fat, blood or amniotic fluid embolism
Sepsis
Addisonian crisis

Neurological
High spinal or epidural block

Surgical
Haemorrhage
Bone cement reaction
Vagal reaction to surgical stimulus (e.g. eyes, cervix, testicles, peritoneum)

Anaesthetic
Local anaesthetic toxicity
Excessive depth of anaesthesia

Top Tips

- **Actively exclude anaphylaxis** (cardiovascular collapse, increased airway pressure, bronchospasm) – in context of hypotension and poor skin perfusion **a rash may not be present.**
- A regular walk around the operating table and inspection of swabs, suction and the operative field helps maintain awareness of ongoing blood losses.
- Common causes of hypotension are hypovolaemia, neuroaxial blockade and unnecessarily deep anaesthesia – these may coexist!
- Consider and plan for the effects of a patient's usual medication – antihypertensives, β-blockers and ACE inhibitors; 50% of hypertensive patients will be on multiple agents.
- Prolonged preoperative fasting or increased insensible losses (nasogastric, vomiting, 'third space' or pyrexia) cause hypovolaemia before the additive effects of anaesthesia and neuroaxial blockade. Consider i.v. fluids before anaesthesia to correct circulating volume.

If blood pressure fails to improve, **call for help** (potentially anaesthetic **and** surgical). Optimise position (head down). Gain additional i.v. access for fluid and consider invasive monitoring. Consider vasopressor infusion if surgical cause excluded.

ACE, angiotensin-converting enzyme; *ALS,* advanced life support; *APL,* adjustable pressure limiting; *FGF,* fresh gas flow; *FiO2,* fraction of inspired oxygen; *PEEP,* positive end-expiratory pressure.

Unexpected hypertension

Mean/systolic blood pressure >20% baseline or systolic pressure >160 mmHg; severe hypertension if systolic blood pressure >180 mmHg

> **Rule out:** *hypoxaemia; hypercapnia; inadequate depth of anaesthesia; inadequate analgesia; raised ICP; drug effect or drug error; measurement error; malignant hyperpyrexia; bladder distension; tourniquet pain.*

Recheck blood pressure, increase depth of anaesthesia and stop surgical stimulus.

1 Increase oxygen delivery
- Increase FGF; give 100% O_2. Confirm measured FiO_2 approaches 100%.
- Confirm breathing circuit connections and that circle valves move freely.
- Verify ventilator bellows or reservoir bag moving and APL valve set correctly.

2 Airway – exclude hypoxia
- Check airway device position and listen for added noise (stridor, spasm, wheeze).
- Confirm end-tidal CO_2 waveform and shape.
- Check airway device is not obstructed (breath sounds, pass a suction catheter).

3 Breathing – exclude hypercapnia
- Confirm equal bilateral air entry.
- Check tidal volume and respiratory rate and feel lung compliance during manual ventilation with reservoir bag.
- Check ventilator settings and confirm adequate minute ventilation/normocapnia.

4 Circulation
- Recheck blood pressure, heart rate and perfusion. Check appropriate cuff size and location.
- Consider invasive arterial monitoring.
- Check arterial transducer height, flush bag pressure and flush line to confirm patency.
- Consider and exclude differential diagnosis.

If a physiological response to surgical stimulus is excluded, consider:
Labetalol 5–10 mg i.v. increments (1:7 α/β activity)
Hydralazine 5 mg slow i.v. (repeat 15 min)
GTN 200 µg bolus, infuse 1–10 mg h^{-1}
SNP 0.5–1.5 µg kg^{-1} min^{-1}
Metoprolol 1–2 mg increments
Esmolol 0.5 mg kg^{-1} loading, then 50–200 µg kg^{-1} h^{-1}

5 Anaesthetic
- Consider remifentanil 0.1–0.5 µg kg^{-1} min^{-1} for managing ongoing intense surgical stimulus.

Differential diagnoses

Airway
Hypoxaemia

Breathing
Hypercarbia

Circulation
Essential or malignant hypertension

Neurological
Raised ICP

Other
Inadequate depth of anaesthesia
Inadequate analgesia
Measurement error (e.g. cuff size, arterial transducer too low, line occluded or calibration error)
Drugs (e.g. vasopressors, ketamine, ergometrine, cocaine and adrenaline containing local anaesthetic preparations).
MAOI reaction
Aortic cross clamping
Bladder distension
Tourniquet pain
TURP syndrome
Compartment syndrome (e.g. prolonged lithotomy position)
Pregnancy induced hypertension/pre-eclampsia
Phaeochromocytoma
Thyroid storm

- Insert temperature probe and treat any pyrexia (may indicate thyroid storm).
- ABG analysis: acidaemia and hyperkalaemia may support diagnosis of malignant hyperthermia; acidaemia, hyperkalaemia and hypocalcaemia support compartment syndrome.
- Insert urinary catheter to relieve bladder distension.
- Bloods: free T4/T3, U&E, CK, troponin.
- If a neurological cause is suspected, check pupils, arrange urgent brain CT, maintain MAP >80 mmHg position with head-up tilt, allow unobstructed venous drainage and ventilate to normocapnia (see Chapter 40). Discuss with neurosurgeons.

Unexpected hypertension

Mean/systolic blood pressure >20% baseline or systolic pressure >160 mmHg; severe hypertension if systolic blood pressure >180 mmHg

Top Tips

- Severe hypoxaemia and hypercapnia cause sympathetic stimulation with tachycardia and hypertension.
- A bolus of alfentanil (10 µg kg^{-1}) can be useful in diagnosing inadequate analgesia.
- Consider failure of regional or neuraxial blockade with unexpected hypertension.
- Unintended administration of vasopressor should be considered – discard and replace drugs.
- After increasing depth of anaesthesia, use of processed EEG can be considered to optimise drug delivery.
- Tourniquet pain and bladder distension are common causes.

- β-blockade particularly useful if hypertension accompanied by tachycardia. Caution in patients with asthma/COPD who may have β-blocker–induced bronchospasm.
- The aim of hypertension management is to reduce myocardial work and reduce risks of perioperative myocardial infarction. A 12-lead ECG and troponin assay are indicated if this is suspected.
- Severe hypertension or surgery where hypertension is deleterious may warrant invasive monitoring and postoperative management in ICU.
- If poorly controlled essential hypertension considered, seek cardiology advice and review medication before discharge.

If blood pressure fails to improve, **call for help.** Optimise position (supine/head up). Insert invasive monitoring. If surgical stimulus excluded, liaise with ICU to plan ongoing and postoperative management.

APL, adjustable pressure limiting; *CK,* creatinine kinase; *COPD,* chronic obstructive pulmonary disease; *CT,* computed tomography; *ECG,* electrocardiogram; *EEG,* electroencephalogram; *FGF,* fresh gas flow; *F$_{IO_2}$,* fraction of inspired oxygen; *GTN,* glyceryl trinitrate; *ICP,* intracranial pressure; *ICU,* intensive care unit; *MAOI,* monoamine oxidase inhibitor; *MAP,* mean arterial pressure; *PEEP,* positive end-expiratory pressure; *SNP,* sodium nitroprusside; *TURP,* transurethral resection of the prostate; *UE,* urea and electrolytes.

Sinus tachycardia
Heart rate >100 beats min^{-1} with a QRS duration <120 ms

Rule out: *hypoxaemia; hypercapnia; inadequate depth of anaesthesia; inadequate analgesia; hypovolaemia and haemorrhage; malignant hyperthermia; anaphylaxis.*

Stop surgical stimulus. Ensure adequate depth of anaesthesia/analgesia. Check pulse, rhythm and blood pressure. If no pulse, commence CPR.

❶ Increase oxygen delivery
- Increase FGF, give 100% O_2. Confirm measured FiO_2 approaches 100%.
- Confirm breathing circuit connections and that circle valves move freely.
- Verify ventilator bellows or reservoir bag moving and APL valve set correctly.

❷ Airway – exclude hypoxia
- Check airway device position and listen for added noise (stridor, spasm, wheeze).
- Confirm end-tidal CO_2 waveform and shape.
- Check airway device is not obstructed (breath sounds, pass a suction catheter).

❸ Breathing – exclude hypercapnia
- Confirm equal bilateral air entry.
- Check ventilator settings and confirm adequate minute volume/normocapnia.
- Check airway pressure using reservoir bag and APL valve (< 3 breaths).

❹ Circulation – exclude haemorrhage/hypovolaemia
- Recheck blood pressure, heart rate and perfusion. Check appropriate cuff size and location.
- Give 250 ml fluid bolus.
- Confirm blood loss with surgical and scrub team. Weigh swabs and check suction bottles, drapes and the floor for occult blood loss.
- Transfuse blood or fluid as indicated.
- Obtain 12-lead ECG to exclude myocardial ischaemia.
- Insert temperature probe; identify sepsis and instigate antibiotic, fluid and/or vasopressor support.

❺ Anaesthetic
- Reconfirm adequate depth of anaesthesia and analgesia. If not hypotensive, alfentanil (250 µg i.v.) is useful to rapidly exclude inadequate analgesia.
- Check extended ABG to exclude electrolyte imbalance, acidaemia and/or anaemia.
- Remifentanil 0.1–0.5 µg kg^{-1} min^{-1} is useful to obtund surgical stimulus if other causes excluded.
- Consider drug error (sympathomimetics, anticholinergics) and replace drug syringes.

If sinus tachycardia excluded, refer to Advanced Life Support tachycardia guidelines (see Chapter 28).

Differential diagnosis

Airway
Hypoxia
Hypoxaemia from any cause

Breathing
Hypercapnia

Circulation
Hypovolaemia from any cause
Sepsis
Primary cardiac arrhythmia (e.g. atrial fibrillation with rapid ventricular response, supraventricular tachycardia, atrioventricular re-entrant tachycardia; see Chapter 28)
Myocardial infarction
Heart failure
Circulatory embolus (fat, amniotic, air or blood)
Recent history of substance abuse (e.g. sympathomimetics)
Electrolyte imbalance
Thyroid storm

Neurological
Early rise in ICP

Anaesthetic
Inadequate anaesthesia/analgesia
Malignant hyperthermia
Anaphylaxis
Local anaesthetic toxicity
Sepsis
CVC or angiography guidewire
Drug effect (ketamine, syntocin, cyclizine) or drug error

Top Tips

- Severe hypoxaemia and hypercapnia cause sympathetic stimulation with tachycardia and hypertension.
- Often caused by inadequate depth of anaesthesia/analgesia or as a sympathetic response to hypovolaemia – cardiogenic narrow complex tachycardia is a diagnosis of exclusion.
- Exclude anaphylaxis and malignant hyperthermia promptly as management of these complications is time critical.

If heart rate fails to improve, **call for help.** Consider invasive blood pressure monitoring.

ABG, arterial blood gas; *APL,* adjustable pressure limiting; *CPR,* cardiopulmonary resuscitation; *ECG,* electrocardiogram; *FGF,* fresh gas flow; *FiO$_2$,* fraction of inspired oxygen; *ICP,* intracranial pressure.

Regurgitation/aspiration of gastric contents
Soiling of the tracheobronchial tree with gastric contents

Rule out: *anaphylaxis, bronchospasm, airway device displacement or disconnection, endobronchial intubation*

Alert team; stop surgery.

Identification:
Tracheal intubation – Direct visualisation of gastric content.
Intraoperative – Coughing, laryngospasm, bronchospasm and hypoxaemia.
Postoperative – Material on suction, unexpected hypoxaemia or tachypnoea. Wheeze and crackles on auscultation.

Immediate actions:
- Stop surgery.
- Tip operating table head-down.
- Remove SAD (if applicable).
- Pharyngeal suction under direct vision.
- Cricoid force to limit further aspiration.
- Intubate the trachea – examine for tracheal soiling.
- Suction trachea via tracheal tube.
- Ventilate with 100% oxygen.

If vomiting continues, turn left lateral, remove cricoid force and call for help.

Secondary actions:
- Perform recruitment manoeuvres and ventilate with PEEP to maintain oxygen saturation.
- Insert nasogastric tube and empty stomach. Leave on free drainage.
- Manage bronchospasm (see later).
- Empirical antibiotic/steroid therapy is not required.
- Bronchoscopy is useful for suctioning particulate aspirate or treating lobar collapse.
- Extubate the trachea with the patient fully awake in the sitting position.

Most patients with minor, non-particulate aspiration can be extubated at the end of the case assuming ventilation/oxygenation are not impaired. Significant soiling may require mechanical ventilation in ICU.

Differential diagnosis

Airway
Foreign body in airway or obstructed airway device

Breathing
Bronchospasm
Endobronchial intubation
Pulmonary oedema
Acute respiratory distress syndrome (ARDS)

Risk Factors
Full stomach (e.g. inadequate fasting, opioids, pain, gastric outlet obstruction, small bowel obstruction)
Gastro-oesophageal reflux disease
Obesity
Pregnancy (particularly > 20/40 gestation)
Diabetic gastropathy (autonomic dysfunction)
Upper gastrointestinal bleeding
Tonsillar haemorrhage, epistaxis (swallowed blood)
Gastric distension as a result of face-mask ventilation
Coughing and straining on SAD
Lithotomy and/or head-down positioning
Impaired airway reflexes (e.g. neurological conditions, topical local anaesthesia)
Oesophageal disease (e.g. stricture, carcinoma, achalasia)

Top Tips
- Limit attempts at ventilation until the trachea is intubated and suctioned to minimise lung soiling.
- A 12F nasogastric tube passes via the gastric port of a second-generation SAD and can be used to drain further gastric content.
- Gastric content may not always be obvious, particularly with a first-generation SAD without a gastric port – remain alert!

If oxygenation fails to improve, **call for help.** Consider bronchoscopy if particulate aspirate. Abandon elective surgery and expedite emergency surgery. Arrange postoperative ventilation on ICU if needed.

ICU, intensive care unit; *SAD,* supraglottic airway device.

Laryngospasm
Uncontrolled muscular contraction of the vocal cords, audible as stridor

Rule out: *aspiration of gastric contents; supra- or infraglottic obstruction from foreign body, tumour, blood or sputum; anaphylaxis; bronchospasm.*

Alert team; stop surgery (if underway)

Identification:
- 'Crowing' or stridor during inspiration indicates partial obstruction. Complete silence is pathognomonic of complete airway obstruction.
- Respiratory distress, tracheal tug and intercostal recession indicate airway obstruction.
- Manual ventilation may be difficult, with no visible trace on the capnograph.
- Aspiration or contamination of the airway may cause laryngospasm.

Immediate actions:
- Perform jaw thrust and stop surgical stimulus.
- Remove airway devices and anything obstructing the airway (perform suction under direct vision).
- Insert oropharyngeal or nasopharyngeal airway.
- Close APL valve to provide CPAP.
- Ventilate with face mask and 100% oxygen, being mindful to avoid gastric distension.
- Observe capnograph trace.

If laryngospasm persists:
- Deepen anaesthesia with propofol.
- Administer NMBA; low-dose suxamethonium (e.g. 25 mg i.v.) may be effective.
- Maintain anaesthesia with sevoflurane or propofol.

Secondary actions:
- Intubate the trachea if evidence of aspiration.
- Decompress stomach distension with a nasogastric tube.
- Consider the best plan, safest location and appropriate support for further attempts at wakening.

Differential diagnosis

Airway
Anaphylaxis
Foreign body in airway
Airway tumour
Epiglottic/supraglottic or deep neck space infections
Subglottic stenosis
Vocal cord paralysis (post-thyroid surgery)
Glottic oedema

Breathing
Anaphylaxis
Bronchospasm
Intrinsic tracheal obstruction or external compression (e.g. thyroid, mediastinal mass)

Top Tips
- Large negative intrathoracic pressures may be generated, causing negative-pressure pulmonary oedema. This can be managed with CPAP. A diuretic is usually not required.
- Laryngospasm occurs in lightly anaesthetised patients exposed to a change in surgical or airway stimulus – be vigilant after 'knife to skin'.
- Sevoflurane is less irritating to the airways than desflurane or isoflurane (see Chapter 3). Similarly, propofol is superior to sodium thiopental in reducing laryngeal reflexes (see Chapter 4).
- The adage 'all laryngospasm breaks eventually' is best forgotten. Be proactive, and communicate the next step in your plan in good time to allow the team to prepare and assist.
- Prolonged surgery in steep head-down or prone position may cause glottic oedema, which can mimic laryngospasm on tracheal extubation.
- If vascular access is unavailable, suxamethonium can be administered i.m. ($2.5\ \text{mg kg}^{-1}$) or sublingually ($2\ \text{mg kg}^{-1}$).
- A mechanically ventilated patient with a correctly positioned tracheal tube will not have laryngospasm.

If oxygenation fails to improve, **call for help** and administer an NMBA. Refractory life-threatening laryngospasm may necessitate a surgical cricothyroidotomy.

APL, adjustable pressure limiting; *CPAP*, continuous positive airway pressure; *NMBA*, neuromuscular blocking agent; *PEEP*, positive end-expiratory pressure.

Difficulty with IPPV, sudden or progressive loss of minute volume
Manifesting a change in airway pressure with an unexpected decrease in minute volume, an increase in $PaCO_2$ and a decrease in SpO_2

Rule out: *displaced airway device; laryngospasm; drug effect (opioid, NMBA); foreign body; bronchospasm; anaphylaxis; ventilator mechanical fault; gas or electrical supply failure.*

Alert team; stop surgery if possible.

❶ Increase oxygen delivery
- Increase FGF; give 100% O_2. Confirm measured FIO_2 approaches 100%.
- Confirm breathing circuit connections and that circle valves move freely.
- Verify ventilator bellows rising to top of bottle.
- Check mains and cylinder oxygen supply pressure. Replace cylinder if < 60 bar (less than ½ full).

❷ Airway
- Check airway device position and listen for added noise (stridor, spasm, wheeze).
- Confirm end-tidal CO_2 waveform and shape.
- Check airway device is patent (breath sounds, pass a suction catheter).
- Consider changing airway device, or tracheal intubation if SAD *in situ*.

❸ Breathing
- Check chest expansion and symmetry.
- Confirm equal bilateral air entry and normal breath sounds.
- Check tidal volume and feel lung compliance during manual ventilation with reservoir bag.
- Consider ventilating with a self-inflating bag to diagnose a circuit or machine problem.
- Ensure mode and ventilator settings are appropriate if controlled ventilation used.

❹ Circulation
- Recheck blood pressure and ensure patient has a perfusing rhythm.

❺ Anaesthesia
- Ensure depth of anaesthesia appropriate.
- Check and optimise neuromuscular blockade.

Differential diagnoses

Airway
Displaced airway device
Foreign body in airway, aspiration
Obstruction in circuit or airway device
Subglottic stenosis

Breathing
Aspiration
Bronchospasm
Pneumothorax
Anaphylaxis
Diaphragmatic splinting (e.g. pneumoperitoneum)
Intrinsic tracheal obstruction or external tracheal compression

Anaesthetic
Drugs: remifentanil ('wooden chest')
Inadequate neuromuscular blockade
Incorrect mode or ventilator settings
Ventilator or gas supply failure

Top Tips:
- Rule out an airway problem before moving on to consider other systems.
- Ventilator or circuit problems can be diagnosed by using a self-inflating bag to assess airway pressure. If normal, a circuit/machine problem is present.
- Return patient to a supine/reverse Trendelenburg position to optimise lung compliance.
- An oxygen supply failure or low pressure should be announced by the whistle and alarm. Ventilation can continue with air.
- Ventilator failures can be managed with manual ventilation with reservoir bag, portable (transfer) ventilator or relocating to the ventilator in the anaesthetic room (if present). Maintain anaesthesia with i.v. agents.

If ventilation not improving, **call for help** and stop surgery. Consider: CXR (tracheal tube position, lung fields), ABG, bronchoscopy. Use alternate means of ventilation and oxygenation.

ABG, arterial blood gas; *CXR,* chest radiograph; *FGF,* fresh gas flow; *FIO₂,* fraction of inspired oxygen; *SAD,* supraglottic airway device.

Bronchospasm
Reversible narrowing of medium and small airways with polyphonic wheeze associated with increased airway pressures, upward sloping capnograph, falling minute volume

> **Rule out:** *anaphylaxis; endobronchial intubation; foreign body or obstruction; aspiration of gastric contents; laryngospasm.*

Alert team, stop surgery, and call for help.

Identification:

- *Spontaneously ventilating:* tachypnoea, wheeze or silent chest, hypoxaemia, lung hyperexpansion, hypotension.
- *Mechanical ventilation:* increased airway pressure, upward sloping capnograph, wheeze or silent chest, prolonged expiratory phase.

Absence of wheeze or capnography indicates airway device misplacement, obstruction or life-threatening bronchospasm.

Immediate actions:

- Give 100% oxygen.
- Expose and examine chest:
  - ° Polyphonic wheeze or silent chest.
  - ° Check expansion (symmetry/hyperexpansion).
- Increase depth of anaesthesia.
- Identify and manage anaphylaxis (hypotension).
- Exclude obstructed/endobronchial airway device.
- Examine for evidence of aspiration.

Subsequent actions:

Drug treatment (adult):
Salbutamol nebuliser 2.5–5 mg nebulised or slow i.v. bolus (4 µg kg^{-1}, max 250 µg) plus infusion (5–20 µg kg^{-1} min^{-1})
Ipratropium bromide nebuliser 500 µg
Magnesium i.v. 50 mg kg^{-1} over 20 min (max 2 g)
Ketamine 20 mg or 1–3 mg kg^{-1} h^{-1}.
Adrenaline 5 ml 1 1000 nebuliser/i.m. 0.5 mg/i.v. 10–100 µg
Hydrocortisone 4 mg kg^{-1} (max 200 mg)
Aminophylline load (if **not** on oral theophylline): 5 mg kg^{-1} over 20 min, then infusion 0.5 mg kg^{-1} h^{-1}.

- Perform a chest radiograph to exclude pneumothorax, endobronchial intubation, hyperexpansion.
- Check ABG (hypercapnia is ominous; hypokalaemia observed with repeated salbutamol administration).
- Plan for safe postoperative care (location, staff, equipment).

Differential diagnosis

Airway
Foreign body obstruction
Laryngospasm

Breathing
Anaphylaxis
Asthma
COPD (with reversible component)
Reactive airway (smokers, recent pulmonary infection)
Carcinoid
Embolus (thrombus, fat, amniotic fluid)
Pulmonary oedema

Anaesthetic
Mechanical airway irritation
Chemical irritation (e.g. pungent vapour, diathermy smoke)
Endobronchial intubation
Drugs (β-blockers, NSAIDs, atracurium, mivacurium morphine, oxytocin, barbiturates)

Top Tips

- Mortality has occurred when a foreign body in the circuit or airway device has been erroneously managed as bronchospasm. A self-inflating bag connected directly to the airway device excludes machine or circuit obstruction.
- Beware 'stacking' of breaths (mechanical breath occurring before a prolonged bronchospastic exhalation is complete); this raises intrathoracic pressure, with potential for hypotension and volutrauma. Temporary disconnection from the circuit and slow manual ventilation (4–5 breaths min^{-1}) may be required.
- Pressure controlled ventilation, prolonged expiratory time and permissive hypercapnia may be needed.
- Nebulised salbutamol during anaesthesia without correct equipment risks volutrauma from unregulated oxygen supply. Seek expert help.
- Adrenaline, administered via the tracheal tube (0.5–1 mg) has been anecdotally beneficial in life-threatening bronchospasm.
- Intravenous lidocaine (1–1.5 mg kg^{-1}) at tracheal intubation or extubation may reduce airway hyperreactivity.

> If ventilation not improving, **call for help** and stop surgery. Consider: bronchoscopy for mucus plugging.
> **ICU assistance will be invaluable.**

ABG, arterial blood gas; *COPD*, chronic obstructive pulmonary disease; *ICU*, intensive care unit; *NSAIDs*, non-steroidal anti-inflammatory drugs.

Simple pneumothorax and tension pneumothorax
Simple = air in the pleural space. Tension = accumulation of air in the pleural space under pressure

Rule out: *endobronchial intubation; airway device obstruction; bronchospasm; aspiration of gastric contents; mucous/blood/tissue plugging causing lobar or lung collapse; unrecognised traumatic diaphragmatic rupture.*

Alert team, stop surgery, and call for help.

Identification:
- *Airway* – high airway pressure.
- *Breathing* – hypercapnia, hypoxia, uneven chest expansion, tracheal deviation, absent or reduced breath sounds, hyper-resonant percussion note, abnormal capnograph shape.
- *Circulation* – hypotension, jugular venous distension.

Immediate actions:
- Give 100% oxygen. **STOP N$_2$O.**
- Expose and examine chest:
  - Check expansion (symmetry/hyperexpansion)
  - Auscultate and percuss for signs of tension.
  - Check tracheal position for evidence of deviation.
- Recheck blood pressure for signs of tension.

If tension suspected:
- **Confirm side.**
- Perform needle decompression in second intercostal space, mid-clavicular line. Listen for hiss of air escaping. Followed by insertion of an intercostal drain with underwater seal.

For post-traumatic tension pneumothoraces or if unable to reach the pleura for needle decompression, perform a finger thoracostomy – a 5-cm incision in the midaxillary line in the fifth intercostal space followed by rapid blunt dissection with forceps through the intercostal muscles and pleura. A finger sweep feeling parietal pleura and lung will confirm entry to the thoracic cavity.

Subsequent actions:
- Chest radiograph can confirm diagnosis of simple pneumothorax or check intercostal drain position.
- Consider inserting an intercostal drain for all ventilated patients with a pneumothorax.
- Re-examine and reassess physiology to confirm clinical improvement.

Differential diagnosis
Airway
Airway obstruction
Endobronchial intubation

Breathing
Anaphylaxis
Bronchospasm

Risk Factors
Mechanical ventilation
CVC insertion (subclavian > internal jugular)
Regional nerve blocks – intercostal, paravertebral, supra- or infraclavicular, cervical plexus
Laparoscopic, thoracic or renal surgery
Trauma – blunt or penetrating
Blast injuries
Post-CPR rib fractures
Asthma/bullous emphysema
Connective tissue diseases (e.g. Marfan's, Ehlers-Danlos)

Top Tips
- Tracheal deviation and jugular venous distension are late signs.
- Needle decompression is best performed with an angiocath – an i.v. cannula will only breach the chest cavity in 50% of patients.
- Differentiate from anaphylaxis and severe bronchospasm (also present with high airway pressure and cardiovascular collapse) as the lung signs will be *bilateral* in these conditions.
- Resonant percussion and unilateral reduced breath sounds may be difficult to identify.
- Beware the ventilated trauma patient who may have an undiagnosed pneumothorax.

If ventilation not improving, **call for help** and stop surgery. Consider: repeating needle decompression, obtaining chest radiograph (pneumothorax, chest tube position).

CPR, cardiopulmonary resuscitation.

Gas, fat or pulmonary embolus
Presence of gas, fat or thrombus in the heart or pulmonary circulation obstructing or preventing blood flow

---

Rule out: *cardiac arrest; anaphylaxis; unrecognised major haemorrhage.*

Alert team, stop surgery, and call for help.

Identification:
Hypotension, tachycardia, decreased end-tidal CO_2, hypoxaemia, loss of cardiac output.

- *PE:* dyspnoea, pleuritic pain, bronchospasm. haemoptysis, hypotension, raised JVP.
- *Fat:* dyspnoea, confusion, seizures, upper body red-brown petechial rash (late sign).
- *Air/gas:* tachycardia, hypotension, cardiac arrest, 'mill wheel' murmur on cardiac auscultation.
- *Amniotic fluid (AFE):* hypotension, hypoxaemia, respiratory failure, DIC, convulsions, coma, circulatory collapse. **Think anaphylaxis of pregnancy.**

Immediate actions:
- Stop surgery – call for cardiac arrest trolley.
- Give 100% oxygen. **STOP N_2O.** Intubate the trachea if necessary.
- If periarrest – start CPR (may break up thrombus/ disperse air).
- Rapid i.v. fluid bolus 500–1000 ml (caution in AFE).
- Inotropes to support cardiac output.

Supportive investigations:
- ABG – increased $PaCO_2$ /end-tidal CO_2 gradient, hypoxaemia, acidaemia.
- Transthoracic or transoesophageal echocardiogram – ventricular bubbles, increased right-sided heart pressure, pulmonary artery emboli.
- Contrast CT of pulmonary arteries (CTPA).
- ECG – sinus tachycardia, right ventricular strain, $S_1Q_3T_3$, anterior T-wave inversion are classically seen with PE.
- Pulmonary artery flotation catheter – raised right-sided heart pressures (insert after treatment commenced).

Specific secondary actions:
Pulmonary embolus:
- Consider systemic or localised thrombolysis by interventional radiologist.
- Surgical thrombectomy
- Radiological percutaneous removal.

Further management will include thromboprophylaxis and screening for deep vein thrombosis. Subsequent procedures may include insertion of an inferior vena cava filter and thrombophilia screening.

Fat embolus:
- Management is supportive: fluid resuscitation, oxygenation and, in severe cases, mechanical ventilation.

Differential diagnosis

Airway
Acute airway obstruction
Breathing circuit disconnection

Breathing
Pneumothorax
Pulmonary oedema

Circulation
Anaphylaxis
Myocardial infarction
Cardiac tamponade
Hypovolaemia
Severe sepsis/cardiogenic shock

Anaesthetic
Bone cement implantation syndrome
Local anaesthetic toxicity

- Cerebral involvement may cause confusion, irritability and require CT scanning and ICP monitoring.
- Subsequent investigations include urine for lipouria.

Air/gas embolus:
- Stop all sources of insufflation. **STOP N_2O.**
- Lower surgical site below heart to increase venous pressure.
- Flood the surgical field with saline and wet packs to prevent further gas embolism.
- Apply bone wax to exposed bone sinuses.
- Place patient in left lateral position if able.
- Attempt to aspirate air if a CVC is *in situ,* ideally with tip in right ventricle. Specfic air aspiration catheters (e.g. Bunegin-Albin catheter) are also available.

Amniotic fluid embolus:
- Management is supportive; treat hypotension and oxygenation to optimise fetal welfare.
- Use i.v. fluids cautiously as pulmonary oedema is common as a result of cardiogenic shock.
- Noradrenaline and dopamine are recommended vasopressors.
- Monitor undelivered fetus.
- Perimortem Caesarean section may be required in catastrophic AFE.
- Treat DIC – liaise with a senior haematologist.

Gas, fat or pulmonary embolus

Presence of gas, fat or thrombus in the heart or pulmonary circulation obstructing or preventing blood flow

Risk Factors

Pulmonary embolism
Prolonged immobility, paralysis, recent air travel
Postoperative patients
Cancer, particularly of pelvic organs
Recent chemotherapy
Thrombophilia/previous DVT
Obesity
Oral contraceptive pill use
Older patients
Heart failure
Pregnancy

Fat embolism
Long bone and pelvic fractures (closed > open fractures)
Rib fractures (including after CPR)
Burns
Liposuction, lipoinjection, fat transplant
Interosseous access, infusion, bone marrow transplant
Pancreatitis
Sickle-cell or thalassaemia crisis
Diabetes mellitus
Intraoperative cell salvage
Cardiopulmonary bypass
Invasive fatty tumour

Air/gas embolism

Surgical positioning with site above heart (e.g. neurosurgery, spinal surgery, intramedullary nailing, major joint arthroplasty, head and neck surgery)
Procedures using gas insufflation (e.g. laparoscopy, endoscopy, thoracoscopy)
Anaesthetic causes (e.g. air in lines, head-up CVC insertion/removal)

Amniotic fluid embolism
Unpredictable and unpreventable
Associated with long, difficult labour, advanced maternal age, grand multiparity, cervical lacerations, eclampsia, medical induction of labour

Top Tips

- The most common ECG signs of a PE are sinus tachycardia and anterior T-wave inversion. $S_1Q_3T_3$ is rarer, seen in 20%–50%.
- Invasive monitoring is helpful but time consuming. Do not delay resuscitation for line insertion.
- Amniotic fluid embolism has 20% mortality, and 85% of survivors have neurological impairment.
- Fat embolism mortality is 5%–15%.
- 10% of patients have a patent foramen ovale leading to a risk of paroxysmal arterial embolism which may have neurological consequences.
- Air embolism from CO_2 has a better outcome than air because of its rapid resorption.

If circulatory embolus suspected, **call for help**; alert ICU colleagues early. ECMO or intra-aortic balloon counter pulsation may be needed for refractory cardiogenic shock.

ABG, arterial blood gas; *AFE,* amniotic fluid embolism; *CPR,* cardiopulmonary resuscitation; *CT,* computed tomography; *DIC,* disseminated intravascular coagulation; *DVT,* deep venous thrombosis; *ECG,* electrocardiogram; *ECMO,* extracorporeal membrane oxygenation; *ICP,* intracranial pressure; *ICU,* intensive care unit; *JVP,* jugular venous pressure; *Paco$_2$,* partial pressure of arterial carbon dioxide; *PE,* pulmonary embolism.

Adverse Drug Reactions
*An unwanted or harmful reaction which occurs after administration of a drug and is suspected,
or known to be, due to the drug*

Rule out: *anaphylaxis; malignant hyperthermia; hypovolaemia; bronchospasm; drug error or interaction.*

Alert team; pause surgery if indicated.

Adverse drug reactions (ADRs) are categorised as type A or type B (see Chapter 26):
- Type A (pharmacological/augmented) result from an exaggeration of a drug's normal pharmacological actions when given at the usual therapeutic dose. These reactions are dose-dependent and therefore readily reversible on reducing the dose of (or withdrawing treatment with) the drug.
- Type B (idiosyncratic/bizarre) cannot be predicted from the known pharmacology of the drug.

Type A adverse reactions are more common than type B reactions and account for more than 80% of all reactions.

Identification:
- Adverse drug reactions can cause many physiological derangements:
  ○ Hypo- and hypertension
  ○ Tachycardia
  ○ Bronchospasm
  ○ Histamine-induced flushing
  ○ Pyrexia
  ○ Cardiac arrhythmia (QT prolongation)

Immediate actions:
- Give 100% oxygen.
- Check cardiac output

If no signs of life, start CPR and treat as anaphylaxis.
- Exclude obstructed/endobronchial airway device.
- Expose and examine chest for symmetry/wheeze.
- Recheck blood pressure, rate and rhythm.
- Identify and manage anaphylaxis (refractory hypotension).
- Identify and manage as MH if symptoms suggest it.
- Manage other problems with an ABC approach.

Secondary actions:
Review drugs given and patient's drug card; if a drug error is possible, quarantine full, part-used and empty syringes and ampoules away from the immediate workplace for later inspection.

Further actions and investigations:
- Complete local and national incident reporting mechanism.
- Explain events to patient and relatives, including importance of further investigations with reference to local duty of candour policy.

Differential diagnosis

Airway
Airway device displacement
Endobronchial intubation

Breathing
Asthma, bronchospasm

Circulation
Hypovolaemia
Myocardial infarction
Arrhythmia

Neurological
Residual neuromuscular blockade
Stroke or intracerebral haemorrhage
Postoperative cognitive dysfunction
High spinal or epidural blockade

Anaesthetic
Carboprost – bronchospasm
Ergometrine – hypertension
Metoclopramide – oculogyric crisis
Dexamethasone – perineal warmth
Gentamicin – temporary deafness
MAOI – hypertension
Serotonergic syndrome

The great medical mimics
Phaeochromocytoma
Carcinoid syndrome
Thyroid storm

Top Tips
- Yellow Card reports should be made for all suspected ADRs that are serious, medically significant or result in harm or are associated with Black Triangle products (as in the BNF), including suspected ADRs considered not to be serious.
- A Yellow Card can be submitted via the MHRA Yellow Card website (www.mhra.gov.uk/yellowcard), using a free Yellow Card mobile app or by post.

If symptoms are not improving, **call for help** and stop surgery. Consider: chest radiograph (tracheal tube position, lung fields), ABG.

ABG, arterial blood gas; *BNF*, British National Formulary; *CPR*, cardiopulmonary resuscitation; *MAOI*, monoamine oxidase inhibitors; *MH*, malignant hyperthermia; *MHRA*, Medicines and Healthcare Products Regulatory Agency.

Anaphylaxis

A severe, life-threatening, generalised or systemic hypersensitivity reaction mediated by Ig-E

Rule out: *airway obstruction; bronchospasm; hypovolaemia; air/gas embolism; tension pneumothorax; cardiac tamponade; septic shock; anaesthetic overdose; bone cement implantation syndrome; amniotic fluid embolism.*

Alert team, stop surgery, and call for help.

Identification:

Commonly (incidence):
- Cardiovascular (75%) – cardiovascular collapse, hypotension, bradycardia, cardiac arrest.
- Bronchospasm (40%).
- Cutaneous (72%) – erythema, pruritus, urticaria.
- Angioedema (12%).

Immediate actions:
- Call for help; get cardiac arrest trolley.
- Stop all infusions and fluids.
- Give 100% oxygen; intubate the trachea if necessary.
- Tip patient head down to elevate legs.
- Check for cardiac output/signs of life.

If no signs of life, start CPR.
- Give adrenaline:

  Adult
  - i.v./i.o: 50 µg (0.5 ml 1 : 10,000 solution)
  - i.m. 0.5 mg

  Child
  - i.v. 1.0 µg kg^{-1} (0.1 ml kg^{-1} 1 : 100 000 solution)
  - i.m. 500 µg (aged >12 years)/300 µg (aged 6–12 years)/150 µg (aged <6 years)
- Several doses may be required – consider adrenaline infusion.
- Give 0.9% saline or Hartmann's solution fast (adult 500–1000 ml, child 20 ml kg^{-1}).

Secondary actions:

Secondary treatment drugs:
- Chlorphenamine i.v.:
  - Adult: 10 mg
  - Child 6–12 years: 5 mg
  - Child 6 months–6 years: 2.5 mg
  - Child <6 months 250 µg kg^{-1}
- Hydrocortisone i.v.:
  - Adult: 200 mg
  - Child 6–12 years: 100 mg
  - Child 6 months–6 years: 50 mg
  - Child <6 months 25 mg
- Take blood for first serum tryptase as soon as practical.
- Insert invasive monitoring depending on patient condition.
- If condition not improving, seek ICU assistance.

Differential diagnosis

Airway
Laryngospasm
Stridor as a result of airway obstruction (e.g. tumour, abscess)

Breathing
Bronchospasm, asthma
Tension pneumothorax
Pulmonary oedema

Circulation
Cardiac arrest
Myocardial infarction
Cardiac tamponade
PE
Hypotension (e.g. major haemorrhage)

Anaesthetic
Anaesthetic overdose/drug error
Fat embolism
Amniotic fluid embolism
Air/gas embolism
Bone cement implantation syndrome
Transfusion reaction

- In absence of other precipitant, remove latex containing products from vicinity of patient (surgeons' gloves, catheter, medications drawn up through latex bung).

Further actions and investigations:
- Tryptase taken at time of anaphylaxis (taken *after* treatment has commenced)
- Tryptase at 1–2 h after onset of symptoms.
- Tryptase at 24 h or during convalescence (baseline).
- Liaise with laboratory about transfer and analysis of samples.
- Record all drugs and infusions given (with times) to facilitate chronological relationship to onset of symptoms.
- Refer patient to clinical immunologist and provide copy of anaesthetic and operation chart. Use local or Association of Anaesthetists referral form.
- Annotate patient's drug card, wrist band and clinical notes to alert others to potential causes.
- Complete MHRA Yellow Card alert system.
- Explain events to patient and relatives, including importance of further investigations, follow-up and consideration of medical alert bracelet after formal diagnosis.

Anaphylaxis

A severe, life-threatening, generalised or systemic hypersensitivity reaction mediated by Ig-E

Top Tips

• Excluding anaphylaxis is a critical step in the management of any episode of unexplained hypotension, bronchospasm, loss of capnograph trace or new erythematous rash.
• A rash may not be present until blood pressure and skin perfusion is restored. **Absence of rash is not reassuring.**
• Anaphylaxis may be delayed with exposure to latex, antibiotics or colloids.
• Tracheal intubation may be difficult because of airway swelling – a surgical airway may be life saving.
• There is no role for a test dose when administering antibiotics; anaphylaxis is an immunological cascade reaction.
• There is no evidence to support the practice of avoiding propofol in patients with egg, soya or nuts. The manufacturing process removes or denatures egg and soya proteins; therefore propofol can be used with usual vigilance.
	• Consider latex allergy in patients with a history of allergy to fruits such as banana, kiwi, avocado and papaya because of their cross reactivity to latex proteins.
	• Agents commonly responsible for anaphylaxis:
	  ◦ Neuromuscular blocking agents
	  ◦ Latex
	  ◦ Antibiotics
	  ◦ Colloids
	  ◦ Chlorhexidine
	• Good history taking is an important part of risk stratification. Be a detective – what was the reaction? Is this anaphylaxis or an expected adverse effect of the drug?

If symptoms are not improving, **call for help** and stop surgery. Involve ICU colleagues.

CPR, cardiopulmonary resuscitation; *Ig-E,* immunoglobulin-E; *ICU,* intensive care unit; *MHRA,* Medicines and Healthcare products Regulatory Agency; *PE,* pulmonary embolism.

Transfusion Reactions
An acute immunological reaction to blood product(s) transfusion

Rule out: *bronchospasm; septic shock; acute respiratory distress syndrome (ARDS)*

Alert team; pause surgery if indicated.

Identification:

A patient who has recently received, or is receiving, a blood transfusion who then develops:

- Anaphylactic shock
- Restlessness or anxiety
- Bronchospasm, tachypnoea
- Flushing or urticarial rash
- Fever
- Chest, flank or lumbar pain
- Haematuria
- Coagulopathy (DIC)

Immediate actions:

STOP BLOOD PRODUCT INFUSION.

- Give 100% oxygen.
- Monitor vital signs including urine output and temperature.
- Respiratory examination: tachypnoea, wheeze, cyanosis.
- Treat anaphylaxis with fluids and adrenaline.
- Treat bronchospasm.
- Check SpO_2 and ABG.
- Check and confirm patient identity and blood product labelling. Return blood bag to laboratory.

Secondary actions:

- Seek expert haematological advice if further blood products needed.
- Send FBC, UE, coagulation and urine samples.
- Liaise with ICU if ongoing support needed; multiorgan failure may ensue.

Further actions and investigations:

- Inform blood bank and on-call haematologist.
- Complete local and national incident reporting mechanism.
- Blood bank will notify hospital transfusion committee, who will complete SHOT (Serious Hazards of Transfusion) notification for MHRA.
- Explain events to patient and relatives, including importance of further investigations with reference to local duty of candour policy.

Differential diagnosis

Breathing
Anaphylaxis (drug)
Bronchospasm
ARDS
Pulmonary oedema

Circulation
Septic shock

Top Tips

- Onset of a major ABO transfusion reaction is rapid and severe. Reactions caused by re-exposure to a minor antigen are often mild and may be delayed.
- Treat a severe reaction as for anaphylaxis.
- If the only reaction is mild pyrexia (<1.5°C), confirm blood compatibility, administer paracetamol and continue the infusion at a slower rate with increased observations.
- Mild urticaria without other signs can be managed as above with chlorphenamine for the itching.
- Transfusion-related acute lung injury (TRALI) is clinically indistinguishable from ARDS and manifests > 4 h post-transfusion with bilateral pulmonary infiltrates, hypoxaemia and pulmonary oedema. It is more common after FFP or platelet transfusion.
- Transfusion-associated circulatory overload (TACO) produces respiratory distress with other signs, including pulmonary oedema, unanticipated cardiovascular system changes *and* evidence of fluid overload (including improvement after diuretic, morphine or nitrate treatment), during or up to 24 h after transfusion.
- A transfusion reaction can occur anywhere in the hospital, and specialist equipment may be limited. Plan ahead and communicate needs early.

If symptoms are not improving, **call for help** and stop surgery. Treat as for anaphylaxis. Involve ICU colleagues.

ABG, arterial blood gas; *DIC,* disseminated intravascular coagulation; *FBC,* full blood cell count; *FFP,* fresh frozen plasma; *ICU,* intensive care unit; *MHRA,* Medicines and Healthcare products Regulatory Agency; *UE,* urea and electrolytes.

Inadvertent arterial injection of irritant fluid(s)

Accidental administration of intravenous drugs into an artery causing endarteritis, vasospasm, thrombosis and potential distal ischaemic necrosis.

Rule out: *pain on induction (propofol, rocuronium) or drug extravasation.*

Alert team; pause surgery if indicated.

Identification:
- Awake patient complaining of burning pain distal to injection site (i.e. fingers).
- Blanching or blistering.
- Oedema, hyperaesthesia or motor weakness may develop within hours.
- Ischaemia is a late sign.

Immediate actions:

STOP INJECTION.
- Leave cannula in place, inject:
  - Heparin sodium (50 IU in 5 ml) or 0.9% saline (as a diluent).
  - 5 ml lidocaine 1%.
  - Papaverine 40 mg (vasodilator).
- If hand well perfused, remove cannula and compress artery to prevent haematoma formation.
- Ensure additional i.v. access available; consider confirming venous placement with ultrasound or measuring $S\text{v}O_2$ via blood gas analysis (< 75%).

Secondary actions:
- Regional blockade can provide prolonged vasodilatation and analgesia – an axillary brachial plexus block ± catheter is ideal for this.
- Systemic heparinisation may be required.
- Elevate the limb to improve venous and lymphatic drainage.
- Discussion with vascular surgical colleagues may be helpful if symptoms and signs persist or if there is any evidence of digital ischaemia.

Further actions and investigations:
- Complete local and national incident reporting mechanism.
- Explain events to patient and relatives, including importance of further investigations with reference to local duty of candour policy.

Risk factors

Cannula inserted in hypotensive patients
Accidental injection into an arterial line
Injection into cannula in the antecubital fossa or the wrist with aberrant radial artery anatomy
Patients who are unable to describe painful symptoms (coma, intoxicated, dementia, neonates)

Top Tips:
- Principles of management: stop injection, dilute, dilate and anticoagulate.
- Intra-arterial sodium thiopental causes severe arterial spasm as a result of local tissue noradrenaline release.
- Sodium thiopental may potentially crystallise in arterioles, obstructing blood flow and leading to ischaemia; fortunately the 5% preparation notorious for this is no longer available.
- Intra-arterial propofol reportedly causes long-lasting extremity blanching.
- Signs of accidental arterial cannulation may not be present, particularly in cannulae inserted some time before anaesthesia.
- Be mindful of (but don't rely on) the following:
  - Cannula insertion more painful than anticipated.
  - Blood running back up drip tubing.
  - Pulsatile blood flow from a new cannula.
  - Flashback appears redder than expected.
  - Distal ischaemia (blanching) on injection.
  - Palpable pulse immediately proximal to cannula.

If symptoms are not improving, **call for help** from senior anaesthetic colleagues. Seek input from vascular and plastic surgeons. Ensure regular observation of the affected limb.

High and total spinal block
Profound local anaesthetic blockade of spinal nerves causing muscle weakness and hypotension, potentially including the brainstem

Rule out: *hypotension from other causes; including aortocaval compression; cardiac arrest; local anaesthetic toxicity; vasovagal episode; drug error (inadvertent neuromuscular blockade).*

Alert team; stop surgery.

Identification:
- *Initially:* hypotension, bradycardia, nausea/vomiting, upper limb motor weakness and respiratory difficulty.
- *Progressing to:* poor respiratory effort leading to respiratory arrest. Cardiovascular collapse. If brainstem affected, loss of consciousness and fixed dilated pupils may result.

Immediate actions:
CALL FOR HELP.
If obstetric spinal, ensure uterine displacement.
- Reassure patient.
- Administer 100% O_2 via non-rebreathing mask.
- Recheck and cycle blood pressure measurement.
- **Start CPR if cardiovascular collapse occurs.**
- Support blood pressure with boluses or infusion of vasopressor as local policy:
  - Ephedrine 6–9 mg
  - Phenylephrine 25–50 µg
  - Metaraminol 0.25–0.50 mg
  - Adrenaline 5–10 µg
- Induce anaesthesia and intubate the trachea if signs of respiratory failure or cardiovascular collapse.
- Use a cardiovascularly stable induction technique.
- Anaesthesia will need to be maintained until the block has resolved.

For obstetric cases:
- Summon senior obstetric and anaesthetic help.
- Transfer to theatre from labour suite.
- Ensure CTG is applied for continuous fetal monitoring.
- Category 1 Caesarean delivery may be needed if evidence of fetal or maternal compromise.

Secondary actions:
- Maintain sedation until spinal blockade resolved to allow adequate spontaneous ventilation; transfer to ICU may be needed.

Further actions:
- These events can be very distressing, particularly for obstetric patients. Senior anaesthetic inpatient and outpatient follow-up will be helpful.

Risk Factors

Spinal
Excessive dose of local anaesthetic
Drug error
Patient of short stature
Multiple pregnancies
Repeated full spinal dose after 'failed' spinal
Spinal anaesthesia after labour epidural
Lithotomy or head-down positioning.

Epidural
Unrecognised dural puncture
Intrathecal migration of epidural catheter

Top Tips
- Presentation may vary from a rapid loss of consciousness to more gradual onset of upper limb weakness and respiratory difficulty.
- Head-down and lithotomy positions will increase height of spinal blockade; caution in urological, gynaecological and colorectal procedures.
- If intubating the trachea, careful induction and maintenance of anaesthesia is important; despite total spinal blockade a patient will still be aware of what is happening.
- Neuromuscular blockade will be required to facilitate tracheal intubation.
- Many cases of 'high' spinal (tingling in fingers) can be managed by slight head-up tilt, reassurance and continued careful monitoring of respiratory function.
- Consider every bolus dose administered via an epidural as a test dose.
- Rapid (< 5 min) onset of *epidural* analgesia or motor block should prompt close neurological examination for evidence of subdural (patchy, high block, Horner's syndrome) or spinal blockade.

If total spinal blockade suspected, **call for help** (include obstetricians if needed). Transfer patient to operating theatre. Have equipment and drugs available to induce and maintain anaesthesia and secure the airway.

CTG, cardiotocogram; *ICU,* intensive care unit.

Local anaesthetic toxicity

Intravenous injection or systemic absorption of local anaesthetic agents leading to high plasma concentrations causing neurological and cardiac signs progressing to unconsciousness and cardiovascular collapse

Rule out: *vasovagal episode; anaphylaxis; cardiac arrest; amniotic fluid embolus; drug error (inadvertent neuromuscular blockade).*

Alert team; stop surgery.

Identification:
- *CNS:* tinnitus, circumoral tingling, diplopia, altered mental state, agitation, seizures, loss of consciousness.
- *CVS:* initially hyperdynamic progressing to conduction blocks, hypotension, bradycardia, ventricular tachycardia, asystole.
- *Airway:* loss of airway reflexes, obstruction, apnoea.

Immediate actions:
> **STOP INJECTING LOCAL ANAESTHETIC.**
> **CALL FOR HELP.**
- Give 100% O_2; maintain airway.
- Induce anaesthesia and intubate the trachea if necessary.
- Hyperventilation may be advantageous as an acidaemia can potentiate local anaesthetic toxicity.
- Recheck and cycle blood pressure measurement.
- Control seizures with small doses of benzodiazepines, sodium thiopental or propofol.

Cardiac arrest:
- Start CPR.
- Perform standard arrhythmia management; may be refractory to treatment.

Give i.v. 20% lipid emulsion (Intralipid):
1.5 ml kg^{-1} over 1 min, THEN infuse 15 ml kg^{-1} h^{-1}.
After 5 min:
If cardiovascular stability not restored, then repeat 1.5 ml kg^{-1} boluses at 5 min intervals (max 3 boluses) **AND** double infusion rate to 30 ml kg^{-1} h^{-1}.
- Continue until cardiovascular stability is restored *or* maximum lipid dose reached (12 ml kg^{-1}).

Without cardiac arrest:
- Lipid emulsion can be considered if seizures occur.
- Use conventional therapies for hypotension, seizures and arrhythmias.

Secondary actions:
- Take blood for plasma level analysis.
- Transfer to appropriate clinical area; ICU may be necessary.
- Check amylase and lipase daily for 2 days to exclude pancreatitis after lipid therapy.

Further actions and investigations:
- Complete local and national incident reporting mechanism.
- Explain events to patient and relatives, including importance of further investigations, with reference to local duty of candour policy.

Risk Factors
Large-volume or high-concentration of local anaesthetic
Surgical infiltration of anaesthesia
Failure to aspirate during injection (intravascular injection)
Landmark techniques of regional anaesthesia
Intravenous lidocaine use for analgesia (dose error)
Drugs with narrow therapeutic window (bupivacaine, prilocaine)

Top Tips
- Local anaesthetic toxicity may occur some time after injection.
- For blocks combined with general anaesthesia, CVS signs will be the presenting feature.
- Local anaesthetic toxicity has been reported with airway topicalisation for awake fibreoptic intubation.
- Refractory cases may need cardiopulmonary bypass if available. Patient transfer likely to be hazardous.
- Bupivacaine binds to myocardium, resulting in prolonged cardiac arrest. Resuscitation should be continued for at least 60 min.
- Aspiration during regional techniques should be gentle to avoid inducing blood vessel collapse with negative pressure.
- Levobupivacaine and ropivacaine are less toxic than bupivacaine. The R-enantiomer binds avidly to myocardium (see Chapter 5).

If symptoms of local anaesthetic toxicity occur, **call for help.** Obtain cardiac arrest trolley and local anaesthetic toxicity kit containing lipid emulsion.

CNS, Central nervous system; *CPR,* cardiopulmonary resuscitation; *CVS,* cardiovascular system; *ICU,* intensive care unit.

Accidental decannulation of tracheostomy or tracheal tube
Accidental removal or displacement of an airway device from the trachea, with potential for hypoxaemia

Rule out: *foreign body or occlusion in the airway; accidental disconnection; ventilator or gas supply failure.*

Alert team; stop surgery.

Identification:
Loss of capnograph trace, collapsing ventilator bellows, hypoxia.

Immediate actions:
- Request tracheal intubation trolley.
- Give 100% O_2.
- Request cricoid force if airway soiling is a risk.
- If good access to the patient's head, reintubate the trachea.
- If access is limited (e.g. prone position), ventilate via face mask or insert SAD.
- Optimise position and attempt tracheal intubation.

For difficult/failed tracheal intubation, follow DAS algorithm (see Chapter 23). For occluded tracheostomy management, see Chapter 37.

Tracheostomy decannulation – patent upper airway:
- Apply 100% O_2 to both mouth *and* tracheostomy.
- Ventilate via face-mask (apply gauze over stoma) *or* ventilate with round paediatric face mask or SAD held over stoma.
- Attempt oral intubation; use uncut tracheal tube advanced beyond the stoma.

In the case of failure to oxygenate:
- Intubate stoma with 6.0-mm ID reinforced tracheal tube.
- If difficult, railroad tracheal tube over a bougie, Cook airway exchange catheter or Aintree catheter directed into the trachea via an intubating fibreoptic scope.

Tracheostomy decannulation – no upper airway (e.g. after laryngectomy):
- Apply 100% O_2 to both mouth *and* tracheostomy.
- Ventilate with round paediatric face mask or SAD held over stoma.
- Intubate stoma with 6.0-mm ID reinforced tracheal tube.
- If difficult, railroad tracheal tube over a bougie, Cook airway exchange catheter or Aintree catheter directed into the trachea via an intubating fibreoptic scope.

Top tips
- Applying oxygen to the face and stoma is the default emergency action for all patients with a tracheostomy, even when the upper airway isn't patent.
- Identify preoperatively whether the tracheostomy patient has a larynx, and perform a full airway assessment – anticipate potential problems.
- A tracheostomy may be relatively inaccessible during surgery; ensure HMEF and circuit are not pulling on the tube.
- Beware the newly formed tracheostomy – the tissue planes can close up, making the stoma difficult to find in the first few days.

Call for help and stop surgery.

DAS, Difficult Airway Society; *HMEF,* heat and moisture exchange filter; *ID,* internal diameter; *SAD,* supraglottic airway device.

Coning as a result of raised intracranial pressure

Forced movement of the brain across fixed intracranial structures due to a pathologically raised ICP (> 25 mmHg)

Call for senior neurosurgical and anaesthetic help.

Identification:

- Patients with persistently low GCS, unreactive pupils or other signs of raised ICP (Cushing's reflex, direct ICP measurement) may require short-term interventions to reduce ICP and the risk of coning.

Immediate actions (see Chapter 40):

Ensure sedation adequate – bolus to reduce $CMRO_2$.

Administer neuromuscular blockade.

Hyperventilate to $PaCO_2$ 4–4.5 kPa.

Administer mannitol 0.25–1.0 g kg^{-1} (can repeat if serum osmolality <320 mOsm kg^{-1}).

Administer hypertonic (3%) saline 2 ml kg^{-1} (can repeat if Na <155 mmol L^{-1}).

Cool to normothermia if febrile.

Administer phenytoin 15–18 mg kg^{-1} i.v. or levetiracetam 20 mg kg^{-1} for seizures.

Obtain urgent CT brain.

Surgery (evacuation of haematoma, CSF drainage).

Secondary actions if ICP remains elevated:

Ensure adequate sedation.

Administer bolus thiopental 250 mg – repeat to burst suppression on pEEG/CFAM.

Cool to 33°C–35°C.

Repeat CT scan.

Surgery (decompressive craniotomy).

Physiological targets after brain injury (adult)

MAP >80 mmHg

PaO_2 >12 kPa

$PaCO_2$ 4.5–5 kPa

Glucose 7–11 mmol L^{-1}

Normothermia (< 37°C)

Top Tips

- Tracheal intubation and ventilation should be instigated for patients with the following:
    - GCS ≤ 8
    - Deteriorating GCS (fall in motor score ≥2 points)
    - Loss of pharyngeal reflexes
    - Hypoxaemia (PaO_2 <13 kPa, hypercapnia $PaCO_2$ >6 kPa)
    - Spontaneous hyperventilation ($PaCO_2$ >4 kPa)
    - Seizures
    - Significant craniofacial trauma
- Close attention to the 'big five': normotension, normoxia, normocarbia, normoglycaemia and normothermia.
- Mannitol should be considered if there are signs of brainstem compression.
- A bolus of sodium thiopental and hyperventilation will rapidly lower the ICP for a short period. Consider it a sticking plaster rather than a solution.

Raised ICP is a neurosurgical emergency. **Call for help** from senior anaesthetic and ICU colleagues.
Talk to neurosurgeons early, and proactively plan for transfer to neurosurgical centre.

CFAM, cerebral function analysing monitor; *CMRO₂*, cerebral metabolic rate for oxygen; *CSF*, cerebrospinal fluid; *CT*, computed tomography; *ICP*, intracranial pressure; *ICU*, intensive care unit; *GCS*, Glasgow Coma Scale; *MAP*, mean arterial pressure; *PaCO₂*, partial pressure of carbon dioxide in arterial blood; *PaO₂*, partial pressure of oxygen in arterial blood; *pEEG*, processed electroencephalogram.

Malignant Hyperthermia
Life-threatening hypermetabolic condition occurring in response to anaesthetic trigger agents (inhalational anaesthetic agents and suxamethonium) with autosomal dominant inheritance

Rule out: *inadequate anaesthesia/analgesia; sepsis; hypoventilation; anaphylaxis; neuroleptic malignant syndrome; thyroid storm.*

Alert team, stop surgery, and call for help.

Identification:
Early signs:
- Raised end-tidal CO_2
- Unexplained tachycardia, arrhythmias
- Increased O_2 consumption
- Mixed metabolic and respiratory acidaemia
- Sweating and mottling of skin
- Muscle rigidity, masseter spasm

Late signs:
- Hyperkalaemia
- Rapid increase in body temperature
- Elevated creatinine phosphokinase and myoglobin
- Dark-coloured urine (myoglobinuria)
- Severe arrhythmias preceding cardiac arrest
- Disseminated intravascular coagulation (DIC)

Initial management:
STOP ALL TRIGGER AGENTS.
CALL FOR HELP – ALLOCATE TASKS.
Hyperventilate (minute volume 2–3 × normal) with 100% O_2 at high flow rate.
Change to TIVA anaesthesia and remove vaporiser.
Instruct surgeons to terminate/expedite surgery.
Do not delay treatment to change anaesthetic circuit.

Administer dantrolene (delegate mixing to second team member):
- Give 2.5 mg kg^{-1} (dilute 20 mg ampoule with 60 ml sterile water).
- Repeat 1 mg kg^{-1} boluses every 10–15 minutes as needed.
- Obtain further supplies from pharmacy.
- May need to exceed the 10 mg kg^{-1} maximum dose.

Monitoring:
Provide continuous core temperature monitoring.
Use CVC, arterial line and urinary catheter.
Obtain blood samples for K^+, CK, ABG, myoglobin, glucose, UE, LFTs and clotting factors.
Check for signs of compartment syndrome.

Hyperthermia:
Administer 2000–3000 ml chilled 0.9% saline i.v.
Provide surface cooling: wet sheets, ice packs to groin/axillae.
Perform bladder, gastric or peritoneal lavage with 10 ml kg^{-1} iced water.
Use other cooling devices as available from ICU.
Stop cooling once core temperature <38.5°C.

Hyperkalaemia:
Administer calcium chloride 0.1 mmol kg^{-1} (7 mmol = 10 ml for 70 kg adult).
Administer insulin/dextrose infusion.
Dialysis may be needed.

Differential diagnosis

Breathing
Insufficient ventilation or fresh gas flow

Circulation
Anaphylaxis

Neurological
Cerebral ischaemia/traumatic brain injury[a]
Neuromuscular disorders

Anaesthetic
Insufficient anaesthesia/analgesia
Anaesthetic machine malfunction
Elevated end-tidal CO_2 during laparoscopic surgery
Sepsis[a]
Ecstasy or other sympathomimetic recreational drugs[a]
Phaeochromocytoma[a]
Thyroid storm[a]
Neuroleptic malignant syndrome[a]
Anticholinergic syndrome[a]
Serotonin syndrome[a]

[a]Causes of perioperative hyperthermia.

Acidaemia:
Hyperventilate to normocapnia.
Administer sodium bicarbonate 8.4% if pH <7.2.

Arrhythmias:
Administer magnesium sulphate.
Administer amiodarone 300 mg (adult).
β-blockers (metoprolol, esmolol, propranolol) can be used for tachycardia. NB. Avoid Ca^{2+} blockers – interaction with dantrolene.

DIC:
Discuss with a senior haematologist.
Consider FFP, cryoprecipitate and platelet replacement as advised by haematologist and/or point-of-care testing.

Urine output
Aim urine output > 1 ml kg^{-1} h^{-1} If evidence of myoglobinuria then consider forced alkaline diuresis (e.g. furosemide 0.5–1.0 mg^{-1} kg^{-1} or mannitol 1 g kg^{-1}).
Transfer to ICU for a minimum of 24 h after resolution of symptoms.

Further actions and investigations:
1. Complete local and national incident reporting mechanism.
2. Explain events to patient and relatives, including importance of further investigations, with reference to local duty of candour policy.
3. Refer patient and family to MH investigation unit for *in vitro* contracture testing and genetic analysis. Include copies of anaesthetic chart and relevant investigations. Give family members written information advising
4. them to inform anaesthetists before surgery whilst awaiting formal test results from the MH centre.

Malignant Hyperthermia

Life-threatening hypermetabolic condition occurring in response to anaesthetic trigger agents (inhalational anaesthetic agents and suxamethonium) with autosomal dominant inheritance

Top Tips

- Start treatment as soon as MH is suspected.
- TIVA techniques and the reduced exposure to trigger agents mean MH is very rare, risking reduced awareness to the condition. However, the *frequency* of events has increased.
- Hyperthermia is a late sign; the diagnosis is made from hypermetabolic symptoms after trigger agent exposure.
- The prevalence of the susceptible genome is 1:3000.
- Onset of symptoms may be immediate or shortly after an anaesthetic (particularly if a short procedure). Previous uneventful trigger agent exposure doesn't rule out MH.
- Call for additional dantrolene from pharmacy or other theatre complexes – **36–50 ampoules may be needed for an adult** (70 kg = 9 vials for initial bolus, then 4 vials subsequently).
- Managing MH is a dynamic and labour-intensive process. Help is critical to start prompt treatment; call for colleagues from other areas (i.e. ICU or obstetric anaesthetists).

First anaesthetist
Declare MH emergency; team leader (or delegate role to most senior anaesthetist).

Second anaesthetist (resuscitation)
Calculate dantrolene dose. Start TIVA anaesthesia.
Manage physiological derangements.

First ODP/theatre nurse
Collect MH kit.
Collect cold saline, ice, and insulin.
Set up invasive monitoring.
Runner for resuscitation drugs; assist third anaesthetist.

Second ODP/theatre nurse (dantrolene)
Reconstitute dantrolene as directed by second anaesthetist.

Third anaesthetist (Procedures/investigations)
Insert arterial line and CVC.
Send samples for:
ABG – repeat every 30 min
FBC, U&Es, LFTs
CK
Coagulation screen (DIC) and cross-matching blood.
Urinary myoglobin.

Surgeons
Abandon or expedite surgery.
Catheterise.
Administer cooling measures.

Remember, MH is very rare; consider more common differentials first. If MH is suspected, **call for help.**

ABG, arterial blood gas; *CK*, creatinine kinase; *FFP*, fresh frozen plasma; *LFTs*, liver function tests; *MH*, malignant hyperthermia; *ODP*, operating department practitioner; *TIVA*, total intravenous anaesthesia; *UE*, urea and electrolytes.

References/Further reading

Flin, R., O'Connor, P., Crichton, M., 2008. Safety at the sharp end: A guide to non-technical skills. Burlington, VT, Ashgate Publishing Co.

Gaba, D.M., Fish, K.J., Howard, S.K., Burden, A.R., 2015. Crisis management in anesthesiology, 2nd ed. Philadelphia, Elsevier.

Chapter | **28** |

Resuscitation

Jerry Nolan

Without intervention, cardiac arrest may lead to permanent neurological injury after just three minutes. The interventions that contribute to a successful outcome after a cardiac arrest can be conceptualised as the 'chain of survival' (Fig. 28.1). The four links in this chain are:
- early recognition – to potentially enable prevention of cardiac arrest – and call for help;
- early cardiopulmonary resuscitation (CPR);
- early defibrillation; and
- post-resuscitation care.

This chapter includes some background to the epidemiology and the prevention of cardiac arrest. It details the principles of initiating CPR in-hospital, defibrillation, advanced life support (ALS), post-resuscitation care and potential modifications to ALS when cardiac arrest occurs intraoperatively.

Science and guidelines

The 2015 International Consensus on Cardiopulmonary Resuscitation and Emergency Cardiovascular Care Science with Treatment Recommendations summarises the current science underpinning CPR. The European Resuscitation Council and Resuscitation Council (UK) Guidelines for Resuscitation 2015 are derived from the 2015 consensus document and have been used as source material.

Epidemiology

Ischaemic heart disease is the leading cause of death in the world. In Europe, sudden cardiac arrest is responsible for more than 60% of adult deaths from coronary heart disease. In Europe, the annual incidence of emergency medical services–treated out-of-hospital cardiopulmonary arrest (OHCA) for all rhythms is 40 per 100,000 population; ventricular fibrillation (VF) arrest accounts for about one third of these. The incidence of VF is declining and has been reported most recently as 23% among treated arrests of cardiac cause. Survival to hospital discharge is 8%–10% for all rhythms and approximately 21%–27% for VF cardiac arrest. Immediate CPR can double or triple survival from VF OHCA. After VF OHCA, each minute of delay before defibrillation reduces the probability of survival to discharge by about 10%.

The incidence of in-hospital cardiac arrest (IHCA) is difficult to assess because it is influenced by factors such as the criteria for hospital admission and implementation of a 'do not attempt cardiopulmonary resuscitation' (DNACPR) policy. The reported incidence of IHCA is in the range of 1–5 per 1000 admissions. Data from the American Heart Association's national registry of CPR indicate that survival to hospital discharge after IHCA is 17.6% (all rhythms). There is some evidence that these survival rates are increasing. Data from the UK National Cardiac Arrest Audit (NCAA) show that survival to hospital discharge after IHCA is 18.4% (all rhythms). The initial rhythm is VF or pulseless ventricular tachycardia (VT) in 16.9% of cases, and 49% of these survive to leave hospital; after pulseless electrical activity (PEA) or asystole, 10.5% survive to hospital discharge. All these individuals received chest compressions, defibrillation, or both, and attendance by a resuscitation team. Many patients sustaining an IHCA have significant comorbidity, and strategies to prevent cardiac arrest are important.

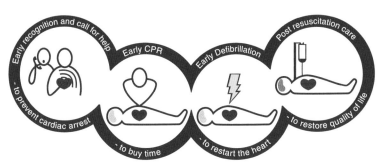

Fig. 28.1 Chain of survival.

Prevention

Out of hospital, recognition of the importance of chest pain enables victims or bystanders to call the emergency medical services and for patients to receive treatment that can prevent cardiac arrest.

Cardiac arrest in hospital patients in unmonitored ward areas is not usually a sudden, unpredictable event caused by primary cardiac disease. These patients often have slow and progressive physiological deterioration, involving hypoxaemia and hypotension that has been unnoticed by staff or recognised but treated poorly. Many such patients have unmonitored arrests, and the underlying cardiac arrest rhythm is usually non-shockable.

Guidelines for the prevention of in-hospital cardiac arrest (Resuscitation Council (UK))

1. Place critically ill patients, or those at risk of clinical deterioration, in areas where the level of care is matched to the level of patient sickness.
2. Monitor such patients regularly using simple vital sign observations (e.g. HR, BP, respiratory rate, conscious level, temperature and SpO_2). Match the frequency and type of observations to the severity of illness of the patient.
3. Use an early warning score (EWS) system or 'calling criteria' to identify patients who are critically ill, at risk of clinical deterioration or cardiopulmonary arrest, or both.
4. Use a patient vital signs chart that encourages and permits the regular measurement and recording of vital signs and, where used, early warning scores.
5. Ensure that the hospital has a clear policy that requires a timely, appropriate, clinical response to deterioration in the patient's clinical condition.
6. Introduce into each hospital a clearly identified response to critical illness. This will vary among sites but may include an outreach service or resuscitation team

(e.g. medical emergency team) capable of responding to acute clinical crises. This team should be alerted, using an early warning system, and the service must be available 24 h.
7. Ensure that all clinical staff are trained in the recognition, monitoring and management of the critically ill patient and that they know their role in the rapid response system.
8. Empower staff to call for help when they identify a patient at risk of deterioration or cardiac arrest. Use a structured communication tool to ensure effective handover of information between staff (e.g. Situation-Background-Assessment-Recommendation or SBAR).
9. Agree on a hospital DNACPR policy, based on current national guidance. Identify patients who do not wish to receive CPR and those for whom cardiopulmonary arrest is an anticipated terminal event for whom CPR would be inappropriate. Increasingly, DNACPR decisions are being incorporated into wider treatment plans such as the Recommended Summary Plan for Emergency Care and Treatment (ReSPECT) – also known in the United States as Physician Orders for Life-Sustaining Treatment. These focus more on what will be done for the patient rather than what will be withheld.
10. Audit all cardiac arrests, false arrests, unexpected deaths and unanticipated ICU admissions using a common dataset. Audit the antecedents and clinical responses to these events. All hospitals should consider joining NCAA (https://www.icnarc.org/Our-Audit/Audits/Ncaa/About).

Cardiopulmonary resuscitation

The division between basic life support and ALS is arbitrary – the resuscitation process is a continuum. The keys steps are that cardiorespiratory arrest is recognised immediately, help is summoned, CPR (chest compressions and ventilations) is started immediately and, if indicated, defibrillation attempted as soon as possible (ideally within 3 min of collapse).

Diagnosis of cardiac arrest

Many trained healthcare staff may not be able to assess a patient's breathing and pulse sufficiently reliably to confirm cardiac arrest. Agonal breathing is common in the early stages of cardiac arrest; it is a sign of cardiac arrest and should not be confused as being a sign of life or circulation. Agonal breathing can also occur during chest compressions as cerebral perfusion improves but is not indicative of a return of spontaneous circulation (ROSC). Delivering chest compressions to a patient with a beating heart is unlikely to cause harm.

High-quality CPR

The quality of chest compressions is often poor, and in particular, frequent and unnecessary interruptions often occur. Even short interruptions to chest compressions may compromise outcome. The correct hand position for chest compression is the middle of the lower half of the sternum. The recommended depth of compression is 5–6 cm and rate 100–120 compressions min^{-1}. The chest should be allowed to recoil completely in between each compression. If available, a prompt or a feedback device should be used to help ensure high-quality chest compressions. The person providing chest compressions should change about every 2 min or earlier if unable to continue high-quality chest compressions. This change should be done with minimal interruption to compressions.

Starting CPR in hospital

The sequence of actions for initiating CPR in hospital is shown in Fig. 28.2.

Advanced life support

Arrhythmias associated with cardiac arrest are divided into two groups: shockable rhythms (VF/pulseless VT); and non-shockable rhythms (asystole and PEA). The principle difference in management is the need for attempted defibrillation in patients with VF/pulseless VT. Subsequent actions, including chest compression, airway management, ventilation, vascular access, injection of adrenaline and the identification and correction of reversible factors, are common to both groups. The ALS algorithm (Fig. 28.3) provides a standardised approach to the management of adult patients in cardiac arrest.

Shockable rhythms (VF/pulseless VT)

The first monitored rhythm is VF/pulseless VT in approximately 25% of cardiac arrests, both in or out of

hospital. Ventricular fibrillation/pulseless VT will also occur at some stage during resuscitation in about 25% of cardiac arrests with an initial documented rhythm of asystole or PEA. Having confirmed cardiac arrest, help (including a defibrillator) is summoned and CPR initiated, beginning chest compressions with a compression/ventilation (CV) ratio of 30:2. When the defibrillator arrives, chest compressions are continued while applying self-adhesive pads. The rhythm is identified and treated according to the ALS algorithm.

Sequence of actions

- If VF/pulseless VT is confirmed, charge the defibrillator while another rescuer continues chest compressions. Choose an energy setting of at least 150 J for the first shock and the same or a higher energy for subsequent shocks, or follow the manufacturer's guidance for the particular defibrillator.
- Once the defibrillator is charged, pause the chest compressions, quickly ensure that all rescuers are clear of the patient, and then give one shock. The person doing compressions or another rescuer may deliver the shock. This sequence should be planned before stopping compressions. This pause in chest compressions should be brief and no longer than 5 s.
- Resume chest compressions immediately (CV ratio 30:2) without reassessing the rhythm or feeling for a pulse.
- Continue CPR for 2 min, then pause briefly to check the monitor.
- If VF/pulseless VT persists:
  - Give a further (second) shock and, without reassessing the rhythm or feeling for a pulse, resume CPR (CV ratio 30:2) immediately after the shock, starting with chest compressions.
- On completion of CPR for 2 min, pause briefly to check the monitor.
- If VF/pulseless VT persists:
  - Give a further (third) shock and, without reassessing the rhythm or feeling for a pulse, resume CPR (CV ratio 30:2) immediately after the shock, starting with chest compressions.
- If i.v./intraosseous access has been obtained, give adrenaline 1 mg and amiodarone 300 mg once compressions have resumed. On completion of CPR for 2 min, pause briefly to check the monitor.
- If VF/pulseless VT persists:
  - Give a further (fourth) shock; resume CPR immediately and continue for 2 min.
  - Give adrenaline 1 mg with alternate cycles of CPR (i.e. approximately every 3–5 min).
- If organised electrical activity is seen during this brief pause in compressions, seek evidence of ROSC (check

Resuscitation Council (UK) **2015** **In-hospital Resuscitation**

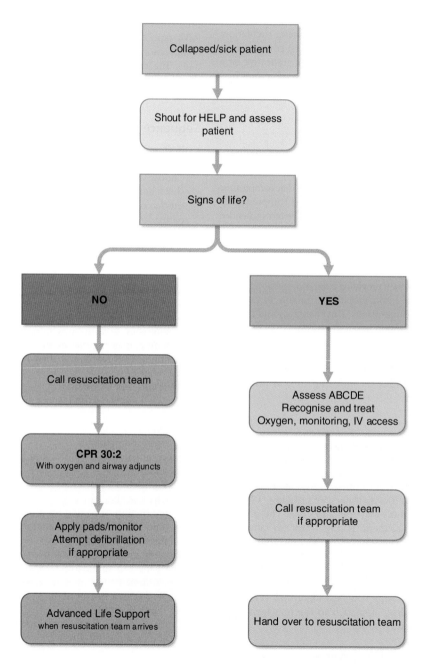

Fig. 28.2 In-hospital resuscitation algorithm. (Adapted from 2015 Resuscitation Guidelines (Resuscitation Council UK), https://www.resus.org.uk/resuscitation-guidelines/in-hospital-resuscitation/.)

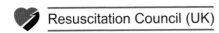 **Adult Advanced Life Support**

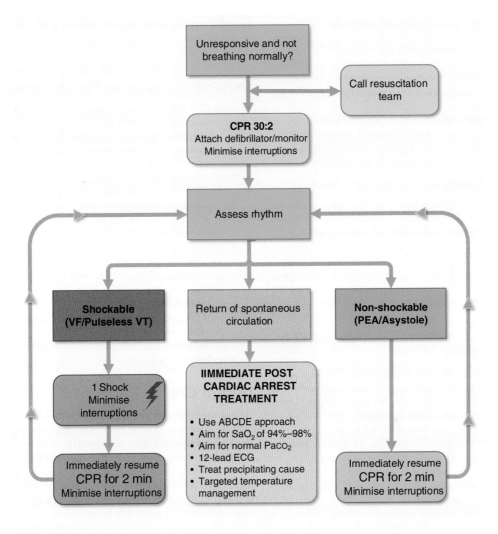

Fig. 28.3 The advanced life support algorithm. (Adapted from 2015 Resuscitation Guidelines (Resuscitation Council UK), https://www.resus.org.uk/resuscitation-guidelines/adult-advanced-life-support/.)

for signs of life, a central pulse and end-tidal CO_2 if available).

- If there is ROSC, start post-resuscitation care.
- If there are no signs of ROSC, continue CPR and switch to the non-shockable algorithm.
- If asystole is seen, continue CPR and switch to the non-shockable algorithm.
- If a rhythm compatible with a pulse is seen during a 2-min period of CPR, do not interrupt chest compressions to palpate a pulse unless the patient shows signs of life suggesting ROSC.
- If there is any doubt about the existence of a pulse in the presence of an organised rhythm, resume CPR.
- If the patient has ROSC, begin post-resuscitation care.

Precordial thump

A single precordial thump has a very low success rate for cardioversion and is only likely to succeed if given within the first few seconds of the onset of a shockable rhythm. There is more success with pulseless VT than with VF. Delivery of a precordial thump must not delay calling for help or accessing a defibrillator. It is reasonable to attempt a precordial thump if VF occurs intraoperatively, but do not delay the call for a defibrillator.

Witnessed and monitored VF/pulseless VT in the cardiac arrest

If a patient has a witnessed and monitored cardiac arrest in the catheter laboratory, coronary care unit (CCU) or critical care area or whilst monitored after cardiac surgery, and a manual defibrillator is rapidly available:

- confirm cardiac arrest and shout for help;
- if the initial rhythm is VF/pulseless VT, give up to three quick successive (stacked) shocks;
- rapidly check for a rhythm change and, if appropriate, check for a pulse and other signs of ROSC after each defibrillation attempt; and
- start chest compressions and continue CPR for 2 min if the third shock is unsuccessful.

This three-shock strategy may also be considered for an initial, witnessed VF/pulseless VT cardiac arrest if the patient is already connected to a manual defibrillator (e.g. intraoperative cardiac arrest where defibrillation pads had been applied before the operation).

Non-shockable rhythms (PEA and asystole)

Pulseless electrical activity is defined as the absence of any palpable pulse in the presence of cardiac electrical activity that would be expected to produce a cardiac output. There

may be some mechanical myocardial contractions that are too weak to produce a detectable pulse or blood pressure; this is sometimes described as pseudo-PEA. Pulseless electrical activity may be caused by reversible conditions that can be treated if they are identified and corrected. A relative overdose of an induction drug is a well-recognised cause of intraoperative cardiac arrest.

Sequence of actions for PEA and asystole

- Start CPR (CV ratio 30:2) and inject adrenaline 1 mg as soon as i.v./intraosseous access is achieved.
- Continue CPR (CV ratio 30:2) until the airway is secured, then continue chest compressions without pausing during ventilation.
- Recheck the patient after 2 min.
- If electrical activity compatible with a pulse is seen, check for a pulse and signs of life:
  - If a pulse or signs of life are present, start post-resuscitation care.
  - If no pulse or no signs of life are present (PEA or asystole):
    - Continue CPR.
    - Recheck the rhythm after 2 min and proceed accordingly.
    - Give further adrenaline 1 mg every 3–5 min (during alternate 2-min loops of CPR).
- If VF/pulseless VT at rhythm check, change to the shockable rhythm algorithm.

During CPR

During the treatment of persistent VF/pulseless VT or PEA/asystole, there should be an emphasis on giving good-quality chest compressions between defibrillation attempts, whilst recognising and treating reversible causes (Table 28.1) and whilst obtaining a secure airway and i.v./intraosseous access. Healthcare providers must practise efficient coordination between CPR and shock delivery. A shock is more likely to be successful if the pre-shock pause is short (less than 5 s).

Table 28.1 Reversible causes of cardiac arrest

4 Hs	4 Ts
Hypoxia	Tension pneumothorax
Hypovolaemia	Tamponade (cardiac)
Hypothermia	Toxic substances
Hyper-/hypokalaemia Hypocalcaemia Acidaemia Other metabolic disorders	Thromboembolism Pulmonary embolism Coronary thrombosis

Optimising the quality of cardiopulmonary resuscitation

Several defibrillator models incorporate CPR feedback systems. These comprise either a puck that is placed on the sternum or modified defibrillator patches, both of which incorporate an accelerometer that enables measurement of chest compression rate and depth. Measurement of the changes in chest impedance enable ventilation rate to be recorded. These modified defibrillators can provide audio feedback in real time, and downloaded data can be used for team debriefing after the event. Use of a CPR feedback device results in CPR performance that is closer to that specified in the guidelines, but this has yet to be shown to improve survival.

Potentially reversible causes

Potential causes or aggravating factors for which specific treatment exists must be sought during any cardiac arrest (see Table 28.1):
- Minimise the risk of **hypoxaemia** by ensuring that the patient's lungs are ventilated adequately with 100% oxygen.
- Pulseless electrical activity caused by **hypovolaemia** is usually due to severe haemorrhage. Restore intravascular volume rapidly with fluid, coupled with urgent surgery to stop the haemorrhage.
- **Hyperkalaemia, hypokalaemia, hypocalcaemia, acidaemia and other metabolic disorders** are detected by biochemical tests or suggested by the patient's medical history (e.g. renal failure). A 12-lead ECG may be diagnostic. Intravenous calcium chloride is indicated in the presence of hyperkalaemia, hypocalcaemia and overdose of calcium channel blocking drugs.
- Suspect **hypothermia** in any drowning incident; use a low-reading thermometer.
- A **tension pneumothorax** may be the primary cause of PEA and may follow attempts at CVC insertion. Decompress rapidly by needle thoracentesis or urgent thoracostomy, and then insert an intercostal chest drain.
- Cardiac **tamponade** is difficult to diagnose because the typical signs of distended neck veins and hypotension are obscured by the arrest itself. Rapid transthoracic echocardiography with minimal interruption to chest compression can be used to identify a pericardial effusion. Cardiac arrest after penetrating chest trauma is highly suggestive of tamponade and is an indication for resuscitative thoracotomy.
- In the absence of a specific history, the accidental or deliberate ingestion of therapeutic or **toxic** substances may be revealed only by laboratory investigations. Where available, the appropriate antidotes should be used, but most often treatment is supportive.

- The most common cause of **thromboembolic** or mechanical circulatory obstruction is massive pulmonary embolus. If cardiac arrest is likely to be caused by pulmonary embolism, consider giving a fibrinolytic drug immediately. Ongoing CPR is not a contraindication to fibrinolysis. Fibrinolytic drugs may take up to 90 min to be effective; give a fibrinolytic drug only if it is appropriate to continue CPR for this duration.

Use of ultrasound imaging during ALS

Several studies have examined the use of ultrasound during cardiac arrest to detect potentially reversible causes. This imaging provides information that may help to identify reversible causes of cardiac arrest (e.g. cardiac tamponade, pulmonary embolism, ischaemia, aortic dissection, hypovolaemia, pneumothorax).

When ultrasound imaging and appropriately trained clinicians are available, use them to assist with assessment and treatment of potentially reversible causes of cardiac arrest. The integration of ultrasound into advanced life support requires considerable training to ensure that interruptions to chest compressions are minimised.

A subxiphoid probe position has been recommended. Placement of the probe just before chest compressions are paused for a planned rhythm assessment enables a well-trained operator to obtain views within 10 s. Pseudo-PEA describes the echocardiographic detection of cardiac motion in the presence of a clinical diagnosis of PEA. The diagnosis of pseudo-PEA is important because it carries a better prognosis than true PEA and will influence treatment.

Resuscitation in the operating room

Patients in the operating room are normally monitored fully, and there should be little delay in diagnosing cardiac arrest. High-risk patients will often have invasive arterial pressure monitoring, which is invaluable in the event of cardiac arrest. If cardiac arrest is considered a strong possibility, apply self-adhesive defibrillation patches before induction of anaesthesia.

Asystole and VF will be detected immediately, but the onset of PEA might not be so obvious; loss of the pulse oximeter signal and end-tidal CO_2 are good clues and should provoke a pulse check.
- If asystole occurs intraoperatively, stop any surgical activity likely to be causing excessive vagal activity if this is the likely cause and give atropine 0.5 mg. Start CPR and immediately look for other reversible causes. The atropine dose can be repeated up to a total of 3 mg. A completely straight line suggests that a monitoring lead has become detached.
- In the case of PEA, start CPR while looking quickly for reversible causes. Give i.v. fluids unless you are certain intravascular volume is adequate. Stop giving the

anaesthetic. Although a vasopressor will be required, in these circumstances adrenaline 1 mg may be excessive. Give a much smaller dose of adrenaline (e.g. 50–100 μg) or another vasopressor (e.g. metaraminol) initially; if this fails to restore the cardiac output, increase the dose.

Cardiac arrest in the prone position

Cardiac arrest in the prone position is rare but challenging. Risk factors include:
- cardiac abnormalities in patients undergoing major spinal surgery;
- hypovolaemia;
- venous air embolism;
- wound irrigation with hydrogen peroxide (no longer recommended); and
- poor patient positioning with occluded venous return.
Consider applying self-adhesive defibrillation patches preoperatively to patients deemed at high risk from cardiac arrest. Chest compression in the prone position can be achieved with or without sternal counter-pressure.

Cardiac arrest caused by local anaesthetic

Patients with cardiovascular collapse or cardiac arrest attributable to local anaesthetic toxicity should be treated with i.v. lipid emulsion in addition to standard ALS (see also Chapter 27). Guidelines for treatment with lipid emulsion have been produced by the Association of Anaesthetists. In general:
- provide initial i.v. bolus 1.5 ml kg^{-1} lipid emulsion 20% over 60 s, followed by an infusion at 15 ml kg^{-1} h^{-1};
- give up to three bolus doses of lipid at 5-min intervals and continue the infusion until the patient is stable or has received up to a maximum of 12 ml kg^{-1} lipid emulsion.

Airway management and ventilation

There are no data supporting the routine use of any specific approach to airway management during cardiac arrest. The best technique depends on the precise circumstances of the cardiac arrest and competence of the rescuer. During CPR with an unprotected airway, two ventilations are given after each sequence of 30 chest compressions. Once a tracheal tube or supraglottic airway device (SAD) has been inserted, the lungs are ventilated at a rate of about 10 breaths min^{-1} and chest compressions continued without pausing during ventilation.

Airway management during cardiac arrest is likely to involve several different interventions delivered stepwise, such as bag-mask ventilation followed by SAD insertion and/or tracheal intubation.

Several alternative airway devices have been considered for airway management during CPR for those not skilled in tracheal intubation or when attempted tracheal intubation fails. Recent randomised controlled trials in out of hospital cardiac arrest patients showed no difference in survival to hospital discharge among patients treated with bag-mask ventilation versus tracheal intubation (physicians in France and Belgium) and among patients treated with an i-gel SADl versus tracheal intubation (paramedics in the UK). However, a randomised controlled trial involving paramedics in the United States showed improved survival to hospital discharge for patients treated with a laryngeal tube compared with those treated with tracheal intubation.

Tracheal intubation should be attempted during cardiac arrest only by trained personnel who are able to carry out the procedure with a high level of skill and confidence. Prolonged attempts at tracheal intubation are harmful; the pause in chest compressions during this time will compromise coronary and cerebral perfusion. No tracheal intubation attempt should interrupt chest compressions for more than 10 s; if tracheal intubation is not achievable within these constraints, bag-mask ventilation should be restarted.

Waveform capnography is the most sensitive and specific way to confirm and continuously monitor the position of a tracheal tube in victims of cardiac arrest and should supplement clinical assessment. Several studies have indicated that exhaled carbon dioxide is detected reliably during CPR, except after prolonged cardiac arrest (>30 min), when pulmonary flow may be negligible. Existing portable monitors make initial confirmation and continuous monitoring of tracheal tube position by capnography feasible in almost all settings where tracheal intubation is performed, including out of hospital, emergency departments, and in-hospital locations. In all locations the standard of care is now that tracheal intubation is attempted only if waveform capnography is available to confirm correct placement of the tracheal tube.

Circulation
Intravascular access

Although peak drug concentrations are higher and circulation times are shorter when drugs are injected into a CVC compared with a peripheral cannula, insertion of a CVC interrupts CPR and is associated with several potential complications; peripheral venous cannulation is quicker, easier and safer. Drugs injected peripherally must be followed by a flush of at least 20 ml fluid and elevation of the extremity for 10–20 s to facilitate drug delivery to the central circulation. If i.v. access cannot be established within the first 2 min of resuscitation, insert an intraosseous device into either the tibia or humerus. Drugs injected via the intraosseous route should achieve adequate plasma concentrations, although a recent observation study suggests that the intraosseous route may be associated with a reduced rate of return of spontaneous circulation. Effective fluid resuscitation can also be achieved via an intraosseous device.

Drugs

Adrenaline

A recent randomised placebo-controlled trial of adrenaline in OHCA showed that it increased the rate of survival to hospital discharge but did not increase the number of survivors with favourable neurological recovery. The optimal dose of adrenaline is not known, and there are no data supporting the use of repeated doses. There are few data on the pharmacokinetics of adrenaline during CPR. The optimal duration of CPR and number of shocks that should be given before giving drugs is unknown. On the basis of current data and expert consensus, for VF/VT, adrenaline is given after the third shock once chest compressions have resumed and then repeated every 3–5 min during cardiac arrest (alternate cycles).

Atropine

Several recent studies have failed to demonstrate any benefit from atropine in out-of-hospital or IHCAs, and it is not recommended for routine use for asystole or PEA.

Antiarrhythmic drugs

No antiarrhythmic drug given during human cardiac arrest has been shown unequivocally to increase survival to hospital discharge after shock-refractory VF/pulseless VT. However, in a large randomised controlled trial, amiodarone and lidocaine were both associated with higher survival to discharge rates in a subgroup of bystander-witnessed OHCA. Based on expert consensus, amiodarone 300 mg should be given by bolus injection (flushed with 20 ml 0.9% sodium chloride or 5% dextrose) after the third shock. A further dose of 150 mg may be given for recurrent or refractory VF/pulseless VT, followed by 900 mg infused over 24 h. Lidocaine 1 mg kg^{-1} may be used as an alternative if amiodarone is not available, but should not be given if amiodarone has been administered already.

Bicarbonate

Cardiac arrest causes combined respiratory and metabolic acid because pulmonary gas exchange ceases and cellular metabolism becomes anaerobic. The best treatment of acidaemia in cardiac arrest is chest compressions; some additional benefit is gained by ventilation. During cardiac arrest, arterial blood gas values may be misleading and bear little relationship to tissue acid–base state; analysis of central venous blood may be better in this regard. Giving sodium bicarbonate routinely during cardiac arrest and CPR, or after ROSC, is not recommended. Give sodium bicarbonate 50 mmol if cardiac arrest is associated with hyperkalaemia or tricyclic antidepressant overdose. Repeat the dose according to the clinical condition of the patient and results of repeated blood gas analysis.

Calcium

There are no data supporting any beneficial action for calcium after most cases of cardiac arrest. High plasma concentrations achieved after injection may be harmful to the ischaemic myocardium and may impair cerebral recovery. Give calcium during resuscitation only when indicated specifically (cardiac arrest caused by hyperkalaemia, hypocalcaemia or calcium channel blocker overdose).

Mechanical CPR

At best, standard manual CPR produces coronary and cerebral perfusion that is only 30% of normal. Several CPR techniques and devices may improve haemodynamics or short-term survival when used by well-trained providers in selected cases. However, the success of any technique or device depends on the education and training of the rescuers and on resources (including personnel). Large prehospital randomised trials have failed to show any benefit for mechanical CPR in comparison with high-quality manual CPR. Current international guidelines recommend the use of mechanical devices for CPR during transport, during primary coronary intervention and during prolonged resuscitation attempts where rescuer fatigue may impair the effectiveness of manual chest compression.

Extracorporeal cardiopulmonary resuscitation

Several observational studies document the successful use of extracorporeal CPR in selected cases of cardiac arrest refractory to standard ALS techniques. It has been generally used for IHCA or for patients admitted in refractory cardiac arrest after OHCA, although there are now case series describing its use in the out-of-hospital setting. Patients are selected for extracorporeal CPR if they have a potentially reversible cause of cardiac arrest (e.g. coronary artery occlusion). The technique involves arteriovenous cannulation during CPR and rapid establishment of the patient on extracorporeal membrane oxygenation (ECMO). The patient can also be rapidly cooled using the extracorporeal circuit, which may provide some neuroprotection. After extracorporeal CPR, good neurological outcomes have been reported in 23% of patients after IHCA and 12% of patients after OHCA.

Periarrest arrhythmias

Cardiac arrhythmias are common in the periarrest period, and treatment algorithms for both tachycardia (Fig. 28.4) and bradycardia (Fig. 28.5) have been developed to enable the non-specialist to initiate treatment safely.

In all cases, oxygen is given, an i.v. cannula inserted and the patient assessed for adverse signs. Whenever possible,

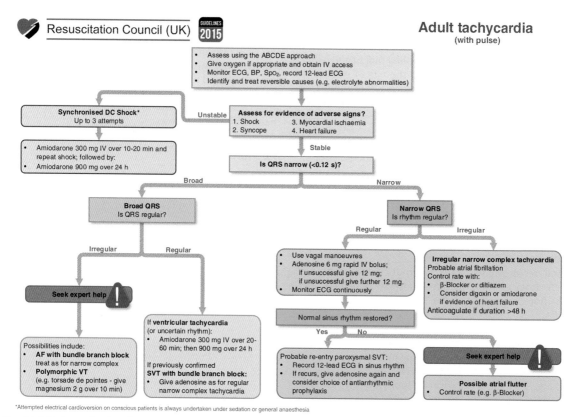

Fig. 28.4 Tachycardia algorithm. (Adapted from 2015 Resuscitation Guidelines (Resuscitation Council UK), https://www.resus.org.uk/resuscitation-guidelines/peri-arrest-arrhythmias/#tachycardia.)

record a 12-lead ECG as this will help determine the precise rhythm. Any electrolyte abnormalities should be corrected.

The presence or absence of adverse signs or symptoms will dictate the appropriate treatment for most arrhythmias. If the patient has adverse factors, electrical therapy is likely to be appropriate. Drugs usually act more slowly and less reliably than electrical treatments and are usually the preferred treatment for the stable patient without adverse signs.

Tachycardia

If the patient is unstable and deteriorating, synchronised cardioversion is the treatment of choice.
- Before cardioversion is attempted, the patient will require anaesthesia or sedation.
- Set the defibrillator to deliver a synchronised shock. This delivers the shock to coincide with the R wave as unsynchronised shock could coincide with a T wave and cause VF.
  - For broad-complex tachycardia or atrial fibrillation (AF), initially start with 120–150 J and increase in increments if this fails.

- Atrial flutter and regular narrow-complex tachycardia will often be terminated by lower-energy shocks; therefore start with 70–120 J.
- If cardioversion fails to terminate the arrhythmia and adverse features persist, give amiodarone 300 mg i.v. over 10–20 min and attempt further synchronised cardioversion.
- The loading dose of amiodarone can be followed by an infusion of 900 mg over 24 h given preferably via a central vein.

The treatment for stable tachycardia is outlined in Fig. 28.4.
- A regular broad-complex tachycardia is likely to be VT or a supraventricular rhythm with bundle branch block; if there is uncertainty about the source of the arrhythmia, give adenosine.
- In general, patients who have been in AF for more than 48 h should not be treated by cardioversion (electrical or chemical) until they have been fully anticoagulated for at least 3 weeks or unless transoesophageal echocardiography has shown the absence of atrial thrombus. If cardioversion is required more urgently, give an i.v. bolus

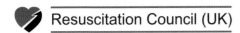 **Adult bradycardia**

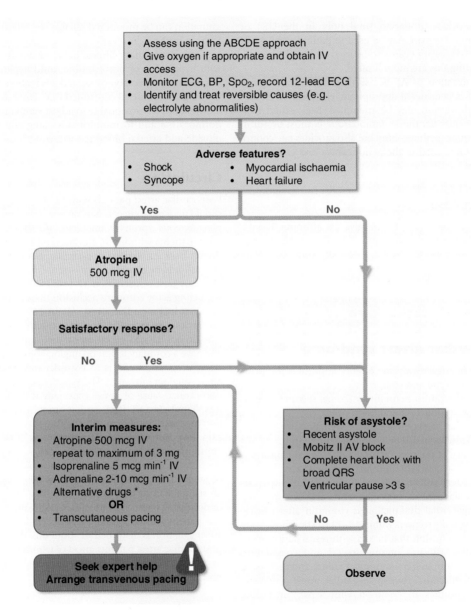

Fig. 28.5 Bradycardia algorithm. (Adapted from 2015 Resuscitation Guidelines (Resuscitation Council UK), https://www.resus.org.uk/resuscitation-guidelines/peri-arrest-arrhythmias/#bradycardia.)

injection of heparin followed by a continuous infusion to maintain the activated partial thromboplastin time (APTT) at 1.5–2 times the reference control value.

- If the aim is to control heart rate, the drugs of choice are β-blockers, diltiazem (oral only in the UK) or verapamil. Digoxin may be used in patients with heart failure. Magnesium can also be used, although the data supporting this are more limited.
- If the duration of AF is less than 48 h and rhythm control is considered appropriate, electrical or chemical cardioversion may be attempted. Seek expert help and consider flecainide. Amiodarone is most useful in maintaining rhythm control but also provides rate control and is often used in the perioperative and critical care settings.

Bradycardia

- If adverse signs are present, give i.v. atropine 500 μg, and, if necessary, repeat every 3–5 min to a total of 3 mg.
- In the intraoperative setting, stop any surgical activity likely to be causing vagal stimulation.

Post-resuscitation care

Post–cardiac arrest syndrome

Post–cardiac arrest syndrome often complicates the post-resuscitation phase and comprises:
- post–cardiac arrest brain injury (coma, seizures, neurocognitive dysfunction and brain death);
- post–cardiac arrest myocardial dysfunction;
- systemic ischaemia/reperfusion response; and
- persistence of the precipitating pathological condition.

Post–cardiac arrest brain injury may be exacerbated by microcirculatory failure, impaired autoregulation, hypercarbia, hyperoxia, pyrexia, hyperglycaemia and seizures. Significant myocardial dysfunction is common after cardiac arrest but typically recovers within 48–72 h. The whole-body ischaemia/reperfusion that occurs with resuscitation from cardiac arrest activates immunological and coagulation pathways contributing to multiorgan failure and increasing the risk of infection. Thus, post–cardiac arrest syndrome has many features in common with sepsis, including intravascular volume depletion and vasodilation.

Airway and breathing

Hypoxaemia increases the likelihood of a further cardiac arrest and may contribute to secondary brain injury. Several animal studies have demonstrated that hyperoxaemia causes oxidative stress and harms post-ischaemic neurons.

Although the lack of robust data is acknowledged, current recommendations are to titrate the inspired oxygen concentration to maintain arterial blood oxygen saturation in the range of 94%–98% as soon as arterial blood oxygen saturation can be monitored reliably (by blood gas analysis, SpO_2 or both).

Some preliminary clinical data indicate that, compared with hypocarbia or normocarbia, mild hypercarbia might improve neurological outcome, and this is about to be studied in a large randomised controlled trial. Until definitive data are available, it is reasonable to adjust ventilation to achieve normocarbia and to monitor this using end-tidal carbon dioxide and arterial blood gas values.

Circulation

Post–cardiac arrest patients with ST elevation on their ECG should undergo early coronary angiography and, if indicated, percutaneous coronary intervention. Those post–cardiac arrest patients without ST elevation on their ECG but who do not have an obvious non-cardiac cause of their cardiac arrest should be considered for urgent coronary angiography. The early post-resuscitation 12-lead ECG is less reliable for predicting acute coronary occlusion than it is in those who have not had a cardiac arrest. About 25% of patients with no obvious extracardiac cause for their cardiac arrest, but who do not have ST elevation on their initial 12-lead ECG, will have a coronary lesion on angiography that is amenable to stenting. The trend is to consider immediate coronary artery angiography in OHCA patients with no obvious non-cardiac cause of arrest, especially if the initial rhythm was VF/pulseless VT. Post–cardiac arrest myocardial dysfunction causes haemodynamic instability, resulting in hypotension, low cardiac index and arrhythmias. If treatment with appropriate fluids and vasoactive drugs is insufficient to support the circulation, an intra-aortic balloon pump may be required. Target the mean arterial blood pressure to achieve an adequate urine output (0.5–1.0 ml kg^{-1} h^{-1}) and normal or decreasing plasma lactate values, taking into consideration the patient's usual blood pressure (if known). Cerebral autoregulation is disturbed in about one-third of comatose post–cardiac arrest patients, most of whom have pre-existing hypertension, and in such patients a higher mean arterial pressure may be optimal.

Disability (optimising neurological recovery)
Seizure control

Seizures occur in 25% of those who remain comatose after cardiac arrest. Although patients with seizures have four times the mortality rate of comatose patients without seizures, good neurological recovery has been documented in 17%

of those with seizures. Seizures increase cerebral metabolism by up to threefold and may cause cerebral injury. There is little evidence for benefit of any specific antiepileptic drug over another in the treatment of post–cardiac arrest seizure, but expert opinion suggests use of benzodiazepines, levetiracetam and sodium valproate.

Targeted temperature management

Treatment of hyperpyrexia

A period of hyperthermia (hyperpyrexia) is common in the first 48 h after cardiac arrest, and this is associated with worse neurological outcome. Treat hyperthermia occurring after cardiac arrest with antipyretics or active cooling.

Mild hypothermia is neuroprotective and improves outcome after a period of global cerebral hypoxia-ischaemia. Cooling suppresses many of the pathways leading to delayed cell death, including apoptosis. Two randomised trials demonstrated improved neurological outcome at hospital discharge or at 6 months in comatose patients who were cooled to 32°C–34°C for 12–24 h after out-of-hospital VF cardiac arrest. In both studies the control groups were not temperature controlled. The use of hypothermia for non-shockable rhythms and after IHCA is supported mainly by observational data, which have a substantial risk of bias. One large observational study has shown an association between use of mild hypothermia and worse outcome among IHCA patients. In the Targeted Temperature Management (TTM) trial, 950 all-rhythm OHCA patients were randomised to 24 h of temperature control at either 33°C or 36°C. There was no difference in neurological outcome at 180 days. An international consensus group has recommended that temperature control is continued for at least 24 h in comatose post–cardiac arrest patients using a constant temperature in the range 32°C–36°C.

Cooling techniques. External or internal cooling techniques, or both, can be used for temperature management. Infusion of 30 ml kg^{-1} crystalloid at 4°C decreases core temperature by approximately 1.5°C, but this should be undertaken with careful monitoring in hospital. The use of prehospital cold fluid i.v. is not recommended because it has been associated with an increased incidence of pulmonary oedema.

Maintenance of target temperature is best achieved with external or internal cooling devices that include continuous temperature feedback to achieve a set target temperature. The temperature is typically monitored from a thermistor placed in the bladder, oesophagus or both. The temperature is maintained in the target range (32°C–36°C) for 24 h followed by controlled rewarming at 0.25°C–0.5°C h^{-1} and strict avoidance of hyperthermia. Plasma electrolyte concentrations can change rapidly during cooling and rewarming; frequent measurement and careful electrolyte replacement is essential.

Prognostication

Two thirds of those dying after admission to ICU after OHCA die from withdrawal of life-sustaining therapy after a diagnosis of severe neurological injury. A quarter of those dying after admission to ICU after IHCA die from neurological injury. A means of predicting neurological outcome that can be applied to individual comatose patients is required, but reliable prognostication cannot be achieved until at least 3 days after return to normothermia. European guidelines on prognostication after cardiac arrest recommend a multimodal approach that includes clinical examination, biochemical markers, neurophysiological studies and imaging (Fig. 28.6).

Clinical examination

There are no clinical neurological signs that predict poor outcome reliably (Cerebral Performance Category 3 or 4, or death) within 24 h after cardiac arrest. In adult patients who are comatose after cardiac arrest (Glasgow Coma Scale (GCS) motor score of 1 or 2) and do not have confounding factors (e.g. hypotension, sedatives or neuromuscular blocking agents), the absence of both pupillary light and corneal reflex at 72 h or later reliably predicts poor outcome. The presence of myoclonic status is associated strongly with poor outcome, but rare cases of good neurological recovery from this situation have been described, and accurate diagnosis is problematic.

Biochemical markers

Serum (e.g. neuron-specific enolase [NSE] or S100 protein) or CSF biomarkers alone are insufficient as predictors of poor outcomes in comatose patients after cardiac arrest. However, serum NSE is being used increasingly as a component of multimodal prognostication; serial values may have better prognostic power than single values.

Neurophysiological studies

No neurophysiological study predicts outcome for a comatose patient reliably within the first 24 h after cardiac arrest. If somatosensory evoked potentials are measured after 72 h in comatose cardiac arrest survivors, bilateral absence of the N20 cortical response to median nerve stimulation reliably predicts poor outcome.

Imaging studies

Many imaging modalities (MRI, CT, single photon emission CT, cerebral angiography, transcranial Doppler, nuclear medicine, near infrared spectroscopy) have been studied to determine their utility for prediction of outcome in adult

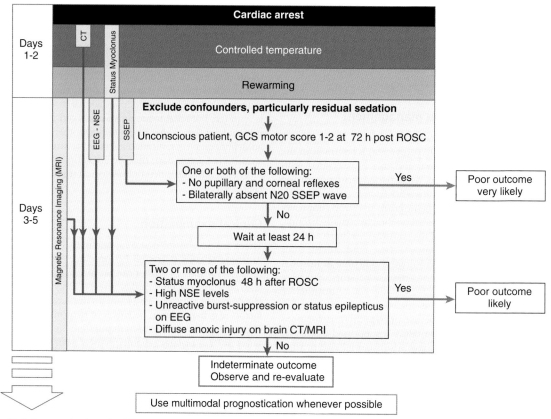

Fig. 28.6 Prognostication algorithm. The algorithm is entered 72 h after return of spontaneous circulation if, after the exclusion of confounders (particularly residual sedation), the patient remains unconscious with a Glasgow Coma Scale (GCS) motor score of 1 or 2. The absence of pupillary and corneal reflexes and/or bilaterally absent N20 somatosensory evoked potentials wave indicates a poor outcome is very likely. If neither of the features is present, wait at least 24 h before reassessing. At this stage, two or more of the following indicate that a poor outcome is likely: status myoclonus for 48 h or less; high neuron-specific enolase values; unreactive burst suppression or status epilepticus on EEG; or diffuse anoxic injury on brain CT and/or MRI. If none of these criteria are met, continue to observe and re-evaluate. (Reprinted from Sandroni, C., Cariou, A., Cavallaro, F., et al. (2014) Prognostication in comatose survivors of cardiac arrest: an advisory statement from the European Resuscitation Council and the European Society of Intensive Care Medicine. *Resuscitation*. 85, 1779–1789, with permission from Elsevier.)

survivors of cardiac arrest. Computed tomography and MRI are an important component of the multimodal approach to prognostication.

Organ donation

Up to 16% of patients who achieve sustained ROSC after cardiac arrest develop clinical brain death and can be considered for organ donation (donation after brain stem death) (see Chapter 48). Data from the UK indicate that 10% of those OHCA patients who are admitted to ICU but who do not survive become solid organ donors; most of these are donation after circulatory death donors. It has

been estimated that 25% of the deceased solid organ donors in the UK are OHCA patients admitted to ICU.

Decisions relating to cardiopulmonary resuscitation

It is essential to identify patients for whom cardiopulmonary arrest represents an anticipated terminal event and in whom CPR is inappropriate. All institutions should ensure that a clear and explicit resuscitation plan exists for all patients. For some patients this will involve a DNACPR decision.

National guidelines from the British Medical Association, Resuscitation Council (UK) Royal College of Nursing (RCN) and General Medical Council, provide a framework for formulating local policy. The main messages are the following:

- Decisions about CPR must be made on the basis of an *individual* assessment of each patient's case.
- Advance care planning, including making decisions about CPR, is an important part of good clinical care for those at risk of cardiorespiratory arrest.
- Communication and the provision of information are essential parts of good quality care.
- It is not necessary to initiate discussion about CPR with a patient if there is no reason to believe that the patient is likely to suffer a cardiorespiratory arrest; however, the patient and/or those close to the patient should be informed of this decision.
- Where no explicit decision has been made in advance, there should be an initial presumption in favour of CPR.
- If CPR would not restart the heart and breathing, it should not be attempted.
- Where the expected benefit of attempted CPR may be outweighed by the burdens, the patient's informed views are of paramount importance. If the patient lacks capacity, those close to the patient should be involved in discussions to explore the patient's wishes, feelings, beliefs and values.
- If a patient with capacity refuses CPR, or a patient lacking capacity has a valid and applicable advance decision refusing CPR, this should be respected.
- A DNACPR decision does not override clinical judgement in the unlikely event of a reversible cause of the patient's respiratory or cardiac arrest that does not match the circumstances envisaged.
- DNACPR decisions apply only to CPR and not to any other aspects of treatment.

DNACPR decisions in the perioperative period

General or regional anaesthesia may cause cardiovascular or respiratory instability that requires supportive treatment. Many routine interventions used during anaesthesia (e.g. tracheal intubation, mechanical ventilation or injection of vasoactive drugs) could be considered to be resuscitative measures. The anaesthetist and the surgeon should review DNACPR decisions with patients, or their representative if they lack capacity, as part of the consent process. The DNACPR decision can be suspended, modified or remain valid during the procedure. The DNACPR management option would normally apply while the patient remains in the operating room and post-anaesthetic care unit.

Recommended Summary Plan for Emergency Care and Treatment

Resuscitation decisions are now much more commonly incorporated into wider treatment plans that include patients' preferences for other aspects of their care, such as organ support in ICU. A multidisciplinary group has recently introduced ReSPECT (www.respectprocess.org.uk). Its aim is to standardise the documentation of patients' wishes in the event of an emergency and is applicable to all healthcare settings.

National Cardiac Arrest Audit

All IHCAs should be reviewed and audited. The NCAA is a UK-wide database of IHCA and is supported by the Resuscitation Council (UK) and the Intensive Care National Audit & Research Centre (ICNARC). The NCAA monitors and reports on the incidence of and outcome from IHCAs attended by a resuscitation team to inform practice and policy. It aims to improve care delivery and outcomes from cardiac arrest.

Acknowledgement

Much of this chapter has been adapted, with permission, from the 2015 Resuscitation Council (UK) Guidelines (www.resus.org.uk).

References/Further reading

Callaway, C.W., Soar, J., Aibiki, M., et al., 2015. Part 4: advanced life support: 2015 international consensus on cardiopulmonary resuscitation and emergency cardiovascular care science with treatment recommendations. Resuscitation 95, e71–e120.

Donnino, M.W., Andersen, L.W., Berg, K.M., et al., 2015. Temperature management after cardiac arrest: an advisory statement by the Advanced Life Support Task Force of the International Liaison Committee on Resuscitation and the American Heart Association Emergency Cardiovascular

Care Committee and the Council on Cardiopulmonary, Critical Care, Perioperative and Resuscitation. Circulation 132, 2448–2456.

Nolan, J.P., Ferrando, P., Soar, J., et al., 2016. Increasing survival after admission to UK critical care units following cardiopulmonary resuscitation. Crit. Care 20, 219.

Nolan, J.P., Hazinski, M.F., Aickin, R., et al., 2015. Part 1: executive summary: 2015 international consensus on cardiopulmonary

resuscitation and emergency cardiovascular care science with treatment recommendations. Resuscitation 95, e1–e31.

Nolan, J.P., Soar, J., Cariou, A., et al., 2015. European resuscitation council and European society of intensive care medicine guidelines for resuscitation 2015 section 5 post resuscitation care. Resuscitation 95, 201–221.

Sandroni, C., Cariou, A., Cavallaro, F., et al., 2014. Prognostication in comatose survivors of cardiac arrest:

an advisory statement from the European Resuscitation Council and the European Society of Intensive Care Medicine. Resuscitation 85, 1779–1789.

Soar, J., Nolan, J.P., Bottiger, B.W., et al., 2015. European Resuscitation Council guidelines for resuscitation 2015: section 3. Adult advanced life support. Resuscitation 95, 100–147.

Chapter | **29** |

Postoperative and recovery room care

Ian Shaw, Jake Drinkwater

In anaesthetic practice the patient is monitored closely and continuously from before induction and throughout the operative procedure. However, many problems associated with anaesthesia and surgery occur in the immediate postoperative period. The 2001 National Confidential Enquiry into Patient Outcome and Death (NCEPOD) report 'Changing the way we operate' stated, 'Immediately after surgery all patients not returning to a special care area (e.g. ICU or HDU) need to be nursed by those trained and practiced in postoperative recovery.'

The anaesthetist retains responsibility for patients during their stay in the postanaesthesia care unit (PACU). With an effective handover they can delegate this responsibility to an appropriately trained and registered PACU practitioner; however, an anaesthetist should be immediately available to review the patient's care if required.

Professional bodies such as the RCoA and Association of Anaesthetists have made recommendations regarding the staffing, monitoring, care and discharge criteria for PACUs.

Staff

The core knowledge and competencies for staff in PACU are:
- assessment and management of airway, breathing and circulation;
- assessment of consciousness;
- monitoring during the immediate postoperative phase;
- i.v. access and fluid balance;
- applied knowledge of pharmacology in perioperative care;
- management of postoperative pain and postoperative nausea and vomiting (PONV); and
- management of surgical and anaesthetic emergencies.

Each patient should receive one-to-one care from an appropriately trained member of staff until the patient has met the following criteria:
- No requirement for any form of airway support
- Breathing spontaneously
- Haemodynamically stable and
- Alert and responding to commands

To maintain this level of care, no fewer than two members of staff should be present in PACU whenever a patient does not meet discharge criteria.

All clinical staff in PACU should have an intermediate life support (ILS) or equivalent qualification, and should an anaesthetist not be immediately available, at least one staff member should be trained in advanced life support (ALS).

Although management of the airway (including simple adjuncts) is a core competency, many PACU staff are specifically trained in the management of patients with supraglottic airway devices (SAD) and their removal. Less commonly, training is extended to include management of tracheal tubes. However, the anaesthetist is responsible for ensuring that the staff member to whom they hand over is capable of taking over care of the patient. Because of the relatively high incidence of airway complications in PACU, a professional with suitably qualified airway skills should always be immediately available. Many units now provide an anaesthetist who is immediately available to attend PACU to enable timely anaesthetic intervention for patients without compromising the efficient running of ongoing operating lists.

After general, epidural or spinal anaesthesia, all patients should be transferred to a dedicated PACU for initial care unless admission to ICU is planned. It is important to recognise that not all high-dependency units (HDUs) are staffed with doctors and nurses with adequate skills in airway management.

Provision should be made for a member of the anaesthetic team to visit patients within 24 h after surgery when one or more of the following applies:

- ASA physical status 3–5
- Epidural analgesia is used on a general ward
- Discharged from PACU with invasive monitoring or
- Request by clinical staff

Facilities

All operating theatre complexes should have a dedicated PACU. Depending on the case load, two PACU beds per theatre are normally required to allow safe recovery of patients and discharge to the ward without delays to theatre schedules. Bed spaces should be adequate to allow unobstructed access for trolleys, x-ray equipment, resuscitation carts and clinical staff.

The principle is that staff members may look after the patient with all equipment and facilities to hand so that they can continue care without needing to leave the bedside. Each bed space should be fitted with 12 electrical socket outlets (six on each side of the bed), one oxygen and one medical air pipeline outlet, two vacuum outlets, an adjustable examination light, an emergency call system, physiological monitors with a display screen and a recording system for patient data. In addition, the PACU should have a fully equipped anaesthetic machine, a defibrillator, means of manual ventilation of a patient's lungs and a selection of airway adjuncts and devices. A comprehensive stock of drugs and equipment is essential, with staff available to deliver these to the bedside. Patient warming devices should be readily available to manage inadvertent perioperative hypothermia.

Patients continue to exhale volatile anaesthetic agents into the environment for some time after they are discontinued and so the ventilation in PACUs must be adequate.

Monitoring

Depending on the condition of the patient and the location of PACU in relation to the operating theatres, the period of transfer from theatre to PACU can be a time of increased risk. A brief interruption of monitoring may be acceptable if PACU is immediately adjacent to the operating theatre. However, where this is not the case, or if the patient is critically ill, appropriate mobile monitoring is required. Minimum monitoring standards (Box 29.1) should be maintained until the patient has fully recovered from anaesthesia. This is to allow the rapid detection of airway, ventilatory and cardiovascular problems. Capnography aids the early detection of airway obstruction and should be used whenever a

---

> **Box 29.1 Minimum standards of monitoring**
>
> **Minimum acceptable monitoring**
>
> Clinical observation (one-to-one)
> Pulse oximetry
> Non-invasive blood pressure
> ECG
> Core temperature
> End-tidal carbon dioxide (if tracheal tube or supraglottic airway device *in situ*)
>
> **Additional monitoring which should be immediately available**
>
> Blood/capillary glucose
> Nerve stimulator
>
> **Additional monitoring which should be available**
>
> Urine output
> Invasive pressure monitoring (arterial line, central venous pressure)
> Cardiac output monitoring
> Access to haematological and biochemical investigations

tracheal tube or SAD is *in situ*. Additional monitoring (e.g. invasive vascular pressures) may be indicated depending upon surgical, patient and anaesthetic factors and is at the discretion of the responsible anaesthetist in conjunction with the surgical and PACU teams.

A contemporaneous record of the measurements from monitoring should be kept and as a minimum should include:

- conscious level;
- patency of airway;
- respiratory rate and adequacy of ventilation;
- SpO_2 and FIO_2;
- BP;
- heart rate and rhythm;
- measure of pain intensity and PONV on an agreed scale;
- any i.v. infusions or drugs administered; and
- core temperature.

Where measured, additional variables such as urine output, central venous pressure, end-tidal CO_2 and surgical drainage volume should also be recorded. The frequency of monitoring depends upon the stage of recovery, nature of the surgery and clinical condition of the patient.

Handover

It is essential that the anaesthetist formally hands over care of the patient to an appropriately qualified PACU practitioner.

Handovers may be optimised through the use of standardised processes such as situation, background, assessment, recommendations (SBAR; an example is shown in Box 29.2) to improve their efficiency, accuracy and completeness. The use of checklists may further enhance the quality of handovers and ensure all relevant information is transferred.

All i.v. lines should be flushed by the anaesthetist to remove any residual drugs and to ensure patency before leaving a patient in PACU.

Postoperative planning

Each patient should have an individualised postanaesthesia care plan, which should be communicated in both written and verbal formats. The extent and detail will depend upon patient, surgical and anaesthetic factors but should be clear and easy to interpret.

Consideration should be given to:

- the management of pre-existing disease;
- the continuation, cessation or review of regular medications;
- the need for and timing of investigations;
- analgesic and fluid requirements;
- the requirement for thromboprophylaxis, antibiotics and glycaemic control;
- the frequency and nature of observations;
- the appropriate level of postoperative care; and
- prescription of oxygen, methods of administration and target SpO_2 (if applicable).

Discharge from PACU

Whilst the responsibility for the safe and appropriate discharge of patients from PACU lies with the anaesthetist, the adoption of strict discharge criteria (Table 29.1) enables this to be delegated to PACU staff.

Patients who do not meet the agreed criteria, or who encounter problems during the recovery period, should remain in PACU and be reviewed by an anaesthetist to decide upon the appropriateness, timing and safety of discharge. Where necessary the patient may require admission to a higher level of care facility (e.g. HDU or ICU).

Levels of postoperative care

There are four recognised levels of postoperative care:

- Level 0: Ward – basic observations.
- Level 1: Enhanced ward – more frequent observations for patients at risk of deterioration or requiring basic resuscitation.
- Level 2: HDU – detailed observation or intervention, and patients requiring single-organ support, excluding tracheal intubation/ventilation.
- Level 3: ICU – complex patients requiring tracheal intubation/ventilation or support of more than one organ system.

Mechanisms for the early identification of patients requiring a higher level of care should be in place, as should the requirement for specialist postoperative intervention.

Several factors may result in the need for higher levels of care or specialist input in the postoperative period (Table 29.2). There are a few absolute indicators for admission to HDU/ICU, but in most cases the decision is based on a combination of factors; early assessment of the patients by senior anaesthetists, followed by discussion with critical care staff, allows care to be offered on an individual basis.

Table 29.1 Association of Anaesthetists minimum PACU discharge criteria

A	Patient has a clear airway and protective airway reflexes.
B	Breathing and oxygenation are satisfactory. Oxygen therapy should be prescribed if appropriate.
C	The cardiovascular system is stable, with no unexplained cardiac irregularity or persistent bleeding. The specific values of pulse and blood pressure should approximate to normal preoperative values (or be at an acceptable level), ideally within parameters set by the anaesthetist, and peripheral perfusion should be adequate. Any i.v. cannulae should be patent, flushed if necessary, and i.v. fluids should be prescribed if appropriate.
D	The patient is fully conscious.
E	Pain and PONV should be adequately controlled and suitable analgesic and antiemetic regimens prescribed. Temperature should be within acceptable limits. All surgical catheters and drains should be checked.
Other	All health records should be complete and medical notes present.

i.v., Intravenous; *PACU,* postanaesthesia care unit; *PONV,* postoperative nausea and vomiting.

Table 29.2 Factors implicated in the need for higher level or specialist postoperative care

Patient	Multiple or complex comorbidities Unstable or newly diagnosed disease Poor functional ability or acute functional decline Cognitive impairment
Surgical	Emergency surgery Prolonged surgery Major surgery (e.g. intra-abdominal, thoracic, vascular) Surgery associated with large fluid shifts Surgical complications or difficulties Specialist postoperative surgical requirements (e.g. cardiac, neurosurgery)
Anaesthetic	Airway complications or difficulties Respiratory or cardiovascular morbidity, complications or instability Reduced conscious level Metabolic derangement Sepsis Anaesthetic complications (anaphylaxis, aspiration) ASA ≥3
Global	Increased perioperative risk score Unexpected failure to meet PACU discharge criteria

ASA, American Society of Anesthesiologists physical status; *PACU,* postanaesthesia care unit.

Common early postoperative complications

Central nervous system

Many patients arrive in PACU with a depressed level of consciousness, ranging from mild disorientation to confusion, agitation, and coma. Usually this is attributable to the residual effects of anaesthetic, sedative, and analgesic medications but may be the result of pathological conditions or deranged physiology. The anaesthetist must be able to differentiate those causes that are benign and self-limiting from those that require investigation and intervention. Regardless of the precipitating cause, the effect on level of consciousness depends on the patient's premorbid condition and cognitive and physiological reserve.

Pathophysiology

Normal CNS function requires a controlled physiological environment. Anaesthesia and other acute or chronic pathological conditions may impair the homeostatic mechanisms responsible for maintaining CNS functions and result in a depressed level of consciousness. Physiological causes of a depressed consciousness level are shown in Table 29.3. It is imperative that physiological derangements are promptly identified as they can cause irreversible CNS injury if not addressed.

Investigation

Clinical examination and an extended arterial blood gas measurement should enable identification of a physiological cause for depressed consciousness level. Infection and sepsis, regardless of source location, may result in confusion, agitation, and depressed consciousness level. This may be due to the global physiological derangements that accompany the condition or a direct effect of infection on the CNS.

Table 29.3 Physiological causes of altered consciousness

Respiratory	Hypoxia Hypercarbia
Metabolic	Acidaemia Hyperglycaemia
Energy substrate	Hypoglycaemia
Temperature	Hypothermia
Cerebral perfusion pressure	Hypotension
Biochemical	Hyponatraemia Uraemia Raised Ammonia

- Physiological observation:
  - HR, BP, SpO_2
  - Temperature
- Extended arterial blood gas measurement
  - Acid–base status
  - PaO_2, $PaCO_2$
  - Haemoglobin
  - Sodium
  - Lactate
  - Glucose
- Targeted investigation based on the patient's medical history
  - Ammonia in liver failure
  - Urea in renal failure

Drugs

A wide range of drugs used in anaesthetic practice result in depression of consciousness level, whether as an intended clinical effect or as an adverse effect, including:

- volatile anaesthetics (particularly those with a high blood/gas solubility coefficient);
- barbiturates;
- benzodiazepines (e.g. midazolam, lorazepam);
- α_2-agonists (e.g. clonidine);
- antimuscarinics (e.g. atropine, hyoscine);
- opioids;
- antiemetics (e.g. droperidol, cyclizine);
- local anaesthetics (e.g. systemic toxicity or total spinal anaesthesia); and
- Neuromuscular blocking agents (NMBAs; e.g. postoperative residual neuromuscular block).

The extent of the effect on level of consciousness depends on the dose, timing and pharmacokinetic profile of the drug. To a degree the CNS effects of a drug may be predictable, but interpatient variability and the presence of acute or chronic pathological conditions may result in significant variation.

Pain

Pain is a potent stimulus to the CNS, but its effect on level of consciousness is complex. In the presence of inadequate analgesia it has the potential to speed recovery of conscious level but can also increase agitation in patients with depressed consciousness. Successful treatment of pain, such as with an effective regional anaesthetic technique, may cause a reduction in the conscious level if long-acting analgesic drugs have already been administered. Distension of the bladder or stomach may cause confusion or agitation or may be interpreted as such in patients who are unable to communicate effectively.

Cerebral pathological conditions

Consciousness may be impaired by functional or structural cerebral damage in the absence of global physiological derangement (Table 29.4). A review of the patient's preoperative condition, surgical and anaesthetic course and clinical examination often aid the diagnosis. A high index of suspicion is essential, and rapid assessment, investigation and intervention may be required to avoid permanent cerebral damage.

Paediatric emergence delirium

Paediatric emergence delirium is most common in children aged 2–5 years and is discussed in detail in Chapter 33. This is a different clinical entity to the delirium that may be seen after the use of ketamine, either for induction of anaesthesia or as analgesic agent (see Chapter 4).

Postoperative delirium

Age-related decline in cerebral and cerebrovascular function contributes to the relatively high prevalence of postoperative delirium (POD) and cognitive dysfunction experienced by older patients, which delays discharge and ongoing functional recovery. The process of identifying and reducing the risk of POD should begin preoperatively and continue into the postoperative period.

Postoperative delirium presents with acute, fluctuating confusion and disorganised thinking. Risk factors for the development of POD include:

- age;
- frailty;
- cognitive impairment;
- previous excessive alcohol or drug consumption;
- cardiovascular and/or cerebrovascular disease; and
- polypharmacy.

Early recognition should be communicated throughout the multidisciplinary care team and facilitate multimodal interventions aimed at reducing the prevalence, severity and/or duration of POD.

Table 29.4 Pathological conditions resulting in altered consciousness

Pathological condition	Causes
Cerebral ischaemia/ infarction	Profound or prolonged global hypoperfusion Profound or prolonged global hypoxia Emboli • Thrombus • Air • Fat Disruption of cerebral blood supply • Surgical (carotid surgery) • Head positioning
Cerebral haemorrhage	Hypertension Trauma Intracranial surgery
Cerebral oedema	Alterations in osmotic balance • Hyper- and hyponatraemia • Hyperglycaemia • Uraemia • TURP syndrome Prolonged Trendelenburg position Trauma
Cerebral mass lesions	Tumour
Cerebral infection	Cerebral abscess Meningitis Encephalitis
Seizure	May be masked by neuromuscular blockade

TURP, Transurethral resection of the prostate.

Recovery room delirium is a strong predictor for POD and so the recovery area can be an appropriate area for delirium testing. The National Institute for Health and Care Excellence (NICE) recommends that CAM-ICU (Confusion Assessment Method for the ICU) is used to diagnose delirium in PACU.

Patients should undergo evaluation for possible underlying triggers (e.g. hypoxaemia, sepsis, hypoglycaemia, or other physiological abnormalities), and these should be treated accordingly. A variety of environmental, supportive and pharmacological interventions may be of value in managing POD:

• Basic steps such as orientation of the patient with their environment, adequate lighting, access to hearing aids and spectacles, hydration, and analgesia are useful in preventing and treating delirium.

• Pharmacological treatment of delirium is indicated to resolve a specific underlying cause (e.g. hypoglycaemia) or, after discussion with a senior clinician, for control of symptoms refractory to basic interventions. The butyrophenone haloperidol is commonly used (p.o., i.m., or i.v. administration).

• Common drugs that may worsen delirium include opioids, benzodiazepines and steroids; therefore all patients who develop POD should undergo a thorough review of their medications.

Postoperative cognitive dysfunction

Postoperative cognitive dysfunction (POCD) can be usefully defined as a 'long-term, possibly permanent, disabling deterioration in cognitive function following surgery'. The incidence of POCD is estimated to be 25% at 1 week and 10% at 3 months. In one study, further follow-up of the affected patients showed that the incidence of cognitive problems eventually fell towards that in matched controls, but 1% still had unresolved POCD 2 years after surgery.

The proposed causes of POCD include emboli, perioperative physiological disturbance and pre-existing cognitive impairment. A number of risk factors for POCD have been identified:
• Early POCD
  • Increasing age
  • General anaesthesia
  • Increasing duration of anaesthesia
  • Respiratory complication
  • Lower level of education
  • Reoperation
  • Postoperative infection
• Prolonged POCD (months)
  • Increasing age

Whilst regional anaesthesia does not appear to be superior to general anaesthesia in preventing prolonged POCD, it may reduce the risk of early POCD, with important implications for physical recovery, co-operation with postoperative therapy and duration of hospital stay.

Respiratory system
Airway obstruction

Obstruction of the upper airway often occurs during recovery from anaesthesia, and the recognition and management of airway compromise is a keystone of good anaesthetic practice. Partial obstruction of the airway is characterised by noisy ventilation, particularly on inspiration (stridor). As the obstruction increases, tracheal tug, indrawing of the supraclavicular areas and use of the accessory muscle of inspiration occur. Total obstruction is signalled by absent sounds of breathing and paradoxical movement of the chest wall and abdomen.

Blood, oral secretions or regurgitated gastric fluids that have accumulated in the pharynx should be aspirated and the patient placed in the recovery position to allow any further fluid to drain. This position should be considered for all unconscious patients who have undergone oropharyngeal surgery and for patients at risk of aspiration of gastric contents.

Airway obstruction caused by the tongue or by indrawing of the pharyngeal tissues may be alleviated by simple airway manoeuvres such as a chin-lift and/or jaw-thrust. In some patients it is necessary also to insert an oropharyngeal airway, although this may stimulate coughing, gagging and laryngospasm during the light planes of anaesthesia. A nasopharyngeal airway is often better tolerated, but there is a risk of causing haemorrhage from the nasopharyngeal mucosa. Occasionally, insertion of a SAD is necessary to maintain the airway until consciousness has returned fully; in extremis, tracheal intubation is required. There may be patient-specific problems; it may be difficult to maintain a patent airway in an unconscious patient with an oral, pharyngeal or laryngeal tumour.

Foreign bodies, such as dentures (particularly partial dentures) or throat packs, may cause airway obstruction. The National Patient Safety Agency (NPSA) have prescribed the standards for management of throat packs to reduce the incidence of their inadvertent retention.

Airway obstruction may result from haemorrhage after surgery to the neck, including thyroid, carotid and spinal surgery; the wound should be opened urgently and the haematoma drained. This may not relieve the obstruction if venous engorgement or tissue oedema are marked. Occasionally, tracheal collapse occurs after thyroidectomy in patients who have developed chondromalacia of the cartilaginous rings of the trachea caused by pressure from a large goitre. Inspiratory stridor may be present or there may be total obstruction during inspiration; the trachea must be reintubated immediately. Rarely, laryngeal obstruction occurs after thyroid surgery if both recurrent laryngeal nerves have been traumatised (see Chapter 39).

Obstructive sleep apnoea (OSA) occurs with the greatest frequency in the first 4 h after anaesthesia, and is more common and severe in patients who receive opioids for postoperative analgesia. Regional anaesthetic techniques are, therefore, often preferred, but do not completely ameliorate the risk. Patients with OSA should be monitored carefully in the postoperative period, preferably in HDU. Patients who normally use a CPAP mask to reduce apnoeic episodes should use the mask at night throughout the postoperative period. If untreated, OSA may produce profound transient, but repeated, decreases in arterial oxygenation to less than 75% (corresponding to a PaO_2 <5 kPa). These repeated episodes of hypoxaemia may cause temporary, and possibly permanent,

defects in cognitive function in older patients and can contribute to perioperative myocardial infarction (MI).

Laryngeal spasm

Laryngeal spasm is relatively common after general anaesthesia, particularly in children and those undergoing oropharyngeal surgery. The common presenting feature is inspiratory stridor that may progress to complete obstruction, and it may be difficult to differentiate this condition from other causes of airway obstruction. It usually results from direct stimulation of the cords or epiglottis during light planes of anaesthesia; consequently, the greatest risk is during induction or emergence. Recommended practice is that tracheal extubation is undertaken when the patient is either in a deep plane of anaesthesia or when fully awake.

Management of laryngospasm is discussed in Chapter 27.

Laryngeal oedema

Laryngeal oedema occurs occasionally after tracheal intubation and may result in severe obstruction, particularly in a child. Treatment depends on the severity of the obstruction; immediate tracheal reintubation may be required if obstruction is complete, but partial obstruction may subside if the patient is treated with heated humidified gases. Dexamethasone may hasten resolution of the oedema.

Bronchospasm

Bronchospasm may result from stimulation of the airway by inhaled material, be secondary to intrinsic airways disease or part of an anaphylactic reaction. It is more common in smokers and patients with asthma or chronic obstructive pulmonary disease (COPD). Several drugs used in anaesthetic practice may precipitate bronchospasm either by a direct effect on bronchial muscle or by releasing histamine; these include barbiturates, morphine, mivacurium, atracurium and carboprost. Treatment comprises the removal of any predisposing factor and administration of oxygen and bronchodilators (e.g. β_2-agonists).

Hypoventilation

Hypoventilation results in an increase in $PaCO_2$ (Fig. 29.1) and a decrease in alveolar oxygen tension (PaO_2). Hypoxaemia may be corrected by increasing the inspired concentration of oxygen.

The risk factors for hypoventilation include:
- older age;
- obesity;
- prolonged surgery;
- intraoperative opioid administration; and
- upper abdominal or thoracic surgery.

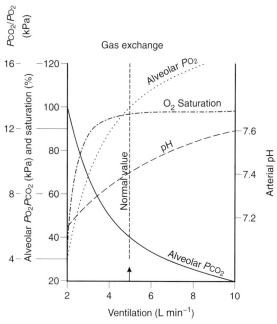

Fig. 29.1 Gas exchange during hypoventilation. Note the relatively rapid increase in the alveolar pressure of carbon dioxide (PCO_2) compared with the slow decrease in arterial oxygen saturation. PO_2, partial pressure of oxygen.

Table 29.5 Causes of postoperative hypoventilation	
Airway factors	Upper airway obstruction • Tongue • Laryngospasm • Oedema • Foreign body • Tumour Bronchospasm
Factors affecting ventilatory drive	Respiratory depressant drugs Preoperative CNS pathological condition Intra- or postoperative cerebrovascular accident Hypothermia Recent hyperventilation ($PaCO_2$ low)
Peripheral factors	Muscle weakness • Residual neuromuscular block • Neuromuscular disease • Electrolyte abnormalities Pain Abdominal distension Obesity Tight abdominal dressings Pneumothorax Haemothorax

Common causes of hypoventilation in the immediate postoperative period are listed in Table 29.5.

Drugs

The most important cause of reduced ventilatory drive during recovery is the effect of drugs administered in the perioperative period.

- All volatile and i.v. anaesthetic agents – with the exception of ketamine – depress the respiratory centre; significant concentrations of these drugs remain in the brainstem during the early postoperative period.
- All opioid analgesics depress ventilation. With most opioids, the effect is dose-dependent, although the agonist-antagonist agents are claimed to have a ceiling effect. In the majority of patients, opioids do not produce apnoea but result in decreased ventilatory drive and increase in $PaCO_2$, which plateaus at an elevated value. Older patients are particularly sensitive to drug-induced ventilatory depression.
- Intrathecal or epidural opioids, particularly lipid-insoluble agents such as morphine, may produce ventilatory depression some hours after administration. Patients who have received intrathecal or epidural opioids should be cared for in areas where specific management protocols have been implemented.

Reduced ventilatory drive is easy to diagnose if the ventilatory rate or tidal volume is clearly reduced. However, lesser degrees of hypoventilation may be difficult to detect, and the signs of moderate hypercapnia (e.g. hypertension and tachycardia) may be masked by the residual effects of anaesthetic agents or misdiagnosed as being pain induced (Table 29.6).

Mild hypoventilation is acceptable provided that oxygenation and clearance of CO_2 remain adequate; this may easily be achieved by a modest increase in the inspired fractional concentration of oxygen (FIO_2). It is recommend that all patients in PACU with a tracheal tube or SAD should have continuous capnography to assess adequacy of respiration.

If ventilatory drive is excessively reduced by opioids, resulting in an increasing $PaCO_2$ or delayed recovery of consciousness, naloxone in increments of 1.5–3 µg kg^{-1} should be administered every 2–3 min until improvement occurs. Administration of excessive doses of naloxone reverses the analgesia induced by systemic (but not to the same extent by spinal) opioids; large doses may cause severe hypertension and have been associated with cardiac arrest on rare occasions. The effects of i.v. naloxone last only for 20–30 min; to prevent recurrence of reduced ventilation

Table 29.6 Symptoms and signs of common problems in the PACU

	Pain	Hypovolaemia	Hypercapnia
Conscious level	May be restless May be quiescent if severe pain	Restless or quiescent depending on extent of analgesia and residual anaesthesia	Comatose
Peripheral perfusion	Vasoconstriction Pallor ± sweating	Vasoconstriction, Pallor ± sweating	Warm Flushed Bounding pulse (if normovolaemic)
Heart rate	Tachycardia	Tachycardia	Tachycardia
Arterial pressure	Systolic increased Diastolic increased Pulse pressure unchanged	Systolic and diastolic may be normal until marked reduction in stroke volume then decreased Pulse pressure decreased	Systolic increased Diastolic increased/decreased Pulse pressure increased

after long-acting opioids, an additional dose (50% of the effective i.v. dose) may be administered i.m. or an i.v. infusion commenced. Artificial ventilation should be started if severe hypercapnia is present or Pa_{CO_2} continues to increase, or if the clinical condition of the patient is deteriorating.

Postoperative residual neuromuscular block

Residual neuromuscular blockade is a common cause of postoperative hypoventilation, with approximately 40% of patients in PACU exhibiting a train-of-four ratio < 0.9. There is a risk of flushing a small residual amount of a neuromuscular blocking agent (NMBA) in the cannula, leading to recurarisation in PACU after staff have administered i.v. analgesia. Systems must be in place to ensure that there is documented flushing of cannulae at handover.

Factors responsible most commonly for difficulty in antagonism of neuromuscular block include:
- excessive NMBA dose;
- omission of antagonist (e.g. anticholinesterase or sugammadex) after intraoperative NMBA use;
- too short an interval between administration of NMBA and anticholinesterase;
- hypokalaemia;
- respiratory or metabolic acidosis;
- administration of agents which affect the neuromuscular muscular junction (e.g. aminoglycoside antibiotics); and
- diseases affecting neuromuscular transmission (e.g. myasthenia gravis).

Delayed elimination of all of the non-depolarising NMBAs (except atracurium and cisatracurium) have been reported and may cause prolonged neuromuscular block. This occurs most often in the presence of renal or hepatic insufficiency or in dehydrated patients with low urine output. Muscle paralysis may recur 30–60 min after administration of neostigmine if elimination of the NMBA is inadequate, even if antagonism appears to be satisfactory initially. A similar phenomenon may occur if acidaemia develops or when patients who have been hypothermic are rewarmed.

Prolonged neuromuscular block after suxamethonium or mivacurium occurs in the presence of atypical plasma cholinesterase or a low concentration of normal plasma cholinesterase (see Chapter 8).

Inadequate reversal of neuromuscular blockade is usually associated with uncoordinated, jerky movements, although these may occur occasionally during recovery of consciousness in patients with normal neuromuscular function. Traditional clinical signs of adequacy of reversal of neuromuscular blockade (such as if the patient is able to lift the head from the trolley for 5 s or maintain a good hand grip) correlate poorly with objective signs of neuromuscular function. Similarly, measurement of tidal volume is not a reliable guide to adequacy of reversal of neuromuscular blockade; a normal tidal volume may be achieved with only 20% return of diaphragmatic power, but the ability to cough remains severely impaired.

In the unconscious or uncooperative patient, peripheral nerve stimulators (see Chapter 8) provide the best means of assessing neuromuscular function, although there are differences among the non-depolarising NMBAs in the relationship between their actions at the diaphragm and at peripheral sites.

If residual non-depolarising blockade is confirmed, further doses of neostigmine may be administered (with glycopyrronium bromide) up to a total of 5 mg; in higher doses, neostigmine can worsen neuromuscular function. Patients who have received rocuronium or vecuronium can be given sugammadex (2 mg kg^{-1} if there are signs of reversal of neuromuscular blockade or 4 mg kg^{-1} if there are no twitches present using train-of-four stimulation). Artificial ventilation of the lungs must be maintained or resumed in any patient who has inadequate neuromuscular function, and anaesthesia should be provided to prevent awareness.

Others

Hypoventilation may also be caused by restriction of diaphragmatic movement resulting from abdominal distension, obesity, tight dressings or abdominal binders. Similarly, pain, particularly from thoracic or upper abdominal wounds, may cause reduced ventilation. The presence of air or fluid in the pleural cavity may result in hypoventilation. Pneumothorax may occur with intraoperative positive pressure ventilation. It is an occasional complication in healthy patients but is a particular risk in those with emphysema (especially if bullae are present), after chest trauma and is a recognised complication of brachial plexus nerve blockade, central venous cannulation or surgery involving the kidney or neck. Haemothorax may result from chest trauma or central venous cannulation. Hydrothorax may be caused by pleural effusions or inadvertent infusion of fluids through a misplaced CVC. These rapidly remediable causes of hypoventilation are often overlooked (see Chapter 27).

Hypoxaemia

Oxygenation of the tissues is a function of arterial oxygenation, oxygen carriage in blood, delivery of blood to the tissues and transfer of oxygen from the blood. It may be impaired by respiratory or cardiovascular dysfunction, severe anaemia or a leftward shift of the oxyhaemoglobin dissociation curve (see Chapter 10).

There are a number of causes of postoperative hypoxaemia that need differentiation.

Ventilation-perfusion abnormalities

Ventilation-perfusion ($\dot{V}/\dot{Q}$) abnormalities are the most common cause of hypoxaemia in the recovery room. Cardiac output and pulmonary arterial pressure may be reduced after general or regional anaesthesia, causing impaired perfusion of some areas of the lungs. Functional residual capacity (FRC) is reduced during and immediately after anaesthesia. Patients who are older or obese or those undergoing thoracic or upper abdominal surgery are particularly at risk. The closing capacity may encroach on tidal breathing range, resulting in reduced ventilation of some lung units, particularly those in dependent regions. Thus the scatter of $\dot{V}/\dot{Q}$ ratios is increased. Areas of lung with increased $\dot{V}/\dot{Q}$ ratios constitute physiological dead space, whilst those with low $\dot{V}/\dot{Q}$ ratios increase venous admixture that results in hypoxaemia unless the inspired oxygen concentration is increased.

Shunt

Physiological shunt increases to 10% with anaesthesia and may persist into the postoperative period. Shunting may also be present in patients with pulmonary oedema of any cause or if there is consolidation in the lung. Shunt may be increased in the later postoperative period as a result of retention of secretions and underventilation of the lung bases because of pain; these changes lead to alveolar consolidation and collapse. Because shunted blood does not perfuse alveoli, hypoxaemia resulting from shunt responds poorly to interventions that increase alveolar oxygen partial pressure (Fig. 29.2), tending instead to increase the alveolar–arterial gradient.

Diffusion defects

Diffusion defects may result from chronic pulmonary disease or arise acutely as a result of interstitial oedema produced by excessive infusion of i.v. fluids or by left ventricular dysfunction. Hypoxaemia results from impairment of oxygen transfer across the alveolar–capillary membrane.

Diffusion hypoxia

Nitrous oxide is 40 times more soluble than nitrogen in blood. When administration of nitrous oxide is discontinued at the end of anaesthesia, nitrous oxide diffuses out of blood into the alveoli in larger volumes than nitrogen diffuses in the opposite direction. Consequently, the alveolar concentrations of other gases are diluted. P_{AO_2} is reduced and arterial oxygenation

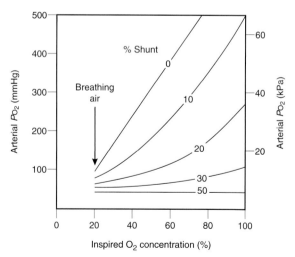

Fig. 29.2 Response of arterial partial pressure of oxygen (P_{O_2}) to increased inspired oxygen concentrations in the presence of various degrees of shunt. Note that, in the presence of shunt, arterial P_{O_2} remains well below the normal value when 100% oxygen is inspired. Nevertheless, useful increases in arterial oxygen occur with a shunt up to 30%.

impaired if the patient breathes air; $PaCO_2$ decreases as a result of effective alveolar hyperventilation. SaO_2 is reduced to values as low as 90% for several minutes in normal individuals after breathing 50% nitrous oxide in oxygen. Arterial desaturation is greater in older patients, if higher concentrations of nitrous oxide have been used or if $PaCO_2$ is initially low because of hyperventilation during anaesthesia. Diffusion hypoxia is avoided by the administration of supplemental oxygen for 10 min after discontinuation of nitrous oxide anaesthesia.

Reduced venous oxygen content

Assuming that oxygen consumption remains unchanged, anaemia or reduced cardiac output result in increased oxygen extraction from circulating arterial blood and consequently in a reduction in mixed venous oxygen content. In the presence of increased $\dot{V}/\dot{Q}$ scatter or intrapulmonary shunt, this causes a variable degree of arterial hypoxaemia. Similarly, if cardiac output remains constant, increased oxygen utilisation by the tissues (as may occur during shivering, restlessness or malignant hyperthermia) causes reduction in mixed venous oxygen content and worsening of arterial hypoxaemia if any shunt is present.

Pulmonary changes after abdominal surgery

Patients with previously normal lungs suffer impairment of oxygenation for at least 48 h after abdominal surgery. The extent of this impairment is related to the site of operation, being less marked after lower abdominal surgery, more severe if there has been a large incision in the upper abdomen, and worst after thoracoabdominal procedures. In these circumstances, the differences between pre- and postoperative PaO_2 may be as much as 4 kPa.

Impairment of oxygenation in the postoperative period is related to a reduction in FRC. After induction of anaesthesia, there is an abrupt decrease in FRC regardless of whether mechanical or spontaneous ventilation is employed. This decrease persists postoperatively because of wound pain, which causes spasm of the expiratory muscles, and abdominal distension, which leads to diaphragmatic splinting. The supine position also reduces FRC.

The reduction in FRC may lead to closing capacity impinging upon the tidal breathing range. This results in small airways closure during normal tidal ventilation. Gas trapping occurs in the affected airways, and subsequent absorption of air may lead to the development of small, discrete areas of atelectasis which are not visible on chest radiograph but may be demonstrated by CT scan very soon after induction of anaesthesia. This occurs mainly in the dependent parts of the lung, and the result is an increase in the number of areas of low $\dot{V}/\dot{Q}$ ratio within the lungs. The relationship between changes in FRC and PaO_2 postoperatively is shown in Fig. 29.3.

In most patients these abnormalities return towards normal by the fifth or sixth postoperative day. However, the areas of low $\dot{V}/\dot{Q}$ ratio may become a focus for infection, particularly in the presence of retained secretions. The following factors contribute to retention of secretions after surgery:

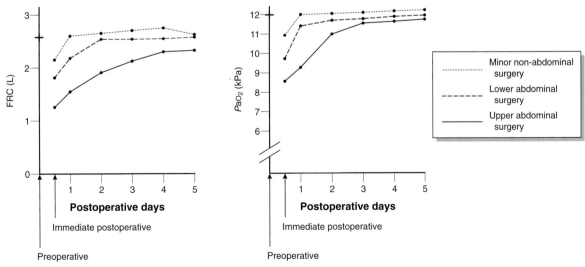

Fig. 29.3 Postoperative changes in functional residual capacity (FRC) and arterial oxygen tension (PaO_2).

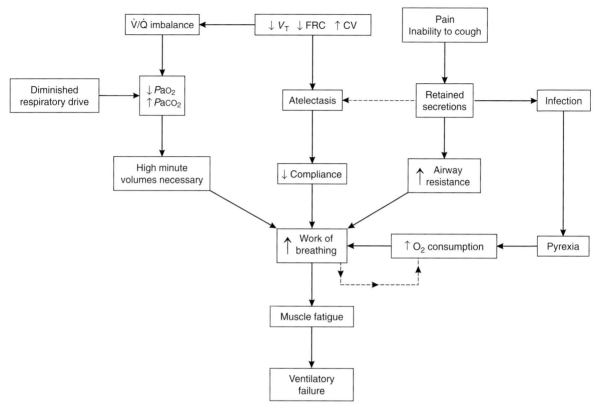

Fig. 29.4 Diagrammatic representation of events that result in postoperative ventilator failure. *CV,* Closing volume; *FRC,* functional residual capacity; *P*aco$_2$, arterial carbon dioxide tension; *P*ao$_2$, arterial oxygen tension; $\dot{V}/\dot{Q}$, ventilation/perfusion; V_T, tidal volume.

- *Inability to cough.* This results most commonly from wound pain. However, excessive sedation may also contribute. Postoperative electrolyte imbalance, especially hypokalaemia or hypophosphataemia, may compound the situation by interfering with muscle function. Patients with pre-existing muscle weakness (cachexia, malnutrition or frailty) are at increased risk.
- *Suppression of bronchial mucosal ciliary activity.* This results from the use of unhumidified anaesthetic gases and also occurs in smokers.
- *Antisialagogue drugs.* When antisialagogue premedicants have been used, the secretions become more viscid. The dry mucosa itself is more prone to inflammatory reaction. If this occurs, the exudate produced increases the problem further.
- *Infection.* If pulmonary infection supervenes, impairment of oxygenation may contribute to a lack of co-operation with physiotherapy.

A combination of these factors may result in retention of secretions, leading to areas of visible pulmonary collapse on chest radiograph and an increase in the work of breathing. Ultimately, oxygenation of the blood may become inadequate despite oxygen therapy, or carbon dioxide retention may occur. The sequence of events that culminate in ventilatory failure is shown in Fig. 29.4. Risk factors for the development of postoperative pulmonary complications and preoptimisation techniques are discussed in Chapters 19 and 30.

Atelectasis

The first signs of atelectasis are usually seen within 24 h of operation. The triad of pyrexia, tachycardia and tachypnoea is often present. Temperature is usually in the range of 38°C–39°C and there is often a productive cough. If atelectasis is extensive, the patient is cyanosed. On physical examination, localising signs are uncommon unless the area of involvement is large. Chest radiograph may reveal patchy areas of atelectasis.

Patients with pulmonary collapse are usually hypoxaemic, but *P*aco$_2$ remains normal or may be low as a result of tachypnoea, at least in the early stages. Usually oxygen in moderate concentrations (30%–40%) is sufficient to correct hypoxaemia. CPAP given via a tightly fitting face mask may be effective in re-expanding collapsed alveoli and improving mechanics of breathing, but there is some evidence that the effects are limited to the duration of CPAP therapy. If the patient fails to respond to these measures, signs of respiratory distress develop; the patient becomes drowsy and ventilation is laboured, with rapid shallow breathing involving the accessory muscles. $PaCO_2$ increases and arterial oxygenation deteriorates despite oxygen therapy; this is an indication for ventilatory support.

Pneumonia

Lobar pneumonia is rare postoperatively. Bronchopneumonia is more common, especially in older adults. The onset of symptoms is not as rapid as in atelectasis. There is usually fever and associated tachycardia, with an increase in the ventilatory rate. Physical examination usually reveals areas of consolidation, predominantly at the lung bases, which are evident on chest radiograph.

Treatment involves antimicrobial therapy and maintenance of oxygenation. A sputum sample (and blood cultures if patient is febrile) should be sent for microbiological analysis. Appropriate antibiotic therapy may then be started. Intensive physiotherapy should be prescribed in an attempt to remove secretions and re-expand atelectatic areas of the lung.

Oxygen therapy

Hypoxaemia may occur to some degree in any patient during the early recovery period as a result of one or more of the mechanisms described earlier. Consequently, *all* patients should receive additional oxygen for at least the first 10 min after general anaesthesia has been discontinued.

Oxygen therapy should be continued for a longer period in the presence of any of the following conditions:

- Hypotension
- Ischaemic heart disease
- Reduced cardiac output
- Anaemia
- Obesity
- Shivering
- Hypo- and hyperthermia
- Pulmonary oedema
- Airway obstruction

The majority of patients recovering after anaesthesia require only a modest increase in FIO_2 to overcome the combined effects of mild hypoventilation, diffusion hypoxia and some degree of increased $\dot{V}/\dot{Q}$ scatter. An inspired concentration of 30% is usually adequate, and this may be achieved in most instances by supplying an oxygen flow rate of 4 L min^{-1} to any of the variable-performance devices

(see later). However, in a small proportion of patients, it is necessary to control the FIO_2 more strictly. All oxygen therapy should be prescribed and with a target SpO_2.

Postoperative oxygen therapy may be administered by a variety of devices.

Oxygen therapy devices

The characteristics of oxygen face-masks depend predominantly on their volume, flow rate of gas supplied and presence of holes in the side of the mask. If no gas is supplied, face-masks act as increased dead space and result in hypercapnia unless minute volume is increased; the increase in dead space is proportional to the volume of the mask. If the mask contains holes, air is entrained readily during inspiration.

When oxygen is supplied, the inspired oxygen concentration increases, but to an extent depending upon the relationship between the oxygen flow rate and ventilatory pattern. If there is a pause between expiration and inspiration, the mask fills with oxygen and a high concentration is available at the start of inspiration; during inspiration, the inspired oxygen is diluted by air drawn in through the holes when the inspiratory flow rate exceeds the flow rate of oxygen. During normal tidal ventilation, the peak inspiratory flow rate (PIFR) is 20–30 L min^{-1}, but it is considerably higher during deep inspiration or in the hyperventilating patient. If there is no expiratory pause, alveolar gas may be rebreathed from the mask at the start of inspiration; this occurs especially when the oxygen flow rate is low or when no holes are present in the mask. A predictable and constant inspired oxygen concentration may be achieved only if the total gas flow to the mask exceeds the patient's PIFR.

Fixed-performance devices. Fixed-performance masks, also termed high air flow oxygen enrichment (HAFOE) devices, provide a constant and predictable inspired oxygen concentration irrespective of the patient's ventilatory pattern. These devices use the Venturi effect, based on the Bernoulli principle. Oxygen is passed through a small aperture resulting in an increase in its kinetic energy and corresponding drop in pressure, which entrains air through side holes (Fig. 29.5).

The mask is designed so that the total flow rate of gas to the mask exceeds the expected PIFR of most patients who require oxygen therapy; the concentration of oxygen delivered is, therefore, predictable according to the rate of oxygen flow and size of the side holes. Various types of HAFOE device are available; an example is shown in Fig. 29.6.

Venturi masks are the most accurate, but a different mask is required for each of the range of oxygen concentrations available. Some manufacturers produce masks in which the side apertures of the jet device can be changed to adjust the oxygen concentration. The recommended oxygen flow rates to achieve the desired inspired oxygen concentration are indicated on the device. Because of the high fresh gas flow rate, expired gas is rapidly flushed from the mask. Thus

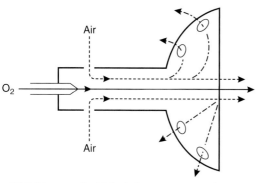

Fig. 29.5 Diagram of a high air flow oxygen enrichment (HAFOE) mask.

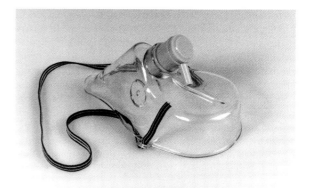

Fig. 29.7 A variable-performance face mask.

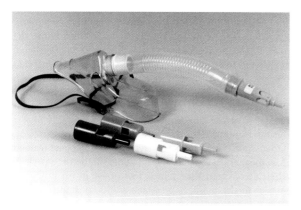

Fig. 29.6 A high air flow oxygen enrichment (HAFOE) mask.

rebreathing rarely occurs; that is, fixed-performance devices rarely act as an additional dead space. There are situations where the flow is not adequate to achieve this, such as hyperventilation.

Variable-performance devices. All other disposable oxygen masks and nasal cannulae provide an oxygen concentration that varies with the oxygen flow rate and the patient's ventilatory pattern (Fig. 29.7). Although there is no increase in dead space when nasal cannulae are used, all variable-performance disposable face masks add dead space, the magnitude of which depends on the patient's pattern of ventilation.

Controlled oxygen therapy

Some patients with chronic bronchitis develop chronic hypercapnia, and their ventilatory drive is produced largely by hypoxaemia. If PaO_2 increases above the concentration which stimulates breathing, ventilatory depression may occur. However, these patients may become dangerously hypoxaemic after anaesthesia, and oxygen therapy is required so that adequate oxygenation of the tissues is maintained. The aim of oxygen therapy in these circumstances is to increase arterial oxygen content without an excessive increase in PaO_2.

This is achieved by a modest increase in FIO_2. In the hypoxaemic patient the relationship between arterial oxygen tension and saturation (and therefore oxygen content) is represented by the steep portion of the oxyhaemoglobin dissociation curve, and a small increase in oxygen tension results in significant increases in saturation and oxygen content. The use of a variable-performance device in these patients is unsatisfactory, as an unacceptably high FIO_2 may be delivered. A fixed-performance device delivering 24% oxygen should be used initially and the response assessed. If the patient remains clinically well, and the $PaCO_2$ does not increase by more than 1–1.5 kPa, 28% oxygen – and subsequently higher concentrations – may be administered if further increases in PaO_2 are desirable.

The aim is not to achieve 'normal' PaO_2 or SaO_2 but to provide acceptable oxygenation for that patient. Patients whose typical SaO_2 is 88%–90% do not need a postoperative SaO_2 greater than 94%. Most patients with chronic bronchitis do not depend on hypoxaemia for respiratory drive and should not be denied adequate inspired concentrations of oxygen.

Cardiovascular system

Hypotension

Although a common event in PACU, there is no agreed definition as to exactly what constitutes postoperative hypotension. Up to 20% reduction in MAP from baseline is tolerated well, except by older patients or those with myocardial disease. It is important to remember that cardiac output and tissue oxygen delivery are often maintained in the presence of mild hypotension (see Chapter 48). No treatment is required in most patients, and the situation usually resolves. Elevation of the legs often increases arterial pressure by increasing venous return. Infusion of $7-10$ ml kg^{-1} i.v. crystalloid (not 5% dextrose) or colloid is usually effective in restoring normotension if there is concern; in patients with limited cardiovascular reserve, urinary catheterisation and strict input/output recordings should be considered.

A systematic approach should be taken to identify the cause. Many of the causes of hypotension are similar to those occurring during anaesthesia (Table 26.1 and Box 26.2). Assuming that MAP $\approx$ (stroke volume [SV] $\times$ HR) $\times$ systemic vascular resistance (SVR) (see Chapter 9), the causes can be divided into the following:

- Decreased SV
  - Decreased preload (e.g. hypovolaemia, tension pneumothorax)
  - Reduced myocardial contractility (e.g. left or right ventricular failure, cardiac tamponade, negatively inotropic drugs)
  - Tachyarrhythmias (supraventricular tachycardia, atrial fibrillation with fast ventricular response etc.)
- Decreased HR (e.g. bradyarrhythmias)
- Decreased SVR (e.g. vasodilatation secondary to sepsis, epidural or spinal anaesthesia).

Decreased preload – hypovolaemia

Decreased preload may result from inadequate or inappropriate replacement of perioperative fluid and blood losses. Hypotension caused by hypovolaemia may be accompanied by signs of poor peripheral perfusion such as cold, clammy extremities and pallor. Tachycardia may be present but is masked, not infrequently, by the effects of drugs (e.g. anticholinesterases, β-blockers). Central venous pressure is a poor guide to volaemic status. Urine output, a better indicator, is reduced (<0.5 ml kg^{-1} h^{-1}).

Surgical bleeding may be obvious from inspection of wounds and drains but may be concealed, particularly in the abdomen, retroperitoneal space or thorax, even when drains are present. Inadequate surgical haemostasis is the usual cause of postoperative bleeding, but coagulation disorders may be present in the following circumstances:

- After massive blood transfusion, which results in decreased concentrations of clotting factors and reduced platelet numbers (dilutional coagulopathy)
- Disseminated intravascular coagulation (consumptive coagulopathy)
- Pre-existing bleeding tendency (e.g. haemophilia)
- If anticoagulant drugs have been administered

The investigation and management of coagulation disorders are discussed in Chapter 14.

The effects of hypovolaemia on arterial pressure are more pronounced in the presence of vasodilatation or reduced myocardial contractility resulting from the effects of residual anaesthetic drugs or antihypertensive, calcium channel or β-blocker therapy. In patients who have undergone prolonged

surgery, and particularly if the core temperature is less than normal, vasoconstriction may be present and hypovolaemia may be unmasked at a relatively late stage as normal vasomotor tone returns with rewarming.

Treatment comprises elevation of the legs and administration of appropriate crystalloid or colloid solutions. In older or high-risk patients, or if hypovolaemia is profound, administration of fluids should be monitored with the assistance of invasive arterial blood pressure and consideration of some form of cardiac output monitoring. Red cells, clotting factors or platelets should be administered if appropriate and surgical bleeding treated by reoperation if necessary.

Reduced myocardial contractility – acute coronary syndrome

Acute coronary syndrome (ACS) is a term that encompasses unstable angina and acute MI. Acute coronary syndrome is the most common cause of reduced myocardial contractility in the postoperative period but can also be caused by other mechanisms, such as arrhythmias or conduction defects. Several factors that may be detected during preoperative assessment are known to increase the likelihood of perioperative ACS; these are discussed in Chapter 19. Acute coronary syndrome is diagnosed by an increase in troponin concentrations with at least one value greater than the 99th percentile of the upper reference limit, plus at least one of the following:

- Symptoms of myocardial ischaemia (e.g. chest pain or angina)
- New (or presumably new) significant ST-segment/T-wave changes or left bundle branch block
- Development of pathological Q waves on ECG
- New loss of viable myocardium or regional wall motion abnormality seen on cardiac imaging
- Identification of intracoronary thrombus on angiography or at postmortem

Increased troponin in isolation is not diagnostic of ACS and may occur in a variety of other cardiac (e.g. cardiac failure, myocarditis, cardiomyopathy, pericarditis) and non-cardiac conditions (e.g. PE, renal failure, sepsis, subarachnoid haemorrhage).

Acute coronary syndrome most commonly occurs in patients with pre-existing coronary artery disease. Coronary artery plaque rupture is often the primary pathological mechanism, but the stability of plaques is affected by high sympathetic activity and the procoagulant state after surgery, both of which increase the risk of rupture. Plaque rupture produces a thrombotic response resulting in a variable reduction in coronary blood flow and subsequent myocardial ischaemia. The coronary artery obstruction is typically complete in ST-elevation MI (STEMI) and incomplete in unstable angina and non–ST-elevation MI (NSTEMI).

Several types of MI are now recognised:

- Type 1: spontaneous, usually secondary to plaque rupture in patients with coronary arterial disease.

- Type 2: induced by an increase in myocardial oxygen demand and/or a decrease in myocardial blood flow rather than an acute coronary artery thrombus (see later).
- Type 3: diagnosed postmortem.
- Type 4a: secondary to percutaneous coronary intervention (PCI).
- Type 4b: secondary to stent thrombosis (may occur if antiplatelet therapy is interrupted for surgical procedures; see Chapter 19).
- Type 4c: secondary to stent restenosis.
- Type 5: related to coronary artery bypass grafting (CABG).

The majority of perioperative MIs are type 2 and may be asymptomatic, particularly in patients with diabetes, or may be associated with ST-segment depression rather than elevation (NSTEMI). This type of non-thrombotic ACS is often caused by myocardial oxygen supply being unable to meet demand rather than an acute coronary artery thrombus. Hypoxaemia, hypotension and anaemia all reduce myocardial oxygen supply, whereas hypertension, tachycardia, pain, and shivering increase myocardial oxygen demand; these conditions are relatively common during and after anaesthesia and often occur in tandem.

The diagnosis may be difficult in the absence of symptoms but should be considered in any patient at risk who develops an arrhythmia or becomes hypotensive in the postoperative period. Premature ventricular contractions occur in 90% of patients who experience MI; sinus bradycardia and the development of any degree of atrioventricular conduction defect are also common.

Any ACS occurring during the recovery period requires prompt treatment; mortality in patients who suffer a perioperative MI is higher than that seen in out-of-hospital MIs.

The immediate treatment of a type 1 MI includes the following:

- Immediate referral to a cardiologist.
- Reduce platelet aggregation and thrombus formation with dual antiplatelet therapy (aspirin and a P2Y12 receptor antagonist, e.g. clopidogrel, ticagrelor or prasugrel) and low molecular weight heparin or fondaparinux. The risk/benefit of platelet inhibition and anticoagulation in the postoperative setting (specifically the increased risk of bleeding) need careful consideration.
- Supplemental oxygen therapy is now considered unnecessary if oxygen saturations are ≥ 90% and may be associated with increased coronary artery resistance and reduced coronary blood flow.
- Glyceryl trinitrate (GTN, s.c. or i.v.) may be used to treat ischaemic chest pain; i.v. morphine is recommended for refractory pain.
- Urgent PCI is the preferred option for revascularisation in the postoperative patient having a STEMI; systemic fibrinolytics are contraindicated.

The management of type 2 MI is slightly different; as there is no plaque rupture and thrombus formation, the benefits of antiplatelet therapy are unproven. The primary treatment

aim is to address the imbalance between myocardial oxygen supply and demand. This may involve: the correction of anaemia, hypovolaemia or hypertension; treatment of sepsis; or rate control of a tachyarrhythmia. The majority of patients who have a type 2 MI will also have coronary artery disease and differentiation from a type 1 MI can be challenging; referral to a cardiologist is essential.

Reduced myocardial contractility – ventricular failure

Left or right ventricular failure may cause hypotension. Right ventricular failure outside of cardiac surgery is uncommon in the postoperative period and is usually secondary to acute pulmonary disease (e.g. PE).

Left ventricular failure in the postoperative period is most commonly associated with perioperative MI, myocardial ischaemia or fluid overload. Signs suggestive of the diagnosis include the following:

- Peripheral circulation is poor
- Tachycardia is usually present
- Clinical and radiological evidence of pulmonary oedema is present
- Jugular venous pulse and CVP are usually elevated, but they may remain normal

Left ventricular failure may be misdiagnosed as hypovolaemia in some patients, and in some patients the two conditions coexist. If there is doubt about the diagnosis, a small i.v. fluid bolus may be administered (<200 ml) and the response of arterial pressure observed; if the diagnosis remains uncertain, echocardiography or cardiac output monitors may be of value.

Treatment comprises administration of supplemental oxygen (if SpO$_2$ is reduced), fluid restriction, diuretics and, if necessary, inotropic support or vasodilator therapy. The possibility of MI and need for PCI should be investigated.

Arrhythmias

Arrythmias are common during and immediately after anaesthesia, although the majority are benign and require no treatment. However, the cause should be sought and its effect on the circulation assessed. Common causes include the following:

- Residual anaesthetic agents
- Hypercapnia
- Hypoxaemia
- Electrolyte or acid–base disturbance
- Vagal stimulation (e.g. by tracheal tube or suction catheters)
- Myocardial ischaemia or infarction
- Pain

The emergency management of arrhythmias is discussed in Chapters 26 and 28.

Sinus tachycardia is common and may be a reflex response to hypovolaemia or hypotension. The most common cause is pain, but sinus tachycardia also occurs in the presence of hypercapnia, anaemia, hypoxaemia or an elevated metabolic rate (e.g. fever, shivering, restlessness or malignant hyperthermia). Tachycardia increases myocardial oxygen consumption and decreases coronary artery perfusion by reducing diastolic time. The combination of arterial hypertension and tachycardia is dangerous in the presence of ischaemic heart disease and should *not* be allowed to persist, as it may result in MI. Sinus tachycardia should only be treated (e.g. with β-blockers) if it persists after therapy for underlying causes has been given.

Decreased SVR – drugs

Hypotension may result from the residual vasodilator effect of i.v. or inhalational anaesthetic drugs. Subarachnoid or epidural anaesthesia may also cause hypotension which persists into the postoperative period. The effects can be assessed by testing the level of blockade; sympathetic blockade may be present two levels above the sensory dermatomal level. Cardiovascular effects of neuraxial blockade are dependent upon the level of the block (<T10: little cardiovascular effect; T6–10: mainly arterial vasodilator fibres with reflex tachycardia; T1–5: cardiac accelerator fibres affected, bradycardia may be seen). This is treated with measured fluid infusion, but with the caution that fluid overload may occur when the blockade recedes.

Decreased SVR – sepsis

Sepsis may occur in the early postoperative period. In this condition, hypotension is accompanied by elevated cardiac output and peripheral vasodilatation in the early stages, followed by vasoconstriction and reduced cardiac output (partly caused by loss of fluid from the circulation). The Surviving Sepsis campaign has led to well-established care bundles (see Chapter 48). Initial management should include the following:

- Measure serum lactate (action if ≥4 mmol L^{-1}).
- Obtain blood cultures before administration of broad-spectrum antibiotics
- Administer fluid bolus 30 ml kg^{-1} i.v.
- Catheterise and assess urine output
- Where hypotension does not respond to fluid bolus, administer vasoconstrictors (aiming for MAP ≥65 mmHg)
- Referral to critical care

Hypertension

Arterial hypertension is a common complication in the early postoperative period. The causes (which may coexist) include the following:

- pain;
- pre-existing hypertension, particularly if controlled inadequately;
- hypoxaemia;
- hypercapnia;
- administration of vasopressor drugs; and

- after aortic surgery, as a result partly of increased plasma concentration of renin.

Hypertension results in increased cardiac work and myocardial oxygen consumption and may result in myocardial ischaemia, MI, left ventricular failure or cerebral haemorrhage. The cause should be elicited rapidly and treated if possible. If no remediable cause is found and the hypertension is felt to be a risk to the patient, careful antihypertensive treatment can be started using appropriate agents (see Chapter 9).

Renal system

Acute kidney injury

The kidney is vulnerable to a wide range of drugs, chemicals and pathophysiological insults (see Chapter 11). It is particularly susceptible to toxic substances for the following reasons:

- large blood flow per unit mass;
- high oxygen consumption;
- non-resorbable substances concentrated by tubules; and
- permeability of tubular cells.

Acute kidney injury (AKI) after surgery is relatively common and is discussed in detail in Chapter 11. Postoperative care should focus on:

- identifying patients at high risk of developing AKI;
- avoiding factors which may increase risk of AKI; and
- close monitoring and intervention in those patients who develop signs of AKI.

There is no single diagnostic criterion for defining postoperative AKI, but a consensus clinical tool is the Kidney Disease: Improving Global Outcomes (KDIGO) diagnostic criteria (see Table 11.4). There is ongoing research into biomarkers of early and ongoing renal injury, but there is no reliable test available yet for clinical practice.

Effects of anaesthesia

All anaesthetic techniques depress renal blood flow and, secondary to this, interfere with renal function. Provided that prolonged hypotension is avoided, the effects are temporary. However, there is the potential for some anaesthetic agents to produce permanent renal damage.

- The administration of the volatile anaesthetic agent methoxyflurane was associated with a relatively high incidence of renal dysfunction. Although now considered an historical agent in anaesthesia, it is available as an analgesic inhaler. The nephrotoxicity of methoxyflurane was dose-dependent and was caused by inorganic fluoride ions produced during its metabolism.
- Fluoride ions are also produced during metabolism of sevoflurane, although to a much smaller extent (2%–3%) compared with methoxyflurane (45%). Concentrations of fluoride ions in blood after administration of sevoflurane may exceed the value associated with renal impairment after anaesthesia with methoxyflurane. However, there has

Table 29.7 Causes of postoperative hepatic dysfunction

Increased bilirubin load (Prehepatic)	Hepatocellular damage (Intrahepatic)	Extrahepatic biliary obstruction (Posthepatic)
Blood transfusion	Pre-existing liver disease	Gallstones
Haemolysis and haemolytic disease	Viral hepatitis	Ascending cholangitis
Abnormalities of bilirubin metabolism	Sepsis	Pancreatitis
	Hypotension/hypoxia	Surgical damage/complication
	Drug-induced hepatitis	
	Congestive heart failure	

been no evidence to suggest that sevoflurane is associated with clinical renal impairment.

Gastrointestinal system

Postoperative hepatic dysfunction

There are many causes of postoperative hepatic dysfunction. Most patients show no evidence of hepatic damage after anaesthesia and surgery. If it occurs, it is usually attributable to one of the causes shown in Table 29.7.

However, if other causes are excluded, consideration should be given to the possibility of hepatotoxicity from anaesthetic drugs. Most of the agents implicated in hepatotoxicity are not clinically available in the UK and are now of historical interest. Halothane hepatitis is discussed in Chapter 3.

Postoperative nausea and vomiting

Nausea and vomiting is the most common complication after general anaesthesia. Estimates of the incidence vary greatly, approximating 30% in untreated patients having an opioid/volatile anaesthetic.

Some patients have a higher risk of developing PONV, and scoring systems have been developed to estimate risk. It has been demonstrated that targeted administration of PONV prophylaxis to those at increased risk of PONV reduces its incidence, and departments should have local management guidelines.

This is discussed in detail in Chapter 7.

Other complications

Pain management

Assessment and management of pain is a core skill for both anaesthetists and PACU staff. This is discussed in depth in Chapter 24.

Headache

The reported incidence of severe headache postoperatively ranges from 12% to 35%, but up to 60% of patients complain of some headache. Individuals who are susceptible to headaches are more likely to complain of postoperative headache. Most investigations have failed to identify any single agent as being responsible for postoperative headache after general anaesthesia. Clinicians should be aware that a severe postural headache may occur after dural puncture during a central neuraxial block; when this occurs, patients should be reassured, information given and management instigated (see Chapter 43).

Sore throat

Postoperative sore throat has a reported incidence of up to 62% after general anaesthesia. Some of the common causes include the following:

- *Trauma during tracheal intubation.* Damage to the pharynx and tonsillar fauces may be caused by the laryngoscope blade.
- *Trauma to the larynx.* This is more likely if the tracheal tube has been forced through the vocal cords. A poorly stabilised tube may cause further frictional damage to the larynx.
- *Trauma to the pharynx.* This may occur during passage of a nasogastric tube or insertion of oropharyngeal or SAD; it is particularly common when a throat pack has been used. Occasionally the pharynx or upper oesophagus may be perforated during insertion of a nasogastric tube or during difficult tracheal intubation, and severe pain in the throat is often the first symptom. Sore throat is likely if a nasogastric tube remains *in situ* during the postoperative period.
- *Other factors.* The mucous membranes of the mouth, pharynx and upper airway are sensitive to the effects of non-humidified gases; the antisialagogue effect of anticholinergic drugs may also contribute to this symptom.

In the absence of a nasogastric tube, postoperative sore throat is usually of short duration; most patients are symptom-free within 48 h. The incidence after tracheal intubation can be minimised by using the smallest tracheal tube possible and by monitoring cuff pressure. Control of cuff pressure also helps reduce sore throat after SAD use. Lidocaine (topical or in a lubricant jelly) and dexamethasone do not appear to be efficacious.

Hoarseness

Hoarseness should not be confused with sore throat. It is almost always associated with tracheal intubation and is caused predominantly by prolonged abduction of, and pressure on, the vocal cords. However, traumatic tracheal intubation can cause direct trauma to the vocal cords, resulting in prolonged hoarseness.

Laryngeal granulomata

Laryngeal granulomata may occur after tracheal intubation and arise from areas of ulceration, usually on the posterior aspect of the vocal cords. The ulcers are caused by excessive pressure and consequent ischaemia. Tracheal cuff pressure monitors should be used intraoperatively to reduce this risk whilst preventing aspiration. Granulomata are reported most commonly after thyroidectomy. If hoarseness persists for longer than 1 week, indirect laryngoscopy should be performed. If ulceration is present, complete voice rest is indicated. Any granulomata present should be excised; untreated granulomata may grow to such a size as to obstruct the airway.

Shivering

This is a common complication in PACU. It may occur in patients who are hypothermic as a result of prolonged surgery or during injection of local anaesthetic solution into the epidural space. However, in most patients the onset of shivering is not related to body temperature, and there is evidence from electromyography that the characteristics of postoperative (or postanaesthetic) shivering differ from those of thermoregulatory shivering. The incidence and severity of shivering are increased in patients who have received an anticholinergic premedication, and women are more likely to shiver in the luteal than in the follicular phase of the menstrual cycle.

Shivering increases oxygen consumption and CO_2 production and may result in hypoxaemia and hypercapnia if the response of the respiratory centre to carbon dioxide is impaired by drugs. Supplemental oxygen should be administered. A small dose of i.v. meperidine (25 mg) is often effective in aborting postoperative shivering, and there is evidence that ondansetron may also be beneficial.

Surgical considerations

During the recovery period, several surgical complications may occur. These include haemorrhage, blockage of drains or catheters, and soiling of dressings. Prosthetic arterial grafts may occlude, resulting in ischaemia of the limbs. Postanesthesia care unit nurses and anaesthetists must be aware of potential surgical complications, as rapid surgical intervention may be required.

Quality assurance

It is difficult to demonstrate quality of care for both an anaesthetist and the anaesthetic departments. The incidence of both pain and PONV are commonly used indicators by which we can measure our care.

Anaesthesia has a long tradition of improving clinical safety and outcome by continuous critical examination of our practice. The RCoA has produced guidance to help the process; the ethos is that compliance against standards should be tracked over a prolonged period. Many aspects of PACU care discussed in this chapter are suggested as topics in RCoA publications.

References/Further reading

Abildstrom, H., Rasmussen, L.S., Rentowl, P., et al., 2000. Cognitive dysfunction 1-2 years after non-cardiac surgery in the elderly. ISPOCD group. International study of post-operative cognitive dysfunction. Acta Anaesthesiol. Scand. 44 (10), 1246e51.

Association of Anaesthetists of Great Britain and Ireland, 2013. UK national core competencies for Post-anaesthesia care 2013. London, AAGBI.

Association of Anaesthetists of Great Britain and Ireland, 2013. Immediate Post-anaesthetic recovery 2013. London, AAGBI.

Association of Anaesthetists of Great Britain and Ireland, 2015. Recommendations for the standards of monitoring during anaesthesia and recovery 2015. London, AAGBI.

Association of Anaesthetists of Great Britain and Ireland, 2014. AAGBI

safety guideline. Peri-operative care of the elderly. London, AAGBI.

Fines, D., Severn, A., 2006. Anaesthesia and cognitive disturbance in the elderly. BJA Education 6(1), 37–40.

NHS England. Patient Safety Alert. Residual anaesthetic drugs in cannulae and intravenous lines. NHS/PSA/W/2014/008.

Reduque, L., Verghese, S., 2013. Paediatric emergence delirium. BJA Education 13 (2), 39–41.

The National Institute for Health and Care Excellence, 2010. Clinical guideline. Delirium: prevention, diagnosis and management. (CG103). London, NICE.

The National Patient Safety Agency, 2009. National Reporting and Learning service. Reducing the risk of retained throat packs after surgery. NPSA/2009/SPN001.

The National Patient Safety Agency, 2009. Rapid Response Report, Oxygen safety in hospitals. NPSA/2009/RRR06.

The Royal College of Anaesthetists, 2011. 4th national audit project of the royal college of anaesthetists and the difficult airway society. Major complications of airway management in the United Kingdom report and findings 2011. London, RCOA.

The Royal College of Anaesthetists, 2017. Guidelines for the provision of anaesthesia services (GPAS). Guidelines for the Provision of Post-operative Care 2017. London, RCOA (Chapter 4).

The Royal College of Anaesthetists, 2017. Guidelines for the provision of anaesthesia services (GPAS). Guidelines for the Provision of Emergency Anaesthesia 2017. London, RCOA (Chapter 5).

Section | 4 |

Clinical anaesthesia

Chapter | **30** |

Managing the high-risk surgical patient

Jonathan Wilson, Alexa Mannings

A high-risk surgical procedure can be considered as one in which there is an accepted postoperative mortality rate of more than 1%. Whether a procedure for a given patient is high risk depends on consideration of the technical hazards of the surgical procedure itself – for example, the construction of a gastrointestinal tract anastomosis and the potential for it to break down – and, secondly, the presence of pre-existing disease in the patient of sufficient severity to significantly affect the patient's response to surgery, particularly when poorly managed.

In most cases poor outcome from major surgery arises from a combination of both of these factors, in which the patient with impaired functional reserve is unable to cope with either the physiological demands of the procedure or the stress of complications. An unrecognised and unchecked sequence of adverse events will lead to multiorgan dysfunction syndrome (MODS), multiorgan failure (MOF), and death in the worst cases.

Emergency anaesthesia and cardiothoracic anaesthesia are considered elsewhere (Chapters 41, 42, and 44), so this chapter will concentrate on the patient undergoing scheduled major non-cardiac surgery. However, the principles of treatment, particularly haemodynamic management, also apply to the patient undergoing an emergency procedure.

What makes an operation high risk?

Major surgery generates a systemic inflammatory response. The magnitude of the inflammatory response, as judged by circulating proinflammatory cytokines, is directly associated with postoperative outcome: higher concentrations of cytokines or other inflammatory markers such as C-reactive protein (CRP) are associated with an increased incidence of postoperative complications. Factors that increase the inflammatory response include surgery involving the gastrointestinal tract, major vascular surgery or cardiac surgery, the need for major blood transfusion, emergency surgery and the presence of decreased tissue perfusion, particularly in the gastrointestinal tract.

The inflammatory response increases oxygen consumption, requiring increases in cardiac output and tissue oxygen extraction. Some patients may not have the physiological reserve to increase cardiac output to the required level, and this group of patients are at higher risk of complications after surgery. Treatment strategies are aimed at identifying high-risk patients early and optimising various aspects of patient care in order to reduce risk and improve outcome.

What makes a patient high risk?

High-risk patients may be elderly with established cardiorespiratory disease, but a significant proportion will not have any documented history of significant comorbidities.

From the 2011 National Confidential Enquiry into Perioperative Deaths (NCEPOD) report 'Knowing the Risk', the approximate increased risk of death after surgery compared with no disease present is:

- twofold for respiratory disease, ischaemic heart disease, non–insulin-dependent diabetes and cancer;
- threefold for cerebrovascular disease, insulin-dependent diabetes, and dysrhythmia; and
- fivefold for congestive cardiac failure and documented cirrhosis.

The list of comorbidities is not exclusive, and other conditions such as renal disease, rheumatoid arthritis, obesity and neurological conditions may adversely affect outcome.

The anaesthetist should be aware that the absence of a recognised chronic disease is no guarantee of a good outcome in the older patient undergoing major surgery, but abnormal cardiorespiratory physiology *per se* generates a high risk.

General risk prediction scoring systems

General (ASA, Surgical Outcome Risk Tool (SORT), and POSSUM) and system-specific (Revised Cardiac Risk Index (RCRI), ARISCAT, PERISCOPE) risk prediction tools are discussed in Chapter 19. Frailty is increasingly recognised as a risk factor for poor surgical outcome (see Chapter 31).

Further investigations for risk assessment

Routine and special investigations

In patients undergoing elective surgery, investigations such as full blood count or urea and electrolytes will not in general be of any significant value in predicting risk, although they may be useful as components of scoring systems such as POSSUM (see earlier) and they may highlight specific abnormalities, such as anaemia, which should be corrected before surgery.

Specialised investigations, including cardiopulmonary exercise testing, are discussed in Chapter 19.

Reducing risk before surgery

Information from preoperative assessment and investigations, particularly cardiopulmonary exercise testing, can help the clinician answer three important questions relevant to an individual patient's perioperative risk:

1. Is the patient fit enough for the proposed surgery, or would a less invasive procedure, or even postponement of surgery, be more suitable?
2. Can the patient's medical condition be improved before surgery, with consequent risk reduction?
3. Does the patient need high-dependency unit (HDU) or ICU care after surgery, or are they fit enough to return directly to the general ward?

Alternatives to major surgery

The availability of different treatment options will depend on the surgical condition. For instance, surgery for an abdominal aortic aneurysm can be performed by open or endovascular repair; alternatively it may be deferred for investigation and optimisation of medical conditions, or surgery may be inappropriate for a particularly high-risk patient where the risks outweigh the benefits. For colorectal cancer disease, the alternatives to curative-intent surgery are limited, but the risks can still be modified – for instance,

by choosing to perform a Hartmann's procedure in a very high-risk patient with a rectal tumour rather than risking an anastomotic leak in a patient with limited reserve. Such decisions have to be taken in conjunction with the patient on a case-by-case basis and with all factors considered.

Fig. 30.1 is an example of a risk assessment and management plan for colorectal cancer surgery patients, based on clinical findings and cardiopulmonary exercise testing (CPET) results. Plans may vary according to local resources.

Preoperative interventions to reduce risk

Beta-blockade

The purpose of cardioselective β-blockade is to reduce risk of myocardial ischaemia after surgery through the prevention of tachycardia and the consequent decrease in myocardial oxygen demand and improvement in myocardial perfusion time.

Retrospective studies have found that the protective effect of β-blockade is greater in those patients who have an increased number of RCRI cardiac risk factors, and there is a suggestion that β-blockade in patients with no cardiac risk factors may be harmful.

Beta-blockers are now also widely used in the treatment of heart failure but have to be established over time for full effect, starting with a low dose. For patients established on long-term β-blockade, it is important that this is continued around the time of surgery as sudden cessation is definitely associated with a worse outcome. Parenteral preparations of atenolol or metoprolol are available for the patient who is nil by mouth; there is some suggestion that the longer-acting atenolol may be more beneficial.

Statin therapy

Many patients are established on long-term statin therapy as part of secondary prevention of cardiovascular disease. If so, it is important that this treatment is continued around the time of surgery as withdrawal can cause a rebound effect.

Long-term statin use has been found to reduce mortality risk after surgery in patients undergoing aortic surgery. Although more evidence is required, introducing statins before surgery may have some beneficial effect, possibly through their anti-inflammatory actions, and is unlikely to cause harm as side effects are rare. There are no parenteral preparations for statins, but it may be useful to use a longer-acting preparation such as fluvastatin, taken on the morning of surgery.

Coronary revascularisation

For patients with new-onset or unstable angina, or severe exercise limitation accompanied with ischaemia, evaluation

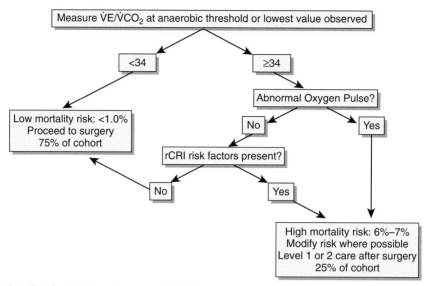

Fig. 30.1 A typical cardiopulmonary exercise testing (CPET)–based management plan for elective colorectal surgery. Example of how data from CPET as well as clinical information can lead to a rational approach to allocation of postoperative critical care. *rCRI*, Revised Cardiac Risk Index.

by a cardiologist is required. These patients are at risk of major adverse cardiac events (see Chapter 20) irrespective of their surgical disease but in practice constitute a small proportion of patients presenting for surgery.

A much larger number of patients are asymptomatic but have cardiac risk factors, in whom coronary lesions can be identified on angiography. Prophylactic revascularisation of such lesions before non-cardiac surgery has no benefit in terms of overall outcome when the morbidity associated with the revascularisation is included.

Surgery may be complicated further in patients who have undergone percutaneous coronary intervention (PCI) with stenting as they will need to be taking dual antiplatelet therapy for a minimum of 6 weeks in the case of bare metal stents and 12 months for drug-eluting stents. In the case of patients who are known to require surgery after their PCI, a bare metal stent should be used to minimise the duration of dual antiplatelet therapy (see Chapter 20).

Smoking cessation

For reducing pulmonary complications, a benefit is only seen 2–3 months after smoking cessation. However, there may be some immediate gains to smoking cessation in the patient at high-risk of cardiovascular complications, as smoking causes a hypercoagulable state which increases myocardial work and decreases oxygen delivery through increased carbon monoxide occupancy of haemoglobin, vasoconstriction and catecholamine release. At the very least,

major surgery should be seen as an opportunity to encourage smoking cessation for further healthcare benefit.

Respiratory therapy

For the patient at risk (PAR) of postoperative pulmonary complications (PPCs) (see earlier) preoperative chest physiotherapy and optimisation of medication may be helpful in reducing atelectasis and pneumonia after surgery. Early postoperative mobilisation is also beneficial.

Correction and management of anaemia

Preoperative anaemia correction is detailed in Chapter 20. It should be part of an overall strategy for perioperative patient blood management, aiming to reserve transfusion only for those in genuine need (see Chapter 14). Other components of the strategy include the use of tranexamic acid, intraoperative cell salvage, permissive hypotension, avoidance of haemodilution of clotting factors and maintenance of normothermia.

Identifying patients in need of post-operative critical care

High-dependency unit beds or ICU beds are expensive resources, and demand usually outstrips supply. Some patients will require critical care as a routine after certain surgery types such as aortic aneurysm repair or upper gastrointestinal cancer surgery. However, for other surgeries, such as colorectal cancer surgery or complex orthopaedic surgery, it is often unclear which patients are more likely to benefit from the extra monitoring and additional supportive measures that critical care can provide.

Cardiopulmonary exercise testing has been found to be accurate in identifying patients who did not need HDU care, irrespective of clinical history or age. This approach is now becoming established in those hospitals with access to preoperative CPET. A typical protocol is shown in Fig. 30.1.

The usefulness of this approach was emphasised by the results from a large audit of surgical outcomes in a UK tertiary centre, which found that using clinical judgement alone does not identify high- or low-risk surgical populations with the same level of accuracy.

Level 1 care

Increasingly an alternative approach to postoperative care for high-risk patients is provided by level 1 care, usually an area of a general surgical ward with increased levels of nursing and continuous monitoring. In some cases, patients can be nursed with arterial lines *in situ*, to provide additional information. This system negates patients having to compete for scarce HDU beds, without any evidence of worse outcomes.

Perioperative management of the high-risk patient

Ideally, high-risk patients will present for surgery having been identified as being at increased risk and having had their medical comorbidities optimised after preoperative assessment.

Choice of anaesthetic and analgesic technique

For patients undergoing major body cavity surgery, general anaesthesia is usually necessary. For peripheral surgery in a high-risk patient, a regional anaesthetic technique may be considered advantageous, although there is little evidence that outcomes are improved by use of regional anaesthesia.

Patients identified as being at risk of PPCs may benefit from thoracic epidural analgesia if having upper abdominal or thoracic surgery.

There is some retrospective evidence that total intravenous anaesthesia using propofol may have some protective effects against the patient developing cancer recurrence at a later date, although this is yet to be confirmed by large prospective trials.

Haemodynamic monitoring and fluid therapy

High-risk patients are more likely to develop complications after surgery if they show signs of impaired tissue perfusion from inadequate oxygen delivery. Clinical signs of impaired end-organ perfusion include poor mentation, increased respiratory rate, tachycardia, hypotension and decreased urine output. In the anaesthetised paralysed patient the clinician generally has to rely on haemodynamic monitoring and blood gas analysis to evaluate perfusion. Particular attention should be paid to increasing lactate concentrations or decreasing central venous oxygen saturations: Both indicate impaired oxygen delivery to the tissues.

There is no 'one size fits all' approach to monitoring the high-risk patient. Invasive arterial access generally has low morbidity and provides easy, repeated blood sampling for blood gases, electrolytes, glucose and assessment of full blood count and coagulation status. It provides beat-by-beat monitoring of arterial blood pressure and hence allows indirect estimation of cardiac output and fluid responsiveness.

There is little evidence that central venous pressure measurement is a useful guide to fluid therapy. However, central access may be helpful for administration of potent vasoactive drugs and measurement of central venous oxygen saturation.

If there is evidence that tissue perfusion is inadequate, oxygen delivery needs to be improved using the following sequence:

- Ensure that the patient has an optimal circulating volume. This is done by giving a carefully measured fluid bolus and assessing its effect on stroke volume, using an appropriate cardiac output monitoring device (Fig. 30.2).
- If volume is optimal yet hypoperfusion persists, use vasoactive medication to optimise stroke volume, ensuring adequate cardiac output and oxygen delivery.
- The highest-risk surgical patients will benefit from measures that aim to optimise oxygen delivery through the careful administration of fluid and vasoactive medication, guided by careful monitoring of circulatory flow and preload.
- It is equally important that intravenous fluid administration is carefully controlled, as too much fluid can also cause problems through development of oedema.

Preload responsiveness to guide fluid therapy

Stroke volume can be measured through analysis of the arterial pulse waveform (pulse contour analysis). This

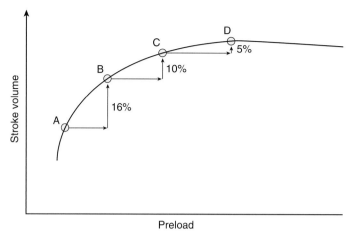

Fig. 30.2 Optimising stroke volume with fluid: the Frank–Starling curve. At point *A* on the curve the patient is significantly hypovolaemic and responds to a fluid bolus with an 18% increase in stroke volume at point *B*. The second bolus (*B* to *C*) produces a lesser but still significant increase, but the third bolus (*C* to *D*) only produces a small (<10%) increase in stroke volume (SV), signifying that the plateau portion of the Frank–Starling curve has been reached and that further fluid boluses will not lead to an increase in stroke volume.

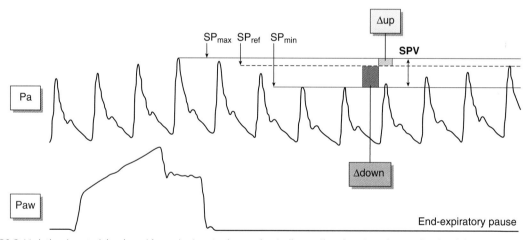

Fig. 30.3 Variation in arterial pulse with respiration. In the mechanically ventilated patient the amplitude of the arterial pulse will vary with the respiratory cycle. Variations in the systolic pressure (*SPV*) greater than 12%–14% will indicate that a patient is hypovolaemic and likely to respond to fluid by increasing stroke volume.

requires the insertion of an arterial line, but this should be considered routine monitoring in the high-risk patient. A patient that has a sustained rise in stroke volume after a fluid bolus can be described as being preload responsive. As an alternative to direct observation of stroke volume responses to a fluid challenge, preload responsiveness can also be estimated by assessing changes in the arterial pressure or plethysmographic waveform during mechanical ventilation (Fig. 30.3). Several variables related to preload responsiveness are available:

- Systolic pressure variation (SPV)
- Pulse pressure variation (PPV)
- Stroke volume variation (SVV)
- Plethysmogram variability index (PVI)

SPV, PPV and SVV all require the insertion of an arterial line, whilst PVI is derived from analysis of the pulse oximetry waveform and is therefore non-invasive.

The ability of these to determine preload responsiveness is based on observation of the cyclical changes that occur in stroke volume in response to mechanical ventilation.

Respiratory variations in stroke volume are the main determinant of the respiratory change in pulse pressure as long as arterial compliance remains the same. In hypovolaemia, SVV and PPV are increased, as the underfilled right atrium and vena cavae are more compliant, and hence collapsible during inspiration and generally more sensitive to changes in preload as they will be on the steeper portion of the contractility–preload response curve. Hence the variation in stroke volume, pulse pressure, and to a lesser extent systolic pressure will increase in hypovolaemic conditions.

A pulse pressure or stroke volume variation greater than 12%–13% is highly sensitive and specific for fluid responsiveness, and patients with these parameters will normally respond to a fluid challenge by moving up their contractility–preload response curve with an increase in stroke volume (Fig. 30.4).

Crystalloids should be used for intravenous fluid therapy until the patient is able to tolerate oral fluid, which should be encouraged as soon as possible after surgery. There is no evidence of benefit from using synthetic colloids (gelatins, starches).

Crystalloids are also a vehicle for electrolyte replacement therapy. Surgical patients will need 1–2 mmol kg^{-1} of sodium daily and 1 mmol kg^{-1} of potassium. Administration of large volumes of solutions containing dextrose only, or a mixture of dextrose and hypotonic saline (0.18%), will lead to hyponatraemia and hypokalaemia and should be avoided.

Crystalloids are also indicated for bolus use to optimise circulating volume. They are as efficacious as synthetic colloids in this respect, as well as being cheaper and safer. High volumes of solutions containing chloride (e.g. 0.9% saline) are associated with hyperchloraemic metabolic acidaemia (see Chapter 12). However, the effects of this on important clinical outcomes are still debated and the advantages of physiologically balanced crystalloids, such as Ringer's lactate, over those containing 0.9% saline are uncertain.

Fluid restriction regimens

Unmonitored administration of crystalloid solutions around the time of surgery can also lead to increased complications by causing tissue oedema, impaired gas exchange in the lungs and gastrointestinal ileus with a delay in return of normal gut function.

Some studies of regimens in which crystalloid use has been restricted have found improved outcomes, but the wide range of regimens used, the lack of the use of goal-directed fluid therapy and the results of other studies showing no benefit have led to uncertainty over the benefits of true restrictive fluid regimes.

In summary, the important considerations are how carefully the administration of intravenous fluids is monitored and the overall effect on end-organ tissue perfusion.

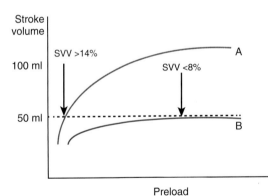

Fig. 30.4 Preload responsiveness in normal and abnormal cardiac function. This graph illustrates the utility of preload responsiveness in assessing the need for fluid bolus administration. A value for stroke volume of 50 ml on its own is not helpful; line A is the response of a healthy individual, where an initial stroke volume reading of 50 ml represents underfilling with a preload responsiveness of greater than 14%. Line B represents the curve of a patient with impaired cardiac function where a stroke volume of 50 ml may mean the patient is optimally filled or even overfilled. Preload responsiveness will be less than 8% in this value. This measure negates the need for unnecessary, and potentially dangerous, fluid challenges to assess response.

Postoperative management

Successful management strategies for the high-risk surgical patient are based on preventing complications where possible through appropriate cardiovascular support as described earlier and through early recognition and treatment of situations where surgical complications or unforeseen medical problems cause deteriorating organ function.

Patients having major surgery but who are not considered as being high risk may be able to be managed in the PACU for a few hours after surgery before returning to the surgical ward. As mentioned earlier, some surgical wards have an enhanced care area (level 1 care) in which patients can have additional continuous monitoring: usually ECG, pulse oximetry, non-invasive blood pressure and occasionally arterial blood pressure, as well as additional nursing support to assist mobilisation and physiotherapy.

Passive leg raise to assess fluid responsiveness

The passive leg raise is a simple manoeuvre to assess fluid responsiveness in the postoperative patient, essentially using the blood pooled in the patient's lower limb as a fluid challenge. Raising the legs to 45 degrees for 1 min increases venous return to the heart, and the clinician can assess the haemodynamic response accordingly. If a sustained rise in cardiac output, stroke volume or blood pressure is identified, then a fluid bolus can be administered i.v. to increase circulating volume. Technique is important, and flow-based measures (e.g. cardiac output) are better than pressure-based measures (e.g. pulse pressure) at predicting fluid responsiveness.

Monitoring on the general ward

General ward monitoring is normally restricted to standard clinical observations. The same principles of monitoring apply to both general ward patients and critical care patients in that the clinician is using the monitoring to detect organ dysfunction and decreased tissue perfusion at the earliest possible stage. Measures to be observed are shown in Table 30.1.

These monitored parameters are usually combined into a scoring system known as a PAR score or early warning system (EWS) score. A particular PAR or EWS score value, or change in value, will be predefined as a trigger point to

alert senior medical assistance, in order that a potentially deteriorating patient can be identified early and appropriate treatment can be given, including transfer to critical care if so indicated. Such scores are not a replacement for clinical assessment and judgement.

Monitoring in the critical care unit

Critical care provides an environment in which the invasive monitoring used in the operating room can continue to be used safely after surgery. Information gained from invasive monitoring in the postoperative critical care unit can be used to detect organ dysfunction at an early stage.

Vasoactive drugs in the high-risk surgical patient

Protocols that target an oxygen delivery value have usually incorporated the use of an inotropic agent to increase cardiac contractility if the oxygen delivery target has not been achieved with fluid loading alone. Some patients may require inotropic or vasoconstrictor drugs if, despite adequate fluid loading, they still have signs of inadequate

Table 30.1 Routine observations for the high-risk surgical patient

	POTENTIAL CAUSES FOR ABNORMALITY	
	Increased	**Decreased**
Level of consciousness	Agitation can be due to poor pain relief or hypoxia.	Hypotension and poor cerebral perfusion Oversedation from opioid analgesia (systemic or epidural) Cerebrovascular accident
Heart rate	Hypovolaemia Dysrhythmia Inadequate pain relief Sepsis	Heart block Drug effect – sedation, beta-antagonist, ACEI
Blood pressure	Inadequate pain relief Omission of antihypertensive medication	Bleeding (until proven otherwise) Hypovolaemia (untreated) Sepsis Sympathetic blockade from epidural or spinal
Respiratory rate	Metabolic acidosis from poor tissue perfusion from bleeding, hypovolaemia or sepsis. Hypoxia from primary pulmonary complication (e.g. infection, atelectasis) Pain	Opioid overdose
Urine output	–	Less than 0.5 ml kg^{-1} h^{-1} of *ideal* body weight suggestive of hypovolaemia

ACEI, Angiotensin-converting enzyme inhibitor.

tissue perfusion (base deficit, raised lactate concentrations decreased central venous oxygen saturation, etc.). In these cases cardiac output monitoring should ideally be used to help guide treatment. Adrenaline (β_1-, β_1- and β_2-agonist) and dobutamine (β_1-agonist) have been used in this context.

Enhanced recovery after surgery

Enhanced recovery after surgery (ERAS) is essentially the application of a series of manoeuvres that supposedly reduce surgical stress, with the aim of reducing complications and speeding up the recovery process. These manoeuvres include the following:

- Explaining the plan to patients before surgery
- Avoiding bowel preparation
- Carbohydrate loading before surgery
- Modifying surgical technique to minimise incision size and avoid drains and nasogastric tubes
- Avoiding opioid analgesia where possible
- Encouraging early oral intake
- Early mobilisation

ERAS can be applied across a range of surgical procedures, including lower-risk surgeries such as joint replacement. The main benefit is that patients follow a plan, where previously there had been a wide variation in practice and lengthy hospital stays. However, like all medical interventions, there are risks as well as benefits. For example, force-feeding patients with undetected ileus can lead to regurgitation and aspiration of gastric contents in otherwise low-risk patients. The overall benefit of ERAS programs remains unclear; though applied widely in colorectal practice, the duration of hospital stay has not been significantly reduced.

References/Further reading

Canet, J., Galart, L., Gomar, C., et al., 2010. Prediction of postoperative pulmonary complications in a population-based surgical cohort. Anesthesiology 113, 1338–1350.

Findlay, G.P., Goodwin, A.P.L., Protopapa, K., et al., 2011. Knowing the risk. National Confidential Enquiry into Perioperative Death (NCEPOD), UK. ncepod.org.uk.

Lee, T.H., Marcantonio, E.R., Mangione, C.M., et al., 1999. Derivation and validation of a simple index for prediction of cardiac risk of major noncardiac surgery. Circulation 100, 1043–1049.

Loftus, I. (Ed.), 2010. Care of the critically ill surgical patient: participant handbook, 4th ed. The Royal College of Surgeons of England.

McConachie, I. (Ed.), 2009. Anaesthesia for the High-risk patient, 2nd ed. Cambridge, Cambridge University Press.

Moran, J., Wilson, F., Guinan, E., et al., 2016. Role of cardiopulmonary exercise testing as a risk-assessment method in patients undergoing intra-abdominal surgery: a systematic review. Br. J. Anaesth. 116, 177–191.

Rawlinson, A., Kang, P., Evans, J., et al., 2011. A systematic review of enhanced recovery protocols in colorectal surgery. Ann. R. Coll. Surg. Engl. 93, 583–588.

Voldby, A.W., Brandstrup, B., 2016. Fluid therapy in the perioperative setting – a clinical review. J. Intensive Care 2016, Open access.

Chapter 31

Surgery under anaesthesia for the older surgical patient

Jugdeep Dhesi, Iain Moppett, Judith Partridge

Increasing numbers of older people are undergoing emergency and elective surgery. This is due to changing demographics, advances in surgical and anaesthetic techniques and changing attitudes and expectations of the older population. Furthermore, degenerative, metabolic and neoplastic conditions, for which surgery is often the definitive management, increase in incidence with age. All these factors contribute to the higher numbers of older patients presenting for surgery, the majority of whom constitute the higher risk surgical population by virtue of age-related physiological decline, increasing prevalence of multimorbidity and frequency of geriatric syndromes. This high-risk group develop adverse postoperative outcomes more often. These include clinician-reported outcomes such as morbidity and mortality, patient-reported outcomes such as impaired cognition and functional dependency, and process-related outcomes such as cancellations, duration of stay and financial cost. It is important for anaesthetists to be aware of the specific needs of the older population and the emerging evidence to optimally manage this cohort in the perioperative period.

Ageing: physiological decline

Organ function declines in all systems with increasing age and with disease. Of particular interest to the anaesthetist are the effects of ageing on the cardiovascular, renal, neurological, and haematological systems and drug metabolism.

Cardiovascular

Cardiovascular disease becomes more prevalent with increasing age. The incidence of heart failure doubles every decade, and the incidence in those aged older than 80 years is approximately 10%. Heart failure can be viewed as a final common pathway for multiple cardiovascular insults.

- *Structural change.* The heart changes shape (more spherical), and although there is no overall change in left ventricular mass, there is relative thickening of the interventricular septum. In the absence of other diseases, systolic function is largely unchanged in healthy ageing; diastolic function is altered, however. Ventricular filling occurs later in diastole, with greater contribution of atrial filling to end-diastolic volume. These changes are compensated for at rest but become unmasked with exercise. Aerobic capacity ($\dot{V}O_2$ max) declines around 50% with ageing. Cardiac output decreases by around 25%, in part because of an inability to increase heart rate. The remainder of the $\dot{V}O_2$ max decline is attributed to alterations in oxygen extraction and redistribution of blood flow with exercise. The vascular tree becomes less compliant with age, resulting in arterial systolic hypertension. Responsiveness to vasoconstrictive (α_1) and vasodilatory (nitric oxide) stimuli reduces with age.
- *Valvular disease.* Moderate to severe mitral or aortic valvular disease affects around 13% of people older than 75 years. Echocardiography demonstrates mild calcification of the aortic valve in around 40% of people aged older than 60 years and 75% of those older than 85 years.
- *Conduction and rhythm abnormalities.* Atrial fibrillation (AF) is more prevalent with ageing. Around 3%–4% of 60–70 year olds have AF; 10%–17% in those aged older than 80 years. Ventricular ectopic beats are also more common, but this may not have clinical significance. Resting heart rate does not change, but peak heart rates decline by around 0.7–1.0 beats min^{-1} year^{-1}. Symptomatic sinus bradycardia is almost exclusively seen in

those aged older than 60 years. Permanent pacemakers (for any indication) are most commonly inserted in older people.

Respiratory

- *Lung mechanics.* Elasticity of the chest wall declines with age because of loss of elastin, degeneration of joints and changes in thoracic shape. There is some decline in diaphragmatic function with age; peak inspiratory pressures are around 20% lower in those older than 65 years compared with young adults. There is enlargement of airspaces and degeneration of elastic tissue in the lung.
- *Lung function.* Measurements of lung function decline steadily from around 20–35 years. Forced expiratory volume in 1 second (FEV_1) declines around 20–30 ml year^{-1}. Functional residual capacity (FRC) and residual volume (RV) increase with age.
- The ventilatory response to hypoxia and hypercapnia is diminished.

Neurological

- Brain volume decreases by around 0.5%–1% year^{-1} after age 60, though the decline may start earlier in adult life. These changes are not uniform across cerebral structures, and age-related changes are probably separate from pathological changes such as Alzheimer's disease.
- Ischaemic damage is common. Around 5% of people aged 60–80 years are survivors of stroke, increasing to 15% of those aged older than 80 years. Subclinical (micro) infarcts are found in around one-third of cognitively intact older people.
- The incidence of dementia increases with age. Reported rates are dependent on the degree of case ascertainment but are around 5%–10% in those aged older than 65 years; the risk may be decreasing (those born more recently may be at a lower risk).
- Mild cognitive impairment, an intermediate spectrum between normal cognition and dementia, is reported to occur in around 15%–20% of people older than 60 years.

Renal

- Glomerular filtration rate (GFR) declines on average by about 8 ml min^{-1} 1.73 m^{-2} decade^{-1} after around the second to fourth decade of life. There is wide interindividual variability, in part because of association with risk factors such as diabetes, smoking, arterial hypertension and so on. Although creatinine clearance declines, so does muscle mass (and hence creatinine excretion). As a consequence, serum creatinine in the elderly may be 'normal' despite markedly reduced GFR.

- The balance of vasoconstriction and vasodilation, which is essential to normal renal function, is precarious in the older kidney. This may explain why even modest insults such as perioperative hypotension and hypovolaemia and the use of non-steroidal anti-inflammatory drugs (NSAIDs) may provoke acute kidney injury (AKI) in the elderly.

Haematological

- Anaemia increases with age. Around 10% of community-dwelling people aged older than 65 years are anaemic; around 50% of nursing home residents are anaemic.
- There is some evidence of hypercoagulability with increasing age.
- There is dysregulation of T-lymphocyte function affecting both cellular and humoral immune responses.
- In common with other systems there may be reduced reserve to respond to increased demands around the time of surgery.

Ageing: multimorbidity

Multimorbidity is the presence of two or more concurrent chronic conditions that collectively have an adverse effect on health status, function or quality of life and require complex healthcare management, decision making and coordination. A chronic condition is one that lasts a year or more, requires ongoing medical attention or limits activities of daily living. These chronic conditions commonly coexist because:
- one is caused by the other (e.g. diabetes can cause chronic kidney disease);
- they share common biological aetiology (e.g. smoking, lung cancer and coronary heart disease);
- they are distinct but both commonly accompany another long-term condition (depression with Parkinson's disease and chronic obstructive pulmonary disease (COPD)); and
- there is a preponderance of particular conditions within a specific socioeconomic class (e.g. 46% of 65 year olds in the highest social class in the UK are likely to have multimorbidity compared with 64% of those in the poorest social class).

Although multimorbidity can occur in the younger population, it is consistently observed to increase with age, with 75% of those aged older than 80 years living with multimorbidity. The complexity of managing multimorbidity is compounded by the associated polypharmacy and inevitable drug interactions. In the perioperative setting, as the surgical population ages, multimorbidity is more commonly encountered, conferring increased perioperative risk in terms of morbidity and mortality. Preoperative identification and optimisation of multimorbidity involves the application of multiple, sometimes conflicting guidelines for single-organ disease delivered using a systematic approach such as the Comprehensive Geriatric Assessment (CGA).

Ageing: geriatric syndromes

Geriatric syndromes are a group of highly prevalent age-related conditions which share common risk factors and confer adverse outcome but have ill-defined pathophysiological aetiology. Of particular relevance in the perioperative setting are frailty and delirium.

Frailty

Frailty is a distinctive health state related to the ageing process in which multiple body systems gradually lose their in-built reserves. This results in the frail individual being vulnerable to an even seemingly minor external stressor such as an uncomplicated infection. With the ageing of the surgical population, frailty is encountered more often; some studies report frailty in up to 50% of patients presenting for surgery. Across cardiac and non-cardiac surgery frailty is consistently reported as an independent risk factor for adverse post-operative outcome, including morbidity, mortality, longer duration of hospital stay and new institutionalisation at hospital discharge.

Two main models of frailty exist: the Frailty Phenotype described in 2001 from data from the Cardiovascular Health Study and the Frailty Index described in 2005 from the Canadian Study of Aging.

The Frailty Phenotype describes a model of five criteria:

- weakness;
- slow gait velocity;
- low activity level;
- exhaustion; and
- weight loss.

Those displaying three or more criteria are described as frail and those with one or two criteria present are described as prefrail.

In contrast the Frailty Index is a measure of the number of deficits an individual has accrued across multiple domains. These domains include physical signs, known medical diagnoses, cognitive or mood issues, falls and so on. For example, if an individual has accrued 11 of a possible 33 deficits, he or she has a Frailty Index of 0.33. At an Index of 0.25 an individual is deemed frail, and at approximately 0.67 few further deficits can be accumulated before death is imminent.

Based on these two models, numerous frailty scores have been designed. Some tools measure a single domain,

such as gait velocity, whilst others are domain based, such as the Edmonton Frail Scale. Pictorial scales exist such as the Clinical Frailty Scale (Fig. 31.1) and more organ specific tools have also been developed, such as the Comprehensive Frailty Score designed for use in cardiac surgical patients. Choosing the most appropriate tool to measure frailty will depend on the surgical setting in which the patients is being assessed. In unwell emergency patients, a pictorial scale which avoids functional assessment may be most appropriate, whereas in preoperative assessment of planned surgery a domain-based tool incorporating functional measures could be used. More recently the Electronic Frailty Index (eFI) has been developed in the UK. This tool uses routinely collected data from primary care electronic records and calculates a Frailty Index. Although not yet universally adopted, it is likely that this will be used in routine clinical care within the UK in the next 5 years.

Although there is no 'cure' for frailty, aspects of the syndrome can be modified, which may result in improvement in frailty status and its clinical consequences. This requires optimisation through multicomponent interventions that can be delivered using the CGA (Table 31.1).

Delirium

Delirium is defined according to fifth edition of the *Diagnostic and Statistical Manual of Mental Disorders* (DSM-V) criteria as 'an acute and fluctuant condition characterised by disturbance of attention, awareness and cognition attributable to an underlying cause'. It is observed commonly in both elective and emergency surgical populations. Patients with hip fracture are often reported as the highest risk group with an incidence more than 30%. Delirium has serious consequences, including higher rates of postoperative morbidity, 12-month mortality and institutionalisation. Evidence is emerging of the adverse impact of an episode of delirium on long-term cognitive trajectory and psychological sequelae, including anxiety and depression.

The aetiology of delirium remains incompletely defined, but it is thought to occur because of the neurotoxicity of proinflammatory cytokine release as result of a precipitating factor in a vulnerable individual with predisposing risk factors. These predisposing and precipitating factors are shown in Table 31.2.

Tools to identify patients at risk of developing postoperative delirium are available but are rarely used in clinical practice as they lack discriminatory power in older surgical patients. In contrast, the diagnosis of delirium should be formally recorded using established tools such as the 4 'A's Test (4AT) or Confusion Assessment Method (CAM).

In terms of management of delirium, no single intervention effectively reduces the incidence, severity or duration of delirium, but evidence does support the role

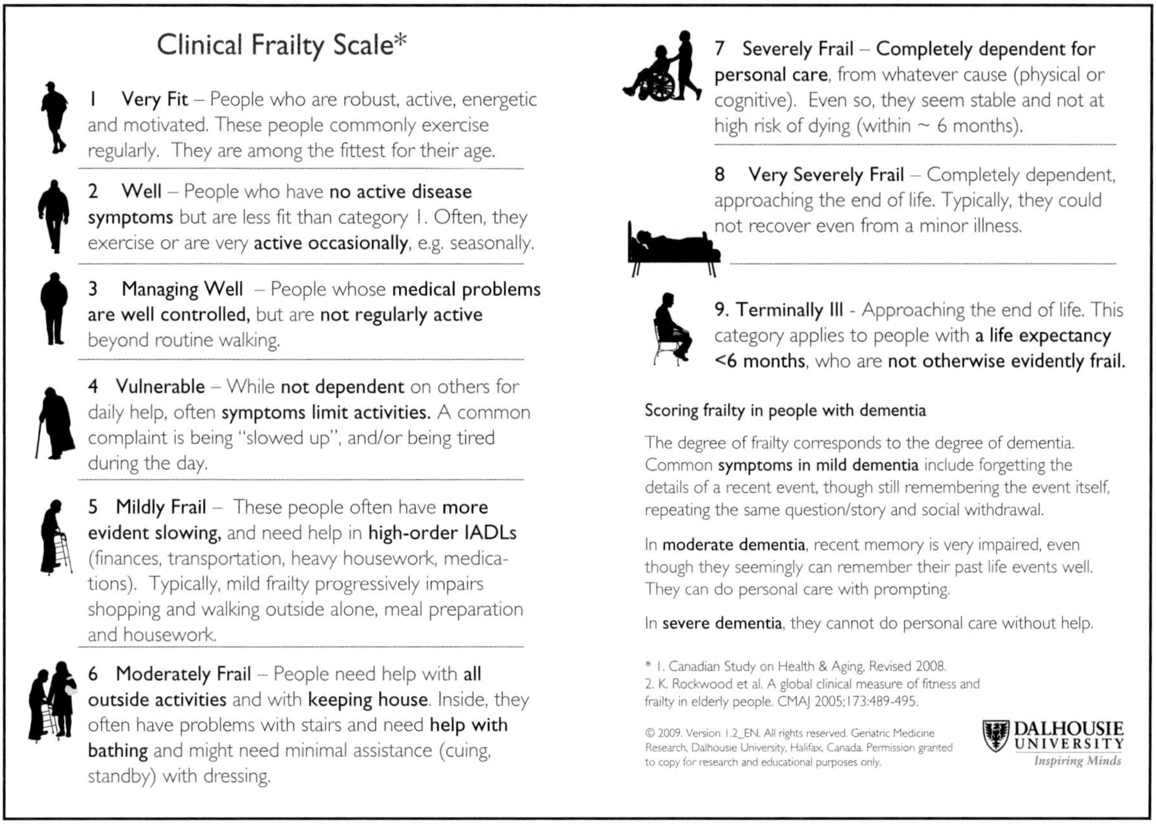

Clinical Frailty Scale*

1 Very Fit – People who are robust, active, energetic and motivated. These people commonly exercise regularly. They are among the fittest for their age.

2 Well – People who have **no active disease symptoms** but are less fit than category 1. Often, they exercise or are very **active occasionally**, e.g. seasonally.

3 Managing Well – People whose **medical problems are well controlled,** but are **not regularly active** beyond routine walking.

4 Vulnerable – While **not dependent** on others for daily help, often **symptoms limit activities.** A common complaint is being "slowed up", and/or being tired during the day.

5 Mildly Frail – These people often have **more evident slowing,** and need help in **high-order IADLs** (finances, transportation, heavy housework, medications). Typically, mild frailty progressively impairs shopping and walking outside alone, meal preparation and housework.

6 Moderately Frail – People need help with **all outside activities** and with **keeping house.** Inside, they often have problems with stairs and need **help with bathing** and might need minimal assistance (cuing, standby) with dressing.

7 Severely Frail – **Completely dependent for personal care,** from whatever cause (physical or cognitive). Even so, they seem stable and not at high risk of dying (within ~ 6 months).

8 Very Severely Frail – Completely dependent, approaching the end of life. Typically, they could not recover even from a minor illness.

9. Terminally Ill - Approaching the end of life. This category applies to people with **a life expectancy <6 months,** who are **not otherwise evidently frail.**

Scoring frailty in people with dementia

The degree of frailty corresponds to the degree of dementia. Common **symptoms in mild dementia** include forgetting the details of a recent event, though still remembering the event itself, repeating the same question/story and social withdrawal.

In **moderate dementia,** recent memory is very impaired, even though they seemingly can remember their past life events well. They can do personal care with prompting.

In **severe dementia,** they cannot do personal care without help.

* 1. Canadian Study on Health & Aging, Revised 2008.
2. K. Rockwood et al. A global clinical measure of fitness and frailty in elderly people. CMAJ 2005;173:489-495.

© 2009. Version 1.2_EN. All rights reserved. Geriatric Medicine Research, Dalhousie University, Halifax, Canada. Permission granted to copy for research and educational purposes only.

DALHOUSIE UNIVERSITY *Inspiring Minds*

Fig. 31.1 Clinical Frailty Scale. (Reproduced with permission from Geriatric Medicine Research, Dalhousie University, Halifax, Canada.)

of multicomponent interventions. These multicomponent interventions are non-pharmacological, with an emphasis on proactively identifying and managing precipitating factors (see Table 31.2) and maintaining a supportive environment, good nursing care and de-escalation strategies with appropriate communication. These interventions described in medical populations have been translated to surgical settings with similar evidence of benefit.

Although there is no evidence to support the use of pharmacological agents to prevent delirium, there is clear guidance on the role of medication in the treatment of postoperative delirium. This is particularly useful in hyperactive delirium when patients are a danger to themselves or others, including through the refusal of essential investigation or treatment. The use of medications to treat a non-capacitous patient with delirium must always be considered within the relevant legal framework. Current guidance differentiates between using dopamine antagonists for the majority of postoperative delirium with benzodiazepine usage reserved for delirium secondary to alcohol withdrawal and those with movement disorders.

Disturbance in cognitive function after surgery is well recognised. Age, pre-existing cognitive impairment and occurrence of delirium are the most consistent associations. Mode of anaesthesia does not seem to influence outcome. There is considerable debate as to how much of a decline in cognition after surgery is simply the progression of pre-existing or subclinical neurocognitive disorders (mild cognitive impairment and dementias). Conversely, there is evidence that some patients' cognition improves after surgery, presumably because of subsequent reduction in pain, inflammation and anxiety.

Using Comprehensive Geriatric Assessment in the preoperative setting

Comprehensive Geriatric Assessment and optimisation is an established and evidenced-based methodology which has been used by geriatricians in various clinical settings

Table 31.1 Using the Comprehensive Geriatric Assessment to preoperatively assess and optimise the older surgical patient

Frailty domain	Specific aspect of frailty	Modification	Compensation
Cognition	*Abnormal clock drawing test*	Vascular risk factor control Onward referral to memory clinic Assessment of capacity	Information provision to patient and carer (diagnosis of cognitive impairment and delirium risk)
Functional independence	*Needs assistance with daily activities*	Referral to occupational therapist and social worker	Pre-emptive assessment of care needs
Social support	*Has no one to help out at home when required*	Referral to social worker for therapeutic interventions	Arrange home care/befriending/day-centre/pendant alarm
Medication use	*Number of medications Forgetting to take medications*	Review/rationalise medications Assess/optimise cognition	Provision of dosette box Arrange carer to prompt medications
Nutrition	*Recent weight loss*	Assess for underlying cause Dietician, speech and language therapy and occupational therapy	Nutritional supplements Highlight to ward / community dietician
Mood	*Self-reported low mood*	Liaise with GP, specialist psychiatric services	Multidisciplinary team input Access to local services
Continence	*Self-reported urinary incontinence*	Medications, exercise strategies, bladder training regimes Referral to continence service	Provision of pads
Functional performance	*'Timed up and go' (TUG) test > 20 s Gait speed < 0.8 m s⁻¹ Grip strength less than norm for age*	Referral for physiotherapy	Provision of walking aids Provision of equipment to assist patients at home (e.g. jar-opening devices)

GP, General practitioner.
The Edmonton Frail Scale can be employed in clinical practice to identify vulnerabilities, to direct assessment and modification and how to ensure the patient is equipped to deal with the day-to-day consequences of the frailty syndrome.

over the last 30 years. It involves a multidomain (medical, functional, psychological and social) assessment, which is usually interdisciplinary and is followed by the planning and implementation of individualised investigations, treatment, rehabilitation and longer-term follow-up. Comprehensive Geriatric Assessment has been found to improve mortality at 18-month follow-up, increase the chance of living independently at home and confer a positive effect on physical function when undertaken in medical inpatients and community-dwelling older people. In the perioperative setting there is good evidence that that CGA has a positive impact on postoperative medical complications and duration of hospital stay in older patients undergoing elective surgery (Table 31.3).

In the perioperative setting CGA provides a systematic approach to the following:
- Preoperative risk assessment:
  - assessment of known comorbidity;
  - identification of previously undiagnosed disease or psychosocial and functional issues; and
  - application of perioperative risk scores tailored to a complex multimorbid population (e.g. lack of discriminatory power of scores such as ASA in a complex multimorbid older population).
- Systematic multidomain modification of risk factors:
  - optimisation of all identified issues using evidence-based guidelines interpreted in the context of multimorbidity;

Table 31.2 Predisposing and precipitating factors for delirium

Predisposing risk factors	Precipitating factors
Increasing age	Severe acute illness
Cognitive impairment or dementia	Surgery under general or regional anaesthesia
Polypharmacy	Trauma
Sensory impairment (e.g. visual or hearing impairment)	Sepsis
Depression	Drug withdrawal (e.g. benzodiazepines or alcohol)
Substance misuse (e.g. alcohol excess)	Pain
Multimorbidity	Opioid analgesia
	Dehydration
	Electrolyte imbalance
	Anaemia
	Constipation
	Acute urinary retention

Table 31.3 Using preoperative the Comprehensive Geriatric Assessment to assess and optimise

Domain	Issue	History / examination	Screening or diagnostic tools	Investigation	Optimisation
Medical	Multimorbidity (e.g. Parkinson's disease)	Known history Reported slowing, falls, tremor, rigidity Proactive assessment for non-motor symptoms Physical examination	Unified Parkinson's Disease Rating Scale (UPDRS)	DAT scan CT/MRI (does not necessarily need to be preoperative)	In established cases plan proactively regards medications when nil by mouth Pre-emptive advice to ward teams about non-motor complications likely at time of surgery (e.g. constipation, delirium, falls) In newly identified cases, consider starting medications preoperatively
Geriatric syndromes	Falls	Previous history History of 'near misses' Bone health screening	Gait speed 'Timed up and go' (TUG) test Fracture Risk Assessment Tool (FRAX)	Bone profile Vitamin D measurement Suggestion to primary care about DEXA and follow-up	Medical management of bone health (e.g. bisphosphate, calcium/ vitamin D supplementation) Medical falls review Strength and balance training referral

Continued

Table 31.3 Using preoperative the Comprehensive Geriatric Assessment to assess and optimise—cont'd

Domain	Issue	History / examination	Screening or diagnostic tools	Investigation	Optimisation
	Cognitive impairment	Self-reported history of cognitive issues Collateral history from relative/carer	4 'A's Test (4AT) Montreal Cognitive Assessment (MoCA)	Cerebral imaging or recommendation to primary care	Delirium risk assessment and optimisation (e.g. cessation of anticholinergics, ensuring normal electrolytes, treating Parkinson's disease) Signposting to standardised postoperative management of delirium Communication with patient and relatives Long-term vascular risk factor management Referral to memory services for long-term follow-up
Psychological	Anxiety and depression	Self-reported history Collateral from family/carer Symptoms	Hospital Anxiety and Depression Score (HADS) Geriatric Depression Score (GDS)	Common medical conditions, e.g. thyroid status Exclusion of cognitive impairment	Referral for psychological support (e.g. talking services) Consider pharmacological treatment
Functional and social	Functional dependency	Self-reported concerns Collateral from family/carer Symptoms	Barthel Index Nottingham Extended Activities of Daily Living (NEADL)	Physical examination and investigation of pathology causing disability (e.g. proximal myopathy secondary to vitamin D deficiency) Prescribe analgesia for osteoarthritis	Preoperative physiotherapy Occupational therapy intervention (e.g. home adaptions) Social worker intervention to proactively identify barriers to discharge Proactive communication regarding anticipated length of stay and access to rehabilitation or care at discharge
	Non-adherence to prescribed medications	Self or family reported concerns Clinical evidence of non-adherence	Screening Tool of Older Persons Prescriptions and Screening Tool to Alert doctors to Right Treatment (STOPP/START)	Assessment of cognition and understanding of medications	Liaising with community pharmacist to assist with dosette box and with care services or telecare to prompt medication

CT, Computed tomography; *DAT,* dopamine transporter single photon emission computed tomographic scan (used for evaluation of patients with suspected Parkinson's disease); *MRI,* magnetic resonance imaging.

- interdisciplinary input to optimise functional and social issues; and (e.g. a pharmacist providing a dosette box for a patient with cognitive impairment to improve adherence or an occupational therapist anticipating falls risk issues in a patient with Parkinson's disease and adapting the environment).
- Shared decision making:
  - formal assessment of cognition;
  - gaining an understanding of the patient's values, judgements;
  - assessment of capacity to consent to the procedure; and
  - discussion of risk and benefit and potential harm of surgical intervention and comparing with other treatment options.
- Anticipation of likely postoperative complications
  - Pre-emptive advice on standardised management of anticipated postoperative complications
  - Pre-emptive anticipation of rehabilitation and discharge needs
- Longer-term medical optimisation to ensure evidence-based management of chronic disease and disability

Intraoperative considerations

The details of the impact of ageing on pharmacokinetics and pharmacodynamics and physiological systems are discussed in the relevant chapters. In summary:
- Older people are all unique. Interindividual variability is often greater than average age-related effects.
- Although basal/resting values may be normal, the ability to respond to stressors (anaesthetic drugs, fluid and blood loss, physiological stress response) may be markedly reduced. Physiological homeostasis in the perioperative period may therefore be harder to achieve.
- Anaesthetic agents tend to have a slower onset and offset of action.
  The concept of 'minimally invasive anaesthesia' has been proposed.
- Anaesthesia should be tailored to the individual to minimise intra- and postoperative derangement.
- The anaesthetist should be aiming to provide a technique that provides:
  - normotension;
  - normothermia;
  - adequate haemoglobin; and
  - pain relief that maximises recovery with minimal adverse effects.

In broad terms, this means using lower doses of drugs, given more slowly, and proactive management of blood pressure and temperature. Choice of agent or general *vs.*

regional anaesthesia probably has far less impact than the care taken by the anaesthetist.

The nadir in blood pressure after induction of anaesthesia is delayed compared with younger adults and often coincides with moving into the operating room or positioning. Blood pressure readings are easily missed or overlooked unless the anaesthetist is vigilant to this risk.

A common trap is to overdose general anaesthesia. Minimum alveolar concentration (MAC) is age dependent (but this is not uniformly adjusted for age if displayed on monitors).

$$MAC_{age} = MAC_{40} \times 10^{-0.00269(age-40)}$$

Care should be taken to adjust agent concentrations to age (Fig. 31.2).

Similarly, sage advice is to draw up syringes of induction agent with less than the 'normal' adult dose to avoid the temptation to give more than necessary.

Patients who are confused must at all times be treated calmly and with dignity. Even the most confused patient can recognise emotions.

Postoperative care in older surgical patients

Older surgical patients are more likely than younger people to develop postoperative complications. These complications are a consequence of age-related physiological decline, multimorbidity and geriatric syndromes such as cognitive impairment and frailty. There is a predominance of medical as opposed to surgical postoperative morbidity in older surgical patients for example: atrial fibrillation, acute coronary syndrome, exacerbation of COPD, acute kidney injury, falls and delirium. These medical issues can contribute to functional deterioration resulting in longer duration of stay, slow rehabilitation and increased care needs at hospital discharge. Despite the medical nature of these complications, postoperative ward care has traditionally been delivered by surgical teams with a reliance on on-call medical input.

Single-organ specialty physicians can provide medical input for patients undergoing surgery on the sister surgical speciality—for example, cardiologists consulting for cardiac surgery patients, gastroenterologists supporting gastrointestinal surgeons. However, the multimorbidity of the older surgical population can result in the involvement of numerous different organ physicians with implications on coordination of care and financial resource. In the United States this has resulted in the development of a hospitalist model of care where general physicians comanage the

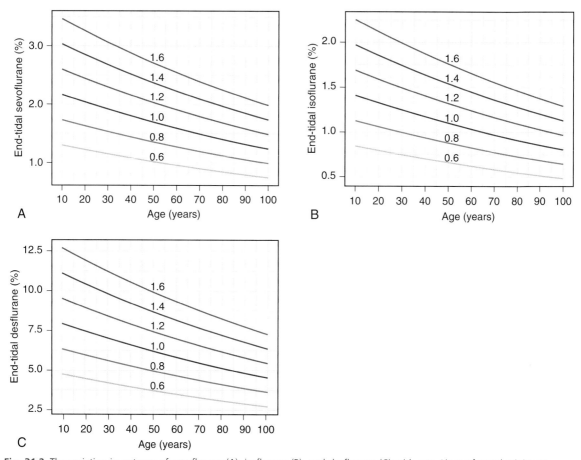

Fig. 31.2 The variation in potency of sevoflurane (A), isoflurane (B), and desflurane (C) with age. Lines of equal minimum alveolar concentration (MAC) (0.6–1.6) are plotted for each agent. (Figures generated using the equation from Mapleson, W. W. (1996) Effect of age on MAC in humans. *British Journal of Anaesthesia*, 76, 179–185.)

whole inpatient stay with surgical colleagues. However, the older surgical population requires management not only of multimorbidity but also of geriatric syndromes. The RCoA in the UK has emphasised the complexity of this population and advocates the importance of teamwork, employing the right expertise to deliver care at the right time in the right place. They advocate the role of perioperative specialists providing input throughout the surgical pathway, with skills in preoperative assessment, optimisation, complex decision making and delivery of postoperative care, including medical management, rehabilitation, discharge planning and end-of-life care. This has resulted in recommendations from a number of organisations to support structured proactive care from geriatricians into the management of older surgical patients. Evidence to support the establishment of such geriatrician-delivered and -led perioperative medicine services is emerging. In practical terms this approach

to postoperative geriatrician-delivered postoperative care involves regular joint medical and surgical ward rounds, multidisciplinary team meetings, board rounds and proactive regular communication with patients and families or carers to ensure consistency throughout the pathway for elective and emergency patients.

Age alone is not a reason to admit or not admit to intensive or high-dependency care. Nor is having a high risk of adverse postoperative outcomes. It is important to consider whether critical care will provide additional benefit for the individual patient over and above ward care. For people who are very frail or have significant multimorbidity, critical care admission may not provide any benefit. Similarly, critical care areas are hostile environments for the person at risk of delirium; ward-based care, particularly on wards with good systems and processes for care of the confused person, may be a better option.

References/Further reading

Braude, P., Partridge, J., Shipway, D., Martin, F., Dhesi, J., 2016. Perioperative medicine for older patients: how do we deliver quality care? Future Hosp. J. 3, 33–36.

Chow, W.B., et al., 2012. Optimal preoperative assessment of the geriatric surgical patient: a best practices guideline from the American college of surgeons national surgical quality improvement program and the American geriatrics society. J. Am. Coll. Surg. 215 (4), 453–466.

Hamel, M.B., et al., 2005. Surgical outcomes for patients aged 80 and older: morbidity and mortality from major noncardiac surgery. J. Am. Geriatr. Soc. 53 (3), 424–429.

Khuri, S.F., et al., 2005. Determinants of long-term survival after major surgery and the adverse effect of postoperative complications. Ann. Surg. 242 (3), 326–341.

Lawrence, V.A., Hazuda, H.P., Cornell, J.E., Pederson, T., Bradshaw, P.T., Mulrow, C.D., et al., 2004. Functional independence after major abdominal surgery in the elderly. J. Am. Coll. Surg. 199 (5), 762–772.

Lee, D.H., et al., 2010. Frail patients are at increased risk for mortality and prolonged institutional care after cardiac surgery. Circulation 121 (8), 973–978.

Lin, H., Watts, J., Peel, N., Hubbard, R., 2016. Frailty and post-operative outcomes in older surgical patients: a systematic review. BMC Geriatr. 16, 157.

Makary, M.A., et al., 2010. Frailty as a predictor of surgical outcomes in older patients. J. Am. Coll. Surg. 210 (6), 901–908.

Mapleson, W.W., 1996. Effect of age on MAC in humans: a meta-analysis. Br. J. Anaesth. 76, 179–185.

Myles, P.S., Grocott, M.P., Boney, O., Moonesinghe, S.R., 2016. COMPAC-StEP Group. Standardizing end points in perioperative trials: towards a core and extended outcome set. Br. J. Anaesth. 116, 586–589.

Nadelson, M., Sanders, R., Avian, M., 2014. Perioperative cognitive trajectory in adults. Br. J. Anaesth. 112 (3), 440–451.

Partridge, J., Harari, D., Martin, F., Dhesi, J., 2014. The impact of pre-operative comprehensive geriatric assessment on postoperative outcomes in older patients undergoing scheduled surgery: a systematic review. Anaesthesia 69 (Suppl. 1), 8–16.

Partridge, J.S.L., et al., 2017. Randomized clinical trial of comprehensive geriatric assessment and optimization in vascular surgery. Br. J. Surg. 104 (6), 679–687. doi:10.1002/bjs.10459.

Rolfson, D.B., Majumdar, S.R., Tsuyuki, R.T., Tahir, A., Rockwood, K., 2006. Validity and reliability of the edmonton frail scale. Age. Ageing 35 (5), 526–529.

Siddiqi, N., Harrison, J.K., Clegg, A., Teale, E.A., Young, J., Taylor, J., et al., 2016. Interventions to prevent delirium in hospitalised patients, not including those on intensive care units. Cochrane Database Syst. Rev. (3), Art. No.: CD005563, doi:10.1002/14651858.CD005563.pub3.

Sündermann, S., Dademasch, A., Praetorius, J., Kempfert, J., Dewey, T., Falk, V., et al., 2011. Comprehensive assessment of frailty for elderly high-risk patients undergoing cardiac surgery. Eur. J. Cardiothorac Surg. 39 (1), 33–37.

Chapter | **32** |

Anaesthesia for the obese patient

Christopher Bouch

Obesity rates have increased from 15% in 1993 to 27% in 2015, and morbid obesity has tripled to affect 2% of men and 4% of women. Figures are projected to rise, with 50% of UK adults expected to be obese by 2030. The scale of demographic changes and associated multisystem comorbidity means that the obese patient presents across the spectrum of healthcare and not simply to the specialist in the bariatric field.

Measuring obesity

A patient's mass varies with size and shape. Absolute mass can be important when considering factors such as equipment safety limits. The most widely used obesity measurement is BMI = (mass in kg) / (height in m)^2. Body mass index was first devised more than 100 years ago and has several limitations:

- It is not representative of certain ethnic groups or those of athletic build.
- It cannot describe the distribution of weight (Fig. 32.1).
- It is unable to discriminate the nature of the excess tissue—that is, muscle or fat.

However, calculation of BMI, from two simple, universal measurements, requires minimum equipment and expertise, and will therefore continue to be used to express degrees of obesity despite its flaws (Table 32.1).

Not all types of fat are the same. Intra-abdominal fat is metabolically active and is associated with a higher incidence of myocardial ischaemia, congestive cardiac failure, sleep-disordered breathing and respiratory problems; it is vital to identify this patient group, and the use of BMI in isolation will not do this. Fat distribution can be described using the fruit analogy of apples and pears (see Fig. 32.1). The apple distribution describes central abdominal obesity, whereas the pear shape describes the peripheral, benign-type buttock

and thigh distribution of fat. Measurement of waist circumference provides a measure of this distribution. A waist circumference greater than 88 cm in women and 102 cm in men identifies individuals with intra-abdominal fat and associated higher risk profiles.

Obesity and the metabolic syndrome

Obesity is a multisystem disorder. The aetiology is complex but in the main is driven by excess nutrient intake (of the wrong type of foods), with little in the way of energy expenditure. There is an associated complex network of contributors, including socioeconomic, ethnic, societal, social and psychological factors. The underlying and acquired pathophysiological changes include the endocrine, cardiovascular, respiratory, gastrointestinal tract, locomotor and psychiatric systems.

The adipose organ

The traditional view of fat tissue has been as a metabolically inert triglyceride energy store that provides protection from physical insults and temperature changes. However, fat tissue is not uniform or benign. Hepatic and intra-abdominal visceral fat tissue is metabolically active and should be considered an endocrine organ; it is known to excrete more than 20 chemical mediators. The observed effects are pro-inflammatory (cytokines, adipsin), procoagulant (plasminogen activator inhibitor 1) and endocrine (leptin, resistin, adiponectin).

The generated underlying biochemical state is probably responsible for the common patterns of accelerated comorbidity observed in morbid obesity. *Metabolic syndrome* is the name applied to the pattern of atherosclerotic disease and diabetes

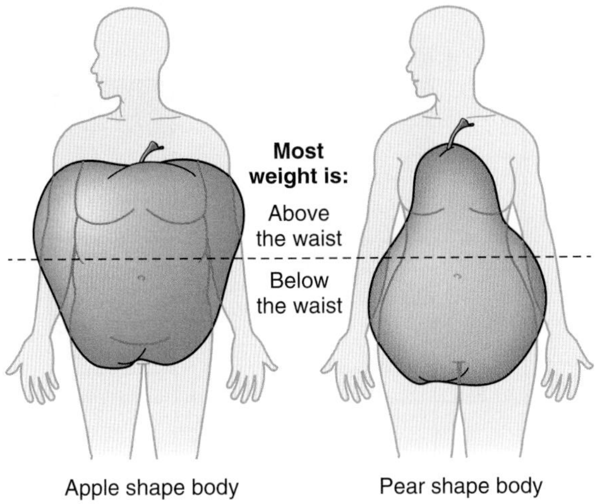
Most
weight is:
Above
the waist
Below
the waist
Apple shape body
Pear shape body

Fig. 32.1 Apples and pears body morphology description. (Reproduced with permission from the Society for Obesity and Bariatric Anaesthesia (SOBA)).

Table 32.1 World Health Organization classification of obesity (other nomenclatures included)

Category	BMI (kg m^{-2})
Underweight	<18.5
Normal	18.5–24.9
Overweight (preobese)	25–29.9
Obese class I	30–34.9
Obese class II (severe to morbid)	35–39.9
Obese class III (morbid to super)	40+
(Super obesity)	45–50+

BMI, Body mass index.

mellitus associated with the presence of at least three of the following:

- Hypertension
- Hyperglycaemia/insulin resistance
- Raised cholesterol
- Visceral obesity
- Low high-density lipoprotein (HDL) concentrations

Development of the metabolic syndrome is associated with a significant increase in perioperative organ dysfunction, resulting in increased mortality. It is vital to identify the presence of the syndrome and optimise each component before surgery to reduce risks. This includes smoking cessation. Cigarette smoking is a powerful catalyst to the development of adverse atherosclerotic events in those with the metabolic syndrome.

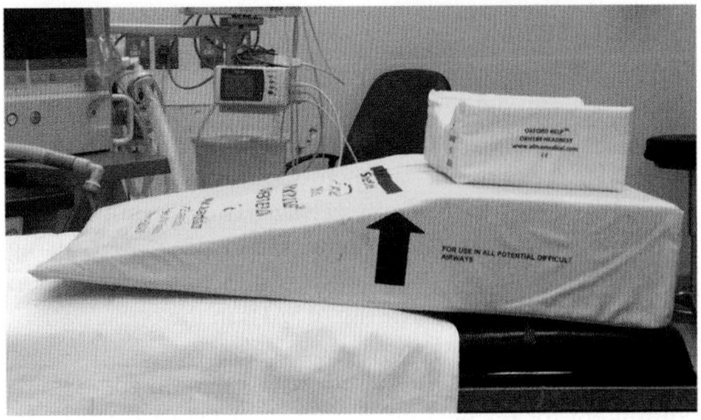

Fig. 32.2 Oxford HELP (head elevating laryngoscopy pillow).

Obesity pathophysiology, comorbidity and anaesthetic management

Airway

The airway of the obese patient should be approached with caution. Traditional teaching and audits of national practice suggest that airway management in obesity is likely to be difficult. However, several studies have demonstrated that tracheal intubation is no more difficult than for normal-weight individuals, but face-mask ventilation is more likely to be difficult. The association of a large abdomen and increased neck circumference with the presence of a beard increases the risk of difficulty. Beard removal before surgery may need to be considered to facilitate safe airway management.

Obesity results in progressive airway infiltration by adipose tissue. This occurs at all levels from oropharynx to vocal cords, causing narrowing and reduction in airway diameter. A reduction of 50% or more from the physiological normal can be encountered. The effect of adipose deposition on airway anatomy is not simply internal; external factors also need to be considered. The presence of a thoracic 'hump' can significantly affect supine posture, resulting in extension of the neck and flexion at the atlanto-occipital joint.

Careful positioning is key to successful management of the bariatric airway. This can be achieved using specifically designed equipment such as the Oxford HELP (Fig. 32.2). However, positioning can also be achieved by ramping with pillows and blankets. The key component of positioning is to place the patient in the reverse Trendelenburg position with the tragus of the ear level with the manubrium sterni. This position facilitates all aspects of airway manoeuvres.

Airway adjuncts

Simple adjuncts such as oral and nasopharyngeal airways should be used routinely. Continuous positive airway pressure during preoxygenation and PEEP during face-mask ventilation can help to splint the airway open. Supraglottic airway devices (SADs) have a role in airway salvage. Their routine use in the morbidly obese patient remains controversial, focusing on concerns around pulmonary aspiration and optimisation of pulmonary function. The use of SADs in the obese patient should be limited to airway rescue.

Standard laryngoscopes and blades remain the default equipment for tracheal intubation in obese patients. Videolaryngoscopes may help if additional risk factors for difficult tracheal intubation are present (see Chapter 23). Many are designed with short-handled bodies which can be useful if a large chest and fixed neck posture limit space.

Respiratory system

Anatomy

The lung fields of obese patients often look small when assessed by chest radiography. This is an artefact of accommodating the patient onto the plate for the radiograph. Obesity results in compromised lung function. This function will change with location of fat mass, patient position and presence of other pathological conditions. Adipose deposition around the chest wall and in breast tissue leads to decreased chest wall compliance and damping of the natural recoil and expansion. Abdominal wall infiltration and raised intra-abdominal pressure with peribronchial and parenchymal fatty infiltration further exacerbate this. Respiratory muscles demonstrate fat infiltration, which, when combined with effects from inflammatory mediators, results in diminished muscle power and respiratory endurance.

Pathophysiology

- Total lung capacity and vital capacity decrease in a linear manner with rising weight. The spirometric observations (Fig. 32.3) reflect the change in the balance between chest wall and parenchymal forces with rising obesity.
- Functional residual capacity (FRC) decreases (Fig. 32.4) and closing volume increases. Resulting atelectatic shunt reduces PaO_2. At higher levels of morbid obesity, tidal ventilation may impinge on closing volume even in the standing position.
- Forced expiratory volume in 1 s (FEV_1) decreases, although the FEV_1/forced vital capacity (FVC) ratio is often preserved, particularly with central obesity patterns.
- Increased metabolic rate is associated with increasing fat and muscle mass. This results in a doubling of meta-

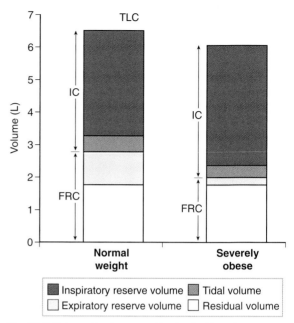

Fig. 32.3 Spirometric changes with obesity. Note the significant reduction in FRC. *FRC*, Functional residual capacity; *IC*, inspiratory capacity; *TLC*, total lung capacity.

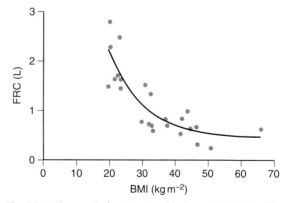

Fig. 32.4 Changes in functional residual capacity (FRC) with increasing body mass index (BMI). (From Pelosi, P., Croci, M., Ravagnan, I., et al. (1998) The effects of body mass on lung volumes, respiratory mechanics, and gas exchange during general anesthesia. *Anesthesia and Analgesia.* 87, 654–660.)

bolic rate compared with lean individuals, causing increased oxygen consumption and carbon dioxide production.
- Work of breathing increases by 70% from low levels of obesity to an energy cost 300% higher in high BMI states. The energy cost of maintaining adequate minute

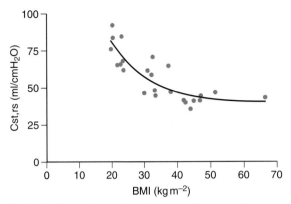

Fig. 32.5 Changes in static respiratory system compliance *(Cst, rs)* with increasing body mass index (BMI). (Adapted from Pelosi, P., Croci, M., Ravagnan, I., et al. (1998) The effects of body mass on lung volumes, respiratory mechanics, and gas exchange during general anesthesia. *Anesthesia and Analgesia.* 87, 654–660.)

ventilation is mitigated by a reduction in tidal volume, resulting in rapid, shallow breathing at rest.
- The elastic load increases (reduced static compliance; Fig. 32.5). This reflects both the reduced elasticity of chest wall and parenchymal tissue and tidal ventilation occurring at lower lung volumes. Dynamic compliance (i.e. resistance to gas movement) also falls.
- In the lower airway there is narrowing of the small conducting airways. This may be due to multiple factors:
  - external compression from parenchymal fat deposition;
  - reduction in the part of the lung volume at which tidal breathing occurs; and
  - chronic inflammatory changes and increased smooth muscle reactivity/bronchospasm.

The consequences of these changes for the anaesthetist include:
- shortened apnoea to desaturation time;
- increased oxygen requirements;
- increased shunt fraction and ventilation/perfusion mismatch;
- increased work of breathing resulting in difficulty with spontaneously breathing general anaesthesia techniques; and
- increased incidence of atelectasis.

Obstructive sleep apnoea

Sleep and associated snoring is a normal physiological process. Snoring occurs as a result of soft tissue collapse of the upper airway and vibration of these tissues and associated turbulent airflow. Snoring becomes abnormal when associated with apnoeas and hypopnoeas to produce obstructive sleep apnoea (OSA). This occurs in up to 25% of the adult population. Obstructive sleep apnoea occurs in up to 60% of obese individuals; the majority of these cases are undiagnosed. Obstructive sleep apnoea is not a benign condition; cyclical occlusion of the upper airway with associated hypoxaemia results in sympathetic nervous system activation, endothelial dysfunction and inflammation. Development of hypertension, myocardial ischaemia and failure, strokes and sudden cardiac death are increased.

Patients in the perioperative period will acquire an abnormal sleep cycle because of anaesthesia, surgery and administered drugs; this has adverse effects. A patient with OSA is at increased risk of respiratory failure and desaturation, emergency tracheal reintubation, delirium, cardiac arrhythmias, unplanned ICU admission and increased duration of hospital stay. Perhaps surprisingly, OSA is not associated with an increase in postoperative mortality.

It is vital to screen for OSA preoperatively to treat and reduce risk. Basic clinical history and examination are poor at identifying OSA. The STOP Bang tool (see Chapter 19) is a simple screening questionnaire designed for use in surgical patients to identify the presence of predictive factors in those with OSA. It is well validated, and its use is supported by experts in bariatric anaesthesia. However, the STOP Bang questionnaire has a greater sensitivity than specificity. Specificity can be improved with measurement of plasma bicarbonate. High STOP Bang scores or the presence of risk factors (large neck, high Mallampati score, bicarbonate concentration > 28 mmol L^{-1} or oxygen saturations of less than 95% on room air) will require referral to a sleep clinic before elective surgery for further investigation and management.

Anaesthetic management points

At induction of anaesthesia, the use of the reverse Trendelenburg position maximises lung function, as the FRC can reduce by up to 50% after induction of anaesthesia. Head-up positioning to ensure the tragus is level with the manubrium (Fig. 32.6) increases apnoea to desaturation time, facilitates face-mask ventilation and assists with tracheal intubation.

Lung ventilation volumes should be based on ideal body weight (IBW; see Pharmacology section later in this chapter) and should be 6–8 ml kg^{-1}. Recruitment manoeuvres (50 cmH_2O for 10 s or a vital capacity volume) and maintenance PEEP concentrations of 10 cmH_2O have been demonstrated to maximise lung function by reducing atelectasis and shunt reduction. The presence of a pneumoperitoneum

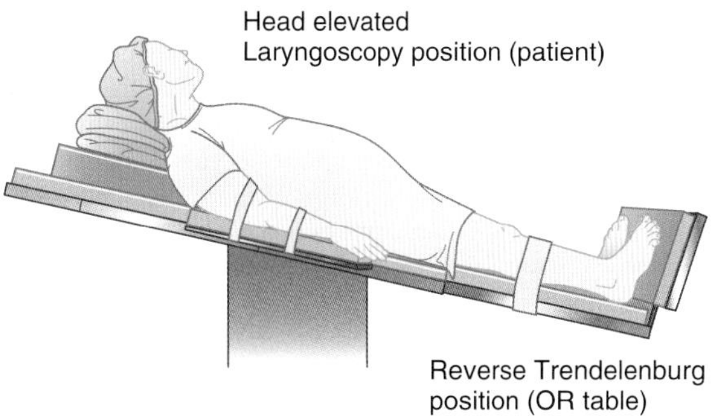

Head elevated
Laryngoscopy position (patient)

Reverse Trendelenburg
position (OR table)

Fig. 32.6 Head-up patient position.

further worsens respiratory function. Optimising patient position, deep neuromuscular blockade and limiting pneumoperitoneum pressures all reduce the adverse consequences. Postoperatively, balanced analgesia (including the use of regional techniques), avoiding long-acting opioid administration, rapid mobilisation, and use of incentive spirometry and physiotherapy may combine to reduce respiratory morbidity.

Cardiovascular system

In common with other organs, cardiovascular changes in obesity are part of a continuum. The nature and extent of the pathophysiology relates to the extent and duration of being overweight and the sequential effects of associated comorbid processes in other organs (Fig. 32.7).

Pathophysiology

- Oxygen demand increases in proportion to the increase in fat-free mass rather than in relation to the patient's BMI. Fat-free mass increases with total body weight (TBW), but with a decreasing curve gradient, to a ceiling of approximately 1 kg per cm of height.
- Blood volume has an inverse hyperbolic relationship with increasing BMI. The blood volume/TBW ratio decreases from around 70 ml kg^{-1} to 40 ml kg^{-1} at a BMI of 70 kg m^{-2}.
- Cardiac output increases with BMI in proportion to the square root of the ratio between actual BMI and ideal BMI. The increase is linear in relation to body surface area and fat-free mass gain. Indexed to adipose tissue mass, fat perfusion decreases as BMI increases. This decrease highlights the relatively poor vascular supply to peripheral adipose tissue (<150 ml kg^{-1} min^{-1}).

- Early in obesity, increases in cardiac output are achieved by blood volume–related preload increases in stroke volume, mediated by β-natriuretic peptide inhibition and aldosterone. The contribution of increased heart rate remains relatively minor.

The heart of the obese patient may exhibit a number of pathological changes. These may be related to either the primary obesity or associated comorbidity (e.g. hypertension, diabetes, hyperlipidaemia or sleep apnoea).

Echocardiographic evidence suggests that three pathological patterns predominate in obesity:
1. Concentric remodelling (left ventricle wall thickening short of hypertrophy)
2. Concentric hypertrophy (ventricular hypertrophy with increased relative wall thickness)
3. Eccentric dilated hypertrophy (thickened hypertrophic left ventricle wall but reduced wall/cavity ratio secondary to dilatation).

The practical application of these states is the recognition of the early existence of reduced ventricular wall compliance and ventricular diastolic dysfunction.

Several ECG changes may be observed in obese patients. These may include the following:
- Atrial fibrillation is the most common arrhythmia associated with obesity, and the prevalence increases exponentially with BMI.
- Voltage magnitudes vary, and QRS complex size is not reliable for diagnosis.
- Conduction axis is often left-shifted, but this may be caused by physical displacement of the heart from the normal position and rotation.

Conduction anomalies are common and relate either to fatty infiltration and fibrosis of the conduction system or underlying coronary artery disease. PR interval and QRS prolongation is common and may be benign, but QTc prolongation appears to have a negative prognostic value. In clinical practice, care must be taken with drug administration that may have a negative impact on conduction defects.

Vascular disease

Arterial disease is associated with both primary obesity and its comorbidities (hyperlipidaemia, diabetes mellitus, etc.). Hypertension is common and contributes to the development of left ventricular hypertrophy and failure. Obesity-associated vascular disease is associated with development of coronary artery disease, myocardial infarction and sudden death. There is an increased risk of progression to cardiac failure as part of this process. Arterial disease is an independent risk factor for the development of stroke.

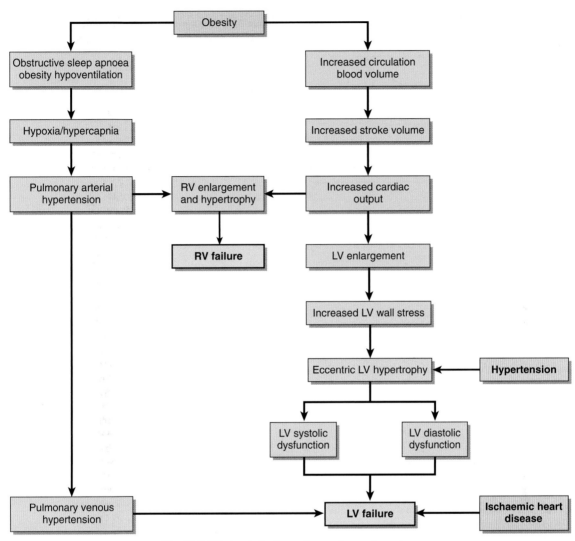

Fig. 32.7 Effects of obesity on the cardiovascular system.

Gastrointestinal

Adipose tissue in the liver is highly metabolically active endocrine and paracrine tissue. There is a close relationship between liver fat content and insulin resistance. In early obesity, insulin sensitivity returns to normal with weight loss. Weight loss of 8% reduces liver fat content by 80%. Non-alcoholic steatohepatitis (NASH) or higher grades of non-alcoholic fatty liver disease (NAFLD) appear to uniformly precede the development of type 2 diabetes. Insulin resistance contributes to dyslipidaemia, hyperglycaemia and eventual pancreatic islet cell burnout. Data suggest that 20% of patients with NASH will progress to cirrhotic liver disease. Non-alcoholic fatty liver disease alone or as part of the metabolic syndrome (see earlier) is associated with accelerated atherogenesis, ischaemic heart disease and increased cardiovascular mortality. Intra-abdominal pressure increases with BMI; resting pressure is usually around twice normal, at 10 mmHg (Fig. 32.8).

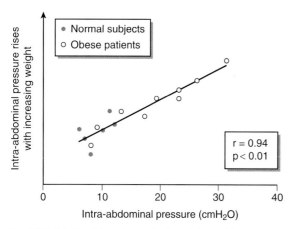

Fig. 32.8 Relationship between body weight and intra-abdominal pressure. (Adapted from Pelosi et al. Anesthesiology. 1999 Nov;91(5):1221-31.)

Pharmacology

There are limited data regarding drug administration in obesity. The majority of drug package inserts recommend dosing based on TBW. Dosing based on TBW in the obese patient is rarely appropriate and will result in overdose of administered drug, along with associated adverse effects.

Different weights can be used to assist with drug dosing in obese patients:
- Total body weight: the actual measured weight of the patient
- Ideal body weight: what the patient should weigh with normal ratio of fat to lean mass
- IBW (kg) = height (cm) − (105 in women and 100 in men)
- Lean body weight (LBW): patient's weight minus fat
  - This rarely exceeds 70 kg in women and 100 kg in men. The formulae for calculating this are complicated. The most commonly used is Janmahasatian:

$$\text{LBW (kg) [Male]} = 9270 \times \text{TBW}/[6680 + (216 \times \text{BMI})]$$

$$\text{LBW (kg) [Female]} = 9270 \times \text{TBW}/[8780 + (244 \times \text{BMI})]$$

- Adjusted body weight (ABW): factors in the increase in lean body mass and hence volume of distribution encountered with obesity

$$\text{ABW (kg)} = \text{IBW} + 0.4\,(\text{TBW} - \text{IBW})$$

Anaesthetic practice is fortunate that titration of pharmacological agents to effect is possible, such as loss of eyelash reflex. Practice amongst bariatric specialists supports dosing many drugs to LBW or adjusted body weight (Table 32.2).

Table 32.2 Dosing guidance for common anaesthetic drugs

Lean body weight	Adjusted body weight	Total body weight
Propofol Induction	Propofol Infusion	Suxamethonium
Thiopental	Alfentanil	
Fentanyl	Neostigmine	
Rocuronium	Sugammadex	
Atracurium	Antibiotics	
Vecuronium	Low molecular weight heparin	
Morphine		
Paracetamol		
Bupivacaine		
Lidocaine		

Reproduced with permission of Society for Obesity & Bariatric Anaesthesia.

Table 32.3 Factors affecting the pharmacokinetic and pharmacodynamic properties of drugs in obesity

Kinetic property	Effect of increasing obesity
Blood volume and cardiac output	Increase
Adipose and lean body mass	Increase
Hepatic blood flow and glucuronidation rate	Increase
GFR and renal excretion	Increase
Cytochrome P450 isoenzymes	Variable
Renal tubular reabsorption	Decrease

GFR, Glomerular filtration rate.

Obese patients display altered pharmacokinetics and pharmacodynamics (Table 32.3). These factors have clinical relevance for drug dosing. Obesity-related increases in cardiac output and blood volume will alter plasma concentrations, drug clearance and half-life of many agents. Pathophysiological changes in obesity (mainly renal and hepatic) result in a higher drug clearance. These effects are not drug specific and are not completely understood.

Intravenous anaesthetic agents

Because of the physiological changes described earlier (particularly blood volume and cardiac output), an i.v. bolus of induction agent based on IBW is likely to achieve a lower peak plasma concentration and a faster redistributive decay – that is, it is less likely to reach effective anaesthetic brain tissue concentrations and will have a shorter duration of effect. This may explain the increased incidence of accidental awareness in obese individuals that was revealed in the UK Fifth National Audit Project (NAP5). An induction dose based on LBW is ideal. If a delay in achieving maintenance anaesthesia is encountered, then further boluses of induction agent should be administered to prevent accidental awareness.

Target-controlled infusions

Controversies surround the ideal pharmacokinetic model to define parameters for TCI administration in the obese patient. This results in a unique pharmacological challenge. Current TCI infusion devices have dosing scalars derived from studies that excluded obese individuals. The Marsh model cannot accept weights greater than 150 kg, and the Schnider model cannot use a BMI greater than 35 kg m^{-2} for women or greater than 42 kg m^{-2} for men. Use of these scalar models may result in either accidental awareness or overdose of agent. Great care should be taken when using this technique and depth of anaesthesia monitoring use is advocated.

Inhalational anaesthetic agents

Theoretical concerns regarding the use of inhalational agents in the obese patient centre on the decreased FRC, increased cardiac output, lipid solubility and adipose mass and possible effects on both wash-in and wash-out curves. However, this does not translate into clinical problems. The majority of bariatric anaesthetists prefer agents that are less lipid soluble, such as desflurane and sevoflurane, which have faster onset and offset than other agents, providing earlier return of airway reflexes (see Chapter 3).

Neuromuscular blocking agents

Suxamethonium
At one time it was routine to facilitate tracheal intubation in obesity with an RSI technique because of concerns about reflux, pulmonary aspiration and difficult airway management. However, these concerns are not supported by evidence, and routine RSI use is not required. Suxamethonium-associated fasciculations will also increase oxygen consumption and result in a shortened apnoea time. Morbidly obese patients have increased pseudocholinesterase activity and a larger immediate distribution volume. Dosing based on 1 mg kg^{-1} TBW provides better tracheal intubating conditions than dose by ideal or lean body weight.

Non-depolarising neuromuscular blocking agents

There is no evidence that any one neuromuscular blocking agent (NMBA) is better than another for use in the obese patient. The presence of a quaternary ammonium group makes non-depolarising NMBAs highly ionised and generally less lipophilic; this limits their distribution to extracellular fluid. Dosing by TBW leads to a prolonged duration of action; LBW dosing allows for more predictable offset.

Sugammadex

Sugammadex provides the ability to rapidly reverse rocuronium and vecuronium and return full neuromuscular function. The availability of this agent may direct the choice of agent administered. Data suggest that a dose based on ABW is acceptable.

Approach to anaesthesia for obese patients

No anaesthetic technique has been found to be safer or to provide better outcomes for obese patients. Optimisation of medical conditions early in the preoperative period will facilitate a smooth perioperative period. Short-acting, easily reversible agents should be administered to facilitate rapid reversal of anaesthesia, return of airway reflexes and early mobilisation. Long-acting opioids should be avoided because of risks of adverse respiratory events, in particular in those with OSA. Regional anaesthesia has been proposed as a safer alternative to general anaesthesia. However, even with ultrasound guidance, regional techniques can be technically challenging, and failure is more common. Surgery itself is a physiological stressor, so it is incorrect and illogical to assume that regional anaesthesia will prevent perioperative complications.

Notable anaesthetic considerations include the following:
- Always perform the chosen anaesthetic technique in the operating room.
- Invasive monitoring is not routinely required.
- Placement of a non-invasive blood pressure cuff on the forearm will provide reliable readings.
- Two i.v. cannulae should be inserted as standard.
- Always plan for postoperative care and have a plan B.

Guidance for anaesthetists has been provided by the Society for Obesity and Bariatric Anaesthesia in the form of the single-sheet guide (http://www.sobauk.co.uk/downloads/single-sheet-guideline).

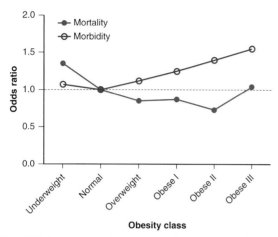

Fig. 32.9 Relationship of obesity class to morbidity and mortality. (Adapted from Mullen, J.T., Moorman, D.W., & Davenport, D.L. (2009) The obesity paradox: Body mass index and outcomes in patients undergoing non-bariatric general surgery. *Annals of Surgery.* 250(1), 166–172.)

Perioperative risk in obesity

Traditionally, obesity is considered a perioperative risk. Evidence demonstrates that this is not the case (Fig. 32.9). Morbidity does prolong operative time and increases the risks of bleeding, venous thromboembolic disease and wound infection. These do not translate into 'serious' morbidity. Mortality after non-bariatric surgery in the overweight and moderately obese patient is paradoxically lower than that of normal-weight individuals (up to a BMI of 45–50) and only then equates to that of ideal-weight individuals. This effect is known as the obesity paradox. The reasons for this paradox may lie partly in the limitations of BMI as a measure of the dangerous central obesity pattern. However, when obesity is assessed by waist circumference and in the presence of the associated metabolic syndrome, perioperative mortality is increased.

Bariatric operations

Dietary measures alone are an ineffective solution to weight loss. Weight-loss surgery encompasses a number of techniques. Some simply restrict the passage of food and create a feeling of gastric fullness; more complicated procedures provide hormonal effects on comorbidity such as diabetes.

Gastric banding

Gastric banding is a restrictive technique. The band restricts the passage of food moving through the oesophagogastric

junction and causes early dilation and stretch of the junction. The stretching of this area sends inhibitory signals to the thalamic satiety centre, inhibiting appetite. At surgery a tract is formed by blunt dissection around the top of the stomach and an inflatable silicone strip is inserted and fixed to form a ring around the fundus. A port site is inserted underneath the skin and attached to the band by tube. Transcutaneous inflation of the band with saline through the port adjusts the degree of restriction to eating and the speed of weight loss can be controlled effectively.

Sleeve gastrectomy

Sleeve gastrectomy achieves approximately 50% loss of excess weight. The operation involves the surgical removal of the greater curve of the stomach, including the fundus. Effects on appetite through stretch of the oesophagogastric junction at low volumes is similar to that of gastric banding. However, there are additional hormonal effects. The removal of 75% of the stomach causes a reduced ghrelin concentration (a hormone that stimulates appetite in the hypothalamus). Reduced ghrelin concentrations shift the arcuate signal balance towards anorexia and increased metabolism.

Malabsorptive procedures

In malabsorptive types of surgery a restrictive 25-ml stomach pouch is formed. Food is diverted away from the pancreas, biliary tree and duodenum mixing with the digestive juices about 100 cm distal to the duodenum. There is thus a short common limb before the colon. The most common of these procedures is a Roux-en-Y gastric bypass. Improvement and resolution of comorbid conditions such as type 2 diabetes and hypertension occur much faster and more often than would simply occur with the expected 70% excess weight loss.

Postoperative care of the bariatric surgery patient

The UK National Bariatric Surgical Register reveals that between 2012–2016, 20 534 bariatric operations were undertaken, with an overall mortality of 0.056% and morbidity of 2.9%. Common complications include infection (wound and urine) and venous thromboembolic disease. Complications associated with the surgical procedure include:
- band slippage, erosion or infection;
- perforation (early and late);
- fistula formation;
- internal hernia; and
- stomal ulceration and bleeding.

Patients who undergo weight-loss surgery must agree to lifelong follow-up. They receive continuing dietetic advice and dietary supplementation. Patients outside follow-up programmes have higher risks of failed weight loss, dietary difficulty and complications.

Management of patients presenting post–bariatric surgery

When dealing with a patient who has undergone bariatric surgery presenting for other surgery, the following points should be considered.

- A careful history should be taken, including information about the procedure performed, follow-up arrangements and weight history.

- Gastric band deflation is not recommended for the perioperative period.
- Care should be taken with oral medication administration in those with malabsorptive procedures.
- Patients with a gastric band are at increased risk of pulmonary aspiration as a result of oesophageal dilatation; this risk persists even with prolonged starvation. Routine RSI with cricoid pressure and tracheal intubation is recommended.
- When concerns are identified, communication with the parent bariatric surgical team is mandatory.

References/Further reading

Chung, F., Nagappa, M., Singh, M., et al., 2016. CPAP in the peri-operative setting: evidence of support. Chest 149 (2), 586–597.

De Baerdemaeker, L., Margarson, M., 2016. Best anaesthetic drug strategy for morbidly obese patients. Curr. Opin. Anaesthesiol. 29 (1), 119–128.

Nightingale, C.E., Margarson, M.P., Shearer, E., et al. Peri-operative management of the obese surgical patient 2015. Guidelines by The Association of Anaesthetists of Great Britain and Ireland and The Society for Obesity and Bariatric Anaesthesia.

Tzimas, P., Petrou, A., et al., 2015. Impact of metabolic syndrome in surgical patients: should we bother? Br. J. Anaesth. 115 (2), 194–202.

Chapter | **33** |

Paediatric anaesthesia

James Ip, Isabeau Walker, Mark Thomas

The delivery of safe paediatric anaesthesia requires an appreciation of the anatomical and physiological characteristics of children at various stages of development, ranging from neonates younger than 44 weeks postconceptional age to infants 1–12 months old to children and young people. Anaesthetic risk is inversely related to age and ASA status with the highest risk in younger, smaller patients. In general terms immature (or impaired) organ systems result in reduced physiological reserve and thus a reduced ability to tolerate the various challenges of anaesthesia and surgery.

This chapter summarises basic sciences relevant to paediatric anaesthesia (organised by physiological system) and provides an overview of the practical conduct of paediatric anaesthesia. The reader is referred to the relevant specialty chapters for management of specific conditions (e.g. bleeding after tonsillectomy is discussed in Chapter 37). Some of the more common conditions affecting neonates are discussed in this chapter, as well as a brief consideration of child protection procedures.

Anatomy and physiology

Respiratory system

Anatomy

Several features distinguish the upper airway anatomy of neonates and infants from that of older children and adults. During normal tidal breathing, the relatively larger tongue tends to occlude the oral cavity by pressing against the soft palate, hence the preference of neonates and young infants for nasal breathing (sometimes termed obligate nasal breathing). This explains their vulnerability to airway obstruction by nasal secretions, oedema, choanal atresia or nasal cannulae. Under anaesthesia and after loss of pharyngeal tone the large tongue tends to obstruct the oropharynx; this is exacerbated by the head being relatively large with a prominent occiput, which encourages head flexion. The larynx is anterior and cephalad (at the level of C3–4 as opposed to C5–6 in adults), and the epiglottis long and U-shaped. The epiglottis may obscure the laryngeal inlet if the tip of a laryngoscope blade is placed in the vallecula using the standard adult technique. In neonates and infants a straight laryngoscope blade often provides a better view of the larynx than a curved blade and can also be used to lift the epiglottis by applying the tip of the blade to the posterior surface of the epiglottis. The trachea is shorter in absolute terms than in older children (~4 cm in a term neonate), with the main bronchi arising at equal angles; inadvertent endobronchial intubation occurs easily and may affect either side.

The cricoid cartilage is the functionally narrowest part of the upper airway up to 8–10 years of age (as opposed to the glottis in adults), and the mucosa in the subglottic region is vulnerable to pressure injury from a tracheal tube. The narrow lumen means that a small amount of mucosal oedema that would be trivial in an adult can cause significant obstruction after tracheal extubation in a small infant. For this reason, uncuffed tracheal tubes with a small leak at 20 cmH_2O airway pressure have been used traditionally in neonates and infants. However, low-pressure, high-volume tracheal tubes have been specifically designed for children of all ages and are increasingly used, particularly for patients with pathological conditions of the lung who require higher ventilation pressures.

The narrow, high-resistance airway is combined with less efficient respiratory mechanics; the horizontal arrangement of the ribs precludes their adult function of increasing the anteroposterior and transverse diameters of the thorax (the so-called pump-handle and bucket-handle movements, respectively). Respiration is therefore largely dependent on the diaphragm, which in children is both less efficient (because of its horizontal attachment) and more prone to fatigue (because of a lower proportion of type 1 muscle fibres until ~8 months of age). Inadvertent distension of the stomach after face-mask ventilation will further impair diaphragmatic excursion. Neonates and infants are thus at risk for respiratory fatigue.

Physiology

Basal oxygen consumption in neonates and young infants is twice that of adults (6–7 ml kg^{-1} min^{-1} vs. 3 ml kg^{-1} min^{-1}) because of the metabolic requirements of growth and temperature homeostasis (the latter as a result of the increased surface area/body mass ratio). To meet this need, alveolar minute ventilation is increased, which is in turn achieved by increasing respiratory rate (respiratory rate is 30–40 breaths min^{-1} in the neonate), as tidal volumes are relatively fixed (7–8 ml kg^{-1}). Higher oxygen consumption contributes to the shorter time to arterial desaturation during apnoea in neonates and infants (e.g. during tracheal intubation).

Increased alveolar minute ventilation results in more rapid uptake (and washout) of inhalational anaesthetic agents during spontaneous ventilation, with faster equilibration between alveolar and brain partial pressures. Apnoea and hypotension can occur readily if high inspired fractions of volatile agents are administered for an extended period.

Neonates and infants are at risk for atelectasis and ventilation-perfusion mismatch. Small airway closure occurs readily under anaesthesia because of a reduced functional residual capacity (FRC) (caused by increased chest wall compliance) combined with a higher closing volume (as a result of reduced elasticity of the lung parenchyma). Application of PEEP helps maintain alveolar recruitment and gas exchange.

Control of breathing is immature in the neonate, with the response to hypoxia reflecting the normal response to low oxygen tension *in utero*. Instead of increasing respiratory drive, hypoxia can provoke bradypnoeic or apnoeic episodes, particularly after general anaesthesia or administration of opioids. This is further exacerbated by a blunted response to hypercarbia. Term neonates are classically considered at risk for postoperative apnoeas up to 1 month of age, with premature neonates at risk up to 60 weeks postconceptional age (5 months corrected age).

The overall picture then is of increased basal oxygen requirements combined with increased work of breathing, reduced efficiency and an impaired response to derangements in blood gas tensions; it is not surprising therefore that neonates and infants are particularly vulnerable to respiratory failure, including in the perioperative period.

Cardiovascular system

Fetal circulation and cardiorespiratory changes at birth

The fetal circulation features several adaptations to the intrauterine environment that preferentially deliver oxygenated blood from the placenta to the developing brain (Fig. 33.1). Significant physiological changes occur at and soon after birth, allowing a transition to the normal adult circulation; an understanding of these processes is fundamental to providing safe anaesthesia for neonates.

In utero

- Oxygenated blood returns from the placenta via the single umbilical vein, passing to the inferior vena cava (IVC). A proportion of this bypasses the liver via the ductus venosus.
- The Eustachian valve lies at the junction of the IVC and right atrium and streams this oxygenated blood across the foramen ovale to the left atrium.
- Oxygen-rich blood then passes via the left ventricle to the ascending aorta and to the brain.
- In contrast, desaturated venous blood from the head and neck returns to the heart via the superior vena cava (SVC); this passes to the right atrium, right ventricle and pulmonary artery.
- Approximately 90% of the right ventricular output is directed via the ductus arteriosus to the descending aorta because of the high pulmonary vascular resistance (PVR) of the non-aerated lungs.
- In this way, relatively oxygenated blood is conserved for the developing brain and coronary circulation, with less oxygenated blood delivered to the rest of the body.
- Fetal haemoglobin (HbF) has a low P50 (see Chapter 10) to reflect the relatively low oxygen tension in utero and to facilitate oxygen uptake at the fetal side of the placenta (Fig. 33.2). However, this is at the cost of HbF being poorer at releasing oxygen to the tissues; to allow adequate tissue oxygen delivery to occur a higher haemoglobin concentration is needed, typically up to 200 g L^{-1} (see later).
- Deoxygenated blood returns to the placenta via the paired umbilical arteries (each arising from the internal iliac arteries).

At birth

- Placental blood flow ceases and systemic vascular resistance (SVR) increases.
- At the same time PVR falls rapidly because of expansion of the lungs, increased oxygen tension and increase in nitric oxide and prostacyclin concentrations.
- As a result, pulmonary perfusion increases dramatically, right-sided heart pressures fall and left-sided heart

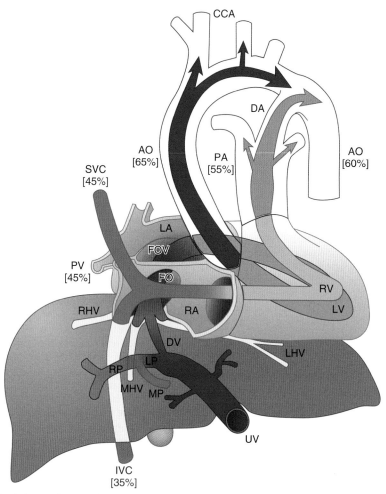

Fig. 33.1 The fetal circulation. Pathways of the fetal heart and representative oxygen saturation values (in brackets). The *via sinistra* (red) directs well-oxygenated blood from the umbilical vein (UV) through the ductus venosus (DV) (or left half of the liver) across the inferior vena cava (IVC), through the foramen ovale (FO), left atrium (LA) and ventricle (LV) and up the ascending aorta (AO) to reach the descending AO through the isthmus aortae. De-oxygenated blood from the superior vena cava (SVC) and IVC forms the *via dextra* (blue) through the right atrium (RA) and ventricle (RV), pulmonary trunk (PA) and ductus arteriosus (DA). *CCA,* Common carotid arteries; *FOV,* foramen ovale valve; *LHV,* left hepatic vein; *LP,* left portal branch; *MHV,* medial hepatic vein; *MP,* portal main stem; *PV,* pulmonary vein; *RHV,* right hepatic vein; *RP,* right portal branch.

pressures increase, which results in closure of the flap valve over the foramen ovale.

- After the initial rapid fall at birth the PVR continues to decline more slowly to reach adult values by 4–6 weeks of age.
- The ductus arteriosus starts to constrict after birth as a result of oxygen-mediated vasoconstriction and metabolism of prostaglandins that maintain ductal patency in utero.

- There is usually no right-to-left shunting across the duct by about day 2 of life in healthy infants, with anatomical closure as a result of intimal fibrosis within 2–3 weeks. Importantly, functional closure of the arterial duct is reversible in the first weeks of life, and neonates may revert to a persistent fetal circulation if the PVR remains high (e.g. because of hypoxia, acidosis, meconium aspiration, sepsis or congenital diaphragmatic hernia), with right-to-left shunting across the ductus arteriosus and reduced pulmonary

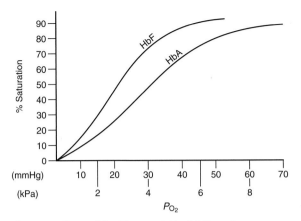

Fig. 33.2 Effects of fetal haemoglobin (HbF) on the oxygen dissociation curve. *HbA*, Adult haemoglobin; *PO₂*, partial pressure of oxygen.

Table 33.1 Normal cardiovascular variables

	Neonate	Child	Adult
Heart rate (beats min⁻¹)	120–200	80–120	50–90
Systolic blood pressure (mmHg)	50–90	95–110	90–140
Diastolic blood pressure (mmHg)	25–50	55–70	60–90
Cardiac output (ml kg⁻¹ min⁻¹)	200–250	100–150	80–100

blood flow. This is termed persistent pulmonary hypertension of the newborn and is demonstrated by the presence of differential cyanosis, with lower oxygen saturations in the lower limbs (postductal) than right upper limb (preductal). This is the basis of oxygen saturation screening for congenital heart disease in newborns.

In some congenital cardiac lesions, continued ductal patency may be required for survival, to allow blood flow to either systemic circulation (e.g. in severe aortic coarctation) or pulmonary circulation (e.g. in pulmonary atresia). A prostaglandin infusion may be required to keep the arterial duct open in these duct-dependent circulations until a more definitive intervention can be performed.

Neonatal and infant circulation

Increased physiological demands combined with reduced reserve seen in the developing respiratory system is mirrored in the cardiovascular system. Oxygen delivery to the tissues is less efficient as 75%–80% of haemoglobin is HbF, which has a higher affinity for oxygen than adult haemoglobin (HbA, HbA₂) at the higher oxygen tensions seen after birth. To compensate for this, haemoglobin concentration is higher in neonates compared with older children (Hb ~ 160 g L⁻¹ at term). The physiological anaemia of infancy occurs as concentrations of HbF fall and before adult concentrations of HbA/HbA₂ are reached. To meet the increased metabolic oxygen requirement for growth and development, the P50 for haemoglobin in neonates and young infants is higher than in adults, and cardiac output is also higher than in adults (200–250 ml kg⁻¹ min⁻¹ vs. 80 ml kg⁻¹ min⁻¹). The high resting cardiac output means that any further increase in demand is limited; by 2–3 months of life cardiac output falls to approximately 150 ml kg⁻¹ min⁻¹, allowing for increased cardiac reserve.

The immature myocardium has fewer contractile elements and is less compliant, resulting in limited preload and afterload reserve, and the stroke volume is relatively fixed. The consequence of this is that any increase in cardiac output is largely achieved by increased heart rate. Conversely, bradycardia (which may occur in response to hypoxia or vagal stimulation) is poorly tolerated in neonates and infants, and cardiac compressions are recommended if the rate falls to less than 60 beats min⁻¹. Normal arterial blood pressure is lower in neonates and infants than older children because of lower resistance presented by the rich systemic vascular beds (Table 33.1).

Central nervous system

Several features of the developing nervous system are of relevance to the anaesthetist. The neonatal blood–brain barrier is anatomically and functionally incomplete; this contributes to increased sensitivity to opioids and other sedatives, as well as to increased vulnerability to local anaesthetic toxicity.

At birth the brain occupies a much larger proportion of total body weight than in the adult (10%–15% vs. 2%). The cerebral metabolic requirement for oxygen (CMRO₂) is also higher (~5 ml 100 g⁻¹ min⁻¹ vs. 3.5 ml 100 g⁻¹ min⁻¹). Autoregulation of blood flow is present at term; however, preterm neonates are vulnerable to changes in blood pressure causing intracranial haemorrhage, particularly affecting the periventricular germinal matrix.

The spinal cord in the fetus initially occupies the entire length of the spinal canal, the termination subsequently moving cranially because of differential growth of the spine and spinal cord. The spinal cord terminates at S1 at 28 weeks gestation, L3 at term, and L1–2 by early adolescence. The sacral hiatus is relatively large in the infant and child and is not ossified, hence allowing ease of access to the epidural space via the caudal route. Furthermore, the epidural fat is less densely packed than in adults, which facilitates spread of local anaesthetic injected into the caudal space to the thoracic region.

The long-term effect of exposure to anaesthetic drugs in infancy and early childhood is an area of active research. Neurotoxicity with persistent cognitive deficit has been demonstrated after exposure to anaesthetic agents in animal studies, but the clinical significance of this in humans is unknown. Initial data from prospective randomised trials suggest that a single short general anaesthetic in infancy has no impact on early cognitive development. At present there is insufficient evidence to alter current anaesthetic and surgical practice, although deferral of non-urgent procedures requiring general anaesthesia (e.g. cosmetic procedures, non-urgent imaging) to older than 3 years of age has been suggested.

Liver function and drug metabolism

Liver function is immature at birth, and hepatic phase I and II processes (except for sulphation) are not fully functional. Immature glucuronidation combined with high red cell turnover in neonates may lead to kernicterus if unconjugated hyperbilirubinaemia is left untreated. Hepatic metabolism and clearance of drugs is reduced, and drugs cleared by this means have a longer duration of effect. Hepatic function accelerates rapidly after birth, reaching adult levels by 2–3 months in normal infants. Relevant examples include morphine and the aminosteroid non-depolarising neuromuscular blocking agents (NMBAs), such as vecuronium and rocuronium. A single dose of these drugs in neonates and young infants will have longer duration of action than in older children because of reduced clearance.

Hepatic synthetic function is also immature in neonates. Vitamin K–dependent clotting factors (II, VII, IX and X) are deficient at birth, and all neonates should receive vitamin K at or soon after delivery. Reduced glycogen stores and impaired gluconeogenesis (combined with a high metabolic rate) increase vulnerability to hypoglycaemia, particularly during starvation. Lower plasma protein concentrations (e.g. albumin and α_1-acid glycoprotein) result in reduced protein binding of drugs (e.g. morphine, lidocaine and bupivacaine) and therefore higher proportion of free drug and increased risk of drug toxicity.

Renal function

Renal blood flow is low in the neonatal period (because of high renal vascular resistance), rising from about 6% of cardiac output to the adult level of approximately 20% by age 1 month. Antidiuretic hormone (ADH) concentrations are high at birth, resulting in low urine output and fluid requirements. A significant diuresis occurs as ADH concentrations fall during the first week of life, and fluid requirements rise. For this reason maintenance i.v. fluids should be

Table 33.2 Neonatal fluid requirements immediately after birth

	Daily fluid requirement (ml kg^{-1})
Day 1 of life	50–60
Day 2	70–80
Day 3	80–100
Day 4	100–120

restricted in the first few days of life until the postnatal diuresis has occurred (Table 33.2).

Although nephrogenesis is complete by 34 weeks gestation, both tubular excretory and concentrating ability are limited in the first few weeks of life. Neonates do not tolerate dehydration, fluid loading and electrolyte or acid–base derangements well. They are particularly at risk for acute kidney injury, hyponatraemia and metabolic acidosis.

Temperature regulation

Thermal homeostasis is immature in neonates and small children, and hypothermia is a particular risk during anaesthesia. Heat losses are high because of increased surface area/body mass ratio, insensible evaporative losses via the respiratory tract and thermal conductance. Compensatory mechanisms such as shivering and vasoconstrictive responses are less effective in neonates and only partially compensated for by non-shivering thermogenesis (metabolism of adipose tissue around the base of the neck, scapulae and back). This situation is reflected in the differing thermoneutral temperature for neonates and adults, the ambient temperature at which metabolic expenditure is minimal – 34°C for a preterm neonate, 32°C for a term neonate and 28°C for an adult.

Conduct of anaesthesia

Preoperative assessment

As with adult practice (see Chapter 19) the goals of preoperative assessment in children include obtaining relevant history and clinical data to anticipate anaesthetic complications (e.g. difficult tracheal intubation), assess the risk of anaesthesia and surgery and inform the appropriate anaesthetic and perioperative plan. In addition, it is important to establish rapport with the patient and parents, to obtain consent for anaesthesia and to agree on a mode of induction; clear and honest communication is crucial, as is providing appropriate reassurance. Where possible, children should be involved in these discussions (see Chapter 21).

History and examination should include assessment of:

- *problems with previous anaesthetics* (e.g. anxiety, nausea and vomiting, airway difficulties).
- *prematurity and its consequences* (e.g. gestational age at birth and current corrected age, previous need for invasive ventilation and evidence of ongoing lung disease). Apnoea monitoring and pulse oximetry are recommended for 24 h after surgery in preterm neonates younger than 60 weeks postconceptual age.
- *respiratory morbidity* (e.g. asthma, including severity and current status; obstructive sleep apnoea; and active upper respiratory tract infection, or URTI).
  - The last of these is a common dilemma for anaesthetists, particularly in elective surgery. On the one hand, perioperative respiratory complications (e.g. laryngospasm, bronchospasm, desaturation or airway obstruction) are more common in children with active symptoms or within 2 weeks of a URTI. On the other hand, mild URTIs are extremely common (and may also be part of the underlying surgical pathophysiology), and deferring surgery until a child is symptom-free may be not be feasible. In practice, minor elective surgery may usually proceed if there are only mild coryzal symptoms without systemic features (e.g. fever, anorexia, difficulty sleeping) or signs of lower respiratory tract infection (e.g. tachypnoea, inspiratory crepitations, purulent sputum). It is sensible to avoid airway surgery in a child with an active URTI. However, these are often not straightforward decisions, and a discussion with the parents, with senior anaesthetic and surgical input, is essential. If you proceed with surgery in a child with airway symptoms the risk of airway complications is lower with i.v. induction of anaesthesia, using inhalational agents for maintenance, use of a face mask rather than tracheal intubation and in the presence of a more experienced anaesthetist. If surgery is deferred because of a URTI the consensus for the minimum period of deferral is 2–4 weeks.
- *cardiovascular morbidity*, particularly high-risk cardiac conditions requiring expert management in a specialist centre, such as cardiomyopathy, pulmonary hypertension, single ventricle circulations and ventricular outflow tract obstruction (left or right). Detection of a previously undiagnosed heart murmur during preassessment is relatively common; in most cases the murmur is innocent, but in some it may indicate significant disease requiring specialist management before surgery. Features suggestive of a significant lesion include signs and symptoms of heart failure, such as failure to thrive; dyspnoea, tachypnoea or diaphoresis during exertion or feeding; recurrent respiratory tract infections; unexplained collapse;

or cyanosis/cyanotic episodes. The index of suspicion should be higher in those with a syndrome associated with cardiac disease (e.g. Down's, DiGeorge's, CHARGE (*c*oloboma, *h*eart defect, *a*tresia choanae, *r*estricted growth and development, *g*enital abnormality and *e*ar abnormality) and VACTERL (*v*ertebral defects, *a*nal atresia, *c*ardiac defects, *t*racheo-oesophageal fistula, *r*enal anomalies and *l*imb abnormalities) associations). Although most congenital cardiac disease is detected before 3 months of age, all infants (<1 year old) with a newly detected murmur should be referred to a paediatric cardiologist for assessment before surgery if possible as significant lesions may be asymptomatic in this age group. An older child who is asymptomatic but has an abnormal 12-lead ECG (e.g. with evidence of left ventricular hypertrophy) should also be referred before surgery. Defer investigation of other children with a murmur until after surgery.

- *other comorbidity, drug history and allergies.* Exacerbation of asthma with NSAIDs is very rare in children, but a history of safe NSAID use is usually sought and documented before prescribing them.
- *family history* of relevant inherited disorders (e.g. plasma cholinesterase deficiency, malignant hyperpyrexia, sickle-cell disease). Children born in the UK are routinely screened for sickle-cell disease at birth.
- *airway assessment.* Clinical features associated with difficult airway management (e.g. micrognathia/retrognathia, reduced mouth opening and thyromental distance) or specific syndromes (e.g. Pierre Robin, Crouzon, Treacher Collins, Down's).
- *weight.* An accurate measure should be obtained to guide drug dosing and fluid management. If this is not possible, weight may be estimated using the formulae in Table 33.3.

Investigations

Most healthy children undergoing minor surgery do not require routine preoperative investigations. For those at risk

Table 33.3 Formulae for estimating children's weights

Age	Estimated weight (kg)
<1 month	~3 kg
1–12 months	(0.5 × age in months) + 4
1–5 years	(2 × age in years) + 8
6–12 years	(3 × age in years) + 7
>12 years	Highly variable

of undiagnosed sickle cell disease (particularly those of African, Mediterranean or Middle Eastern descent), a rapid Sickledex screening test may be performed in children older than 6 months (high concentrations of HbF in infants younger than 6 months may lead to false-negative results); this does not differentiate between sickle-cell trait and disease. Children with a positive result and those younger than 6 months require formal haemoglobin electrophoresis to establish or quantify their disease. A full blood count is usually performed in children presenting for major surgery with the potential for significant bleeding; blood biochemistry may be indicated if the child has relevant comorbidity (e.g. renal or endocrine) or is acutely unwell (e.g. with vomiting or diarrhoea or receiving i.v. fluids).

Preoperative fasting

Similar fasting times to adult practice are used in paediatrics to minimise the risk of regurgitation and aspiration of gastric contents. These are:

- more than 6 h for food and formula milk;
- more than 4 h for breast milk (which has a shorter gastric transit time than formula milk); and
- 1–2 h for clear fluids.

Excessive fasting should be avoided as it increases discomfort, thirst and irritability for the child; is distressing for parents; and may make i.v. cannulation more difficult. Neonates are at risk of hypoglycaemia, and i.v. maintenance fluids containing 10% glucose with 0.45% sodium chloride and 0.15% potassium chloride may be required during preoperative fasting.

Premedication

An important part of the preoperative visit is to agree to a plan for induction of anaesthesia and to identify children who may benefit from anxiolytic or sedative premedication. The latter can be difficult to achieve; not uncommonly children who appear cooperative and cheerful during preassessment can become extremely anxious and uncooperative in the anaesthetic room. Benzodiazepines are commonly used, such as oral midazolam (0.5 mg kg^{-1} up to 20 mg p.o.) and temazepam (10–20 mg p.o. in children aged 12–18 years). Buccal midazolam has the advantages of faster onset (~10 min vs. ~30 min) and smaller drug volume (0.2–0.3 mg kg^{-1} buccal up to 5 mg if <10 years old and 6–7 mg if >10 years old). Alternatives are ketamine (p.o. or, rarely, i.m.) and intranasal dexmedetomidine. In addition to drugs, interventions by play specialists and clinical psychologists may help to reduce anxiety in the anaesthetic room, but this approach may not always be available.

Other potential premedication agents include antisialagogues/vagolytics (e.g. glycopyrronium bromide, atropine), which may be useful in airway surgery, or analgesics (e.g. paracetamol, ibuprofen). Topical local anaesthetics should be used if i.v. induction is planned. Options include tetracaine 4% gel (Ametop), which is effective within 30–45 min and lasts 4–6 h, or eutectic mixture of local anaesthetic (EMLA), a mixture of lidocaine (2.5%) and procaine (2.5%), which requires 1–2 h to be effective, with a duration of action of 2–4 h.

Induction of anaesthesia

All the usual safety precautions should be completed before induction of anaesthesia (see Chapters 18 and 22).

A calm induction is the aim, whether administered via i.v., inhalational or (rarely) i.m. routes. Developmentally appropriate interaction and distraction techniques should be used; toys, books and electronic devices (e.g. tablets, smartphones) are often useful adjuncts. Parental presence in the anaesthetic room helps alleviate the child's anxiety, but parents should be warned of what to expect (e.g. excitation phenomena during inhalational induction, loss of motor tone after i.v. induction). Infants and toddlers are often anaesthetised sitting on a parent's lap. Older children may exhibit varying degrees of resistance to intervention. Demonstration of the loss of sensation to cold may help boost confidence that topical local anaesthetics are working, or use of a scented face mask with nitrous oxide may improve acceptability of inhalational induction (see later). Forcible restraint of an uncooperative or cognitively impaired child should be avoided as this risks lasting psychological harm. In general it is sensible to adopt a friendly non-confrontational approach, to involve parents to provide comfort or distraction and to avoid negative suggestions. Very rarely, physical constraint may be necessary (e.g. when urgent treatment is required to prevent significant harm).

Intravenous induction offers theoretical safety advantages: It allows rapid transition through the excitation phase of anaesthesia (during which the child is vulnerable to breath holding and laryngospasm) and having venous access in place before induction allows fluids, emergency drugs and NMBAs to be given immediately if required. However, in patients with difficult veins or extreme anxiety around cannulation this may not be feasible, and inhalational induction is routinely used. As already mentioned, inhalational induction is faster in babies and small children than adults because of the relatively higher alveolar minute ventilation. Sevoflurane is most commonly used because of its combination of a low blood/gas partition coefficient and non-irritant properties (see Chapter 3). The addition of nitrous oxide speeds up induction via the second gas effect (see Chapter 3). Nitrous oxide also has the advantage of being odourless; allowing a child to breathe only nitrous oxide and oxygen for a few seconds before slowly introducing sevoflurane may be better tolerated than starting at a high concentration of volatile agent, particularly with older children. Care must be taken not to stimulate the child with venous cannulation, airway instrumentation or an over-vigorous jaw thrust until adequate depth of anaesthesia has been achieved as this may provoke laryngospasm, particularly during the excitation phase of anaesthesia.

Propofol is the most common i.v. induction agent used, although injection may be quite painful. Cannulation of a larger vein (e.g. at the antecubital fossa rather than dorsum of the hand) and addition of 1% lidocaine have been shown to mitigate this. Unpremedicated children typically require higher doses of propofol than adults (e.g. 3–5 mg kg^{-1}), and coinduction with an opioid (e.g. fentanyl) is usual. Ketamine (1–2 mg kg^{-1} i.v.) provides haemodynamic stability in patients with reduced cardiovascular reserve (e.g. in acute hypovolaemia, cardiomyopathy). Etomidate (0.3 mg kg^{-1} i.v.) may be used as an alternative, with coinduction with fentanyl and/or benzodiazepine (e.g. midazolam).

The place of the traditional RSI in children (see Chapter 23) is controversial, in part because of the practical difficulties associated with RSI in this population. For example, venous cannulation may not be possible, and inhalational induction may be necessary. Effective preoxygenation may be difficult to achieve and only provides a short apnoea time in small children because of their higher oxygen consumption to FRC ratio. Finally the value of cricoid force is unclear, given the propensity for cricoid pressure to make laryngoscopy and tracheal intubation more difficult. For these reasons many advocate a modified or controlled RSI, involving gentle face-mask ventilation while waiting for the NMBA to take effect. Gentle cricoid force may be applied, but most apply a low threshold for removing it if it appears to impair laryngoscopy.

Airway and ventilation management

As mentioned younger children are at risk for upper airway obstruction under anaesthesia, and an appropriately sized oropharyngeal airway is often useful after induction and during emergence. The stomach is easily insufflated during face-mask ventilation; in neonates and infants this can cause significant diaphragmatic splinting and difficulty in ventilation. A nasogastric tube should always be available to decompress the stomach if needed.

Equipment dead space and resistance should be minimised in the anaesthetic breathing system. In the UK the Ayre's T-piece (Mapleson-E system) with the Jackson Rees modification (Mapleson-F) is widely used in children weighing less than 25 kg (see Chapter 15). This has the benefit of low resistance to spontaneous ventilation, and the open-ended bag can be used to provide a variable amount of CPAP or positive pressure ventilation; during the latter, it provides immediate tactile information reflecting changes in lung compliance or airway resistance. A disadvantage of the Mapleson-F system is that it requires high gas flow rates to prevent rebreathing during spontaneous ventila-tion: 2.5–3 times the alveolar minute volume, equating to 300–400 ml kg^{-1} min^{-1}, with a minimum of flow of 4 L min^{-1}. It is much more efficient during positive pressure ventilation, requiring a flow rate of 1000 ml plus 100 ml kg^{-1} min^{-1} to prevent rebreathing. As there is no pressure-limiting valve in the system care must be taken not to completely occlude the end of the bag; airway pressure may build up to dangerous levels, causing barotrauma. The open-ended bag also makes it difficult to scavenge inhalational anaesthetic agent.

Appropriately sized laryngoscope blades are used, with straight blades typically used in children younger than 1 year, for reasons discussed earlier. Five blade sizes are commonly available for different age groups: neonates/small infant, 0; infant, 1; child, 2; adult, 3; large adult, 4. A wide range of tracheal tubes are available, and various formulae/ranges have been suggested as a guide to sizing and appropriate depth of insertion (Table 33.4). Uncuffed tracheal tubes have traditionally been used in children younger than 7–8 years old, but high-volume, low-pressure tracheal tubes are increasingly being used in children of all ages, particularly in situations requiring higher ventilation pressures (e.g. during laparoscopic surgery or in patients with parenchymal lung disease). Other potential advantages of cuffed tracheal tubes include reduced trauma from repeated laryngoscopy when selecting the correct tube size, greater protection against aspiration of gastric contents and secretions, and more accurate capnography/nasopharyngeal temperature

Table 33.4 Uncuffed tracheal tube size and length estimations according to age

Age	Internal diameter (mm)	Length oral (cm)	Length nasal (cm)
Neonate (3 kg)	3.0–3.5	9–10	11–12
6 months	4.0	11–12	13
1 year	4.5	13	15
>1 year	(Age in years / 4) + 4	(Age in years / 2) + 12	(Age in years / 2) + 15

measurement. If using a cuffed tracheal tube, it is essential that cuff pressure is monitored regularly and is not allowed to exceed 20 cmH_2O. An important disadvantage of a cuffed paediatric tracheal tube is the reduced internal diameter compared with an uncuffed tracheal tube of equivalent external diameter; the reduced airway calibre may impede effective ventilation and suctioning of airway secretions.

Paediatric tracheal tube introducers (bougies) and malleable stylets are widely used to aid tracheal intubation in children as the laryngeal inlet is often more anteriorly placed than in adults. These adjuncts must be used carefully to avoid tracheobronchial trauma, and malleable stylets should not protrude beyond the tip of the tracheal tube. Tracheal tubes are routinely secured with tape in infants and children rather than the ribbon ties used in adults. Nasal tracheal intubation is often preferred in young children and infants who will remain intubated postoperatively, as nasal tracheal tubes are usually more secure and better tolerated by the child during weaning from ventilation. It is essential to avoid pressure on the nares as this can result in damage to the nasal cartilage and unsightly scarring.

If tracheal intubation is not required the airway may be maintained using a supraglottic airway device (SAD) with either spontaneous or positive pressure ventilation. A wide range of SADs are available in paediatric sizes, determined according to body weight (Table 33.5). Although in theory size 1 SADs may be used for infants weighing less than 5 kg, in practice their propensity for displacement means that their use is reserved for the shortest of procedures or as part of management of the difficult airway or resuscitation. It is important to note that in SADs with inflatable cuffs, inflation to the maximum cuff volume stated by the manufacturer may lead to cuff pressures that exceed the maximum recommended pressure (60 cmH_2O), increasing the risk of mucosal injury and airway morbidity. As with cuffed tracheal tubes, it is best practice to inflate the laryngeal mask cuff in small increments to the lowest volume required to achieve an adequate seal and to measure cuff pressure using an appropriately sensitive manometer.

Table 33.5 Estimated sizes for supraglottic airway devices (SAD) and oropharyngeal airways

Weight (kg)	SAD size	Oropharyngeal airway size
<5	1	00
5–10	1½	0
10–20	2	0 or 1
20–30	2½	1
30–50	3	1 or 2

The approach to ventilatory support during anaesthesia varies according to indication and available equipment. In infants and small children, pressure-controlled ventilation (PCV) is traditionally used as it delivers a constant inspiratory pressure pattern while limiting peak pressure. In contrast, volume-controlled ventilation (VCV) modes may be difficult to use if there is a variable tracheal tube leak or high circuit compliance relative to the size of the child. More modern ventilators may offer a pressure-regulated volume-controlled mode (PRVC), which delivers a combination of the benefits of both standard modes. In spontaneously breathing patients (e.g. via a SAD) pressure support ventilation (PSV) may be useful to reduce the work of breathing. It is usual to provide PEEP of 4–5 cmH_2O to prevent small airway closure (thereby improving compliance and reducing atelectasis). Whichever ventilation strategy is used it is important to set appropriate maximum inspiratory limits to prevent barotrauma or volutrauma.

Intraoperative management

Intraoperative management in children follows similar general principles to adult practice.

Monitoring and temperature control

Usual essential monitoring is applied to all cases; specific adaptations are required for children, such as adhesive plaster pulse oximeter probes, neonatal ECG electrodes and paediatric blood pressure cuffs. Neonates and infants are at risk for bradycardia (heart rate < 100 beats min^{-1}) because of vagal stimulation and hypoxia; ECG monitoring may detect the latter earlier and more reliably than the pulse oximeter. Minimum monitoring devices are supplemented as indicated by clinical and operative factors. In all but the shortest cases, temperature (ideally core temperature via a nasopharyngeal or rectal probe) should be measured and active measures taken to prevent hypothermia, including raising the ambient temperature of the operating room. Commonly used warming devices include forced air warmers, heating mattresses and fluid warmers.

Maintenance

Maintenance of anaesthesia is via either inhalational or i.v. routes. Sevoflurane, isoflurane, desflurane and nitrous oxide are the inhalational agents most commonly used (see Chapter 3). Of note is that the minimal alveolar concentration (MAC) of the volatile agents varies with age during childhood, and this pattern of variation differs between agents. For example, the MAC of sevoflurane in neonates and young infants is 3.3% (vs. 2.1% in adults) and decreases to 2.5% in late infancy, reaching adult levels in adolescence. In contrast, the MAC of isoflurane is 1.6% in neonates, rising to a peak of 1.9% in young infants and then falling with increasing age. The physiological reasons for these variations are unclear.

Total intravenous anaesthesia techniques, typically using propofol and remifentanil, are well established in paediatric practice and are used particularly in children undergoing airway procedures, intracranial surgery (to control intracranial pressure) and spinal surgery (as volatile anaesthetic agents interfere with evoked potentials). Total intravenous anaesthesia is also indicated in those at risk of malignant hyperthermia and those with muscular dystrophy (because of the risk of volatile anaesthetic-induced rhabdomyolysis). Manual infusion regimens are commonly used, but syringe drivers programmed with target-controlled infusion (TCI) models derived from paediatric pharmacokinetic data (e.g. Paedfusor) are also widely available. These are discussed in detail in Chapter 4.

Neuromuscular blocking agents used in adult practice are also used in children, in similar doses on a per weight basis. Although the volume of distribution in neonates is larger, resulting in lower effective tissue concentrations for a given dose, the immature neuromuscular junction is more sensitive to the effects of NMBAs (because of lower acetylcholine concentrations). These factors seem to mitigate each other such that dosing does not change with age. However, as already mentioned, immature hepatic metabolic pathways in neonates result in a longer duration of action of aminosteroid NMBAs.

A balanced anaesthetic technique includes appropriate intraoperative analgesia usually extending into the postoperative period. The multimodal approach to analgesia advocated in adult anaesthesia remains applicable. Intravenous paracetamol should be considered for all, carefully observing appropriate dose reductions in smaller children. Inadvertent overdosing or double-dosing of i.v. paracetamol is a relatively common source of medication error in paediatrics. NSAIDs offer a useful synergistic analgesic effect with paracetamol and should be considered for all children outside the neonatal period. Similarly, use of local anaesthetic agents via regional or peripheral block or wound infiltration should be employed wherever possible. Finally, for procedures likely to cause moderate to severe pain, i.v. opioids are the mainstay of management; commonly used options include fentanyl, remifentanil and morphine.

Fluid management

Hypovolaemia is common in children who are acutely unwell and should be treated before surgery where possible. Fluid deficit is traditionally defined clinically as:

- *mild* (5% body weight loss equating to 50 ml kg^{-1} deficit): reduced skin turgor and dry mucus membranes;
- *moderate* (10% body weight loss and 100 ml kg^{-1} deficit): sunken fontanelle, tachycardia, lethargy; or
- *severe* (15% body weight loss and 150 ml kg^{-1} deficit): hypotension, shock, sunken eyes.

Mild dehydration may be corrected with oral fluids if time allows; moderate to severe hypovolaemia is treated with intravenous isotonic crystalloid solution. Hypotonic solutions (e.g. 5% glucose, or 5% dextrose 0.45% saline) should not be used as resuscitation fluid because of the risk of iatrogenic hyponatraemia (which may cause life-threatening encephalopathy). Intravenous resuscitation should be with an initial bolus of isotonic crystalloid 10–20 ml kg^{-1}, repeated according to response; the current consensus is that if more than 60 ml kg^{-1} of fluid is given, then the airway should be secured with a tracheal tube and inotropic support considered.

Caution is necessary in children with hyponatraemia or hypernatraemia as rapid correction of sodium imbalance may result in central pontine myelinolysis or cerebral oedema, respectively.

Maintenance i.v. fluid requirements are calculated according to the regimen described by Holliday and Segar, the '4, 2, 1' formula (Table 33.6). Maintenance fluid requirements in the intraoperative period are very low, and replacement fluid only is usually required (isotonic crystalloid or blood).

In routine elective surgery it is unusual to encounter significant dehydration unless the patient has been fasted excessively. Thus after induction of anaesthesia a 10–20 ml kg^{-1} bolus of a balanced salt solution (e.g. Hartmann's, Plasmalyte) is usually sufficient to replace the fasting deficit and manage the anaesthesia-induced vasodilatation and reduces the requirement to drink early, therefore reducing postoperative nausea and vomiting (PONV).

Intraoperative fluid replacement (e.g. because of evaporation during laparotomy) is traditionally estimated according to the type of surgery:

- Minor surgery: 1–2 ml kg^{-1} h^{-1}
- Moderate surgery: 2–5 ml kg^{-1} h^{-1}
- Major surgery with large fluid losses: 6–10 ml kg^{-1} h^{-1}

This is only an approximate guide, and in practice fluid replacement is usually administered via intermittent boluses of 10–15 ml kg^{-1} with close observation of clinical effect. Once more than 75 ml kg^{-1} of crystalloid has been given (one blood volume), significant dilution of clotting factors

Table 33.6 Estimated fluid maintenance requirements	
Weight (kg)	**Maintenance fluid requirement (ml kg^{-1} h^{-1})**
<10	4
10–20	40 + 2 for each kg >10 kg
>20	60 + 1 for each kg >20 kg[a]
[a]To a maximum of 2.5 l day^{-1} (boys) or 2 l day^{-1} (girls).	

and platelets may occur and consideration given to replacement with the relevant blood products, guided by near-patient and laboratory tests.

The haemoglobin threshold for transfusing packed red cells is generally accepted at concentrations of less than 70 g L^{-1}. The decision to transfuse should be tailored to the individual patient, and higher thresholds are advocated when there is active bleeding or comorbidity (e.g. cyanotic cardiac disease) and in neonates requiring ongoing ventilatory support or supplemental oxygen. The circulating volume decreases with age, progressing from approximately 90 ml kg^{-1} in the term neonate and approximately 80 ml kg^{-1} in the infant to 70–75 ml kg^{-1} (adult levels) by age 7–8 years. In theory, using the following formula, it is possible to estimate the maximum tolerated blood loss before transfusion is indicated:

Maximum tolerated blood loss = estimated blood volume
  × (starting haemoglobin − transfusion threshold
    haemoglobin) / starting haemoglobin

It is good practice to measure the haemoglobin concentration before transfusing (e.g. with a blood gas analyser or Hemocue device) and to estimate the volume of transfusion required. In general it is ideal to limit the number of donors the child is exposed to, particularly for a small infant, where a single donor unit can be fractionated to give multiple top-ups. As a guide, 4–5 ml kg^{-1} of packed red cells (~60% haematocrit) will raise the patient's haemoglobin concentration by 10 g L^{-1}. Tranexamic acid (an antifibrinolytic lysine analogue) should be considered for any child at risk of significant bleeding. The management of major haemorrhage is discussed in detail in Chapter 14.

Postoperatively, increased concentrations of ADH reduce the ability of the kidneys to excrete free water for up to 24–48 h, and only isotonic fluids should be administered during this time. Children younger than 6 years require additional dextrose (e.g. 5% dextrose Plasmalyte) to avoid hypoglycaemia and ketosis. The volume of i.v. fluid administered is controversial; some advocate 50%–60% of standard maintenance to reduce postoperative tissue oedema; others suggest that hypernatraemia is more common if isotonic fluids are given with volume restriction. In any case, any child receiving i.v. fluids in the perioperative period should have fluid balance and electrolytes monitored carefully.

Of note, term neonates are fluid-restricted during the first few days of life (see Table 33.2) as ADH concentrations, and hence total body water, are increased for the first few days of life before the postnatal diuresis occurs. The type of solution used varies according to institution, but isotonic fluid containing glucose is commonly advocated; if hypotonic fluid is administered (e.g. 0.45% sodium chloride with 10% glucose), plasma sodium and should be measured regularly.

Emergence, recovery and postoperative care

Towards the end of surgery, administration of anaesthetic agents is reduced and neuromuscular blockade is assessed and appropriately reversed or antagonised. All cannulae and infusion lines must be flushed properly to avoid the risk of subsequent inadvertent drug administration. The spontaneous ventilation rate can be used to titrate i.v. analgesia during this time. Before emergence, the usual airway equipment (face mask with or without Mapleson-F, suction) is made immediately available and the inspired oxygen concentration switched to 100%. Management of emergence is primarily focussed on the airway and ventilation. As with adults, there are two general approaches, each with its own merits: allowing the child to fully wake (and regain normal airway reflexes) before extubating the trachea/removing the SAD, or doing so with the child deeply anaesthetised (and breathing spontaneously). Deep tracheal extubation prevents coughing and straining on the tracheal tube; however, the absence of a secure airway during emergence may increase the risk of laryngospasm or aspiration of gastric contents. If extubating the child's trachea awake, it is important to ensure that the child is not in the early stages of emergence (intermittent gagging/coughing, non-purposeful movement), as tracheal extubation during this time may provoke dense laryngospasm.

Transfer to the PACU may therefore occur with the child awake with an intact airway or anaesthetised; clearly the latter requires greater ongoing vigilance with respect to the airway and breathing. Supplemental oxygen and routine essential monitoring are applied in all cases until the child is fully awake. Common complications seen in recovery include pain, PONV, airway obstruction and laryngospasm (see Chapter 27) and emergence delirium (see later).

Delayed or failed emergence occurs rarely but may result from residual drug effects (e.g. opioids, anaesthetic agents, NMBAs), carbon dioxide narcosis, hypothermia, hypoglycaemia or severe electrolyte or acid-base disturbance. If it occurs, the underlying cause should be identified and treated.

Postoperative pain is managed along similar principles to adult practice (i.e. assessment, rapid control followed by a maintenance strategy with monitoring and management of adverse effects; see Chapter 6). Assessing children can be challenging. Self-reporting is recognised to be more valid than assessment of physiological parameters, and in older children and adolescents, the usual adult visual or verbal analogue pain scales may be appropriate methods. In younger children a pictorial representation of pain (e.g. FACES pain scale) may be used (see Chapter 24). In infants and toddlers, behavioural scoring systems aggregating features such as posture, consolability, crying or facial expression and sleep disturbance are useful. Some neonatal pain assessment tools also integrate physiological parameters such as heart rate and blood pressure. Pain management in recovery should be a continuation of the analgesic strategy initiated in theatre; the child should receive a combination of simple analgesics and opioid (most commonly morphine). The latter is titrated intravenously either by manual bolus injection or patient- or nurse-controlled analgesia (PCA/NCA) infusions. Codeine was previously widely used but since 2013 has been contraindicated in children younger than 12 years (and all children undergoing adenotonsillectomy for obstructive sleep apnoea). This change was due to fatalities attributed to excessive respiratory depression in children who were ultra-fast metabolisers of codeine to morphine.

Postoperative nausea and vomiting is common in children, with a cited incidence of 15%–40% (approximately double that seen in adults). It is the leading cause of unanticipated admission after day-case surgery. Risk factors include: age older than 3 years, previous history of PONV, strabismus surgery or adenotonsillectomy, exposure to opioids and inhalational anaesthesia. Ondansetron and dexamethasone are commonly used for prophylaxis and are more effective in combination than either alone. Repeat administration of ondansetron is unlikely to be effective at treating established PONV if it has already been given. Droperidol may be an effective agent, particularly in those unable to receive dexamethasone. Despite a lack of evidence of efficacy, cyclizine is still commonly administered as a third-line antiemetic. Management of PONV is discussed in detail in Chapter 7.

Emergence delirium is a behavioural disturbance occurring in the immediate postoperative period characterised by thrashing, inconsolable crying and dissociation (appearing unable to recognise familiar surroundings or people, including parents). It can be difficult to distinguish from pain and therefore can be distressing for parents to witness. Unlike pain, it is self-resolving after 10–15 min. It is most common in children aged 2–6 years (with a cited incidence of 10%–50%) and after anaesthesia with sevoflurane and desflurane. The risk may be lower with isoflurane and appears lowest with TIVA using propofol. The underlying mechanism is unclear, as is the optimum method of preventing it. Premedication with midazolam has yielded conflicting results; however, there is evidence that premedication with α_2-agonists (e.g. clonidine or dexmedetomidine) or fentanyl given 10–20 min before the end of surgery reduces the risk of emergence delirium without increasing PONV or time to discharge from recovery. When it occurs, very severe agitation (e.g. causing physical harm to child at the surgical site) may be treated with propofol (0.5–1 mg kg^{-1} i.v.), midazolam (0.02–0.1 mg kg^{-1} i.v.) or opioids (e.g. fentanyl 1–2 µg kg^{-1} i.v.).

Some studies have demonstrated an association between high levels of preoperative anxiety, emergence delirium and longer lasting behavioural disturbances. Thus if emergence delirium does occur, parents should be warned that mild developmental regression (e.g. bedwetting) and maladaptive behaviour (e.g. poor appetite, difficulty concentrating) may occur in the weeks after surgery.

Regional anaesthesia/analgesia

A comprehensive review of the use of regional anaesthesia is beyond the scope of this chapter and can be found in Chapter 25. The general principles used in adult practice apply to children, namely patient assessment and selection; informed consent; preparation of drugs; equipment and monitoring; and safe, aseptic technique grounded in detailed knowledge of the relevant anatomy with anticipation and management of complications, including local anaesthetic toxicity.

The full range of regional blocks using anatomical landmarks and ultrasound guidance has been described in children. In contrast to adults most blocks used to provide intra- and postoperative analgesia are performed under general anaesthesia rather than awake or under sedation, with no evidence of increased complication rates. Indications for using regional anaesthesia as a sole technique in the awake patient include ex-premature neonates (e.g. undergoing inguinal hernia repair), to avoid the risk of apnoea after general anaesthesia, and children with severe myopathy or respiratory disease in whom weaning from ventilatory support would be difficult. The most commonly used regional techniques in children are caudal epidural injection, supraclavicular and axillary brachial plexus blocks for upper extremity surgery, femoral/sciatic blocks for lower extremity surgery and ilioinguinal/iliohypogastric blocks for inguinal hernia repair. Levobupivacaine is the most commonly used local anaesthetic, with a maximum safe dose of 2 mg kg^{-1}.

There are important age-related variations in the pharmacodynamics and pharmacokinetics of local anaesthetics. First, lower concentrations of drug provide effective blockade in infants and neonates (e.g. levobupivacaine 0.125%–0.25% vs. 0.375%–0.5% in adults). Pharmacodynamic reasons for this include smaller diameter nerve fibres, incomplete development of perineural fibrous sheaths and myelination and less subcutaneous fat than adults, facilitating local anaesthetic spread. Lower concentrations of plasma binding proteins (predominantly α_1-acid glycoprotein) increase the unbound (free) fraction of drug. Lower hepatic clearance renders infants and neonates more vulnerable to local anaesthetic toxicity, particularly if continuous infusions or repeated boluses are given. For this reason some have advocated halving the maximum dose in infants younger than 6 months old and/or limiting the duration of continuous infusions. In practice, many anaesthetists will allow a similar maximum safe dose in all age groups (e.g. 2 mg kg^{-1} levobupivacaine) on the basis that the larger volume of distribution in infants prevents high plasma concentrations being reached after a single injection.

Caudal injection is the most commonly used regional technique in children because of its technical ease, low complication rate and high efficacy. It provides high-quality analgesia for any operation below the umbilicus (e.g. hypospadias repair, orchidopexy). In addition to the usual contraindications of neuraxial blocks, signs of spinal dysraphism (e.g. sacral pit, midline haemangioma, anorectal malformation) should prompt neuraxial imaging to confirm normal anatomy of the spine before a caudal injection is performed. The anatomy and technique of caudal injection are described in Chapter 25. Paediatric-specific considerations include the following:

- The sacrum (and therefore the sacral hiatus) is higher relative to the iliac crests, descending as the pelvis grows to reach the adult position by 3–4 years.
- The dural sac ends at S3–4 level at birth, ascending to S2 by age 3 years; inadvertent intrathecal injection resulting in a total spinal is a risk particularly in neonates and infants.
- Ossification of the posterior vertebral arches of the sacrum progresses with age, so the sacral hiatus becomes more difficult to access in older children and adolescents.
- The epidural veins are small and prone to collapse under negative pressure. Aspiration with a syringe may therefore not reveal i.v. needle/cannula placement; opening the needle/cannula to air for a few seconds may be more effective.
- Epidural fat is loculated and less densely packed, facilitating cranial spread of local anaesthetic solution in children. A dose of 0.5 ml kg^{-1} is used to block sacral roots, whereas 1 ml kg^{-1} is used to cover high lumbar roots.

Commonly used adjuncts to prolong the duration of analgesia include preservative-free clonidine (1–2 μg kg^{-1}) and morphine (30–50 μg kg^{-1}), although morphine-related adverse effects such as itching and urinary retention may be troublesome. Ketamine is no longer advocated as an adjunct to epidural analgesia because of concerns about neurotoxicity.

Anaesthetic and perioperative management of a child may bring additional stressors to the anaesthetist because of unfamiliarity, anxiety and emergency presentations, as well as the problem of age and size adjustments for drugs, fluids and equipment. Many departments now provide personal or location-based cognitive aids to reduce cognitive load for the anaesthetist and their assistants. Smartphone apps and data sources are also available, though quality varies. Use of cognitive aids should be considered part of good paediatric practice.

Airway emergencies

Epiglottitis

Widespread vaccination against *Haemophilus influenzae* B, the most common causative organism, has dramatically reduced the incidence of epiglottitis in children. It does still occur, with group A β-haemolytic streptococci the most common cause. Classically the child presents with rapid-onset severe sore throat, drooling, fever and tachypnoea and is 'toxic'. Often the child will be more comfortable sat up or leaning forward; stridor is a late sign. If acute epiglottitis is suspected, then the airway should be secured early.

It is important to avoid upsetting the child. This includes not attempting i.v. access, not forcing oxygen masks on the face and not inserting tongue depressors. Tracheal intubation has a high risk of difficulty, and the team should prepare for this. If the child is more comfortable sat up, then induction should be in the upright position. Placing the child supine may precipitate airway obstruction. Inhalational induction is used, but this may be slow because of partial airway obstruction. Spontaneous ventilation is maintained until successful tracheal tube placement is confirmed. The view at laryngoscopy may be very poor with only a bubble to direct the anaesthetist. Expect to use a smaller diameter tracheal tube than normal.

Croup

Croup (viral laryngotracheobronchitis) classically presents in the winter with a barking cough, stridor and a hoarse voice. Management for most patients is medical with nebulised adrenaline, dexamethasone and humidified oxygen. Symptoms and signs of impending respiratory failure include sternal retraction (though this may paradoxically lessen as respiratory failure progresses), lethargy or decreased level of consciousness. As with epiglottitis, care should be taken to avoid additional distress to the child.

Inhaled foreign body

Often, but not always, there is a clear history of an inhaled foreign body. Exactly where it lodges is a function of the object size and shape and the relative airway dimensions. Bronchus obstruction may be suspected by unilateral respiratory signs. Emergency tracheal intubation is usually avoided because of the risk of worsening impaction.

Anaesthesia may be induced via the inhalational or i.v. route; there are advantages and disadvantages to both. Topical anaesthesia to the vocal cords is provided with lidocaine and a rigid bronchoscope (e.g. Storz ventilating bronchoscope) inserted by the experienced ear, nose and throat surgeon. Oxygenation, ventilation and delivery of inhalational anaesthetic agent can be provided whilst the eyepiece is on. Good communication between surgeon and anaesthetist is essential.

Neonatal emergency surgery

Laparotomy for necrotising enterocolitis

Necrotising enterocolitis (NEC) is common, particularly in preterm infants, affecting 5%–15% of neonates weighing less than 1.5 kg at birth. Neonates present with abdominal distension, bilious aspirates and signs of sepsis. They may be managed conservatively with i.v. fluids and antibiotics or by insertion of a peritoneal drain, or they may require a laparotomy for stoma formation or excision of necrotic bowel for control of sepsis. Perioperative mortality is high and anaesthesia challenging. Surgery may be associated with significant blood loss and requirement for blood, blood products, and inotropic support and may be performed in the neonatal intensive care unit (NICU) if the patient is very unstable.

Inguinal hernia repair

Inguinal hernia repair is one of the most commonly performed surgical procedures in infants, affecting up to 5% of term neonates and 30% of preterm neonates. Patients may present for emergency surgery as a result of bowel obstruction or infarction or for semi-elective repair, often before discharge from the neonatal unit to minimise the risk of surgical and anaesthesia complications. Surgery may be laparoscopic or open and dictates the anaesthetic options to a certain extent, the choices being general anaesthesia with or without caudal, ilioinguinal nerve block or local infiltration or an awake regional technique using spinal, caudal or a combination of the two. General anaesthesia is usually performed for laparoscopic repair. Regional techniques are more commonly used in ex-premature infants to reduce the risk of postoperative apnoea (seen in 20%–30% of preterm neonates undergoing hernia repair under general anaesthesia). To date, there have been no identifiable differences in neurodevelopmental outcome between neonates managed using sevoflurane anaesthesia and those managed with awake regional techniques.

Pyloromyotomy

Hypertrophic pyloric stenosis (idiopathic thickening of the pyloric smooth muscle) has an incidence of 1 in 300–400 live births (commoner in boys), presenting between the third and eighth week of life with projectile, non-bilious vomiting. This causes progressive dehydration with the classic electrolyte disturbance of a hypokalaemic, hypochloraemic metabolic alkalosis. Diagnosis is confirmed by ultrasound, and initial management consists of intravenous fluid resuscitation and nasogastric drainage. A key management point is that pyloric stenosis is not a surgical emergency; surgery is urgent but should not proceed until hypovolaemia and acid–base or electrolyte disturbance abnormalities have been corrected. A fluid bolus of 10–20 ml kg^{-1} 0.9% saline may be required if the baby is shocked, followed by rehydration with maintenance 5% glucose in 0.45% saline with potassium (provided the plasma sodium is in the normal range). Rehydration usually takes 24–48 h, depending on the severity of dehydration, and is signalled by a good urine output, plasma bicarbonate of less than 26 mmol L^{-1}, chloride greater than 100 mmol L^{-1} and normal sodium and potassium concentrations. It is important to delay surgery if there is ongoing metabolic alkalosis as this increases the risk of postoperative apnoeas.

Before induction of anaesthesia, the nasogastric tube should be suctioned while tilting the patient in different directions to facilitate complete gastric emptying; some advocate performing saline lavage until the aspirate is clear of particulates. Induction techniques vary from a modified rapid sequence induction to a standard inhalational induction followed by muscle relaxant and tracheal intubation on the basis that the stomach has been emptied, and depends on the preference and experience of the anaesthetist. During surgery the surgeon may ask for air to be injected via the nasogastric tube to exclude mucosal perforation. Surgery is performed open or laparoscopically. In either case the procedure is short, not associated with significant bleeding and minimally painful. Intravenous paracetamol with local anaesthetic infiltration of the wound usually provides adequate postoperative pain relief. The child should be extubated when fully awake and recovered in the usual way, and most infants can return to a general surgical ward with postoperative oxygen saturation and apnoea monitoring. Maintenance fluid is continued until oral feeding is established (usually 4–8 h postoperatively).

Oesophageal atresia/ tracheo-oesophageal fistula repair

Oesophageal atresia/tracheo-oesophageal fistula is associated with discontinuity of the oesophagus and/or a fistulous connection with the trachea. There are six subtypes, the most common being Gross type C. This consists of proximal oesophageal atresia with the oesophagus ending as a blind pouch above the sternal angle and a fistulous connection between the distal oesophagus and the posterior aspect of the mid-trachea in two thirds of patients, or close to the carina in the remainder. Up to 50% of patients have other congenital abnormalities, such as cardiac lesions (e.g. ventricular septal defect) or VACTERL association. All patients should have a preoperative echocardiogram and renal ultrasound if they have not passed urine. Infants with a duct-dependent systemic or pulmonary circulation have a significantly higher perioperative mortality risk.

The diagnosis may be suspected antenatally because of polyhydramnios with a small or absent gastric bubble. Most cases present postnatally, with 'bubbling' as a result of difficulty in swallowing secretions and choking and cyanosis if a feed is attempted. Diagnosis is confirmed by failure to pass a nasogastric tube and plain chest radiograph showing coiling of the nasogastric tube in the upper oesophageal pouch. Before surgery, a specialised double-lumen suction/irrigation tube (Replogle tube) is passed into the pouch for continuous drainage of saliva and secretions and to prevent aspiration.

Anaesthesia should be induced carefully, with the tracheal tube positioned to minimise ventilation of the fistula, massive gastric distension and desaturation. Intravenous or inhalational induction can be used, with NMBAs and gentle face-mask ventilation before tracheal intubation. A common technique is to deliberately intubate the right main bronchus keeping the bevel of the tracheal tube facing anteriorly and then withdraw the tracheal tube gently until air entry becomes bilateral, at the same time obstructing the fistula in the posterior wall of the trachea. Some surgeons may perform a rigid bronchoscopy before tracheal intubation to assess the anatomy and location of the fistula or to identify a proximal fistula. If severe gastric distension does occur, the tracheal tube should be disconnected briefly to allow gastric decompression via the tracheal tube. Performing a gastrostomy before ligating the fistula may render the child becoming unventilatable. The surgical approach is usually via a right thoracotomy; gentle manual ventilation is performed until the fistula is ligated. Provided the oesophageal gap is short, a primary end-to-end anastomosis is performed, and a transanastomotic tube (TAT) is passed by the surgeon to allow enteral feeding postop. In long-gap oesophageal atresia, a cervical oesophagostomy is formed and a feeding gastrostomy sited, with a view to delayed formation of the oesophageal anastomosis. A period of postoperative mechanical ventilation is indicated if the oesophageal anastomosis is under tension or if there is significant cardiorespiratory comorbidity.

Abdominal wall defects (exomphalos and gastroschisis)

Abdominal wall defects have an incidence of 1 in 3000 live births. Gastroschisis is herniation of viscera through a defect in the abdominal wall lateral to the umbilicus. The intestine is exposed to the amniotic fluid in utero and is usually thickened and functionally abnormal, and there may be associated intestinal atresia or malrotation. However, other congenital abnormalities are rarely present. In contrast, exomphalos is herniation of the abdominal viscera into the base of the umbilical cord. The viscera are covered by a membrane, and the bowel is largely normal. Significant comorbidity is common in exomphalos, and this may include cardiac lesions, chromosomal abnormalities (e.g. trisomy 21) and bladder exstrophy. Initial management is supportive to avoid hypothermia, hypovolaemia and sepsis. Gastroschisis requires urgent reduction, either with primary closure or (if the defect is large) a staged reduction over several days using a Prolene mesh 'silo' covering, with subsequent closure of the defect 3–5 days later. The presence of the protective membrane in exomphalos means that reduction is less urgent, which may allow time for investigations to identify potential comorbidities.

Anaesthetic considerations for the two conditions are similar and follow the usual principles of neonatal anaesthesia. A modified RSI may be used, or inhalational induction (without nitrous oxide) with subsequent neuromuscular blockade and tracheal intubation in the normal way. Care must be taken to avoid gaseous distension of the bowel. The anaesthetist should monitor any increase in intra-abdominal pressure during reduction of the viscera as this may profoundly impair ventilation and venous return. Patients are at risk of abdominal compartment syndrome, and close communication with the surgeon is required. The child is usually returned to the NICU for a period of postoperative ventilation.

Diaphragmatic hernia repair

Congenital diaphragmatic hernia (CDH) has an incidence of 1 in 3000–5000 live births. Approximately 50% of patients with CDH have cardiac or chromosomal anomalies. The abdominal contents herniate through a defect in the diaphragm, most commonly on the left side (80% of cases). This causes hypoplasia of the ipsilateral lung, although the contralateral lung can also be affected if there is significant mediastinal shift. This results in a reduced number of functional lung units and alveolar surface area, as well as pulmonary hypertension as a result of pulmonary arteriolar smooth muscle hypertrophy. Diagnosis may be made via antenatal ultrasound, or patients may present after birth with varying degrees of respiratory compromise and pulmonary hypertension.

Initial management involves stabilisation and ventilatory support. This may include conventional ventilation with nitric oxide and inotropes, high-frequency oscillatory ventilation or extracorporeal membrane oxygenation, depending on the severity of pulmonary hypertension and hypoxia. Permissive hypercapnia is usually employed to minimise barotrauma. Surgical repair is carried out once there is physiological stability and the child is on conventional ventilation and requiring only minimal inotropic support. The approach is usually via a left thoracoabdominal incision. The intrathoracic abdominal viscera are reduced into the abdomen and the diaphragmatic defect closed with a patch. Surgery may be performed with thoracoscopic assistance. Specific anaesthetic challenges include maintaining adequate ventilation; achieving adequate carbon dioxide clearance, particularly if a thoracoscopic technique is used; and preventing or managing pulmonary hypertensive crises.

Child protection and safeguarding

The safeguarding of children, defined as action to protect them from maltreatment or neglect, is a statutory duty of all health professionals. The signs of maltreatment or neglect and the referral processes and possible interventions should be considered core knowledge. All organisations must have local safeguarding processes in place that are to be followed whenever maltreatment or neglect is suspected; these processes are grounded in statutory guidance (e.g. Working Together to Safeguard Children), which are in turn drawn from statute law, most notably the 1989 and 2004 Children Acts. The single overarching principle is that the child's best interests are paramount at all times.

Instances in which anaesthetists may be involved in safeguarding procedures include an incidental finding of suspicious signs during elective or emergency surgery, when a child or relative makes a disclosure suggestive of abuse or neglect, when a child is admitted as an emergency for illness or injury where the aetiology is unclear and/or maltreatment is suspected, or when a child is admitted specifically for investigation of safeguarding concerns. The myriad signs of neglect, abuse and non-accidental injury are beyond the remit of this chapter; however, certain features should raise suspicion and may be as simple as the child appearing to be unusually dirty or smelly. Important signs include a mechanism of injury that is inconsistent with the developmental age of the child (such as a fracture in a non-ambulant infant); an unusual clinical picture (such as symmetrical burns in liquid scalds); delayed presentation; injury to inaccessible places (such as inside the mouth); and cigarette burns and bite marks.

If there is cause for concern regarding a child's welfare the anaesthetist has a duty to discuss these with the designated doctor or nurse for child protection. The child should be assessed jointly with a consultant paediatrician and an explanation sought for suspicious features. If concerns remain, a formal assessment by the child protection team should be carried out. This results in one of three possible outcomes:

1. No further action is taken.
2. The child is placed under a voluntary plan of support, described as a 'child in need' plan.
3. A compulsory child protection plan is put in place based on the assessment that the child is at risk of actual or likely significant harm.

Emergency cases may require the police and social services to be involved urgently. Clear, accurate contemporaneous recordkeeping is essential.

References/Further reading

Association of Paediatric Anaesthetists of Great Britain and Ireland, 2016. Guidelines on the Prevention of Post-operative Vomiting in Children. http://www.apagbi.org.uk/sites/default/files/images/2016%20APA%20POV%20Guideline-2.pdf. (Accessed 25 August 2017).

Dept for Education, HM Government, 2015. Working together to safeguard children. https://www.gov.uk/government/uploads/system/uploads/attachment_data/file/592101/Working_Together_to_Safeguard_Children_20170213.pdf. (Accessed 25 August 2017).

Gregory, G.A., Andropolous, D.B. (Eds.), 2012. Gregory's pediatric anaesthesia. Wiley-Blackwell, West Sussex.

Habre, W., Disma, N., Virag, K., et al., 2017. Incidence of severe critical events in paediatric anaesthesia (APRICOT): a prospective multicentre observational study in 261 hospitals in Europe. Lancet Respir. Med. 5, 412–425.

National Institute for Health and Care Excellence, 2015. Intravenous fluid therapy in children and young people in hospital. NICE guideline. https://www.nice.org.uk/guidance/ng29/resources/intravenous-fluid-therapy-in-children-and-young-people-in-hospital-pdf-1837340295109. (Accessed 25 August 2017).

Shah, R.D., Suresh, S., 2013. Applications of regional anaesthesia in paediatrics. Br. J. Anaesth. 111 (Suppl. 1), i114–i124.

von Ungern-Sternberg, B.S., Boda, K., Chambers, N.A., et al., 2010. Risk assessment for respiratory complications in paediatric anaesthesia: a prospective cohort study. Lancet 376 (9743), 773–783.

Walker, I., James, I. (Eds.), 2013. Core topics in paediatric anaesthesia. Cambridge University Press, Cambridge.

Chapter | 34 |

Anaesthesia for day surgery

Rachel Tibble

Introduction

Day surgery is defined as surgery where patient discharge occurs on the same day as admission. Twenty-three-hour discharge and enhanced recovery have the same underlying principles as day surgery but are considered separately.

Organisations such as the British Association for Day Surgery (BADS), working with the RCoA and the Association of Anaesthetists, have been central in moving day surgery services forward to encompass more operations and include more complex patients. Their ethos is to change the mindset towards offering day surgery to all until proven otherwise.

The benefits of day surgery for the patient include reduced hospital-acquired infection rates, improved recovery in familiar surroundings and earlier postoperative mobilisation, thereby reducing thromboembolic complications. The benefits for health services include reduction in cost per patient episode and more inpatient bed availability for patients needing major operations and longer hospital stays. Some healthcare systems incentivise day surgery through collection of higher tariffs for same-day surgery patients than inpatients.

Success in day surgery requires a multidisciplinary approach with dedicated teams applying day surgery techniques in surgery, anaesthesia, preoperative and postoperative care to promote same-day discharge by minimising complications. Patients should follow a day surgery pathway to enhance efficiency (Fig. 34.1). Anaesthetic involvement in each step along the pathway promotes success.

Anaesthetic involvement in each step along the pathway promotes success.

Preoperative assessment

If efficiently carried out early in the patient pathway, preoperative assessment has a key role in the success and safety of day surgery.

A nurse-based team in the day-case unit, coordinated by a consultant anaesthetist, allows development of robust local protocols for the investigation and management of complex patients. Specific training for staff and a consultant with specialty interest in day surgery maintains quality and can improve patient outcomes. Access to specialty support services such as pharmacy, laboratory analysis and radiology is essential.

Preoperative assessment is covered in detail in Chapter 19. Particular issues pertinent to day surgery include identification of patient or surgical factors that make day surgery unsuitable, diagnosis of new conditions such as obstructive sleep apnoea that if managed preoperatively can still allow successful day surgery and addressing postoperative expectations and postdischarge care.

Patient suitability for day surgery

The final aim is a decision on patient suitability for day surgery. Suitability for day surgery now avoids narrow prescriptive limits like age, ASA physical class and BMI and uses individual approaches to expand the number of patients offered day surgery.

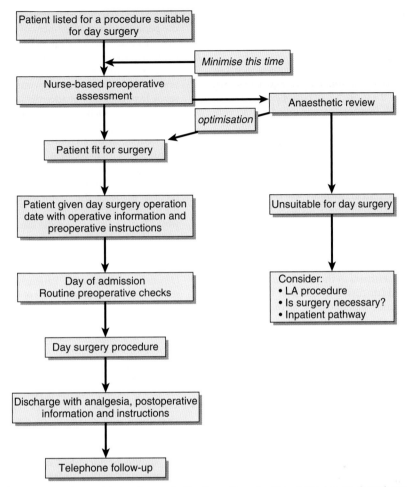

Fig. 34.1 An ideal day surgery pathway. *LA,* Local anaesthetic. (From Quemby, D.J., & Stocker, M. (2013) Day surgery development and practice: key factors for a successful pathway. *Continuing Education in Anaesthesia Critical Care & Pain.* 14(6):256–261.)

Criteria can still be divided into social, medical and surgical factors.

Social factors

- The patient needs suitable conditions at home for postoperative care and access to a telephone in case of complications.
- A responsible adult carer is recommended to escort the patient home and remain with the patient for 24 h after a general anaesthetic.
- Travelling distance from hospital less than 60 min is recommended for operations where serious postoperative haemorrhage may be a risk, such as tonsillectomy.

- The patient (and/or carer) should understand the nature of the surgery and its implications, including complications which may occur at home.

Medical factors

Offering day surgery to patients with complex medical needs is now well established. Intense preoperative management with involvement of a consultant anaesthetist may be necessary but can produce good outcomes for same-day discharge. Anaesthetic involvement in patient selection is recommended to develop local protocols and management strategies for complex patients and communicate with other specialties including surgical consultants to improve the

683

efficiency of the process and minimise cancellation on the day of surgery.

A detailed history and examination should determine suitability for day surgery.

- *Patients who are ASA physical class 3.* Patients with stable, optimised disease have no contraindication to day surgery, with no increase in the incidence of postoperative complications, unplanned admissions or unplanned contact with healthcare services. Appropriate anaesthetic techniques help to maximise the chance of discharge home. Local anaesthetic techniques may give the best outcome.
- *Obesity (BMI > 30 kg m⁻²).* Obesity does not preclude successful day surgery. Assessment of associated comorbidities, rather than BMI in isolation, will define suitability. Postoperative complications increase with central obesity and the metabolic syndrome. Case reports exist for successful day surgery in patients with a BMI greater than 60 kg m⁻² with careful preplanning, availability of specific equipment and good team communication. Guidelines for anaesthesia in the obese surgical patient should be applied (discussed in detail in Chapter 32). Patients need to understand postoperative expectations and the necessary procedures for success.
- *Cardiovascular disease.* Stable ischaemic heart disease may be managed in day surgery. Careful review of functional capacity and symptoms is necessary preoperatively, with further investigations and optimisation of disease if appropriate (see Chapter 19). Preoperative assessment should aim to identify cases of severe aortic valve stenosis, cardiomyopathies, severe ventricular dysfunction, pulmonary hypertension and arrhythmias, as these may lead to perioperative critical incidents if undiagnosed. Atrial fibrillation, once rate control is achieved, is not a contraindication to day surgery. Patients taking anticoagulants and antiplatelet therapy should be managed in the usual way (see Chapter 19). Patients at high risk of thrombotic events who require bridging therapy with low-molecular-weight heparin (LMWH) can often have this organised via day surgery in conjunction with primary care. Pacemakers are not a contraindication to day surgery if the team and anaesthetist are aware and a plan in case of failure is prepared.
- *Respiratory disease.* Patients with severe chronic obstructive pulmonary disease (COPD) may be managed in day surgery, especially if the operation is amenable to a regional or nerve block technique. Pulmonary function tests can help to quantify severity of disease and current exacerbations should be excluded preoperatively. Patients with mild obstructive sleep apnoea (OSA) and those with severe OSA on established CPAP therapy can usually be managed in day surgery.
- *Endocrine disease.* Patients with well-controlled diabetes mellitus, even those on insulin, can be safely managed as day cases. Diabetic control should be assessed by glycosylated haemoglobin levels; National guidance for the perioperative management of diabetes recommends that elective surgery should be postponed if HbA1$_C$ concentrations are greater than 69 mmol mol⁻¹. Communication with the primary care team or diabetologists may be necessary to improve control, and patients with severe hypoglycaemic attacks may not be suitable. Diabetic complications such as renal disease should be identified early. Precise patient information (verbal and written) is essential, with an individual patient plan for the perioperative management of diabetic medication and postoperative effects on blood sugars clearly documented. Many regimens are available for the perioperative management of diabetes; the simplest puts the patient first on the morning list, omitting his or her morning medication whilst fasting, then taking the usual diabetic medication with a light breakfast after the operation. Perioperative diabetic management is discussed in greater detail in Chapter 20.
- *Hepatic/renal dysfunction.* Patients with cirrhosis are not suitable for day surgery because of increased perioperative mortality rates. Milder liver function test abnormalities are usually not a problem. Renal dysfunction does not prohibit day surgery, but careful assessment of associated comorbidities is required and appropriate anaesthetic agents used (see Chapters 11 and 20). Regional techniques have been used to allow vascular access procedures for dialysis to be done as a day case.
- *Rheumatoid disease.* The issues regarding preoperative assessment and cessation of disease-modifying antirheumatic drugs are discussed in Chapters 19 and 20.
- *Chronic pain.* Patients with chronic pain (see Chapter 24) should be identified early in the pathway and a perioperative analgesic plan determined in conjunction with the patient.
- *Dementia.* Patients with dementia often make a better postoperative recovery in their own home. A perioperative plan should be agreed on during preoperative assessment so carers are clear about the proposed pathway.
- *Paediatrics.* Children are often suitable for day surgery. They should be aged 60 weeks and older postconceptual age without significant lung disease or apnoeas (see Chapter 33).

Surgical factors

Operations deemed suitable for day surgery are ever expanding. The BADS directory now contains more than 200 recommended operations, and more complex operations in specialties such as breast surgery, otolaryngology and orthopaedic and endocrine surgery are also being developed as day surgery procedures. A team approach is necessary to introduce new operations to day surgery to minimise surgical complications and produce guidelines for optimal

1. Should have the ability to control haemorrhage.
2. Low risk of postoperative bleeding or cardiovascular instability.
3. Surgery should not produce large fluid shifts.
4. Allows rapid return to oral intake after surgery.
5. Patient is able to mobilise safely postoperatively.
6. No prolonged period of observation is required.
7. Postoperative pain controllable with oral analgesics.
8. If abdominal or thoracic cavities are entered, minimally invasive techniques should be used.

management. The principles guiding surgical suitability are outlined in Box 34.1.

Emergency surgery is also moving into the day surgery arena. Designated lists for abscesses or minor hand surgery are produced where patients are discharged after initial presentation but rapidly return for scheduled surgery. Other pathways are evolving for acute cholecystitis treated with day surgery laparoscopic cholecystectomy and for patients with uncomplicated laparoscopic appendectomy to be allowed home on the same day as their surgery.

Anaesthetic techniques

Although preoperative assessment should produce a patient ready for surgery, each patient should be seen by the anaesthetist on the day of admission to discuss anaesthetic techniques, assess the airway, provide postoperative instructions (including analgesia) and address any anxiety issues the patient may have.

Anaesthetic techniques influence successful patient outcomes. The aim is for a rapid return of full cognitive function, oral intake and mobilisation, taking into account the patient's comorbidities, predicted difficulties and patient wishes where possible.

Techniques include sedation, general anaesthesia and regional techniques, which may include peripheral nerve or plexus blocks. Combinations work well in certain circumstances.

General anaesthesia

Facilities for anaesthesia should be equivalent to those for inpatient anaesthesia, with standard monitoring and equipment available and the same trained anaesthetic assistance and recovery care available for any general anaesthetic, regional technique or sedation performed.

Anaesthetic agents for general anaesthesia should have rapid onset and offset for clear-headed emergence, with minimal drowsiness, nausea, vomiting or dizziness in the postoperative period. The aim is to get back to street fitness for home discharge.

Inhalational anaesthetic agents

When used as part of a balanced anaesthesia regimen, volatile agents with a rapid offset such as sevoflurane or desflurane (see Chapter 3) can lead to more rapid recovery of consciousness and thus avoid bottlenecks and delays in stage 1 recovery. Low-flow techniques should be applied as a routine to reduce costs.

Intravenous anaesthetic agents

Propofol is a widely used induction agent because of useful properties such as reduction of laryngeal reflexes for SAD insertion, antiemetic properties and reasonably rapid offset with little hangover effect (see Chapter 4). Total intravenous anaesthesia with propofol, which is discussed in detail in Chapter 4, is useful for many day surgery procedures, especially when the risk of PONV is high. Appropriate equipment, such as target-controlled infusion (TCI) pumps and processed EEG monitors, should be available.

Analgesia

Multimodal approaches are widely advocated for day surgery to achieve good analgesia for discharge and minimise the use of long-acting opioids. Use of multiple non-opioid drugs with diverse modes of action, including NSAIDs, paracetamol and local anaesthetics, make this possible.

Simple analgesics

Premedication protocols have become a popular way of beginning the multimodal approach to analgesia. The administration of oral paracetamol and a modified-release NSAID (e.g. diclofenac 75 mg or ibuprofen 800 mg) have a synergistic opioid-sparing effect. A loading dose of paracetamol (2 g orally) may achieve greater efficacy in reaching therapeutic plasma concentrations.

Opioids

Judicious use of opioids is appropriate in day surgery. Indiscriminate use of long-acting opioids causes adverse effects that may prevent discharge; nausea and vomiting, sedation and respiratory depression are all problematic.

More complex operations will need opioids as part of the multimodal analgesia to prevent excessive postoperative pain. Set protocols for anaesthesia and analgesia (e.g. for laparoscopic cholecystectomy) may help achieve this. Short-acting opioids such as fentanyl are often used, as these are associated with reductions in PONV.

Local anaesthetics

Longer-acting local anaesthetic agents for infiltration or specific nerve blocks, including ilioinguinal nerve block for inguinal hernia repair or penile block for circumcision, can reduce postoperative pain and promote early discharge.

Analgesia after discharge

Some operations may cause pain that may last for several days, so the anaesthetist should prescribe stronger analgesics (e.g. tramadol, codeine phosphate) for discharge according to local protocols. Written and verbal information regarding the postoperative use of over-the-counter analgesics should be given during preoperative assessment.

Adjuncts

Ketamine (N-methyl-D-aspartate receptor antagonist), gabapentin (gabapentinoid) and clonidine (α_2-adrenergic agonist) have been found to work as part of the multimodal analgesia regimen. However, adverse effects such as dizziness, hypotension and sedation limit their use in patients having day surgery. Intravenous lidocaine has been found to reduce pain in laparoscopic cholecystectomy patients, but robust evidence in the day-case setting is lacking. Small i.v. doses of ketamine may be useful in patients with chronic pain. Dexamethasone (0.1 mg kg^{-1} or greater i.v.) has analgesic properties in addition to its antiemetic effect.

Postoperative nausea and vomiting

Postoperative nausea and vomiting is a common reason for unplanned overnight admission and is discussed in detail in Chapter 7. General measures to reduce PONV should be adopted for all patients having surgery, including consideration of the use of regional anaesthesia and avoidance of nitrous oxide. In addition to the standard risk factors, gynaecological surgery and laparoscopic cholecystectomy may also be associated with a greater incidence of PONV.

Adoption of risk-related protocols has been found to reduce rates of PONV, so local policies should be drawn up and be visible within the day surgery unit. In addition to the use of pharmacological prophylaxis, the use of intraoperative i.v. fluids also reduces PONV. Avoidance of PONV is particularly important for diabetic patients to allow resumption of usual oral intake after surgery.

Airway management

Standard tests to predict difficulty with airway management and tracheal intubation should be performed at preoperative assessment (see Chapter 23). The presence of a difficult airway should not necessarily mean exclusion from day surgery, and standard equipment for difficult airway management should be available in day surgery units, including videolaryngoscopy and fibreoptic endoscopes for awake tracheal intubation.

Second-generation supraglottic airway device (SAD) use should be considered for appropriate day surgery patients who do not need a tracheal tube placed, but there is concern about a small increased risk of regurgitation.

Regional anaesthesia
Spinal anaesthesia

Spinal anaesthesia has now gained a central role in day surgery anaesthesia with the development of newer techniques (e.g. low-dose spinal anaesthesia) and advent of short-acting local anaesthetics. Spinal anaesthesia is useful to minimise morbidity for patients with cardiorespiratory disease, high BMI, acid reflux disease, OSA, potentially difficult airways or a history of severe PONV.

Delays in discharge secondary to the adverse effects of spinal anaesthesia (e.g. hypotension, delayed return of motor power and ambulation, urinary retention and post–dural-puncture headache) have previously limited its use in day surgery. Lidocaine, as a shorter-acting agent, had unacceptable rates of transient neurological symptoms. Low-dose bupivacaine techniques were then devised and successfully used to allow early ambulation and minimise adverse effects. Successful day surgery regimens have used 5–10 mg hyperbaric bupivacaine 0.5% (with or without fentanyl 20–25 µg) for lower limb, inguinal hernia and pelvic operations.

Shorter-acting agents are now available reducing time to ambulation and discharge with minimal side effects. Hyperbaric prilocaine 2% solution is widely available; the hyperbaricity accelerates onset and offset times compared with the isobaric formulation previously used. Suggested doses are 40–60 mg for lower extremity (duration approximately 90 min) and lower abdominal procedures and 10–30 mg for perineal surgery. To avoid the previous neurotoxicity issues, 2-chlorprocaine is now available as a preservative-free 1% solution. Block duration is related to the dose administered; 30–60 mg is acceptable for procedures less than 60 min in duration, with the addition of fentanyl prolonging surgical block without increasing time to discharge. Written and verbal patient information is essential about complications (which may occur at home) and actions to take.

Plexus or nerve blockade

For certain operations (e.g. shoulder surgery) the use of nerve plexus blocks can allow more complex operations and patients access to day surgery. The individual nerve blocks are discussed in detail in Chapter 25. Ultrasound-guided blocks are used to reduce amount of local anaesthetic required and increase efficacy. Advantages include improved patient satisfaction, better postoperative analgesia and reduced incidence of PONV. Interscalene, supraclavicular, infraclavicular and axillary blockade have all been used for upper limb day surgery. For hand surgery, ultrasound-guided peripheral sensory blocks using long-acting local anaesthetics are often useful. For lower limb surgery, residual motor blockade is a concern. Specific sensory blocks such as adductor canal blockade may therefore be used where appropriate.

The patient may be discharged home with residual block but should be fully informed of the dangers of injury to the insensate limb and given written information about protection from pressure, heat and extremes of movement. Advice to commence oral analgesia before the block recedes will be necessary in conjunction with the prescription of appropriate analgesics. Continuous perineural catheters for postoperative analgesia after orthopaedic operations involving osteotomy (e.g. ankle surgery) allow same-day discharge with good pain relief.

Sedation

Sedation may be employed for short procedures on patients with serious comorbidities who cannot tolerate regional or general anaesthesia (e.g. suprapubic catheter change in patients with end-stage multiple sclerosis). TIVA-based techniques allow rapid reversal of sedation and same-day discharge.

Recovery in day surgery

Stage 1 recovery

Stage 1 is the immediate postanaesthetic recovery area. Stage 1 recovery staff should be trained to a defined standard in airway management and treatment of postoperative complications. Teamwork and training promote early treatment of pain and PONV which might otherwise delay discharge. Intravenous fentanyl protocols are common in stage 1 recovery for rapid pain control, with simultaneous administration of oral analgesics for smooth transition of analgesia. Criteria to leave first-stage recovery are shown in Box 34.2.

Stage 2 recovery

Stage 2 is the ward area that patients reside in before discharge home. Stage 2 recovery should have all patients visible to staff

---

> **Box 34.2 Criteria for stage 1 recovery discharge**
>
> The patient is conscious and orientated.
> The patient has control of his or her own airway.
> No continued haemorrhage is present.
> Pain and PONV are minimised.
> ___
> *PONV*, Postoperative nausea and vomiting.

> **Box 34.3 Typical criteria for nurse-led discharge from day surgery**
>
> 1. Patient is awake and conscious.
> 2. Patient is orientated.
> 3. Pain is controlled with oral analgesics. Has supply of appropriate analgesics.
> 4. Patient has minimal or acceptable nausea.
> 5. No dizziness is present.
> 6. Patient has the ability to mobilise
> 7. Vital signs are stable (BP, pulse).
> 8. Patient is able to eat and drink
> 9. Patient has passed urine if high-risk patient or operation.
> 10. Blood sugars are stable.
> 11. Patient received venous thromboembolism prophylaxis if needed.
> 12. Outpatient follow-up date has been scheduled.
> 13. Patient has 24-h emergency phone numbers in case of complications. This should be for an acute surgical area out of hours.
> 14. Relevant patient information (verbal and written) has been provided for the effects of surgery, anaesthetic complications and analgesia at home, with clarity on when to drive and the level of care needed from relatives/carers.
> 15. Advice on dressings or sutures has been provided.
> 16. Appropriate documentation for primary care physician has been provided.

and easy access to inpatient beds if needed. Isolated units should have agreed protocols for overnight admission. Nurse-led discharge is accepted as the most efficient way of discharging day surgery patients using locally agreed criteria (Box 34.3).

Management and organisation of the day surgery unit

The RCoA recommends that it is essential to have a clinical director or lead consultant to promote day surgery and lead the team towards development of new practice and review current practice. A nurse manager should support everyday unit activity. The anaesthetic service should be consultant led, as should the preoperative assessment clinics, with specifically trained nursing staff.

Facilities should be fully maintained and operating theatres equipped to the same standard as inpatient theatres, with full monitoring and resuscitation equipment available. Equipment should be available to assist regional anaesthesia (e.g. ultrasound machines). Day surgery units should ideally be purpose built, with their own recovery, ward and operating theatres. Poorer outcomes are seen when inpatient and day-case procedures are mixed or day surgery cases recovered on normal inpatient wards.

Children should have facilities and equipment as appropriate for any paediatric unit. Recovery in a separate area from adults with appropriately trained staff is essential.

Audit

Audit allows improvement in anaesthetic quality and patient experience in day surgery. The RCoA recommends audit should cover unplanned admissions from day surgery, cancellations on the day of surgery, preoperative assessment provision, patient satisfaction and patient analgesia at home.

Unplanned admissions may be surgery or anaesthesia related. Anaesthetic factors such as pain and PONV are common reasons for overnight stay, and anaesthetic practice should be audited to improve this if possible. Other reasons include excess sedation, retention of urine, dizziness, inability to mobilise, vasovagal symptoms and hypotension.

Education and training

Education is vital in dissemination of good practice for future anaesthetists and improvement and development of day surgery. Techniques in preoperative assessment, anaesthesia and patient follow-up should be taught.

Controversies in day surgery

- A carer for 24 h after a general anaesthetic may not be essential for short non-invasive procedures with minimal haemorrhage risk or complications. This is currently being debated.
- Some day surgery units do not insist on a patient eating and drinking before discharge, as this may precipitate nausea.
- Regional anaesthesia for all procedures has been advocated in some units, whereas the general anaesthesia debate about the superiority of TIVA vs. volatile agents continues.
- Some major surgery has been attempted as day surgery, including carotid endarterectomy, open craniotomy and laparoscopic nephrectomy, which creates controversy over the safety of patients at home after surgery where major haemorrhage is a possibility. However, the boundaries will continue to be pushed as we develop new and less invasive techniques.

References/Further reading

Allen, J., Watson, B., April 2007. Upper Limb Plexus and Peripheral Nerve Blocks in Day Surgery—A Practical Guide. BADS.

Ansell, G.L., Montgomery, J.E., 2004. Outcome of ASA III patients undergoing day case surgery. Br. J. Anaesth. 92, 71–74.

British Association of Day Surgery. BADS Directory of Procedures 2007. London: available from www.bads.co.uk, 2007.

Claxton, A.R., McGuire, G., Chung, F., Cruise, C., 1997. Evaluation of morphine versus fentanyl for postoperative analgesia after ambulatory surgical procedures. Anesth. Analg. 84, 509–514.

Davies, K.E., Houghton, K., Montgomery, J.E., 2001. Obesity and day-case surgery. Anaesthesia 56, 1112–1115.

Day case and short stay surgery 2. AAGBI and BADS, London 2011.

Elvir-Lazoa, O.L., White, P.F., 2010. The role of multimodal analgesia in pain management after ambulatory surgery. Curr. Opin. Anesthesiol. 23, 697–703.

Manassero, A., Fanelli, I., 2017. Prilocaine hydrochloride 2% hyperbaric solution for intrathecal injection: a clinical review. Local Reg. Anesth. 10, 15–24.

Mayell, A.C., Barnes, S.J., Stocker, M.E., 2009. Introducing emergency surgery to the day case setting. Journal of One-Day Surgery 19, 10–13.

Organisational issues in pre-operative assessment for day surgery. BADS, London 2010.

Philip, B.K., Kallar, S.K., Bogatz, M.S., Scheller, M.S., Wetchler, B.V., 1996. A multicentre comparison of

maintenance and recovery with sevoflurane or isoflurane for adult ambulatory anaesthesia. Anesth. Analg. 83, 314–319.

Royal College of Anaesthetists. Guidelines for the provision of anaesthesia services (GPAS): Guidance on the Provision of Anaesthesia Services for Day Surgery; 2016.

Tibble, R., Carrick, L., 2015. The difficult airway and videolaryngoscope use in day surgery. The Journal of One Day Surgery 25, 48–50.

Watson, B., Howell, V., 2007. Spinal anaesthesia: the saviour of day surgery? Curr. Anaesth. Crit. Care 18, 193–199.

Chapter | **35** |

Anaesthesia for general, gynaecological and genitourinary surgery

Martin Beed

One-third of all anaesthetics delivered are for general, gynaecological or genitourinary surgery. In all three disciplines there are increasing numbers of frail or older patients. There is also widespread adoption of endoscopic techniques as well as emphasis on anaesthetic techniques which allow day-case surgery or fast-track recovery programmes.

Anaesthetic considerations

Patient positioning

Patient positioning is also discussed in detail in Chapter 22.

Head-down

Many abdominal operations are performed with the patient supine, but the addition of 20-degree head-down tilt (Trendelenburg) improves access to the pelvis. Some procedures, such as laparoscopic prostate surgery or hysterectomy, may require steep Trendelenburg positioning (30–45 degrees) for prolonged periods (see Fig. 22.8). Head-down positioning is associated with several complications, summarised in Table 35.1. As a result, careful assessment for preoperative conditions such as glaucoma or respiratory disease is necessary.

Tracheal intubation is required in most patients who require prolonged head-down positioning in order to maintain adequate ventilation and protect the airway. Positive end-expiratory pressure may minimise the risk of lung atelectasis. In patients at high risk of passive regurgitation, tracheal intubation should be considered even for short procedures. If passive regurgitation occurs in the head-down position, gastric acid can pool around the eyes leading to corneal burns. Where there is significant risk of this occurring (e.g. prolonged steep head-down position or bariatric patients), further measures may also be required, such as the use of a throat pack to prevent soiling, or a nasogastric tube inserted to empty the stomach. Ideally the patient should be positioned such that the anaesthetist is able to see the face, and if the eyes are affected they should be washed out rapidly.

Animal studies suggest prolonged, steep Trendelenburg positioning raises ICP, especially if combined with hypercapnia and/or raised intraperitoneal pressure from laparoscopic surgery. Patients may be at risk of developing delirium on emergence, but there is little evidence to support the prophylactic treatment for raised ICP used by some centres (i.v. dexamethasone or mannitol). Reassuringly, studies measuring intraoperative cerebral oxygenation in urological patients positioned in this way suggest that it is well preserved.

Various methods may be employed to prevent the patient sliding on the table during head-down positioning. One option for steep Trendelenburg is to use specialist vacuum beanbags (placed under the patient's torso) combined with Lloyd-Davies positioning (see Fig. 22.8). Any technique must avoid the risk of pressure injury to load-bearing areas. Lloyd-Davies positioning alone can result in calf compression; poorly positioned shoulder braces can put undue pressure on the superior aspect of the brachial plexus.

Lloyd-Davies and lithotomy

Access to the anus, perineum and genitals can be facilitated by use of the Lloyd-Davies or lithotomy positions

Table 35.1 The physiological effects and risks associated with steep Trendelenburg positioning and/or pneumoperitoneum[a]

Area of the body	Pneumoperitoneum effect	Trendelenburg effect
Airway		Tracheal tube displacement Airway swelling
Respiratory	Decreased functional residual capacity and vital capacity Decreased compliance $\dot{V}/\dot{Q}$ mismatch	As with pneumoperitoneum – and will act synergistically to further worsen the effects on $\dot{V}/\dot{Q}$, FRC and compliance Hypercapnia
Cardiovascular	Increased venous return at low pneumoperitoneum pressures Decreased venous return at higher pressures Occasional bradycardia at initial insufflation Increased systemic vascular resistance Decreased splanchnic perfusion Risk of air embolism	Increased venous return Increased systemic vascular resistance
Neurological	Raised intracranial pressure Cerebral perfusion pressure maintained or decreased	Raised intracranial pressure Cerebral perfusion pressure maintained
Renal	Decreased renal function Increased renin-angiotensin production	Poor bladder drainage
Eyes	Raised intraocular pressure	Raised intraocular pressure Risk of ocular burns if gastric contents pool in eye Optic nerve ischaemia
Other	Passive regurgitation	Passive regurgitation Facial swelling Accidental movement if patient not adequately secured Risk of neuropraxia from shoulder supports

FRC, Functional residual capacity.
[a]Many of the effects of pneumoperitoneum and steep Trendelenburg are synergistic and additive.

(see Fig. 22.3). Both have the patient supine with the hips flexed and abducted with bent knees. Lithotomy uses a greater hip flexion (typically close to 90 degrees). Prolonged extreme hip flexion can result in femoral nerve compression, or sciatic/ obturator nerve stretching (see Fig. 22.4). Care should be taken to avoid prolonged pressure against the femoral and tibial condyles (common peroneal or saphenous nerve compression). Typically the patient's legs are put into the leg attachments, which are raised to achieve the desired position. If patients' hands are by their sides, fingers may be trapped in the operating table mechanism (Fig. 35.1). Patients with prosthetic joints should be identified and care taken to avoid accidental dislocation.

Low-pressure calf muscle compartment syndrome is a rare complication of prolonged leg-up positioning – often appearing several hours after surgery. The cause is unknown but may relate to direct calf pressure or femoral vein obstruction as a result of hip flexion. The use of intermittent calf compression devices (e.g. Flowtron therapy) whilst in the leg-up position may increase the risk. Periodic lowering of the legs during prolonged procedures may help.

Absolute or relative hypovolaemia from blood loss or regional anaesthesia may be masked when legs are raised, only becoming apparent only after they are lowered.

Lateral and prone positioning

Lateral positioning is required for access to the lower back or flank—for instance, during pilonidal sinus surgery or nephrectomy operations. A 'break' may be applied to the middle of the table to extend the flank. Patient supports may be applied to the back or the abdomen, with the upper arm on a Carter Braine support to stop the upper torso

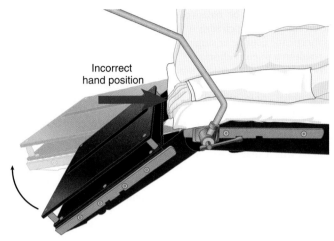

Fig. 35.1 Incorrect placement of the hands in the lithotomy position places the fingers at risk of crush injury. (With permission from Rothrock, J. C. (2015) *Alexander's care of the patient in surgery,* 15th ed. St. Louis, Elsevier.)

rotating (see Fig. 22.5). Leg and arm padding is required to avoid peroneal, saphenous and ulnar nerve damage, and lateral neck flexion should be avoided as it can result in brachial plexus injuries. Profound wrist flexion should be avoided in the arm resting on the Carter Braine support.

Corneal abrasions are a risk in the lateral position because of the dependent eye pressing against the pillow or from inadvertent contact with apparatus near the head.

Prone positioning is only needed for a few general or urological/gynaecological procedures (e.g. percutaneous nephrolithotomy; see Fig. 22.6D). Prone positioning requires tracheal intubation with the tracheal tube carefully secured, as reintubation will inevitably require turning the patient supine. Careful attention should be paid to head position, eye-padding, avoidance of abdominal compression and pressure-point protection (e.g. nose, chin, genitals, knees). The neck should remain as neutral as possible, and specialist head supports are available that distribute pressure away from areas such as the eyes and nose.

Turning a patient lateral or prone requires enough staff to safely rotate the patient whilst protecting the head and airway, guarding i.v. lines and preventing injury. Typically four to six staff are required. Cardiorespiratory stability is maintained in most patients, although temporary hypotension sometimes occurs as a result of decreased venous return or the sudden transfer of blood to newly dependent areas. Tracheal tubes can move during patient positioning, resulting in cuff leaks or endobronchial intubation.

Prolonged (>5 h) prone and steep Trendelenburg positioning are both independently associated with the risk of ischaemic optic neuropathy (see Chapter 26). The exact cause is unknown, but hypotension, anaemia and large-volume crystalloid use may be contributory factors.

Surgical techniques

Laparoscopic surgery

Laparoscopic surgery is associated with lower intraoperative blood loss and heat loss, reduced postoperative analgesia requirements and faster recovery times.

Most laparoscopic surgery requires a pneumoperitoneum produced by the insufflation of carbon dioxide. Exceptions include renal surgery, in which a retroperitoneal approach is possible, and some radical prostate surgery using an anteroperitoneal approach.

The pneumoperitoneum is typically held at pressures of 10–15 mmHg. This can be achieved by surgically inserting a laparoscopic port or by using a Veress needle. During insertion, inadvertent damage to bowel or major blood vessels can occur. Subcutaneous insufflation can result in surgical emphysema, whilst i.v. insufflation can cause venous gas embolism. Gas insufflation or port insertion can sometimes cause peritoneal stimulation, triggering a vagal bradycardic response requiring rapid deflation; occasionally, anticholinergic treatment is needed.

Peritoneal insufflation increases venous return, cardiac output and systemic vascular resistance. If higher pressures are used, compression of the vena cava may occur. It also decreases functional residual capacity, and when combined with the Trendelenburg position, there is an increased risk of atelectasis and ventilation/perfusion ($\dot{V}/\dot{Q}$) mismatch (Table 35.1).

Tracheal intubation and ventilation with PEEP may minimise effects of pneumoperitoneum, but patients with marked respiratory disease may not tolerate a prolonged pneumoperitoneum (although this should be balanced against the risk of inadequate breathing after open surgery). On occasion, congenital diaphragmatic fistulae or surgical diaphragmatic breaches can result in a pneumothorax.

Carbon dioxide is absorbed through the peritoneum during laparoscopic surgery, resulting in elevated $PaCO_2$, tachycardia and increased myocardial contractility. Pneumoperitoneum will often result in significant pain in the first few postoperative hours, until the carbon dioxide is absorbed. Retro- or anteroperitoneal insufflation often results in a faster onset of hypercapnia, which may persist after surgery, as well as sometimes causing surgical emphysema in the scrotum and/or chest and face. Nitrous oxide diffuses into gas-filled cavities and so is often avoided during laparoscopic surgery.

Conversion from laparoscopic to open surgery is a potential but infrequent risk that should be borne in mind during anaesthetic planning.

Robotic surgery

After inserting laparoscopic ports in the standard manner, robotic surgery involves 'docking' a surgical telemanipulator, which manoeuvres the laparoscopic camera and instruments. A three-dimensional image is transmitted to the operator, who remotely controls instruments which have a much wider range of movement than standard laparoscopic equipment. At present, robotic radical prostatectomy is the most common procedure, but major colorectal and gynaecological surgeries are increasingly using robotic equipment.

Radical prostatectomy requires the patient to be placed in steep Trendelenburg position (see Fig. 22.8), with its attendant risks (see table 35.1). Furthermore, robots do not tolerate operating table or patient movement, and neuromuscular blockade is advised until the robot is undocked. Whilst the robot is docked, patient access is limited, so tracheal tube and i.v. line positions should be checked before surgery. In the event of an emergency, access for treatment would require the robot to be rapidly undocked; it is recommended that rapid undocking is practised as a safety drill.

Communication between surgeon and anaesthetist is significantly altered during robot surgery. The surgeon sits in a booth, distant to the surgery, unable to directly view the anaesthetist or operating table. The surgeon's voice is projected by speakers, and allowances must be made for the inherent decrease in non-verbal communication, which will alter the whole dynamic of crisis resource management in an emergency situation.

Other endoscopic surgery

Flexible endoscopes are used for many diagnostic procedures, including oesophagogastroduodenoscopy (OGD), colonoscopy/sigmoidoscopy and surveillance cystoscopy.

Flexible biopsy forceps, snares or injection needles may be inserted down the endoscope for certain treatments. Endoscopy can often be performed using topical anaesthesia with or without sedation, but a GA may be required in situations where there is significant risk to the airway (e.g. OGD for major haemorrhage).

Rigid endoscopes allow the use of rigid instruments (e.g. resection diathermy loops) and fluid irrigation. Irrigation allows surgical field visualisation in enclosed spaces (e.g. bladder or uterus) and washes away blood and resected tissue. Rigid scopes mostly require GA or regional anaesthesia.

The choice of irrigation fluid depends on the surgical technique. Monopolar diathermy equipment requires a relatively non-conducting irrigating fluid so that current is not dissipated away from the diathermy loop when it touches the body. Until recently, most diathermy equipment used by urologists was monopolar using glycine, which combines good optical properties with poor conduction. In contrast, newer bipolar resectoscopes require saline irrigation, which conducts a charge from the active part of the instrument to the nearby return electrode.

Endoscopic resection with continuous irrigation requires the fluid to be under pressure, achieved by hanging the fluid reservoir from a drip stand. Fluid can be forced under pressure into tissue planes as well as veins opened by diathermy. Large amounts of fluid can be absorbed, causing fluid overload in susceptible patients. If the irrigating fluid is glycine, transurethral resection (TUR) syndrome may also develop (see later and Box 35.1).

Patient factors

Obese and bariatric patients

Increasing numbers of obese and bariatric patients are being operated on in all fields of surgery. The anaesthetic implications of obesity are described in Chapter 32, but in the context of general, urological and gynaecological surgery obese patients present specific problems in relation to airway, positioning and recovery.

Because of the attendant risks of lung atelectasis and hypoventilation, there is a preference for regional anaesthesia in obese patients. If a GA is required, there is a lower threshold for tracheal intubation and mechanical ventilation, even though airway manoeuvres will be more difficult, and hypoxic desaturation more rapid.

Elderly and frail patients

Many patients requiring surgery are elderly or frail, especially where any pathological condition is associated with advancing age, such as prostatic disease or cancer of the bowel or

Box 35.1 Risk factors and clinical features of transurethral resection (TUR) syndrome

Risk factors

- Only occurs with monopolar diathermy requiring hypotonic irrigation fluids (e.g. glycine)
  - Glycine should be switched for saline as soon as surgery complete
- High irrigation pressures
  - May be reduced by limiting the height of the reservoir to 60–80 cm above the operating field
- Large prostate/prolonged resection time
  - Surgery may need to be cut short
  - Diuretics may reduce risk if surgery is prolonged
- Prostatic capsule perforation during surgery

Symptoms in the awake patient

- Vertigo
- Nausea and/or vomiting
- Abdominal pain
- Visual disturbance/blurred vision
- Dyspnoea
- Chest tightness

Clinical signs and investigation results

- Confusion or agitation
- Decreased consciousness
- Seizures
- Pupillary dilatation
- Papilloedema
- Bradypnoea/hypopnoea
- Pulmonary oedema
- Cyanosis
- Oliguria
- Hypotension (although there may be initial hypertension)
- Bradycardia or other dysrhythmias
- Widened QRS and/or ST-segment changes on ECG
- Cardiac arrest
- Hyponatraemia
- Decreased serum osmolality
- Hyperammonaemia

bladder. Although the anaesthetic considerations for age and frailty are described in Chapter 31, it should be noted that coexisting chronic diseases can contribute to frailty. Urology operations are strongly associated with prior renal dysfunction, whilst patients having bowel and gynaecological surgery often have poor nutrition or advanced cancer. These factors, and any associated polypharmacy, increase the risk of biochemical or haematological abnormalities. For example, hyponatraemia and anaemia will affect the ability to tolerate

TUR syndrome and haemorrhage, respectively. As a rule, regional techniques are often better tolerated than GA in frail patients.

Cancer and chemotherapy

Anaesthetic assessment for cancer surgery should take into account the possibility of metastatic spread, particularly to the lungs.

Neoadjuvant chemotherapy (chemotherapy given before surgery) is increasingly being used to improve the likelihood of cure, or to reduce tumour burden and facilitate surgery; where patients require surgery for tumour recurrence, it is likely that they will have had intervening chemotherapy. Some chemotherapy regimens can produce systemic effects which may be identifiable preoperatively (e.g. anthracyclines and taxols, used in ovarian, breast and gastric cancers, can reduce cardiac reserve).

Bleomycin, used for germ cell tumours, is implicated in severe pulmonary toxicity, especially in the presence of high inspired oxygen fractions. Reducing delivered oxygen concentrations, targeting saturations of 88%–92%, is recommended.

Anaesthetic techniques

Regional anaesthesia

In combination with GA, regional techniques can also be used to provide excellent intraoperative and postoperative analgesia for larger operations. Where patients have significant comorbidities, it may decrease the risks of respiratory and airway dysfunction. Laparoscopic techniques typically do not benefit from additional regional anaesthesia and analgesia, whilst regional anaesthesia alone is often preferred for genitourinary procedures.

Sympathetic nerve blockade is associated with spinal and epidural anaesthesia, and hypotension can result when this is combined with the cardiovascular effects of sedative or hypnotic agents. This is particularly true of 'one-shot' techniques such as spinal anaesthesia performed immediately before a GA. Inserting epidurals or spinals *before* induction of anaesthesia is advisable to minimise the risk of inadvertent nerve damage.

Epidural analgesia

Epidurals are often combined with GA in procedures where there is likely to be prolonged postoperative abdominal pain, such as open surgery for cystectomy, bowel resection, ultraradical hysterectomy or nephrectomy. Larger incisions, particularly those involving the upper midline of the abdomen, result in pain on inspiration, and it is possible that epidural analgesia may reduce the risk of postoperative pneumonia. Epidurals have a significant failure rate (15%–40%) and need to be carefully monitored postoperatively, both to ensure efficacy and to be watchful for complications such as epidural haematoma formation (see Chapter 26).

Spinal anaesthesia

Spinal anaesthesia may be combined with GA for procedures where postoperative pain is less severe, such as operations involving Pfannenstiel or lower-midline abdominal incisions. The addition of an intrathecal opioid to the local anaesthetic can extend the duration of spinal analgesia further into the postoperative period, but there is increased incidence of nausea, vomiting and pruritus. Larger doses also increase the risk of delayed respiratory depression, particularly if a parenteral opioid is also prescribed. Spinal anaesthesia is also associated with urinary retention, most often in older men. Prophylactic catheterisation may need to be considered if spinal anaesthesia is used for procedures not routinely requiring catheters, such as inguinal hernia surgery.

Occasionally, spinal anaesthesia results in penile tumescence, which complicates penile surgery and urethral instrumentation. Intravenous ketamine can be used to treat tumescence, but it has adverse effects and limited efficacy. Intracorporeal administration of low-dose phenylephrine 100–200 µg is more effective, with less systemic adverse effects.

Other regional and local anaesthetic techniques

Local anaesthetic infiltration is often used during perineal surgery, and the addition of a vasoconstrictor reduces bleeding, but it has the potential to be absorbed, causing systemic effects.

Other techniques include the use of caudal block to provide saddle analgesia, and transversus abdominis plane (TAP) blocks to provide analgesia of the abdominal wall. Penile ring blocks provide excellent analgesia for penile operations such as circumcision but should be performed using plain local anaesthetic solution to avoid vasoconstriction.

Although many techniques offer only short-term analgesia, 'nerve-sheath' catheters or wound infusors are increasingly used to continuously deliver local anaesthetic solutions directly to nerves supplying the incision, such as paravertebral infusions for open nephrectomy or breast surgery or rectus sheath catheters for midline abdominal incisions. Additional opioid-based analgesia is often required, albeit at reduced doses.

Conduct of anaesthesia

Anaesthetic agents

Because of the previously mentioned effects of pneumoperitoneum and Trendelenburg positioning, it is preferable to use an anaesthetic with a fast 'wash-out'. This enables patients to rapidly awaken, protect their own airways and reverse any respiratory compromise. This can be achieved by newer volatile agents (e.g. sevoflurane and desflurane) or TIVA with propofol. Other than propofol being less emetogenic than volatiles, there is little to choose between the two agents. However, the possibility that TIVA use may reduce rates of cancer recurrence is being investigated.

Day-case and enhanced recovery surgery (see Chapter 34)

Many general, gynaecological and urological operations are suitable for day-case surgery, where the following principles apply:
- Rapid emergence from anaesthesia to an ambulatory state as a result of rapid 'wash-out' anaesthetic agents
- Good control of pain, nausea and vomiting; the ability to eat, drink and pass urine before discharge (especially after urological procedures)
- No requirement for prolonged monitoring, either as a result of the surgery, the anaesthetic, or because of pre-existing disease
- The ability to rapidly access appropriate health care in the event of unexpected delayed deterioration

Spinal anaesthesia is no longer a barrier to day-case surgery, as short-acting intrathecal agents are available (e.g. chloroprocaine, hyperbaric prilocaine).

For patients who require admission, enhanced recovery after surgery (ERAS; 'fast-track' surgery) programmes may reduce duration of stay. Enhanced recovery after surgery promotes recovery using a package of measures, the exact content of which varies between different centres and according to the surgical procedure. Typical elements include:
- preoperative optimisation, avoidance of prolonged fasting, carbohydrate loading and planned discharge date;
- minimally invasive surgical techniques (laparoscopic, small incisions or single-dermatome incisions);
- opioid-sparing anaesthetic technique (using regional or non-opioid analgesia);
- goal-directed fluid management using cardiac output monitoring, aiming to minimise fluid and sodium loading;
- avoidance or early removal of drains, catheters and nasogastric tubes; and
- early postoperative feeding and mobilisation.

Nausea, vomiting and postoperative feeding

Postoperative nausea and vomiting (PONV) occurs after approximately 20% of anaesthetics and is discussed separately in Chapter 7.

Where possible, PONV should be controlled and eating and drinking re-established as soon as possible after surgery. The routine placement of nasogastric tubes is discouraged as it is thought to delay normal feeding; these may be placed later if ileus is suspected. Some surgeries may still require a period of postoperative fasting and the siting of a nasogastric tube for drainage, including gastric surgery, emergency surgery for bowel obstruction and some small bowel surgery.

Heat loss

Keeping patients warm maintains cardiovascular stability, avoids coagulopathy, and improves postoperative recovery. Active warming measures are often necessary, particularly in open procedures or those requiring fluid irrigation. Large blood transfusions also put patients at risk of inadvertent cooling.

Warming can be achieved by using fluid warmers and over- or underbody warming blankets. Temperature is mostly monitored using oesophageal thermistor probes. Urinary catheter probes may also be used but may be inaccurate if the abdomen is opened (and are not possible if the urethra is instrumented).

Perioperative antimicrobial and venous thromboembolic prophylaxis

Antimicrobial prophylaxis is required where there is potential for bowel perforation (e.g. bowel surgery, cystectomy or radical prostate surgery). The choice of antibiotic depends on local protocols but should include gram-positive, gram-negative and anaerobic cover (see Chapter 18).

There is a high incidence of infection in patients with urinary obstruction, urinary tract stones or an indwelling catheter. Antimicrobial prophylaxis is required for surgery where the urinary tract mucosa may be breached (e.g. stone extraction, bladder tumour or prostate resection). The choice of antibiotic depends on local protocols and the sensitivity of any recent infections.

Prophylaxis may also be required to minimise the risk of postoperative implant infection (e.g. testicular prosthesis or hernia mesh).

Venous thromboembolic events are strongly associated with cancer surgery and renal, abdominal or pelvic procedures. Appropriate perioperative prophylaxis should always be considered and is likely to consist of lower leg pressure compression devices and low molecular weight heparin (LMWH). If neuraxial regional anaesthesia is used, then prophylactic doses of LMWH should be withheld for 12 h before the procedure (see Chapter 19).

Blood transfusion and conservation

Major surgery will require pre-emptive cross-matching. Alternatively, if recent group-and-screen samples have been sent, it may be possible to rapidly issue 'computer cross-matched' blood, provided there are no atypical antibodies. Further details on the transfusion of blood and blood products can be found in Chapter 14.

Blood conservation strategies should be considered for major operations associated with blood loss. This may include the use of antifibrinolytic medications such as tranexamic acid. However, tranexamic acid is typically avoided if intraluminal bladder surgery is planned, because of the risk of bladder clot retention.

Cell salvage technology may also be of benefit but is limited in cancer surgery because of the theoretical risk of haematogenous metastasis. Currently, many centres infuse cell-salvaged blood through white cell filters for cystectomy and radical prostate operations but not for gynaecological malignancies. Cell salvage should be stopped immediately before planned bowel incision in order to avoid contamination (e.g. at the time of ileal conduit formation).

Critical care

Planned critical care admission is often required for patients with significant comorbidities, for planned major surgery or for emergency laparotomies. Elective cases that are likely to be prolonged, associated with major haemorrhage or physiological disturbance should be considered for admission. Examples include ultraradical debulking of ovarian cancer and cystectomy operations. In some centres the use of a postoperative epidural requires critical care admission. Although there are exceptions, most laparoscopic procedures do not require critical care admission.

The National Emergency Laparotomy Audit (NELA) has recommended that all high-risk emergency laparotomy patients should be considered for critical care admission. They recommend using the P-POSSUM scoring system to estimate mortality (see Chapters 30 and 44) and that, as a minimum, patients with a risk of more than 10% should be admitted to critical care postoperatively.

Anaesthetic implications of specific operations

Emergency abdominal surgery

Emergency abdominal surgery is discussed in detail in Chapter 44.

Elective abdominal and pelvic surgery

Abdominal operations, especially cancer operations, are often performed on elderly adults. Preoperative assessment should encompass the potential comorbidities present within this group. Patients may also be malnourished because of poor oral intake or recent critical illness (e.g. patients undergoing reversal of Hartmann's procedure). Some patients may have incipient bowel obstruction and delayed gastric emptying.

Chronic blood loss relating to diseases requiring cystectomy, hysterectomy or bowel cancer surgery may mean the patient is anaemic before surgery. Other preoperative considerations include the potential for renal dysfunction caused by chemotherapy or ureteric obstruction or compression. Large pelvic tumours can cause abdominal mass effects such as abdominal compartment syndrome, vena caval compression and diaphragmatic splinting.

All patients are positioned supine, with lower abdominal and pelvic procedures requiring Lloyd-Davies and/or Trendelenburg, whilst upper abdomen procedures, such as cholecystectomy, can require head-up positioning. Examples of pelvic surgery include rectal or sigmoid surgery (e.g. abdominoperineal (AP) or anterior resection, Hartmann's procedure, sigmoid colectomy), cystectomy and some hysterectomy operations. For both abdominal and laparoscopic approaches, tracheal intubation and mechanical ventilation are required.

The choice of postoperative analgesia depends on the premorbid condition of the patient and the incision used. Low open approaches (e.g. lower-midline or Pfannenstiel) are often managed with PCA, sometimes supplemented by preoperative spinal anaesthesia containing opiates. Midline incisions extending past the umbilicus can also be managed this way, although epidurals are commonly used. Alternatively, postoperative local anaesthetic wound infusion catheters may be used. Upper abdominal incisions may benefit from an epidural, with high midline or subcostal ('rooftop', 'clamshell') incisions being the most painful.

Laparoscopic and minimal access approaches (e.g. laparoscopic bowel operations or cholecystectomy) require less analgesia postoperatively, although this depends on the risk of converting to an open procedure as well as on any final incision required to remove resected viscera.

Pelvic operations are often prolonged and carry the risk of substantial blood loss. Extensive resection has the potential for marked physiological derangement, and invasive monitoring combined with postoperative critical care admission is advisable. Examples include cystectomy, ovarian cancer debulking and extensive bowel tumour resection. Ultraradical debulking of extensive gynaecological cancers may require the excision of multiple structures, and any peritoneal stripping can cause a profound inflammatory response requiring large-volume fluid resuscitation and/or vasopressors.

All bowel operations carry a risk of postoperative ileus. Cystectomy operations, where the ureters are diverted into a newly formed ileal conduit, are especially prone to this complication.

Vaginal hysterectomy causes less trauma and postoperative pain than open abdominal surgery. Depending on the patient, a GA with a supraglottic airway device (SAD) or spinal anaesthesia alone may be sufficient. Perioperative occult bleeding is possible because of the impaired surgical view.

Laparoscopic sterilisation is often performed using a GA with a SAD. The degree of postoperative pain as a result of placing fallopian tube clips is hard to predict, but most patients require only oral analgesics.

Prostate surgery

Prostate surgery may be required for cancer or benign prostatic hypertrophy. Both are strongly associated with increasing age, and patients may be frail or have comorbidities. In addition, patients with benign prostatic hypertrophy often present with acute urinary retention triggered by a medical insult such as recent surgery. As a result, acute urinary retention is associated with a high 1-year mortality, especially if comorbidities are present. Preoperative assessment should particularly aim to identify cardiovascular, respiratory or renal illnesses. In addition to the anaesthetic risks from cardiovascular disease, the fluid shifts involved in transurethral prostate resection (TURP) may cause fluid overload in susceptible individuals. Pre-existing metabolic derangements, in particular hyponatraemia, are also likely to be exacerbated by surgery. Almost all prostate surgery has the potential for major haemorrhage.

Curative prostatic cancer surgery (radical prostatectomy) requires transperitoneal or anteroperitoneal resection performed using open, laparoscopic, or robotic techniques. A GA with tracheal intubation is required, with or without spinal or epidural analgesia. During laparoscopic radical prostatectomy, the urethra is resected at the bladder base, and causing diuresis by fluid-loading may obscure the surgical field.

Complications of TURP for benign prostatic hypertrophy include blood loss, hypothermia, sepsis and TUR syndrome. Blood loss during TURP is difficult to quantify because of dilution from irrigation fluid. Although a GA with a SAD can be used, spinal anaesthesia is often the preferred anaesthetic technique for TURP because of the decreased risks of respiratory and airway dysfunction. It can also allow earlier identification of TUR syndrome when monopolar techniques are used because confusion and agitation are amongst the earliest clinical signs (see Box 35.1). A sensory block to at least the T10–12 dermatomes is needed to prevent discomfort caused by bladder irrigation.

Very large prostates may require a retropubic prostatectomy (Millen's procedure) using a Pfannenstiel-type incision. Because of the size of the prostate, there is an increased risk of major blood loss.

Holmium and GreenLight lasers can be used for TUR and prostatic resection, resulting in minimal blood loss with faster postoperative recovery times. For selected cases, flexible endoscopic lasering without anaesthetic may be possible.

TUR syndrome (a.k.a. TURP syndrome)

As the name implies, TUR syndrome is most commonly associated with endoscopic prostatic surgery during which opened prostatic sinuses and veins can absorb hypotonic irrigating fluid. It is not exclusive to transurethral surgery, however, and has been reported after bladder tumour resection, cystoscopy, lithotripsy and transcervical endometrial resection.

Glycine solution is the most commonly used hypotonic irrigation (approximately 200 mOsmol L^{-1}), and absorption of more than 2 L results in rapid lowering of serum osmolality and sodium concentration. In addition, glycine exhibits toxic effects on the cardiovascular and central nervous systems (including retinal neurotransmission). Acute haemolysis has been associated with TUR syndrome but is unlikely to occur with modern glycine solutions.

The risk factors and clinical findings associated with TUR syndrome are shown in Box 35.1. The most obvious clinical features and biochemical abnormality are altered consciousness, cardiovascular compromise and acute hyponatraemia. Spinal anaesthesia may allow earlier identification of TUR syndrome, as most common initial signs are agitation and restlessness. Unfortunately, delayed absorption from perivesicular tissue sometimes results in presentation after surgery.

If TUR syndrome is suspected, the operation should be rapidly concluded and supportive measures initiated, combined with diuretics such as furosemide or mannitol. Hypertonic saline is required for patients with extreme neurological or myocardial dysfunction. Relatively rapid sodium correction of acute TUR syndrome is unlikely to result in pontine demyelination. A commonly quoted formula is (body weight × 1.2) ml h^{-1} 3% saline, which increases the serum sodium concentration by about 1 mmol L^{-1} h^{-1}. High-dependency monitoring is required.

Bipolar diathermy with saline irrigation eliminates the risk of TUR syndrome but still has a risk of fluid overload.

Nephrectomy and renal surgery

Indications for nephrectomy include renal tumour, intractable infection, trauma, calculous disease and renovascular hypertension or being a living donor. Renal tumours are associated with preoperative renal tract blood loss and anaemia.

Paraneoplastic syndromes occasionally occur in patients with renal tumours, causing hypercalcaemia, hypertension, polyneuropathy or fever. Preoperative renal function should be assessed, although nephrectomies do not necessarily affect postoperative renal function, particularly if the kidney was functioning poorly beforehand. Nephrotoxic drugs (e.g. NSAIDs and aminoglycosides) may be used, provided renal function is adequate and perioperative hypotension avoided. If the only functioning kidney is being removed, dialysis is required postoperatively and care should be taken to avoid infusions of drugs likely to accumulate, such as morphine. Care should also be taken to avoid placing cannulae in forearm veins, which are likely to be needed for future fistulae. Partial nephrectomies may preserve some renal function, but these have a lower rate of tumour clearance and a higher incidence of perioperative haemorrhage.

Large or vascular tumours may require radiological endovascular embolisation up to 24 h before surgery, and an epidural block is often inserted for procedural analgesia.

Depending on the size of the tumour and complexity of resection, renal surgery may be performed using open or laparoscopic surgery. In both eventualities the patient will be lateral, requiring tracheal intubation. Epidural or paravertebral blockade usually provides good postoperative analgesia for open surgery. Parenteral opioids are generally sufficient for laparoscopic procedures.

Haemorrhage is the most common complication, and tumour may impinge on the inferior vena cava, requiring it to be clamped during surgery. Occasionally, renal surgery can result in pneumothorax. Pneumothoraces are generally self-limiting and resolve after laparoscopic insufflation is discontinued. Insertion of an intrapleural drain is rarely required.

The anaesthetic requirements for nephroureterectomy are similar to those for nephrectomy except that patients initially require Lloyd-Davies positioning whilst the ureter is disconnected.

Intrauterine and transurethral bladder surgery

Cervical and transcervical surgery includes resection of tumours, endometrial ablation for menorrhagia, hysteroscopy and cervical dilatation and uterine curettage. Most bladder surgery is for transurethral resection of bladder tumours (TURBT). Patients with a bladder tumour are often elderly and may have a history of cigarette smoking; cardiorespiratory comorbidities should be identified preoperatively.

Anaesthesia for cystoscopy or uteroscopy has to facilitate irrigation but not always resection. Bladder tumours often require regular surveillance cystoscopy with only intermittent resection; it is often difficult to predict the extent of surgery preoperatively. General anaesthesia using a SAD is usually sufficient as these procedures are often short.

Spinal anaesthesia is a good alternative for higher-risk patients, although patients with respiratory disease may be more prone to coughing when lying in the Lloyd-Davies position, which can make surgery potentially hazardous. Resection of lateral bladder wall tumours can stimulate the obturator nerve, resulting in sudden leg movements, increasing the risk of bladder perforation. If GA is used, the administration of a neuromuscular blocking agent can avoid this complication.

Complications include TUR syndrome, haemorrhage and bladder perforation. Bladder perforation may not be immediately obvious postoperatively, as spinal anaesthesia may mask any pain. Blood clots may cause postoperative catheter obstruction and urinary retention, even if irrigation is used. Care should be taken to avoid undue catheter tension and accidental displacement when moving patients. Bladder spasm is common postoperatively, often in catheter-naive patients who may benefit from i.v. hyoscine butylbromide.

Postoperative pain associated with TURBT and transcervical surgery is often controlled with simple analgesics, with intermittent opioid administration if required.

Brachytherapy may be used to insert radioactive sources directly into cancerous areas such as the prostate, uterus or cervix. Anaesthesia is usually required for gynaecological brachytherapy, along with spinal, epidural or caudal analgesia if prolonged postoperative pain relief is required. Institutions undertaking brachytherapy have specific protocols designed to protect staff from ionising radiation.

Breast, hernia, perineal, penile and testicular surgery

Surface operations where no body cavity is entered (e.g. breast and hernia surgery) have fewer associated anaesthetic risks, and elective surgery is often performed using GA with a SAD. Alternatively, spinal anaesthesia is both appropriate for most penile, perineal, inguinal, or anal procedures.

Analgesic requirements are relatively low, although opioids may still be required. Supplemental nerve blocks may be used (see Chapter 25), such as:
- paravertebral or PECS (pectoral nerves) for breast surgery;
- ilio-inguinal block for hernia or orchidectomy (similar incisions);
- penile ring block for circumcision.

Infiltration of local anaesthetic may provide additional analgesia, and in patients unfit for any anaesthetic, circumcisions and hernia repairs may be performed just using ring blocks or surgical infiltration, respectively.

Radical vulvectomy and penile amputation are both cancer resections and are likely to include additional lymph node dissection. Both have the potential for severe blood loss.

Antibiotics are not routinely required unless implants (penile, breast, testes) or mesh are inserted.

Emergency operations include abscesses, testicular torsion, penile fracture, strangulated or irreducible hernias (where bowel ischaemia or obstruction may be present). Gastric emptying may be delayed in such cases, and sepsis may occur.

Fournier's gangrene (fasciitis of the perineum) is an emergency operation requiring extensive debridement. Patients are often septic, requiring broad-spectrum antimicrobial treatment and critical care admission. Postoperative pain may be quite severe and significant blood loss may occur.

Continence surgery

Pelvic floor repair operations can be performed under general or spinal anaesthesia, with supplemental local anaesthetic infiltration as required. Postoperative analgesia requirements are generally low.

Abdominal procedures, such as colposuspension, require open or laparoscopic approaches. Clam cystoplasty requires the bladder to be incised and a bowel 'patch' sutured to the incision edges increasing bladder volume. Cystoplasty anaesthetic requirements are similar to those of cystectomy.

Surgery for renal tract stones

Stones within the bladder or ureter are often removed during cystoscopy or ureteroscopy using mechanical or laser instruments. Ureteric stents (JJ stents) may be inserted during surgery, under radiographic guidance. General or spinal anaesthesia may be used. All renal tract stone surgery carries the risk of postoperative sepsis.

Percutaneous nephrolithotomy/lithotripsy (PCNL) requires tracheal intubation and mechanical ventilation. After cystoscopy and ureteric balloon insertion, the patient is placed in the prone position and a nephroscope is inserted into the renal pelvis. Ultrasonic fragmentation or nephroscopic forceps are used to break up the stone, with saline irrigation to flush out stone fragments. Fluid can be forced into retroperitoneal or peritoneal spaces, occasionally resulting in a 'tense abdomen' with diaphragmatic splinting.

Early pregnancy

Donor egg retrieval (as part of fertility treatment) is performed using ultrasound-guided transvaginal aspiration. This is performed under sedation or using GA with a SAD. Complications during egg retrieval are rare (e.g. haemorrhage or damage to intervening structures).

Suction termination of pregnancy (STOP) requires cervical dilatation and instrumentation of the uterus. The procedure is often quick and intermittent propofol TIVA can be used, accompanied by short-acting opioids. Volatile agents may cause uterine relaxation and so are avoided by some anaesthetists. Cervical dilatation occasionally results in a profound vagal response or laryngospasm.

Evacuation of retained products of conception (ERPC) has similar anaesthetic requirements to STOP. Both procedures are associated with the risk of haemorrhage and uterine perforation. Oxytocin is often administered after these procedures to promote uterine contraction and decrease postoperative bleeding. The administration of oxytocin can cause transient hypotension and tachycardia. Oral analgesics are usually sufficient postoperative analgesia.

Emergency ectopic pregnancy surgery may be either urgent (as a result of early detection) or immediate (if rupture and haemorrhage have occurred). Young, fit patients may not exhibit many signs of haemorrhage, but if bleeding is suspected, surgery should be rapidly expedited. Wide-bore venous access is required for resuscitation with fluids or blood. Patients can rapidly become hypovolaemic, requiring fluids or vasopressors after induction.

If there is no evidence of haemorrhage, a laparoscopic technique may be used, but in both cases an RSI technique is advised because of delayed gastric emptying.

Chapter | 36 |

Anaesthesia for orthopaedic surgery

David Hewson, Nigel Bedforth

One in five operations in the UK is for orthopaedic, spinal or trauma surgery. This chapter provides a framework for the conduct of anaesthesia for orthopaedic surgery.

The patient population

A large proportion of patients presenting for orthopaedic surgery are young and healthy. Sporting injuries and disease processes without systemic impact are common, and these patients are at low risk of complications relating to anaesthesia or surgery. However, several systemic disease processes are over-represented in patients presenting for orthopaedic surgery, including rheumatoid arthritis, systemic lupus erythematosus and ankylosis spondylitis. Drug therapies used to treat such conditions, including NSAIDS, corticosteroids, opioids and disease-modifying antirheumatic drugs (DMARDS), may affect the conduct of anaesthesia and surgery. These conditions are discussed in more detail in Chapter 20.

Techniques of anaesthesia

General anaesthesia

General anaesthesia is appropriate for some types of orthopaedic surgery, but regional anaesthesia is the preferred technique for many procedures, for reasons discussed later. Patients undergoing procedures of long duration (e.g. hip revision) often require general anaesthesia because of the discomfort incurred by remaining in the same position for a prolonged time. In many countries, including the UK, patients often expect to receive general anaesthesia and may not have been aware in advance of their surgery that regional anaesthesia represents a viable option. The implementation of preoperative patient education about their anaesthetic options, often undertaken during routine nurse-led assessment clinics, leads to better patient understanding of the benefits of regional anaesthesia in orthopaedic surgery. General anaesthesia causes the greatest loss of control for the patient, and many patients are pleasantly surprised to find that regional anaesthesia is an option for their operation.

Regional anaesthesia

Central neuraxial block (intrathecal or epidural anaesthesia) reduces the stress response to surgery and has been shown to reduce some serious complications after many types of surgery. Benefits may include a reduction in the incidences of deep vein thrombosis, blood loss, myocardial infarction, respiratory and renal complications and possibly pulmonary embolism. There is a high incidence of thromboembolic events in patients undergoing major lower limb arthroplasty, which makes this type of anaesthesia an attractive option.

Lower limb arthroplasty and minor lower limb procedures are often carried out using central neuraxial block alone. For longer procedures, such as hip arthroplasty, the use of sedation may be preferable.

After central neuraxial block, the patient is usually pain free in the immediate postoperative period. Careful thought should be given to administration of analgesia after the block has worn off. There is a higher incidence of urinary retention in patients who have undergone joint arthroplasty under central neuraxial block, particularly when long-acting intrathecal opioids have been coadministered. Patients may be managed by prophylactic urethral catheterisation or increasingly by monitoring of bladder volume postoperatively using ultrasound. If an intrathecal opioid has not been used, routine prophylactic urethral catheterisation is no longer routinely mandated.

Peripheral nerve block is commonly used as a sole technique for many procedures, with the advantages of excellent early pain relief, reduction of surgical stress, avoidance of complications of general anaesthesia and earlier discharge in the day-case setting. Orthopaedic surgery in patients at high risk of complications from general anaesthesia may also be carried out under peripheral nerve block. Patients report a high degree of satisfaction after surgery carried out using this form of anaesthesia. Table 36.1 shows the sites at which surgery may be performed in association with specific nerve blocks. This form of anaesthesia requires a high level of expertise and an understanding of the issues of managing a conscious patient during surgery.

Intravenous regional anaesthesia (IVRA) is suitable for manipulation of fractures and brief operations (less than 30 min) on the forearm and lower leg. It is technically easy to perform, but fatalities have occurred as a result of large doses of local anaesthetic reaching the systemic circulation. Before performing IVRA, it is essential to understand how the risk of complications may be minimised and how they may be treated if they occur. Details of the technique and safety precautions are described in Chapter 25.

Postoperative analgesia

Oral and intravenous agents

Many patients are already taking regular analgesics for pre-existing bone and joint pain. Paracetamol is very useful in reducing the dose requirements of other analgesics and may occasionally be sufficient analgesia alone. It is virtually free from adverse effects in standard doses and is contraindicated only in patients with hepatocellular insufficiency. Caution should be used when dosing paracetamol in elderly and frail patients who weigh less than 50 kg and should therefore receive less than the standard adult dose. The addition of NSAIDs, in the absence of contraindications, is often beneficial and further reduces the requirement for opioid analgesia.

NSAIDs inhibit the formation of prostaglandins and are widely used as analgesics in the treatment of acute bone-related pain. Selective cyclo-oxygenase-2 (COX-2) inhibitors potentially widen the number of patients who could benefit from NSAIDs by reducing the potential for gastroduodenal ulceration, but their use has been severely curtailed because of the increased incidence of myocardial infarction and stroke in patients taking long-term COX-2 inhibitors; this led to the withdrawal of rofecoxib in September 2004. The only COX-2 inhibitors currently licensed in the UK are celecoxib, parecoxib and etoricoxib.

Prostaglandins are known to have an important role in bone repair and homeostasis. Animal studies have demonstrated that NSAIDs impair fracture healing. This has raised concerns regarding their use as anti-inflammatory or analgesic drugs in patients undergoing orthopaedic procedures; however, the clinical implications of this are probably minimal and they remain extremely important analgesic agents for orthopaedic patients.

NSAIDs also affect platelet function and therefore could be expected to increase perioperative blood loss. The clinical evidence for increased blood loss in major arthroplasty surgery patients receiving NSAIDs is minimal.

Opioids are often used after major joint arthroplasty. Orthopaedic procedures, unlike many other forms of surgery, do not usually result in disruption to the enteral route of drug delivery, and therefore oral opioids are commonly used for severe postoperative pain. These can be prescribed on an 'as required' basis as immediate-release preparations, dosed regularly as modified-release capsules or a combination of the two. Patient-controlled analgesia systems using i.v. opioids are relatively rarely required in orthopaedic surgery. The doses of opioid required are reduced by the use of other

Table 36.1 Peripheral regional anaesthesia and analgesia

Site of Surgery	Block
Shoulder	Interscalene brachial plexus
Upper arm	Interscalene or supraclavicular brachial plexus, plus intercostobrachial after either of these
Elbow	Supraclavicular, infraclavicular or axillary brachial plexus
Forearm and hand	Infraclavicular or axillary brachial plexus, IVRA, elbow or wrist
Fingers	Metacarpal or digital nerve
Hip	Posterior lumbar plexus (psoas compartment), femoral nerve, proximal sciatic nerve, fascia iliaca block
Knee	Femoral and sciatic nerve (popliteal fossa or above) ± obturator nerve
Ankle	Sciatic (popliteal fossa) ± saphenous nerve or IVRA
Foot	Sciatic (popliteal fossa) ± saphenous nerve or ankle or IVRA
Toes	Ankle, metatarsal or digital nerve

IVRA, Intravenous regional anaesthesia.

analgesic agents and regional techniques, thus minimising the risk of adverse effects. For operative procedures undertaken using central neuraxial or peripheral regional anaesthesia, adequate systemic analgesia should be prescribed to provide adequate pain relief when the block recedes.

Central neuraxial drugs

Single-dose intrathecal or epidural anaesthesia using local anaesthetic alone usually provides analgesia for relatively short periods after operation. An adjuvant, such as an opioid agent, administered into the intrathecal or epidural space with the local anaesthetic improves the quality of the block and extends the duration of analgesia. These benefits must be weighed against the increased incidence of intrathecal opioid-related adverse effects such as pruritus, nausea and urinary retention.

Epidural infusions may be used for up to 5 days after major orthopaedic surgery. Careful observation for signs of inadequate analgesia (often a result of catheter migration) and infection is required. The involvement of an acute pain team is very useful in this regard. Many units manage these patients in an extended recovery or high-dependency setting to increase the level of nursing care and to facilitate early detection and prompt management of complications.

Peripheral nerve blocks

Peripheral nerve block, with or without a central neuraxial block or general anaesthesia, provides excellent pain relief for several hours postoperatively, allowing transition to oral or intravenous analgesia. Analgesic regimes should be commenced before peripheral nerve blocks wear off after painful procedures to avoid onset of severe rebound pain.

More recently, early rehabilitation after orthopaedic surgery has led to the development of motor-sparing blocks such as adductor canal blockade for knee surgery. Periarticular infiltration of high-volume, low-concentration local anaesthetic agents and an emphasis on early mobilisation after surgery as part of orthopaedic enhanced recovery programmes have reduced the use of more traditional peripheral nerve blocks to reduce prolonged motor blockade after lower limb arthroplasty.

Single-dose peripheral nerve blocks using a long-acting local anaesthetic such as levobupivacaine may last for more than 16 h. Additives such as dexamethasone may be used to prolong the duration of single-dose blocks, although the magnitude of this effect seems similar regardless of whether the dexamethasone is given perineurally or intravenously. Alternatively, a perineural catheter may be inserted, allowing an infusion of a low-concentration local anaesthetic drug (e.g. ropivacaine 0.2%) for several days postoperatively.

Nerve injury as a result of peripheral nerve block is rare (see Chapter 26), and patients with concurrent comorbidity such as diabetes or vascular disease may have an increased risk. However, the incidence of nerve injury secondary to orthopaedic surgery (direct trauma, tourniquet or positioning) is more common and often occurs in the sensory distribution of the nerve block.

Surgical considerations

Positioning

A patient's ability to assume the position required for operation must be assessed carefully; it is often useful to ask the patient to adopt that position before induction of anaesthesia if there is concern that mobility of joints may be an issue. Patients with arthritis often have restricted mobility of joints, and positioning at the extremes of the range of movement may cause severe postoperative pain in addition to the pain resulting from the operation. Orthopaedic surgery often requires the use of unusual positions, some of which carry risks of nerve damage, soft tissue ischaemia, electrical and thermal injury and joint pain. Care must be taken in protecting areas at risk of injury. These include bony promontories, sites of poor tissue viability and locations where nerves run close to the skin or close to the surface of a bone.

Forceful movement of the patient by the surgeon is often inevitable during orthopaedic surgery. When such movement occurs, it is advisable to recheck the patient's position, ensuring that soft tissues, nerves, eyes and venous access sites are protected.

Some positions adopted during orthopaedic surgery are associated with venous air embolism. These postures include the lateral position for hip surgery, the sitting position for shoulder surgery and the prone position for spinal surgery. Monitoring for and treatment of air embolism are discussed in detail in Chapter 27.

Prophylaxis against infection

Prophylactic i.v. antibiotics are often used during orthopaedic surgery. Infection of bone is particularly threatening to the patient and is very difficult to eradicate; consequently, prevention is a high priority. Allergic reactions to antibiotics may occur, and facilities must be available to treat such a reaction when antibiotics are used.

Laminar flow is used commonly in orthopaedic theatres to provide a constant flow of microscopically filtered air over the surgical field and to minimise the risk of wound infection by environmental pathogens. The evidence for laminar flow in the antibiotic era is controversial. This high flow of air over the patient's body surface greatly speeds convective heat loss, and precautions should be taken to avoid hypothermia.

Various in-theatre rituals exist for the prevention of cross-infection. These include the wearing of face masks and hats; however the evidence supporting their use is scant.

Prophylaxis against hypothermia

After induction of general or regional anaesthesia, heat is redistributed from the core to the peripheries. After induction of general anaesthesia, there is typically a reduction in core temperature of $1\,°C$ in the first 30 min of anaesthesia. Core temperature reduces more slowly after this initial redistribution phase, typically by approximately $0.5\,°C$ per hour, although the rate of fall is heavily dependent on ambient temperature, exposure and insulation, and the use of warming devices (see Chapter 13).

Hypothermia is known to be associated with increased blood loss because of the narrow temperature range in which enzyme-dependent systems work and perhaps because of platelet sequestration in the spleen. Hypothermia is also associated with poor postoperative wound healing and postoperative hypoxaemia.

The most effective method of reducing heat loss is forced air warming. However, warmed intravenous and surgical irrigation fluids and impermeable surgical drapes to reduce heat loss by evaporation are also useful.

Prophylaxis against thromboembolism

Deep venous thrombosis may complicate any surgery but is associated particularly with surgery involving the pelvis, hip and knee. Pulmonary embolism may be fatal and accounts for 50% of all deaths after surgery for hip replacement. There is evidence that heparin reduces the incidence of fatal PE in high-risk groups, including patients who undergo surgery on the pelvis, hip or knee. Low molecular weight heparins (LMWHs) have replaced unfractionated heparin (UFH) in the perioperative thromboprophylaxis regimens of most hospitals but are themselves being superseded by newer oral agents. Early mobility after lower limb surgery reduces the risk of venous thromboembolism.

Dehydration and immobility increase the risk of the development of postoperative DVT; consequently, adequate hydration, with minimal fasting times and encouragement of early postoperative mobilisation are advisable. Good analgesia improves mobilisation, and regional anaesthesia may be particularly helpful in this regard.

Epidural anaesthesia reduces fibrinolysis and activation of clotting factors and therefore reduces the risk of DVT and may reduce the risk of PE. These advantages, and the very small risk of epidural haematoma in patients who have received heparin, must be considered in an overall risk–benefit assessment when considering the use of epidural anaesthesia or analgesia during and after surgery. Current practice is to wait at least 12 h after the administration of prophylactic subcutaneous LMWH before insertion of an epidural catheter. A similar interval should be used between administration of LMWH and removal of the epidural catheter.

Correctly applied graduated stockings and intermittent calf compression devices reduce the incidence of DVT, but there may be no additional benefit for patients who receive heparin.

Limb tourniquets

Effective exsanguination of a limb and application of an arterial tourniquet greatly improve the visibility of the surgical field, as well as minimising intraoperative surgical blood loss. Exsanguination may be performed by elevation of the limb or by wrapping it in a rubber bandage or purpose-designed limb exsanguinator. The tourniquet cuff should be 20% wider than the diameter of the limb; this correlates to approximately one third of the circumference of the limb. To avoid damage by shearing and compression of skin, nerves and other tissues, the tourniquet should be lined with padding and applied over muscle bulk. Entry of spirit-based sterilising solutions under the tourniquet, including chlorhexidine in alcohol, may cause chemical burns and must be prevented. This is usually achieved by wrapping adhesive tape round the distal edge of the tourniquet and the adjacent skin.

The pressure in the arterial tourniquet should, in all cases, exceed arterial pressure; however, for reasons explained later, pressures are required that significantly exceed arterial pressure if arterial ooze is to be prevented. For the lower limb, this pressure is typically 300 mmHg (or 150 mmHg above systolic arterial pressure) and for the upper limb, 250 mmHg (or 100 mmHg above systolic arterial pressure). These rather wide margins are used for two reasons. First, the pressure on the measuring gauge is not the same as the effective tourniquet pressure; the narrower the cuff, the greater is the difference. Second, blood pressure commonly increases about 30 min after the tourniquet is inflated. This is not caused by the autotransfusion during exsanguination or by the increased systemic vascular resistance caused by tourniquet inflation, but results probably from activation of C fibres by ischaemia (mediating 'slow' pain). This pain may be difficult to relieve, and patients whose operation is conducted under regional anaesthesia may eventually find the pain intolerable and therefore require general anaesthesia. Some temporary tolerance may be achieved by administration of a short-acting intravenous opioid (e.g. alfentanil; titrate 100 mcg boluses), inhaled nitrous oxide or intravenous ketamine (e.g. titrate $0.1\ \mathrm{mg\ kg^{-1}}$ boluses). Dense regional anaesthesia, whether spinal, epidural or nerve block, may prevent tourniquet pain. However, despite an apparently adequate block, occasions may arise in which the patient becomes intolerant of the tourniquet after some time. The noxious stimulation of tourniquet pain is also apparent during general anaesthesia, when the patient's systolic arterial pressure often increases progressively until the tourniquet is deflated.

Electromyographical and histological changes which follow prolonged application of a tourniquet reverse after deflation. The maximum period of safe ischaemia is unknown. Lasting damage is unlikely if a tourniquet time of 90–120 min is not exceeded. Current practice is that 2 h represents the absolute upper limit of tourniquet inflation time. Brief deflation followed by reinflation of a tourniquet that has been in place for 2 h is not adequate rest for the limb; several hours are required for restoration of metabolic normality.

When the tourniquet is deflated, the products of anaerobic metabolism in the limb are released. A bolus of cold, acidic, hypercapnic and hypoxic blood is returned to the circulation. The systemic vascular resistance suddenly decreases, and venous volume increases. This may result in transient cardiovascular changes, including cardiac arrhythmias, myocardial ischaemia and changes in arterial pressure. There may also be an increase in intracranial pressure. Bleeding may also occur at the operative site. Tourniquets on more than one limb should not be deflated (or inflated) simultaneously.

Tourniquets may cause damage to peripheral tissues, to the tissue underlying the cuff and to the whole patient as result of the release of altered blood once the tourniquet is deflated. They are contraindicated to differing degrees in patients with poor peripheral circulation, crush injuries, infection and sickle-cell disease or trait. The use of a tourniquet in a patient with sickle-cell disease may result in within-limb sickling and subsequent ischaemia or thrombosis.

Blood conservation

An arterial tourniquet is used during a large proportion of orthopaedic operations. Consequently, intraoperative blood loss is often slight. However, tourniquets cannot be used for some procedures, such as hip arthroplasty and shoulder surgery, which may result in significant blood loss. Spinal surgery in particular is often associated with very extensive blood loss; bleeding from epidural veins is often responsible, and the techniques of blood conservation described later have made possible several spinal surgical procedures which were previously too dangerous to contemplate. Transfusion of donated blood carries significant risks, including cross-infection, hypothermia, clotting dysfunction, electrolyte disturbances, mismatched transfusion and allergic reactions. Donor blood is also a very expensive and rapidly dwindling resource. For these reasons, it is considered appropriate to avoid blood transfusion where possible. Various techniques are in popular use.

Avoidance of red cell loss

The use of a tourniquet significantly reduces blood loss associated with limb surgery. Isovolaemic and hypervolaemic haemodilution have been proposed as methods of reducing the requirement for donor blood, but the evidence for these practices is tenuous. Careful positioning may reduce venous bleeding through the assurance of adequate venous drainage at the surgical site. The maintenance of normothermia avoids hypothermia-induced clotting dysfunction. Epidural and spinal anaesthesia are associated with reduced intraoperative blood loss; this association is probably related to reductions in both arterial and venous pressures.

Cell salvage

The collection and retransfusion of blood lost during surgery has become popular in recent years. Few contraindications exist, although some of these are relevant in patients presenting for orthopaedic surgery.

- Cell salvage from a wound containing malignant cells is contraindicated because of the risk of dissemination of tumour cells. Malignant cells are incompletely removed by washing and filtration.
- Contamination with bowel contents or infected debris at the site of blood retrieval is a contraindication to salvage and retransfusion.
- Salvaged blood which contains topical haemostatic agents such as collagen, cellulose, gelatine and thrombin should not be retransfused, as it may result in intravascular coagulation.
- Salvaged blood which contains surgical irrigants, liquid methylmethacrylate or antibiotics not licensed for parenteral use (e.g. neomycin) should not be retransfused.

Pharmacological control of fibrinolysis

Increased fibrinolytic activity is a contributing factor in blood loss after major orthopaedic surgery. Tranexamic acid is a synthetic lysine derivative that competitively binds to lysine binding sites on plasminogen. In doing so it prevents fibrin degradation by the plasminogen–plasmin tissue activator complex. Much of the evidence to support the perioperative use of tranexamic acid in reducing blood loss is derived from lower limb surgery, and it is commonly given as a single i.v. dose for such surgery. Tranexamic acid is contraindicated in patients with a history of venous or arterial thrombosis, acute renal failure and seizures.

Modified transfusion triggers

Most clinical practice guidelines recommend restrictive red blood cell transfusion practices with the goal of minimising transfusion-related complications. The haemoglobin concentration used as a trigger for transfusion has reduced progressively in recent years as awareness has increased that patients are relatively tolerant of anaemia if they do not have any organs with perfusion or oxygenation problems and if an adequate cardiac output (and therefore an adequate circulating intravascular volume) is present. The context of the patient's anaemia is also of importance; if the patient is still losing blood, a haemoglobin concentration of 80 g L^{-1} is less tolerable than if bleeding has ceased. Independent of the patient's coexisting pathological condition, anaemia is less acceptable halfway through a hip arthroplasty than it would be at the end of a knee arthroscopy. Thus the patient's haemoglobin concentration is relevant but must be considered together with coexisting organ function and oxygenation (e.g. ischaemic heart disease, renal dysfunction, transient ischaemic attacks), the nature of the operation and the timing of the measurement in relation to the progress of the procedure.

Healthy patients tolerate a haemoglobin concentration of 70 g L^{-1} well if they have no additional requirements for physiological reserve. It may be safer to use a higher trigger than this for patients with known organ malperfusion. The adoption of lower transfusion triggers for patients undergoing surgery mandates that intravascular volume is maintained meticulously, because anaemia is tolerated poorly in the presence of a reduced cardiac output. It is also necessary to check the patient's haemoglobin concentration frequently during the operation and in the early postoperative period; this is performed easily using a point-of-care testing device such as the Hemocue haemoglobinometer.

Hypotensive anaesthesia

Intentional reduction of the systemic arterial pressure is rarely indicated in orthopaedic surgery. The risk of poor perfusion of vital organs makes this a potentially dangerous technique, and other options exist to avoid donor blood transfusion and to maintain a clear surgical field.

Specific surgical procedures

Primary hip arthroplasty

The operation is performed in either a supine or a modified lateral position. The femoral head is removed, and the new cup and femoral components are fixed to prepared bone with polymethylmethacrylate cement. Application and hardening of the cement, particularly after its insertion into the femoral shaft, are sometimes accompanied by sudden reductions in end-tidal CO_2 concentration and arterial pressure. Although attributable in part to toxic monomers released as the cement polymerises, the high incidences of these changes reported when the technique was relatively new were probably related to a high frequency of air embolism; air was forced into the circulation as the prosthesis was pushed into the femoral shaft. Techniques such as placing of cement restrictors, filling the shaft with cement from the

bottom upwards, or venting the shaft with a cannula have dramatically reduced the incidence of adverse events. However, insertion of cement may still cause embolism of marrow, fat or blood clots. Embolisation of air is also possible if the intramedullary pressure increases above venous pressure. Intramedullary pressure reaches its highest values when intact bone is first opened and reamed. Bone cement implantation syndrome, air and fat embolism are dealt with in more detail in Chapter 27.

Neuraxial anaesthesia with or without intraoperative sedation is regarded by many anaesthetists as the preferred technique for hip arthroplasty. Blood loss is rarely large during primary replacement, but vigilance is required, as assessment is made difficult by the large volumes of irrigation fluid used during the operation. Temperature homeostasis should be maintained using active warming devices such as a forced-air warming blanket.

To reduce the risk of dislocation of the new joint, the patient is placed supine in an abduction splint at the end of the procedure. This device makes it difficult to move the patient, and extra assistance is needed if the patient needs to be turned during the immediate recovery phase. After the first few postoperative hours, analgesic requirements are usually low irrespective of the anaesthetic technique employed. The complex innervation of the hip joint and the overlying skin means no single peripheral nerve block can provide totally effective analgesia after hip arthroplasty. The sciatic, femoral and obturator nerves all supply the joint, but blockade of these nerves leads to postoperative motor weakness that delays early mobilisation and increases the risk of falls. Many locally implemented enhanced recovery programmes recommend the periacetabular infiltration of large volumes of dilute local anaesthetic to facilitate postoperative analgesia, early mobilisation and encourage rapid recovery after surgery. Local anaesthetic agents of prolonged action, usually ropivacaine 0.2%, are used either alone or in combination with additives such as NSAIDs, adrenaline and opioids. Vigilance is required to ensure maximum recommended doses of local anaesthetic are not exceeded using this technique.

Hip resurfacing arthroplasty

Hip resurfacing is a more recently developed surgical technique for primary hip arthroplasty with the advantage that only the joint surfaces are removed during surgery. Most of the normal bone is preserved, including the femoral head and neck. The medullary canal is not opened, and no femoral stem prosthesis is necessary. It is an operation designed to postpone definitive joint replacement in younger patients with progressive disease. The operation is intended to interfere minimally with the normal mechanics of the joint, and it is also anticipated that the longevity of the prosthesis should be greater than when a rigid stem prosthesis is placed in elastic bone. The anaesthetic management for this procedure is essentially the same as for traditional primary hip arthroplasty. The risk of embolic events is low because of the reduced bone destruction and lack of exposure of the femoral medullary canal.

Dislocation of a prosthetic hip

Prosthetic hip dislocation needs manipulation and reduction to relieve pain and is more urgent if posterior dislocation threatens the sciatic nerve; this is more likely after trauma. Usually a brief general anaesthetic without neuromuscular blockade suffices; if reduction is difficult, muscle relaxation may be required. It is often unrealistic to move the patient from the bed before inducing anaesthesia, but precautions against regurgitation and aspiration of gastric fluid, including antacids and rapid sequence induction, may be indicated if urgent reduction is required or if the patient has been receiving systemic opioid analgesics (which delay gastric emptying). Usually the patient wakes up with considerably less pain than before manipulation.

Hip fracture

The effective treatment of patients with hip fracture, a life-threatening injury, requires the anaesthetist to combine meticulous preoperative assessment with evidence-based intraoperative anaesthetic techniques.

Approximately 98% of fractures are fixed surgically because non-operative management typically involves prolonged immobility with lower limb traction and consequently high risks of systemic infection, venous thromboembolism, pressure ulceration and muscle deconditioning. Surgery should be performed within 36 hours of hospital admission because delayed surgery results in higher mortality, and should be conducted with the minimum disturbance to baseline physiological and mental functions. Early fixation provides the best analgesia for patients with hip fracture, but anaesthetists will often be asked to assist in the preoperative analgesia regimen of patients awaiting surgery. Femoral nerve or fascia iliaca plane blocks, either as single-shot or catheter techniques, are effective in providing analgesia to patients. All patients should be offered regular analgesia and assessment of treatment efficacy. Ninety percent of hip fractures occur after a fall from standing height, but anaesthetists should be vigilant to contributory factors such as infection, arrhythmia, neuropathy, postural hypotension or valvular heart disease. Approximately 70% of hip fracture patients will be classified as ASA 3 or 4, and in addition to an anaesthetic history and focused clinical examination, a laboratory full blood cell count, urea and electrolytes and a 12-lead electrocardiogram should be undertaken in all patients before surgery. Further investigations should be determined on an individual basis, and a balance must be struck between the need for targeted

investigations to safely conduct anaesthesia and the resultant delay that these investigations may cause to surgery. In the absence of uncontrolled or acute-onset heart failure, it is rarely appropriate to delay surgery while awaiting investigations such as echocardiography, and it is unacceptable to delay on the basis of minor haematological or biochemical abnormalities. Estimation of risk of mortality is possible using validated risk scoring tools such as the Nottingham Hip Fracture Score (Table 36.2AB), and these may assist

Table 36.2A The Nottingham Hip Fracture Score (NHFS)

Domain		Score
Age	66–85 years	3
	≥86 years	4
Haemoglobin	<100 g L⁻¹	1
Residential status	Living in an institution	1
Mental state	Abbreviated mental test score ≤6/10	1
Comorbidities	≥2	1
Malignancy	Active in last 20 years (excluding skin)	1

Points are ascribed for the six domains. The total score can be used to estimate 30-day mortality.

Table 36.2B The Nottingham Hip Fracture Score (NHFS)

Total NHFS	Predicted 30-day mortality
0	0.4
1	0.6
2	1.0
3	1.7
4	2.8
5	4.6
6	7.4
7	11.8
8	18.2
9	27.0
10	38.0

Points are ascribed for the six domains. The total score can be used to estimate 30-day mortality.

the multiprofessional team in care planning and realistic discussions with patients and their families. Undisplaced intracapsular fractures are typically associated with only modest blood loss at the time of injury and can be fixed by cannulated screws or a dynamic hip screw. Displaced intracapsular fractures place the femoral head at risk of avascular necrosis and are usually managed by hemiarthroplasty, although younger and more active patients may benefit from total joint replacement. Cementation offers benefits in terms of long-term joint function and pain but may place the patient at risk of intraoperative bone cement implantation syndrome (BCIS). The aetiology of BCIS is complex, involving cardiovascular effects of the cement polymers; bone, fat and marrow emboli; and effects of anaesthesia, surgery and blood loss. Extracapsular fractures (including inter- or subtrochanteric types) usual result in more preoperative pain and blood loss than intracapsular injuries. They are usually treated surgically with a dynamic hip screw or proximal femoral intramedullary nailing. Surgery can be conducted using either neuraxial or general anaesthesia. Nerve blockade (femoral, fascia iliaca) provides a useful preoperative adjunct in both cases. It provides effective analgesia to allow positioning of the patient for spinal anaesthesia and has an opioid-sparing analgesic effect if a general anaesthetic technique is planned. More than 90% of hip fractures occur in patients older than 60 years and therefore, regardless of which particular anaesthetic technique is used, a knowledge of the special perioperative requirements of this age group is required to safely conduct this surgery. Intraoperative hypotension is associated with a worse outcome and should be avoided. High doses of spinal anaesthetic are not required – typically less than 10 mg bupivacaine is sufficient. Similarly, general anaesthesia must be titrated in accordance with the age of the patient. There is little evidence to suggest superiority of spinal or general anaesthesia – anaesthetists must be able to perform both to a high standard in this challenging group of patients.

Primary knee arthroplasty

Spinal or general anaesthesia are appropriate techniques for primary knee arthroplasty. Knee replacement is performed with the patient in the supine position. Pain after knee replacement is more severe than after most other major joint replacements. A variety of techniques can be employed to assist with postoperative analgesia, including intrathecal administration of opioids, femoral and sciatic nerve blockade and the infiltration of the joint capsule and surrounding tissues with a large volume of dilute local anaesthetic agent. The priority of enhanced recovery programmes to promote early mobilisation and avoid idiopathic complications means intrathecal opioids and traditional sciatic and femoral nerve blocks are used less often for knee arthroplasty than previously. Evidence exists that selective blockade of the

predominately sensory components of the femoral nerve in the adductor canal may offer analgesic benefit with relatively preserved quadriceps muscle strength, but whether this technique is superior to high-volume joint capsule infiltration is debated. Regardless of the intraoperative technique, all patients should have paracetamol and an NSAID prescribed on a regular basis (if there are no contraindications) together with an opioid. It is common to prescribe a short course of modified-release oral opioid, together with immediate release tablets for breakthrough pain. Coadministration of regular GI ulcer prophylaxis and antiemetic medication is common given the potential adverse effects of NSAID and opioid consumption.

There is less risk of thromboembolism after knee replacement than after other major joint replacements. Close observation for evidence of hypotension and cardiac arrhythmias, particularly in frail patients, is required after deflation of the tourniquet as the products of cellular metabolism are washed out of the tissues into the circulation. Significant blood loss may occasionally occur when the tourniquet is deflated requiring reassessment of fluid and blood transfusion needs in the early recovery period. Specialised drains which collect postoperative blood loss and allow immediate retransfusion may be inserted by the surgeon.

Manipulation under anaesthesia is sometimes needed in the postoperative period to improve mobility of the implanted joint. Neuromuscular blockade is not required. Depending on the extent of manipulation, i.v. opioid analgesia may be required to control pain, especially in the first hour after the procedure. Nerve blocks may be given to aid passive mobilisation of the joint after the procedure.

Revision of hip/knee arthroplasty

Increasing numbers of patients present for removal of the original prosthesis and insertion of a new one; this can be due to age-related wear and loosening of the primary prosthesis or infection. This procedure is of longer duration and usually involves greater blood loss than primary hip replacement. General anaesthesia is therefore commonly used. In addition to the precautions for primary arthroplasty, central venous and invasive arterial pressure monitoring may be considered. A urinary catheter should be inserted to monitor urine output. Greater heat loss is experienced because of the increased length of the procedure, and attention needs to be paid to maintenance of core temperature to reduce intraoperative coagulation abnormalities and postoperative complications. The use of blood conservation techniques such as intraoperative cell salvage should be considered, and all patients should have allogenic blood readily available for transfusion if required. Replacement of clotting factors may be required to correct abnormalities of coagulation if major blood loss occurs. Patients who have undergone arthroplasty revision may require a period of high dependency care postoperatively and will typically experience more postoperative pain than patients who have undergone primary replacement. Continuous epidural or continuous peripheral regional blocks such as posterior lumbar plexus block or femoral nerve catheters may be considered for postoperative analgesia.

Shoulder replacement

Patients undergoing shoulder replacement are often younger than those requiring hip or knee arthroplasty. They usually mobilise more rapidly in the postoperative period and rarely require a prolonged infusion of i.v. fluids or blood transfusion.

During surgery, the patient is placed in a lateral or 'deckchair' position, and general anaesthesia is typically required. Depending on the operating room layout, the patient's head may be relatively inaccessible during surgery, and decisions on how to safely secure the patient's airway should be made with this in mind. Surgery often involves vigorous manipulation of the arm, so the patient's head needs to be firmly secured, with adequate padding and regular checks during the operation. Elevation to the deckchair position should be undertaken with a freely running i.v. fluid infusion and with vasopressors available to manage any resulting hypotension. Because the shoulder is above the heart during surgery, there is a risk of air embolism. Shoulder surgery is associated with significant postoperative pain, but interscalene brachial plexus block with insertion of a perineural catheter provides effective analgesia after joint replacement surgery; indeed, it is possible to carry out the whole procedure under this block in combination with judicious sedation. Transient neuropraxia may be attributed to these blocks but, as with lower limb surgery, this is more likely to be caused by the surgical procedure.

Arthroscopic shoulder surgery

Arthroscopic shoulder surgery lends itself well to ambulatory regional anaesthesia using single-shot interscalene brachial plexus block. Most arthroscopic surgery can be performed with this as the sole anaesthetic technique, although posterior port sites will routinely require additional preoperative infiltration of local anaesthetic by the surgeon. Unexpected intraoperative discomfort responds effectively to a small dose of short-acting opioid such as alfentanil. As with shoulder replacement surgery, arthroscopic surgery is usually performed in a deckchair position, and the anaesthetist must be vigilant for the occasional profound bradycardic vasovagal episode, particularly in younger patients. Such episodes require prompt treatment with atropine or glycopyrronium bromide and ephedrine. Postoperatively, patients may experience severe pain when the block wears off. Multimodal analgesic regimes

including perineural catheter infusions of local anaesthetic are necessary to manage postoperative pain.

Spinal surgery

Spinal surgery is a major orthopaedic subspecialty. It provides several challenges for the anaesthetist; these include massive blood loss, difficult airway management, coexisting respiratory pathological conditions, one-lung ventilation and consideration of a variety of pathological conditions seldom seen outside this surgical population. Spinal surgical procedures include vertebral stabilisation after trauma or degeneration, decompressive surgery such as laminectomy, correction of spinal deformities such as scoliosis and excision of spinal tumours. Patients present for spinal surgery at any age; most scoliosis surgery occurs in the first two decades of life, decompressive surgery occurs most commonly in middle age and the majority of stabilisation procedures are undertaken in the elderly.

Most spinal surgery is performed with the patient prone, and significant time is spent ensuring safe positioning. Some procedures, however, require anterior approaches (e.g. via laparotomy incision to access the lumbar vertebral bodies) or lateral approaches (e.g. via thoracotomy to access the thoracic vertebral bodies). Sometimes surgery is undertaken using more than one approach, either as a single or a staged procedure.

Spinal anaesthetists must be confident in the management of the ventilatory requirements, intraoperative complications (including massive blood loss and use of cell salvage techniques) and postoperative analgesic needs of these disparate surgical approaches.

Airway management may be difficult in patients with cervical spine instability or underlying conditions such as ankylosing spondylosis. Awake video- or fibreoptic intubation allows neurological assessment before induction of general anaesthesia in patients with the most unstable injuries. Communication between anaesthetist and surgeon on the precise cervical injury and a mutually agreed plan for airway management is needed in such cases. Patients with a cervical cord injury may develop autonomic hyperreflexia and cardiovascular instability.

Scoliosis is associated with neuromuscular diseases in some patients. There is some evidence that such diseases (e.g. muscular dystrophies) may be associated with an increased risk of malignant hyperthermia or a malignant hyperthermia–like syndrome of abnormal metabolism in muscles, with a rapid and progressive increase in core temperature. There may also be increased difficulty with spontaneous ventilation in the postoperative period because of muscle weakness.

Patients with scoliosis may have severely limited respiratory function (e.g. restrictive defect because of scoliosis) and may be at risk of increased intraoperative bleeding. One-lung ventilation is sometimes required to achieve adequate surgical access during the correction of thoracic scoliosis.

Spinal cord function may be compromised during correction of spinal deformity because of ischaemia caused by excessive straightening of the spine. Spinal cord integrity may be tested using an intraoperative wake-up test. This requires preoperative psychological preparation of the patient and a suitable anaesthetic technique. However, the wake-up test has been largely superseded by advances in spinal cord monitoring techniques including somatosensory and motor evoked potential recording, which give an early warning of compromised spinal cord blood supply during surgery to correct scoliosis. Such monitoring will be instituted by specialist neurophysiologists and requires avoidance of volatile inhalational agents and neuromuscular blocking agents during the monitoring phase.

Peripheral surgery

Most peripheral orthopaedic surgery to either upper or lower limbs may be carried out in the day-case setting. Regional techniques provide excellent analgesia postoperatively and reduce the degree of disability which the patient suffers. Regional techniques obviate the need for general anaesthesia, leading to earlier discharge from hospital and a high level of patient satisfaction. Specific peripheral nerve blocks are described in Chapter 25. Certain patterns of orthopaedic injury (e.g. tibial shaft fractures) are associated with a risk of postoperative compartment syndrome. Peripheral or neuraxial nerve blockades have been implicated as a possible cause of delayed diagnosis of raised compartment pressures; however, examination of the literature offers many alternative explanations for diagnostic delay in such cases, often related to failures in communication and decision making. The use of a low concentration of local anaesthetic in suitably monitored patients and with the agreement of surgical colleagues are prerequisites for safe peripheral nerve blockade in patients at risk of compartment syndrome. Similarly, peripheral nerves are sometimes at particular risk of damage, either by the underlying orthopaedic injury or by the surgical approach required to provide fixation to that injury. A common example is the risk to the radial nerve after fractures of the humeral shaft. Early postoperative bedside assessment of nerve function to exclude intraoperative injury may be required, and peripheral nerve blockade in such circumstances is unhelpful.

It is easy to underestimate the degree of pain and disability that the patient may experience after peripheral orthopaedic operations. Analgesia should be prescribed on a regular basis postoperatively and additional 'as required' analgesia should be made available. Regular paracetamol, NSAIDs and opioids, if required and not contraindicated, should be prescribed.

References/Further reading

Gibbs, D.M., Green, T.P., Esler, C.N., 2012. The local infiltration of analgesia following total knee replacement: a review of current literature. J Bone Joint Surg Br 94, 1154–1159.

Grevstad, U., Mathiesen, O., Valentiner, L.S., Jaeger, P., Hilsted, K.L., Dahl, J.B., 2015. Effect of adductor canal block versus femoral nerve block on quadriceps strength, mobilization, and pain after total knee arthroplasty:

a randomized, blinded study. Reg. Anesth. Pain Med. 40 (1), 3–10.

Griffiths, R., White, S.M., et al., 2015. Safety guideline: reducing the risk from cemented hemiarthroplasty for hip fracture 2015: Association of Anaesthetists of Great Britain and Ireland, British Orthopaedic Association, British Geriatric Society. Anaesthesia 70, 623–626.

Marufu, T.C., White, S.M., Griffiths, R., Moonesinghe, S.R., Moppett, I.K.,

2016. Prediction of 30-day mortality after hip fracture surgery by the Nottingham Hip Fracture Score and the surgical outcome risk tool. Anaesthesia 71, 515–521.

Soffin, E.M., YaDeau, J.T., 2016. Enhanced recovery after surgery for primary hip and knee arthroplasty: a review of the evidence. Br. J. Anaesth. 117 (Suppl. 3), iii 62–iii 72.

Chapter 37

Anaesthesia for ENT, maxillofacial and dental surgery

Nicholas Chesshire

Ear, nose and throat (ENT), maxillofacial and dental surgical procedures account for a significant proportion of work in most anaesthetic departments. Recent cost–benefit and evidence-based analyses have reduced the number of common procedures performed, such as tonsillectomy, insertion of grommets and removal of impacted wisdom teeth. Other trends in surgical practice have offset this reduction, such as the prevalence of alcohol-related facial trauma and the increasing use of surgery in the treatment and palliation of cancer of the head and neck. The incidence of these cancers, particularly of the oral cavity, presents a significant and increasing global burden of disease.

The development of anaesthetic practice in these areas has therefore been concentrated on increasing the use of day-case surgery for more minor procedures and facilitating long and technically challenging operations to remove tumours and reconstruct defects. The effect of surgical pathological conditions on the upper airway requires meticulous attention to airway management and has led to the proliferation of new devices and techniques to overcome difficult tracheal intubation.

Airway management for shared airway surgery

Surgical pathological conditions and the fact that the airway is shared by the anaesthetist and surgeon can create challenges in managing the airway (Box 37.1). Tumours, abscesses, facial trauma, bleeding, anatomical variation such as receding mandible, obstructive sleep apnoea and other inflammatory conditions affecting the head and neck can all contribute difficulties. Meticulous planning of airway management must take place in consultation with the surgical team when the

airway is shared to enable safe and appropriate surgical access. This planning should take place during the WHO team brief so all staff are aware of the airway management plan. If bleeding is anticipated, the airway *must* be protected and the oropharynx may be packed to avoid contamination of the larynx with blood, pus and other debris. The decision to use a throat pack should be justified by the anaesthetist or surgeon for each patient. This person should assume responsibility for ensuring the chosen safety procedures are undertaken, and all staff should be fully informed of the chosen procedures; at least one visually based and one documentary-based procedure should be applied. At the end of the procedure the throat pack, if present, must be removed and the pharynx cleared of blood and debris before the trachea is extubated once full control of airway reflexes is present. Deep extubation can be achieved with the patient in the lateral head down position. The fact that a throat pack was used and has been removed should be recorded.

The anaesthetic circuit connections are usually hidden under the surgical drapes and are at risk of being dislodged by the surgeon during the procedure. Circuit disconnections are therefore a constant threat. It is important to realise that disconnections on the machine side of the capnograph sampling tube in a patient who is breathing spontaneously does not lead to a loss of the capnograph trace, and so careful observation of the reservoir bag is mandatory.

ENT surgery

Tonsillectomy

The number of tonsillectomy operations has decreased, but there are still approximately 50,000 procedures performed annually in England, just less than half of which are in

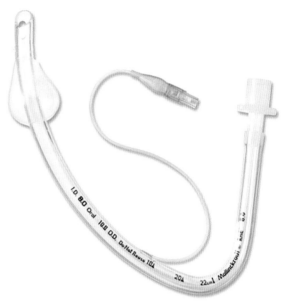

Fig. 37.2 South-facing moulded Ring-Adair-Elwyn (RAE) tracheal tube. (With permission from http://www.medtronic .com/covidien/en-us/products/intubation/shiley-taperguard -oral-nasal-endotracheal-tube.html.)

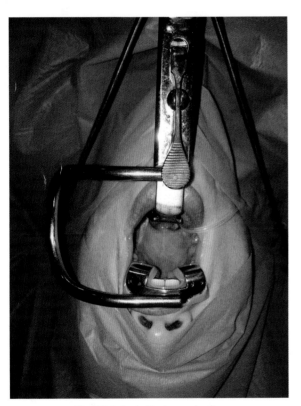

Fig. 37.1 Boyle-Davis gag *in situ*.

children. Almost all are performed under general anaesthesia, with one third undertaken as day-case surgery. Premedication is often impractical with modern admission practices, but robust preoperative assessment is mandatory (see Chapters 19 and 33), in particular to obtain any history of obstructive sleep apnoea or other airway problems. Often the patient is young and otherwise fit and routine investigations are unnecessary.

Surgical access to the pharynx requires the insertion of a Boyle-Davis gag (Fig. 37.1). To facilitate this, a secure

airway is usually maintained with a south-facing Ring, Adair and Elwyn (RAE) moulded tracheal tube (Fig. 37.2). Alternatively, a reinforced supraglottic airway device (SAD) (Chapter 23; see Fig. 23.5C) can be used successfully provided that the surgeon carefully avoids displacement of the SAD during the insertion and removal of the gag.

Spontaneous ventilation after the use of a short-acting neuromuscular blocking agent (NMBA) can be used to facilitate deep tracheal extubation in the lateral head-down position to protect the airway from soiling during emergence. Alternatively, positive pressure ventilation can be maintained throughout the procedure, with tracheal extubation fully awake in the sitting position. Various surgical techniques can be employed including cold steel dissection, electro-diathermy, laser and coblation. Blood loss can be significant, and vigilance must be maintained regarding fluid replacement; however, blood transfusion is rarely necessary.

Tonsillectomy is painful and requires adequate post-operative analgesia. This often involves a multimodal approach with an initial dose of i.v. morphine together with paracetamol and an NSAID. The latter can be given orally before surgery or parenterally during the procedure. Some evidence may point towards an increased risk of bleeding associated with the use of NSAIDs, but this is not clear-cut and most centres use this combination of drugs to facilitate early discharge. Multimodal antiemetic therapy should also be used because postoperative nausea and vomiting (PONV) is a common cause of delay in discharge. There is also evidence to support the use of steroids for control of emesis and pain, usually as a single dose of dexamethasone. Some evidence supports the use of topical or locally infiltrated local anaesthetic. The early establishment of oral intake of food, fluids and analgesia encourages early discharge and should enable most operations to be performed as a day case.

Adenoidectomy

Adenoidectomy is a commonly performed operation in children to improve the symptoms of otitis media with effusion and chronic rhinosinusitis. It is often combined with tonsillectomy and insertion of grommets. Recent systematic reviews have questioned the evidence of efficacy of adenoid surgery, and therefore the frequency of the procedure is decreasing. Adenoidectomy is also performed occasionally for glue ear in adults.

As in tonsillectomy, good access to the pharynx is required, usually with a Boyle-Davis gag, and therefore airway control with a south-facing tracheal tube or reinforced SAD is employed. Adenoidectomy as a sole procedure is usually rather quicker and less painful than tonsillectomy and may not require long-acting opioid pain control.

Rigid endoscopy and microlaryngoscopy

Rigid endoscopy is performed commonly in ENT to facilitate examination, biopsy and treatment of abnormalities of the upper aerodigestive tract. General anaesthesia is required, usually with tracheal intubation to provide a safe airway during surgery. Provided that no difficulty with tracheal intubation is predicted, i.v. or gaseous induction is followed by the administration of an NMBA, depending on the anticipated duration of the procedure. Examination, with or without biopsy, is usually short, and mivacurium or suxamethonium are often used (see Chapter 8). Increasingly, however, the operating microscope is used to resect neoplasms of the upper airway, especially laryngeal carcinoma, allowing less damage to voice function. These operations may be prolonged, requiring attention to normothermia and fluid balance. In general a small cuffed (microlaryngoscopy) tracheal tube (ID 4–6 mm) (Fig. 37.3) is inserted into the trachea to allow the surgeon greater access to the pharynx. This should be placed in the left side of the mouth to allow passage of the rigid endoscope down the right.

Microlaryngeal tumour resection is often carried out using a precision laser cutting tool. The use of laser in airway surgery creates the risk of airway fire, which can be catastrophic where flammable material exists in combination with oxygen and a means of ignition. The use of a metallic tracheal tube with cuffs inflated with saline (Fig. 37.4)

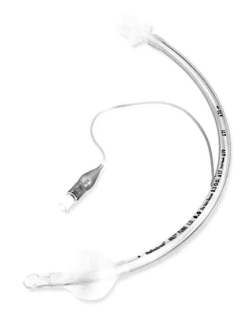

Fig. 37.3 Microlaryngeal tracheal (MLT) tube. (With permission from http://www.medtronic.com/covidien/en-us/products/intubation/shiley-microlaryngeal-oral-nasal-endotracheal-tube.html.)

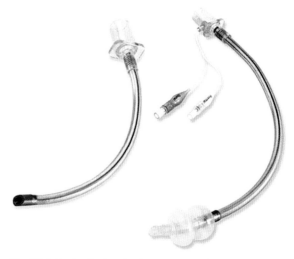

Fig. 37.4 Tracheal tubes for laser surgery. These can be uncuffed or have double cuffs that are inflated with saline. (With permission from http://www.medtronic.com/covidien/en-us/products/intubation/shiley-laser-oral-endotracheal-tubes.html.)

can minimise the risk but may not always be practical. All laser safety protocols must be implemented, such as eye protection, access to extinguishers, laser smoke masks and the use of reduced oxygen concentrations in the ventilating mixtures if possible. Short-acting opioids provide balanced anaesthesia, but morphine may be required for longer operations. Blood loss is not usually significant and is often controlled by the topical application of adrenaline with or without local anaesthetic. Safe tracheal extubation is normally achieved with full emergence and recovery of airway reflexes and careful pharyngeal suction before the removal of the tracheal tube.

Occasionally the surgeon requires access to the larynx without the presence of a tracheal tube. In this situation oxygenation can be provided by jet insufflation of the lungs via a subglottic catheter or an attachment to the endoscope (Chapter 23; see Fig. 23.52). The catheter can be inserted into the trachea either down the endoscope or through the cricothyroid membrane. Anaesthesia is maintained using an i.v. agent, usually propofol.

Thyroid and parathyroid surgery

Thyroid surgery is increasingly performed by specialist ENT surgeons, although some general surgeons still undertake the operation. Thyroidectomy may be partial or total and is performed for indications including thyroid cancer, toxic thyroid nodule, multinodular goitre and Graves' disease. Safe anaesthesia for thyroid surgery requires preoperative assessment accounting for specific hazards, an effective plan for intraoperative care and an awareness of the potential postoperative complications. Specific issues include the following:

- *Thyroid function.* Patients should be prepared so they are euthyroid both clinically and biochemically (as indicated by thyroid function testing) before surgery (see Chapter 20). Resting tachycardia and poorly controlled atrial fibrillation may indicate inadequate control of hyperthyroidism.
- *Airway compression and displacement.* A large goitre may displace or compress the trachea. The central position of the trachea above the sternal notch should be confirmed. Hard goitres are suggestive of malignancy. Infiltrating thyroid carcinoma may make neck movement and tracheal intubation difficult. An inability to feel below an enlarged thyroid may be due to retrosternal extension of a goitre. In severe cases the upper end of the sternum may have to be split at surgery to enable resection. Stridor and an inability to lie flat suggest airway compression. A chest radiograph may show tracheal narrowing or deviation. If there is more than 50% narrowing of the trachea, then a CT scan to fully explore the extent of airway compromise is advisable.

- *Superior vena cava obstruction.* This is uncommon but may be seen with extensive disease. The neck veins are distended and do not collapse on sitting up.
- *Vocal cord palsy.* Nasendoscopy to identify pre-existing vocal cord palsy is advisable before surgery.
- *Blood tests.* Preoperative tests should include thyroid function and corrected serum calcium concentrations.

Thyroidectomy is generally performed under general anaesthesia. Although most cases are uneventful the anaesthetist should be prepared for airway problems, and the patient's lungs should be preoxygenated before induction. If there are particular concerns regarding the airway, anaesthesia may be induced with the patient in a semirecumbent position. In cases where there is evidence of incipient airway obstruction, tracheostomy under local anaesthesia may be performed. Where there is obstruction of the mid-trachea after induction of anaesthesia the situation may be rescued with ventilation of the lungs through a rigid bronchoscope.

For surgery the patient is positioned supine with a sandbag between the shoulders to extend the neck. Particular care must be taken to protect the eyes where there is exophthalmos. Tracheal extubation should be performed with the patient awake. Rarely, prolonged compression by a large goitre may cause tracheomalacia leading to tracheal collapse and postoperative airway obstruction.

The surgeon often infiltrates the operative site with local anaesthetic and adrenaline. This may be supplemented with a superficial cervical plexus block for postoperative pain relief. Thyroidectomy is associated with a number of potential postoperative complications. Postoperative haemorrhage may lead to neck swelling and airway compromise. Clip removers or stitch cutters should be kept by the patient's bedside to allow expeditious release of a neck haematoma in the event of airway obstruction. Unilateral or bilateral recurrent laryngeal nerve injury may lead to vocal cord palsy, stridor or airway obstruction. With modern surgical techniques and fastidious identification of the nerves this is uncommon, but with severe airway obstruction, tracheal reintubation may be required. Temporary hypocalcaemia may be seen, especially after surgery for a large goitre. It may present with twitching, facial tingling, tetany and prolongation of the QT interval. Mild hypocalcaemia may be treated with oral calcium supplements, whereas severe hypocalcaemia requires i.v. calcium.

Parathyroid surgery is most often performed for primary hyperparathyroidism caused by adenoma. The traditional operation of exploration of all four parathyroid glands requires general anaesthesia, and surgery may be protracted. Technetium-99m or sestamibi scanning now allows the preoperative localisation of the adenoma in most patients, allowing surgery through a small incision to be performed under local anaesthesia.

713

Tracheostomy

The indications for tracheostomy include:

- loss of upper airway;
- prolonged mechanical ventilation;
- tracheobronchial toilet; and
- airway protection.

Tracheostomy may be performed percutaneously, usually in the ICU, or surgically in the operating theatre. Patients are usually already sedated or anaesthetised, although upper airway emergency management may require a tracheostomy to be placed under local anaesthetic (see airway emergencies section later). If surgical tracheostomy is required the patient is stabilised and the lungs ventilated in the operating theatre with the head and neck extended to allow access. When the surgeon has dissected down to the trachea, the lungs are ventilated with 100% oxygen, and the tracheal tube is withdrawn carefully into the proximal trachea to allow the tracheal window to be excised without perforating the cuff. At this point, positive pressure ventilation of the lungs becomes impossible, but in the event of surgical failure to insert the tracheostomy tube the anaesthetic tracheal tube can be advanced back down the trachea past the defect to allow ventilation to be reinstituted. After the tracheostomy tube has been inserted the breathing system is connected to it and ventilation confirmed with visualisation, auscultation and capnography. The anaesthetic tracheal tube may be removed and discarded after the tracheostomy tube has been secured. Early complications of tracheostomy include bleeding, loss of airway as a result of malposition, pneumothorax/pneumomediastinum and injury to surrounding structures. Later complications such as blockage of the tube as a result of secretions, infection, secondary haemorrhage and accidental decannulation; postoperatively patients require careful nursing and monitoring in an appropriate environment. Delayed complications can occur, such as stoma stenosis and tracheomalacia. Patients with tracheostomies should be managed by a multidisciplinary team including expert physicians, physiotherapists and speech/swallowing therapists. Many different types of tracheostomy tube may be encountered, including double lumen, which incorporate an outer and inner tube to facilitate speech and cleaning, adjustable flange for the obese patient and various long-term tracheostomy tubes. These should be regularly cleaned and changed according to the type of tube. The National Tracheostomy Safety Project has developed guidelines and resources for the management of tracheostomy emergencies, which should be embedded in organisations that care for these patients (Fig. 37.5).

Nasal and sinus surgery

Various operations are performed on the nose and sinuses to treat and prevent epistaxis, to improve the nasal airway, to reduce the symptoms of chronic rhinosinusitis or to improve the external appearance of the nose.

Most nasal procedures in the UK are performed endoscopically under general anaesthesia as a day case and range from simple diathermy of the inferior turbinates to prolonged cosmetic external rhinoplasty. The application of a mixture of topical local anaesthetic agents and other adjuncts (e.g. Moffett's solution, a mixture of cocaine, adrenaline and bicarbonate) provides vasoconstriction before surgery. The airway must be secured to protect the trachea from soiling by blood from the operative site. This can be achieved satisfactorily by the use of a reinforced SAD if there are no specific indications for tracheal intubation such as obesity or the expectation of a prolonged operation. Special attention must be paid to avoid disconnection or occlusion of the breathing system by the surgeon or soiling of the trachea. Balanced anaesthesia is achieved using increments of a short-acting opioid or a longer-acting drug for prolonged or painful procedures. Careful pharyngeal suction is performed at the end of surgery to ensure the removal of blood and other debris which may have accumulated. The use of a pharyngeal pack is generally unnecessary, but if used, it is vital to ensure that it has been removed before emergence. The usual principles applying to day-case anaesthesia are adhered to, including preoperative assessment and postoperative care (see Chapter 34).

Ear surgery

Examination under anaesthetic, suction clearance and myringotomy with insertion of grommets are common operations, particularly in children, and are performed to relieve the symptoms of chronic otitis media with effusion and to improve hearing. They may be combined with adenoidectomy and tonsillectomy for recurrent tonsillitis or chronic rhinosinusitis. In general, these are quick operations requiring attention to the principles of paediatric day-case anaesthesia. Postoperative pain is usually managed with a combination of paracetamol and NSAIDs to allow early discharge.

More complex procedures performed on the structures of the ear using a microscope, such as tympanoplasty, mastoidectomy and stapedectomy, are performed under general anaesthesia. Deliberate hypotension has been employed to minimise bleeding in the operative field, but agents such as β-blockers and vasodilators have largely been superseded by the use of short-acting narcotic agents given by intermittent bolus or infusion. These provide smooth anaesthesia without variations in blood pressure associated with surgical bleeding, which can obscure the surgeon's view through the microscope. If hypotensive anaesthesia is to be used, care should be taken to maintain vital organ perfusion and keep the MAP above the lower limit of autoregulation of about 55 mmHg. In general, these techniques require

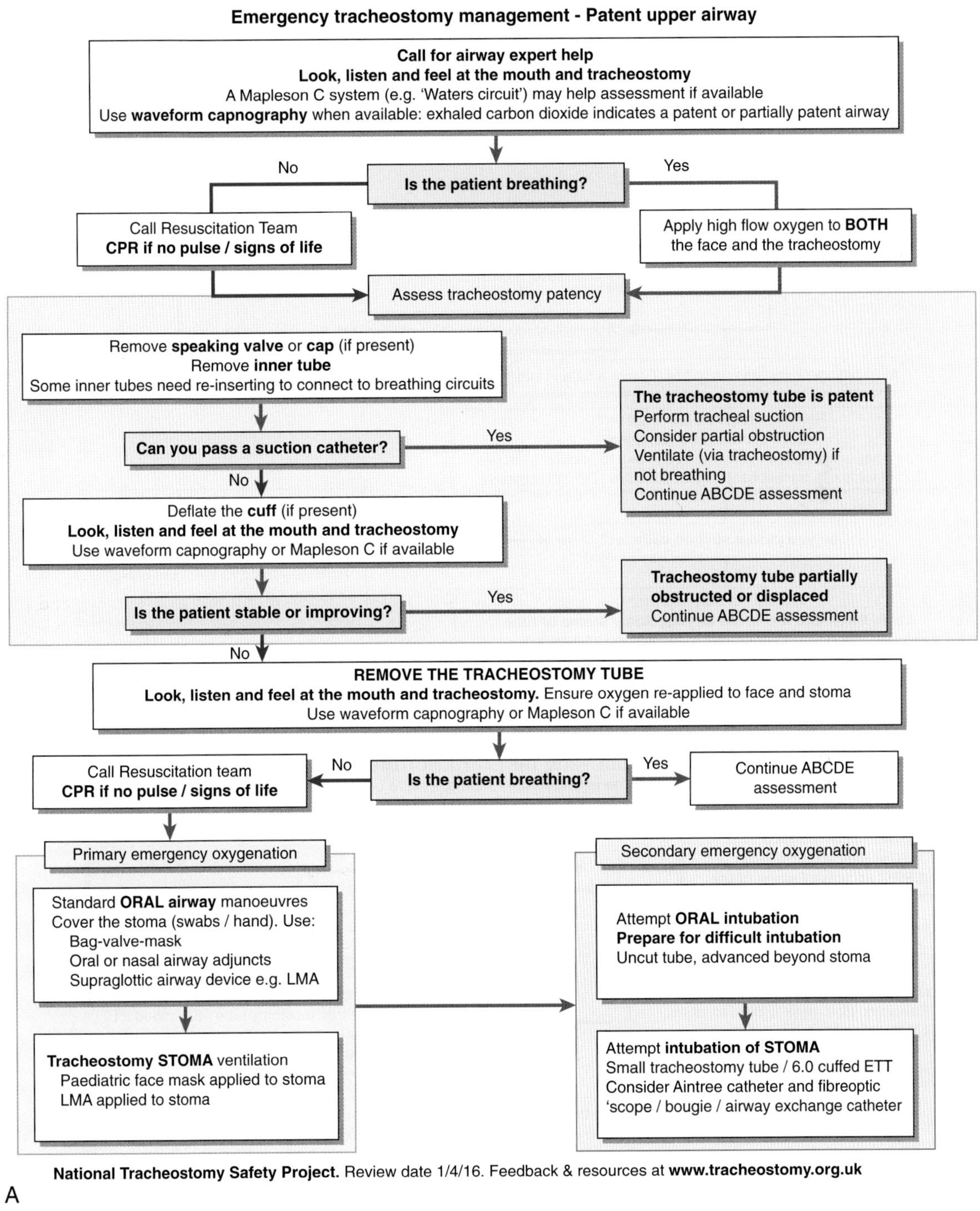

Emergency tracheostomy management - Patent upper airway

Call for airway expert help
Look, listen and feel at the mouth and tracheostomy
A Mapleson C system (e.g. 'Waters circuit') may help assessment if available
Use **waveform capnography** when available: exhaled carbon dioxide indicates a patent or partially patent airway

Is the patient breathing?

No → Call Resuscitation Team **CPR if no pulse / signs of life**

Yes → Apply high flow oxygen to **BOTH** the face and the tracheostomy

Assess tracheostomy patency

Remove **speaking valve** or **cap** (if present)
Remove **inner tube**
Some inner tubes need re-inserting to connect to breathing circuits

Can you pass a suction catheter?

Yes → **The tracheostomy tube is patent**
Perform tracheal suction
Consider partial obstruction
Ventilate (via tracheostomy) if not breathing
Continue ABCDE assessment

No → Deflate the **cuff** (if present)
Look, listen and feel at the mouth and tracheostomy
Use waveform capnography or Mapleson C if available

Is the patient stable or improving?

Yes → **Tracheostomy tube partially obstructed or displaced**
Continue ABCDE assessment

No → **REMOVE THE TRACHEOSTOMY TUBE**
Look, listen and feel at the mouth and tracheostomy. Ensure oxygen re-applied to face and stoma
Use waveform capnography or Mapleson C if available

Is the patient breathing?

No → Call Resuscitation team **CPR if no pulse / signs of life**

Yes → Continue ABCDE assessment

Primary emergency oxygenation

Standard **ORAL airway** manoeuvres
Cover the stoma (swabs / hand). Use:
Bag-valve-mask
Oral or nasal airway adjuncts
Supraglottic airway device e.g. LMA

Secondary emergency oxygenation

Attempt **ORAL intubation**
Prepare for difficult intubation
Uncut tube, advanced beyond stoma

Tracheostomy STOMA ventilation
Paediatric face mask applied to stoma
LMA applied to stoma

Attempt **intubation of STOMA**
Small tracheostomy tube / 6.0 cuffed ETT
Consider Aintree catheter and fibreoptic
'scope / bougie / airway exchange catheter

National Tracheostomy Safety Project. Review date 1/4/16. Feedback & resources at **www.tracheostomy.org.uk**

A

Fig. 37.5 Emergency tracheostomy management algorithm for (A) patients with a patent upper airway and (B) after laryngectomy. *ABCDE*, Airway, breathing, circulation, disability, exposure; *ETT*, endotracheal tube; *LMA*, laryngeal mask airway. (With permission from http://www.tracheostomy.org.uk/healthcare-staff/emergency-care.) *Continued*

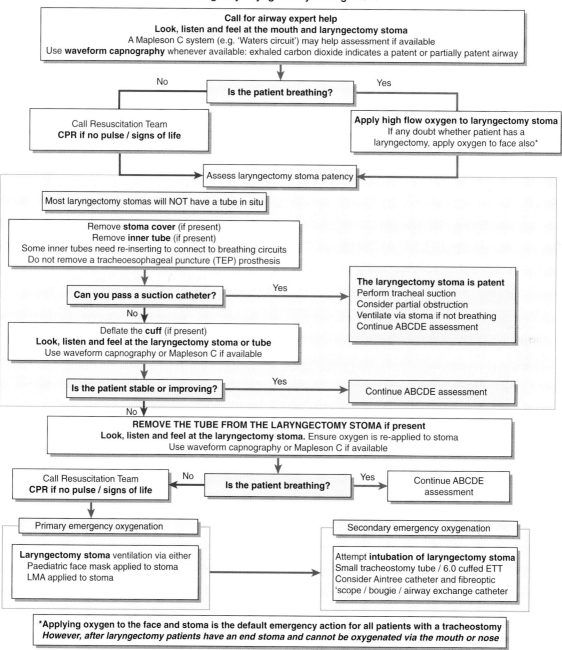

Emergency laryngectomy management

Call for airway expert help
Look, listen and feel at the mouth and laryngectomy stoma
A Mapleson C system (e.g. 'Waters circuit') may help assessment if available
Use **waveform capnography** whenever available: exhaled carbon dioxide indicates a patent or partially patent airway

Is the patient breathing?

No → Call Resuscitation Team
CPR if no pulse / signs of life

Yes → **Apply high flow oxygen to laryngectomy stoma**
If any doubt whether patient has a
laryngectomy, apply oxygen to face also*

Assess laryngectomy stoma patency

Most laryngectomy stomas will NOT have a tube in situ

Remove **stoma cover** (if present)
Remove **inner tube** (if present)
Some inner tubes need re-inserting to connect to breathing circuits
Do not remove a tracheoesophageal puncture (TEP) prosthesis

Can you pass a suction catheter?

Yes → **The laryngectomy stoma is patent**
Perform tracheal suction
Consider partial obstruction
Ventilate via stoma if not breathing
Continue ABCDE assessment

No → Deflate the **cuff** (if present)
Look, listen and feel at the laryngectomy stoma or tube
Use waveform capnography or Mapleson C if available

Is the patient stable or improving?

Yes → Continue ABCDE assessment

No → **REMOVE THE TUBE FROM THE LARYNGECTOMY STOMA if present**
Look, listen and feel at the laryngectomy stoma. Ensure oxygen is re-applied to stoma
Use waveform capnography or Mapleson C if available

Is the patient breathing?

No → Call Resuscitation Team
CPR if no pulse / signs of life

Yes → Continue ABCDE
assessment

Primary emergency oxygenation

Secondary emergency oxygenation

Laryngectomy stoma ventilation via either
Paediatric face mask applied to stoma
LMA applied to stoma

Attempt **intubation of laryngectomy stoma**
Small tracheostomy tube / 6.0 cuffed ETT
Consider Aintree catheter and fibreoptic
'scope / bougie / airway exchange catheter

***Applying oxygen to the face and stoma is the default emergency action for all patients with a tracheostomy**
However, after laryngectomy patients have an end stoma and cannot be oxygenated via the mouth or nose

National Tracheostomy Safety Project. Review date 1/4/16. Feedback & resources at **www.tracheostomy.org.uk**

B

Fig. 37.5, cont'd

positive pressure ventilation and neuromuscular blockade. A south-facing moulded tracheal tube or reinforced SAD can be used. Nitrous oxide is avoided because it can increase the pressure in the middle ear, thereby increasing the risk of graft failure. Postoperative pain is not usually severe and can usually be managed using oral analgesia, often allowing same-day discharge.

ENT emergencies

Bleeding tonsil

Primary haemorrhage occurs in the immediate postoperative period, usually in the recovery room, whereas secondary haemorrhage occurs at home some days later and may present via the emergency department. Blood loss may be profound, and fatalities can occur. Initial treatment involves attention to the primary goals of life support with the establishment of good i.v. access and volume resuscitation as well as the administration of oxygen. A blood sample must be sent for urgent cross-match. Emphasis has been placed on restoration of blood volume and pressure before induction of anaesthesia, but in the face of profuse active bleeding, urgent surgical haemostasis is of paramount importance. Most experienced practitioners advocate an RSI of anaesthesia with cricoid pressure because the stomach may be full of blood. Preoxygenation of the lungs is often difficult with the patient sitting up regularly spitting out blood, but it is vital. As soon as loss of consciousness has been achieved the patient is placed in the supine position and the trachea is intubated as quickly as possible, with suction readily available. Alternatively, gaseous induction can take place in the left lateral head-down position and the trachea intubated under deep inhalational anaesthesia. However, this is a technique rarely used outside of this situation, and the axiom of using familiar techniques when faced with emergency situations applies. When haemostasis has been achieved, full resuscitation takes place. Restoration of normal blood pressure must be ensured to reveal all potential bleeding points. Consideration can then be given to postoperative management, which will depend on the condition of the patient.

Epistaxis

Common causes of epistaxis include surgery and trauma, and spontaneous epistaxis can also occur, the last particularly in elderly hypertensive patients. Blood loss can be profound, and resuscitative measures may be necessary. General anaesthesia may be required to facilitate anterior or posterior packing of the nose, ligation of the sphenopalatine or anterior ethmoid arteries (often done endoscopically) and occasionally exploration of the neck to tie off the external carotid artery. Elderly patients are often on long-term anticoagulant

therapy which may require urgent reversal using vitamin K and/or prothrombin complex concentrates, and blood samples must be sent for cross-matching. The patient has usually ingested significant amounts of blood, and RSI with tracheal intubation is mandatory. If haemorrhage is swift and ongoing, preoxygenation may take place in the sitting position with immediate transition to the supine position with the application of cricoid pressure as soon as consciousness is lost. When surgical control has been achieved, normal blood pressure must be restored to reveal any further bleeding points before emergence and tracheal extubation fully awake. Occasionally, if surgical control is incomplete or tenuous, it may be prudent to keep the patient sedated with the trachea intubated to allow for full correction of clotting abnormalities and for clots to form and organise before tracheal extubation.

Epiglottitis and stridor

Epiglottitis is an acute life-threatening illness characterised by inflammation of the epiglottis and surrounding structures which can progress rapidly to complete airway obstruction. Previously it was considered to be primarily a disease of childhood, but since the introduction of routine *Haemophilus influenzae* type B (Hib) vaccination, it is now seen less often in children (discussed in detail in Chapter 33) and is more common in adults. Presentation commonly involves a combination of one or more of drooling, dysphagia and distress, often with other signs of systemic illness such as fever. The onset of respiratory symptoms such as breathlessness or stridor indicates an extreme emergency, and action should be taken to secure the airway. The cause is usually Hib bacterial infection (even in previously immunised individuals), and treatment involves airway support and i.v. antibiotics. If progression of airway compromise is anticipated, intubation of the trachea is indicated. Airway management may be very difficult, and senior anaesthetic and ENT support must be summoned urgently. Tracheal intubation should take place, if possible, in an operating theatre environment with ENT surgical support and equipment immediately available, including facilities for rigid bronchoscopy and emergency tracheostomy. Tracheal intubation may be difficult because of distortion of the laryngeal anatomy, and equipment for difficult tracheal intubation should be readily to hand. In the adult, fibreoptic–assisted tracheal intubation has been recommended. The patient's trachea must remain intubated in the ICU until it is confirmed that the swelling has largely subsided, usually by fibreoptic nasendoscopy. If ventilation becomes compromised before tracheal intubation, creation of an emergency surgical airway may be necessary.

Stridor, defined as a harsh high-pitched noise of breathing usually on inspiration, may also be due to other pathological conditions. Treatment is aimed at resolving the cause, but in the face of worsening respiratory distress emergency intubation of the trachea may be required. The anaesthetic management principles are as earlier; senior anaesthetic and ENT personnel must be available, and tracheal intubation should take place in an operating theatre environment. In general, supraglottic stridor caused by neoplasm or abscess may cause extreme difficulty in rigid laryngoscopy, and specialised methods must be available such as flexible fibreoptic endoscopy or retrograde tracheal intubation. In the event of failure, rapid surgical access to the airway may be necessary. In the presence of periglottic stridor (e.g. caused by laryngeal neoplasia) or subglottic stridor (e.g. as a result of thyroid disease), tracheal intubation can usually be achieved using a rigid laryngoscope under deep inhalational anaesthesia. Intravenous hypnotics or NMBAs must *never* be administered to a stridulous patient before securing the airway.

Oral and maxillofacial surgery

Oral surgery

The scope of modern oral surgical practice under anaesthesia continues to encompass primarily the removal of impacted teeth and treatment of associated dental pathological conditions which cannot be dealt with under local anaesthesia because of the severity of the disease or the inability of the patient to tolerate dental procedures.

Consideration must be given to the principles of management of the shared airway (see Box 37.1), and often nasotracheal intubation is required to allow a safe airway with good surgical access to the mouth. Careful attention is paid to the correct length of tube (Fig. 37.6) and visualisation of the reservoir bag and capnography. The NMBA used is determined by the anticipated length of the procedure and whether the anaesthetist prefers to use a spontaneous breathing technique or positive pressure ventilation. In simple surgery the anaesthetist and surgeon may elect to work around a SAD, but vigilance is required to avoid displacement or disconnection, leading to ventilation problems. The use of a throat pack is largely historical because the surgeon should pay close attention to pharyngeal toilet at all times, and the airway used should protect the trachea from soiling.

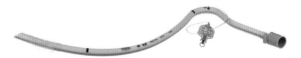

Fig. 37.6 North-facing moulded nasotracheal tube. (Used with the permission of Smiths Medical ASD, Inc. https://catalogue.bunzlhealthcare.co.uk/product/portex-clear-pvc-oralnasal-soft-seal-cuff-tracheal-tubes/.)

Tracheal extubation may occur either under deep anaesthesia in the lateral head-down position or fully awake with the patient upright. Most procedures are undertaken as a day case and the principles of pain control involve a multimodal combination of local anaesthetic infiltrated by the surgeon, simple analgesics and NSAIDs. Strong opioids are rarely required.

Orthognathic surgery

Patients with severe facial architecture abnormalities or bite asymmetry problems may present for treatment requiring mandibular or maxillary osteotomy and advancement procedures. This occurs generally at a young age with minimal comorbidities but requires a general anaesthetic, usually lasting for several hours. Difficult laryngoscopy may be anticipated in patients with a severely retrognathic mandible and can require flexible fibreoptic tracheal intubation. Nasotracheal intubation is necessary, and attention must be paid to fluid balance and intraoperative temperature control. Prophylactic i.v. antibiotics are given because microplates and screws are inserted to fix the skeleton into the new position. Postoperative pain and swelling can be severe, and patients are often monitored on a high-dependency unit and given ice packs and morphine if required. Postoperative jaw wiring is rarely indicated, but multimodal antiemetic therapy is still important, including dexamethasone, which may reduce swelling as well as emesis. Paediatric orthognathic surgery, such as for cleft lip or palate repair, may also be performed by oromaxillofacial surgeons.

Facial trauma and fractures

In the field of maxillofacial trauma, the anaesthetist may be called on to provide help in the treatment of the acutely injured patient in the emergency department or, more commonly, in the operating theatre for scheduled repair of facial fractures.

The initial management of facial trauma follows the principles of 'airway, breathing and circulation', and these are the primary goals particularly in victims of polytrauma. In facial trauma, airway difficulties may result from obstruction, bleeding, disruption of normal anatomy, intoxication and cervical spine immobilisation. Emergency tracheal intubation may be required if the clinical features of respiratory obstruction, hypoxaemia or coma are progressing and also if the anticipated course of events is likely to lead to airway compromise (e.g. facial burns). In these circumstances, RSI of anaesthesia with preoxygenation and cricoid pressure is the technique of choice if tracheal intubation via the oral route is feasible. Equipment must be available for difficult laryngoscopy, such as the gum elastic bougie, videolaryngoscopes and McCoy laryngoscope (see Chapter 23). Senior anaesthetic personnel familiar with these techniques must be present. In the event of failure to intubate the trachea, a plan must be in place to maintain oxygenation if bag-mask ventilation is difficult; this is discussed in detail in Chapter 23. If tracheal intubation using direct laryngoscopy is predicted to be extremely difficult or impossible, awake tracheal intubation may be necessary, or tracheostomy can be performed under local anaesthesia. Either technique can be challenging in the intoxicated and combative individual. Some advocate the 'awake look', which involves gentle insertion of the laryngoscope before anaesthesia to ascertain whether a good view of the posterior pharyngeal structures can be obtained. If this is satisfactory, i.v. induction of anaesthesia may be attempted safely.

Patients with facial fractures usually present for reduction and fixation 24–48 h after injury, when swelling has subsided, intoxication is no longer present and the presence of a significant head injury has been excluded. Depending on the mechanism of injury, the fracture may be mandibular, mid-face or isolated fractures of the zygoma or orbit. General anaesthesia is required, and tracheal intubation is necessary. Attention must be paid to the principles of the shared airway and consideration given to the optimal route of access to allow surgical intervention to proceed. Rarely, difficult tracheal intubation may be encountered because of anatomical disruption or residual swelling. Reduced mouth opening is usually caused by pain and stiffness. Most repairs of the mandible or mid-face involve intraoperative intermaxillary fixation to optimise postoperative function, and nasotracheal intubation is required. Isolated orbital or zygomatic repairs can be managed with a south-facing oral tracheal tube. Occasionally, nasotracheal intubation is not possible if complex repairs involving the nasoethmoidal bony skeleton are also to be undertaken or if a fracture of the base of the skull is suspected (which may occur in Le Fort III fractures of the mid-face). In these circumstances tracheostomy may be required or, alternatively, submental intubation in which the tube is passed via an incision in the floor of the mouth through the oral cavity and into the trachea.

When the operation has been completed, the tracheal tube can be removed safely, and the patient should be nursed in an environment in which postoperative pain and swelling can be monitored and treated.

Anaesthesia for head and neck cancer surgery

Tumours of the head and neck can arise from the lips, oral cavity, salivary glands, nose or nasal sinuses, oropharynx, hypopharynx or larynx. Worldwide, cancer of the mouth and oropharynx is the tenth most commonly occurring form of cancer. The tumours are most commonly squamous cell carcinomas which metastasise to lymph nodes in the neck.

Neck disease may present with an unknown primary cancer which can often be identified by examination or radiological scanning. Squamous cell carcinomas are known to be associated with alcohol and tobacco use and increase in incidence with age. Surgical resection may be performed by ENT surgeons or maxillofacial surgeons depending on the site of the tumour, and the expertise of plastic surgeons may be used for the reconstruction of defects. Anaesthesia must create conditions that allow surgery to take place safely, ensuring physiological support of all systems, lack of awareness, pain control and excellent surgical access.

Laryngectomy

Small superficial tumours of the larynx are treated surgically by laser microlaryngoscopy (see earlier) or by partial or hemilaryngectomy. Total laryngectomy is performed for more advanced disease, usually without neck dissection because tumours of the glottis rarely metastasise to the neck. Preoperative assessment of patients for laryngectomy must establish whether there is any evidence of respiratory compromise, which may be due to airway obstruction by the tumour or concurrent smoking-related illness. Flexible endoscopic examination of the glottis and CT staging of the neck can be used to predict difficulty in direct laryngoscopy. Tumours at the glottic level rarely present difficulty in tracheal intubation, and if no respiratory obstruction exists, i.v. induction followed by tracheal intubation can be performed. A smaller non-cuffed tube may be required if there is significant glottic or subglottic stenosis. If respiratory obstruction with stridor is present, inhalational induction and laryngoscopy under deep inhalational anaesthesia should be performed. Fibre optic tracheal intubation may be necessary if difficult laryngoscopy is encountered or predicted, such as because of radiation-induced scarring of the floor of the mouth. During surgery, an end-tracheostomy is fashioned, and a tracheostomy tube is inserted after the trachea has been divided below the larynx. To facilitate the division the oral tracheal tube must first be withdrawn proximally and the lungs ventilated with 100% oxygen. The operation usually lasts for several hours, and attention must be paid to intraoperative warming, monitoring and fluid balance.

Excision of salivary glands

Access may be intra- or extraoral; in the former, nasotracheal intubation may be required. Otherwise, standard general anaesthesia using an oral tracheal tube is appropriate. Operations on the parotid gland may be prolonged, and it may be necessary to avoid neuromuscular blockade during surgery so that the surgeon can use a peripheral nerve stimulator to identify branches of the facial nerve. An infusion of a potent short-acting opioid analgesic such as remifentanil can facilitate this.

Neck dissection

Neck dissection may be performed as a curative procedure or for local control of disease. It is usually combined with excision of the primary lesion, which may be oropharyngeal or nasal, but it is performed occasionally as a sole procedure if the primary is unknown or has been treated using another modality such as radiation. Cervical lymph tissue is dissected out, preserving blood vessels and nerves if possible. The tissue can then be examined microscopically to stage the disease and guide further treatment and prognosis. The neck dissection is often followed by creation of a free tissue graft pedicle with anastomoses to the blood vessels in the neck. General anaesthesia with tracheal intubation is required, using a reinforced tube facing away from the neck to allow access. A long procedure should be anticipated. In radical neck dissection the internal jugular vein may be ligated; if this is performed bilaterally, severe oedema of the face and neck may develop and tracheostomy may be necessary to protect the airway.

Surgery for oral, nasal and oropharyngeal cancer

If surgery is used, it generally consists of wide excision of the primary tumour, dissection of the cervical lymph nodes (depending on the staging of the disease) and reconstruction of the resulting defect. Procedures include glossectomy, pharyngectomy, maxillectomy and mandibular resection. Operations can be extremely prolonged (up to 15 h), particularly if microvascular tissue transfer is performed.

Preoperative assessment may reveal significant comorbidities, particularly in the older patient, and these may influence the anaesthetic technique and postoperative care. Supraglottic tumours can cause difficult tracheal intubation, and this should be anticipated by careful examination of the patient and radiological investigations. Techniques such as awake fibreoptic tracheal intubation or the use of other difficult airway devices may be required (see Chapter 23).

The functions of airway control and ingestion are usually secured by insertion of a tracheostomy and gastrostomy feeding tube, which can be removed after bleeding and swelling have resolved and healing has produced a stable and secure tract. Prolonged operations require careful attention to fluid balance and warming, and blood loss may be significant.

Reconstruction of defects is an important element of surgery. This commonly involves the insertion of a tissue graft into the defect. The graft may be swung on a vascular pedicle (e.g. pectoralis major flap), or a free tissue graft may be anastomosed with the blood vessels of the neck. A free flap tends to give a more favourable cosmetic and functional result but is extremely time consuming. Grafts may be soft tissue only (e.g. radial forearm skin) or composite for bony defects (e.g. fibula). A free jejunal graft or a pull-up of the stomach from the abdomen may be required to restore integrity of the GI tract if total pharyngectomy has been performed. Both will require laparotomy. Consideration should be given to allowing adequate rest breaks for the entire theatre team, including the anaesthetist. Postoperatively the patient should be nursed on a high-dependency unit where monitoring can continue and pain can be controlled effectively.

Dental anaesthesia

Anaesthesia and dentistry have a strong historical association. The development of both disciplines and the increasing awareness of the benefits of dental care and oral hygiene resulted in the uncontrolled proliferation of the use of anaesthesia in dental practice, often by dentists themselves, who had had minimal training in anaesthesia, sedation and resuscitation. At its peak in the 1950s, more than 2 million outpatient dental anaesthetics were given annually in the UK. Disquiet relating to the possible risks of death associated with the use of anaesthesia in dentistry resulted in the Department of Health commissioning a report in 1990, which recommended that general anaesthesia should be avoided if possible and that pain and anxiety associated with dental procedures should be ameliorated by local anaesthesia and conscious sedation. Further reports and guidelines since then have reinforced this viewpoint, and general anaesthesia is now reserved almost exclusively for small children and for adults with learning difficulties. General anaesthesia for dental procedures must be administered in a hospital setting with full theatre resources and anaesthetic support. Conscious sedation can be used in dental surgery if anxiolysis is required. This is administered by an anaesthetist or trained sedationist. The traditional dental chair anaesthetic has ceased to exist.

General anaesthesia

In paediatric practice the vast majority of procedures are for the extraction of carious teeth. There is a low incidence of systemic disease, but upper respiratory tract infections are common. Premedication may consist of topical local anaesthetic cream together with an oral analgesic and, if necessary, a sedative such as oral midazolam. Psychological preparation is an important element and is best carried out in a specialised paediatric environment. The majority of procedures are extremely short. Induction may be i.v. or inhalational, and airway support is commonly provided using a face mask, nasal mask or SAD delivering a combination of oxygen, nitrous oxide and a volatile anaesthetic agent.

The principles of care of the shared airway must be observed, and good communication between the anaesthetist and dentist is essential. Full anaesthetic monitoring is required, although it may be necessary to wait until after induction of anaesthesia in uncooperative patients. A combination of paracetamol and NSAIDs is generally used for pain control and allows early discharge.

In the adult, general anaesthesia for simple dentistry is indicated only for patients who are unable to tolerate local anaesthesia with sedation for psychological reasons or those unable to co-operate (e.g. because of severe learning difficulties). The vast majority of dental procedures under general anaesthesia in adults are performed when it is technically difficult to achieve the result without general anaesthesia (e.g. severely impacted third molar teeth or roots) or if poorly controlled carious disease has resulted in significant infection or anatomical derangement. These operations take place on oral surgery lists, commonly as day-case procedures. Nasotracheal intubation may be required for more difficult operations (see earlier). Patients are generally young and fit, but concurrent disease may be present in patients undergoing a total dental clearance before treatment for head and neck cancer or cardiac valve surgery.

Sedation

The greatly reduced use of general anaesthesia in dental surgery has resulted in an increase in the use of sedative techniques to allow surgery to take place comfortably in anxious patients or when complex dental work is undertaken. Sedation is defined as the use of a drug or drugs to render a state of reduced consciousness to allow treatment to be carried out but in which verbal contact is maintained with the patient throughout the period of sedation. The drugs and techniques used should carry a margin of safety large enough to make loss of consciousness unlikely. In the UK, intercollegiate working parties from dentistry and anaesthesia have developed guidance relating to the safe conduct of sedation in dental surgery, stressing the need for adequate equipment, training and documentation. It is recognised that potentially life-threatening complications may occur rarely.

Common techniques involve the administration of an i.v. benzodiazepine or the use of nitrous oxide. Sedation may be administered by the operator before surgery, or there may be a dedicated sedationist. Anaesthetists are often asked to take on this role and may use more complex techniques such as a continuous infusion of propofol using a target-controlled infusion device.

References/Further reading

Ahmed-Nusrath, A., 2017. Anaesthesia for head and neck cancer surgery, BJA Education, 17 (3), 383–389. https://doi.org/10.1093/bjaed/mkx028.

McGrath, B.A., Bates, L., Atkinson, D., Moore, J.A., 2012. Multidisciplinary guidelines for the management of tracheostomy and laryngectomy airway emergencies. Anaesthesia 67, 1025–1041.

Chapter 38

Ophthalmic anaesthesia

Chandra M. Kumar, Alfred Chua

Patients who present for eye surgery are often at the extremes of age. Neonatal and geriatric anaesthesia both present special problems (see Chapters 33 and 31, respectively). Some eye surgery may last many hours, and repeated anaesthetics at short intervals are often necessary. The anaesthetic technique may influence intraocular pressure (IOP), and skilled administration of either local or general anaesthesia contributes directly to the successful outcome of the surgery. Close co-operation and clear understanding between surgeon and anaesthetist are essential. Risks and benefits must be assessed carefully and the anaesthetic technique selected accordingly.

Anatomy and physiology of the eye

The perception of light requires function of both the eye and its central nervous system connections. The protective homeostatic mechanisms of the eye are interfered with by anaesthesia in a similar way to the effects of anaesthesia on the central nervous system. The sclera and its contents are analogous to the skull and its contents.

Control of intraocular pressure

The factors influencing IOP are complex, including external pressure, volume of the arterial and venous vasculature (choroidal volume) and the volumes of the aqueous and vitreous humour. Intraocular pressure is affected by a variety of systemic and ophthalmic factors (Table 38.1).

Intraocular pressure depends on the rigidity of the sclera as well as any external pressure. Functionally it is a balance between the production and removal of aqueous humour (approximately 2.5 μl min⁻¹). Chronic changes in IOP (normally 10–25 mmHg, mean 15 mmHg) may result in loss of ocular function.

Pressure is distributed evenly throughout the eye and is generally the same in the posterior vitreous body as it is in the aqueous humour, although the pressure is generated in the anterior segment. Each eye may have a different pressure. The aqueous humour is produced by an active secretory process in the non-pigmented epithelium of the ciliary body. Large molecules are excluded by a blood–aqueous barrier between the epithelium and iris capillaries. The sodium-potassium ATPase pump is involved in the active transport of sodium into the aqueous humour. Carbonic anhydrase catalyses the conversion of water and carbon dioxide to carbonic acid, which passes passively into the aqueous humour. Acetazolamide, an inhibitor of carbonic anhydrase used in the treatment of raised IOP, reduces bicarbonate and sodium transport into the aqueous to produce its therapeutic effect. There is a less important hydrostatic element dependent on ocular perfusion pressure. Aqueous humour production is related linearly to blood flow. Flow and vascular pressure are controlled by the autonomic nervous system, and autoregulation exists, similar to cerebral blood flow. Aqueous humour removal is inhibited by pressure within the pars plana, and episcleral venules restrict the vascular outflow, as does the IOP.

The aqueous humour flows from the ciliary body through the trabecular meshwork into the anterior chamber before exiting through the angle of Schlemm (Fig. 38.1). The sum of the hydrostatic inflow and the active aqueous humour production minus the active resorption and passive filtration must equal zero to achieve balance. Alteration of any individual feature can lead to changes in IOP.

Ocular blood flow

Ocular blood flow and IOP are intrinsically linked. The control mechanisms are similar to cerebral blood flow, although there are differences in the anatomy. Ocular perfusion pressure (OPP) equals the MAP minus the intraocular

Table 38.1 Factors affecting intraocular pressure

Increased intraocular pressure	Decreased intraocular pressure
Systemic factors	
Elevated venous pressure	Reduced venous pressure
Elevated arterial blood pressure	Reduced arterial blood pressure
Elevated $PaCO_2$	Reduced $PaCO_2$
Decreased PaO_2	Head-up position
Valsalva manoeuvre	Pregnancy
Head-down position	Hypothermia
Age	Acidosis
Increased carotid blood flow	Adrenalectomy
Carotid-cavernous fistula	Parasympathetic stimulation
Plasma hypo-osmolality	Plasma hyperosmolality
Sympathetic stimulation	General anaesthesia
Ophthalmic factors	
Increased episcleral venous pressure	Decrease in episcleral venous pressure
Blockage of ophthalmic vein	Decrease in ophthalmic artery blood flow
Blockage of trabecular meshwork	Prolonged external pressure
Contraction of extraocular muscles	Retrobulbar anaesthesia
Restricted extraocular muscle	Ocular trauma
Acute external pressure	Intraocular surgery
Forced blinking	Retinal detachment
Relaxation of accommodation	Choroidal detachment
Prostaglandin release (biphasic)	Inflammation
Hypersecretion of aqueous humour	Prostaglandins (biphasic)
	Accommodation
	Increased aqueous outflow
Anaesthetic drugs	
Suxamethonium	Intravenous anaesthetic agents
Ketamine	Volatile anaesthetic agents
	Opioids

pressure. This is subject to autoregulation within the range 60 to 150 mmHg. Ocular blood flow is affected to some degree by local anaesthetic injections.

Oculocardiac reflex

The oculocardiac reflex is a triad of bradycardia, nausea and syncope. Classically precipitated by muscle traction, it may also occur in association with stimulation of the eyelids or the orbital floor and pressure on the eye itself. Apnoea may also occur. The ophthalmic division of the trigeminal nerve is the afferent limb, passing through the reticular formation to the visceral motor nuclei of the vagus nerve.

The risk of development of the oculocardiac reflex is highest in children undergoing squint surgery and in retinal detachment surgery. Treatment requires either a cessation of the stimulus or an appropriate dose of an anticholinergic drug such as atropine or glycopyrronium bromide.

Cornea

The normal cornea is about 520 μm thick. It consists of five layers: epithelium, Bowman's membrane, stroma, Descemet's membrane and endothelium. The stroma comprises 80%–85% of the corneal thickness and provides the main structural framework. Corneal endothelium is a single sheet of hexagonal cells with poor regenerative capacity. Its main function is pumping fluid out of the cornea.

Conditions for intraocular surgery

For most intraocular operations, the eye must be insensate, preferably immobile, with intraocular pressure reduced and pupil dilated. In a few operations, such as glaucoma, corneal transplantation and insertion of iris-clipped intraocular lens, the pupil is constricted to protect structures behind the iris or for centring purposes.

Expulsive haemorrhage

In the presence of markedly raised IOP, sudden reduction in pressure on incision of the globe may lead to the expression of the contents. The balance between venous and intraocular pressure is crucial. An increase in venous pressure causes fluid to pool in the choroid and may progress to cause rupture of the ciliary artery with prolapse of the iris. On rare occasions, disastrous expulsive haemorrhage may result in the loss of the entire contents of the eyeball. The overall incidence is 0.19% in all intraocular procedures, with the highest incidence of 0.54% in penetrating keratoplasty.

Drugs

- *Premedication.* Drugs used for premedication have little effect on intraocular pressure, and commonly used anxiolytic and antiemetic drugs may be used as preferred.
- *Intravenous anaesthetic agents.* Most of the i.v. induction agents, with the exception of ketamine, reduce IOP and may be used as indicated clinically. Ketamine should be avoided if intraocular surgery is planned.

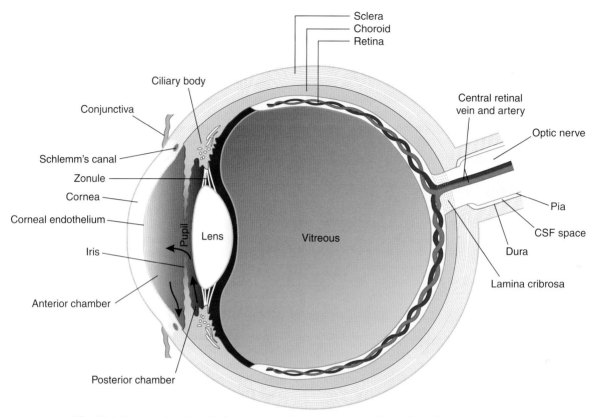

Fig. 38.1 Cross-section through the eye and optic nerve. *Arrows* indicate flow of aqueous humour.

- *Neuromuscular blocking agents (NMBAs.)* Suxamethonium increases intraocular pressure, with a maximal effect 2 min after administration, but the pressure returns to baseline values after 5 min. This effect is thought to be caused by the increase in tone of the extraocular muscles and intraocular vasodilatation. Pretreatment with a small dose of a non-depolarising NMBA does not obtund this response reliably. Non-depolarising NMBAs have no significant direct effects on IOP.
- *Volatile anaesthetic agents.* All the volatile anaesthetic agents in current use decrease IOP. Nitrous oxide has no effect on IOP in the absence of air or a therapeutic inert gas bubble in the globe.
- *Opioids.* All opioid agents cause a moderate reduction in IOP in the absence of significant ventilatory depression. They contribute to postoperative nausea and vomiting (PONV) and are not often required for postoperative analgesia after eye surgery.

Choice of anaesthesia

The type of surgery, its urgency and the age and fitness of the patient influence the choice of anaesthesia. Local anaesthesia is preferred for older and sicker patients because the stress response to surgery is diminished and complications such as postoperative delirium, PONV and urinary retention are mostly eliminated. Younger patients may sometimes be too anxious for local anaesthesia and are usually managed with general anaesthesia.

There is a need to maintain homeostasis in the eye if intraocular surgery is planned. For the purposes of patient comfort, it may also be necessary to consider the duration of the procedure and the patient's ability to stay still for a longer period. However, all types of ophthalmic surgery have been carried out with local anaesthesia in compliant patients, including repair of ocular trauma.

General anaesthesia

General anaesthesia is indicated when the patient is unwilling or unable to tolerate local anaesthesia (e.g. adults with special needs). The length and complexity of the operation are also important determinants. Patients with dementia, irrespective of the stage of the disease, are generally scheduled for general anaesthesia. The majority of patients in the early stages of the disease tolerate locoregional anaesthesia for routine cataract surgery. It is not uncommon for patients with serious comorbidities which cannot be improved preoperatively to accept the increased risk of death associated with proceeding with surgery and general anaesthesia when the desired outcome is maintenance or improvement of vision.

Assessment and preparation

Standard preoperative assessment for patients undergoing general anaesthesia should be carried out for all patients (see Chapter 19). It is important that the preoperative preparation includes consideration of whether the patient will be able to lie flat for up to an hour without having problems related to cognitive function; becoming uncomfortable, claustrophobic or hypoxaemic; developing myocardial ischaemia; or coughing. Concurrent upper respiratory infection should prompt a cancellation, as coughing and sneezing during the surgery can cause serious difficulties. Long-term anticoagulation presents potential complications that are more relevant to the surgeon or those practising local anaesthesia; however, there are a number of ophthalmic procedures that can be safely carried out without the need to interrupt anticoagulation or antiplatelet therapy. Warfarin therapy is not considered an absolute contraindication to local anaesthesia provided that the preoperative international normalised ratio (INR) is in the therapeutic target range; a sub-Tenon's block or topical anaesthesia is preferred in these cases.

Patients receiving only local anaesthesia are usually not fasted, and this is particularly helpful in managing patients with diabetes mellitus who can receive all their normal medications and achieve better glycaemic control. The blood sugar concentration should still be checked.

Ophthalmic drugs relevant to the anaesthetist

Oral, intravenous and topical ophthalmic drugs can all have systemic effects relevant to the anaesthetist; a careful drug history is needed (Table 38.2).

Table 38.2 Ophthalmic drugs used during surgery and anaesthesia

Drugs	Use	Adverse effects
Carbonic anhydrase inhibitors (e.g. acetazolamide)	Reduce aqueous formation orally or intravenously to treat or prevent increases in IOP	Allergic cross-reaction with sulphonamides Renal acidosis (renal loss of bicarbonate) and diuresis
Phenylephrine	Topical mydriatic	Increased blood pressure Cerebrovascular accidents Pulmonary oedema Ventricular arrhythmias Reflex bradycardia
		Adverse effects increased in the presence of:
		Disturbed corneal epithelial barrier (e.g. intraoperative/trauma/inflammation) Decreased lacrimation (e.g. with general anaesthesia)
Cyclopentolate	Topical mydriatic	Drowsiness Disorientation Agitation Cerebellar dysfunction (incoherent speech, ataxia) Visual and tactile hallucinations GI symptoms

Continued

Table 38.2 Ophthalmic drugs used during surgery and anaesthesia—cont'd

Drugs	Use	Adverse effects
Pilocarpine	Topical miotic	Headache Brow ache Salivation Sweating Increased GI motility Relaxation of urethral and anal sphincters Bronchospasm in susceptible patients
Brimonidine	Treatment of glaucoma and ocular hypertension	Dry mouth Fatigue Drowsiness Shortness of breath Dizziness Headache Low mood
Beta-blockers (e.g. timolol)	Treatment of glaucoma; decreases IOP by reduction of production of aqueous humour	Bradycardia Hypotension Bronchospasm Fatigue Depression
Mannitol	Decreases IOP by increase in aqueous outflow	Numbness and tingling of extremities/perioral region Metallic taste Weakness, drowsiness, lethargy GI irritation Metabolic acidaemia Relative hypokalaemia, hyponatraemia Formation of renal stones Blood dyscrasias
Intravenous mannitol	Decreases IOP by increase in aqueous outflow	Dehydration Hypernatremia Metabolic acidaemia Heart failure Thrombophlebitis Skin necrosis if extravasation occurs

IOP, Intraocular pressure.

Induction of anaesthesia

Smooth induction is particularly important in the ophthalmic setting. Coughing, straining and increases in intrathoracic pressure should be avoided as these cause venous congestion and elevate IOP. The choice of induction agent is of much less importance than how it is used (see Chapter 4). In equipotent doses, propofol has a greater depressant effect on IOP than thiopental but also causes more hypotension. Suxamethonium in isolation causes an immediate increase in IOP. Short-acting opioids (e.g. fentanyl or alfentanil) act synergistically with anaesthetic induction agents and obtund cardiovascular responses to airway manipulation.

Airway management

The airway may remain inaccessible throughout surgery, and any need to adjust or reposition an airway device during surgery could cause disruption to surgery. The use of supraglottic airway devices (SADs) has become popular, particularly for short ophthalmic procedures. The administration of an NMBA in conjunction with a SAD may aid mechanical ventilation and tighter control of ocular physiology but is considered by some anaesthetists to carry an increased risk of aspiration. If there is any doubt about maintaining the airway with a SAD, it should be changed to a tracheal tube before surgery commences. If tracheal intubation is used, it is important to avoid increases in IOP both at intubation (e.g. because of the pressor response to laryngoscopy) and extubation (laryngospasm, coughing/straining on tracheal tube); this is of much greater importance in open eye surgery. These responses can be attenuated with short-acting opioids (e.g. remifentanil) or topical/intravenous lidocaine. Tracheal tube ties are avoided, with tape used in preference.

Maintenance of anaesthesia

There are, in practice, few clinical differences between the effects of different volatile anaesthetic agents or between inhalational and intravenous anaesthesia (see Chapters 3 and 4, respectively). The use of nitrous oxide depends on local availability of medical air and personal preference. Two particular risks of nitrous oxide must be considered in relation to ophthalmic anaesthesia: the increased risk of PONV, and the effect on IOP when intraocular gases are used for vitrectomy.

Relative hypotension during anaesthesia combined with normoxia and normocapnia provide a soft, well-perfused eye. A 15-degree head-up tilt may improve surgical conditions. However, excessive hypotension may prompt questions from the ophthalmologist because of the absence of flow in the retinal arteries during some ocular procedures. Maintenance of an adequate blood pressure is a greater challenge in elderly patients in the absence of significant surgical stimulation.

Avoidance of increases in IOP is necessary to avoid loss of ocular contents during open surgery. The systemic physiological disturbance associated with most eye surgery is low. There is little, if any, alteration in body fluid status, and care should be taken not to be too liberal with i.v. fluids to avoid overloading the myocardium or inducing urinary retention in the older patient. Ophthalmic surgery is performed commonly on patients with diabetes because of complications of the disease. If general anaesthesia is required, local protocols must be followed (see Chapter 20). Analgesia requirements are based on the intraoperative use of a short-acting opioid and paracetamol. NSAIDs may be useful if there are no contraindications. Local anaesthesia with a longer-acting local anaesthetic drug is particularly useful intraoperatively. Ophthalmic patients are particularly at risk for PONV despite the absence of long-acting opioids. The combination of antiemetic agents from different classes is more effective than a single antiemetic agent (see Chapter 7).

Local anaesthesia for ophthalmic surgery

An experienced ophthalmic surgery team can achieve a safe and efficient service with prompt patient turnaround and excellent operating conditions based on the use of local anaesthesia. However, although rare, serious complications of ophthalmic local anaesthesia can and do occur. A detailed knowledge of the anatomy of the eye and the relevant pharmacology is important.

Relevant anatomy for ophthalmic regional techniques

The orbit is a four-sided irregular pyramid with its apex pointing posteromedially and its base anteriorly. The annulus of Zinn is a fibrous ring which arises from the superior orbital fissure. Eye movements are controlled by rectus muscles (inferior, lateral, medial and superior) and the superior oblique and inferior oblique muscles (Fig. 38.2). These muscles arise from the annulus of Zinn and insert on the globe anterior to the equator to form an incomplete cone. The distance from annulus to inferior temporal orbital rim ranges from 42–54 mm. It is very important that the needle should not be inserted too far, close to the annulus, where the vital nerves and vessels are tightly packed.

The optic nerve (II), oculomotor nerve (III, containing superior and inferior branches), abducent nerve (VI), nasociliary nerve (a branch of the trigeminal nerve), ciliary ganglion and vessels lie in the cone. The ophthalmic division of the oculomotor nerve divides into superior and inferior branches before emerging from the superior orbital fissure. The superior branch supplies superior rectus and levator palpebrae superioris muscles. The inferior branch divides into three to supply the medial rectus, inferior rectus and inferior oblique muscles. The abducent nerve emerges from the superior orbital fissure beneath the inferior branch of the oculomotor nerve to supply the lateral rectus muscle. The trochlear nerve (IV) courses outside the cone but then branches and enters the cone to supply the superior oblique muscle. An incomplete block of this nerve leads to retained activity of the superior oblique muscle. Squeezing and closing of the eyelids are controlled by the zygomatic branch of the facial nerve (VII), which supplies the motor innervation to the orbicularis oculi muscle. This nerve emerges from the foramen spinosum at the base of the skull, anterior to the mastoid and behind the earlobe. It passes through the parotid gland before crossing the condyle of the mandible and then passes superficial to the zygoma and malar bone before its terminal fibres ramify to supply the deep surface of the orbicularis oculi. The facial nerve also supplies secretomotor parasympathetic fibres to the lacrimal glands and glands of the nasal and palatine mucosa.

Tenon's capsule, or bulbar fascia, is a membrane which envelops the eyeball from the optic nerve posteriorly to the sclera anteriorly, separating it from the orbital fat and forming a socket in which it moves (Fig. 38.3). The capsule extends 5–8 mm behind the limbus and extends posteriorly to the optic nerve and as sleeves along the extraocular muscles.

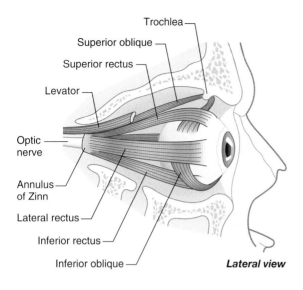

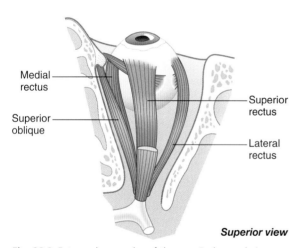

Fig. 38.2 Extraocular muscles of the eye. Each muscle is indicated by an *arrow*. (Adapted from Gray, H. (1918) *Anatomy of the human body.* Philadelphia, Lea & Febiger; and Bartleby.com, 2000.)

Tenon's capsule is divided arbitrarily by the equator of the globe into anterior and posterior portions. The anterior Tenon's capsule is adherent to episcleral tissue from the limbus posteriorly for about 5–8 mm and is fused with the intermuscular septum of the extraocular muscles and overlying bulbar conjunctiva. The conjunctiva fuses with Tenon's capsule in this area, and the sub-Tenon space can be accessed easily through an incision 5–8 mm behind the limbus. The posterior sub-Tenon's capsule is thinner and passes round

to the optic nerve, separating the globe from the contents of the retrobulbar space. Posteriorly the sheath fuses with the openings around the optic nerve.

Sensation to the eyeball is supplied through the ophthalmic division of the trigeminal nerve (V). Just before entering the orbit, it divides into three branches: lacrimal, frontal and nasociliary. The nasociliary nerve provides sensation to the entire eyeball. It emerges through the superior orbital fissure between the superior and inferior branches of the oculomotor nerve and passes through the common tendinous ring. Two long ciliary nerves give branches to the ciliary ganglion and, with the short ciliary nerves, transmit sensation from the cornea, iris and ciliary muscle. Some sensation from the lateral conjunctiva is transmitted through the lacrimal nerve and from the upper palpebral conjunctiva via the frontal nerve. Both nerves are outside the cone. Intraoperative pain may be experienced if these nerves are inadequately blocked.

The superomedial and superotemporal quadrants have abundant blood vessels, but the inferotemporal and medial quadrants are relatively avascular and are safer places to insert a needle or cannula. The globe occupies almost 50% of the orbital volume at birth and 33% at 4 years, whereas the adult globe only fills 22% of the orbital volume. As a result of these anatomical differences, sharp needle blocks carry more potential risks in children than in adults.

Nomenclature of blocks

The terminology used for ophthalmic block varies, but the widely accepted nomenclature is based on the anatomical location of the needle tip. The injection of local anaesthetic agent into the muscle cone behind the globe formed by the four rectus muscles is known as an intraconal (retrobulbar) block (Fig. 38.4), whereas in the extraconal (peribulbar) block, the needle tip remains outside the muscle cone (Fig. 38.5). Multiple communications exist between the two compartments, and it is difficult to differentiate whether the needle is intraconal or extraconal during insertion. Injected local anaesthetic agent diffuses easily across compartments and, depending on its spread, anaesthesia and akinesia may occur. A faster onset of akinesia suggests intraconal block. A combination of intraconal and extraconal block is described as a combined retroperibulbar block. In sub-Tenon's block, local anaesthetic agent is injected under the Tenon's capsule and this block is also known as parabulbar block, pinpoint anaesthesia or medial episcleral block.

To achieve adequate anaesthesia and akinesia, the cranial and sensory nerves described earlier must be blocked. However, it is very difficult to target these nerves individually, and an adequate volume of local anaesthetic should be injected safely either into the retrobulbar or peribulbar space; subsequent diffusion will ultimately block most nerves.

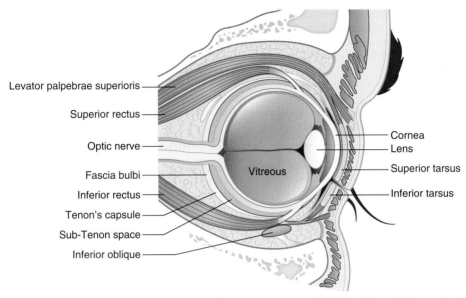

Levator palpebrae superioris
Superior rectus
Optic nerve
Fascia bulbi
Inferior rectus
Tenon's capsule
Sub-Tenon space
Inferior oblique
Vitreous
Cornea
Lens
Superior tarsus
Inferior tarsus

Fig. 38.3 A sagittal section through the right orbital cavity, showing Tenon's capsule indicated by pink line on the hind surface of the globe and the sub-Tenon space is between the globe and Tenon capsule containing connective tissue bands. (Adapted from Gray, H. (1918) *Anatomy of the human body.* Philadelphia, Lea & Febiger; and Bartleby.com, 2000.)

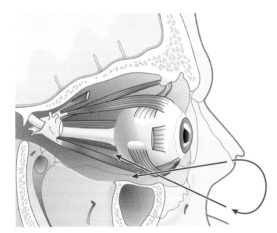

Fig. 38.4 Intraconal injection (*arrow* is shown to illustrate a needle placed between the lateral and inferior orbital margins and advanced slightly upwards and inwards to enter the intraconal space).

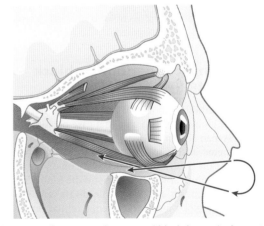

Fig. 38.5 Inferotemporal extraconal block (*arrow* is shown to illustrate needle inserted at the junction of lateral and inferior orbital margin and advanced along the floor of the orbit).

Patient selection

The preferred technique varies from topical anaesthesia through cannula-based block to needle-based blocks. There is conflicting evidence about whether there are real differences in effectiveness of blocks, suggesting that peribulbar and retrobulbar anaesthesia produce equally good akinesia and equivalent pain control. Sub-Tenon's block is very effective for sensory block, but achievement of akinesia takes longer. The technique chosen depends on a balance between the patient's wishes, the operative needs of the surgeon, the skills of the anaesthetist and the type of surgery.

The axial length of the eye is usually measured before cataract surgery, and caution in the use of needle blocks is required if the axial length exceeds 26 mm or if the axial length is unknown. If the axial length is not readily available for cataract surgery, it can also be estimated from the inserting intraocular lens power except in patients who have had previous refractive eye surgery, such as laser-assisted *in situ* keratomileusis (LASIK).

Ophthalmic regional blocks

Insertion of an i.v. cannula is good practice and must be established if a sharp-needle technique is planned. Appropriate cardiorespiratory monitoring should be used.

Modern retrobulbar block

Surface anaesthesia of the eye is obtained with local anaesthetic drops (e.g. oxybuprocaine 0.4%). The conjunctiva is cleaned with aqueous 5% polyvidone iodine. The eye should be kept in the neutral (primary) gaze position at all times, and a needle length less than 31 mm is inserted through the skin or conjunctiva in the inferotemporal quadrant as far lateral as possible below the lateral rectus. The needle is directed upwards and inwards, with the needle always tangential to the globe (see Fig. 38.4), and then 4–5 ml of the local anaesthetic agent of choice is injected. A separate facial nerve block is not required.

Inferotemporal peribulbar block (see Fig. 38.5)

Surface anaesthesia and asepsis are obtained as described earlier. The globe is kept in a neutral gaze position, and a needle less than 31 mm in length is inserted as far as possible in the extreme inferotemporal quadrant through the conjunctiva or skin. A peribulbar block is essentially similar to a modern retrobulbar block, but the needle is not directed upwards and inwards and the needle always remains tangential to the globe along the inferior orbital floor (Fig. 38.6); 5–6 ml local anaesthetic agent is injected. However, more than 60% of patients require a supplementary injection in the form of a medial peribulbar block.

Medial peribulbar block (Fig. 38.7)

A needle is inserted between the caruncle and the medial canthus to a depth of 1–1.5 cm and 3–5 ml local anaesthetic is injected. A single medial peribulbar block with 6–8 ml local anaesthetic has been advocated if akinesia is essential in patients with myopic eyes. The gauge of needle should be the finest that can be used comfortably, but this is usually limited to a 25G–27G needle. Finer needles are difficult to

manipulate, but larger needles may cause more pain and damage. Sharp needles are used because blunt needles are painful to insert. Gentle digital pressure and massage around the globe help to disperse the anaesthetic and reduce IOP. Alternatively, a pressure-reducing device such as Honan's balloon can be used. The maximum pressure should be limited to 25 mmHg to avoid compromise to the globe's blood supply.

Sub-Tenon's block (Fig. 38.8)

Sub-Tenon's block markedly reduces the incidence of complications of needle blocks, but its use is associated with some specific minor problems such as chemosis and subconjunctival haemorrhage. Surface anaesthesia and asepsis are obtained as described earlier. The lower eyelid is retracted. The patient is asked to look upwards and outwards. The conjunctiva and Tenon's capsule are gripped together with a non-toothed forceps 5–8 mm from the limbus in the inferonasal quadrant. A small incision is made through these layers with Westcott scissors until the white sclera is seen. A blunt sub-Tenon cannula (19G, curved, 2.54 cm long, metal, opening at the end) is inserted gently along the curvature of the globe and should pass easily without resistance; 3–5 ml of the local anaesthetic of choice is injected slowly. The injected local anaesthetic agent diffuses around and into the intraconal space, leading to anaesthesia and akinesia. Inferotemporal, superotemporal and medial quadrants may also be used to access the sub-Tenon's space. A variety of cannulae, both flexible and shorter lengths, are available. This method reduces the risk of central nervous system spread, optic nerve damage and global puncture, but akinesia may take longer to achieve.

Ultrasound-guided ophthalmic blocks

Ultrasound-guided ophthalmic blocks have been performed. However, it requires an ophthalmic-rated ultrasound transducer that has reduced mechanical and thermal index output. There are additional procedural skills that need to be learned and practised, visualisation of the needle-tip may be difficult, and displacement of the globe posteriorly from the transducer pressure on the eye may increase the risk of globe puncture. A preblock eye scan can provide important information on the globe size and shape and its axial length. These may be invaluable in high myopic eyes with increased axial length and high prevalence of staphyloma and therefore at higher risk of globe puncture. The ultrasound can track the spread of injected local anaesthetic solution as there is a positive correlation between failure to identify local anaesthetic within episcleral or intraconal space and failure of the block. The use of ultrasound in eye blocks has not been taken up readily among ophthalmic anaesthetists.

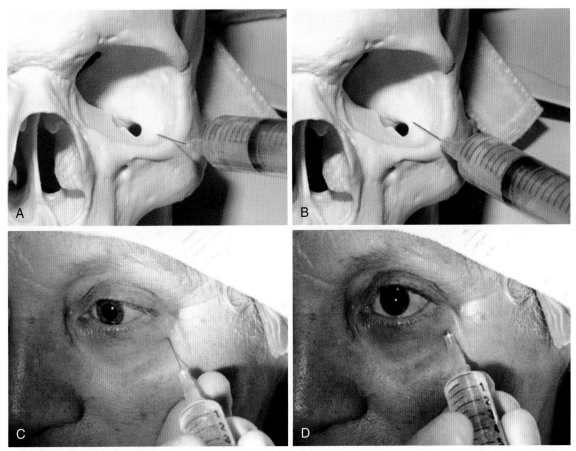

Fig. 38.6 Inferotemporal percutaneous extraconal block: (A and C) The needle is inserted in the extreme inferotemoral quadrant of the bony orbit (B and D) The needle is advanced along the floor of the orbit tangentially in the inferotemporal quadrant of the bony orbit.

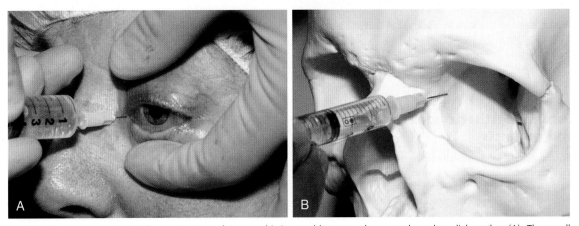

Fig. 38.7 Medial peribulbar block. A 10–15 mm long need is inserted between the caruncle and medial canthus (A). The needle is shown along the nasal bone in a bony orbit (B).

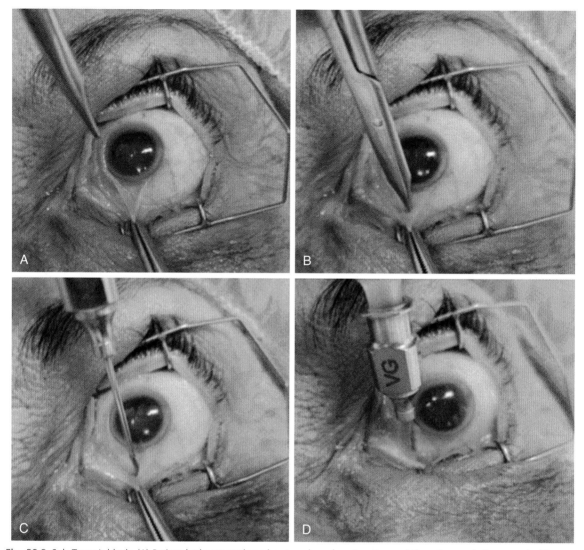

Fig. 38.8 Sub-Tenon's block. (A) Patient looks upwards and outwards and conjunctiva and Tenon's capsule is grasped with a blunt Moorfields (non-toothed) forceps; (B) a small nick is made in the conjunctiva and Tenon's capsule; (C) a blunt 19G curved metal cannula is inserted; (D) cannula is advanced along the curvature of the globe.

Local anaesthetic agents and adjuncts

Most available local anaesthetic agents either alone or in combination have been used with varying success, and it is up to the clinicians to choose the appropriate agent for surgery. The ideal local anaesthetic agent should be safe and painless to inject; it should block motor and sensory nerves quickly. The duration of action should be long enough to perform the operation but not so long as to cause

persistent postoperative diplopia. Lidocaine 2% remains the gold standard. It is safe and produces effective motor and sensory blocks.

Hyaluronidase is an enzyme which reversibly liquefies the interstitial barrier between cells by depolymerisation of hyaluronic acid to a tetrasaccharide, thus enhancing diffusion of molecules through tissue planes. The amount of hyaluronidase powder mixed with the local anaesthetic varies from 5–150 IU ml^{-1}. The use of hyaluronidase for ophthalmic blocks is controversial, and its use for sub-Tenon's block is questioned for a short operation such as cataract surgery. Adverse effects are rare but include allergic reactions, orbital cellulitis and formation of pseudotumours.

A vasoconstrictor such as adrenaline can be added to local anaesthetic solutions to increase the intensity and duration of block and minimise bleeding from small vessels. Absorption of local anaesthetic is reduced, which avoids surges in plasma concentrations. Adrenaline may cause vasoconstriction of the ophthalmic artery, compromising the retinal circulation, and has also been implicated in complications in older patients with cardiovascular and cerebrovascular comorbidities. Except in oculoplastic surgery, its use is generally not recommended.

Alkalinisation of local anaesthetic solutions decreases onset time and prolongs the duration of action after needle blocks, but its use in clinical practice is probably unwarranted.

Complications of ophthalmic regional blocks

Reported complications of needle blocks range from mild to serious and may affect the eye or be systemic (Table 38.3). Systemic complications such as local anaesthetic agent toxicity, brainstem anaesthesia and cardiorespiratory arrest may occur because of i.v. injection or spread or misplacement of drug in the orbit during or immediately after injection.

Sub-Tenon's block is considered a safe alternative to needle block, but minor and common complications such as pain during injection, reflux of local anaesthetic, chemosis and subconjunctival haemorrhage occur. Anterograde reflux and loss of local anaesthetic on injection occurs if the dissection is oversized relative to the gauge of the cannula. Inadequate access into the sub-Tenon's space can also promote chemosis. The incidence of chemosis varies with the volume of local

Table 38.3 Complications of ophthalmic regional blocks	
Orbital	**Systemic**
Incorrect eye blocked	Oculocardiac reflex
Failure of the block	Allergic reaction
Corneal abrasion	Local anaesthetic toxicity
Chemosis	Brainstem anaesthesia
Subconjunctival haemorrhage	Cardiorespiratory arrest
Orbital haemorrhage	
Globe damage	
Optic nerve damage	
Extraocular muscle malfunction	

anaesthetic, dissection technique and choice of cannula. Shorter cannulae are associated with an increased likelihood of conjunctival chemosis. Subconjunctival haemorrhage is common and inevitable, and no method is known to reduce it significantly.

Orbital haemorrhage

Orbital haemorrhage is a sight-threatening complication of intraconal, extraconal and, rarely, sub-Tenon's block. It occurs with a frequency of 0.1%–3% after needle-based blocks. The haemorrhage may be venous or arterial in origin and may be concealed or revealed. Venous bleeding is slow and usually stops. Severe venous haemorrhage usually presents as markedly bloodstained chemosis and slightly raised IOP. It may be possible to reduce the IOP by digital massage and cautious application of an IOP-reducing device to such an extent that surgery can proceed safely. Before the decision is made to proceed with surgery or postpone it for a few days, it is advisable to measure and record IOP. Arterial bleeding is rapid, with blood filling the periorbital tissues, increasing tissue volume and pressure. This is transmitted to the globe, raising the IOP significantly. Urgent measures must be taken to stop the haemorrhage and reduce IOP. Firm digital pressure usually stops the bleeding, and when it has been arrested, consideration must be given to reducing the IOP so that the blood supply to the retina is not compromised. Lateral canthotomy, acetazolamide or mannitol, or even paracentesis may need to be considered in consultation with the ophthalmologist.

Prevention of haemorrhage
Straining because of anxiety during the block leads to engorgement and potential puncture of vessels around the eye. Sedation may help, and the patient should be encouraged to breathe quietly through an open mouth and so prevent a Valsalva manoeuvre. The fewer injections that are made into the orbit, the less are the chances of damaging a blood vessel. Cutting and slicing movements at the needle tip should be avoided. Fine needles are less traumatic than thicker ones. Deep intraorbital injections must be avoided. The inferotemporal quadrant has fewer blood vessels and is less hazardous.

Central spread of local anaesthetic agent

Mechanism
The cerebral dura mater provides a tubular sheath for the optic nerve as it passes through the optic foramen. This sheath fuses to the epineurium of the optic nerve, providing a potential conduit for local anaesthetic to pass subdurally to the brain. Central spread can occur on injection if the needle tip has entered the optic nerve sheath. Central spread, although very rare after sub-Tenon's block, has also been

reported. Even an injection of a small volume of local anaesthetic may enter the central nervous system or cross the optic chiasm to the opposite eye and may cause life-threatening sequelae such as catastrophic cardiorespiratory collapse. The time of onset of symptoms is variable, but they usually appear in the first 15 min after injection. Central spread may occur on rare occasions if an orbital artery is cannulated by the needle tip, resulting in retrograde spread up the artery until it meets a branch where it can then flow in a cephalad direction; in addition to orbital haemorrhage, systemic collapse is almost instantaneous.

Signs and symptoms

The symptoms of central spread are varied and depend on which part of the central nervous system is affected by the local anaesthetic. Because of the anatomical proximity of the optic nerve to the midbrain, it is usual for this area to be involved. Signs and symptoms involving the cardiovascular and respiratory systems, temperature regulation, vomiting, temporary hemiplegia, aphasia and generalised convulsions have been described. Palsy of the contralateral oculomotor and trochlear nerves with amaurosis (loss of vision) is pathognomonic of central nervous system spread and should be sought in any patient whose response to questions after block are not as crisp as they were beforehand.

Treatment

The management is the same as that for a high or total spinal block (see Chapter 27).

Prevention

Intra- or extraconal injections should always be undertaken with the patient looking in the neutral or the primary gaze position. The optic nerve is a C-shaped structure, and there is slackness in the primary gaze position. If the needle encounters the optic nerve in this position, it is unlikely to damage or perforate its sheath because slackness in the structure allows the nerve to be pushed aside. The most dangerous position is when the patient looks upwards and inwards, as this presents the stretched nerve to a needle directed from the inferotemporal quadrant. The injection should not be made deep into the orbit, where the optic nerve is likely to be tethered.

Damage to the globe

Global puncture is a serious complication of ophthalmic blocks. It has been reported after both intraconal and extraconal blocks and even after sub-Tenon's and subconjunctival injection. Perforation of the globe has entry and exit wounds, whereas penetration of the globe has only the wound of entry. With appropriate care, it should be a very rare complication because the sclera is a tough structure and, in most patients, is not perforated easily. Puncture of the eyeball is most likely to occur in patients with high myopia, previous scleral band, posterior staphyloma or a deeply sunken eye in a narrow orbit. Not all globes are the same length, and not all orbits are the same shape. In most patients who present for cataract surgery, axial length of the eyeball is measured with ultrasound. Patients with high myopia have much thinner sclera, and extreme caution is needed for needle blocks in these patients.

Puncture of the globe is usually recognised at the time of surgery and presents as an exceptionally soft eye with a loss of red reflex. In cataract surgery, if the block is good, the surgeon should be encouraged to proceed with the lensectomy but to stitch up the eye with twice as many sutures as normal. Without lensectomy, it may not be possible to observe the damage to the posterior segment of the eye. It can be expected that the needle track through the vitreous humour will form a band of scar tissue. If this is not excised, it contracts and detaches the retina, sometimes causing sudden total blindness in the affected eye.

Optic nerve damage

Optic nerve damage is a rare but late complication of ophthalmic blocks which usually results from obstruction of the central retinal artery or direct trauma after retrobulbar block with a long needle. The central retinal artery is the first and smallest branch of the ophthalmic artery arising from that vessel as it lies below the optic nerve. It runs for a short distance within the dural sheath of the optic nerve and, about 35 mm from the orbital margin, pierces the nerve and runs forward in the centre of the nerve to the retina. Damage to the artery may cause bleeding into the confined space of the optic nerve sheath, compressing and obstructing blood flow. If the complication is recognised early then surgical decompression of the optic nerve is performed.

Extraocular muscle malfunction

The inadvertent injection of a long-acting local anaesthetic into any extraocular muscle mass may result in muscle damage manifesting as prolonged weakness, fibrosis or even necrosis of the muscle. The addition of hyaluronidase to the local anaesthetic agent helps disperse the agent before lasting damage can be done. Persistent diplopia after local anaesthesia should be investigated.

Sneezing

Reflex sneezing after sharp needle block can occur and is attributed to the irritation of branches of the trigeminal nerve. This may lead to inadvertent injury to the ocular structure if it happens while the needle is *in situ*. Sedation with propofol has been associated with a higher incidence of sneezing (around 35%); it may be related to the initial neuroexcitatory phase of anaesthesia with propofol. Addition of an opioid to the sedation regime suppresses the sneezing reflex.

Ophthalmic procedures requiring general anaesthesia

Penetrating eye injury

Eye injuries may be difficult to inspect in detail because of swelling and pain, and exploration under general anaesthesia may be required at the earliest opportunity. The potential for loss of intraocular contents exists even if penetration is not obviously present preoperatively. Eye injury may also coexist with other major head injuries or polytrauma. As with any trauma, there may be a short fasting time before the injury and subsequent delay in gastric emptying, especially if alcohol was consumed before the injury or if an opioid was administered in the emergency department. Therefore the situation may exist of the need for anaesthesia in a patient with a potentially full stomach.

General anaesthesia is the typical for patients with a penetrating eye injury. Loss of vision in one or both eyes after accidental injury in the young population understandably heightens preoperative anxiety. Increases in IOP secondary to injection of local anaesthetic solution for a regional technique may precipitate extrusion of ocular contents. However, orbital regional anaesthesia has been used successfully in some centres. The anaesthetist must choose the technique which minimises the risk of pulmonary aspiration of gastric contents most effectively throughout the perioperative period, but consideration should be given to reducing the IOP until the eye is made safe. Most patients will require RSI; rocuronium, with its fast onset of action and lack of effect on IOP, may be the NMBA of choice. However, some studies have shown that suxamethonium can also be used safely despite its effect on IOP.

The urgency of surgery has the greatest influence on the anaesthesia decision making process. Ophthalmologists are currently more likely to choose to wait for 6 h after the last meal or often, because of the time of day, until the next morning before exploring the eye. This is dependent on the severity of the injury as well as the potential to produce a good ocular outcome. There is little incentive to risk aspiration and death if there is little likelihood of preserving vision as the benefit. Surgery may be bilateral and lengthy; subsequent return to theatre for repeated procedures is also common.

Cataract surgery

Phacoemulsification surgery with small-gauge probes is the norm. The procedure can be performed under topical anaesthesia, although many ophthalmologists prefer a block technique. The use of sub-Tenon's block is common, and needle-based block is avoided in many countries. General anaesthesia is a rarity.

Vitreoretinal surgery

Vitreoretinal surgery covers a range of intra- and extraocular procedures which may involve lengthy periods in the dark. Both needle- and cannula-based blocks are used. General anaesthesia is used in younger patients or if surgery is expected to exceed the patient's ability to remain comfortable. Vitrectomy removes all the vitreous from the eye with the purpose of clearing cloudy or bloody vitreous, as well as performing intraocular procedures on the retina. The integrity and pressure of the vitreous cavity is determined by the surgeon throughout the procedure whilst the structured jelly-like apparatus is removed. The cavity may then be filled with an air/gas mixture (commonly perfluoropropane or sulphur hexafluoride) or silicone. The surgeon may make a decision on which of these to use towards the end of surgery, and therefore it is sensible to avoid the use of nitrous oxide for vitrectomy surgery. If an air/gas mixture is used by the surgeon, nitrous oxide in equilibrium in the eye cavity may diffuse out quickly at the end of the procedure, leaving a lower pressure in the eye than intended surgically. This can cause detachment of the retina. If nitrous oxide has been used, it should be switched off well before the insertion of surgical gas into the vitreous cavity. Gases may persist in the eye for up to 3 months postoperatively, and the non-ophthalmic anaesthetist needs to be aware of the relevance of ophthalmic gases. A wristband is placed on the patient after surgery to alert any subsequent anaesthetist to avoid nitrous oxide; nitrous oxide would diffuse into the cavity faster than nitrogen would diffuse out and the IOP could increase, with serious consequences. The gas diffuses out of the eye slowly over time. Silicone oil used for the same purpose needs to be removed surgically at a later stage. Nitrous oxide use is of no relevance if silicone oil has been used.

Retinal surgery can also be performed from outside the sclera. Buckling, bands, cryotherapy and laser therapies are used to repair breaks. There is a risk of precipitating the oculocardiac reflex.

Subsequent repeated operations are very common. General anaesthetic considerations remain the same. Regional anaesthesia techniques (both needle- and cannula-based blocks) are also used.

Corneal transplant surgery

Donor corneas can be stored up to 7–10 days. This allows corneal grafts to be performed largely as scheduled surgery. Penetrating keratoplasty is a full-thickness corneal transplant where all five layers of the cornea are replaced with donor cornea. Visual recovery is often slow and unpredictable. It can be performed under regional block, though general anaesthesia is the preferred method in longer and more complicated cases.

In selective lamellar keratoplasty, only the diseased layers are replaced with donor tissue, whereas the healthy layers of the cornea are retained. This is the current preferred surgical procedure. The important considerations are the duration of surgery and the high risk of graft displacement.

Keratoprosthesis (artificial cornea) is considered as the last therapeutic option for patients in whom conventional corneal transplant procedures have failed. The surgical time is long, and it is usually performed under general anaesthesia.

Strabismus surgery

Strabismus surgery is the most commonly performed paediatric ophthalmic procedure and is usually undertaken as a day case. Airway considerations of head and neck procedures apply, but a SAD is the most commonly selected technique, particularly in older children. Long-acting opioids are not required and are likely to increase an already high risk of PONV. Surgery itself requires tension to be applied to the extraocular muscles. Steady deep anaesthesia with or without neuromuscular blockade (to guarantee immobility) allows the surgeon to gauge how much muscle repositioning is required. However, it is the tension applied by the surgeon to the muscle which can cause severe bradycardia, especially in the vagally responsive child. Prophylaxis with glycopyrronium bromide or atropine may be given as a premedication or at induction. A supplementary regional block can suppress the oculocardiac reflex. Contrary to previous belief, strabismus surgery is not associated with a higher risk of malignant hyperthermia.

In cooperative adults, strabismus surgery may be performed under regional block. However, patients often experience pain especially during resection of muscle. In some adults adjustable-suture strabismus surgery may achieve more accurate results, especially for those who have had previous surgery. This is commonly performed as a two-stage operation. Most of the surgical correction is completed in first stage under general or regional anaesthesia, with the final muscle fixation suture tied in a bow only. In second stage the patient is awake, eye alignment checked and adjustment made if needed. This is usually performed under topical anaesthesia only. Some patients may experience mild discomfort during the adjustment of suture.

Botulinum toxin injection to the extraocular muscle has also been used in the treatment of strabismus. It can be performed transconjunctivally with an electromyograph-guided injection needle under topical anaesthesia in adults. If general anaesthesia is required, NMBAs should be avoided. Direct injection to the extraocular muscle under open exposure may be preferred in children. General anaesthesia is required for all paediatric patients.

Glaucoma surgery

Glaucoma surgery can be performed under regional block or general anaesthesia. If regional block is used, particular attention should be given to avoid exacerbating ocular ischaemia, such as addition of vasoconstrictor, large volume of injectate and prolonged ocular compression. If general anaesthesia is required most of the considerations are the same as for cataract surgery. However, unlike most ocular surgery, intraoperative miosis is required; this is not a contraindication to the use of i.v. atropine. A still, soft eye makes the surgical procedure easier to perform. Neuromuscular blockade and good anaesthetic control over IOP produce ideal conditions.

Patients with glaucoma, who already have a compromised optic nerve, are at risk of complete or partial loss of vision after surgery ('wipe-out'). This can occur after general or regional anaesthesia. There are many proposed mechanisms, but the exact cause is unclear. Tiny stents can also be inserted into the angle between the iris and cornea to bypass the trabecular meshwork and allow aqueous humour to flow directly to Schlemm's canal at the time of cataract surgery in glaucoma patients. Anaesthesia for the additional stent insertion is the same as for the cataract operation.

Dacryocystorhinostomy

Dacryocystorhinostomy (DCR) is a procedure performed for watery eyes. There is surgical exposure of the tear duct and a new opening is created into the nasal cavity. This is a relatively stimulating procedure. General anaesthesia is suitable, although local anaesthesia (with or without sedation) has gained popularity. The operation may be performed with an open technique or through a nasal endoscope. There is a risk of blood in the airway during and immediately after the procedure. The patient should be kept conscious with minimal sedation if a local anaesthetic technique is employed. Tracheal intubation and the safe use of a throat pack offer better airway protection. Measures to prevent blood ooze at the site of surgery can aid the surgeon, and these include controlled hypotension, head-up positioning and the use of vasoconstriction in the surgical field. Xylometazoline or cocaine provides vasoconstriction in the nose. Endoscopic laser DCR necessitates training in laser safety (see Chapter 37).

Other oculoplastic procedures

The range of surgery for this subspecialty relates to the lid, socket or adnexae. Many procedures are short, and lid surgeries are performed under local anaesthesia. Longer procedures such as enucleation and tumour surgery are generally performed under general anaesthesia. Bilateral blepharoplasties for cosmetic reasons are increasingly common and, as with all oculoplastic surgery, the requirements for a bloodless field are best met with controlled relative hypotension and surgical site vasoconstriction.

Paediatric procedures

In addition to strabismus surgery, children, including infants and neonates, may require other ophthalmic procedures. The airway is commonly maintained with a reinforced SAD in older children, whereas a tracheal tube may be required in infants and neonates. Although the majority of children are fit and well and may be managed as day cases, there are a number of patients with associated comorbidities who require detailed examinations or ocular surgery. Congenital cataracts, glaucoma, vascular and lens disorders can occur in diseases such as Down's syndrome, mucopolysaccharidoses and craniofacial and connective tissue disorders. Retinopathy

of prematurity may require treatment in sick neonatal patients outside the theatre suite. Anaesthetic considerations relevant to the condition balanced with the surgical requirements guide anaesthesia choices. An infant with airway anomalies may require a complex anaesthetic skill set simply to undergo ophthalmoscopy.

Sedation and ophthalmic blocks

Selected patients in whom explanation and reassurance have proved inadequate may benefit from sedation. Minimal doses of short-acting benzodiazepines, opioids and small doses of i.v. anaesthetic induction agents may be used. The routine use of sedation is discouraged because of an increased incidence of adverse intraoperative events. A means of providing supplementary oxygen along with equipment and skills to manage any life-threatening events must be immediately accessible. Sedation is not a substitute for an inadequate block. The quality of the block should be assessed before the surgery commences.

References/Further reading

Kumar, C.M., Seet, E., 2017. Stopping antithrombotics during regional anaesthesia and eye surgery: crying wolf? Br. J. Anaesth. 118, 154–158.

Kumar, C.M., Seet, E., Eke, T., Dhatariya, K., Joshi, G.P., 2016. Glycaemic control for cataract surgery under locoregional anaesthesia – we are none the wiser. Br. J. Anaesth. 117, 687–691.

Kumar, C.M., Seet, E., 2016. Cataract surgery in patients with dementia-time to reconsider anaesthetic option. Br. J. Anaesth. 117, 421–425.

Kumar, C.M., Dodds, C., 2006. Sub-tenon's anesthesia. Ophthalmol. Clin. North Am. 19, 209–219.

Kumar, C.M., 2011. Needle-based blocks for the 21st century ophthalmology.

Acta Ophthalmol. 89, 5–9. doi: 10.1111/j.1755-3768.2009.01837.

Local anaesthesia for ophthalmic surgery: Joint guidelines from the Royal College of Anaesthetists and the Royal College of Ophthalmologists 2012 (https://www.rcophth.ac.uk/wp-content/uploads/2014/12/2012-SCI-247-Local-Anaesthesia-in-Ophthalmic-Surgery-2012.pdf).

Chapter | **39** |

Anaesthesia for vascular, endocrine and plastic surgery

Jonathan Thompson, Simon Howell

Major vascular surgery

Many aspects of vascular surgery have changed during the last two decades, largely as a result of advances in radiological practice and cardiology. Examples include improvements in the treatment of myocardial infarction, the development of endovascular aortic surgery and lower limb angioplasty; such progress is likely to continue. However, anaesthesia for major vascular surgery remains a challenging area of practice. In addition to general considerations, the specific features of the more common vascular procedures are described in this chapter: elective and emergency open and endovascular repair of abdominal aortic aneurysm (AAA), thoracic endovascular aortic repair (TEVAR) and hybrid procedures, lower limb revascularisation and carotid endarterectomy.

General considerations

Peripheral vascular disease is a manifestation of generalised cardiovascular disease, and therefore coronary artery disease is present to some degree in almost all patients presenting for major vascular surgery. Most are elderly and have a high incidence of coexisting medical diseases, in particular:
- ischaemic heart disease
- hypertension
- congestive cardiac failure
- chronic obstructive pulmonary disease
- renal disease
- diabetes mellitus

Most of these are risk factors for perioperative cardiac complications after major surgery (see Chapters 19 and 29).

The broad aims of preoperative evaluation before vascular surgery are to:
- assist risk assessment, permit further investigation if appropriate and allow optimisation of coexisting medical conditions;
- evaluate and discuss the risks with the patient and surgical team;
- establish the best surgical options (e.g. non-invasive or endovascular surgery) for an individual; and
- plan the anaesthetic technique, perioperative monitoring and postoperative care, and allow required facilities (e.g. ICU) to be organised.

Vascular surgery is associated with high morbidity and mortality, resulting mostly from cardiac complications (myocardial infarction, arrhythmias and heart failure) (see Chapters 29 and 30). It is therefore vital that cardiac function is assessed preoperatively and that the risks of surgery are evaluated and discussed with the patient. Although the outcome of subsequent vascular surgery is improved in those who have previously undergone coronary revascularisation by coronary artery bypass grafting (CABG), this is associated with additional risks. Percutaneous coronary interventions (PCIs) are increasingly used in preference to CABG in suitable patients. The perioperative management of antiplatelet medication in patients who have undergone PCI is discussed in Chapters 19 and 30. Coronary revascularisation should be performed only if indicated because of severe coronary disease; it is not justified simply to improve outcome from subsequent vascular surgery.

Preoperative medical therapy in vascular surgical patients

The preoperative assessment clinic is an ideal opportunity to assess concurrent medication. Drugs particularly relevant to the patient with vascular disease are β-blockers, antiplatelet drugs and statins (see also Chapters 9, 20 and 30).

Beta-blockers are used extensively in patients with angina and improve long-term survival after myocardial infarction and in patients with heart failure. The perioperative discontinuation of β-blockers may be harmful, and they should be continued when already being used to control angina, arrhythmias or hypertension. However, there is now evidence that the de novo initiation of sympatholytic drugs such as β-blockers in the immediate preoperative period is associated with perioperative hypotension, stroke and perioperative death.

All patients undergoing major vascular surgery should be receiving cardiovascular secondary prevention, including antiplatelet therapy, unless there is a contraindication. Clopidogrel is recommended as first-line treatment for patients with peripheral arterial disease. Aspirin is recommended as first-line treatment for patients with abdominal aortic aneurysm. Some clinicians consider that clopidogrel should be stopped 5 days before aortic surgery, but this should be discussed with the surgeon and prescribing physician. Aspirin should be continued throughout the perioperative period. Statin therapy should also be considered in all vascular surgical patients, and if prescribed, it should be continued throughout the perioperative period.

Minimum investigations before major vascular surgery should include ECG, chest radiograph, FBC, and U&Es, but more invasive or specialised tests may be required (see Chapter 19), including cardiopulmonary exercise testing where available. Some assessment of exercise tolerance should be made in all patients because it is a useful indicator of functional cardiac status, although many vascular patients are limited by intermittent claudication, musculoskeletal diseases, frailty or deconditioning associated with a sedentary lifestyle. In this case a patient with severe coronary artery disease may have no symptoms of angina and a normal resting ECG. In some patients (e.g. those with limited functional capacity or life expectancy because of severe intractable coexistent medical conditions), the risks of elective vascular surgery may outweigh the overall potential benefits, and invasive surgery may not be appropriate.

Abdominal aortic aneurysm

Abdominal aortic aneurysms (AAA) occur in 2%–4% of the population aged older than 65 years, predominantly in men. Approximately 90% of AAAs arise below the origin of the renal arteries, and they tend to expand over time. The risk of rupture increases exponentially when the aneurysm exceeds

5.5 cm in diameter, and elective surgery is usually then indicated. The in-hospital mortality from elective AAA repair is decreasing and is now 3%–5%, but overall mortality from a ruptured AAA is up to 90% and is 50% in those who survive until emergency surgery can be performed. Consequently, screening programmes are in place to identify patients with a small asymptomatic aneurysm and to offer intervention when the aneurysm reaches a diameter of 5.5 cm. Aortic aneurysm screening has been shown to be cost effective in men but not women. Open surgery involves replacing the aneurysmal segment with a tube or bifurcated prosthetic graft, depending on the extent of iliac artery involvement. In all cases the aorta must be cross-clamped (see later) and a large abdominal incision is required. Surgery is prolonged and blood loss may be substantial. Patients are usually elderly, with a high prevalence of coexisting disease. These factors contribute to the high morbidity and mortality of open AAA surgery. Endovascular AAA procedures avoid some of these problems (see later).

Elective open AAA repair

Preoperative evaluation and risk assessment are paramount. All vasoactive medication (except perhaps angiotensin-converting enzyme (ACE) inhibitors and angiotensin II receptor blockers) must be continued up to the time of surgery, and an anxiolytic premedication may be advantageous. Patients may have recently undergone arteriography, and the injection of large volumes of high-osmolar radiopaque dye may cause kidney injury. Maintenance of hydration using oral and/or intravenous regimens before surgery decreases the risk of kidney injury. Some patients with severe chronic obstructive pulmonary disease may benefit from regular nebulisers and chest physiotherapy before surgery to decrease the incidence of postoperative respiratory complications.

An intra-arterial and two large intravenous cannulae should be inserted before induction of anaesthesia, with monitoring of ECG and pulse oximetry. Cardiovascular changes at induction may be diminished by preoperative hydration and careful titration of the intravenous induction agent. After neuromuscular blockade, the trachea is intubated (see later) and anaesthesia continued using a balanced volatile/opioid or total intravenous technique. Perioperative epidural analgesia is useful and may be undertaken before or after induction of anaesthesia.

Several important considerations apply to patients undergoing open aortic surgery (Box 39.1). The following are required:
- Two large (14G) cannulae for infusion of warmed fluids
- Arterial catheter for intra-arterial pressure monitoring and blood sampling for acid–base and blood gas analysis
- Multilumen CVC for drug administration and determination of right atrial pressure

- Continuous ECG monitoring for ischaemia (CM_5 position) preferably with ST-segment analysis
- Oesophageal or nasopharyngeal temperature probe
- Urinary catheter
- Nasogastric tube

In the more compromised patient, such as with ischaemic heart disease and poor left ventricular function, an additional cardiac output monitor (e.g. transoesophageal echocardiography or other non-invasive device) may be used to monitor cardiac index and guide fluid management. All possible measures should be undertaken to maintain body temperature, including heated mattress and overblanket, warmed intravenous fluids, and warmed and humidified inspired gases. However, care should be taken to avoid active warming of the lower body whilst the aorta is cross-clamped. The ambient temperature should be warm, and the bowel may be wrapped in clear plastic to minimise evaporative losses.

Three specific stimuli may give rise to cardiovascular instability during surgery:

- *Induction of anaesthesia.* Careful titration of intravenous anaesthetic agents is important to avoid hypotension at induction. In some cases blood pressure may have to be supported by short-acting vasopressor agents. Laryngoscopy and tracheal intubation may be accompanied by marked increases in arterial pressure and heart rate, which may precipitate myocardial ischaemia in susceptible individuals. This response should be attenuated, ensuring an adequate depth of anaesthesia, before laryngoscopy.

- *Cross-clamping of the aorta.* Clamping of the aorta causes a sudden increase in aortic impedance to forward flow and hence left ventricular afterload. This increases cardiac work and may result in myocardial ischaemia, arrhythmias and left ventricular failure. Arterial pressure proximal to the clamp increases acutely even though left ventricular ejection fraction and cardiac output are reduced. The effects on preload are variable. The degree of cardiovascular disturbance is greater when the clamp is applied more proximally (supracoeliac > suprarenal > infrarenal levels). A vasodilator, such as glyceryl trinitrate (GTN), is often infused just before clamping (and continued up to clamp release) to obviate these problems. Deepening of volatile anaesthesia or an additional dose of an opioid may also be used at aortic clamping. While the aorta is clamped, blood flow distal to the clamp decreases, and distal organ perfusion is largely dependent on the collateral circulation. The lower limbs and pelvic and abdominal viscera suffer variable degrees of ischaemia during which inflammatory mediators are released from white blood cells, platelets and capillary endothelium. These mediators include oxygen free radicals, neutrophil proteases, platelet-activating factor, cyclo-oxygenase products and cytokines.

- *Aortic declamping.* Declamping of the aorta causes sudden decreases in aortic afterload, systemic vascular resistance and venous return with reperfusion of the bowel, pelvis and lower limbs and redistribution of blood. Inflammatory mediators flow into the systemic circulation, causing vasodilatation, metabolic acidosis, increased capillary permeability and sequestration of blood cells in the lungs. This is a critical period of anaesthesia and surgery because hypotension after aortic declamping may be severe and refractory unless circulating volume has been well maintained. The aim is to maintain the patient in at least a euvolaemic state during cross-clamping. The use of intravenous fluids to achieve mild to moderate hypervolaemia before declamping is thought to limit declamping hypotension and the subsequent metabolic acidosis. It has been standard practice to target a CVP of greater than 12–14 mmHg before declamping. This can be difficult to achieve, and it is now recognised that CVP is an unreliable monitor of circulatory filling. Other monitors of fluid responsiveness, such as pulse pressure variability, may be used, but there are limited data specific to their use in aortic surgery. Glyceryl trinitrate may be administered to achieve a degree of venodilatation and discontinued before clamp release, helping to produce a state of hypervolaemia and a rise in blood pressure before the clamp is removed. Declamping hypotension usually resolves within a few minutes, but vasopressors or positive inotropes are often required; these can be given before clamp release in anticipation. Good communication with the surgeon and slow or sequential clamp release helps the anaesthetist to manage aortic declamping. Renal blood flow decreases even when an infrarenal cross-clamp is used, and steps to maintain renal function are often required. The single most important measure is the maintenance of extracellular fluid volume. A number of drugs have been used to provide renal protection. These include dopamine, mannitol, furosemide, and *N*-acetylcysteine. None has been demonstrated to be effective, and there are concerns that loop diuretics may increase the risk of injury by increasing renal tubular oxygen demand. Although both furosemide and mannitol can increase urine production, this does not equate to renal protection.

Bleeding is a problem throughout the operation, often after aortic clamping, when back-bleeding from lumbar vessels occurs, but may be particularly severe at aortic declamping as the adequacy of vascular anastomoses is tested. A red cell salvage device should be used routinely in aortic surgery. It is now well understood that even mild anaemia is associated with an increased risk of complications after major surgery. Preparation for elective aortic surgery, and indeed for vascular surgery generally, should include the identification, diagnosis and treatment of preoperative anaemia (see Chapter 20). The use of parenteral iron for the treatment of preoperative anaemia is being examined in a number of studies. In addition to red cells, specific clotting factors are often required. It is often preferable to reserve the use of clotting factors until the anastomoses are complete and most of the anticipated blood loss has occurred. Unfractionated heparin is administered before aortic cross-clamping. A standard dose may be used (usually 5000 units i.v.) or the dose may be titrated to weight (50–70 units kg^{-1}). The response to heparin shows considerable intraindividual variation. Whichever approach is used, the monitoring of coagulation using activated clotting time (ACT) or thromboelastography is valuable to confirm adequate anticoagulation, diagnose coagulopathy and guide the use of clotting products.

Epidural analgesia is usually provided through a catheter placed at the mid-thoracic level unless there is a contraindication. At least an hour should elapse between placement of the epidural and the administration of heparin. There is some debate as to whether epidural local anaesthetics are best administered during surgery (to attenuate cardiovascular and stress responses) or at the end of surgery (because sympathetic blockade may cause hypotension and make cardiovascular management more difficult during the procedure). A popular technique is to use combined volatile general anaesthesia with boluses of fentanyl or an infusion of remifentanil for intraoperative analgesia; epidural analgesia is then established after aortic declamping and once cardiovascular stability is ensured, using a combination of local anaesthetic and fentanyl.

Most patients are elderly and are unable to tolerate the large heat loss occurring through the extensive surgical exposure, which necessitates displacement of the bowel outside the abdominal cavity. Hypothermia causes vasoconstriction, which may cause myocardial ischaemia, delayed recovery and difficulties with fluid management during rewarming because large volumes of intravenous fluid may be required. Therefore all measures should be taken to prevent hypothermia.

The postoperative period

Postoperatively the patient should be transferred to a high-dependency unit or ICU. The decision to continue artificial ventilation or to extubate the trachea after surgery depends on the patient's previous medical condition and physiological stability during and at the end of surgery. Artificial ventilation should be continued until body temperature and acid–base status are normalised, cardiovascular stability restored and effective analgesia provided. Patients have a high incidence of postoperative cardiovascular and respiratory complications; renal dysfunction and ileus are also common. Close monitoring is required for several days.

Emergency open repair

The principles of management for emergency open repair are similar to those discussed earlier. However, the patient may be grossly hypovolaemic, and arterial pressure is often maintained only by marked systemic vasoconstriction and the action of abdominal muscle tone on intra-abdominal capacitance vessels. Resuscitation with intravenous fluids before the patient reaches the operating theatre should be judicious; permissive hypotension (maintaining systolic pressure at 80–100 mmHg) limits the extent of haemorrhage and improves outcome. The patient is prepared and anaesthesia induced on the operating table. While 100% oxygen is administered by face mask, an arterial and two large-gauge i.v. cannulae are inserted under local anaesthesia. The surgeon then prepares and drapes the patient ready for surgery, and it is only at this point that anaesthesia is induced using a rapid-sequence technique. When muscle relaxation occurs, systemic arterial pressure may decrease precipitously and immediate laparotomy and aortic clamping may be required. Thereafter, the procedure is similar to that for elective repair.

The prognosis is poor for several reasons. There has been no preoperative preparation and most patients have concurrent disease. There may have been a period of severe hypotension resulting in impairment of renal, cerebral or myocardial function. Blood loss is often substantial, and massive transfusion of red cells and clotting factors is usually required. Postoperative jaundice is common because of haemolysis of damaged red cells in the circulation and in the large retroperitoneal haematoma that usually develops after aortic rupture. In addition, postoperative acute kidney injury and ileus often occur. Artificial ventilation and organ support are required for several days, and the cause of death is usually multiorgan failure.

Endovascular aortic aneurysm repair

Endovascular aortic aneurysm repair (EVAR) is now an established alternative to open surgery. In conventional EVAR

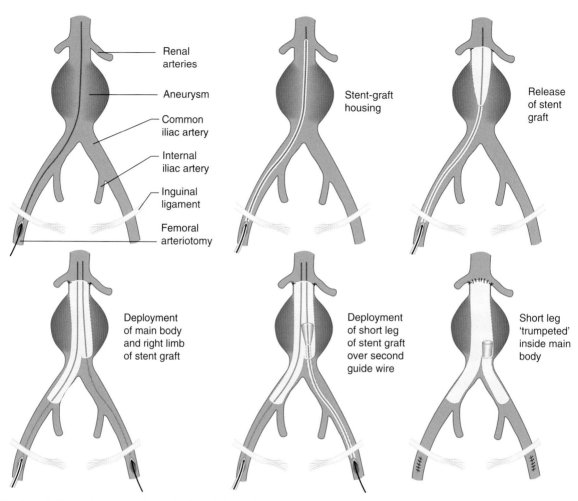

Fig. 39.1 Endovascular stent-graft repair of an abdominal aortic aneurysm. (From Bradbury, A. W., & Cleveland, T. J. (2012) *Principles and practice of surgery.* 6th ed. Edinburgh, Elsevier.)

an expandable stent graft is inserted under radiological guidance via the femoral or iliac arteries into the aneurysm to exclude it from the circulation (Fig. 39.1). Endovascular repair is generally performed via groin incisions, and the aortic lumen is temporarily occluded from within rather than being cross-clamped. The cardiovascular, metabolic and respiratory consequences are reduced compared with conventional open surgery. Perioperative blood loss, transfusion requirements, postoperative pain, hospital stay and morbidity are lower compared with open surgery. In 2016 two thirds of patients undergoing intervention for AAA in the UK underwent EVAR. In-hospital mortality after EVAR was 0.4% in the UK in 2016, whereas that for open repair was 3%. Long-term follow-up data suggest that beyond 8 years, patients who undergo open repair have better survival.

However, it must be remembered that many patients die from coexisting disease in the years after repair, with approximately half of patients in one major study surviving beyond 8 years. Patients who undergo EVAR have a significant incidence of late aneurysm rupture. They require lifelong surveillance and may require interventions to treat stent-graft leaks (endoleaks). Despite advances in stent-graft technology, the morphology of the aneurysm in some patients renders it unsuitable for EVAR (based on the site, shape, degree of angulation and the size of iliac arteries). Repeated radiological procedures (e.g. angioplasty) are required in up to 20% of patients. The procedure usually takes 1–2 h and may be performed by radiologists or surgeons, but the patients have the same coexisting diseases and some of the anaesthetic considerations are similar.

In some cases EVAR may be preferred as a less invasive technique in patients judged unfit for open surgery. Access to the iliac vessels is generally possible through infra-inguinal incisions in the groin. The use of low-profile devices with a relatively small diameter allows many cases to be performed under local anaesthetic infiltration. The presence of an anaesthetist is considered essential for such percutaneous access cases both for cardiovascular monitoring and in case of difficulty with the procedure. EVAR is generally performed in the radiology suite, and vascular centres often have a dedicated hybrid suite. Although these are equipped for both anaesthesia and surgery the suite may be remote from the main operating theatres, and considerations for anaesthesia in remote locations apply.

EVAR may be performed under general, regional or local anaesthesia with or without sedative adjuncts. In all cases, direct arterial pressure monitoring is mandatory because rapid fluctuations in arterial pressure may occur during stent-graft deployment. In awake patients, hyoscine butylbromide 20 mg i.v. may be useful to decrease bowel motility during stent-graft placement. CVP monitoring is not usually necessary unless dictated by the patient's medical condition (e.g. moderate/severe cardiac disease). Short periods of apnoea are needed during insertion of the device; this is easy when ventilation is controlled but requires the patient's co-operation if a regional or local anaesthetic technique is used. The devices are positioned under angiographic control, and large volumes of radiocontrast may be used, predisposing to contrast-induced nephropathy (CIN). It is important to avoid hypotension and hypovolaemia, both of which can contribute to CIN. The importance of maintaining hydration before, during and after the case is well recognised. Oral or intravenous prehydration may be used in patients with pre-existing renal impairment, and renal function should be monitored in the postoperative period. As with open repair, there is limited evidence to support interventions such as sodium bicarbonate, N-acetylcysteine or mannitol. Brisk haemorrhage is unusual during EVAR and although bleeding may be significant it is usually insidious. However, large-diameter cannulae should be inserted and vasoactive drugs readily available.

EVAR is now widely used for the repair of leaking and ruptured AAA. In these cases the procedure is performed under local anaesthesia if possible. If the patient is haemodynamically unstable or cannot cooperate with the procedure under local anaesthesia alone, general anaesthesia may be required. An intra-aortic balloon may be placed to act as an internal aortic cross-clamp and provide cardiovascular stability until the stent graft is deployed.

Endovascular graft placement is challenging if there is no normal aorta between the proximal end of an AAA and the renal arteries (a juxtarenal aneurysm), if the length of normal aorta is short or if the neck of the aneurysm is conical in shape. A number of solutions have been developed to address this. A conical-necked aneurysm may be treated with a graft whose top end is sealed in place with polymer-filled rings. Juxtarenal aneurysms may be treated with fenestrated grafts. These have holes (fenestrations) which overlie the position of the renal arteries. The graft is opposed to the aortic wall with the fenestrations opposite the relevant arteries, and stents are placed through the fenestrations into the renal arteries to complete the repair at the top end of the aneurysm. Such procedures may be performed under regional or general anaesthesia.

Thoracic endovascular aortic repair

Endovascular grafts are used to treat disease of the thoracic as well as the abdominal aorta. Aneurysms of the descending thoracic aorta, acute type B dissection (involving the descending aorta or the arch of the aorta distal to the left subclavian artery), penetrating aortic ulcers, intramural haematomas within the aortic wall and traumatic aortic transection may all be treated with thoracic aortic stents. Such repairs may be carried out under regional or general anaesthesia. Many anaesthetists, surgeons and radiologists prefer general anaesthesia to facilitate the delivery of induced hypotension whilst the top end of the stent is being placed. Patients with severe peripheral vascular disease may also require additional surgery with the placing of temporary grafts (conduits) to facilitate the insertion of the stent.

Thoracic endovascular aortic repair (TEVAR) carries risks of acute kidney injury and stroke. A particular concern is the risk of spinal cord injury and consequent paraplegia. The spinal cord receives its blood supply from a (usually single) anterior spinal artery and paired posterior spinal arteries (Fig. 39.2). These arise superiorly from the left subclavian and vertebral arteries and inferiorly from the hypogastric artery. They are supplied throughout their length by a rich anastomotic network of vessels. Classical teaching was that flow from the artery of Adamkiewicz arising on the left between T8 and L1 was of particular importance. It is now understood that there may be multiple segmental feeding vessels contributing to the blood supply of the spinal cord. Stent coverage of a length of 20 cm or more of the thoracic aorta and stent graft exclusion of blood supply in the T8 to L2 region of the aorta pose a particular risk of spinal cord ischaemia and paraplegia. Spinal cord monitoring may be used during surgery, including direct communication with the awake patient or the use of sensory or motor evoked potentials. Paraplegia may present after surgery as well as arising during the intraoperative period, and rigorous postoperative monitoring is paramount. Key manoeuvres to mitigate and reverse cord ischaemia include blood pressure maintenance and CSF drainage. The latter involves placing a catheter into the subarachnoid space, allowing CSF to be drained to reduce pressure in the space to less than 10 mmHg. Spinal cord perfusion pressure depends on the

743

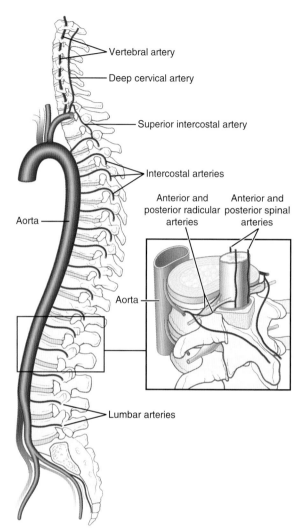

Vertebral artery

Deep cervical artery

Superior intercostal artery

Intercostal arteries

Anterior and posterior radicular arteries

Anterior and posterior spinal arteries

Aorta

Aorta

Lumbar arteries

Fig. 39.2 Arterial blood supply to the spinal cord. (From Macfarlane, A. J. R., Brull, R., & Chan, V. W. S. (2017) Spinal, epidural, and caudal anesthesia. In: Pardo, M. & Miller, R. (eds.) *Basics of anesthesia*. 7th ed. Philadelphia, Elsevier.)

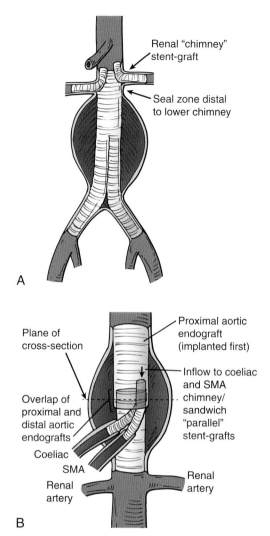

Renal "chimney" stent-graft

Seal zone distal to lower chimney

A

Plane of cross-section

Proximal aortic endograft (implanted first)

Inflow to coeliac and SMA chimney/sandwich "parallel" stent-grafts

Overlap of proximal and distal aortic endografts

Coeliac

SMA

Renal artery

Renal artery

B

Fig. 39.3 (A) Stent grafting of abdominal aortic aneurysm with additional 'chimney' grafting of renal arteries (upper pane). (B) Lower pane shows suprarenal aortic aneurysm stent graft with parallel stent grafts to superior mesenteric and coeliac arteries. (Adapted from Fillinger, M. (2014) Technique: managing branches during endovascular aortic aneurysm repair. In: Cronenwett J. L., & Johnston, K. W. (eds.) *Rutherford's vascular surgery.* 8th ed, Philadelphia, Elsevier, pp. 1357–1380.e2.)

difference between the arterial pressure in the spinal arteries and the CSF pressure. Reducing the latter therefore increases cord perfusion pressure.

Branched grafts and hybrid procedures

A number of alterative graft designs are available to treat anatomically challenging aneurysms. Stenting of a long segment of the aorta may exclude key vessels including the renal arteries, coeliac axis and superior mesenteric artery.

Fenestrations, branched grafts (which incorporate side arms) or additional grafts (parallel or chimney grafts) to feed these vessels may be used to overcome this problem (Fig. 39.3). Branch grafts differ from fenestrated grafts in that the side arms cross the aortic lumen, whereas fenestrations are opposed to the aortic wall. In some cases surgery may be performed to preserve the blood supply to vessels that are

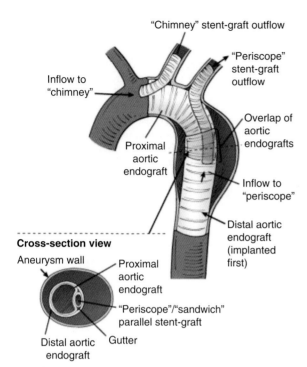

"Chimney" stent-graft outflow

"Periscope" stent-graft outflow

Inflow to "chimney"

Overlap of aortic endografts

Proximal aortic endograft

Inflow to "periscope"

Distal aortic endograft (implanted first)

Cross-section view

Aneurysm wall

Proximal aortic endograft

"Periscope"/"sandwich" parallel stent-graft

Distal aortic endograft

Gutter

Fig. 39.4 Multiple stent grafting of aortic arch aneurysm with additional 'chimney' and 'periscope' grafts to carotid and subclavian arteries. (Adapted from Fillinger, M. (2014) Technique: managing branches during endovascular aortic aneurysm repair. In: Cronenwett J. L., & Johnston, K. W. (eds.) *Rutherford's vascular surgery.* 8th ed, Philadelphia, Elsevier, pp. 1357–1380.e2.)

to be covered by a stent graft. Such hybrid procedures are of particular importance to allow endovascular repair of the ascending aorta and the aortic arch (Fig. 39.4). The treatment of aneurysmal disease or of type A dissection by stent grafting alone would result in the great vessels supplying the head and neck being covered, with potentially catastrophic results. So-called debranching operations which may involve anastomoses between the carotid and subclavian arteries maintain blood supply to the great vessels supporting stent repair or combined stent and surgical repair to the proximal aorta. Such procedures require general anaesthesia and in some cases cardiopulmonary bypass and circulatory arrest.

Surgery for occlusive peripheral vascular disease

Peripheral reconstructive surgery is performed in patients with severe atherosclerotic arterial disease causing ischaemic rest pain, tissue loss (ulceration or gangrene), severe claudication with disease at specific anatomical sites (aortoiliac, femoropopliteal, popliteal or distal) or after failure of non-surgical procedures. Most patients are heavy smokers, suffer from chronic pulmonary disease, have widespread arterial disease and present initially with intermittent claudication. Consequently, exercise tolerance is limited and severe coronary artery disease may be present despite few symptoms. Surgical revascularisation is performed to salvage the ischaemic limb, but arterial angioplasty is a less invasive alternative and is generally performed as a first-line procedure in suitable patients. Patients presenting for surgical reconstruction are often those in whom angioplasties have failed and who may have more severe vascular disease. In-hospital mortality (3% in the UK in 2016) after lower limb revascularisation is comparable to that after elective AAA repair, and long-term outcome is worse as a consequence of associated cardiovascular disease. Acute limb ischaemia that threatens limb viability requires rapid intervention comprising full anticoagulation; intravascular thrombolysis after arteriography; analgesia; revascularisation via embolectomy; angioplasty or bypass surgery as indicated. The clinical findings of sensory loss and muscle weakness necessitate intervention within 6 h, and therefore preoperative evaluation and correction of risk factors may be limited.

Bypass of aortoiliac occlusion

Aortic bifurcation grafting is performed to overcome occlusion in the aorta and iliac arteries and to restore flow to the lower limbs. Because the disease evolves gradually, considerable collateral circulation usually develops. Normal surgical practice is to side-clamp the aorta, maintaining some peripheral flow, and to declamp the arteries supplying the legs in sequence. Thus the cardiovascular and metabolic changes are less severe than those seen during open AAA surgery, but the anaesthetic considerations and management are similar.

Peripheral arterial reconstruction

The most common procedures involve the insertion of an autologous vein or synthetic vascular graft between the axillary and femoral, or femoral and popliteal, arteries. Axillofemoral bypass surgery is performed in those not considered fit for open aortic surgery, and these patients are often particularly frail. All these operations are prolonged, and an intermittent positive-pressure ventilation/relaxant balanced anaesthetic technique is suitable. A meticulous anaesthetic technique is paramount, with particular attention to the maintenance of normothermia and administration of i.v. fluids. Hypothermia, hypovolaemia or pain may cause peripheral vasoconstriction, compromising distal perfusion and postoperative graft function. Blood loss through the walls of open-weave grafts may continue for several hours after surgery, and

745

cardiovascular status should be monitored closely during this time. Epidural analgesia may be used alone or as an adjunct to general anaesthesia for lower limb procedures. Despite theoretical advantages, epidural anaesthesia has no effect on graft function *per se*, but it does provide effective postoperative analgesia. However, i.v. heparin is usually administered during and after surgery (see later), and the risks of epidural haematoma should be considered. Oxygen therapy should be continued for at least 24 h after surgery, and monitoring in a high-dependency unit is often required.

Carotid artery surgery

Despite advances in the medical treatment of patients with stroke, it remains a significant cause of death and disability. Carotid endarterectomy is performed to prevent disabling embolic stroke in patients with atheromatous plaques in the common carotid bifurcation or internal or external carotid arteries (Fig. 39.5). Most patients are elderly, with generalised vascular disease. Cerebral autoregulation may be impaired, and cerebral blood flow is therefore much more dependent upon systemic arterial pressure. The main risk of surgery is the production of a new neurological deficit (which may

be fatal or cause permanent disability), although cardiovascular complications account for 50% of the overall morbidity and mortality.

The recommendations for carotid endarterectomy are based on an extensive body of research regarding the best management of stroke and transient ischaemic attack. Carotid endarterectomy is recommended in patients with symptoms of embolic carotid artery disease and a 70%–99% carotid stenosis so long as the risk of periprocedural death or stroke is considered to be less than 6%. It should be considered in symptomatic patients with a stenosis of 50%–69% whose surgical risk is considered to be less than 6%. There is also evidence to support carotid endarterectomy in asymptomatic patients with a 60%–99% carotid stenosis. However, the benefit is less marked than in symptomatic disease, and practice is more variable in this setting. Carotid artery angioplasty and stenting is a less invasive alternative to surgical endarterectomy. It is often considered for patients in whom neck surgery may be challenging – for example, after previous radiotherapy or in the patient at particular risk of perioperative cardiac complications. The risks of major stroke are highest within the first few days after a transient ischaemic attack (TIA) or minor stroke. Consequently, carotid

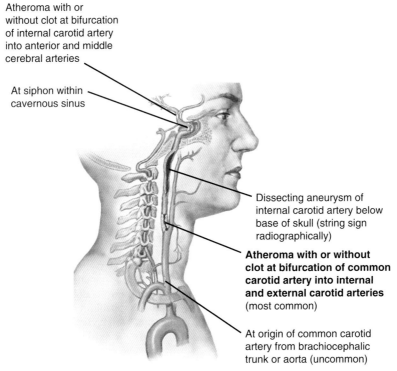

Atheroma with or without clot at bifurcation of internal carotid artery into anterior and middle cerebral arteries

At siphon within cavernous sinus

Dissecting aneurysm of internal carotid artery below base of skull (string sign radiographically)

Atheroma with or without clot at bifurcation of common carotid artery into internal and external carotid arteries (most common)

At origin of common carotid artery from brachiocephalic trunk or aorta (uncommon)

Fig. 39.5 Common sites of atheroma within carotid arteries. (Adapted from Goldstone, J. (2014) Exposure of the carotid bifurcation. In: Delaney, C. *Netter's surgical anatomy and approaches.* Philadelphia, Saunders, pp. 389–398.)

endarterectomy should be performed as soon as is feasible (within 14 days and ideally within 48 h) after a minor stroke or TIA when indicated (embolic stroke, significant carotid stenosis). This limits the time available for preoperative preparation, investigation and risk reduction.

During surgery, the internal, external and common carotid arteries are clamped and the atheromatous plaque removed. During application of the clamps, cerebral perfusion is dependent on collateral circulation via the circle of Willis. Many surgeons insert a temporary shunt to bypass the site of obstruction, minimising the period of potential cerebral ischaemia. Several methods are available to assess cerebral blood flow during clamping before proceeding with the endarterectomy; if flow is adequate, some surgeons prefer not to use a temporary shunt. Monitoring of neurological status in an awake patient is considered by many to be the gold standard, but other methods used in practice include the following:

- Transcranial Doppler ultrasonography of the middle cerebral artery flow velocity
- Measurement of arterial pressure in the occluded distal carotid segment (the stump pressure)
- EEG monitoring

Although most strokes related to surgery are associated with thromboembolism rather than hypo- or hypertension, and the majority of these are caused by technical surgical issues, the anaesthetist has a crucial role in the maintenance of cardiovascular stability before, during and after surgery. Rapid swings in arterial pressure are common because of the direct effects of surgical manipulation, plaque removal and carotid cross-clamping in patients with impaired baroreceptor function as a result of carotid atheroma and cardiovascular disease.

The main aims of anaesthesia for carotid endarterectomy are maintenance of oxygen delivery to the brain, cardiovascular stability, airway protection, provision of neurological protection and rapid recovery. Most intraoperative strokes are apparent on recovery from anaesthesia, and early postoperative neurological assessment is important. Any residual postoperative effects of anaesthesia may confuse the diagnosis of intraoperative embolism or ischaemic change, so a technique that permits rapid return of function is required. These aims may be achieved using general, local or regional anaesthetic techniques, with or without sedative or analgesic adjuncts. In all cases an intra-arterial cannula is mandatory for monitoring of arterial pressure, which should be maintained particularly during carotid clamping, and attention paid to maintaining normothermia.

Local infiltration of the surgical field may be used alone or in combination with superficial and intermediate or deep cervical plexus blockade. Cervical plexus block can be performed using landmark- or ultrasound-guided techniques. Superficial cervical plexus block is performed by infiltration of local anaesthetic along the entire length of the posterior border of the sternomastoid muscle, using 10–15 ml local anaesthetic (e.g. levobupivacaine 0.25%). The intermediate block involves injection of 5 ml local anaesthetic 1–2 cm deep to the midpoint of the sternomastoid. Additional infiltration of local anaesthetic by the surgeon may be required and should be anticipated. Advantages of locoregional techniques include definitive neurological monitoring (therefore allowing selective use of shunts), preservation of cerebral and coronary autoregulation and the maintenance of higher cerebral perfusion pressures during the procedure (Table 39.1). These techniques rely on good cooperation among the patient, the surgeon and the anaesthetist. Many patients find it difficult to lie still and supine for the duration of the procedure, particularly those with heart failure or respiratory disease; this may be compounded by diaphragmatic compromise because phrenic nerve paralysis may accompany deep cervical plexus blockade. Sudden loss of consciousness or seizures may occur if cerebral perfusion is inadequate after clamping, and subsequent airway control may be very difficult because access is limited.

Performing surgery under general anaesthesia avoids these problems. Both propofol and volatile agents (at low doses) preserve cerebral and coronary autoregulation, reduce cerebral oxygen requirements and, in theory, may provide some degree of neuroprotection. General anaesthesia with artificial ventilation allows $PaCO_2$ to be manipulated, but hypotension may be more common compared with regional anaesthesia. The airway is not accessible during surgery, and tracheal intubation with a well-secured reinforced tracheal tube is advisable. Anaesthesia should be induced cautiously using an i.v. agent and maintained with a balanced inhalational or total intravenous technique using an inspired oxygen concentration of 50% in air or nitrous oxide (100% inspired oxygen produces cerebral vasoconstriction). All anaesthetic agents should be short acting, and remifentanil, alfentanil or low-dose fentanyl (100–200 μg) are useful adjuncts. Hypotension may potentially occur after induction and during the placement of cerebral monitoring, but it should be treated promptly. Vasopressors (e.g. ephedrine 3–6 mg or phenylephrine 25–50 μg increments) are often required and should be prepared before induction of anaesthesia. A high PaO_2, normocapnia and normothermia should be maintained. Blood loss and fluid requirements are usually modest. Postoperatively, significant pain is unusual and the combination of wound infiltration with local anaesthetic with a nonsteroidal anti-inflammatory analgesic during surgery is effective.

Data from the GALA trial (general anaesthesia vs. local anaesthesia) and systematic reviews have shown no difference in overall outcome with any specific anaesthetic technique.

Patients should be monitored in a high-dependency environment or PACU for several hours postoperatively. Hypertension is common in the early postoperative period

Table 39.1 Suggested advantages and disadvantages of local or general anaesthesia for carotid surgery

Advantages	Disadvantages
Local anaesthesia	
Definitive CNS monitoring	Technical difficulties
Maintenance of higher cerebral perfusion pressure	Patient discomfort lying supine during prolonged procedure
Maintenance of cerebral autoregulation	Sedative or analgesic supplementation usually required
Allows selective shunting	Lack of airway protection
Arterial pressure usually higher, so less vasopressors required compared with GA	Difficult access to patient if intraoperative neurological or cardiac complications occur
Avoids 'minor' complications of general anaesthesia	
General anaesthesia	
Patient comfort	Some method of monitoring of cerebral blood flow required
Airway protection	'Minor' complications of general anaesthesia (e.g. sore throat, sedation, nausea, vomiting)
Reduced $CMRO_2$ and theoretical cerebral protection	Tendency towards intraoperative hypotension, requiring treatment with vasopressors
Cerebral autoregulation maintained using low doses of volatile agents	
Therapeutic manipulation of arterial CO_2 possible	

$CMRO_2$, Cerebral metabolic rate for oxygen.

because of impaired circulatory reflexes; pain from the wound or from bladder distension may also contribute. Hypertension is associated with adverse neurological outcomes because it may compromise the graft or cause intracranial haemorrhage. Arterial pressure should be controlled to achieve systolic pressures less than 165 mmHg and diastolic pressures less than 95 mmHg, accounting for the range of individual preoperative values. Intravenous α- or β-blockers or an infusion of a vasodilator (e.g. GTN or hydralazine) may be required as prophylaxis or treatment.

The other main postoperative complication is the development of a haematoma. Initial treatment involves local pressure and reversal of heparin with protamine. However, local oedema and the presence of a large haematoma may cause airway compromise and hypoxaemia requiring urgent surgical exploration. Induction of general anaesthesia in these circumstances is particularly hazardous, and evacuation of the haematoma under local infiltration is usually preferable. Recurrent laryngeal nerve damage is a recognised complication of carotid endarterectomy. In most cases this simply causes a hoarse voice, but in patients who have had a previous contralateral carotid endarterectomy, specific preoperative evaluation of vocal cord function should be performed before surgery.

Cardioversion

Direct current (DC) cardioversion is an effective treatment for some re-entrant tachyarrhythmias. Atrial fibrillation of less than 6 months duration, atrial flutter, supraventricular tachycardia and ventricular tachycardia may be converted to sinus rhythm, although maintenance of sinus rhythm depends usually on subsequent antiarrhythmic drugs. Cardioversion has little effect on contractility, conductivity or excitability of the myocardium and has a low incidence of side effects or complications.

Modern defibrillators (see Chapter 15) use a number of different current waveforms. The key distinction is between monophasic and biphasic defibrillators. In the latter the polarity of the electrodes reverses after 5–10 ms, reversing current flow between the pads. This is associated with fewer complications and a better success rate for defibrillation. Modern defibrillators are generally biphasic. The defibrillator pads are usually positioned on the anterolateral chest with the patient supine, but the anteroposterior arrangement, with the patient in the lateral position, is sometimes used. The anteroposterior position is better for temporary pacing in the event of asystole. The pads should not be sited over the scapula, sternum or vertebrae and must be placed at least 10 cm from any pacemaker or implantable defibrillator. These devices must be checked after the procedure.

The ECG monitoring lead chosen should demonstrate a clear R wave to synchronise the discharge away from the T wave and thus reduce the risk of development of ventricular fibrillation. The shocks delivered by biphasic defibrillators are about half those used in monophasic defibrillators. For atrial fibrillation, an initial shock of 120 J is generally used. Supraventricular tachycardia and atrial flutter may be cardioverted with energy settings of 70–120 J.

Despite the use of synchronised discharge, ventricular fibrillation may be produced in the presence of hypokalaemia, ischaemia, digoxin toxicity and QT prolongation (e.g. caused by quinidine or tricyclic antidepressants).

Preanaesthetic assessment

Patients may present with a chronic arrhythmia for elective cardioversion or as an emergency *in extremis* with a life-threatening arrhythmia. They may have other serious cardiovascular pathological conditions such as rheumatic disease, ischaemic heart disease, recent myocardial infarction or cardiac failure. Digoxin therapy predisposes to postcardioversion arrhythmias; it is often withheld for 48 h before cardioversion. In some patients there is a significant risk of embolic phenomena. Anticoagulation to an international normalised ratio of more than 2 is essential in all patients with atrial fibrillation of greater than 48 hours' duration to avoid the risk of embolic events even if no intra-atrial thrombus is visible on echocardiography.

Anaesthesia

Treatment should be carried out only in areas specifically designed for the purpose and with a full range of drugs, resuscitation and monitoring equipment available (see Chapter 46). These must be checked by the anaesthetist and patients prepared as for a surgical procedure.

Electrocardiographic monitoring, pulse oximetry and measurement of arterial pressure are instituted. A vein is cannulated, and the patient's lungs are preoxygenated before i.v. induction of deep sedation or anaesthesia (see Chapter 4). The choice of drug is determined by the cardiovascular stability and recovery period required. If the patient is clinically shocked, precautions to prevent aspiration of gastric contents should be taken, and RSI with cricoid pressure and tracheal intubation should be used. However, many patients are admitted for elective cardioversion on a day-case basis, and a technique using i.v. propofol and spontaneous ventilation is suitable.

As soon as the patient is unconscious, the airway is secured and oxygenation maintained with a suitable breathing system. Before activation of the defibrillator, it is important to check that the patient is not in contact with any person or metal object. If repeated shocks are required, incremental doses of the anaesthetic may be given. The patient should be monitored carefully both during anaesthesia and after recovery of consciousness, in particular for evidence of recurrent arrhythmia, hypotension, pulmonary oedema or systemic or pulmonary embolism.

Surgery for tumours of the endocrine system

Amine precursor uptake and decarboxylation (APUD) cells originate from neuroectoderm and are distributed widely throughout the body. They synthesise and store neurotransmitter substances, including serotonin, adrenocorticotropic hormone (ACTH), calcitonin, melanocyte-stimulating hormone (MSH), glucagon, gastrin and vasoactive intestinal polypeptide (VIP). Neoplastic change within these cells produces the group of tumours termed apudomas, such as carcinoid, pancreatic islet cell tumour, pituitary and thyroid adenoma, medullary carcinoma of thyroid and small cell carcinoma of the lung. These may be orthoendocrine or paraendocrine – the former produce amines and polypeptides associated normally with the constituent cells, whereas the latter secrete substances produced usually by other organs. Two orthoendocrine apudomas in particular may produce significant problems for the anaesthetist.

Carcinoid tumour

Carcinoid tumours are rare tumours derived from enterochromaffin cells of the intestinal tract, most commonly the small bowel or appendix. However, they may arise at any site in the gut and rarely in the gall bladder, pancreas or bronchus. They are usually benign. Malignant change occurs in 4% and may produce hepatic metastases. Carcinoid tumours may secrete a number of vasoactive peptides and amines (e.g. serotonin, histamine, kinins and prostaglandins) that have a variety of effects on vascular, bronchial and GI smooth muscle. These compounds are normally metabolised in the liver, and carcinoid tumours are usually asymptomatic unless the mediators reach the systemic circulation from hepatic metastases or an extra-abdominal primary (e.g. bronchus) tumour or if the tumour is large and hepatic metabolism is exceeded. In these cases the clinical symptoms of carcinoid syndrome occur; these are variable but include flushing, increased intestinal motility, abdominal pain, bronchospasm and dyspnoea. Flushing, bronchospasm, increased intestinal motility, hypotension and oedema are related to the production of kallikrein, which is metabolised to bradykinin, a potent vasodilator. Adrenergic stimulation and alcohol ingestion increase the production of bradykinin. Serotonin (5-hydroxytryptamine, 5-HT) causes

749

abnormal gut motility, diarrhoea and bronchospasm. It has positive inotropic and chronotropic effects and produces vasoconstriction. The 5-HT may cause endocardial fibrosis, leading to pulmonary and tricuspid stenosis or regurgitation (although bronchial carcinoid tumours may lead to left-sided cardiac valvular lesions). Histamine secretion may cause bronchoconstriction and flushing. Acute attacks of carcinoid syndrome may also be precipitated by fear or hypotension.

Diagnosis is confirmed by high urinary excretion of 5-hydroxyindoleacetic acid (5-HIAA), a metabolite of 5-HT. Urinary 5-HIAA concentrations correlate with tumour activity and perioperative complications.

Primary and secondary tumours are localised by CT, MRI, ultrasound, combined positron emission tomography (PET)/CT scans or radionuclide scans. Although medication may alleviate some symptoms, the definitive treatment of carcinoid tumours is surgery, including excision of the primary tumour and resection or radiofrequency ablation of hepatic metastases. The main anaesthetic considerations are perioperative prevention of mediator release and preparation for control of carcinoid crises. Systemic release of carcinoid mediators can be exacerbated or precipitated by anxiety, tracheal intubation, inadequate analgesia, tumour manipulation or the administration of catecholamines or drugs which cause histamine release. In severe cases, acute intraoperative cardiovascular instability (arrhythmias and extreme fluctuations in arterial pressure) and resistant bronchospasm may occur.

Medical management

Patients may be taking drugs for symptomatic relief from diarrhoea, flushing and bronchospasm, but specific agents are used to inhibit synthesis, prevent release or block the actions of the mediators released by the tumour. The most important drug is the somatostatin analogue octreotide, which improves both symptoms and biochemical indices and is useful in the prevention and management of perioperative hypotension and carcinoid crisis. Somatostatin (half-life 1–3 min) is secreted naturally by the pancreas and regulates GI peptide production by inhibiting the secretion of growth hormone, thyroid-stimulating hormone (TSH), prolactin and other exocrine and endocrine hormones. Octreotide, the octapeptide analogue of somatostatin, has a longer half-life, high potency and low clearance and may be given i.v. or s.c. The usual s.c. dose is 50–200 μg every 8–12 h. It is useful for symptom relief in other conditions, notably acromegaly, VIPoma and glucagonoma. It may cause GI side effects, gallstones and impaired glucose tolerance.

The 5-HT antagonists (ketanserin, methysergide) and antihistamines, such as ranitidine and chlorphenamine, are also used. Cyproheptadine has both antihistamine and anti-5-HT actions.

Anaesthesia

Perioperative management should be in close cooperation with both physician and surgeon, and the patient's regular medication should be continued up to the time of surgery. The possibility of cardiac valvular lesions should be considered. Hypovolaemia and electrolyte disturbance should be corrected before operation. Anxiolytic premedication with minimal cardiovascular disturbance is desirable; an oral benzodiazepine is often used alone or together with an antihistamine, although oversedation should be avoided. Octreotide must be continued as premedication 50–100 μg s.c. 1 h preoperatively. It may also be administered during surgery as an i.v. infusion at 50–100 μg h^{-1}. A smooth anaesthetic technique is essential, and techniques that may cause hypotension, including epidural and subarachnoid block, should be used with extreme caution. Drugs that cause histamine release (e.g. thiopental, morphine, meperidine, atracurium, mivacurium) should be avoided.

Continuous monitoring of ECG and direct arterial pressure should be started before careful induction of anaesthesia with etomidate or propofol, accompanied by measures to obtund the potentially exaggerated pressor response to tracheal intubation. Suxamethonium is best avoided because it may cause peptide release, and non-depolarising neuromuscular blocking drugs with minimal histamine release (e.g. rocuronium or vecuronium) are preferable. Anaesthesia should be maintained with opioids (e.g. fentanyl or remifentanil), inhaled nitrous oxide and a volatile agent. Total intravenous anaesthesia with propofol has also been used. Bronchospasm may be severe and should be treated with octreotide or aminophylline rather than adrenaline. Major fluid shifts may occur during surgery, and the effects of circulating peptides may distort the physiological response to hypovolaemia. Central venous pressure measurement is advisable when large blood loss is likely, and pulmonary artery catheterisation may be occasionally required in patients with cardiac complications. Intraoperative hypotension may be severe and should be treated with intravenous fluids and octreotide 100 μg i.v. Sympathomimetic drugs may cause α-mediated peptide release and are not recommended for the treatment of bronchospasm or hypotension. Hypertension is usually less severe and usually responds to increased depth of anaesthesia, β-blockade or ketanserin.

Close cardiovascular monitoring and good analgesia are required postoperatively, and the patient should be observed in a high-dependency or intensive therapy unit. The use of epidural analgesia is controversial, but an epidural infusion of fentanyl alone or with bupivacaine 0.1% has been used successfully.

Phaeochromocytoma

Phaeochromocytomas are derived from chromaffin cells that secrete catecholamines (predominantly noradrenaline but also adrenaline and occasionally dopamine) and occur in less than 0.1% of hypertensive patients. The majority present in middle-aged adults, but they may be found in childhood. Most are found as a single benign tumour of the adrenal medulla, but 10% occur in ectopic sites, such as the paravertebral sympathetic ganglia. Approximately 10% of phaeochromocytomas are malignant, and 10% are bilateral. Genetic factors are often involved, and they may be associated with multiple endocrine neoplasia (MEN) and other syndromes (Box 39.2).

The clinical features depend on the quantity of hormones secreted and on which is predominant, although episodes may be paroxysmal and clinical findings may be normal between attacks. Noradrenaline-secreting tumours tend to cause severe refractory hypertension, headaches and glucose intolerance; circulating blood volume is reduced and vasoconstriction occurs. Adrenaline-secreting tumours trigger palpitations, anxiety and panic attacks, sweating, hypoglycaemia, tachycardia, tachyarrhythmias and occasionally high-output cardiac failure. Malaise, weight loss, pallor and psychological disturbances may occur, and end-organ damage (e.g. retinopathy, nephropathy, dilated cardiomyopathy) may arise as a consequence of hypertension. They present several problems for the anaesthetist (Box 39.3).

Diagnosis

Diagnosis is important because the mortality of patients undergoing unrelated surgery with an unsuspected phaeochromocytoma is up to 50%. Diagnosis is confirmed by measurement of metanephrine and normetanephrine in blood or urine. Plasma tests are more sensitive and convenient, whereas urine tests are more specific. An MRI of the abdomen is probably the investigation of choice to localise tumours greater than 1 cm in diameter. Computed tomography (performed without intravenous contrast media, which may precipitate release of hormone) is an alternative. Confirmation of the identity and position of an adrenal mass is by uptake of $[^{131}I]$ *m*-iodobenzylguanidine (MIBG) monitored by gamma camera. Either MIBG scanning or $[^{18}F]$-fluorodopamine PET may be useful for the localisation of small or extra-adrenal tumours not detected by other means.

Preoperative preparation

Medical treatment of the effects of the tumour must be achieved before surgery. α-Adrenergic antagonists counteract the increased peripheral vascular resistance and reduced circulating volume, and phenoxybenzamine (non-competitive, non-selective antagonist), prazosin and doxazosin ($α_1$-selective, competitive antagonists) have been used successfully. Non-competitive α-antagonists are preferable because surges of catecholamine concentrations, occurring particularly during tumour handling, do not overwhelm the effects of a non-competitive drug. Phenoxybenzamine is given in increasing titrated doses over 2–3 weeks before surgery, starting from 10 mg b.d. up to a usual dose of 40–50 mg b.d. In this way the circulating volume expands gradually with normal oral intake of fluid. Adverse effects include initial postural hypotension, tachycardia, blurred vision and nasal congestion. A β-adrenergic antagonist may be required later to control tachycardia, but acute hypertension, cardiac failure and acute pulmonary oedema may occur if β-blockade is introduced first because of unopposed α-mediated vasoconstriction. Propranolol, metoprolol and atenolol are useful agents if beta-blockade is required. Labetalol is favoured by some physicians, but its β effect predominates and α-antagonists should be administered first. Occasionally, phenoxybenzamine or phentolamine may be given by i.v. infusion (e.g. for 48–72 h preceding surgery). In this event, intravascular volume must be monitored by measurement of CVP, and i.v. colloids are often required to maintain a normal circulating volume. Alternatively, catecholamine synthesis may be suppressed actively by administration of α-methyl-*p*-tyrosine, a tyrosine hydroxylase inhibitor. This drug may be very successful in controlling catecholamine effects but may cause severe side effects, including diarrhoea, fatigue and depression, and is usually reserved for long-term medical treatment in patients considered unsuitable for surgery.

Preoperative investigations depend on the patient's physical condition; the presence of end-organ damage should be determined. Nephrectomy may be required to remove the tumour completely, and renal function should be assessed preoperatively. Echocardiography is also useful.

Anaesthesia

Sudden, severe hypertension (as a result of systemic release of catecholamines) may occur during tumour mobilisation and handling, particularly if preoperative preparation has been inadequate. Severe hypotension may occur after ligation of the venous drainage of the tumour (when catecholamine concentrations decrease acutely). Marked fluctuations in arterial pressure may also occur during induction of anaesthesia and tracheal intubation.

Sedative and anxiolytic premedication is useful, and both α- and β-adrenergic antagonists should be continued up to the day of surgery. Monitoring of ECG, CVP and direct arterial pressure must be started before induction of anaesthesia. Intraoperative monitoring should include temperature, blood gas tensions and glucose concentration; transoesophageal echocardiography may be required if significant cardiomyopathy is present. Anaesthetic drugs should be selected on the basis of cardiovascular stability, and agents which have the ability to provoke histamine (and hence catecholamine) release are best avoided (Box 39.4). The exact choice of individual anaesthetic drugs is less important than careful conduct of anaesthesia, which may be induced by slow

Box 39.4 **Drugs that should be avoided in patients with phaeochromocytoma**

Atropine	Pancuronium
Suxamethonium	Droperidol
d-Tubocurarine	Morphine
Atracurium	Halothane

administration of thiopental, etomidate or propofol and maintained with nitrous oxide in oxygen, supplemented by sevoflurane or isoflurane. Desflurane has the theoretical disadvantage of causing sympathetic stimulation if the inspired concentration is increased too rapidly. Moderate doses of an opioid (e.g. fentanyl 3–5 μg kg^{-1}) may aid cardiovascular stability. Drugs should be immediately available to treat acute hypertension (e.g. sodium nitroprusside, phentolamine or nicardipine), tachycardia or arrhythmias (e.g. esmolol). Hypotension is treated with fluids initially, but vasopressors (e.g. ephedrine, phenylephrine or noradrenaline) may be required. Intravenous magnesium sulphate may be useful; it suppresses catecholamine release from the tumour and adrenergic nerve endings, is a direct-acting vasodilator and has antiarrhythmic effects. However, it has a narrow therapeutic window, and plasma Mg^{2+} concentration should be monitored. Perioperative epidural analgesia may attenuate some of the cardiovascular responses, except during tumour handling, and is useful for postoperative analgesia. It should be used judiciously to avoid hypotension. Postoperative problems may include hypoglycaemia, somnolence, opioid sensitivity, hypotension and hypoadrenalism. Invasive monitoring should be continued for 12–24 h after surgery, and the patient must be nursed in a high-dependency unit or ICU.

Laparoscopic adrenalectomy is now the surgical treatment of choice for adrenal phaeochromocytoma. It is performed via the transperitoneal or retroperitoneal routes. Laparoscopic techniques are associated with less postoperative pain, earlier mobilisation and faster recovery compared with open surgery. Overall, cardiovascular disturbance may be less, but the creation of a pneumoperitoneum during transperitoneal laparoscopy may cause large surges in catecholamine concentrations in addition to those occurring during tumour mobilisation. Consequently, similar anaesthetic considerations apply as for open surgery.

Surgery for adrenal cortical disorders

Adrenalectomy (open or laparoscopic) is indicated for adrenal carcinoma or for the removal of hormone-secreting adenomas. Open surgery is associated with significant postoperative pain and atelectasis, and patients may benefit from epidural analgesia. Many of the challenges of adrenalectomy relate to the endocrine disorder for which surgery is being performed. Mineralocorticoid-secreting adenomas cause Conn's syndrome: patients present with hypertension, refractory hypokalaemia and in some cases metabolic alkalosis. Blood pressure should be controlled and hypokalaemia corrected (as far as possible) before surgery. Spironolactone is valuable both to manage the metabolic effects of hyperaldosteronism and to correct hypervolaemia. Additional treatment with ACE inhibitors may also be required. Invasive arterial pressure monitoring is essential. Undercorrection of hypervolaemia before surgery may predispose the patient to hypertension, whereas manipulation of the adrenal gland during surgery may cause catecholamine release. Hyperventilation and hypocapnia have the potential to exacerbate hypokalaemia. Hypokalaemia alone may prolong the action of non-depolarising neuromuscular blocking agents (NMBAs). After surgery, patients who have undergone bilateral adrenalectomy require corticosteroid and mineralocorticoid replacement therapy; this treatment may also be needed in patients who have undergone unilateral adrenalectomy,

Cushing's syndrome is caused by excessive glucocorticoid production. In the majority of cases this is due to excess ACTH production by a pituitary adenoma (Cushing's disease), but 20%–30% of patients have an adrenal adenoma. Patients have hypertension, impaired glucose tolerance or diabetes and may be hypokalaemic. They can display the classic stigmata of Cushing's syndrome, including obesity, muscle weakness and atrophy, thin skin and poor wound healing. These patients have a high incidence of gastro-oesophageal reflux and may require RSI. They may require reduced doses of NMBAs because of existing muscle weakness, and neuromuscular monitoring is required.

Thyroid and parathyroid surgery

Thyroid and parathyroid surgery are discussed in Chapter 37.

Plastic surgery

Plastic surgery includes the reconstitution of damaged or deformed tissues (congenital abnormalities or resulting from trauma, burns or infection), removal of cutaneous tumours or cosmetic alteration of body features. Division or removal of the abnormality often necessitates skin grafting. Major plastic surgery includes the formation and repositioning of free and pedicle grafts and the movement of skin flaps.

General considerations

Many of these procedures have important common features. Patients may be physically deformed, and attention should be directed to their psychological state. This is influenced by long periods of confinement and rehabilitation, concern over disfigurement or loss of limb function, and occasionally chronic pain. The presence of local or generalised infection and the patient's state of nutrition are important factors in postoperative outcome and should be considered. Conversely, cosmetic surgery of the face, tattoo removal, breast augmentation and removal of unwanted adipose tissue are usually performed on healthy patients. Surgery is often prolonged, requiring special attention to blood and fluid replacement therapy, and maintenance of body temperature. Pain is usually peripheral in origin but may be severe, particularly from donor skin graft sites; local anaesthetic techniques (nerve or plexus blockade, or local infiltration) are very effective.

Anaesthesia for prolonged procedures should be administered in a warmed theatre environment, employing a technique which minimises protracted recovery from anaesthesia. A remifentanil-based technique supplemented by an insoluble volatile agent (e.g. isoflurane, desflurane or sevoflurane) is effective. Alternatively, a total intravenous technique may be employed, although the vasodilatation produced by volatile agents may be beneficial to surgical outcome. Nitrous oxide may produce bone marrow depression with exposure of more than 8 h duration and an oxygen/air mix should be substituted. Fluid balance should be maintained scrupulously. Significant haemorrhage is common during plastic surgery, and blood transfusion may be required. Volatile anaesthetic agents and regional or sympathetic blockade cause vasodilatation, which may be helpful. Measures should be taken to prevent DVT formation. When surgery has been completed, wound dressing and bandaging may be lengthy procedures. Bandages may be applied around the trunk, and the patient must be lifted carefully to avoid injury.

Head and neck

Tracheal intubation using a reinforced tube is recommended for surgery in the head and neck area. Tumours or scarring of the neck, deformity of facial bones and cleft palate can make tracheal intubation particularly difficult. The airway should be assessed carefully before anaesthesia and any difficulties anticipated, and a complete range of equipment should be available (see Chapter 23). The administration of NMBAs in such patients may be unwise before the airway is secured by intubation; awake fibre-optic intubation under local anaesthesia or an inhalational technique should be considered. The method of maintenance is determined by the condition of the patient, the type and duration of surgery (often prolonged) and the experience and preference of the anaesthetist. Venous drainage is improved and bleeding reduced in head or neck surgery if the patient is positioned in a 10- to 15-degree head-up tilt. Hypotensive techniques may also be indicated, in which case an arterial cannula is advisable for measurement of arterial pressure. It is important to protect the eyes from pressure, the ears from blood and other fluids and the tracheal tube and anaesthetic tubing from dislodgement. It may be difficult to monitor chest movement, and access to the arms may be impossible. An i.v. infusion with extension tubing is essential; there should be access to a three-way tap for injection of drugs.

Anaesthesia for pedicled and free flap surgery

Reconstructive surgery may require the transposition of flaps of skin, fat and muscle from one part of the body to another. These may be pedicled flaps that remain connected to their blood supply through a vascular pedicle throughout the operation (e.g. the pectoralis major myocutaneous flap is often used in head and neck reconstruction) or free flaps where the vascular pedicle supplying the flap is disconnected from its original blood supply and anastomosed to vessels at the site of reconstruction (e.g. the transverse rectus abdominis myocutaneous (TRAM) free flap and the deep inferior epigastric perforator (DIEP) free flap, both used in breast reconstruction procedures). The considerations are similar for both types of surgery, with the integrity of the blood supply across the new anastomoses being a particular concern in free flap surgery. Surgery is generally prolonged, and there are a number of concerns for the anaesthetist.

- Careful attention to positioning and padding to avoid pressure injury is essential. Some types of flap surgery may require the patient to be repositioned after the flap has been harvested, and care must be taken to ensure that all pressure areas are protected in the new position.
- Normothermia is important to support flap perfusion. The patient's temperature should be monitored and appropriate warming devices used.

- A haematocrit of 0.3–0.35 should be targeted as an appropriate compromise between maintaining a low blood viscosity and ensuring adequate oxygen delivery.
- The aim should be to maintain a hyperdynamic circulation with a high cardiac output and peripheral vasodilatation to support the microcirculation. This was traditionally achieved with aggressive fluid therapy. However, tissue oedema because of aggressive fluid administration is a cause for concern, and targeted fluid therapy guided by cardiac output or stroke volume variability monitoring may help to avoid this. Many anaesthetists and surgeons eschew the use of vasoconstrictors, although the evidence to support this is equivocal.

Limbs

Local anaesthesia (e.g. by blockade of nerve plexuses in the neck, axilla or groin) may be an advantage in terms of analgesia and vasodilatation for surgery on upper or lower limbs. The duration of some plastic surgical operations and the use of a surgical tourniquet to provide a bloodless field may preclude some techniques, but prolonged neural blockade may be achieved using a catheter technique and by selection of an agent with a prolonged duration of action (e.g. bupivacaine or ropivacaine). Intravenous sedative drugs or light general anaesthesia are useful adjuncts to help the patient tolerate a prolonged procedure. Specific nerve blocks may be useful; for example, blockade of the femoral and lateral cutaneous nerve of the thigh provides good analgesia for skin graft donor sites during and after operation. Bier's block is of limited value because of tourniquet pain, and cuff deflation may be required by the surgeon to identify bleeding points.

Surgical techniques of reimplantation and microsurgical repair of the limbs are well established and make specific demands upon the anaesthetist. These include maintenance of general anaesthesia for up to 24 h, control of vascular spasm and provision of optimum conditions for postoperative recovery.

References/Further reading

Kasten, K.R., Makley, A.T., Kagan, R.J., 2011. Update on the critical care management of severe burns. J. Intensive Care Med. 26 (4), 223–236.

Mancuso, K., Kaye, A.D., Boudreaux, J.P., et al., 2011. Carcinoid and perioperative anesthetic considerations. J. Clin. Anesth. 23, 329–341.

Thompson, J.P., Telford, R.J., Howell, S.J. (Eds.), 2013. Oxford specialist handbook of vascular anaesthesia. OUP, Oxford.

Thompson, J.P., 2017. Anaesthesia for vascular surgery. In: Hardman, J.G., Hopkins, P.M., Struys, M.R.F. (Eds.), Oxford textbook of anaesthesia. OUP, Oxford.

Chapter | 40 |

Neurosurgical anaesthesia

Michael Nathanson

Neurosurgical procedures include elective and emergency surgery of the CNS, its vasculature and the CSF, together with the surrounding bony structures, the skull and spine. Almost all require general anaesthesia; however, some procedures require an awake patient. In addition to a conventional anaesthetic technique which pays meticulous attention to detail, the essential factors are the maintenance of cerebral perfusion pressure and the facilitation of surgical access by minimising blood loss and preventing increases in central nervous tissue volume and oedema.

Applied anatomy and physiology

Anatomy

Brain

The brain comprises the brainstem, cerebellum, midbrain and paired cerebral hemispheres. The brainstem is formed from the medulla and the pons, with the medulla connected to the spinal cord below and to the cerebellum posteriorly. The medulla contains the ascending and descending nerve tracts, the lower cranial nerve nuclei and the respiratory and vasomotor (or 'vital') centres. Running through the brainstem is the reticular system which is associated with consciousness. A lesion or compression of the brainstem secondary to raised intracranial pressure produces abnormal function of the vital centres, which is rapidly fatal ('coning'). The cerebellum coordinates balance, posture and muscular tone.

The midbrain connects the brainstem and cerebellum to the diencephalon (the major components of which are the hypothalamus and thalamus) and the cerebrum (the two cerebral hemispheres and the subcortical structures such as the basal ganglia). The thalamus contains the nuclei of the main sensory pathways. The hypothalamus coordinates the autonomic nervous system and the endocrine systems

of the body. Below the hypothalamus is the pituitary gland. Pituitary tumours may produce the signs of a space-occupying lesion, restrict the visual fields by compressing the optic chiasma, or give rise to an endocrine disturbance.

The cerebral hemispheres comprise the cerebral cortex, basal ganglia and lateral ventricles. A central sulcus or cleft separates the main motor gyrus (or fold) anteriorly from the main sensory gyrus posteriorly. Each hemisphere is divided into four areas, or lobes. The function of the different lobes is incompletely understood. The frontal lobe contains the motor cortex and areas concerned with intellect and behaviour. The parietal lobe contains the sensory cortex, the temporal lobe is concerned with auditory sensation and the integration of other stimuli and the occipital lobe contains the visual cortex. Lesions of the cerebral hemispheres give rise to sensory and motor deficits on the opposite side of the body.

Spinal cord

The spinal cord is approximately 45 cm long and passes from the foramen magnum, where it is continuous with the medulla, to a tapered end termed the conus medullaris at the level of the first or second lumbar vertebrae. At each spinal level, paired anterior (motor) and posterior (sensory) spinal roots emerge on each side of the cord. Each posterior root has a ganglion containing the cell bodies of the sensory nerves. The two roots join at each intervertebral foramen to form a mixed spinal nerve.

Cerebrospinal fluid

Cerebrospinal fluid fills the cerebral ventricles and the subarachnoid space around the brain and spinal cord. The CSF acts as a buffer, separating the brain and spinal cord from the hard bony projections inside the skull and the vertebral canal. It is produced by the choroid plexus in

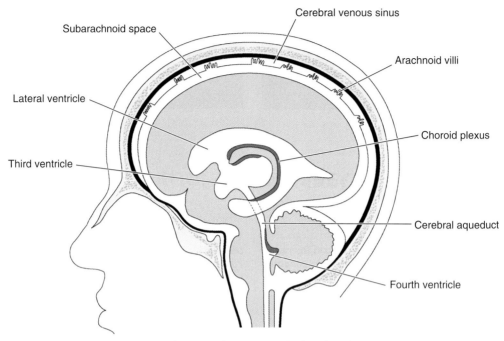

Fig. 40.1 The ventricular system and subarachnoid space.

the lateral, third and fourth ventricles by a combination of filtration and secretion (Fig. 40.1). The total volume of CSF is 150–200 ml. Cerebrospinal fluid passes back into the venous blood through arachnoid villi. Obstruction of the normal flow of CSF through the ventricular system, or reduction in reabsorption, leads to a build-up in ICP, producing intracranial hypertension, dilatation of the ventricles and hydrocephalus.

Meninges

Three meninges (or membranes) surround the brain and the spinal cord. These are the dura, arachnoid and pia mater. Around the brain the dura mater is a thick, strong double membrane which separates into its two layers in parts to form the cerebral venous sinuses. The outer or endosteal layer is adherent to the skull bones and is the equivalent of the periosteum. The inner layer is continuous with the dura which surrounds the spinal cord. The major artery supplying the dura mater in the head is the middle meningeal artery, which may be damaged in a head injury or skull fracture, leading to the formation of an extradural (epidural) haematoma (Fig. 40.2). The arachnoid mater is a thin membrane normally adjacent to the dura mater. Cortical veins from the surface of the brain pass through the arachnoid mater to reach dural venous sinuses and may be damaged by relatively minor trauma, leading to the formation of a

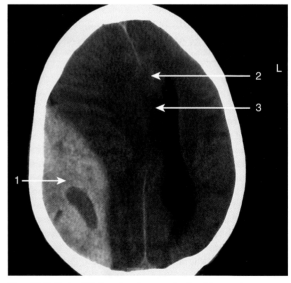

Fig. 40.2 Brain CT showing large extradural haematoma. (From Kelly, B. E., & Bickle, I. (2007) *Crash course: imaging*. St. Louis, Mosby, p. 154.)

each hemisphere. The majority of cerebral aneurysms are of vessels that are part of, or very close to, the circle of Willis. Other important vessels supplying the brainstem and the cerebellum branch from the basilar artery. Venous blood drains into the cerebral venous sinuses, whose walls are formed from the dura mater. These sinuses join and empty into the internal jugular veins.

The blood supply to the spinal cord comes from the single anterior spinal artery formed at the foramen magnum from a branch from each of the vertebral arteries and the paired posterior spinal arteries derived from the posterior inferior cerebellar arteries. The anterior artery supplies the anterior two thirds of the cord. There are additional supplies from segmental arteries and also a direct supply from the aorta, often at the level of the eleventh thoracic intervertebral space. The blood supply to the spinal cord is fragile, and infarction of the cord may result from even minor disruption of the normal arterial supply.

Autonomic nervous system

The autonomic nervous system is classified on anatomical and physiological grounds into the functionally opposing sympathetic and parasympathetic nervous systems. The central areas responsible for coordinating the autonomic nervous system are mostly in the hypothalamus and its surrounding structures and in the frontal lobes. The sympathetic nervous system cells arise from the lateral horn of the thoracic and first two lumbar segments of the spinal cord. The neurons of the parasympathetic nervous system exit the central nervous system with the third, seventh, ninth and tenth cranial nerves and from the second to the fourth sacral segments of the spinal cord.

Physiology
Intracranial pressure

With normal cerebral compliance (note: the correct physiological parameter is *elastance*, the reciprocal of compliance, as the variable of interest is the change in pressure for a given change of volume; however, the parameter *compliance* is more commonly used), ICP is 7–15 cmH$_2$O (5–11 mmHg) in the horizontal position. When moving to the erect position, ICP decreases initially, but then, because of a decrease in reabsorption of CSF, the pressure returns to normal. Intracranial pressure is related to intrathoracic pressure and has a normal respiratory swing. It is increased by coughing, straining and PEEP. In the presence of reduced cerebral compliance, small changes in cerebral volume produce large changes in ICP. Such critical changes may be induced by drugs used during anaesthesia (e.g. volatile anaesthetic agents; see Chapter 3), elevations in Paco$_2$ and posture, as well as by surgery and trauma (Fig. 40.5).

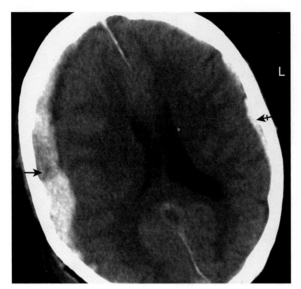

Fig. 40.3 CT scan showing acute subdural haematoma. (From Kelly, B. E., & Bickle, I. (2007) *Crash course: imaging.* St. Louis, Mosby, p. 153.)

subdural haematoma (Fig. 40.3). The pia mater is a vascular membrane closely adherent to the surface of the brain and follows the contours of the gyri and sulci. The space between the pia and arachnoid maters is the subarachnoid space and contains CSF.

The dura mater forms a sac which ends below the cord, usually at the level of the second sacral segment. The dura extends for a short distance along each nerve root and is continuous with the epineurium of each spinal nerve. Around the spinal cord there is an extensive subarachnoid space between the arachnoid mater and the pia mater. The space between the dura and the bony part of the spinal canal (the extradural or epidural space) is filled with fat, lymphatics, arteries and an extensive venous plexus.

Vascular supply

The arterial blood supply to the brain is derived from the two internal carotid arteries and two vertebral arteries. The vertebral arteries are branches of the subclavian arteries and pass through foramina in the transverse processes of the upper six cervical vertebrae. The vertebral arteries join together anterior to the brainstem to form the single basilar artery, which then divides again to form the two posterior cerebral arteries. These vessels and the two internal carotid arteries form an anastomotic system known as the circle of Willis at the base of the brain (Fig. 40.4).

The main arteries supplying the cerebral hemispheres are the anterior, middle and posterior cerebral artery for

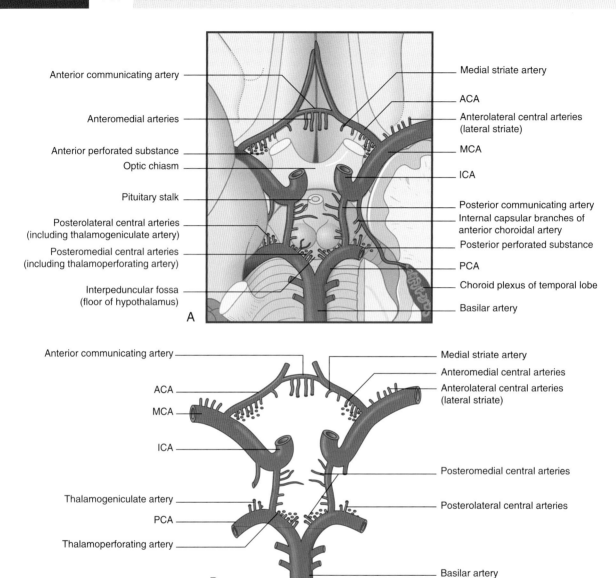

Fig. 40.4 Brain viewed from below showing the Circle of Willis. *ACA,* Anterior cerebral artery; *ICA,* internal carotid artery; *MCA,* middle cerebral artery; *PCA,* posterior cerebral artery. (From Fitzgerald, M. J., Gruener, G., & Mtui, E. (2012) *Clinical neuroanatomy and neuroscience,* 6th ed. Philadelphia, Saunders, p. 56.)

Cerebral blood flow

Under normal conditions, the brain receives about 15% of the cardiac output, which corresponds to a cerebral blood flow (CBF) of approximately 50 ml 100 g^{-1} tissue min^{-1}, or 600–700 ml min^{-1}. The cerebral circulation is able to maintain an almost constant blood flow between a MAP of 60 and 140 mmHg by the process of autoregulation. This is

mediated by a primary myogenic response involving local alteration in the diameter of small arterioles in response to changes in transmural pressure. Above and below these limits, or in the traumatised brain, autoregulation is impaired or absent so that CBF is closely related to cerebral perfusion pressure (CPP) (Fig. 40.6).

Cerebral perfusion pressure may be reduced as a result of systemic hypotension or an increase in ICP; CBF is

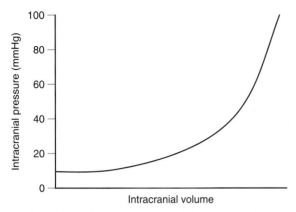

Fig. 40.5 The intracranial pressure/volume relationship.

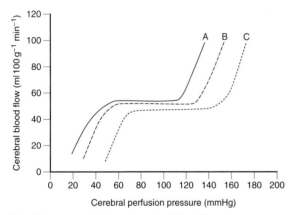

Fig. 40.6 Autoregulation of cerebral blood flow: (A) drug-induced vasodilatation; (B) normal; (C) hypertension or haemorrhagic hypotension.

maintained until the ICP exceeds 30–40 mmHg. The Cushing reflex increases CPP in response to an increase in ICP by first producing reflex systemic hypertension and tachycardia and then bradycardia, despite these compensatory mechanisms also contributing to an increase in ICP. In the treatment of closed head injuries, when both ICP and MAP are monitored, it is essential to maintain the calculated CPP with vasopressor therapy if cerebral perfusion is borderline as even transient absence of flow to the brain may produce focal or global ischaemia with infarction.

Fig. 40.6 also demonstrates that haemorrhagic hypotension associated with excess sympathetic nervous activity results in a loss of autoregulation at a higher CPP than normal, whereas the use of vasodilators to induce hypotension shifts the curve to the left, maintaining flow at lower levels of perfusion pressure.

Cerebral blood flow is closely coupled to cerebral metabolic rate. Local increases in cerebral metabolic rate are associated with very prompt increases in CBF. The increased electrical activity associated with convulsions produces an increase in lactic acid and other vasodilator metabolites. This, together with an increase in CO_2 production, produces an increase in CBF. Conversely, cerebral metabolic depression, in association with either deliberate or accidental hypothermia or induced by drugs, reduces CBF.

It is important to understand that these descriptions of autoregulation are of the 'average' person. There are differences between individuals and within the brains of individuals. Modern neurointensive care management attempts to target therapy to individual behaviours.

Cerebral metabolism

The energy consumption of the brain is relatively constant, whether during sleep or in the awake state, and represents approximately 20% of total oxygen consumption at rest, or 50 ml min^{-1}. General anaesthesia results in a decrease in cerebral metabolic rate. Cerebral metabolism relies on glucose supplied by the cerebral circulation as there are no stores of metabolic substrate. Other substrates which the brain can use are ketone bodies, lactate, glycerol, fatty acids and some amino acids including glutamate, aspartate and γ-aminobutyric acid (GABA). The brain can tolerate only short periods of hypoperfusion or circulatory arrest before irreversible neuronal damage occurs.

The energy production of the brain is related directly to its rate of oxygen consumption, and the cerebral metabolic rate for oxygen ($CMRO_2$) is often used to quantify cerebral activity. By Fick's principle:

$$CMRO_2 = CBF \times \text{arteriovenous oxygen content difference}$$

Barbiturates have been used to reduce cerebral metabolic rate, and propofol and benzodiazepines have a similar, although less profound, effect. All have been used in the sedation of patients with head injury, and the choice is related more to the anticipated duration of sedation than to differences in the effects of the drugs, with the exception of prolonged barbiturate coma induced by infusion of thiopental.

Hypothermia is associated with a reduction in cerebral metabolic rate, with a decrease of approximately 7% for every 1°C decrease in temperature.

Effects of oxygen and carbon dioxide on cerebral blood flow

Physiologically, carbon dioxide is the most important cerebral vasodilator. Even small increases in $PaCO_2$ produce significant

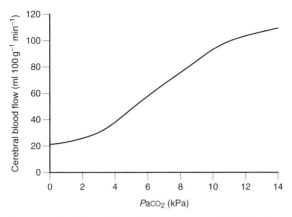

Fig. 40.7 The effect of increasing $PaCO_2$ on cerebral blood flow.

increases in CBF and therefore ICP. There is an almost linear relationship between $PaCO_2$ and CBF (Fig. 40.7). Over the normal range an increase of $PaCO_2$ by 1 kPa increases CBF by 30%. Conversely, hyperventilation to produce a $PaCO_2$ of 4 kPa produces cerebral vasoconstriction and a decrease in ICP. This is compensated for by an increase in CSF production over a more prolonged period of hyperventilation, such as that used in the treatment of head injuries. Thus, there is no advantage in aggressive hyperventilation regimens in head injury management. Hypocapnia below a $PaCO_2$ of 4 kPa to lower ICP should be avoided, except as a last resort, because the vasoconstriction induced may be associated with increased areas of hypoperfusion and ischaemia. At a $PaCO_2$ of 10 kPa or greater, the vessels are maximally dilated and there is little, if any, further increase in CBF.

A reduction in blood oxygen content also leads to cerebral vasodilation such that cerebral oxygen delivery remains approximately constant. In the normal physiological range, alterations in PaO_2 have little effect on CBF. It is only when PaO_2 decreases below approximately 7 kPa that cerebral vasodilatation occurs. Reduction in cerebral blood oxygen content as a result of anaemia has similar effects.

General principles of neurosurgical anaesthesia

Most intracranial operations require access to the meninges and brain substance beneath. This may be achieved through craniotomy (removal and replacement of a piece or flap of bone), craniectomy (removal of bone without replacement) or burr-hole craniectomy (essentially a single drill hole). The size and site of cranial access varies by indication from single burr-holes for biopsies, subdural haematoma drainage, and insertion of ventricular drainage devices (shunts and external ventricular drain (EVD)) through moderate-sized craniotomies for tumour excisions, and very large craniotomies for trauma. Some operations can be undertaken with local anaesthesia alone (e.g. evacuation of chronic subdural haematoma in very frail patients), whereas others require an awake patient for part of the procedure (e.g. awake craniotomy for resection of tumours near eloquent areas such as the motor strip and insertion of deep brain stimulation electrodes in patients with Parkinson's disease).

A smooth anaesthetic technique is essential, avoiding increases in arterial and venous pressures and abrupt changes in $PaCO_2$ concentration while at the same time avoiding a decrease in cerebral oxygenation. Most anaesthetists maintain anaesthesia with either an inhalational anaesthetic agent, usually sevoflurane, or with a continuous infusion of propofol. Intraoperative analgesia is provided by a short-acting opioid such as remifentanil by infusion or intermittent doses of fentanyl (for short or minor procedures). Neuro-muscular blockade and intermittent positive-pressure ventilation (IPPV) are usually employed. It is extremely important to ensure adequate fixation of the tracheal tube and intravascular cannulae and to protect the eyes, as access to the head and limbs is restricted during the operation. Continuous monitoring of the electrocardiograph and arterial pressure is essential; direct arterial pressure and temperature monitoring are normally used, together with continuous measurement of oxygen saturation, end-tidal carbon dioxide concentration and end-tidal anaesthetic agent concentration/processed EEG. At the end of the procedure, the patient must be transferred to the recovery room with no residual neuromuscular blockade or opioid-induced respiratory depression because both may produce critical increases in ICP related to hypercapnia and hypoxaemia. Long-acting drugs with a marked sedative action are used with caution perioperatively so that a pathological failure of return to consciousness is not masked. Craniotomy can be painful, and morphine (or similar) is an appropriate analgesic in most cases.

Monitoring during neurosurgical anaesthesia

Standard monitoring should be started before induction of anaesthesia (see earlier). In patients in whom cardiovascular instability may be a problem, including the frail or after subarachnoid haemorrhage, this should include direct arterial pressure monitoring. Direct arterial pressure monitoring is now used routinely in the majority of patients undergoing an intracranial operation, for some surgeries on the cervical spine and in other situations in which rapid fluctuations in arterial pressure may occur. This also facilitates sampling for arterial blood gas analysis. Use of CVCs varies greatly among practitioners and neurosurgical units. They are used when major blood loss is expected, such as surgery for very vascular meningiomas or when there is a high risk of air embolism. Cerebral oximetry, transcranial Doppler, electro-encephalography and evoked potentials are used in specific situations.

Induction of anaesthesia

For major procedures, an i.v. infusion of an isotonic electrolyte solution should be started through a large-gauge i.v. cannula before induction. Although fluid loading to prevent hypotension on induction is not evidence-based, a primed infusion can be used as needed for maintenance of normal haemodynamics. Intravenous induction should be used whenever possible; however, inhalational induction may be appropriate in children if the risk of a crying, distressed child is more likely to increase ICP than the vasodilator effects of a high inspired concentration of a volatile anaesthetic agent. Although both thiopental and propofol reduce ICP and are suitable induction agents, propofol is the most commonly used agent. The i.v. anaesthetic should be given with an appropriate dose of short-acting opioid. For craniotomy or when TIVA is used, a remifentanil infusion is standard practice. Boluses of fentanyl can be used for shunt insertion, drainage of chronic subdural haematoma or insertion of an EVD. A neuromuscular blocking agent (NMBA) is used to facilitate tracheal intubation. A nerve stimulator should be used to ensure complete neuromuscular blockade before attempting direct laryngoscopy to prevent coughing or straining causing increases in ICP.

Cerebral perfusion may be reduced when the ICP is raised, and an induction technique which produces significant hypotension may critically reduce cerebral perfusion in patients with an intracranial space-occupying lesion (SOL) or subarachnoid haemorrhage associated with vasospasm. The most commonly used techniques to reduce the hypertensive response to laryngoscopy and tracheal intubation are supplementary short-acting opioids (fentanyl, alfentanil, remifentanil) or short-acting β-adrenoceptor blockade (e.g. esmolol). If remifentanil is used as a coinduction agent, an infusion is usually started immediately after the induction dose and acts to control the hypertensive response; alternatively, a target-controlled infusion (TCI) is used for induction, during tracheal intubation, and during maintenance.

The tracheal tube used should be appropriate to avoid kinking of the tube by drapes, instruments or surgeons; this may require preformed or reinforced tubes. Careful positioning of the tracheal tube is vital because any intraoperative flexion of the neck may result in endobronchial intubation if the tip of the tube is initially placed too close to the carina. After the tracheal tube has been secured, the neck should be flexed gently while listening for the presence of breath sounds in both axillae. The tracheal tube should be secured in place with several layers of sticky tape to prevent it peeling away after application of surgical prep solution to the scalp. Cotton ties should not be used because they may compress the internal jugular veins, increasing venous pressure and leading to a reduction in CPP and increased intraoperative haemorrhage. A throat pack is may be placed if transnasal surgery (e.g. trans-sphenoidal hypophysectomy) is planned.

Positioning

Skin cleaning (prep) solutions must be prevented from entering the eyes. For cranial or cervical spine surgery, the eyes are protected by applying paraffin gauze, padding with a folded swab and then covering with a waterproof tape.

Many neurosurgical operations are long, and positioning of the patient to facilitate optimal access, while preventing hypothermia, pressure sores and peripheral nerve injury, is important. Supratentorial cranial surgery involving the frontal or frontotemporal areas is performed with the patient supine, whereas parietal and occipital craniotomies are carried out in the lateral or three three-quarters ('park bench') position. In all cases, care must be taken to avoid neck positions such as marked rotation or flexion which might impede venous drainage. The fully prone position is used for surgery on the posterior fossa, around the foramen magnum and the spine. The prone position is discussed in more detail in the section on spinal surgery (see later). For some procedures it is necessary to tilt or roll the table during the operation. The patient must be positioned securely with supports to prevent slipping if the table is moved. Whatever position is used, it is essential that all pressure points are protected adequately. During long operations, the pulse oximeter probe should be moved at least every 4 h.

Maintenance of anaesthesia

The basis of anaesthesia for neurosurgery is ventilation of the lungs with air and oxygen to produce a $PaCO_2$ of 4.5–5.0 kPa, using either a volatile anaesthetic agent or a propofol infusion supplemented by an opioid analgesic (remifentanil infusion or fentanyl boluses). Unless used carefully, remifentanil may produce hypotension, and when it is stopped, there may be rebound hypertension and the sudden onset of pain or agitation. Sevoflurane is the volatile agent of choice, given that its effects on the cerebral vasculature are much less than those of isoflurane (see Chapter 3). At clinical concentrations, sevoflurane has no effect on cerebral autoregulation and causes only a minimal increase in ICP. Alternatively, TIVA with propofol may be used. There is no evidence that one technique is associated with a better outcome compared with any other. If TIVA is used along with neuromuscular blockade, then depth of anaesthesia should be monitored by processed EEG.

The choice of NMBA depends usually on personal preference. In most cases these drugs should be given by infusion. A peripheral nerve stimulator should be used and the infusion rate titrated to maintain an adequate degree of block (one twitch of the train-of-four stimulus pattern should be present), while preventing overdosage so that the block can be completely reversed shortly (10–15 min) after stopping the infusion and administering a reversal/ antagonist agent.

The initial part of a craniotomy is painful, but after the bone flap has been reflected and the dura incised, pain is not a significant feature again until closure of the wound. For this reason, supplementary intraoperative opioids in large doses are unnecessary. Use of opioids during mainte- nance does allow use of less hypnotic agent. Reflex vagal stimulation can occur, particularly after stimulation of the cranial nerve roots or during vascular surgery around the circle of Willis and the internal carotid artery. This may necessitate immediate administration of an anticholinergic agent to avoid severe bradycardia or even asystole.

Use of techniques permitting rapid recovery (e.g. sevo- flurane, propofol, remifentanil) are particularly valuable in situations in which the patient is required to wake up and move to command intraoperatively, such as trigeminal nerve radiofrequency lesion generation.

Blood pressure management

Maintenance of normal arterial pressure is important in all patients but may be a particular problem in very sick or frail patients. Hypotension, with the consequent reduction in cerebral perfusion, should be treated promptly by judicious use of i.v. fluids and vasopressors such as ephedrine.

Induced hypotension was formerly one of the mainstays of cerebrovascular surgery, but its use for intracranial surgery is now rare because of the appreciation that cerebral perfusion is all-important. Most open aneurysm surgery in now carried out at normotension; indeed, if the patient has an element of cerebral vasospasm, any reflex hypertension should be maintained. Hypotension is now a therapy of last resort if bleeding is torrential and it is otherwise impossible for the surgeon to regain control. The alternatives are a short-acting β-adrenoceptor blocker such as esmolol or increasing the depth of anaesthesia. Direct vasodilators are rarely used because of the risk of 'steal' away from areas of poor perfusion and the possibility of increasing cerebral blood volume and affecting the ICP.

Hypotensive anaesthesia is used more often in spinal surgery, although the risks of inducing ischaemia in the cord substance are the same as in the brain. In this situation, evoked potentials may be used to assess spinal cord function during periods of hypotension.

Fluid replacement therapy

Most patients who present for elective intracranial operations are satisfactorily hydrated preoperatively. Patients with acute conditions such as trauma, those with a high ICP associated with nausea and vomiting and patients with general debility and cachexia may be dehydrated. Cerebral tumours are associated with oedema and raised ICP, and therefore such patients may have been fluid-restricted preoperatively. However, to avoid intraoperative hypotension, careful perioperative fluid administration is necessary.

Cerebrovascular surgery can be associated with vasospasm, and maintaining an adequate CBF is the prime prerequisite. A normal circulating blood volume is essential if the perfu- sion pressure is to be maintained, and although a slight reduction in haematocrit to about 0.30 is optimal for perfu- sion, adequate fluid replacement must be given.

Hypotonic fluids are avoided. Isotonic crystalloids are the standard maintenance fluids. There is no evidence for a specific role for colloid solutions, although blood is used if the haemoglobin falls below 80–90 g L^{-1}. During significant haemorrhage or in patients with multiple injuries, careful attention to haemostasis is essential.

Supplementary drug therapy

Patients with a tumour or some other lesions may already be receiving an oral anticonvulsant, and others may require i.v. anticonvulsant, depending on the site of surgery. Patients receiving high-dose steroids need peri- and postoperative dexamethasone; the normal dose is 4 mg every 6 h with 8–16 mg as an intraoperative bolus. Steroids should not be given to patients undergoing tumour biopsy without discussing it with the surgeon first because of possible effects on the histological diagnosis of cerebral lymphoma.

Antibiotics

For most procedures, antibiotics are given (the exact choice is subject to local guidelines; see Chapter 18). Deep-seated infections are feared after both cranial and spinal surgery, and some operations involve implantation of foreign material (e.g. a shunt).

Heat loss

Temperature should be monitored and normothermia maintained using a forced warm air blanket. It is important to prevent heat loss during prolonged surgery. However, hyperthermia should be avoided.

Venous thromboembolism

Low molecular weight heparin is not used preoperatively but started 1–2 days after surgery when the risk of perioperative haemorrhage has reduced. There is, however, a significant risk of DVT in this group of patients, and thromboembolism (TED) stockings and intermittent pneumatic compression devices should be used perioperatively in accordance with local guidelines.

Techniques for reducing intracranial pressure

The methods used commonly to reduce ICP (or to limit increases) are drugs, ventilation of the patient's lungs, posture and drainage. Adequate cerebral venous drainage must be assured by ensuring the neck veins are not compressed by ties, tapes or excessive neck rotation or flexion. Diuretics such as mannitol 10% or 20% ($0.5–1.0$ g kg^{-1}) or furosemide (20–40 mg) deplete the intravascular fluid volume and subsequently reduce CSF production. A bolus of i.v. anaesthetic agent (e.g. propofol or thiopental) may be used to reduce the cerebral metabolic rate, causing a temporary reduction in CBF and therefore decreases in cerebral blood volume and ICP. Direct drainage of CSF may be accomplished either by lumbar puncture, lumbar drain or by direct puncture of the cisterna magna or lateral ventricles. A move to an increased head-up position reduces venous congestion and ICP, but arterial hypotension must be avoided. Hypercapnia must be prevented by the use of IPPV, whereas short-term use of moderate hyperventilation produces cerebral vasoconstriction and a reduction in cerebral blood volume. If in doubt, an arterial blood gas analysis should be performed to verify adequate lung ventilation.

Recovery from anaesthesia

The majority of patients are allowed to wake up as usual at the end of operation, preferably in a dedicated neurosurgical recovery room. The Glasgow Coma Scale (Table 40.1) or an equivalent for children is recorded. Patients should return rapidly to at least their preoperative level of consciousness. A failure to achieve this, or a deterioration after an initial awakening, should alert clinicians to possible ischaemia or raised ICP. Reimaging or immediate wound exploration is then required. Seizures after elective intracranial neurosurgery are surprisingly rare; if they occur, they should be treated immediately and the cause identified. However, they may be difficult to detect and are a one cause of depressed consciousness after the end of surgery.

Complete reversal of neuromuscular blockade must be achieved; judicious use of intraoperative opioids should remove the need for administration of naloxone. Paracetamol is used, but NSAIDs are avoided because of the risk of inhibiting platelet function and precipitating a postoperative intracranial bleed.

Table 40.1 The Glasgow Coma Scale

Clinical sign	Response	Score
Eyes opening	Spontaneous	4
	To sound	3
	To pressure	2
	None	1
Verbal response*	Orientated	5
	Confused	4
	Words	3
	Sounds	2
	None	1
Motor response	Obeys commands	6
	Localising	5
	Normal flexion	4
	Abnormal flexion	3
	Extension	2
	None	1

Scores range from 15 (normal) to 3 (deeply unconscious with no response).
*Replace the numerical value with 'T' if the patient has a tracheal tube *in situ* or 'A' if aphasic.

Postoperative care

Although many patients who have undergone spinal or intracranial surgery are awake and conscious in the immediate postoperative period, some still require active, intensive treatment. This is important particularly in patients who have raised ICP (or when ICP is liable to rise) and in those who have undergone cerebral aneurysm surgery, when postoperative vasospasm may be a problem. Ideally all patients who have undergone intracranial surgery should be cared for in level 1 or 2 environments (see Chapters 29 and 48). Elective postoperative sedation and lung ventilation with continuous monitoring of both arterial and intracranial pressures is rarely necessary unless severe oedema is likely or when there is damage to critical structures such as the respiratory centre.

Fluid therapy is required to replace ongoing losses and while the patient is not drinking only isotonic fluids should be used. Patients who have undergone craniotomy or major spinal surgery often have a urinary catheter in place.

Historically, long-acting opioids were used very cautiously after craniotomy or upper cervical spine surgery. However, moderate to severe pain is common, and most patients can be given an opioid intravenously or orally in addition to paracetamol. Surgery of the thoracic and lumbar spine is associated with significant postoperative pain, and NSAIDs and PCA are used.

Anaesthesia for intracranial surgery

The preoperative condition of patients who present for craniotomy varies enormously. Elective, planned surgery is common for many conditions. Some patients, such as those with rapidly expanding tumours, are confused, disorientated, euphoric or aggressive, and surgery is not truly elective.

Intracranial tumours

Gliomas usually grow quickly and the history is often short (days or weeks) (Fig. 40.8); meningiomas are slow growing and the history may be slow and insidious. Unlike gliomas, the volume effect of a meningioma is often minimal because a reduction in the volume of the other intracranial contents compensates. However, the volume effects may eventually become apparent, especially if there is bleeding into it.

Patients with an intracranial tumour are usually taking steroids (normally large doses of dexamethasone), which may precipitate a diabetic state requiring insulin during the acute episode. Most patients have some symptoms of raised ICP, such as headache, nausea, vomiting or visual disturbances. Anticonvulsant therapy may have been prescribed to patients who have presented with seizures or who are thought to be at risk. Some patients may be frankly dehydrated, and although it is important to avoid aggressive preoperative

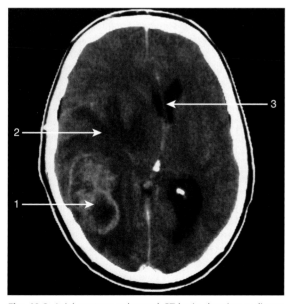

Fig. 40.8 Axial contrast-enhanced CT brain showing a glioma causing mass effect. (From Kelly, B. E., & Bickle, I. (2007) *Crash course: imaging*. St. Louis, Mosby, p. 151.)

fluid therapy, hypovolaemia must be treated before induction of anaesthesia.

For slowly growing tumours such as meningiomas and less aggressive gliomas, as near a total excision as possible is attempted. However, total excision of all the macroscopically identifiable glioma tissue is now considered futile for fast-growing lesions. Large portions of tumours are excised if pressure symptoms are the main presenting feature. For aggressive tumours, the greatest need is for a tissue diagnosis. If lesions are small, deep-seated or near critical areas (such as the motor strip or speech centre) a radiologically guided biopsy or awake surgery is appropriate. Frameless image-guided surgery is now the method of choice for biopsy and tumour excision. A scan of the brain (and skull) is compared with topographical features of the head in theatre to guide a biopsy needle or small craniotomy biopsy and excision. The head is usually kept in a constant position relative to the registration using three-pin fixation. Registration of the image guidance system can take some time, and the anaesthetist should be alert to the problems of the anaesthetised but unstimulated patient.

Stereotactic biopsy involves a CT scan with a rigid metal frame firmly attached to the skull. Trigonometry is then used to find coordinates relative to the frame which describe the exact site of the lesion (to within 1 mm). A biopsy needle is then passed through the brain to sample tissue from this site. The frame is applied after induction of anaesthesia, and because small changes in brain volume cause the lesion to move, the Pa_{CO_2} should be maintained at a constant concentration for both the CT scan and the biopsy.

There is a small ($\sim$1%) risk of haemorrhage after a biopsy. After surgery, patients should be assessed for neurological defects related to the excised tissue. There is a risk of postoperative haemorrhage after any craniotomy, and a deterioration in conscious state should be investigated urgently. After retraction of normal brain tissue to access a tumour (e.g. retraction of the frontal lobes to excise an olfactory groove meningioma), reperfusion injury can lead to swelling and infarction during the first 24 h.

Pituitary surgery (hypophysectomy)

The pituitary fossa is most commonly approached through the nose and sphenoid sinus (trans-sphenoidal). Less commonly it requires a frontotemporal craniotomy for large suprasellar tumours. The majority of pituitary adenomas are non-functioning and cause pressure symptoms, usually on the optic chiasm leading to a bitemporal hemianopia. However, there may be preoperative endocrine abnormalities such as acromegaly or Cushing's disease. Acromegalic patients who present for pituitary surgery may pose difficulties in tracheal intubation and are at risk of obstructive sleep apnoea.

Glucocorticoid replacement is required in the immediate perioperative period; mineralocorticoid requirements increase only slowly over the subsequent days. Diabetes insipidus may present in the immediate postoperative period and requires stabilisation with vasopressin until the degree of the imbalance is known. It usually resolves over the first few days. If the nasal approach is used, a pharyngeal pack should be inserted and the airway protected to prevent aspiration of blood and CSF.

CSF shunt insertion

The majority of patients who present for insertion or revision of a ventriculoperitoneal shunt are children with congenital hydrocephalus, often resulting from spina bifida or from intraventricular haemorrhage after premature birth. Older patients may require a permanent shunt after intracranial haemorrhage or head injury or to treat normal pressure hydrocephalus. These procedures range from elective to emergency (the latter for acute hydrocephalus).

The major anaesthetic considerations lie in the presentation of a patient with severely raised ICP who may be drowsy, nauseated and vomiting, with resultant dehydration. Compensatory systemic hypertension to maintain cerebral perfusion may also be present. Rapid-sequence induction may be indicated to avoid aspiration; the increase in ICP caused by suxamethonium is of secondary importance. Artificial ventilation to control $PaCO_2$ is essential to prevent further increases in ICP, and a volatile anaesthetic agent should be used with care for the same reason. When the ventricle is first drained, a rapid decrease in CSF pressure may result in an equally rapid reduction in systemic arterial pressure which no longer needs to be elevated to maintain cerebral perfusion. Adequate venous access is important to allow rapid resuscitation in response to this severe but temporary hypotension. Shunt surgery may be painful, particularly at the site of insertion into the peritoneum or from the tunnelling of the catheter under the skin. Use of long-acting opioids has to be balanced against the need to have the patient achieve at least the preoperative level of consciousness.

Alternatively, an endoscopic technique may be used to create a new passage for the flow of CSF. The endoscope is passed through a small burr-hole into the lateral and then the third ventricles. The sudden changes in ICP from the use of irrigating fluid and the passage of the neuroendoscope near to vital structures may result in dramatic changes in heart rate and arterial pressure.

Awake craniotomy

Surgery to remove slow-growing or benign tumours from 'eloquent', or critical, areas near the main motor and sensory gyri may be performed in an awake patient to guide the surgeon and avoid damage. The initial exposure is usually performed under general anaesthesia, and then the patient is awoken and repeated tests, for example of motor function

or speech, are performed to assess surgical encroachment on healthy critical areas of cortex. Careful assessment, selection and preparation of patients are essential to ensure that the patient knows what to expect and can cooperate during long periods of awake surgery. Careful positioning (to avoid neck strain), urethral catheterisation and temperature control are required.

Surgery for Parkinson's disease and epilepsy are also performed in an awake patient. After creating the opening in the skull, mapping of the brain and the surgery itself (e.g. inducing a lesion in the basal ganglia) are performed awake.

Treatment of trigeminal neuralgia

Trigeminal neuralgia, an extremely debilitating condition, is usually treated pharmacologically (see Chapter 24). However, surgical lesions of the trigeminal ganglion are performed when the adverse effects of medical treatment become unacceptable. A lesion of the ganglion is induced by radiofrequency ablation or injection of either phenol or alcohol. All these techniques are very painful and require general anaesthesia. The patient is anaesthetised while the ganglion is identified radiologically, awakened to allow identification of correct positioning of the needle, and then reanaesthetised for generation of the lesion or neurolytic injection. If the CSF is encountered during localisation of the ganglion, nausea often occurs and vomiting with the patient in the supine position should be anticipated.

Some cases of trigeminal neuralgia are caused by an abnormal vascular loop compressing the trigeminal nerve in the posterior fossa. A small craniectomy and decompression of the nerve by placing a Teflon pad between the nerve and vessel is often successful in curing the symptoms; the problems of anaesthesia and surgery in this area are highlighted next.

Posterior fossa craniotomy

Surgery in the posterior cranial fossa is undertaken for lesions of the cerebellum and fourth ventricle. The lateral, or 'park bench', position may be used for lateral lesions such as vestibular schwannoma (acoustic neuroma) (Fig. 40.9). The prone position facilitates operations on the cerebellum, foramen magnum and upper cervical spine. Bone is usually removed as a craniectomy (permanent removal) in the posterior fossa rather than by raising a bone flap.

Sitting position

In the past some surgeons favoured the sitting position because this produced good venous drainage, relative hypotension and excellent operating conditions (see Fig. 22.9). The patients were often allowed to breathe a volatile

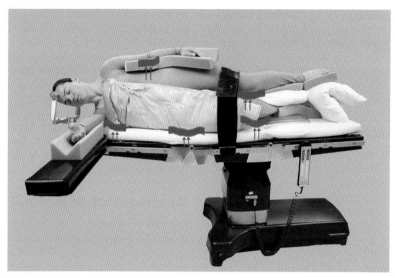

Fig. 40.9 Lateral position with vacuum mattress and head secured in Mayfield pins. Pressure areas are highlighted in red. (From Rothrock, J. C. (2015) *Alexander's care of the patient in surgery,* 15th ed. St. Louis, Elsevier, p. 183.)

anaesthetic agent (usually trichloroethylene) spontaneously so that changes in the respiratory pattern could be used to monitor the progress of fourth ventricular surgery in the region of the respiratory centre. This posed several major anaesthetic problems. Patients in the sitting position are at risk for hypotension, which results inevitably in poor cerebral perfusion. Air embolism is also a potential severe problem because when the skull is opened; many of the veins within the bone are held open, and if the venous pressure at this point is subatmospheric air may enter the veins, leading to systemic air embolism. For these reasons the sitting position is no longer used other than in exceptional circumstances. Although this change has diminished the risks of cerebral hypoperfusion and consequent hypoxia, air embolism is still a potential problem. The operative site, particularly with a moderate head-up tilt, is still above the level of the heart, and the veins are held open by the surrounding structures.

Detection and treatment of air embolism

The mainstay of detection is vigilance and a high index of suspicion. The main period of risk during surgery in the prone position is when the posterior cervical muscles are cut and the craniectomy is being performed. Air embolism may occur in the supine position because the patient is often placed slightly head-up to encourage venous drainage. Surgery near the dural venous sinuses may result in a sinus being opened. This may lead to torrential bleeding, but if the head is raised it may alternatively lead to air

entrainment as the walls of the sinuses, formed by the dura, are held apart.

The severity of the effects of air embolism depends upon the volume of air entrained and the time course of the accumulation of the air in the central circulation.

The main practical method of detection is by end-tidal carbon dioxide monitoring because the airlock produced in the pulmonary circulation results in a rapid reduction in CO_2 excretion (usually together with a reduction in peripheral blood oxygen saturation). Arterial pressure decreases, and cardiac arrhythmias are often seen. The use of an oesophageal stethoscope permits auscultation of the classic mill wheel murmur with large quantities of air but requires continuous listening. Doppler ultrasonography is probably the most sensitive method of early detection before the embolus leaves the heart but often suffers from interference. Unfortunately, there are many false positives with more sensitive techniques such as Doppler ultrasonography. In practice, provided that the sitting position is not used, large air emboli are uncommon. Management of venous air embolism is discussed in Chapter 27.

Anaesthesia for interventional neuroradiology

In addition to coiling of intracranial aneurysms, radiologists treat a variety of other lesions including arteriovenous malformations (AVMs), carotid-cavernous sinus fistulae and dural arteriovenous fistulae in the head or spine. These procedures use several techniques, including detachable coils and glue placed within vessels to interrupt blood supply. The blood vessels supplying some tumours (e.g. meningiomas) may also be occluded before surgical excision. This is discussed further in Chapter 46.

Anaesthesia for surgery of the spine and spinal cord

Many neurosurgical procedures involve surgery around or on the spinal cord, usually either for decompression of nerves or the cord itself as a result of a prolapsed intervertebral disc or degenerative arthritis, or for decompression of the cord when the spinal canal is occupied by tumour or other masses. Compression of the spinal cord, like any other part of the central nervous system, can lead to poor perfusion. Because its blood supply is fragile the cord can become ischaemic from compression, low perfusion pressure or a combination of the two. The thoracic cord is particularly susceptible.

Some cervical spine surgery is performed supine, but most spinal procedures require the patient to be positioned prone. The patient can be supported on a Montreal mattress, on bolsters or blocks placed under the upper chest and iliac crests or on a purpose-built frame, all of which allow unimpeded respiratory movements and avoid abdominal compression (see Fig. 22.6). In the prone position, pressure areas may develop over the facial bones, particularly around the eyes; careful padding is vital. There is a risk of postoperative visual loss in patients undergoing prolonged prone surgery, usually in those with significant blood loss. Protection of the eyes is of paramount importance. The neck should be kept in a neutral position to avoid stretching the brachial plexus, and if it is necessary to have the arms up above the head, they should not be abducted excessively nor should there be anything pressing into the axillae.

Anaesthesia for cervical spine surgery

The cervical spine may be approached from either the anterior or the posterior route, depending largely upon the site of cord or root compression. Although the posterior approach is less likely to damage vital structures, the patient must lie prone, and hypotension, blood loss and patient access, particularly in a large individual, may cause problems.

In most patients the neck is relatively stable, even if bony degeneration from osteoarthritis has resulted in cord compression. However, rheumatoid arthritis can produce neck instability, particularly in flexion. It is essential to assess the range of neck movement in addition to the assessment of the ease of tracheal intubation. It is doubly unlucky to have a difficult intubation in a patient with an unstable neck! If problems are anticipated the standard difficult tracheal intubation plan should be followed, using the methods with which the anaesthetist is most familiar (see Chapter 23). Severe ankylosing spondylitis involving the neck probably presents the most awkward problem, caused by the rigid immobility of the cervical spine. Additional factors which apply particularly in patients with rheumatoid disease include anaemia, steroid therapy, fragile skin and renal and pulmonary problems (see Chapter 20).

Anterior cervical decompression

Anterior cervical decompression involves exposing the anterior aspect of the cervical vertebral bodies and their interposing discs through a collar incision, removing the intervertebral disc and decompressing the cord while distracting the disc space mechanically. The vertebral bodies are then kept separated with a prosthetic spacer or artificial disc, or sometimes a bone graft taken from the iliac crest. Single or multiple levels may be involved, and the neck may be quite rigid for future tracheal intubation if several adjacent levels are decompressed.

Apart from the potential problems of tracheal intubation, anaesthesia is often relatively straightforward. Pneumothorax is a potential problem with operations at the C7–T1 level. Retraction of the oesophagus and more particularly the carotid sheath and sinus may produce severe temporary cardiovascular disturbance (usually sinus bradycardia). Postoperative haemorrhage may lead to acute airway obstruction.

Posterior cervical laminectomy

Patients are usually placed prone, with the neck flexed and in a slightly head-up posture to reduce haemorrhage. Bleeding from the nuchal muscles is often a problem, and air embolism is a risk. The main difficulties, as in all spinal surgery in the prone position, arise from epidural venous bleeding, and the changes in intrathoracic pressure from IPPV can have a significant effect. In addition, prolonged cord compression can result in an autonomic neuropathy, which may produce significant hypotension both at induction and when the patient is turned into the prone position. Cervical laminectomy may be accompanied by posterior fusion with either bone or metal.

Anaesthesia for thoracic and lumbar spine surgery

Lumbar microdiscectomy for sciatica and one-level laminectomy are usually relatively minor procedures.

767

Patients with severe sciatica may gain immediate pain relief postoperatively. However, multiple-level laminectomies are more major operations, and direct arterial blood pressure measurement may be required in elderly or debilitated patients. Thoracic discs and tumours such as neurofibromata may be approached by an anterior transthoracic route involving thoracotomy and a combined approach with the patient in the lateral position. Bronchial intubation and one-lung anaesthesia (see Chapter 41) may be needed to facilitate access in this situation.

Correction of spinal deformities such as scoliosis and surgery to stabilise vertebrae damaged by trauma or destroyed by metastatic tumour are often associated with significant bleeding and the need for massive blood transfusion. Hypotensive anaesthesia is used occasionally to decrease bleeding, particularly the venous ooze in the operative field. Cell salvage reduces the need for blood transfusion, although its role in tumour surgery is unclear.

Spinal cord monitoring using somatosensory- or motor-evoked potentials allows identification of spinal cord ischaemia during surgery. These potentials are affected by many anaesthetic agents, particularly the volatile anaesthetic agents, and a TIVA-based technique is preferred. Children with congenital scoliosis associated with other conditions (such as Duchenne muscular dystrophy) represent a significant anaesthetic challenge because of their comorbidities, in particular lung function, and the volume of blood loss.

Chronic pain procedures

Some patients with chronic pain benefit from spinal cord stimulation. Apart from therapeutic tests, most of the procedures (e.g. electrode implantation through a laminectomy, generator implantation and lead tunnelling) require general anaesthesia.

Anaesthesia for emergency intracranial surgery

Most emergency surgery is performed for a rapidly expanding haematoma resulting from either trauma or spontaneous haemorrhage. Other indications are infection (e.g. an abscess), bony injuries from trauma, and acute hydrocephalus. The conscious state in patients with intracerebral haemorrhage ranges from lucid to unconscious. Those in the older age group may be receiving drugs with cardiovascular effects and are also often receiving aspirin or oral anticoagulants, which may be a contributory factor. Some patients with an intracerebral haemorrhage have an identifiable underlying aneurysm or AVM, but many do not.

Cerebrovascular lesions

Patients with a vascular lesion such as an intracranial aneurysm or AVM may present acutely with a subarachnoid or intracerebral haemorrhage. Subarachnoid haemorrhage is graded using the World Federation of Neurosurgeons' (WFNS) scale (Table 40.2). Most intracranial aneurysms are treated by interventional neuroradiological coiling (see Chapter 46). Some aneurysms are found coincidentally, or multiple aneurysms are found, some of which are treated electively after the initial injury and bleed has been dealt with.

Open aneurysm surgery

Radiologically inaccessible aneurysms and those associated with an intracerebral clot and pressure symptoms are dealt with by craniotomy, clot evacuation (if present) and clipping of the neck of the aneurysm. Although application of clips (clipping) should prevent the risk of further bleeding, significant perioperative morbidity and mortality can result from vasospasm, which may occur pre- or postoperatively. The calcium channel blocker nimodipine is used to reduce or prevent vasospasm. By preference, it is given orally although i.v. preparations are available.

As flow is more pressure dependent in areas with vasospasm, it is necessary to avoid both hypotension and hypertension. A normal CPP should be maintained, and hypocapnia should be avoided. Although fluid replacement therapy may be all that is required, the careful use of a vasopressor may be necessary in the interval between induction and incision. Nimodipine therapy interacts with inhalational anaesthetic agents to enhance their hypotensive effects. Postoperatively, nimodipine therapy is continued for 21 days until the risk of vasospasm has passed. Blood entering the CSF either as a result of the initial haemorrhage

Table 40.2 World Federations of Neurosurgeons (WFNS) grading of subarachnoid haemorrhage

WFNS grade	GCS	Motor deficit
1	15	Absent
2	13–14	Absent
3	13–14	Present
4	7–12	Present or absent
5	3–6	Present or absent

GCS, Glasgow Coma Scale.

or during operation is an extreme irritant. Its presence may cause large increases in plasma catecholamine concentrations, with consequent hypertension and vasospasm. Blood which clots in the aqueduct of Sylvius causes obstruction to CSF flow and non-communicating hydrocephalus, necessitating temporary external ventricular drainage.

Intraoperative temporary clipping of feeding vessels (or to prevent anastomotic backflow from tributaries) may be required to allow safe application of the permanent clip to the neck of the aneurysm. Temporary clips may also be required if the aneurysm bursts to allow the surgeon to stop the haemorrhage. These clips cause temporary ischaemia in the territory supplied by that vessel. Attempts may be made to reduce the risk of permanent ischaemic damage via metabolic suppression with i.v. anaesthetic agents or mild hypothermia. There is, however, no evidence that these techniques have any beneficial effect on outcome.

Traumatic lesions

Acute intracranial haematoma may be extradural (epidural) (see Fig. 40.2), subdural (see Fig. 40.3) or intracerebral. Patients receiving oral anticoagulants may develop a subdural haematoma after a very minor head injury.

Many patients who present for anaesthesia and surgery are unconscious or semiconscious and irritable as a result of raised ICP and cerebral compression. Many will have undergone tracheal intubation and ventilation of the lungs after their initial assessment or after a CT scan and are kept anaesthetised and transferred to a neurosurgical unit and taken straight to the operating theatre for surgery to decompress the brain. It is important to remember that with an expanding intracranial haematoma speed is of the essence if cerebral damage is to be minimised or avoided. Although adequate anaesthetic time must be taken to ensure safety, excessive delays may seriously affect the overall result of decompression and make the difference between a good and a merely a moderate recovery.

The anaesthetic maintenance technique is similar to that used for elective intracranial surgery, consisting of careful use of a hypnotic, a short-acting i.v. opioid, neuromuscular blockade and IPPV to a $PaCO_2$ of 4.5 kPa. Tracheal intubation in patients at risk of regurgitation and aspiration of stomach contents should be facilitated with suxamethonium or a rapid-onset non-depolarising agent. If the patient is unconscious, the initial anaesthetic requirements may be small. Most acute haematomata are evacuated through a full craniotomy because, if necessary, the bone flap may be left out or allowed to float free, providing a method of decompression in the case of severe oedema. It is important to avoid long-acting opioid analgesics because these may mask the level of consciousness, which is used to follow the progress of cerebral trauma postoperatively.

Chronic subdural haematoma

Chronic subdural collections often have an insidious onset. They are usually evacuated via burr-holes. Many patients with a chronic subdural haematoma have significant chronic comorbidities, and it is unlikely that delaying surgery for investigation or treatment of these will improve outcome. Preadmission oral anticoagulation is common and should be reversed (see Chapter 14) regardless of the indication for anticoagulation. The risks of haematoma expansion outweigh the risks of thrombosis.

Evacuation of subdural haematoma is usually performed under general anaesthesia but may be undertaken with local anaesthesia alone in frail, older patients. Many chronic subdural haematomas recur. As the patient's brain is decompressed the level of consciousness may lighten considerably, and it may be necessary to deepen anaesthesia to prevent the patient becoming aware.

Management of the brain-injured patient

Brain-injured patients' treatment and subsequent rehabilitation represent a considerable proportion of neurosurgical practice. The immediate management requires meticulous attention to the prevention of secondary brain injury from ischaemia; little can be done about the primary insult to the brain or spinal cord. The resuscitation and immediate care of all brain-injured patients uses the same ABC principles taught on courses for care of all trauma victims and other seriously ill patients (see Chapter 44). Although isolated traumatic brain injury is common, many patients will present with other significant trauma.

Key management points

1. *Initial airway maintenance* is crucial, remembering that patients with craniofacial injuries often have associated damage to the cervical spine. Tracheal intubation is usually necessary, should be accomplished without excessive neck manipulation and should be performed by an experienced person. It is important to make tracheal intubation as atraumatic as possible; consequently sedation and neuromuscular blockade should be used irrespective of the level of consciousness except in the most severe situation. Nasotracheal intubation is contraindicated because of the possibility of a basal skull fracture.
2. *Maintain adequate ventilation* with oxygen-enriched air. Avoidance of hypoxaemia and hypercapnia is essential.
3. *Maintain adequate circulating volume and arterial pressure.* Hypotension after head injury greatly worsens outcome.

Other injuries which may affect the circulatory state must be identified while resuscitation is being performed.

4. *Sedation, analgesia and neuromuscular blockade* are usually continued to allow management of other injuries, CT scanning and possible interhospital transfer (see Chapter 48).

5. *Detailed assessment of thoracic, abdominal and limb injuries* and appropriate therapy to stabilise the patient's cardiovascular and respiratory systems are required before, during and after transfer to the CT scanner. Other life-threatening injuries must be dealt with to prevent secondary brain injury caused by hypoxaemia or hypotension.

6. *Invasive arterial pressure monitoring* together with ECG, capnography and pulse oximetry are all important in the early detection of a fall in CPP, cardiovascular instability or failing respiratory function. A contused, oedematous and non-compliant brain tolerates only minimal changes in oxygen supply or carbon dioxide tension before ICP increases still further. However, definitive treatment (i.e. removal of the clot) should not be delayed just to facilitate placement of arterial or CVCs. The priority is to remove the cause of the raised intracranial pressure and improve perfusion of the brain tissue.

7. *After a CT scan,* many patients are transferred directly to the neurosurgical operating theatre for evacuation of haematoma or insertion of an intraventricular catheter or pressure transducer. Patients who are scanned in peripheral hospitals have their scans relayed to the main neurosurgical centre. The patient is then transferred directly by ambulance to the neurosurgical operating theatre, but both cardiovascular and neurological stability must be achieved before the journey. Realistically, this involves the transfer of an anaesthetised patient, often pretreated with mannitol to minimise acute increases in ICP.

Intensive care management of head-injured patients

The main benefits of intensive care are in the provision of optimal conditions to allow recovery from the primary cerebral injury while minimising secondary damage.

General care
Sedation

Sedation is usually achieved with an infusion of either propofol or midazolam together with an opioid (usually morphine or alfentanil). Thiopental may be beneficial in the presence of severely compromised CBF and metabolism

or status epilepticus. Neuromuscular blockade is often used in addition to sedative drugs.

Lung ventilation

Mechanical lung ventilation is particularly important in patients suffering from multiple trauma, especially with the combination of head and chest injuries, to ensure optimal oxygenation in the face of pulmonary contusion. This is normally achieved by the use of IPPV and PEEP. There is evidence to suggest that hyperventilation worsens outcome, and the main benefits of mechanical ventilation are the prevention of hypercapnia and the provision of adequate cerebral oxygenation.

Fluid therapy and nutrition

Although otherwise healthy patients with an isolated brain injury have very low metabolic requirements, many fail to absorb from the GI tract because of the effects of sedative and opioid drugs or simply secondary to trauma; associated hypoxaemia exacerbates the problem. As with elective patients at risk from elevated ICP caused by cerebral oedema, brain-injured patients are also at risk from excessive i.v. fluid therapy, particularly if hypotonic solutions are used. Mild fluid restriction may be appropriate, and if large amounts of fluid have been given during initial resuscitation, gradual drug-induced diuresis with furosemide to create an overall negative fluid balance (or at least to prevent a positive balance) may be appropriate. Fluid overload also impairs oxygenation further in potentially hypoxaemic patients with combined head and chest injuries or after aspiration at the time of brain injury. The use of mannitol tends to be reserved for the emergency treatment of raised ICP rather than the treatment of simple fluid overload.

Neurological care
Assessment

The Glasgow Coma Scale (see Table 40.1), which is based upon eye opening and verbal and motor responses, is used in non-sedated patients. Brain function may also be assessed by use of the EEG (or a processed EEG monitor such as the cerebral function analysing monitor [CFAM]), transcranial Doppler and near-infrared spectroscopy.

ICP monitoring

It is very helpful to be able to monitor the effectiveness of therapy used to manage intracranial hypertension, and in particular to achieve an effective cerebral perfusion pressure. The ICP is monitored using a transducer inserted either extradurally, subdurally or into the brain parenchyma itself. This may be undertaken in the ICU or in the operating theatre. Intracranial pressure often increases in response to stimulation, physiotherapy, tracheal suction and so on but should return to the prestimulation value within 5–10 min. Frequent and prolonged increases in ICP demonstrate a low cerebral compliance and the need for further sedation and ventilation. If weaning from mechanical ventilation is started and the ICP increases and remains elevated, the patient should be resedated and the lungs ventilated for a further 24-h period. It is beneficial to nurse head-injured patients in a 15-degree head-up tilt to assist in control of ICP, provided that coexisting conditions permit.

Anaesthesia for CT and MRI scanning

Anaesthesia for CT and MRI is discussed in Chapter 46.

Chapter | 41 |

Anaesthesia for thoracic surgery

Alexander Ng, Nguk Hoon Tan

In thoracic anaesthesia there are a number of key areas that require specific consideration in the preoperative, intraoperative and postoperative phases of care. They include understanding of pulmonary anatomy, assessment of fitness for lung surgery, understanding the indications and methods of lung isolation, management of hypoxaemia during one-lung ventilation, and provision of pain relief after thoracotomy. Oesophagectomy is also performed as a thoracic procedure.

Anatomy

The trachea leads from the cricoid cartilage below the larynx at the level of the sixth cervical vertebra (C6) and passes 10–12 cm in the superior mediastinum to its bifurcation at the carina into the left and right main bronchi at the sternal angle (T4–5). During inspiration, the lower border of the trachea moves inferiorly and anteriorly. The trachea lies principally in the midline but is deviated to the right inferiorly by the arch of the aorta. The oesophagus is immediately posterior to the trachea, and behind it is the vertebral column. The wall of the trachea is held patent by 15–20 cartilaginous rings deficient posteriorly where the trachealis membrane, a collection of fibroelastic fibres and smooth muscle, lies. It is wider in transverse (20 mm) than anteroposterior diameter (15 mm). The trachea passes from neck to thorax via the thoracic inlet at T2.

The right main bronchus is larger and less deviated from the midline than the left. The origin of the right upper lobe bronchus arises laterally 2.5 cm from the carina, whereas the origin of the left upper lobe arises laterally after 5 cm. These dimensions determine the relative ease of isolating and ventilating each lung independently using double-lumen endobronchial tubes (DLTs).

The right lung comprises three lobes, each with the following segments (Fig. 41.1):
- Right upper lobe – apical, anterior, posterior
- Right middle lobe – medial, lateral
- Right lower lobe – superior, anterior basal, posterior basal, medial basal, lateral basal

In the left lung there are two lobes with the following segments:
- Left upper lobe – apical, anterior, posterior, superior lingual, inferior lingual
- Left lower lobe – superior, anterior basal, posterior basal, lateral basal

The lingual lobe, which looks like a tongue, is part of the left upper lobe and is not a lobe in its own right, compared with the right lung, which has a distinct middle lobe. The right middle lobe has lateral and medial segments, in contrast with the left lingual lobe, which has superior and inferior segments. This difference may be explained by the position of the heart, which can be considered to elevate the vertical separation between two segments to make it horizontal on the left. On the right there is absence of the heart, and so the vertical separation remains, resulting in the presence of lateral and medial segments.

The asymmetrical structure of the bronchial tree gives rise to characteristic bronchoscopic views at the various branches (Fig. 41.2). There is significant interindividual variation. Of particular anaesthetic relevance is where the right upper lobe bronchus arises.

The oesophagus is a continuation of the pharynx at the level of the lower border of the cricoid cartilage (C6) 15 cm from the incisor teeth. It passes immediately anterior to the thoracic spine and aorta and descends through the oesophageal hiatus of the diaphragm at T10, to the left of the midline at the level of the seventh rib. There are four slight constrictions: at its origin, as it is crossed by the aorta and left main bronchus, and at the diaphragm, at 15 cm, 25 cm, 27 cm and 38 cm from the incisors.

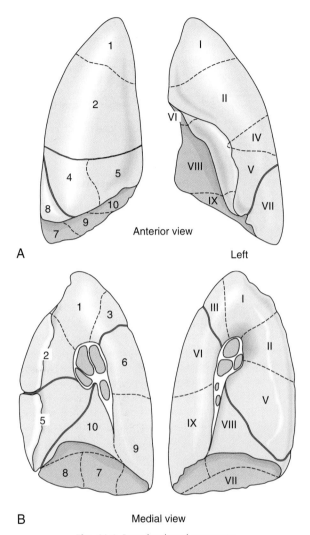

B

Anterior view

A   Left

Medial view

B

Fig. 41.1 Bronchopleural segments.

Radiographic surface markings

The apices of the lungs extend 2.5 cm above the point at which the middle and inner third of the clavicle meet. Lung borders descend behind the medial end of the clavicle to the middle of the manubrium. The lung border is behind the body of the sternum and xiphisternum before sweeping inferiorly and laterally down to the level of the eleventh thoracic vertebra. On the left, at the level of the horizontal fissure at the fourth costal cartilage (T7), the medial border of the lung is displaced to the left of the sternal edge in the cardiac notch. The oblique fissure descends from 3 cm lateral to the midline at T4, inferiorly and anteriorly to the sixth costal cartilage 7 cm from the midline. The diaphragmatic

reflection of the pleura extrudes below the lung to the lower border of T12.

Preoperative assessment

There are several considerations to acknowledge when providing an anaesthetic for patients who require thoracic procedures. They include the procedure and its indication, the underlying diagnostic process, and the fitness for surgical intervention as well as one-lung ventilation for many procedures. In combination with rigid bronchoscopy after induction of general anaesthesia, typical procedures are:

- lobectomy or pneumonectomy for treatment of non–small cell lung cancer;
- reduction of lung volume in patients with emphysema;
- lung biopsy for diagnosis of lung cancer and other diseases such as sarcoidosis;
- cervical mediastinoscopy for staging of lung cancer;
- pleurectomy with bullectomy for recurrent spontaneous pneumothorax;
- decortication for empyema; and
- closure of bronchopleural fistula.

Of these procedures, there is loss of lung tissue during lobectomy, pneumectomy and lung-volume reduction. Compared with general anaesthesia with two lungs, these three procedures require specific preoperative anaesthetic assessment.

Lobectomy or pneumonectomy
Staging of lung cancer

Other than a chest radiograph, patients will have had a CT scan of their thorax to demonstrate radiological evidence of size, number and location of a tumour either in the right lung or the left lung. In addition, there may be mediastinal lymphadenopathy (Fig. 41.3). Before lung resection, a separate general anaesthetic for lung biopsy and cervical mediastinoscopy is often required for diagnosis and staging of suspected lung cancer.

There are four stages of lung cancer, dependent on the size, location and number of tumour, nodes and metastases. In addition to a CT scan, metabolic activity and hence location and spread of the tumour may have been assessed by positron emission tomographic (PET) scanning. This test is based on accumulation of phosphorylated ^{18}F-fluoro-2-deoxy-D-glucose (FDG). There is increased uptake of FDG and phosphorylation by hexokinase and decreased dephosphorylation by glucose-6-phosphatase in malignant cells compared with normal cells. Standard uptake values greater than 2.5 are suggestive of the presence of tumour cells. In general, surgical treatment and hence anaesthesia for lung

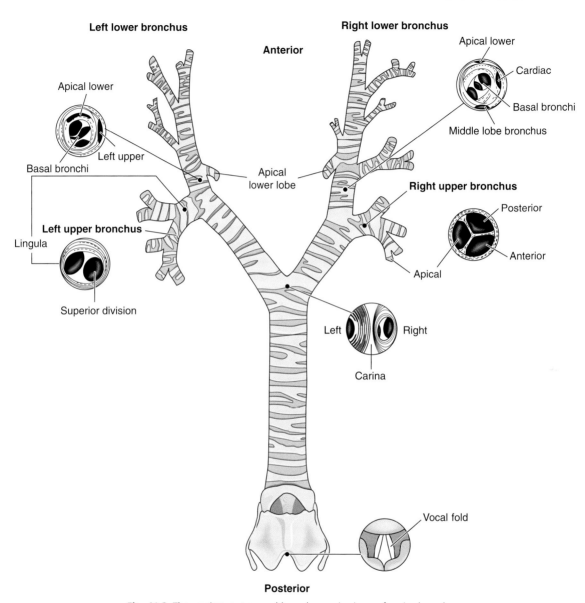

Fig. 41.2 The respiratory tree and bronchoscopic views of major branches.

resection are indicated in patients with stage 1 or 2 non–small cell lung cancer.

General anaesthetic considerations

Patients who present for lung surgery may not only have lung cancer but may have other medical conditions which should be assessed for both severity and for possible preoperative optimisation (see Chapters 19 and 20). There may

be respiratory disease such as chronic obstructive pulmonary disease (COPD) with infection and a history of smoking. From the cardiac perspective, there may be a history of ischaemic heart disease, atrial fibrillation, anticoagulation with warfarin, heart failure, valvular heart disease, hypertension, diabetes mellitus and obesity.

The Eastern Cooperative Oncology Group (ECOG) performance status score (used by the WHO and also called the Zubrod score) provides a general assessment of functional

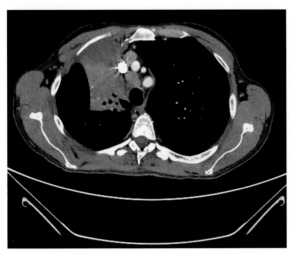

Fig. 41.3 Computed tomographic scan showing mediastinal lymphadenopathy in the pretracheal area and obstruction of the right upper lobe bronchus.

Table 41.1 Eastern Cooperative Oncology Group (ECOG) performance status	
0	Fully active, able to carry on all predisease performance without restriction
1	Restricted in physically strenuous activity but ambulatory and able to carry out work of a light or sedentary nature (e.g., light housework, office work)
2	Ambulatory and capable of all self-care but unable to carry out any work activities; up and about more than 50% of waking hours
3	Capable of only limited self-care; confined to bed or chair more than 50% of waking hours
4	Completely disabled; cannot carry on any self-care; totally confined to bed or chair
5	Dead

capacity before thoracic surgery (Table 41.1). The majority of operable patients are grade 2 or less.

Predicted postoperative lung function

Other than general anaesthetic considerations, many surgical procedures require one-lung ventilation and lung resection. The issue is whether the patient will tolerate one-lung ventilation and possible postoperative complications. Of the measurements of lung function, forced expiratory volume in 1 second (FEV_1) and transfer factor (diffusing capacity for carbon monoxide (DL_{CO}) and carbon monoxide transfer coefficient (K_{CO})) are recommended and cited at multidisciplinary meetings for lung cancer; FEV_1 assesses lung mechanics, whereas transfer factor measurements estimate the effect of cardiopulmonary disease on reduction in gas transfer. These measurements are generally quoted as a percentage of the predicted value for each patient. Ventilation or perfusion scintigraphy may be used to predict postoperative lung function if a ventilation-perfusion mismatch is suspected.

To calculate predicted postoperative lung function, it is necessary to know the number of bronchopulmonary segments in each lobe of lung before and after lung resection (see Fig. 41.1). Overall, the right lung has 10 segments, whereas the left lung has 9 segments, giving a total of 19 segments. After a simple right lower lobectomy, there will be 5 segments removed (19 − 5 = 14 segments), and so the predicted postoperative FEV_1 or transfer factor will be the preoperative value multiplied by 14 divided by 19. However, if 2 segments in the right lower lobe are obstructed by tumour and so do not contribute to the lung function measurements, then they would have to be deducted from the denominator (i.e. 19 − 2 = 17 segments). So, after right lower lobectomy, the predicted postoperative FEV_1 or transfer factor would be multiplied by 14 divided by 17. The predicted postoperative FEV_1 and transfer factor proportions are used to define severity of lung disease. There are differing definitions:

The British Thoracic Society has two levels of risk:
- Low risk (≥40% predicted)
- High risk (<40% predicted)

The American College of Chest Physicians has three levels of risk:
- Low risk (>60% predicted)
- Medium risk (30%–60% predicted)
- High risk (<30% predicted)

Exercise testing

According to UK and American guidance, the shuttle-walk test is recommended for patients at moderate risk, as suggested by the lung function results (see Chapter 19). The perioperative risk is considered to be high if the test of 25 sets of 10 m is not completed. Patients seem to be at a low risk if they can walk 400 m. The stair-climbing test has also been recommended; patients are at high risk if they cannot climb 22 m. Both the stair-climbing and the shuttle-walk tests are low-technology assessments of exercise tolerance.

In contrast, cardiopulmonary exercise testing (CPET; see Chapter 19) involves the use of special equipment and is recommended in both the UK and American guidelines, with peak oxygen consumption ($\dot{V}O_2$) used to estimate fitness. In the UK, a peak $\dot{V}O_2$ >15 ml kg^{-1} min^{-1} indicates good function. However, the American guidance defines three thresholds for peak $\dot{V}O_2$:

- Low risk: >20 ml kg^{-1} min^{-1} or 75% predicted
- Medium risk: 10–20 ml kg^{-1} min^{-1} or 35%–75% predicted
- High-risk: <10 ml kg^{-1} min^{-1} or <35% predicted

Prediction of mortality

In addition to an assessment of fitness for lung cancer surgery, it is possible to use a scoring system (Thoracoscore, Table 41.2) to estimate the global risk of death. In this way the operative risk can be stratified. Many of the Thoracoscore factors apply to other types of patients who present for a general anaesthetic. They provide the basis for:

- providing patient information and obtaining consent (see Chapter 21);

Table 41.2 Thoracic Surgery Scoring System (Thoracoscore)

Variable	Value	Score
Age (years)	55–65	0.7679
	≥65	1.0073
Sex	Male	0.4505
ASA	≥3	0.6057
Performance status classification	≥3	0.689
Dyspnoea score	≥3	0.9075
Priority of surgery	Urgent or emergency	0.8443
Procedure class	Pneumonectomy	1.2176
Diagnosis group	Malignant	1.2423
Comorbidity score	1–2	0.7447
	≥3	0.9065

Dyspnoea score is graded using the Medical Research Council score:
0: None
1: Slight (troubled by shortness of breath when hurrying on the level or walking up a slight hill)
2: Moderate (walks slower than people of the same age on the level because of breathlessness)
3: Moderately severe (has to stop because of breathlessness when walking at own pace on the level)
4: Severe (stops for breath after walking about 100 yards or after a few minutes on the level)
5: Very severe (too breathless to leave the house or breathless when dressing or undressing)
Performance status is the Eastern Cooperative Oncology Group performance status scale used by the WHO (see Table 41.1). The probability of in-hospital mortality is estimated as: $P_{\text{in-hospital mortality}}$ (%) = 100 / (1 + e$^{(7.3737 + \text{Total Score})}$).

- determining anaesthetic technique and level of intraoperative monitoring; and
- planning postoperative management (ICU vs. high-dependency unit vs. ward).

Lung volume reduction

Some patients with severe emphysema may present for reduction of lung volume. There are two types: traditional surgery and bronchoscopic surgery, which involves the placement of endobronchial valves at the entrance of appropriate bronchopulmonary segments. Currently, bronchoscopic lung-volume reduction surgery is in vogue as it reduces perioperative complications and hence mortality. Appropriate anatomical targets for lung-volume reduction include the following:

- High residual volume (150%–180% predicted)
- High total lung capacity (>100% predicted)
- Reduced predicted FEV$_1$ (but still >20% predicted)
- Presence of target lobe (heterogeneous, upper-lobe disease rather than homogeneous disease is preferred)
- Presence of a fissure between lobes of the lung (a complete fissure between lobes of a lung provides anatomical evidence to predict absence of collateral air flow)
- Evidence of the location of ventilation-perfusion mismatch

Intraoperative considerations

In this section there are general and specific issues that need to be discussed. As with any anaesthetic, the following general considerations should be reviewed:

- *Preoperative preparation.* This includes factors such as smoking cessation, physiotherapy, and optimisation of any active cardiac conditions.
- *Marking of side of procedure.* Many thoracic procedures are unilateral, with no external distinguishing features, and so the side of the operation must be marked and checked to prevent wrong-side surgery.
- *Patient information, options and agreement for specific procedures.* Many thoracic procedures are associated with moderate to severe pain, and so information regarding epidural, spinal and paravertebral block should be provided.
- *Individualised requirements for monitoring.* Major procedures generally require invasive arterial blood pressure monitoring and central venous access.
- *Temperature.* Patients should be normothermic before arrival in the anaesthetic room.
- *Cross-matching.* Blood should be cross-matched for major procedures.

Specific issues regarding thoracic procedures relate to positioning, rigid bronchoscopy, cervical mediastinoscopy, unilateral procedures involving lung isolation, hypoxaemia during one-lung ventilation and postoperative analgesia.

Positioning

In thoracic anaesthesia, patients are usually positioned supine or in the lateral decubitus position. The supine position is required for rigid bronchoscopy, cervical mediastinoscopy and other midline procedures such as thymectomy. For cervical mediastinoscopy, there is neck extension similar to a tracheostomy. This position opens a space for placement of a video mediastinoscope beneath the suprasternal notch. The standard position for unilateral operations such as lobectomy, pneumonectomy, surgical lung-volume reduction, pleurectomy and decortication is the lateral decubitus position. The non-dependent side of the chest is elevated so that the rib spaces are maximised for surgical access and the non-dependent lung allowed to collapse for surgery, while the dependent lung is ventilated.

Rigid bronchoscopy

Almost all thoracic patients undergo rigid bronchoscopy, which can occur on its own or followed by another thoracic procedure. Rigid bronchoscopy is an example of a shared airway between surgeon and anaesthetist. With advances in digital technology bronchoscopy is now video-assisted and allows the surgeon to:

- assess the trachea and bronchial tree before transection during lung resection;
- provide tracheobronchial toilet, particularly when there are retained secretions (this intervention benefits the anaesthetist as it clears the airway for subsequent endobronchial tube placement and ventilation);
- biopsy an airway tumour in a palliative procedure;
- debulk a proximal tumour and place a stent for airway obstruction; and
- assess and place an airway stent for closure of a bronchopleural fistula.

After induction of general anaesthesia and neuromuscular blockade, anaesthesia is maintained intravenously with propofol and a short-acting opioid (e.g. remifentanil). It is important to ensure adequate depth of anaesthesia during placement of the rigid bronchoscope in the trachea. Given the brevity of rigid bronchoscopy, ventilation may be provided by a jet ventilator (see Fig. 16.37) attached to the proximal side port of the bronchoscopy. The anaesthetist insufflates the lungs in a fashion similar to high-frequency jet ventilation (small volumes at a high rate). During retrieval of tumour tissue or lung biopsy, insufflation should stop transiently. This manually controlled technique of jet ventilation has the following features:

- *Driving pressure 100–200 kPa.* The inspiratory phase is active, in contrast to the expiratory phase, which is passive

by elastic recoil of the chest. Observation of chest movement during the respiratory cycle is needed as airway pressure is not measured.
- *Rate 100–200 breaths min^{-1},* as determined by the operator's hand.
- *Tidal volume 2–5 ml kg^{-1}.* It is not possible to measure the tidal volume, as a variable flow of room air is entrained by the jet of oxygen through the rigid bronchoscope. However, tidal volumes are small compared with those obtained by conventional mechanical ventilation.
- *No humidification.* Humidification to some extent is possible only with a high-frequency jet ventilator rather than a manual jet ventilator. However, as the procedure is brief, humidification is not usually required.

The mechanism of gas exchange contrasts with that of conventional mechanical ventilation, which is related to bulk flow of gas. Additional mechanisms of gas exchange during jet ventilation include the following:

- Augmented longitudinal dispersion of gas which, moving by convection, mixes with gas in the alveoli
- Streaming of gas in the smaller airways: Inspiratory flow occurs in the centre of the airway, whilst expiratory flow happens in the periphery
- Pendelluft effect: Gases mix when they flow from alveoli of short time constant to those of long time constant
- Cardiogenic mixing of gas in the distal airway as a result of movement of the heart

Cervical mediastinoscopy

Cervical mediastinoscopy necessitates a single-lumen tracheal tube and ventilation of both lungs. Complications are related to damage by the surgeon to any of the mediastinal structures, such as the trachea, oesophagus, aorta, pulmonary artery and pleura.

Unilateral lung procedures and lung isolation

Midline procedures such as rigid bronchoscopy and cervical mediastinoscopy do not require lung isolation, which is usually reserved for unilateral procedures. The indications for lung isolation are:

- to facilitate surgical access during lobectomy, pneumonectomy, surgical lung-volume reduction, pleurectomy and decortication;
- to minimise contamination of the contralateral lung (e.g. from haemorrhage, abscess, bronchiectasis and lavage); and
- to control distribution of ventilation (e.g. in patients with bronchopleural fistula).

Lung isolation is usually provided by DLTs or endobronchial blockers.

Double-lumen endobronchial tubes

Double-lumen endobronchial tubes have the following features:

- Laterality – left- (Fig. 41.4) and right-sided (Fig. 41.5) DLTs are not mirror images.
- Two narrow lumens – one is long for placement in the bronchus, and the other is short for placement in the trachea. The two lumens allow separate lung ventilation and toileting.
- Two cuffs, one endobronchial Fig. 41.6 and the other tracheal.

The choice of DLT depends on the following:

- *Patient size.* Sizes 35, 37, 39 and 41 French (F; 1F is equivalent to an external diameter of 0.33 mm) are available for adult patients. In general, 37F is suitable for female patients, and 39F is suitable for male patients.
- *Side of surgery.* Generally it is most appropriate to select a left-sided DLT for right-sided lung resection and a right-sided DLT tube for a left-sided lung resection. If the operation extends from a lobectomy to a pneumonectomy, then the endobronchial side of the tube will not obstruct the surgical field. However, right-sided DLTs have to be placed accurately because of the proximal location of the right upper lobe bronchus compared with the distal left upper lobe bronchus. Therefore some anaesthetists prefer to place left-sided DLTs, particularly during peripheral procedures such as lung biopsy, pleurectomy or decortication, only using right-sided DLTs when absolutely necessary (e.g. during left pneumonectomy).

Correct placement of a DLT is of paramount importance. The clinical method involves three main steps.

Step 1

The anaesthetist verifies placement of the DLT in the trachea and ventilates the lungs via both lumens. During two-lung ventilation, the anaesthetist then:

- checks for excretion of carbon dioxide, which should be present provided the DLT is in the trachea;
- observes for bilateral chest movement and checks the airway pressure; and

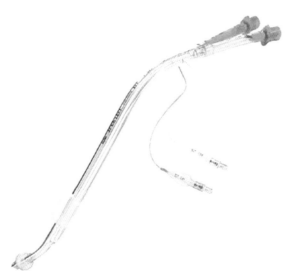

Fig. 41.4 Left-sided double lumen endobronchial tube. (Image from http://www.sumi.com.pl/produkty-katalog/double-lumen-bronchial-tube-left-sided/.)

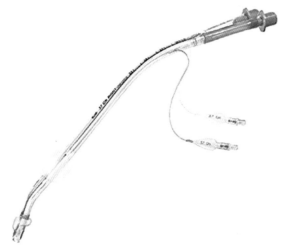

Fig. 41.5 Right-sided DLT. (Image from http://www.sumi.com.pl/produkty-katalog/double-lumen-bronchial-tube-right-sided/.)

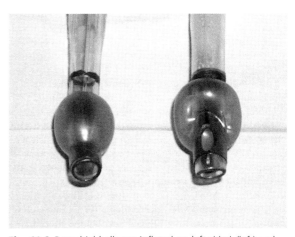

Fig. 41.6 Bronchial balloons inflated on left-sided *(left)* and right-sided *(right)* bronchial DLTs. The right tube is eccentric and shows the side lumen to allow inflation of the right upper lobe.

- auscultates and listens for absence of air leak, which, if present, indicates inadequate sealing of the airway by the tracheal cuff.

Step 2

The anaesthetist checks for unilateral ventilation through the endobronchial lumen after occluding the tracheal lumen of the Y-connector to the DLT. During ventilation through the endobronchial lumen, the anaesthetist:

- listens for air leak after opening the cap of the tracheal side of the DLT connector and during inflation of the endobronchial cuff (provided there is sufficient inflation of the endobronchial cuff, no air leak should be detected);
- observes for chest movement on the endobronchial side of the chest; and
- auscultates for air entry on the endobronchial side of the chest.

Step 3

The anaesthetist checks for unilateral ventilation through the tracheal lumen (i.e. the contralateral side to the endobronchial side). To do this manoeuvre, the endobronchial lumen rather than the tracheal lumen of the Y-connector is occluded. During ventilation through the tracheal lumen, after closure of the tracheal cap of the Y-connector attached to the DLT, the anaesthetist:

- listens for absence of air leak after opening the endobronchial cap of the Y-connecter (air leak should not occur if the endobronchial cuff is inflated sufficiently);
- observes for chest movement on the tracheal side of the chest; and
- auscultates for chest movement on the tracheal side of the chest.

In addition, correct placement of the DLT should be checked using a flexible bronchoscope. This method is especially useful:

- when a right-sided DLT is placed; the orifice in the slotted endobronchial cuff should be facing the orifice of the right upper lobe and cannot be determined by auscultation and observation of chest movement;
- for checking correct inflation of the endobronchial cuff, which should not herniate at the carina; and
- when clinical signs of chest expansion and auscultation may be equivocal, such as in patients with pleural effusion, emphysema and pneumothorax.

After checking placement of the DLT, it may be unnecessary to ventilate one lung until surgery commences. However, in some circumstances it is necessary to collapse the lung immediately after isolation:

- In the presence of a pneumothorax. Patients who present with a pneumothorax are often tall and slim. They have an inflated lung field and require pleurectomy and resection of associated blebs or bullae (Fig. 41.7). They may have a preoperative intercostal drain that can become

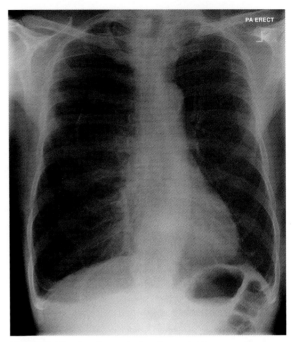

Fig. 41.7 Chest radiograph showing a right pneumothorax requiring pleurectomy and bullectomy. The air in the pleural space has no vascular bed surrounding the visceral pleura.

kinked. Thus air trapping and a tension pneumothorax can occur.
- After surgical removal of an intercostal drain before aseptic skin preparation by the surgeon.
- When there is a bronchopleural fistula in which losses of ventilator gases occur during positive pressure ventilation.

Complications of DLT are largely the same as those encountered with single-lumen tracheal tubes and may be traumatic (see Chapter 26) or a consequence of placement. These include:

- failure to ventilate the lungs (may be fatal);
- pneumothorax;
- endobronchial aspiration;
- laryngeal obstruction;
- vocal cord paralysis;
- submucosal haemorrhage; and
- diffuse fibrosis in the glottic area.

Endobronchial blockers

Endobronchial blockers may also be used for lung isolation in patients having procedures such as pleurectomy and lung biopsy. Endobronchial blockers are generally not suitable for patients who require pneumonectomy and lobectomy, as a DLT allows transection of the airway and airway toilet,

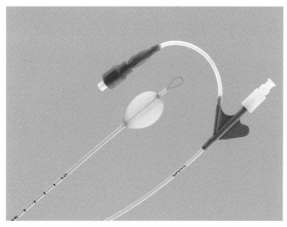

Fig. 41.8 The tip and proximal ends of the Arndt endobronchial blocker. (Image from https://www.cookmedical.com/products/cc_aebs_webds/.)

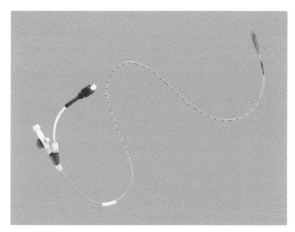

Fig. 41.9 The Cohen endobronchial blocker. (Image from https://www.cookmedical.com/products/cc_aebts_webds/.)

whereas the endobronchial blocker would interfere with surgery. Typical endobronchial blockers include:

- Arndt endobronchial blocker, which has a tip with a loop for placement of a bronchoscope (Fig. 41.8);
- Cohen endobronchial blocker, which has a steerable tip (Fig. 41.9); and
- Coopdech endobronchial blocker, which has a flexed tip.

Using a bronchoscope placed via a three-way connector on the tracheal tube, the endobronchial blocker is directed to the side that requires absence of ventilation. The endobronchial blocker is then withdrawn so that its cuff is located

just distal to the carina. The cuff is visualised during inflation, which should be sufficient to provide lung isolation, but without herniation. The endobronchial blocker is then fixed in position on a special connector attached to the tracheal tube.

Lung-volume reduction

The anaesthetic for surgical reduction of lung volume is similar to that of a lobectomy (i.e. lung isolation and the lateral decubitus position). For endobronchial valve placement, however, the patient remains supine, and tracheal intubation is achieved with a single-lumen tracheal tube. Anaesthesia is maintained either by volatile anaesthetic agents or by a propofol infusion. Both lungs are ventilated and flexible bronchoscopy is carried out; a large-diameter bronchoscope is required for administration of a measurement catheter with a balloon and, later, a deployment device for the endobronchial valve. After placement of a measurement catheter, collateral air flow is assessed after balloon occlusion of the orifice to the target lobe. If air flow from the target lobe is maintained, then collateral flow is deemed to occur. However, if there is a continuous decrease in air flow over time, then collateral flow from another lobe is unlikely to be present. Provided there is no collateral flow, endobronchial valve deployment would be appropriate. The orifice of the target-specific lobe is also assessed for suitability of deployment of endobronchial valves so that the landing zone is identified before deployment. These valves should be located so that they occlude ventilation to the target lobe but without movement, particularly when coughing. After the procedure, there should be reduction in lung volume.

Tracheal surgery

Unless cardiopulmonary bypass is used (see Chapter 42), there must be a changing sequence of the means of ventilating the lungs during surgery. In addition, measures must be employed to keep the neck flexed after surgery to avoid tension on the tracheal repair before it heals. Carinal surgery is one of the few remaining indications for a single-lumen endobronchial tube.

Until the tracheal lesion is resected, airway obstruction must be overcome during the early stages of anaesthesia. Maintaining spontaneous ventilation initially allows assessment of the adequacy of assisted ventilation under anaesthesia. With the lesion exposed, ventilation of one or both lungs through an incision in the trachea distal to the lesion allows resection of the lesion and repair of the posterior wall of the trachea. A narrow tracheal or bronchial tube is passed through the larynx beyond the anastomotic site and must allow space for repair of the anterior wall of the trachea. Suturing the chin to the skin over the sternum keeps the neck in flexion until the tracheal anastomosis heals.

Oesophageal surgery

Oesophagectomy is often preceded by oesophagoscopy with all the attendant risks of pulmonary aspiration. Thoracic approaches to the oesophagus may require one-lung ventilation to provide access for surgery. Oesophagectomy may take some hours and be associated with considerable fluid loss into the wound and surrounding tissues. The anaesthetist may be asked to pass a nasogastric tube that the surgeon pass across the anastomosis. It is very important that this is secured. After surgery, effective analgesia is necessary to enable the patient to expand the chest and cough effectively. Patients should be nursed sitting or supported on pillows to avoid regurgitation of GI fluid and subsequent aspiration. Total parenteral nutrition is not required as a routine but may be necessary in the presence of postoperative complications such as mediastinitis from an anastomotic leak. Judicious use of i.v. fluids after surgery is required.

Hypoxaemia during one-lung ventilation

There are various changes that occur with both the lateral position and having the thoracic cavity open to atmospheric pressure, in addition to the effects of anaesthesia and positive pressure ventilation (see Chapter 10).

- The lateral position converts the normal superior-inferior (upright) or anteroposterior (supine) gradients of pressures and volumes into top lung (non-dependent) to bottom lung (dependent). The non-dependent lung therefore exists on the steep part of the compliance curve, whereas the opposite is the case for the dependent lung. Compression of the dependent lung by mediastinal contents, jack-knife position and cephalic movement of the abdominal contents pushing on the diaphragm all contribute.
- Blood flow, conversely, preferentially flows to the dependent lung (60%). The end result is worsened ventilation-perfusion matching.
- Once the chest is open, the non-dependent lung is no longer constrained by the chest wall, so compliance increases further and leads to more relative overventilation. At the same time, atelectasis of the dependent lung results in more shunting. Distribution of perfusion remains largely unchanged.
- One-lung ventilation results in more shunt – the non-dependent lung is markedly hypoventilated but still has blood flow. Transmitted pressure changes from the (ventilated) dependent lung do result in a small amount of ventilation of the non-dependent lung (c. 150 ml).

$PaCO_2$ is less affected than PaO_2 as the quasi-linear relationship between $PaCO_2$ and $CaCO_2$ means that CO_2 can be excreted by blood flow to the dependent, ventilated lung.

In practice the fall in PaO_2 is rather less than expected for several reasons.

- Hypoxic pulmonary vasoconstriction (see Chapter 10) reduces blood flow to the non-dependent lung, from the expected 50% of cardiac output to around 20%.
- PEEP applied to the dependent lung has contrasting effects. The increase in pulmonary vascular resistance may increase blood flow to the non-dependent lung (worsening shunt), but it may also reduce atelectasis in the dependent lung (reducing shunt).
- Pulmonary vascular resistance in the dependent lung has a U-shaped relationship with lung volume (see Chapter 10). Ventilating the lung with moderate airway pressures therefore reduces diversion of blood to the non-dependent lung.
- Collapse of the non-dependent lung, alongside surgical manipulation, will tend to reduce blood flow to that lung.
- By definition the non-dependent lung is diseased, so areas of lung may already have existing ventilation-perfusion abnormalities.

During thoracic surgery in the lateral decubitus position, the patient's oxygen saturation may decrease beyond what would be expected given the shunt in the collapsed, non-dependent lung. In this situation, general and specific causes should be identified and managed accordingly.

General causes relate to gas delivery as with any anaesthetic:

- Faulty oxygen supply needing the anaesthetist to check the pipeline pressure and gas analyser
- Problems with the breathing system such as disconnection or obstruction

Specific causes relate to either high airway pressure or to intrapulmonary shunt. High airway pressure occurs in the presence of:

- Malposition of the DLT. The anaesthetist should check for correct positioning. If the view via the bronchoscope does not look like that seen during surgical rigid bronchoscopy, then it is likely to be incorrect. It is possible to misidentify the carina by viewing a distal bifurcation of the tracheobronchial tree. The position of the DLT should be checked after induction of general anaesthesia rather than waiting for hypoxaemia or high airway pressure to occur.
- Malposition of the endobronchial blocker. The anaesthetist should check for occlusion of the airway by the blocker cuff, which can move from one of the bronchi into the trachea.
- Sputum and blood which require airway toileting, particularly after surgical dissection.

- Bronchospasm and pneumothorax in the dependent ventilated lung, which can occur but are rare. Pneumothorax is difficult to diagnose in the lateral decubitus position. A high index of suspicion is needed particularly if bullae are seen on preoperative CT scans.

To reduce shunt and hence improve oxygenation during one-lung ventilation, the anaesthetist may perform any of the following strategies:

- Check ventilator settings and give 100% oxygen.
- If not already applied, apply PEEP to the ventilated dependent lung to counteract atelectasis.
- Increase cardiac output by a small fluid challenge and/ or use of vasopressors.
- Insufflate oxygen to the non-dependent collapsed lung, without or with CPAP.
- Inflation and ventilation of both lungs.
- Surgically clamp the pulmonary artery to the collapsed lung.

Continuous airway pressure to the non-dependent lung, ventilation of two lungs and clamping of the pulmonary artery to the collapsed lung make the procedure more difficult from a surgical perspective. Generally, hypoxaemia during one-lung anaesthesia is caused by malposition of the airway device. The airway pressure is a barometer of the cause; if the airway pressure is high, then the problem is likely to be related to the airway device, and if the airway pressure is consistent with ventilation of one lung, then the causes are likely to be related to intrapulmonary shunting of blood. The latter cause can be rectified by optimisation of lung recruitment of the dependent ventilated lung and an increase in cardiac output.

Postoperative analgesia

The analgesic requirements after thoracic surgery are largely dependent on the magnitude of the operation. For relatively minor operations such as cervical mediastinoscopy, a combination of routine multimodal analgesia is sufficient (e.g. local anaesthetic infiltration and other analgesics such as i.v. opioids and paracetamol). For more major surgery, additional analgesia is required depending upon the incision. In thoracic surgery, access to the lungs is by video-assisted thoracoscopy alone or followed by thoracotomy.

- Thoracoscopy allows the surgeon to perform lobectomy, lung biopsy, pleurectomy and decortication. In general, three short incisions are made anteriorly in the fourth intercostal space, posteriorly in the fifth intercostal space and inferiorly in the eighth intercostal space.
- Thoracotomy may be necessary for the procedures listed above plus pneumonectomy. A posterolateral thoracotomy is performed in the fifth intercostal space.

Other than an individual patient's pain risk and wishes, analgesia depends not only on type of surgical access but also on the degree of internal dissection. For example, pain can be expected to increase in the following order: thoracoscopic lung biopsy < thoracoscopic pleurectomy, decortication, lobectomy < thoracotomy for any operation.

Compared with thoracoscopy, thoracotomy is associated with greater incisional pain as a result of intercostal nerve damage from the rib retractor and sutures that close the thoracotomy. In addition, shoulder pain occurs on the ipsilateral side. This pain is referred and occurs as a consequence of phrenic nerve conduction after tissue dissection close to the diaphragm and mediastinal structures.

Various strategies have been considered with some evidence of benefit:

- Local anaesthetic block (e.g. intercostal block or intrapleural administration)
- Intravenous opioid by PCA
- Thoracic epidural
- Thoracic paravertebral block/catheter
- Intrathecal morphine

The latter three options are the main analgesic strategies, particularly for any thoracotomy and major thoracoscopic operations.

Epidural

Epidural analgesia is discussed in detail in Chapter 25. Thoracic epidural catheters are placed at a midthoracic interspace as the surgical incision is approximately at these dermatomes. The spinous processes of the thoracic spine are at an acute angle compared with that of the lumbar spine; as a result, the epidural needle has to be advanced obliquely in the narrow interspace between the spinous processes, in the midline. This approach is not always straightforward and so the paramedian method may be preferred:

- Insert the epidural needle approximately 1 cm lateral to the spinous process.
- Advance the epidural needle to the transverse process and then angle towards the midline to seek the ligamentum flavum.
- Once there is confirmed loss of resistance via the epidural syringe, insert and secure the epidural catheter in the usual way.

Compared with lumbar epidural analgesia, the thoracic level of administration of local anaesthetic, even of a low concentration and dose, results in a greater incidence of hypotension. The complications of epidural analgesia are discussed in Chapters 25 and 26.

Paravertebral

Thoracic paravertebral analgesia, ipsilateral to the side of surgery, can be instituted either before skin incision by the anaesthetist or intraoperatively by the surgeon. For anaesthetic placement, the needle is placed about 2.5 cm lateral to the spinous process and advanced to the transverse process, where it is guided over the upper border towards the superior costotransverse ligament, at a level similar to that for a thoracic epidural. There should be a subtle loss of resistance, which, along with ultrasound imaging, guides catheter placement and administration of a large volume of local anaesthetic. In contrast to anaesthetic administration, which occurs at the time of induction, surgical placement of a paravertebral catheter occurs under direct vision either during thoracoscopy or during thoracotomy.

Paravertebral analgesia is as effective as epidural analgesia. However, compared with epidural analgesia, paravertebral analgesia is unilateral and has a reduced incidence of block failure, hypotension and urinary retention. Complications of paravertebral analgesia are associated with the trauma and the effect of local anaesthetic to adjacent structures. They include pneumothorax; vascular puncture; dural puncture; Horner's syndrome; and Harlequin syndrome (unilateral flushing and sweating).

Intrathecal morphine

Intrathecal administration of preservative-free morphine can be performed through the standard lumbar interspace such as at L3–4 or L4–5. The dose of morphine used is variable, but approximately 300–500 µg results in effective analgesia, even after thoracotomy. Compared with epidural and paravertebral analgesia, patients do not experience shoulder pain if they receive intrathecal morphine. However, the duration of single dose intrathecal morphine is limited to less than 24 h and so it should be combined with another form of analgesia such as paravertebral block or PCA.

Postoperative considerations

After thoracic surgery, the majority of patients undergo tracheal extubation so that the lungs are not subjected to further positive pressure ventilation. Most patients do not require ICU admission and return to a monitored area in the thoracic ward. However, in addition to routine observations, thoracic patients require some specific interventions:

- *Monitoring of the efficacy and complications related to the method of analgesia* (e.g. respiratory depression, sedation, hypotension, inadequate analgesia and limb weakness).
- *Enhanced recovery interventions* involving physiotherapy and mobilisation, provided there are no significant intraoperative complications impairing progress.
- *Fluid balance.* Patients should drink but must not be fluid overloaded particularly after pneumonectomy. Some surgeons prefer a mild fluid restriction in the first 24 h after surgery (e.g. 1500 ml).
- *Chest radiographs and CT scans* if complications occur. Other than ensuring lung expansion, these can demonstrate:
  - the expected absence of lung markings and fluid accumulation after pneumonectomy; and
  - complications such as subcutaneous emphysema, loculated pneumothorax, loculated pleural effusion and pulmonary infiltrates.
- *Intercostal drainage for air leak and haemorrhage.* The intercostal drain system is a one-way valve system that has an underwater seal on the side of the patient. The water level in the drain set must be well above the tube connected the patient but below the other tube which is open to air. The tube that is open to air allows lung re-expansion and application of mild wall suction, which may be appropriate if there is inadequate lung re-expansion. Excessive suction can promote an air leak. The intercostal drain is removed provided there is no air leak and the lung has re-expanded.

References/Further reading

Brunelli, A., Kim, A.W., Berger, K.I., Addrizzo-Harris, D.J., 2013. Physiologic evaluation of the patient with lung cancer being considered for resectional surgery. Diagnosis and management of lung cancer, 3rd ed: American college of chest physicians Evidence-based clinical practice guidelines. Chest 143 (Suppl. 5), e166S–e190S.

Detterbeck, F.C., Postmus, P.E., Tanoue, L.T., 2013. The stage classification

of lung cancer. Diagnosis and management of lung cancer, 3rd ed: American college of chest physicians Evidence-based clinical practice guidelines. Chest 143 (Suppl. 5), e191S–e210S.

Howington, J.A., Blum, M.G., Chang, A.C., et al., 2013. Treatment of stage I and II Non-small cell lung cancer diagnosis and management of lung cancer, 3rd ed: American college of chest physicians evidence-based clinical

practice guidelines. Chest 143 (Suppl. 5), e278S–e313S.

Lim, E., Baldwin, D., Beckles, M., et al., 2010. Guidelines on the radical management of patients with lung cancer. Thorax 65 (Suppl. III), iii1–iii27.

Ng, A., Swanevelder, J., 2010. Hypoxaemia during one lung anaesthesia. Cont Educ Anaes Crit Care Pain (10), 117–122.

Ng, A., Russell, W., 2004. High frequency jet ventilation. CPD Anaesthesia 6 (2), 68–72.

Silvestri, G.A., Gonzalez, A.V., Jantz, M.A., et al., 2013. Methods for staging non-small cell lung cancer. Diagnosis and management of lung cancer. 3rd ed: American college of chest physicians. Evidence-based clinical practice guidelines. Chest 143 (5 Suppl.), e211S–e250S.

Chapter | 42 |

Anaesthesia for cardiac surgery

Andrew A Klein, Joseph Arrowsmith

In the UK and much of the developed world, more than half of all cardiac surgical procedures are undertaken to revascularise ischaemic myocardium. Of the remainder, surgery for acquired valvular disease, congenital anomalies and disorders of the great vessels comprise the majority. Impaired ventricular function is not uncommon in this group of patients, the severity of which may greatly affect the conduct of anaesthesia and surgery as well as outcome. The combination of underlying cardiac pathological conditions, comorbid conditions and concomitant medications make many patients with cardiac disease susceptible to the adverse haemodynamic effects of anaesthetic agents, particularly peripheral vasodilatation. Regardless of the disease process or state, all efforts should be made to maintain haemodynamic stability and promote a positive myocardial oxygen balance during anaesthesia and throughout the postoperative period.

Undoubtedly, there is more equipment and technology on show in the cardiac surgical theatre than in other operating theatres, and the number of staff present is often large. This makes familiarity with equipment and multidisciplinary teamwork imperative, as well as a specialist knowledge of cardiovascular and respiratory physiology. The replacement of the functions of the heart and lungs by cardiopulmonary bypass (CPB) is often required, although some coronary surgery can be performed on the beating heart (off pump). Indeed, novel minimally invasive methods may allow repair of various structures within the heart and even valve replacement or repair without CPB, and this is an exciting area of development.

The number of older patients undergoing cardiac surgery of all types has increased over recent years such that patients older than age 75 now make up more than 20% of the cardiac surgical population, and more than 5% are older than 80.

Ischaemic heart disease

Since being popularised in the late 1960s, revascularisation by coronary artery bypass grafts (CABG) has become the most commonly performed cardiac operation. The internal mammary artery is used routinely as a graft conduit, and there is good evidence that this provides good survival benefit. Improved surgical techniques have increased the popularity of off-pump coronary revascularisation, but its precise role remains uncertain, and any advantages over surgery using CPB have not yet been proven. Technological advances in coronary stent technology, especially coated (drug-eluting) stents, have led to a huge expansion in the use of percutaneous coronary intervention (PCI), such as angioplasty, atherectomy and stenting of coronary arteries (Fig. 42.1), in the cardiac catheter laboratory. However, the long-term efficacy of stenting has recently been called into question, and traditional CABG, once thought to be in terminal decline, remains a popular procedure.

Valvular disease

Stenosis or incompetence (regurgitation or insufficiency) most commonly involves the mitral and aortic valves. The most common diseases are calcific degeneration (causing aortic stenosis, with or without regurgitation), chronic rheumatic disease (affecting mitral and aortic valves) and myxomatous disease (most often causing mitral regurgitation). It should be borne in mind that valve dysfunction may occur as the result of systemic disease (e.g. carcinoid syndrome, infective endocarditis) and disruption of nearby

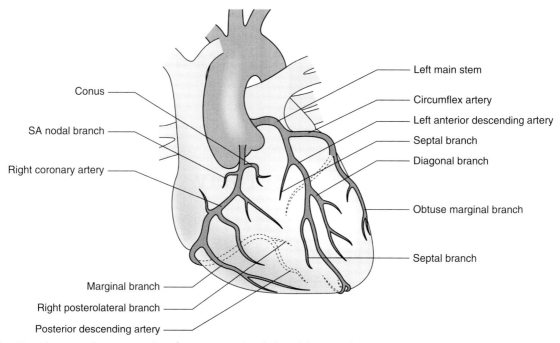

Fig. 42.1 Diagrammatic representation of coronary arteries. (Adapted from Mackay, J. H., & Arrowsmith, J. E. (2012) *Core topics in cardiac anesthesia.* Cambridge, Cambridge University Press.)

anatomical structures (e.g. aortic regurgitation in acute dissection of the ascending aorta and mitral regurgitation after papillary muscle rupture).

Surgery usually entails repair or prosthetic replacement guided by intraoperative transoesophageal echocardiography (TOE). The use of bioprosthetic or tissue (porcine, bovine, cadaveric homograft) valves obviates the necessity for, and risks associated with, lifelong anticoagulation but exposes the patient to the prospect of reoperation within 15–20 years. In contrast, mechanical (tilting disc) valves tend to last longer than bioprostheses and are therefore better suited to younger patients and those already anticoagulated for other reasons (e.g. chronic atrial fibrillation). Improvements in technology have led to some prostheses lasting more than 20 years, especially in patients aged older than 70 years at the time of surgery.

Transcatheter aortic valve replacement (TAVR; also known as transcatheter aortic valve implantation, TAVI) has become much more common in the last few years. It allows replacement of the aortic valve without sternotomy or CPB, and the prosthetic tissue valve is rolled up and crimped into a tube-like shape before deployment. The most common approach is transfemoral, during which the femoral artery is accessed and a wire passed up into the ascending aorta under fluoroscopic control. The aortic valve is crossed, and the prosthetic valve is then inserted before

being deployed; exact positioning is crucial to minimise the risk of valve embolism. The most common complication of the procedure is damage to, or dissection of, the femoral or iliac artery. If the femoral/iliac artery is not suitable because of small size or excessive calcification, alternative approaches, including transapical (mini-thoracotomy) or transaortic (mini-sternotomy), are possible. Anaesthetic management for transfemoral TAVR commonly involves conscious sedation and regional blockade, because this is associated with greater haemodynamic stability and reduced procedure and recovery time.

Arrhythmias

Most ablation procedures undertaken to treat arrhythmias are minimally invasive and undertaken by cardiologists in the cardiac catheter laboratory. Until recent times, the majority of these were facilitated by sedation administered by the cardiologist and/or cardiac catheter nurses. However, recent studies have demonstrated improved 'cure' rates and longevity when facilitated by general anaesthesia, leading to an increase in the demand for anaesthetic services in cardiac catheter labs. The majority of procedures are for recurrent atrial fibrillation or flutter or supraventricular tachycardias. Mapping the heart for electrical activity and subsequent ablation takes 2–3 hours on average but can last up to 4

Box 42.1 **Potential adverse events and outcomes in patients with implantable cardiac defibrillators (ICDs)**

Damage to the device, the leads or site of lead implantation
Failure to deliver pacing, defibrillation or both
Changes in pacing behaviour
Inappropriate delivery of a defibrillatory shock
Inadvertent electrical reset to backup pacing modes

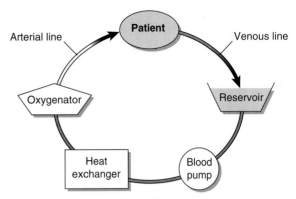

Fig. 42.2 Components of a cardiopulmonary bypass circuit. (Adapted from Mackay, J. H., & Arrowsmith, J. E. (2012) *Core topics in cardiac anesthesia.* Cambridge, Cambridge University Press.)

or 5 hours. Haemodynamic instability is more of a feature during ablation for ventricular tachycardia, during which invasive arterial monitoring is recommended. Processed EEG monitoring is recommended for all ablation treatments, as excessively deep anaesthesia (e.g. bispectral index <25) is associated with failure to map electrical currents.

Implantable rhythm management devices

Sedation or general anaesthesia may be required for pacemaker or implantable cardioverter defibrillator (ICD) insertion, especially if tunnelled deep under the pectoral muscles or if ventricular arrhythmias are to be induced to check function. In patients with cardiomyopathy or severely impaired left ventricular (LV) function, ICDs may be implanted prophylactically to prevent sudden death. Implantable cardioverter defibrillators are now the definitive therapy for patients at high risk for malignant ventricular arrhythmias (primary prophylaxis) and for patients who have survived a malignant arrhythmia (secondary prophylaxis). Consideration should be given to suspending the defibrillator function of ICDs during surgery, as diathermy may prompt unnecessary defibrillation (Box 42.1).

Congenital heart disease

Congenital heart disease has an incidence of 6–8 per 1000 live births. The majority of lesions requiring surgery are repaired during childhood in specialist paediatric cardiac surgical centres. Conditions such as a small atrial septal defect, partial anomalous pulmonary venous drainage or a bicuspid aortic valve may not present until adulthood. As a result of improvements in paediatric surgical and medical care, many patients now survive well into adulthood and may require repeat surgery or other cardiac procedures. Specialist adult congenital heart disease (ACHD) centres have been created to cater to the often complex needs of this group of patients. A further description of these procedures is beyond the scope of this chapter.

Cardiopulmonary bypass

The essential components of a CPB circuit (Fig. 42.2) are:
- venous reservoir;
- pump;
- oxygenator;
- heat exchange unit;
- cardioplegia delivery system; and
- connecting tubes and filters.

Full anticoagulation of the patient, typically with unfractionated heparin, is required to prevent coagulation in the CPB circuit caused by contact between the blood and the plastic components, which would otherwise lead to potentially lethal CPB/oxygenator blockage and failure. Despite anticoagulation, blood or plastic contact leads to the release of a number of active substances which cause vasodilatation, consumption of clotting factors and fibrinolysis. These include cytokines, thromboxane-A_2 and leukotrienes, and they are responsible for the hypotension and increased bleeding associated with CPB.

Blood from the venae cavae or right atrium is drained by gravity to a venous reservoir, from where it is pumped into a gas exchange unit (oxygenator) where oxygen is delivered to, and carbon dioxide removed from, the blood. The blood can also be cooled or warmed efficiently at this point, using water pumped through a countercurrent heat exchanger located within the oxygenator. Oxygenated or 'arterialised' blood is then delivered into the systemic circulation, usually via a cannula in the ascending aorta. The heart and lungs are thus bypassed or isolated and their function maintained temporarily by mechanical equipment remote from the body. Any blood in or around the bypassed heart (whether spilt or drained) may be aspirated and returned to the venous (cardiotomy) reservoir for filtration, oxygenation and subsequent return to the circulation.

Venous reservoir

A 500–2000 ml reserve of circulating volume permits the delivery of a constant systemic flow during times when venous drainage is inadvertently reduced or deliberately impeded. Clinical systems are described as being 'open' (blood in contact with air) or 'closed' (blood in a soft, flexible container not in contact with air). To prevent air entrainment, most systems incorporate a critical level alarm which automatically stops the CPB pump if the reservoir becomes empty.

Pumps

Roller pumps displace blood around the circuit by intermittent, semiocclusive compression of the circuit tubing during each rotation. Intermittent acceleration of the roller head can be used to produce a pulsatile pressure waveform, although there is little evidence that a more physiological flow pattern improves outcome. Alternatively, a centrifugal pump may be used. Movement of a disc at very rapid speeds (>3000 revolutions per min) leads to exertion of gravitational force on blood and results in propulsion at a flow which is dependent on the resistance (afterload) offered by the arterial tubing and the patient's systemic vascular resistance. There is some evidence that centrifugal pumps cause less blood component damage and activation, but this has not translated into improved outcome, and their use is usually confined to prolonged or complex surgery. Unlike roller pumps, which impede all flow when stopped, centrifugal pumps permit passive retrograde blood flow when switched off.

Oxygenator

Membrane oxygenators comprise a semipermeable membrane which separates gas and blood phases and through which gas exchange occurs. Commercially available devices have an effective exchange area of around 7 m^2 – one-tenth of the alveolar surface area of an adult.

Connecting tubes, filters, manometer, suction

Tubes, filters, manometer and suction must be sterile and non-toxic and should damage blood as little as possible. A filter should also be incorporated in the arterial line to remove particulate and gaseous emboli which would otherwise pass directly to the aorta and cause blood vessel occlusion. Low-pressure suction pumps are supplied to vent blood collecting in the pulmonary circulation or left ventricle during bypass and also to remove shed blood from the surgical field. The blood is collected in the cardiotomy

reservoir, filtered and returned to the main circuit. Cardiotomy suction causes damage to blood components.

Fluid prime

The CPB circuit must be primed with fluid (de-aired) before use. When CPB is commenced and the patient's blood is mixed with the clear fluids which prime the bypass circuit, the haematocrit decreases by approximately 20%–25%. Although oxygen content is reduced, oxygen availability may be increased by improved organ blood flow resulting from reduced blood viscosity. In some patients (those with low body weight, children or patients with preoperative anaemia, when dilution would reduce the haematocrit to <20%), blood may be added to the prime. In the normal adult, clear primes are used almost exclusively (usually a crystalloid/colloid mixture). Most units have individual recipes for addition to the prime (e.g. mannitol, sodium bicarbonate and potassium) to achieve an isosmolar solution at physiological pH.

Preoperative assessment

In recent years there has been a trend towards the assessment of elective patients in pre-admission clinics, typically 1–2 weeks before surgery. Despite undergoing an extensive array of specialised investigations to diagnose and quantify cardiac disease, there is evidence that a significant number of cardiac surgical patients have additional and hitherto undocumented pathological conditions. Thorough preoperative evaluation by the anaesthetist remains an essential component of perioperative care (see Chapter 19).

Exercise electrocardiography

Exercise (treadmill) testing is often used as a screening test before coronary angiography. Various stress protocols are used in which a standard exercise test provokes ischaemic changes and symptoms. Changes in rhythm, rate, arterial pressure and conduction are recorded. Although it has relatively low sensitivity and specificity (60%–70%) for coronary artery disease, it does provide some indication of effort tolerance.

Cardiac catheterisation

Left-sided heart catheterisation typically comprises coronary angiography, aortography, left ventriculography and manometry. This provides the following information:
• Site and severity of coronary artery disease
• Mitral and aortic valve function
• Left ventricular morphology and function

Table 42.1 Measurements obtained during cardiac catheterisation

	Parameter	Normal values
Left side of the heart	Systemic arterial/aortic pressure	<140/90 (mean 105) mmHg
	LV pressure	<140/12 mmHg
Right side of the heart	RA pressure	<6 (mean) mmHg
	RV pressure	<25/5 mmHg
	PA pressure	25/12 (mean 22) mmHg
	PAWP	12 mmHg
	Cardiac index	2.5–4.2 L min^{-1} m^{-2}
	PVR	100 dyne s cm^{-5}
	SVR	800–1200 dyne s cm^{-5}

LV, Left ventricle; *PA,* pulmonary artery; *PAWP,* pulmonary artery wedge pressure; *PVR,* pulmonary vascular resistance; *RA,* right atrium; *RV,* right ventricle; *SVR,* systemic vascular resistance.

The efficiency of ventricular contraction (ejection fraction, EF) can be estimated using the following formula:

$$\text{(end-diastolic volume – end-systolic volume)} / \text{end-diastolic volume}$$

Right-sided heart catheterisation allows measurement of right-sided heart and pulmonary artery pressures. When combined with measurements of cardiac output, these can be used to determine pulmonary and systemic vascular resistances (Table 42.1).

Echocardiography

Transthoracic echocardiography (TTE) is often used to define cardiac anatomy and assess ventricular and valvular function. It is non-invasive and can be performed at intervals to monitor disease progression and to optimise the timing of surgical intervention before irreversible ventricular damage has occurred. It may also assist planning of the type of intervention required. Doppler techniques allow recognition of the direction and velocity of blood flow and are valuable in the diagnosis of valvular disease.

Unfortunately, TTE is of limited use in obese patients and patients with chronic lung disease (because of poor ultrasound windows caused by tissue or air). In addition, certain parts of the heart may not be visualised adequately because of their distance from the probe (such as the left atrium and interatrial septum). Therefore TOE may be required preoperatively (usually performed under sedation); TOE may also be indicated in mitral valve pathological conditions to aid surgical decision making between valve replacement and repair.

Radionuclide imaging

By imaging the activity of an appropriate radioisotope as it passes through the heart or into the myocardium, ventricular function and myocardial perfusion can be assessed. Technetium images blood volume and can be used to demonstrate abnormal wall motion and EF. Thallium, which is taken up by the myocardium, may be used to assess regional blood flow. These techniques can be used before and after exercise or pharmacologically induced stress (e.g. dobutamine infusion).

CT/MRI

Electrocardiogram-gated, multislice scanning, real-time motion and 3-dimensional reconstruction have led to the incorporation of CT and MRI in the preoperative assessment of many cardiac surgical patients. Computed tomography can demonstrate coronary anatomy and disease less invasively than traditional angiography, and MRI can be used to assess valvular lesions, especially in complex cases or when previous surgery has taken place.

Additional investigations

Respiratory function tests, arterial blood gas analysis, carotid ultrasonography, creatinine clearance and evaluation of a permanent pacemaker or cardio-defibrillator should be conducted as appropriate.

Preoperative drug therapy

Care is required to balance the risks of discontinuation of medication in the perioperative period against the risk of major adverse cardiovascular events (e.g. withholding antiplatelet agents such as aspirin and clopidogrel).

- *Beta-blockers.* Continued administration of these drugs up to the time of surgery is desirable because discontinuation may increase the risk of perioperative myocardial infarction.
- *Calcium channel antagonists.* Have a negative inotropic effect, but it is preferable to continue therapy.

- *Nitrates.* Should be continued to prevent rebound angina.
- *Digoxin.* Discontinued 24–48 h before surgery to diminish digoxin-associated arrhythmias after surgery.
- *Diuretics.* Should be continued until the day before surgery.
- *Antiplatelet agents.* Aspirin and clopidogrel are usually stopped up to 1 week before surgery to permit platelet function to return towards normal. However, there is recent evidence that stopping aspirin is associated with increased morbidity, and it is continued throughout the perioperative period in many centres.
- *Anticoagulants.* Management is discussed in Chapter 19. The international normalised ratio (INR) should be 1.5 or less in patients taking warfarin, with a target INR of 2.5.
- *Angiotensin-converting enzyme (ACE) inhibitors/angiotensin receptor blockers (ARBs).* May produce significant vasodilatation and hypotension intra- and postoperatively. Perioperative use varies from unit to unit; they may be stopped up to 1 week before surgery or continued until the day of operation.
- *Potassium channel activators.* May be continued up to the day of operation.

Investigations

Investigations are generally identical to non-cardiac surgery (see Chapter 19). Specific differences include the following:
- Chronic anaemia (Hb <130 g L^{-1}) should be investigated and treated because it is associated with blood transfusion and worsened outcomes, including complications, prolonged ICU and hospital stay and increased mortality.
- Quantitative platelet or leucocyte abnormalities should also be excluded.
- Clotting studies should be performed before surgery. In the absence of anticoagulant administration, the finding of a seemingly trivial prolongation of the activated partial thromboplastin time (APTT) should prompt further investigation because it may indicate the presence of a factor deficiency.

Risk assessment

Despite advances in surgical techniques, anaesthesia and critical care, cardiac surgery still carries a finite risk of death and serious complications. Although this risk has decreased steadily over the last 10 years (<1% for isolated CABG or aortic valve replacement in young male patients), outcomes vary from centre to centre and from surgeon to surgeon. Although helping the patient to understand the benefits (symptomatic and prognostic) and risks of surgery during the consent process is the responsibility of the surgeon, it is essential that the anaesthetist understands how risk is assessed so that the patient is not given contradictory information.

The European System for Cardiac Operative Risk Evaluation (EuroSCORE) provides a robust risk assessment and can be calculated easily at the bedside (Table 42.2). The EuroSCORE has been validated in the UK, Europe and North America and has been found to be predictive of major complications, duration of ICU stay and resource utilisation.

Monitoring

Extensive and accurate physiological monitoring is essential throughout the perioperative period for the safe practice of cardiac surgery. Instrumental monitoring should be considered an adjunct to, rather than a replacement for, routine clinical observation of the patient.

Electrocardiography

The ECG should be monitored throughout the perioperative period. The ideal system is one which allows simultaneous multiple-lead monitoring, or at least switching between leads II and V5, for accurate identification of ischaemia.

Systemic arterial pressure

Arterial cannulation is mandatory, and the arterial line should normally be sited before induction of anaesthesia. It not only permits direct measurement of blood pressure but also facilitates sampling of arterial blood for analysis. Bilateral radial arterial monitoring should be considered in patients undergoing aortic arch surgery. Radial and femoral arterial pressure monitoring should be considered in patients likely to undergo deep hypothermic circulatory arrest (DHCA).

Central venous pressure

Right-sided filling pressure should be monitored by a catheter placed into a central vein. In selected cases, a flow-directed pulmonary artery catheter (PAC) may be inserted at induction to monitor left heart filling pressure.

Cardiac output

Cardiac output (CO) can be measured by thermodilution using a PAC. This, together with the derivatives of stroke work, pulmonary and systemic vascular resistances and tissue oxygen flux, allows titration of vasoactive infusions. Modified

Table 42.2 The European System for Cardiac Operative Risk Evaluation (logistic version II) risk stratification model (EuroSCORE)

Factor	Description	Coefficient
Age	≤60 years >60 years	0.0285181 (Age −60) × 0.0285181
Sex	Female	0.2196434
Renal impairment	CC 50–85 ml min^{-1} CC <50 ml min^{-1} On dialysis	0.303553 0.8592256 0.6421508
Chronic lung disease	Bronchodilators or steroids	0.1886564
Extracardiac arteriopathy	Claudication, carotid stenosis >50%, abdominal aortic, limb artery or carotid surgery planned or undertaken	0.5360268
Diabetes mellitus	On insulin therapy	0.3542749
Poor mobility	Severe impairment of mobility secondary to musculoskeletal or neurological dysfunction	0.2407181
Previous cardiac surgery	Pericardium opened	1.118599
Active endocarditis	On antibiotics	0.6194522
Critical preoperative state	VT, VF, cardiac massage, invasive ventilation, inotropic support, IABP, acute renal failure	1.086517
Unstable angina	Angina at rest requiring i.v. nitrates (CCS class IV)	0.2226147
Functional status	NYHA class II NYHA class III NYHA class IV	0.1070545 0.2958358 0.5597929
LV function	Moderate (LV EF 31%–50%) Poor (LV EF 21%–30%) Very poor (LV EF ≤20%)	0.3150652 0.8084096 0.9346919
Recent myocardial infarction	Within 90 days	0.1528943
Pulmonary hypertension	Moderate (PAP systolic 31–55 mmHg) Severe (PAP systolic >55 mmHg)	0.1788899 0.3491475
Urgency	Urgent (intervention or surgery on the current admission for medical reasons) Emergency (operation before the beginning of the next working day) Salvage (external cardiac massage) en route to the operating theatre or before induction of anaesthesia	0.3174673 0.7039121 1.362947
Other than isolated CABG	Single non-CABG procedure Two procedures Three procedures	0.0062118 0.5521478 0.9724533
Surgery on thoracic aorta		0.6527205
Mathematical constant		−5.324537

CABG, Coronary artery bypass graft; *CC,* creatinine clearance; *CCS,* Canadian Cardiovascular Society; *EF,* ejection fraction; *IABP,* intra-aortic balloon pump; *LV,* left ventricle; *NYHA,* New York Heart Association; *PAP,* pulmonary artery pressure; *VF,* ventricular fibrillation; *VT,* ventricular tachycardia.
Predicted mortality = e$^{(sum\ of\ coefficients)}$ / 1 + e$^{(sum\ of\ coefficients)}$.
(From Nashef, S. A. M., Rogues, F., & Sharples, L. D., et al. (2012) EuroSCORE II. *European Journal of Cardio-Thoracic Surgery.* 41, 734–745.)

PACs allow real-time measurement of CO and mixed venous oxygen saturation. Cardiac output may also be measured by techniques such as oesophageal Doppler and pulse contour analysis, but these have not replaced thermodilution in routine practice because of concerns about accuracy and bias.

Echocardiography

Transoesophageal echocardiography is indicated whenever valve surgery is undertaken, in cases of impaired LV function or when the underlying diagnosis is uncertain. Performed immediately before surgery, it may be used to help guide the surgeon in the choice of procedure (e.g. valve repair). In addition, it may identify lesions which have not been detected or diagnosed correctly during preoperative evaluation and may change surgical practice in up to 15% of cases. Immediately after CPB, TOE is useful for detecting intracardiac air and the need for further deairing manoeuvres. In addition, the adequacy of surgery can be judged and the need for reoperation in case of failure identified. After valve repair, persistent regurgitation (moderate or severe) should prompt consideration of reinstitution of CPB and an attempt at further surgical repair or replacement. After valve replacement, paravalvular leak should also prompt consideration of further surgical intervention. Abnormal motion of the ventricular wall (dyskinesia or akinesia) detected at this time but not present before surgery may indicate myocardial ischaemia, prompting further surgical revascularisation or inotropic support. The TOE probe is inserted with care after induction of anaesthesia and tracheal intubation. Complications include damage to structures in the mouth (including the teeth) and palate and to the oesophagus, including perforation, which is rare (approximately 1 in 1000 to 1 in 10,000).

Cerebral monitoring

Despite being available for many years, monitors of cerebral function and cerebral substrate (oxygen) delivery are rarely used during routine cardiac surgery. In recent years, however, cerebral near-infrared spectroscopy (NIRS) has gained popularity. This non-invasive technique allows measurement of tissue oxygen saturation in the frontal cortex throughout the perioperative period and may prompt titration of haemodynamic and respiratory indices to improve cerebral oxygen delivery or reduce consumption (cooling). The effect of such measures on outcomes remains unproven and is the subject of ongoing research.

Temperature

Core temperature should be monitored in the nasopharynx, which approximates to brain temperature, or the bladder.

Biochemistry and haematology

Facilities should be available for immediate blood gas analysis. Many systems also measure the concentrations of sodium, potassium, calcium, lactate, haemoglobin and glucose. Measurement of coagulation status should also be available. Activated clotting time (ACT) can be measured quickly in the operating theatre (normal 100–120 s), but rapid access to a central laboratory is required for additional testing. Thromboelastography (TEG) assesses viscoelastic changes in blood during clotting and may usefully assess haemostatic function at or near the point of care.

Pathophysiology

The anaesthetist should have a clear understanding of the fundamental principles of cardiac and cardiovascular physiology to manipulate factors which ensure adequate CO and myocardial blood supply (also discussed in Chapter 9).

Preload and contractility determine the work performed by the heart (Fig. 42.3). In the failing heart, afterload determines the work expended in overcoming aortic pressure compared with that used to provide forward flow. Thus CO may be increased by increasing preload or contractility or by reducing afterload. Any increases in heart rate, contractility, preload or afterload result in increased myocardial oxygen consumption. For this reason, augmentation of CO by increasing preload or contractility may have a detrimental effect on oxygen balance. Reducing afterload may increase CO whilst simultaneously reducing oxygen demand.

Adequate coronary perfusion demands the maintenance of an adequate diastolic aortic pressure. Oxygen supply to the myocardium occurs predominantly during diastole and is dependent on the gradient between diastolic aortic pressure and intraventricular pressure and on the duration of diastole. The portion of myocardium most at risk of developing ischaemia is the LV endocardium. Fig. 42.4 illustrates how these variables affect oxygen supply and demand in the myocardium and how a satisfactory supply/demand ratio may be preserved.

Care of the patient with valvular heart disease depends on the type, severity and consequences of the valvular lesion. In general, patients with valvular heart disease are intolerant of extremes in heart rate. In patients with valvular regurgitation, reducing afterload tends to reduce the regurgitant fraction and increases forward flow. In contrast, patients with valvular stenosis often require increased preload and are intolerant of acute reductions in peripheral resistance (afterload). This is particularly true of patients with aortic stenosis, when most of the afterload to LV ejection is caused

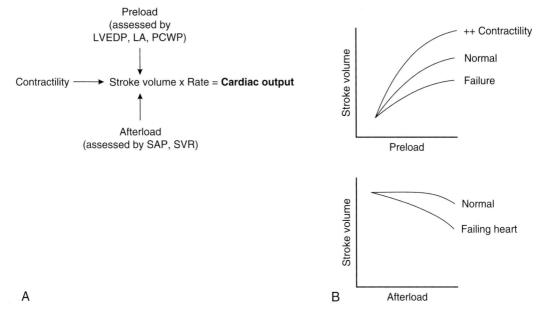

Fig. 42.3 Important aspects of mechanical function. *LA*, Left atrium; *LVEDP*, left ventricular end-diastolic pressure; *PCWP*, pulmonary capillary wedge pressure; *SAP*, systolic arterial pressure; *SVR*, systemic vascular resistance.

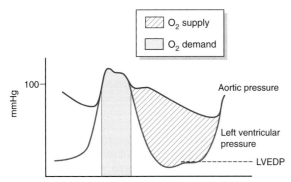

Fig. 42.4 The factors determining myocardial oxygen supply and demand. *LVEDP*, Left ventricular end-diastolic pressure.

by the stenosed valve itself. This afterload is fixed and cannot be reduced simply by lowering peripheral resistance. Vasodilatation in these patients produces marked hypotension and results in failure of perfusion of the hypertrophied myocardium with no increase in forward flow through the stenosed valve. Furthermore, diastolic dysfunction secondary to LV hypertrophy dictates that the majority of ventricular filling occurs later in diastole as a consequence of atrial

systole. For this reason, atrial fibrillation and nodal (junctional) rhythms may be tolerated poorly.

Anaesthetic technique

There is no single preferred anaesthetic technique for cardiac surgery. The choice of specific drugs is less important than the care with which they are administered and their effects monitored. The techniques described here are suitable for standard CABG with cardiopulmonary bypass. Anaesthesia for off-pump coronary surgery may be complicated by significant haemodynamic disturbances whilst the heart is positioned by the surgeon and by intraoperative myocardial ischaemia when coronary arteries are cross-clamped during anastomosis of the grafts. The reader is directed to more specialised texts for details of management.

Premedication

In the particularly anxious patient, sedation can be beneficial and may prevent increases in heart rate and arterial pressure before surgery. When deemed appropriate, preoperative sedation can be achieved with either an oral benzodiazepine (lorazepam 2–4 mg or temazepam 20–50 mg) or intramuscular opioid (morphine 10–20 mg), with or without an antisialagogue (hyoscine 0.4 mg).

Induction of anaesthesia

All drugs and equipment should be ready and the theatre and bypass circuit available for immediate use before the patient arrives in the anaesthetic room. Cross-matched blood should also be available immediately in case of rapid deterioration or surgical misadventure. Arterial and large-gauge venous cannulae should be inserted under local anaesthesia along with adequate sedation to reduce stress (e.g. midazolam 1–2 mg i.v.). External defibrillation electrodes should be applied in patients undergoing minimally invasive or repeat cardiac surgery. The lungs should be preoxygenated.

Induction may be achieved in a variety of ways. Most often, a large dose of an opioid analgesic (e.g. fentanyl 5–15 µg kg^{-1}) is administered with a benzodiazepine (e.g. midazolam 0.05–0.1 mg kg^{-1}) to obtain unconsciousness. Alternatively, a small dose of propofol (0.5–2 mg kg^{-1}) together with opioid or benzodiazepine may be used; consciousness is obtunded by an opioid in moderate dose, and hypnosis is then produced by a small dose of i.v. induction agent. An alternative is a target-controlled infusion of propofol, with the target concentration increased in small steps, accompanied by an infusion of a short-acting opioid such as alfentanil or remifentanil (0.04–0.15 µg kg^{-1} h^{-1}).

As consciousness is lost, a neuromuscular blocking agent (NMBA) is administered and ventilation supported when necessary. Almost all currently available NMBAs have been used during cardiac surgery, although pancuronium remains a popular choice. The objective is to undertake tracheal intubation without cardiovascular stimulation, and thus adequate analgesia and anaesthesia are required. Positive pressure ventilation is continued, usually with an oxygen/air mixture. Nitrous oxide, which may depress myocardial function and increase the volume of gaseous emboli, tends to be avoided in cardiac anaesthesia.

Induction of anaesthesia and institution of controlled ventilation often causes vasodilatation, decreased venous return and hypotension. In patients with critical coronary artery lesions or valvular disease (most particularly severe aortic stenosis), hypotension may precipitate myocardial ischaemia, which can very rapidly spiral into further cardiac depression, hypotension and malignant arrhythmias such as ventricular fibrillation, as well as infarction and myocardial damage. Hypotension (MAP <60 mmHg) in such patients should be promptly treated with vasopressors, hence the need for continuous arterial pressure monitoring during induction. Cardiac arrest is not uncommon if hypotension is not actively managed, and without prompt institution of CPB it may be irrecoverable. Central venous cannulation is performed using a multilumen catheter to allow monitoring

and i.v. infusions. A nasopharyngeal temperature probe and a urinary catheter should be inserted.

Previously identified high-risk patients, such as those with poor ventricular function or severe pulmonary hypertension, may require more extensive monitoring, such as a PAC. In the critical or emergency situation the CVC can be inserted under local anaesthesia, and induction of anaesthesia can be undertaken in theatre with the full team ready for immediate surgery.

Anaesthesia before cardiopulmonary bypass

After the patient is prepared and draped, the sternum is opened and, if required, the left internal thoracic (mammary) artery is harvested. Many surgeons request discontinuation of mechanical ventilation whilst actually performing sternotomy to reduce the risk of direct injury to the lungs. The pericardium is then opened and the heart inspected. Heparin is administered (usually 300 IU kg^{-1}) to prolong the ACT. The target ACT depends on local protocols but is typically more than 400 s. The surgeon then places cannulae in the aorta and the vena cava. Cannulation is commonly undertaken via the right atrium into the inferior vena cava (IVC) using a two-stage cannula, allowing drainage of both lower body (IVC) and upper body (right atrium). Alternatively, if the heart chambers are to be opened (e.g. mitral valve surgery), the cavae are cannulated separately.

The goals of haemodynamic management are to maintain a stable heart rate and arterial pressure during this period, particularly at moments of profound stimulation, notably skin incision, sternotomy and sternal retraction. If a technique based on opioids or volatile anaesthetics has been chosen, additional analgesia or inhalational anaesthesia should be given before stimulation. Alternatively, the opioid infusion rate can be increased temporarily as necessary, perhaps accompanied by increased target concentrations of propofol. The tendency of isoflurane to produce 'coronary steal' (the diversion of blood away from ischaemic muscle) is considered not to be of clinical importance. There is evidence that volatile anaesthetic agents increase myocardial tolerance to ischaemia by a mechanism known as preconditioning, thought to be mediated via adenosine triphosphate–dependent potassium channels.

If arterial pressure decreases during the period before institution of CPB, small doses of a vasopressor (e.g. metaraminol or phenylephrine) should be administered to maintain a sufficient MAP to maintain vital organ perfusion. This will obviously depend on the individual patient, but in most patients a MAP greater than 70 mmHg is sufficient. During aortic cannulation, hypertension should be avoided to reduce the risk of aortic dissection. Many surgeons request a maximum MAP at this delicate point in the procedure (typically <70 mmHg). Manipulation of the arterial pressure is required at frequent intervals to achieve different goals.

Cardiopulmonary bypass

Two factors complicate the provision of anaesthesia during CPB. First is the impact of haemodilution, hypotension, non-pulsatile blood flow and hypothermia on the pharmacokinetics of anaesthetic agents. Second is the inability to administer volatile inhalational agents via the lungs – mechanical ventilation is discontinued when full pump flow is reached and ventricular ejection ceases. Temporary loss of the lungs as a route for drug administration can be circumvented by use of total intravenous anaesthesia or the addition of a volatile agent to the CPB oxygenator 'sweep' gas. It should be borne in mind that the solubility of volatile agents in blood increases as temperature falls and that the time to achieve steady-state concentration may be significantly prolonged.

Surgery is usually preceded by placing an aortic cross-clamp proximal to the arterial cannula to isolate the coronary circulation. During CABG surgery the distal anastomoses are usually fashioned first and the cross-clamp then removed to permit restoration of myocardial perfusion. Application of a side-biting aortic clamp then allows the proximal (aortic) anastomoses to be fashioned without interfering with perfusion of the native coronary arteries.

Myocardial preservation

Most surgical techniques require that the heart be immobile. During CPB, the aorta is cross-clamped between the aortic cannula and the aortic valve, thus isolating the heart from the flow of oxygenated blood. Ischaemic damage to the myocardium can be reduced by hypothermia and the institution of diastolic cardiac arrest. The latter is typically achieved by instilling 500–1000 ml crystalloid cardioplegic solution, often mixed with the patient's blood, into the coronary arteries. Many cardioplegic solutions are available; the majority contain potassium and a membrane-stabilising agent, such as procaine.

Myocardial cooling is achieved by using ice-cold cardioplegia and by pouring cold saline (4 °C) into the pericardial sac. Depending on surgical preference, the patient may also be cooled systemically. This is most often carried out when more complex or prolonged surgery is proposed, to allow better organ preservation due to reduced metabolic rate. Administration of cardioplegia is usually repeated at regular intervals (e.g. every 20–30 min).

Perfusion on bypass

At normothermia, a pump flow of 2.4 L min^{-1} m^{-2} of body surface area is required to prevent inadequate perfusion of

the tissues. Mean systemic (arterial) pressure is dependent on pump flow and systemic vascular resistance. Controversy exists regarding the optimum perfusion pressure because essential organs, particularly the brain, may be damaged if MAP is <45 mmHg. Unfortunately, perfusion is difficult to assess clinically, especially in the hypothermic patient.

Following the onset of CPB, haemodilution causes marked decreases in peripheral resistance and arterial pressure, which in most instances resolve spontaneously in 5–10 min. If this does not occur, arterial pressure may be increased by raising systemic resistance with a vasopressor. Frequently, peripheral resistance and arterial pressure increase during hypothermic CPB as a result of increasing concentrations of catecholamines and then decrease during active rewarming because of profound vasodilatation.

Cell salvage

Cell salvage is commonly employed during cardiac surgery, most often before and after CPB (during CPB, blood is usually suctioned straight back into the bypass reservoir) (see Chapter 14). Cell salvage has been shown to reduce the requirement for and amount of allogeneic transfusion during cardiac surgery. It can also be used in ICU to process blood collected from the chest drains.

Coagulation control

Adequate anticoagulation must be maintained during CPB; ACT should be measured every 30 min and extra doses of anticoagulant administered as necessary.

Oxygen delivery

Arterial blood samples should be taken at regular intervals for measurement of blood gas tensions, acid–base status and haematocrit. Tissue oxygen delivery is dependent on pump flow, haemoglobin concentration and oxygen tension. The haematocrit can usually be permitted to fall to 20%, but further reduction should be prevented by the addition of packed cells or blood to the bypass circuit.

Acid–base balance

The development of a metabolic acidaemia suggests that perfusion is inadequate and, if necessary (base deficit >6–8 mmol L^{-1}), sodium bicarbonate may be administered.

When systemic hypothermia is used during CPB, consideration needs to be given to the effect of hypothermia on the solubility of gases in blood and how these affect values obtained from arterial blood gas analysis. As temperature decreases, the solubility of gases in liquids increases, and the proportion of gas in equilibrium with the gas phase (partial pressure) decreases, although the total content of each

795

gas remains the same. The net result of this phenomenon is a metabolic acidaemia secondary to reduced $PaCO_2$. There are two strategies for dealing with this issue. Not correcting arterial blood gas measurements for temperature allows a normal pH to be maintained. This is known as alpha-stat, because this maintains the degree of ionisation of alpha-histidine. Alternatively, adding additional CO_2 to maintain a normal pH on the basis of corrected blood gas measurements is known as pH stat. In most centres, alpha-stat is used, but pH-stat offers a number of theoretical benefits in patients undergoing procedures requiring deep hypothermia.

Serum potassium concentration

Serum potassium concentration should be maintained at approximately 4.5–5.5 mmol L^{-1} by the administration of potassium chloride (10–20 mmol) into the CPB circuit as required. It should be borne in mind that repeated administration of cardioplegic solutions may cause a significant rise in serum potassium concentration.

Weaning from cardiopulmonary bypass

Following removal of the aortic cross-clamp, oxygenated blood flows into the coronary arteries again, washing out cardioplegia and repaying the oxygen debt. In many cases the heart regains activity spontaneously. In a minority of patients it starts to beat in sinus rhythm but reverts usually to ventricular fibrillation; internal defibrillation is required to convert fibrillation to sinus rhythm and is successful only if pH, serum potassium concentration, oxygenation and temperature are approaching normal values. The heat exchanger in the oxygenator is used to increase the temperature of blood, but peripheral temperature is often depressed for some time. If a spontaneous heartbeat cannot be maintained, external pacing via epicardial wires should be started.

When core body temperature exceeds 36 °C, metabolic indices are normal and a regular heartbeat is present, the establishment of spontaneous CO is attempted. By gradually restricting venous drainage to the venous reservoir, venous blood is diverted to the right atrium. When the pulmonary circulation has been restored, mechanical ventilation is restarted; 100% oxygen is given because the efficiency of pulmonary gas exchange is unknown at this stage, and any gas bubbles which have not been vented may enlarge in volume if nitrous oxide or nitrogen (air) is introduced.

Left ventricular ejection produces an upward deflection on the arterial pressure trace after a QRS complex. If the myocardium is contracting satisfactorily, pump flow is reduced cautiously, and the heart, now receiving all the

venous return, achieves normal output. Although arterial pressure is the most easily measured index of successful termination of CPB, it is merely the product of CO and peripheral resistance. If there is doubt about efficiency of the heart, CO should be measured and peripheral resistance derived.

After successful termination of CPB, preload can be adjusted by retransfusing any blood left in the CPB circuit, by altering the patient's posture and by administering a vasodilator or vasoconstrictor.

Low cardiac output state

Failure to wean a patient from extracorporeal support should prompt the resumption of CPB whilst the cause is identified and supportive treatment initiated. Transoesophageal echocardiography may be particularly helpful in this situation, permitting continuous assessment of preload, ventricular wall motion and valvular function. Attention should be focused on cardiac contractility and afterload. Coronary aeroembolism, which may occur during and after separation from CPB, causes myocardial ischaemia manifesting as a regional ventricular wall motion abnormality and rhythm disturbance. The problem usually resolves when arterial pressure is elevated and the heart permitted to eject on CPB.

The choice of inotrope in this setting is largely a matter of personal preference; there is little evidence to suggest that one drug is superior to another. Despite the theoretical risk of worsened myocardial reperfusion injury, calcium salts (e.g. $CaCl_2$ 250–1000 mg) are commonly used first. Other drugs commonly used (either alone or in combination) include adrenaline (0.05–0.2 μg kg^{-1} min^{-1}), dobutamine (2–20 μg kg^{-1} min^{-1}) and dopamine (2–20 μg kg^{-1} min^{-1}); all increase myocardial oxygen demand and tend to precipitate tachyarrhythmias. Both adrenaline and dopamine cause vasoconstriction at high doses. Quite often, an infusion of vasoconstrictor is required, such as noradrenaline or vasopressin, to increase MAP and counter vasodilatation after CPB.

Phosphodiesterase III inhibitors, such as milrinone and enoximone, may be a suitable alternative or adjunct to conventional inotropes, particularly in patients with right ventricular dysfunction and pulmonary hypertension. By inhibiting the breakdown of cytosolic cyclic adenosine monophosphate (cAMP), they improve myocardial performance and dilate both arterioles and veins. By reducing afterload, they reduce myocardial oxygen demand and augment ventricular ejection. Arterial hypotension, more commonly seen with milrinone, can be treated with vasoconstrictor infusion, as earlier.

Failure to achieve an adequate spontaneous circulation by pharmacological means alone is an indication for mechanical support such as intra-aortic balloon counterpulsation.

Intra-aortic balloon pump

An intra-aortic balloon pump is inserted through a femoral artery and positioned in the descending aorta, just distal to the left subclavian artery. The balloon is inflated during diastole immediately after closure of the aortic valve, and deflated before ventricular ejection. Inflation displaces blood in the aorta, simultaneously promoting distal flow and augmenting coronary perfusion. After deflation of the balloon, proximal aortic pressure (afterload) is reduced, favouring improved ventricular ejection and lowering LV end-diastolic pressure.

Extracorporeal mechanical support

Often referred to as extracorporeal membrane oxygenation (ECMO), extracorporeal mechanical support is similar in many respects to CPB in that a pump (usually centrifugal) and oxygenator (membrane) are used to support the circulation and provide oxygenation and carbon dioxide removal. Failure to wean from CPB should prompt consideration for ECMO after discussion and careful consideration of patient risk factors and prognosis. In this setting, ECMO is usually arterial and central, with cannulae placed in the right atrium and aorta. However, in the setting of acute hypoxia (usually in the ICU), ECMO is most often venovenous and peripheral, with cannulae placed (most commonly percutaneously) in the femoral and/or internal jugular veins. Continuous anticoagulation using heparin by infusion is usually required but may be omitted for up to 24–48 h if the patient is actively bleeding or is at excessive risk of bleeding.

Bleeding

After decannulation of the heart, it is necessary to restore normal coagulation and achieve haemostasis. In the case of heparin anticoagulation, protamine sulphate (~1 mg for each 100 U heparin given) is administered cautiously. Protamine typically produces a transient and occasionally profound fall in arterial pressure because of peripheral vasodilatation. Rarely, protamine may cause acute pulmonary vasoconstriction. In excessive dosage, protamine may itself act as an anticoagulant.

The use of antifibrinolytic drugs in cardiac surgery is routine and ubiquitous. The most commonly used drug in UK practice is the lysine analogue, tranexamic acid, and this has been found to reduce bleeding, reoperation and transfusion. Dosing practice is variable; the authors recommend a loading dose of 2 g in most patients. In patients at increased risk of bleeding, a dose of 1g followed by an infusion at 5–10 mg kg^{-1} h^{-1} (~500 mg h^{-1} in a 70-kg patient). Aprotinin, a serine protease inhibitor, has not been used in recent years after the withdrawal of its licence because of concerns about increased risk of acute kidney injury and mortality. However, the regulators have now relicenced aprotinin for myocardial revascularisation only. Most centres have started using aprotinin again but in patients where there is at increased risk of bleeding, such as resternotomy, valve replacement for endocarditis or repair of aortic dissection.

Excessive bleeding after cardiac surgery is associated with increased resource utilisation, morbidity and mortality. Coagulopathic bleeding may be caused by residual anticoagulation or the consumption of clotting factors and platelets during CPB. Failure to achieve adequate haemostasis within 45 min of separation from CPB should prompt a full blood count, coagulation screen and, where available, thromboelastography (TEG) or thromboelastometry (ROTEM). The results should then be used to guide the selection of blood component therapy.

Whilst assisting the surgeon to achieve haemostasis, the anaesthetist must maintain adequate anaesthesia, maintain haemodynamic stability and correct any metabolic or biochemical abnormalities.

Haemodynamics after cardiopulmonary bypass

Myocardial injury and a degree of cardiac dysfunction are inevitable consequences of cardiac surgery and CPB. Virtually all patients exhibit brief increases in serum troponin and cardiac enzyme concentrations in the early postoperative period. The net result is reduced contractility (depressed Frank–Starling curve), reduced sensitivity to adrenergic agonists (endogenous and exogenous) and increased sensitivity to myocardial depressants (e.g. β-blockers). In the normal course of events, myocardial contractility tends to improve in the week after surgery.

Peripheral vasoconstriction may persist for several hours after CPB. This may lead to hypertension in patients with preserved ventricular function (particularly after surgery for aortic stenosis) or a low CO state in patients with impaired ventricular function. The treatment of hypokalaemia and hypomagnesaemia, and administration of a vasodilator such as sodium nitroprusside, decrease myocardial oxygen demand, improve peripheral perfusion and may increase CO. In addition, blood pressure control reduces the stress placed on vascular anastomoses.

In some patients, however, a profound systemic inflammatory response produces excessive vasodilatation and hypotension. Having excluded hypotension secondary to low CO, it may be necessary to initiate treatment with phenylephrine, noradrenaline or vasopressin.

Other aspects

In addition to maintaining cardiac function and oxygen supply to the tissues during this period, the anaesthetist should ensure that normality is regained as soon as possible and maintained in respect of the following.

Temperature

The thermal gradient between body core and peripheral tissues limits both the rate and efficiency of cooling and rewarming during CPB. The rate of transfer of thermal energy is largely governed by patient weight, muscle mass, vascular tone, perfusion pressure and pump flow. The inevitable fall in core temperature secondary to redistribution after CPB (so-called after-drop) can be mitigated by using external warming devices.

Biochemical monitoring

Essential monitoring includes arterial blood gas tensions, acid–base status, serum electrolyte concentration and haematocrit.

Cardiac rhythm

Heart block
Heart block may follow aortic valve surgery and operations on the ventricular septum, or as a consequence of right coronary aeroembolism. Atrioventricular (sequential; D00, DDD) pacing using epicardial pacing wires ensures an adequate ventricular rate and maintains late diastolic ventricular filling, which is particularly important if ventricular compliance is poor.

Supraventricular arrhythmias
Synchronised direct current cardioversion is the most convenient treatment when the chest is open. After chest closure, options include amiodarone, β-blockade, verapamil or adenosine.

Ventricular arrhythmias
The threshold for arrhythmias is reduced by hypokalaemia, hypomagnesaemia and hypocalcaemia. The abrupt onset of ventricular tachycardia or ventricular fibrillation after moving the patient from the operating table to the bed may herald coronary aeroembolism.

Postoperative care

In most centres, intraoperative support and monitoring are extended into the postoperative period. The duration of this care depends on institutional practice and the patient's speed of recovery. In some centres, patients are routinely cared for in the ICU. However, there may be some advantages to managing these patients on separate extended recovery units. In such instances the interval between admission and weaning from mechanical ventilation can usually be considerably shortened. This so-called fast-track approach may be associated with earlier discharge and reduced morbidity from unnecessarily prolonged sedation and mechanical ventilation of the lungs.

Transferring patients from the operating theatre is not without risk. Care must be taken to prevent inadvertent injury and avulsion of indwelling tubes, catheters and cannulae. Mechanical ventilation, drug therapy and haemodynamic monitoring should be continued throughout transfer.

Regardless of location, there should be a well-practised routine for the care of patients after surgery. Usually, ventilation of the lungs and full cardiovascular monitoring are recommended immediately. The principles of care in this phase are similar to those described for the period of anaesthesia after termination of bypass.

The principles underpinning the management of patients in the first few hours after cardiac surgery are the maintenance of haemodynamic stability, adequate pulmonary gas exchange, normal acid–base homeostasis, haemostasis and renal function.

In the uncomplicated patient, sedation can be discontinued 3–4 h after admission and the patient weaned from mechanical ventilation. In a significant minority of patients, however, haemodynamic instability, poor gas exchange, bleeding, hypothermia or agitation may necessitate prolonged sedation.

Criteria for tracheal extubation include the following:
- Awake, orientated, responds to commands
- Temperature greater than 35.5°C with core–peripheral gradient less than 6°C
- Intercostal drainage less than 100 ml h^{-1}
- Satisfactory blood gases with an inspired oxygen concentration less than 50%
- Haemodynamic stability

Bleeding

Bleeding after cardiac surgery is normal and to be expected. However, excessive bleeding (>150 ml h^{-1}) should be considered abnormal and prompt further assessment. Coagulopathic bleeding may be due to thrombocytopenia or impaired platelet function, clotting factor deficiency, or residual effects of heparin and should be treated actively on the basis of laboratory and point-of-care investigations (TEG or ROTEM). Blood component administration is often required (fresh frozen plasma, cryoprecipitate or platelet concentrate). The use of factor concentrates such as prothrombin complex concentrate (instead of fresh frozen plasma) or fibrinogen concentrate (instead of cryoprecipitate) may also be considered, especially in patients who are already fluid overloaded.

Temperature and acid–base balance should be normalised and anaemia corrected, as low haemoglobin concentration is also associated with increased bleeding. A further dose (e.g. 1 g) of tranexamic acid may be administered, and if the ACT is prolonged, further protamine (e.g. 50 mg) may also be given. In contrast, bleeding in the setting of normal coagulation should prompt consideration of early surgical re-exploration. However, it should be borne in mind that both resternotomy and massive transfusion are associated with significantly increased morbidity and mortality.

In some instances in which chest tube drainage is inadequate, the accumulation of blood within the chest may lead to haemodynamic collapse secondary to cardiac tamponade. Falling arterial blood pressure and rising central venous pressure should be considered to be due to tamponade until proved otherwise. If deterioration occurs rapidly, resternotomy must be undertaken in the ICU.

Analgesia

Pain after sternotomy is limited because surgical wiring of the sternum during closure prevents excessive bone movement and muscle injury is not a feature. Patients tend to complain more about pain from chest drain sites and leg or arm wounds (from harvesting of the saphenous vein or radial artery). Regular paracetamol should be administered, and morphine by infusion or nurse-administered bolus is often required. Morphine can often be replaced by a strong oral analgesic such as tramadol or codeine soon after extubation of the trachea, but PCA may be required by some patients. Intercostal drains are usually removed on the day after surgery, and analgesia for their removal can be provided by nitrous oxide/oxygen (Entonox) inhalation.

References/Further reading

Besser, M.W., Ortmann, E., Klein, A.A., 2015. Haemostatic management of cardiac surgical haemorrhage. Anaesthesia 70, 87–95, e29–31.

Hensley, F.A., Gravlee, G.P., Martin, D.E. (Eds.), 2012. A practical approach to cardiac anesthesia, 5th ed. Lippincott Williams & Wilkins, Philadelphia.

Klein, A.A., Collier, T.J., Brar, M.S., et al., 2016. The incidence and importance of anaemia in patients undergoing cardiac surgery in the UK – the first association of cardiothoracic anaesthetists national audit. Anaesthesia 71, 627–635.

Klein, A.A., Vuylsteke, A., Nashef, S.A.M. (Eds.), 2008. Core topics in cardiothoracic critical care. Cambridge University Press, Cambridge.

Ludman, P.F., British Cardiovascular Intervention Society. BCIS Audit Returns. Adult Interventional Procedures Jan 2015 to Dec 2014. http://www.bcis.org.uk/wp-content/uploads/2017/01/BCIS-audit-2014.pdf. Accessed July 2017.

Mackay, J.H., Arrowsmith, J.E. (Eds.), 2012. Core topics in cardiac anesthesia, 2nd ed. Cambridge University Press, Cambridge.

Muñoz, M., Acheson, A.G., Auerbach, M., et al., 2017. International consensus statement on the peri-operative management of anaemia and iron deficiency. Anaesthesia 72, 233–247.

Ortmann, E., Besser, M.W., Klein, A.A., 2013. Antifibrinolytic agents in current anaesthetic practice. Br. J. Anaesth. 111, 549–563.

Society for Cardiothoracic Surgery in Great Britain & Ireland. Blue Book Online. http://www.bluebook.scts.org. Accessed July 2017.

Chapter 43

Obstetric anaesthesia and analgesia

Arani Pillai

Obstetric anaesthesia and analgesia involve caring for women during childbirth in three situations:
- Provision of analgesia for labour, usually by epidural or spinal analgesic techniques
- Anaesthesia for peripartum operative procedures such as instrumental (e.g. forceps or Ventouse) or caesarean delivery
- Care of the critically ill parturient

The obstetric anaesthetist is involved in the care of the parturient as part of a multidisciplinary team including obstetricians, midwives, health visitors, physicians and intensive care specialists, necessitating excellent communication skills and record-keeping. Successive reports from the triennial confidential enquiries into maternal mortality currently conducted by the National Perinatal Epidemiology Unit (NPEU), and formerly by the Centre for Maternal and Child Enquiries (CMACE), have highlighted the problems of women with intercurrent medical disease, including obesity, and the importance of the obstetric anaesthetist in their care. This has led to the establishment of obstetric anaesthetic assessment clinics in many hospitals.

Many anaesthetists in training are wary of their obstetric modules. Remote site work in a dynamically changing environment can be challenging, however obstetric anaesthesia offers the opportunity to make a key difference to safety and the overall experience of women around labour and delivery.

Anatomy and physiology of pregnancy

The obstetric anaesthetist must understand maternal adaptation to pregnancy in order to manipulate physiological changes after general anaesthesia or regional analgesia and anaesthesia in such a way that the condition of the neonate at delivery is optimised.

The physiological changes of pregnancy are exaggerated in multiple pregnancy, which is increasing in incidence after the success of assisted conception.

Progesterone

Progesterone is the most important hormone in pregnancy. It is secreted in increasing amounts during the second half of the menstrual cycle to prepare the woman for pregnancy. After conception, the corpus luteum ensures adequate blood concentrations until placental secretion is adequate. The key physiological role of progesterone is its ability to relax smooth muscle. All other physiological changes stem from this pivotal function (Fig. 43.1).

Haemodynamic changes (Table 43.1)

- Blood volume increases from 65–70 to 80–85 ml kg^{-1} mainly by expansion of plasma volume (maximal at 30–32 weeks) (Fig. 43.2).
- By the third trimester, cardiac output has increased by about 40%–50% as a result of significant increases in heart rate and stroke volume.
- Pulmonary capillary wedge pressure and central venous pressure do not increase because of the relaxant effect of progesterone on the smooth muscle of arterioles and veins and dilatation of the left ventricle.
- Systemic and pulmonary vascular resistance are markedly decreased; this allows the increased blood volume to be accommodated at normal vascular pressures.

Aortocaval compression

When a pregnant woman lies supine, arterial pressure decreases because the gravid uterus compresses the inferior

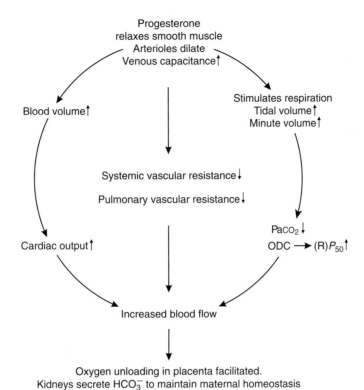

Fig. 43.1 Summary of the main actions of progesterone. It establishes the maternal physiological adaptation to pregnancy. *ODC*, Oxyhaemoglobin dissociation curve; *PaCO₂*, arterial carbon dioxide tension; *P₅₀*, partial pressure of oxygen when haemoglobin is 50% saturated at pH 7.4 and temperature 37°C; HCO_3^- bicarbonate.

Table 43.1 Cardiovascular changes in pregnancy

Variable	Change	Proportional change
Heart rate	Increased	20%–30%
Systolic blood pressure	Decreased	10%–15% second trimester
Diastolic blood pressure	Decreased	
Stroke volume	Increased	20%–50%
Cardiac output	Increased	40%–50% by third trimester
Systemic vascular resistance	Decreased	20%
Central venous pressure	Unchanged	
Pulmonary vascular resistance	Decreased	30%
Pulmonary capillary wedge pressure	Unchanged	

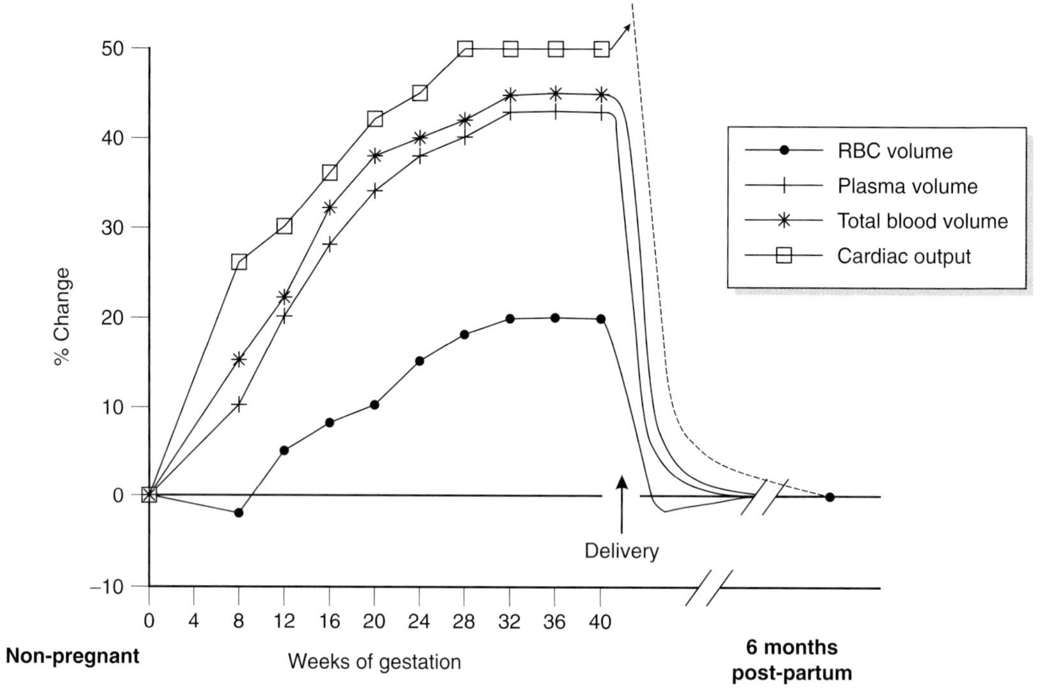

Fig. 43.2 Changes in blood, plasma and red cell volumes and cardiac output during pregnancy. *RBC*, Red blood cell.

vena cava, reducing venous return and therefore cardiac output. At term the vena cava is completely occluded in 90% of pregnant women, and stroke volume may only be 30% of that of a non-pregnant woman. The aorta is also often compressed, so femoral arterial pressure may be lower than brachial arterial pressure; this is the main cause of a reduction in uterine blood flow. The combination of both effects is known as aortocaval compression, which becomes clinically significant from around 20 weeks. Physiological compensation occurs via sympathetic stimulation and collateral venous return via the vertebral plexus and azygous veins. The effect of aortocaval compression varies from asymptomatic mild hypotension to cardiovascular collapse and is usually prevented or relieved by left tilt or wedging, although complete lateral position is required in some cases. In the event of cardiac arrest the uterus may be manually displaced to the left if a wedge or tilting table is not present.

Regional blood flow

Blood flow to various organs increases, especially the uterus and placenta, where it rises from 85 to 500 ml min^{-1} (Fig. 43.3).

Blood flow to the nasal mucosa is increased. Nasal intubation may be associated with epistaxis.

There is a considerable increase in blood flow to the skin, resulting in warm, clammy hands and feet. This vasodilatation, together with that in the nasal mucosa, helps dissipate heat from the metabolically active fetoplacental unit.

Respiratory changes (Table 43.2)

Respiratory function undergoes several important modifications as a result of the actions of progesterone.
- The larger airways dilate, and airway resistance decreases.
- There are increases in tidal volume (from 10–12 weeks' gestation) and minute volume (by up to 50%).
- Progesterone exerts a stimulant action on the respiratory centre and carotid body receptors.
- Alveolar hyperventilation leads to a low arterial carbon dioxide tension (Pa_{CO_2}) during the second and third trimesters. By the 12th week of pregnancy, Pa_{CO_2} may be as low as 4.1 kPa.
- The respiratory alkalosis is accompanied by a decrease in plasma bicarbonate concentration resulting from renal excretion (base deficit increases from 0 to −3.5 mmol L^{-1}). Arterial pH does not change significantly.
- The oxyhaemoglobin dissociation curve is shifted to the right because the increase in red cell 2,3-diphosphoglycerate (2,3-DPG) concentration outweighs the effects of a low

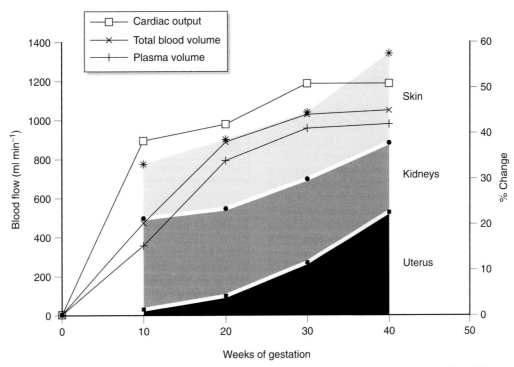

Fig. 43.3 Diagrammatic representation of changes in blood flow to various organs during pregnancy, together with percentage changes in cardiac output and blood and plasma volumes.

Table 43.2 Changes in respiratory function in pregnancy

Variable	Non-pregnant	Term pregnancy
Tidal volume ↑	450 ml	650 ml
Respiratory rate	16 min^{-1}	16 min^{-1}
Vital capacity	3200 ml	3200 ml
Inspiratory reserve volume	2050 ml	2050 ml
Expiratory reserve volume ↓	700 ml	500 ml
Functional residual capacity ↓	1600 ml	1300 ml
Residual volume ↓	1000 ml	800 ml
PaO_2 slight ↑	11.3 kPa	12.3 kPa
$PaCO_2$ ↓	4.7–5.3 kPa	4 kPa
pH slightly ↑	7.40	7.44

PaO_2, Arterial oxygen tension; $PaCO_2$, arterial carbon dioxide tension.

PCO_2, which would normally shift the curve to the left. The P_{50} increases from about 3.5 to 4.0 kPa. The oxy-haemoglobin dissociation curve of haemoglobin F (HbF) is to the left of that for HbA. The loading–unloading advantages of HbF are at *low* oxygen tensions. Placental exchange of oxygen is regulated mainly by a change in oxygen affinities of HbA and HbF caused principally by altered hydrogen ion and carbon dioxide concentrations on both sides of the placenta.

- The double Bohr and double Haldane effects maintain efficiency of gas transfer.
- The functional residual capacity (FRC) and residual volume are reduced at term because of the enlarged uterus (Table 43.2). This substantial reduction, combined with the increase in tidal volume, results in large volumes of inspired air mixing with a smaller volume of air in the lungs. The composition of alveolar gas may be altered with unusual rapidity and alveolar and arterial hypoxia develop more quickly than normal during apnoea or airway obstruction. In normal pregnancy, closing volume does not intrude into tidal volume.
- Oxygen consumption ($\dot{V}O_2$) increases gradually from 200 to 250 ml min^{-1} at term (up to 500 ml min^{-1} in labour). Carbon dioxide production parallels oxygen consumption. In the intervillous space the diffusion gradient for oxygen

Interstitial oedema of the upper airway, especially in pre-eclampsia
Enlarged tongue and epiglottis
Enlarged, heavy breasts that may impede laryngoscope introduction
Increased oxygen consumption
Restricted diaphragmatic movement, reducing FRC

FRC, Functional residual capacity.

Table 43.4 Liver function and enzyme changes in pregnancy

Measure	Change in pregnancy
Albumin	Decreased
Alkaline phosphatase	Increased (from placenta)
ALT/AST	No change
Plasma cholinesterase	Decreased

ALT, Alanine aminotransferase; *AST,* aspartate aminotransferase.

Table 43.3 Renal changes in pregnancy

Measure	Non-pregnant	Pregnant
Urea (mmol L^{-1})	2.5–6.7	2.3–4.3
Creatinine (μmol L^{-1})	70–150	50–75
Urate (μmol L^{-1})	200–350	150–350
Bicarbonate (mmol L^{-1})	22–26	18–26
24-h creatinine clearance	Increased	

Table 43.5 Haematological changes associated with pregnancy

Variable	Non-pregnant	Pregnant
Haemoglobin (g dl^{-1})	140	120
Haematocrit	0.40–0.42	0.31–0.34
Red cell count (L^{-1})	4.2×10^{12}	3.8×10^{12}
White cell count (L^{-1})	6.0×10^{9}	9.0×10^{9}
Erythrocyte sedimentation rate	10	58–68
Platelets (L^{-1})	$150–400 \times 10^{9}$	$120–400 \times 10^{9}$

is approximately 4.0 kPa, and for carbon dioxide is approximately 1.3 kPa.

Overall several changes occur in pregnancy that contribute to airway difficulty and an increased rate of development of hypoxaemia during apnoea (Box 43.1).

Renal changes

Renal changes are shown in Table 43.3.

Renal blood flow is increased (see Fig. 43.3). By 10–12 weeks, glomerular filtration rate (GFR) has increased by 50% and remains at that concentration until delivery. Glycosuria often occurs because of decreased tubular reabsorption and the increased load. The renal pelvis, calyces and ureters dilate as a result of the action of progesterone and intermittent obstruction from the uterus, especially on the right.

Gastrointestinal changes

Gastrointestinal changes also stem from the effects of progesterone on smooth muscle.

A reduction in lower oesophageal sphincter pressure occurs before the enlarging uterus exerts its mechanical effects (an increase in intragastric pressure and a decrease in the gastro-oesophageal angle). These mechanical effects are greater when there is multiple pregnancy, hydramnios or morbid obesity. A history of heartburn denotes a lax gastro-oesophageal sphincter.

Placental gastrin increases gastric acidity. Together with the sphincter pressure changes, this makes regurgitation and inhalation of acid gastric contents more likely to cause pneumonitis in pregnancy.

Gastrointestinal motility decreases but gastric emptying is not delayed during pregnancy. However, it is delayed during labour but returns to normal by 18 h after delivery. Thus women are at risk of regurgitation of gastric contents during this time. Pain, anxiety and systemic opioids (including epidural and subarachnoid administration of opioids) aggravate gastric stasis. Small and large intestinal transit times are increased in pregnancy and may result in constipation.

Changes in liver function and blood tests are summarised in Table 43.4. Liver blood flow is *not* increased.

Haematological changes (Table 43.5)

- Red cell volume increases linearly but not as much as plasma volume, which results in decreased haematocrit (physiological anaemia of pregnancy).

- Haemoglobin concentration decreases from 140 to 120 g L^{-1}.
- Decreased haematocrit promotes blood flow by reducing the blood viscosity.
- Cell-mediated immunity is depressed.
- There is an increase in platelet production, but the platelet count falls because of increased activity and consumption. Platelet function remains normal.
- Haematological changes return to normal by the sixth day after delivery.

Coagulation

Pregnancy induces a hypercoagulable state. Coagulation and fibrinolysis generally return to pre-pregnant levels 3–4 weeks postpartum. These changes are summarised in Box 43.2.
- There is an increase in the majority of clotting factors, a decrease in the quantity of natural anticoagulants and a reduction in fibrinolytic activity.
- Fibrinolysis decreases as a result of decreased tissue plasminogen activator (t-PA) activity because of inhibitors produced by the placenta.
- Bleeding time, prothrombin time and partial thromboplastin time remain within normal limits. Thromboelastography may be useful to assess platelet function and clot stability, but its use in pregnancy is unproven.
- The increase in clotting activity is greatest at the time of delivery, with placental expulsion releasing thromboplastic substances. These substances stimulate clot formation to stop maternal blood loss.

Box 43.2 Coagulation changes in late pregnancy

Fibrinogen increased from 2.5 (non-pregnant value) to 4.6–6.0 g L^{-1}
Factor II slightly increased
Factor V slightly increased
Factor VII increased 10-fold
Factor VIII increased – twice non-pregnant state
Factor IX increased
Factor X increased
Factor XI decreased 60%–70%
Factor XII increased 30%–40%
Factor XIII decreased 40%–50%
Antithrombin IIIa decreased slightly
Plasminogen unchanged
Plasminogen activator reduced
Plasminogen inhibitor increased
Fibrinogen-stabilising factor decreases gradually to 50% of non-pregnant value

---

The epidural and subarachnoid spaces

The epidural space in pregnancy

In pregnancy the epidural veins are dilated by the action of progesterone. These valveless veins of Batson form collaterals and become engorged as a result of aortocaval compression during a uterine contraction or secondary to raised intrathoracic or intra-abdominal pressure (e.g. coughing, sneezing or expulsive efforts of parturition). The dose of local anaesthetic for epidural analgesia or epidural/subarachnoid anaesthesia is reduced by about one third for the following reasons:
- Spread of local anaesthetic in either the subarachnoid or epidural space is more extensive as a result of the reduced volume.
- Progesterone-induced hyperventilation leads to a low $PaCO_2$ and a reduced buffering capacity; thus local anaesthetic drugs remain as free salts for longer periods.
- Pregnancy itself produces antinociceptive effects. The onset of nerve block is more rapid, and human peripheral nerves have been shown to be more sensitive to lidocaine during pregnancy. Increased plasma and CSF progesterone concentrations may contribute towards the reduced excitability of the nervous system.
- Increased pressure in the epidural space facilitates diffusion across the dura and produces higher concentrations of local anaesthetic in CSF.
- Venous congestion of the lateral foramina decreases loss of local anaesthetic along the dural sleeves.

During contractions, particularly in the second stage, the pressure in the subarachnoid and epidural space becomes very high. Consequently, it is advised not to advance an epidural needle, insert epidural catheters or administer epidural top-ups at that time.

Even if precautions are taken to prevent it, intermittent aortocaval compression always occurs in association with maternal movement. Consequently the epidural veins become intermittently and unpredictably engorged.

Pain pathways in labour and caesarean section

The afferent nerve supply of the uterus and cervix is via Aδ and C fibres, which accompany the thoracolumbar and sacral sympathetic outflows. The pain of the first stage of labour is referred to the spinal cord segments associated with the uterus and the cervix, namely T10–12 and L1. Pain of distension of the birth canal and perineum is conveyed via S2–4 nerves (Fig. 43.4). When anaesthesia is required for caesarean section, all the layers between the skin and the uterus must be anaesthetised. It is important to remember that the most sensitive layer is the peritoneum, and therefore the block

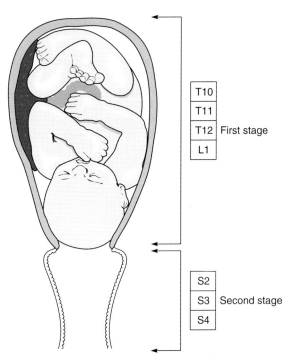

Fig. 43.4 Nerve supply to the uterus and birth canal.

T10
T11
T12 First stage
L1

S2
S3 Second stage
S4

should extend up to at least T4 and also include the sacral roots (S1–5) to cold and T5 to touch.

The placenta

The placenta is both a barrier and link between the fetal and maternal circulations. It consists of both maternal and fetal tissue – the basal and chorionic plates, separated by the intervillous space.

The two circulations are separated by two layers of cells – the cytotrophoblast and the syncytiotrophoblast. Fetal well-being depends on placental blood flow. Placental blood flow depends on the perfusion pressure across the intervillous space and the resistance of the spiral arteries. The spiral and uterine arteries possess α-adrenergic receptors. Placental perfusion is reduced by a reduction in cardiac output (e.g. haemorrhage) or uterine hypertonicity (e.g. overstimulation with Syntocinon).

Functions of the placenta

Transport of respiratory gases

Transport of respiratory gases is the most important function of the placenta and was described earlier.

Hormone production

Human chorionic gonadotrophin (hCG) is secreted by placental syncytiotrophoblasts. Production commences very early in pregnancy and peaks at 8–10 weeks. It stimulates the corpus luteum to secrete progesterone. The hCG concentrations increase again near term gestation, but its role in late pregnancy is unclear.

Human placental lactogen (hPL) has similar effects to growth hormone and causes maternal insulin resistance.

Oestrogens are secreted by the placenta and have a role in breast and uterus development. Progesterone is secreted by the placenta (see earlier).

Immunological

The placenta modifies the fetal and maternal immune system so that the fetus is not rejected.

Immunoglobulin G (IgG) is transferred across the placenta and confers some passive immunity but may also produce disease.

There is a reduction in cell-mediated immunity.

Placental transfer of drugs

The barrier between maternal and fetal blood is a single layer of chorion united with fetal endothelium. The surface area of this is vastly increased by the presence of microvilli. Placental transfer of drugs occurs, therefore, by passive diffusion through cell membranes, which are lipophilic. However, this membrane appears to be punctuated by channels that allow transfer of hydrophilic molecules at a rate that is around 100,000 times lower.

Drugs cross the placenta by simple diffusion of unionised lipophilic molecules. Fick's law of diffusion applies. The rate is directly proportional to the materno–fetal concentration gradient and the area of the placenta available for transfer, and inversely proportional to placental thickness.

Factors determining placental transfer

Materno–fetal concentration gradient

Drug transfer occurs down a concentration gradient in either direction. The maternal drug concentration depends on the route of administration, dose, volume of distribution, drug clearance and metabolism. The highest concentration is achieved after intravenous administration, although epidural and intramuscular administration result in similar concentrations. Fetal drug concentration depends on the usual factors of redistribution, metabolism and excretion. The fetus eliminates drugs less effectively because its enzyme systems are immature. The distribution differs because of the anatomical and physiological organisation of the fetal circulation; for example, drugs accumulate in the liver because of the umbilical venous flow to the liver and are metabolised before distribution. The relatively high extracellular fluid volume explains the large volumes of distribution of local anaesthetics and muscle relaxants.

Molecular weight and lipid solubility

The placental membrane is freely permeable to lipid-soluble substances, which undergo flow-dependent transfer. The majority of anaesthetic drugs are small (molecular weights of less than 500 Da) and lipid soluble and so cross the placenta readily. The main exceptions are the neuromuscular blocking drugs.

Protein binding

A dynamic equilibrium exists between bound (unavailable) and unbound (available) drug. Reduced albumin concentration increases the proportion of unbound drug. Many basic drugs are bound to α_1-glycoprotein, which is present in much lower concentrations in the fetus than in the adult.

Degree of ionisation

The placental membrane carries an electrical charge; ionised molecules with the same charge are repelled, whereas those with the opposite charge are retained within the membrane. The rate of this permeability-dependent transfer is inversely proportional to molecular size. Size limitation for polar substances begins at molecular weights between 50 and 100 Da. Ions diffuse much more slowly. Factors affecting the degree of ionisation alter the rate of transfer.

Maternal and fetal pH

Changes in maternal or fetal pH alter the degree of ionisation and protein binding of a drug and thus its availability for transfer. This has most significance if the pKa is close to physiological pH (local anaesthetics) and is clinically relevant in the acidotic fetus. Fetal acidosis increases the ionisation of the transferred drug, which is then unable to equilibrate with the maternal circulation, resulting in accumulation of the drug. This is known as ion trapping.

The degree of ionisation of acidic drugs is greater on the maternal side and lower on the fetal side. The converse applies for basic drugs.

Placental factors and uteroplacental blood flow

Placental drug transfer depends on the area of the placenta available for transfer. Physiological shunting occurs, and in pre-eclampsia the placenta itself may present an increased barrier to transfer.

Effects of drugs on the fetus

Drugs may have a harmful effect on the fetus at any time during pregnancy. In the early stages of pregnancy (at a stage when the woman may be unaware that she is pregnant), the conceptus is a rapidly dividing group of cells and the effect of drugs at that stage tends to be an all-or-nothing phenomenon, either slowing cell division if no harm is done or causing death of the embryo. Drugs may produce congenital malformations (teratogenesis), and the period of greatest risk is from weeks 3–11. In the second and third trimesters, drugs may affect the functional development of the fetus or have toxic effects on fetal tissues. Drugs given in labour or near delivery may adversely affect the neonate after delivery. Hence, drugs should be prescribed in pregnancy only if the perceived benefit of the therapy to the mother outweighs the possible detrimental effects on the fetus.

Effects of drugs on the neonate

The ratio of maternal vein to umbilical vein concentration is commonly quoted but indicates the situation at delivery only and gives little information about the effects or distribution of the drug in the neonate.

- *Inhalational anaesthetics.* Provided that the induction–delivery interval is short, the fetus is minimally affected. Neonatal elimination is dependent on ventilation.
- *Neuromuscular blocking drugs.* These cross the placenta very slowly. Bolus doses of suxamethonium and rocuronium are safe.
- *Thiopental.* Crosses the placenta rapidly, with umbilical vein concentration closely following the relatively rapid decrease in maternal blood concentration. Fetal plasma concentration continues to increase for around 40 min after single exposure. However, because of the relatively large fetal volume of distribution, fetal and neonatal tissue concentrations are lower than maternal. Doses of thiopental greater than 8 mg kg^{-1} have been shown to produce neonatal depression. Lower inductions doses do not affect Apgar score or umbilical cord gas tensions but may produce subtle changes in the neuroadaptive capacity score (NACS), such as reduction in muscular tone, decreased excitability and a predominant sleep state in the first day of life.
- *Propofol.* There is conflicting evidence concerning the effects of propofol on the neonate. Induction doses as low as 2–3 mg kg^{-1} and maintenance doses as low as 5 mg kg^{-1} h^{-1} have been found to cause significant neonatal depression. Neonatal elimination of propofol is slower than that in adults. Several comparative studies of propofol and thiopental have shown no difference in neonatal outcome.
- *Diazepam.* Should be avoided if possible. The neonate may suffer from respiratory depression, hypotonia, poor thermoregulation and raised bilirubin concentrations.
- *Opioids.* Opioids or other sedative drugs may cause a flat cardiotocograph (CTG) trace with loss of beat-to-beat variability. Meperidine and its metabolite norpethidine depress all aspects of neurobehaviour in the neonate. Neonatal elimination is slow, resulting in prolongation of the effects. Transfer of meperidine is increased in the

presence of fetal acidosis. Depressant effects are maximum if administration to delivery time is 2–3 h. Fentanyl rapidly crosses the placenta. Apgar scores are low after administration of i.v. fentanyl. Epidural administration of fentanyl in doses of less than 200 µg is not associated with any adverse effect on the fetus. Theoretically, Apgar and neurobehavioural scores should be less affected with alfentanil.

- Remifentanil crosses the placenta readily but appears to have few adverse effects on the fetus/neonate because it is rapidly metabolised. It can be used for PCA in labour (see later).
- NSAIDs should be avoided in pregnancy because they can result in premature closure of the ductus arteriosus and premature birth.

Lactation and drugs in obstetric anaesthesia

Many women wish to suckle their infant immediately after delivery and are encouraged to do so.

The effects of a drug administered to the mother on a breastfeeding neonate are determined by peak plasma concentration of the drug, its transfer into milk, composition of milk, volume ingested, metabolism (including first-pass metabolism by the neonate), pharmacokinetics and action in the neonate. Colostrum is more likely to be contaminated by water-soluble drugs, whereas lipid-soluble drugs are secreted into mature milk. The pH of mature human milk is 7.09. Therefore weak acids are less easily transferred than weak bases.

The pharmacokinetics of drugs in the neonate may differ markedly from those in adults. Lipophilic and acidic drugs are bound to albumin and may displace unconjugated bilirubin. Metabolic and excretory pathways are immature, so elimination may be delayed.

- *Opioids.* Morphine appears safe with conventional administration. Patient-controlled analgesia may increase maternal plasma concentration. It is transferred readily to breast milk but does not appear to cause neonatal depression, possibly because of first-pass metabolism. A European review of the safety of codeine-containing medicines licensed for pain relief in children began after cases of respiratory depression in children given codeine after adenoidectomy and tonsillectomy. As a result codeine has been restricted in its use in children and is contraindicated in breastfeeding mothers because of the potential harm to babies. Meperidine is associated with neurobehavioural depression of the neonate. Short-acting opioids such as fentanyl and alfentanil are safe, even by continuous epidural infusion.
- *Non-steroidal anti-inflammatory drugs.* The NSAIDs ibuprofen, ketorolac and diclofenac are safe. The neonate has immature biotransformation and excretory pathways. Aspirin should be avoided because high concentrations

have been observed after a single oral dose. Neonates may be at risk of developing Reye's syndrome.

- *Paracetamol.* Paracetamol is minimally secreted into breast milk. However, it is cleared by the neonatal liver more slowly than in adults. It is considered safe.
- *Thiopental and propofol.* These drugs are detectable in milk and colostrum. However, the dose received by the neonate after a single induction dose is insignificant.
- *Diazepam.* Diazepam and its metabolites are excreted in breast milk. As with placental transfer, there is the possibility of adverse effects on the neonate, especially with continuous administration.
- *Lidocaine and bupivacaine.* The amounts excreted in breast milk are small or undetectable.

Pharmacology of relevant drugs

The detailed pharmacology of the drugs used during pregnancy is covered elsewhere, but the following are of particular relevance to the obstetric anaesthetist.

Uterotonic drugs

Syntocinon (oxytocin)

Syntocinon is a synthetic analogue of the posterior pituitary hormone oxytocin, which is responsible for effective uterine muscle contraction. It is used during labour to augment progress, at delivery to aid placental delivery and closure of uterine vasculature and in the postpartum period to reduce postpartum haemorrhage. For augmentation or induction of labour, Syntocinon is usually administered via a syringe or volumetric pump using an increasing dose. The usual dose at delivery is 5 IU, and 40 IU may be infused over 4 h to maintain myometrial contraction and reduce bleeding.

Syntocinon may cause vasodilatation and tachycardia and so boluses should be administered cautiously in the presence of hypovolaemia and in patients with significant cardiac disease. Lower bolus doses (0.3–1 IU) may be equally effective with fewer side effects. Syntocinon also has an antidiuretic hormone effect, so care should be taken if infused in dilute dextrose solution, as hyponatraemia may occur.

Carbetocin

Carbetocin is a long-acting oxytocin analogue that can be given as a single dose to prevent postpartum haemorrhage as an alternative to an infusion of Syntocinon. The optimal dose is probably 100 µg intravenously at caesarean section. It has a plasma half-life between four and ten times that of Syntocinon.

Ergometrine

Ergometrine is also given to stimulate uterine contraction, usually in a dose of 500 µg. Ergometrine causes peripheral vasoconstriction, which may be severe, leading to hypertension and pulmonary oedema; thus it should be avoided in women with hypertensive disease. It can cause nausea and vomiting as a result of its action on other types of smooth muscle, and it is usually reserved for more severe cases of uterine atony.

Syntometrine

Syntometrine is a combination of ergometrine 500 µg and Syntocinon 5 units. Until recently, it was administered routinely by intramuscular injection at the delivery of the anterior shoulder to assist in placental separation and to reduce postpartum haemorrhage; however, Syntocinon alone is now favoured because of its reduced side effect profile.

Prostaglandins

Prostaglandins are a group of endogenous short polypeptides with a wide diversity of physiological functions. Prostaglandins are commonly used to 'ripen' the cervix on induction of labour but may cause bronchospasm and hypertension.

Carboprost

Carboprost is prostaglandin $F_2\alpha$. It has an important role in the treatment of severe uterine atony unresponsive to Syntocinon or ergometrine. It is administered intramuscularly (250 µg) at 15 min intervals to a maximum dose of 2 mg. It should **not** be given intravenously or intramyometrially. It may induce bronchospasm and hypertension and should be avoided in patients with asthma.

Misoprostol

Misoprostol is a prostaglandin E_1 analogue. It may be used to induce labour and is given vaginally. It may be given as third or fourth line treatment of postpartum haemorrhage (600 µg p.r.). It produces pyrexia, shivering, nausea and vomiting and diarrhoea.

Dinoprostone

Dinoprostone is prostaglandin E_2 given as a gel, tablets or pessary to induce labour by ripening the cervix before rupture of membranes and intravenous infusion of Syntocinon.

Mifepristone (RU486)

Mifepristone is a prostaglandin antagonist that causes luteolysis and trophoblastic separation. It is given orally with prostaglandins to induce labour after intrauterine death of the fetus and when labour is induced for a non-viable fetus. It is associated with headache, dizziness and gastrointestinal upset.

Tocolytic drugs

β₂-adrenergic receptor agonists (terbutaline, salbutamol, ritodrine)

β_2-Adrenergic agonists act on uterine β_2-receptors, causing relaxation of the myometrium. They can be given orally, subcutaneously or by intravenous infusion for premature labour. The effects should be monitored carefully because severe tachycardia, hypotension, pulmonary oedema, hypokalaemia and hyperglycaemia may occur.

The drugs may also be given by slow i.v. bolus injection (salbutamol or terbutaline 100–250 µg) as part of an *in utero* fetal resuscitation regimen before emergency caesarean section.

Oxytocin antagonists (atosiban)

Atosiban is an oxytocin antagonist used to decrease uterine contractions; it has few adverse effects but it is expensive.

Glyceryl trinitrate

Glyceryl trinitrate (GTN) acts directly on uterine smooth muscle and can be given intravenously (50 µg) or sublingually (200–400 µg) to produce rapid but short-term uterine relaxation. It can be used as part of intrauterine resuscitation, or in cases of uterine hypertonicity, retained placenta and uterine inversion. It causes hypotension and headache.

Indomethacin

Indomethacin is an NSAID and a prostaglandin synthetase inhibitor. It may be given orally or rectally to inhibit contractions after cervical cerclage. It can cause premature closure of the fetal ductus arteriosus and therefore should not be used after 32 weeks' gestation.

Basic obstetrics

Labour

A large number of pregnant women are assessed as being low risk and are predicted to have an uncomplicated labour, though this can only be confirmed in retrospect. The features of good progress in labour are:
- contractions occurring every 3 min and lasting 45 s;
- progressive dilatation of the cervix (approximately 1 cm h⁻¹);

- progressive descent of the presenting part;
- vertex presenting with the head flexed and the occiput anterior;
- labour not less than 4 h (precipitate) or more than 18 h (prolonged);
- delivery of a live healthy baby;
- delivery of a complete placenta and membranes; and
- no complications.

The first stage of labour

Initially the cervix effaces (i.e. becomes thin along its vertical axis and soft in consistency) and then cervical dilatation begins. The rate of cervical dilatation should be about 1 cm h^{-1} for a nulliparous woman and 2 cm h^{-1} for a multiparous woman. It is standard practice to examine the woman every 4 h, or more frequently if there is cause for concern. Indications for continuous electronic fetal monitoring (EFM) include insertion of an epidural, meconium-stained liquor, oxytocin for augmentation, abnormal fetal heart rate on auscultation, maternal pyrexia, fresh vaginal bleeding and maternal request.

The second stage of labour

The second stage of labour starts at full dilatation of the cervix and ends at the delivery of the baby. At full dilatation of the cervix, the character of the contractions changes and they become associated with a strong urge to push. In normal labour, Ferguson's reflex occurs, in which there is an increase in circulating oxytocin secondary to distension of the vagina from the descending presenting part of the fetus, with consequent increased strength of uterine contractions at full dilatation. Epidural analgesia may attenuate the effect of this reflex. The second stage of labour may be classified into passive and active stages, and this is particularly relevant when epidural analgesia is used. With epidural analgesia, the labouring woman does not have the normal sensation at the start of the second stage of labour produced by Ferguson's reflex, and therefore the active stage of pushing should start only when the vertex is visible or the woman has a strong urge to push. If the active second stage is prolonged, the fetus may become acidotic. A diagnosis of delay is made after 2 h in nulliparous women and 1 h in primiparous and multiparous women.

The third stage of labour

The third stage of labour is the complete delivery of the placenta and membranes and contraction of the uterus. An uncomplicated delivery can have physiological management of the third stage involving no prophylactic uterotonics and no clamping or cutting the cord until the placenta is delivered. Gravity and maternal effort assist placental delivery. Active management shortens the duration of the third stage

of labour and reduces the risk of postpartum haemorrhage. It involves prophylactic uterotonics, cord clamping and controlled cord traction. Delayed cord clamping, after at least 1 min, is currently the National Institute for Health and Care Excellence (NICE) recommended practice and has been found to improve the iron status of neonates. The cord may be clamped earlier if there is a need for neonatal resuscitation or concerns regarding cord integrity.

During the third stage of labour, there is redistribution of the former placental blood flow (about 15% of cardiac output). This results in an increase in circulating blood volume, which is potentially dangerous to women who have cardiac disease because it may precipitate heart failure immediately postpartum.

Fetal monitoring

Recent developments have made it possible to assess fetal well-being in the antenatal period. An obstetric anaesthetist is often involved when a decision to deliver the baby early is made on the outcome of these assessments. The most commonly used tests are:
- serial ultrasonography
- serial umbilical artery Doppler flow studies; and
- CTG monitoring.
   Fetal well-being during labour may be monitored using the following methods:
- Fetal heart auscultation
- Fetal heart cardiotocography
- Colour of the liquor
- Fetal blood sampling
   When the fetus becomes hypoxic, there is an accumulation of lactic acid and a reduction in fetal pH. Fetal blood sampling allows more accurate assessment of fetal well-being than is afforded by the CTG and should be performed whenever there is anxiety about the CTG or when there is meconium in the liquor. Fetal blood sampling should be performed in the left lateral position to avoid aortocaval obstruction.
   Values for fetal pH are as follows:
- pH >7.25: normal
- pH 7.21–7.24: borderline result, and sampling should be repeated 30 min later
- pH ≤7.20: abnormal result requiring urgent delivery of the baby

Urgency of caesarean section

Urgency of delivery is guided by the results of fetal monitoring (Table 43.6).

Umbilical cord blood analysis

Umbilical cord blood gases may be of value in auditing outcomes of labour and predicting future development of

Table 43.6 Classification relating the degree of urgency of caesarean section to the presence or absence of maternal or fetal compromise

Urgency	Definition	Category
Maternal or fetal compromise	Immediate threat to life of woman or fetus	1
	No immediate threat to life of woman or fetus	2
	Requires early delivery	3
No maternal or fetal compromise	At a time to suit the woman and maternity services	4

the newborn, although opinion on their prognostic value varies. If the fetus is deprived of adequate oxygenation during labour – for example, through placental malfunction, cord compression or excessive uterine contractions – anaerobic metabolism is activated and lactic acid is produced, causing the pH to drop and base deficit to increase. Fetuses with limited metabolic reserve, such as those that are growth restricted or preterm, are less able to withstand the effects of hypoxaemia. Umbilical cord *arterial* (A) blood normally reflects fetal acid–base balance, whereas *venous* (V) blood reflects a combination of maternal acid–base status and placental function. Both should be taken as it ensures that an arterial sample has definitely been obtained. The combination of results also provides further information. A large A–V difference may suggest an acute reduction in fetal blood flow, whereas both venous and arterial acidaemia suggest fetal hypoxia is not acute in onset, especially in the case of metabolic acidaemia.

Physiologically significant values below which long-term sequelae are more likely are:

- arterial pH ≤ 7.00 base deficit ≥ 12 mmol L^{-1}
- venous pH ≤ 7.10 base deficit ≥ 10 mmol L^{-1}

Feeding and antacid prophylaxis in labour

Mendelson first described the syndrome of aspiration of gastric contents in 1946. He described the pathological changes seen when solid food or liquid gastric contents are inhaled during anaesthesia in pregnancy. The chemical pneumonitis resulting from inhalation of acidic gastric contents in pregnancy prompted a number of recommendations, some of which still hold true today, such as increased use of local anaesthesia, alkalinisation of stomach contents before general anaesthesia and adequate delivery room equipment, including transparent masks, suction and a tilting table.

Oral intake in labour remains an area of controversy but can be managed on the basis of risk. Women at low risk of intervention are allowed to eat and drink, whereas those at high risk are allowed only clear fluids and are given regular antacids. NICE guidelines on intrapartum care produced in 2007 recommended that women may drink during established labour and be informed that isotonic drinks may be more beneficial than water. Women may eat a light diet in established labour unless they have received opioids or they develop risk factors that make a general anaesthetic more likely.

Because acid aspiration causes chemical pneumonitis, various methods are used routinely to reduce the acidity of the stomach contents. This includes non-particulate antacids such as 30 ml sodium citrate 0.3 M administered orally less than 30 min before general anaesthesia. In addition, H_2-antagonists have now become standard gastric acid prophylaxis. NICE guidelines recommend that neither H_2-receptor antagonists nor antacids should be given routinely to low-risk women, but that H_2-receptor antagonists and antacids should be considered for women who receive opioids or who have, or develop, risk factors that make a general anaesthetic more likely; for example, ranitidine 150 mg may be administered orally every 6 h throughout labour. It is routine practice to administer oral ranitidine before elective caesarean section, for example, in two doses – one the night before and the second on the morning of operation.

Pain and pain relief in labour

Many women have strong views about the pain relief they want during labour, shaped by previous experience, culture and social inputs. It is important to facilitate choice in conjunction with the presentation of accurate facts when discussing options for analgesia. Meeting women antenatally in a more relaxed setting is often invaluable in a woman with complex needs and worries.

The effect of pain and analgesia on the mother and fetus

Pain has multiple physiological and emotional effects that can affect both mother and fetus. Pain compromises

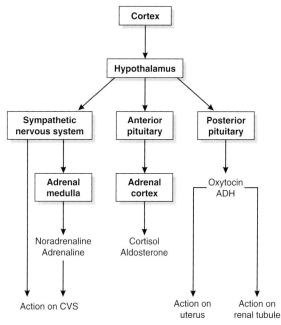

Fig. 43.5 The adverse effects of pain in labour on mother and fetus. *ADH*, Antidiuretic hormone.

placental blood flow and renders uterine contractions less effective. Increased catecholamine secretion results in increased arterial pressure and myocardial work and may also compromise blood flow to the placenta by peripheral vasoconstriction. Activation of the adrenocortical hormones may adversely affect electrolyte, carbohydrate and protein metabolism. These effects are summarised in Fig. 43.5.

The ideal analgesic

The ideal analgesic for labour should provide excellent rapid-onset pain relief in both first and second stages without risk or side effects to the mother or fetus and should also retain the mother's ability to mobilise and be independent during labour. Many women do not wish complete pain relief, and therefore the analgesic should be easy to control. There is no ideal analgesic at the present time, but it is perhaps most closely approached by low-dose central neuraxial (spinal or epidural) techniques that provide effective analgesia in more than 90% of cases while preserving motor function to a large degree. Effective epidural (or spinal) analgesia reverses the adverse physiological effects of labour pain listed earlier by blocking the psychological and biochemical stress response, resulting in improved maternal well-being and placental perfusion.

Analgesia during labour

Analgesia for labour may be classified broadly into the following areas:
- Non-pharmacological
- Parenteral
- Inhalational
- Regional

Non-pharmacological analgesia

Birth preparation classes
The goals of childbirth preparation are to inform women fully about what to expect in labour and to enhance their ability to cope without analgesia. Although there are few controlled studies on outcome, published observations do not indicate any benefits in terms of outcome of labour and reduced maternal morbidity from childbirth preparation.

Environment and the management of labour
Continuous support in labour is associated with shorter labours and reduced requirement for analgesia. Traditional cultures have always had the support of experienced women to be with the woman in labour. Midwifery (literally 'with woman') has its roots in this role of emotional support. There is a trend in the USA and UK towards the use of professional birth partners, or doulas.

Mobility in labour is helpful in maintaining the dignity and independence of the woman. Although it is thought to be helpful, there are no randomised controlled trials to support the view that pain is easier to cope with when ambulant.

Most would accept that a bath or shower is relaxing, and use of the birthing pool is increasing in popularity. The evidence regarding the first stage of labour suggests a reduction in labour pain and analgesic requirements with current evidence showing no effect on labour outcome or neonatal status. Because of difficulties managing medical emergencies in the pool, it remains an option for otherwise healthy mothers in uncomplicated labour.

Transcutaneous electrical nerve stimulation
The transcutaneous electrical nerve stimulation (TENS) electrodes should be applied at the appropriate dermatomal levels involved with the transmission of pain in labour (see Fig. 43.4). The TENS machine then emits a low background stimulus, which may be boosted with each contraction. There is little evidence that use of TENS reduces the need for analgesics, duration of labour or incidence of instrumental delivery; however, it is widely accepted by mothers and midwives because of its lack of side effects on the mother and fetus.

Complementary therapies

Hypnosis may provide reliable analgesia for a small number of women. However, they need considerable antenatal preparation and it has not proved suitable on a large scale for labour analgesia.

Acupuncture has only recently received attention for labouring women. In volunteer parturients, it was found to be ineffective in almost 80% of cases.

Aromatherapy and reflexology are also practised in labour and, although there is no trial evidence to support their use, many women gain emotional support and satisfaction from them.

Parenteral (systemic) analgesia

Many opioids have been used to provide obstetric analgesia, but the most popular have been meperidine, morphine and diamorphine. Meperidine has become established in obstetric practice without good scientific data to support its use, and in the UK two doses of 100 mg may be prescribed for a labouring woman by a midwife. Meperidine is given by intramuscular injection, and the maximum effect is seen about 1 h after administration. Subcutaneous diamorphine in doses of 2.5–10 mg is used increasingly. Diamorphine has a more rapid onset of action than meperidine and, when the two were compared, diamorphine was found to be more likely to provide some pain relief and had a lower incidence of nausea and vomiting. However, the analgesic effects of the opioids are variable and they cause significant side effects, including maternal sedation, nausea and vomiting, dysphoria and inhibition of gastric emptying. They may also have adverse effects on the fetus (see earlier) as they freely cross the placenta, potentially causing CTG abnormalities and respiratory and neurobehavioural depression of the newborn. It is standard practice for paediatric staff to be available at delivery of an infant whose mother has received meperidine within 3 h of delivery.

Several i.v. opioids have been used in PCA for labour. Remifentanil is probably the most suitable in terms of its pharmacological profile, being the most rapidly acting opioid available, with the shortest half-life. Various dosing regimens exist, such as doses of 30–50 μg with a lockout period of 2 min. However, serious maternal side effects such as respiratory depression can occur, necessitating close monitoring and continuous one-to-one care. In most units, remifentanil PCA is used only if there are contraindications to epidural analgesia.

Inhalational analgesia

The ideal inhalational agent should be a good analgesic in subanaesthetic doses, have a rapid onset of action and recovery and not accumulate. Nitrous oxide is relatively insoluble in blood and has these properties. Other inhalational agents such as isoflurane and sevoflurane have been found to be effective but have not gained widespread use because of concerns about maternal sedation and environmental pollution. In the UK, nitrous oxide is supplied as Entonox, which is 50% nitrous oxide and 50% oxygen under pressure in a cylinder (see Chapters 14 and 15). Entonox is administered usually via a demand valve with a face mask or mouthpiece. Administration needs to be timed for the maximum analgesic effect to coincide with the peak of the contraction. Most women tend to hyperventilate while breathing Entonox, and therefore there are often alternating phases of hyperventilation and then hypoventilation, especially if the Entonox is administered after meperidine. Although Entonox is a reasonably effective analgesic, many women feel faint and nauseated and may vomit or become disinhibited.

Regional analgesia for labour

Epidural and subarachnoid analgesia

Epidural and subarachnoid analgesia are the most effective forms of analgesia in labour, with up to 90% of women reporting complete or near-complete pain relief. However, they are invasive, and patients require careful monitoring.

In addition to the relief of pain and distress there are other benefits to epidural analgesia in labour. Factors that support and contraindicate the use of epidural analgesia are summarised in Table 43.7.

Technique of regional analgesia

The insertion method of epidurals and combined spinal-epidurals are discussed elsewhere in the text; however, we highlight some key aspects of importance in obstetrics. Neuraxial access can be achieved in the sitting or lateral position. The relative merits of each approach are outlined in Table 43.8.

Consent

Information should be given to the woman in the antenatal period about regional analgesia and anaesthesia. It is often difficult to explain the risks and benefits of epidural analgesia to a woman who is distressed and under the effects of opioids and Entonox. However, there is a legal, ethical and professional requirement to obtain consent before performing a procedure on a patient. Women should be presumed to have capacity to make these decisions, including refusal of treatment, except in very exceptional circumstances. Verbal consent should be obtained and the main elements of the discussion documented. Essential information should probably include partial or complete failure of the technique, dural puncture and headache, increased risk of instrumental delivery and neurological complications. Other complications are listed later in this chapter and may be discussed if time allows and the patient requires.

Table 43.7 Factors that support or contraindicate the use of epidural analgesia

Support epidural analgesia	Contraindicate epidural analgesia
Maternal request	Maternal refusal
Occipitoposterior presentation	Bleeding disorders – seek haematology advice or local guidelines (acquired or congenital)
Pregnancy-induced hypertension or pre-eclampsia	Sepsis – seek senior advice regarding risk vs. benefit (local or systemic)
Prematurity or intrauterine growth retardation	
Intrauterine death	
Induction or oxytocin augmentation of labour	
Instrumental or caesarean delivery likely	
Previous caesarean delivery	
Presence of significant concurrent disease (e.g. heart disease, diabetes, hypertension)	
Twin pregnancy	
Maternal obesity	

Table 43.8 Comparison of sitting and lateral positions for performing spinal or epidural procedures

Sitting	Lying (left lateral)
Advantages	
Midline easier to identify in obese women	Can be left unattended without risk of fainting
Obese patients may find this position more comfortable	No orthostatic hypotension Uteroplacental blood flow not reduced (particularly important in the stressed fetus)
Disadvantages	
Orthostatic hypotension may occur	More difficult to find the midline in obese patient
Increased risk of orthostatic hypotension if Entonox and meperidine have been administered	
Patient sitting on edge of bed may be too far away from a small anaesthetist for good manual dexterity	
Assistant (or partner) needed to support patient	
May be more difficult to monitor CTG	
CTG, Cardiotocograph.	

Combined spinal-epidural for labour and the 'walking' epidural

The combined spinal-epidural (CSE) was described in 1993 by anaesthetists in Queen Charlotte's Hospital in London. It was used to minimise motor block to the extent that a small proportion of their patients walked around the delivery suite. Some units use CSE routinely for labour analgesia, but in most it is reserved for women in whom rapid onset of analgesia is desirable.

Intrathecal injection of 1 ml bupivacaine 0.25% with fentanyl 25 µg was originally used, now modified to use a larger volume of low-dose mixture such as 3–3.5 ml levo-bupivacaine 0.1% and fentanyl 2 µg ml⁻¹. The intrathecal injection usually produces a rapid onset of analgesia (<5 min), and approximately 70% of patients have normal or near-normal leg power and can walk. The intrathecal injection has an analgesic duration on the order of 90 min, after which the epidural component of the CSE is used, usually starting with a bolus of 10–15 ml bupivacaine 0.1% with fentanyl 2 µg ml⁻¹, without a test dose, as described earlier. Similar degrees of mobility have been achieved using epidural boluses or infusions of low-concentration bupivacaine and fentanyl mixtures without the need for the initial intrathecal injection.

Management of the labouring woman with epidural analgesia

Posture

A labouring woman who wishes to remain supine should be positioned with at least a 15-degree left lateral tilt to prevent aortocaval compression; alternatively, and preferably, she may sit upright at an angle of 45 degrees or more. The reduction in systemic vascular resistance in women with epidural analgesia decreases the ability of the woman to maintain her arterial pressure, and therefore she is more likely to faint. In addition, the lumbosacral spine should be supported, as the epidural may allow unnatural positions to be adopted, which would usually produce discomfort in the back. Prolonged abnormal posture may contribute to low back pain after the epidural has worn off; in the past, this has been ascribed incorrectly to the epidural itself.

Mobility

The preservation of motor function and reduced need for bladder catheterisation have increased maternal satisfaction with epidural analgesia, although there have been concerns that proprioception may be affected even with this low dose of local anaesthetic, potentially making walking hazardous. The medicolegal position of the anaesthetist in the event of a fall of a parturient during a walking epidural is unclear. Nonetheless, if visual and vestibular functions are intact, proprioceptive impairment seems to have a minimal effect on walking. Many parturients do not wish to walk, and moreover, clinical trials to date have not shown that walking significantly alters outcome of labour.

Monitoring of mother and baby

NICE guidelines recommend continuous EFM for at least 30 min during establishment of regional analgesia and after administration of each further bolus of 10 ml or more.

Analgesia for the first stage of labour requires a sensory block extending from T10 to L1, whereas for the second stage, a block from S2 to S5 is desirable. The aim is to provide effective analgesia with minimal side effects. Local anaesthetics injected into the epidural space affect all nerves to some degree, in the following order: sympathetic fibres, pain fibres, proprioception fibres and finally motor fibres. The volume of local anaesthetic solution governs the spread of the block, whereas the concentration of local anaesthetic governs the density of block, with an increased risk of motor block at higher concentrations.

Maintenance of analgesia

Epidural analgesia for labour may be maintained by the following methods.

Repeated bolus administration

After the first dose has been given by the anaesthetist, boluses are usually administered as required by a midwife trained in the use of epidural analgesia. The volume and concentration need to be high enough to provide adequate analgesia, but large volumes may cause too great a spread of block, with attendant toxicity and hypotension. Bupivacaine 0.25% given in 5–10 ml boluses was standard practice until relatively recently, but in most units this has been replaced by the use of more dilute mixtures using 0.1% bupivacaine, levo-bupivacaine or ropivacaine and 2 µg ml⁻¹ fentanyl in 10–15 ml boluses. The lower concentration of local anaesthetic reduces the incidence of hypotension and increases the ability of the woman to mobilise. The disadvantage of boluses is the possibility of intermittent pain if top-ups are not administered at appropriate intervals, and the requirement for two midwives to check and administer each top-up can cause problems in busy delivery suites.

Continuous infusion by syringe pump

A mixture of local anaesthetic and fentanyl is infused epidurally at a constant rate (e.g. levobupivacaine 0.1%–0.125% or ropivacaine 0.1% containing fentanyl 2 µg ml⁻¹ at a rate of 10 ml h⁻¹). The sensory level and the analgesia should be checked regularly to maintain good pain relief. The infusion method is indicated particularly when there is a need for cardiovascular stability (e.g. the patient with cardiac disease or pre-eclampsia). It is associated with the administration of greater amounts of local anaesthetic solution and increasing motor block as labour progresses.

Patient-controlled epidural analgesia

Patient-controlled epidural analgesia (PCEA) involves establishing analgesia with an initial bolus dose and maintaining analgesia by allowing the mother to self-administer boluses of analgesic solution as required by depressing a button on a computer-controlled volumetric syringe. There may or may not be a low-dose background infusion, although background infusion does not improve the effectiveness of the epidural. The advantage of this method is that it gives more control to the mother.

Programmed intermittent epidural bolus

A programmable pump delivers a fixed epidural bolus at a set interval. This is usually combined with the facility to allow patients to self-administer additional boluses; this is then fed back to the pump to adjust the interval until next timed bolus. Multiple studies have shown this to achieve better or equivalent analgesia with smaller total doses of local anaesthetic compared with continuous infusions. Benchtop and cadaveric studies have shown that the speed of administration of a bolus compared with continuous infusion aids the spread of local anaesthetic; this is the likely cause of this effect. The smaller total dose of local anaesthetic used in programmed intermittent epidural bolus has been linked to better preserved motor function and reduced instrumental delivery rates.

Problems maintaining epidural analgesia

- *Epidural is not effective.* If the epidural is not providing good analgesia within 20 min with 15–20 ml bupivacaine 0.1% and fentanyl 2 μg ml⁻¹ or 10 ml bupivacaine 0.25%, the catheter is probably not central in the epidural space and it should be partially withdrawn. If this fails, it should be resited.
- *Missed segment or unilateral block.* Groin pain is the most common manifestation of a missed segment (i.e. L1), and it is important to ensure that the bladder is empty and the block is not unilateral. A bolus of dilute levo-bupivacaine and fentanyl or a small bolus (e.g. 5 ml levobupivacaine 0.25%) often provides analgesia. If there is persistent groin pain between contractions, the possibility of uterine dehiscence should be excluded.
- *Hypotension.* If the mother feels faint or her arterial blood pressure decreases, she should be turned on to her side to exclude aortocaval compression. Intravenous fluids and oxygen should be administered while extensive regional block is excluded. Catheter migration may occur and an accidental spinal may manifest itself at any stage of the epidural. If hypotension persists, ephedrine or phenylephrine should be administered.

Regional anaesthesia for the parturient

The common indications for anaesthesia for parturients are caesarean section, forceps delivery, retained placenta and repair of trauma to the birth canal. Regional anaesthesia is the technique of choice.

Elective caesarean section

Regional anaesthesia is the technique of choice for elective caesarean section. Though most hospitals admit women on the day of surgery, it is still important to discuss the procedure and potential risks preoperatively. It is advisable to have an information sheet for the woman before admission to hospital to support this communication. As a minimum, the woman should be informed about partial or complete failure of the regional technique, the possibility of discomfort, pain and conversion to general anaesthesia, and the risk of neurological damage. Other side effects that should be discussed are hypotension, post–dural puncture headache, motor block, and nausea and vomiting. The techniques available are:

- spinal anaesthesia;
- epidural anaesthesia; and
- combined spinal-epidural anaesthesia.

Spinal anaesthesia is the most popular choice for elective caesarean section. The CSE may be particularly useful in complex cases where the operative duration is foreseen to be longer than normal. The Third National Audit Project (NAP3) of the Royal College of Anaesthetists showed that overall obstetric neuraxial blockade had an extremely low incidence of complications; however, it is worth noting that although less than 6% of all neuroaxial blocks were CSEs, they were associated with more than 13% of the reports of harm.

As with many operative procedures there is risk of postoperative infection, and as such NICE recommends prophylactic antibiotics be given before skin incision.

Spinal anaesthesia

The method of performing spinal anaesthesia is covered elsewhere in the book; however, we highlight some key aspects of importance in obstetrics.

Most spinal anaesthetics are performed with the patient on the operating table because this reduces the need to move the patient after establishment of the block.

Hyperbaric bupivacaine 0.5% is the drug of choice, and 2.5 ml (12.5 mg) is usually sufficient. An opioid should be added to the local anaesthetic because this improves the quality of anaesthesia and provides postoperative analgesia. Fentanyl 25 μg, morphine 0.1 mg or diamorphine 0.25–0.4 mg may be used. NICE recommends diamorphine 0.3–0.4 mg, although 0.25 mg may be an easier amount to prepare, especially in an emergency. Arterial pressure should be measured at frequent intervals and the patient placed supine, ensuring that aortocaval compression is prevented by lateral tilt. The block should be tested for loss of sensation to a combination of cold and touch. It is good practice to test the block from the sacral roots to the thoracic dermatomes, even though it is unusual for a spinal block to be patchy or to miss the sacral roots. The height of the block should be T4 bilaterally to cold and T5 to touch. The level of sensory block as well as the degree of motor block should be documented.

Phenylephrine has now replaced ephedrine as the preferred vasopressor in obstetric anaesthesia because it has been shown that ephedrine causes a decrease in umbilical arterial pH and hence neonatal pH. A phenylephrine infusion is more effective than intermittent boluses in preventing hypotension after spinal anaesthesia for caesarean section. A suggested regimen starts at 40 µg min^{-1} and the infusion is then titrated according to the blood pressure. However, 100 µg phenylephrine boluses may still be used in addition to or instead of a titratable infusion. Vasopressor infusions may mask the cardiovascular changes associated with haemorrhage, and the anaesthetist should be vigilant to monitor on-table loss, remembering that vaginal losses may be hidden during surgery.

Surgery can start when the anaesthetist is content that there is good anaesthesia. Peritoneal traction and swabbing of the paracolic gutters are the most stimulating parts of the operation and the times when pain or discomfort is most likely to be experienced. Exteriorisation of the uterus is to be discouraged because this is challenging even to the most perfect block. Pain or discomfort should be treated promptly. Nitrous oxide, ketamine and/or small doses of a rapidly acting i.v. opioid such as alfentanil are all useful to control breakthrough pain. If the pain is severe, general anaesthesia should be offered and administered if appropriate. Syntocinon 5 IU as a bolus is normally administered intravenously after the delivery of the baby to assist myometrial contraction, usually followed by an infusion of 40 IU Syntocinon to maintain uterine tone, which has been shown to reduce the need for further uterotonics. Routine postoperative care should take place in a well-equipped recovery area.

Epidural anaesthesia

Epidural anaesthesia achieves greater cardiovascular stability than a single-shot spinal anaesthetic; this benefits patients with heart disease or pre-eclampsia. The disadvantages are that the onset of the block is slower than that for spinal anaesthesia and that the spread of the block may be patchy, often giving poor anaesthesia of the sacral roots. When the epidural catheter is in place, anaesthesia can be achieved by local anaesthetic, often combined with an opioid. Epidural anaesthesia for caesarean section is most commonly used when there is already an epidural catheter *in situ* for labour analgesia and the epidural is 'topped up'.

The following are standard prescriptions for an epidural anaesthetic:

- 15–20 ml bupivacaine or levobupivacaine 0.5% with or without 1 in 200,000 adrenaline – this should be given in divided doses;

- 15–20 ml lidocaine 2% with 1 in 200,000 adrenaline – this should be given in divided doses;
- a combination of bupivacaine and lidocaine;
- addition of 2 ml sodium bicarbonate 8.4% to a 20 ml top-up mixture (lidocaine + bupivacaine) is advocated by some and may speed onset;
- fentanyl 50 µg at establishment of anaesthesia or diamorphine 2.5 mg after delivery may be administered in addition to the local anaesthetic and has been shown to improve the quality of the anaesthesia;
- 10–15 ml ropivacaine 0.75%.

It is essential to test the block by testing each dermatome in a systematic way that the woman understands from the thoracic level down to the sacral roots to ensure that good anaesthesia has been produced before surgery starts.

Combined spinal-epidural anaesthesia

There are various techniques for CSE; 'needle through needle' is probably the most popular. The CSE allows increased flexibility by combining epidural and spinal blocks.

In the CSE technique, the spinal is usually conducted using the same dose of drugs as listed in the spinal section and the epidural is placed as insurance. The CSE may also be used as a sequential block, with a smaller intrathecal dose of local anaesthetic being given (e.g. bupivacaine 5–7.5 mg), followed by an epidural top-up to achieve full anaesthesia. This method provides greater cardiovascular stability because the onset of the block is slower, whereas an excellent sacral block is achieved with the spinal anaesthetic. This technique has extended the use of regional anaesthesia in pre-eclampsia.

Emergency caesarean section

Regional anaesthesia has increased in frequency for emergency caesarean section partly because of the increased use of spinal anaesthesia and the use of epidural analgesia in labour.

Topping up an existing epidural

A labour epidural may be topped up to achieve anaesthesia within 10–20 min using the prescriptions described previously under epidural for elective caesarean section. The epidural should be topped up incrementally while the patient is monitored continuously. Between 10 and 20 ml local anaesthetic solution are usually needed. While the epidural is being topped up, it is important to explain what is going to happen, to ensure that the woman understands what she is likely to feel and that help is available if pain or discomfort is experienced. There is some controversy over where the top-up should be administered; if started in the labour room, the anaesthetist must stay with the patient continuously and monitor her closely.

Spinal anaesthesia for an emergency

Spinal anaesthesia is to be encouraged for the woman who has no epidural *in situ* and who requires an emergency caesarean section. There are times when general anaesthesia is indicated, but these decrease as experience with spinal anaesthesia increases. Spinal anaesthesia may be used in the same manner as for an elective caesarean section; however, it is important to explain the procedure to the woman as fully as possible in the time available and to be present after the caesarean section to provide a better retrospective explanation of events. Follow-up is particularly important in the emergency situation. Continuous communication with the obstetric team is vital to ensure that they are assured with the state of the fetus, and the anaesthetist must be prepared to abandon the procedure and give a general anaesthetic if the obstetric team are concerned.

Rapid-sequence spinal anaesthesia aims to reduce some of the steps in the procedure and decrease the time taken, thereby increasing access to spinal anaesthesia in an emergency. The technique is controversial as its proposers advocate reduced aseptic precautions. Again, continuous communication is vital.

Forceps and ventouse delivery

Surgical anaesthesia is required for any operative delivery, except for a simple lift-out by forceps or Ventouse. For a simple lift-out, the labour epidural should be well topped up. Ideally, time to achieve good perineal anaesthesia should be allowed before the woman is placed in the lithotomy position for the assisted delivery. Bupivacaine 0.5% or lidocaine 2% with adrenaline 1 in 200,000 in a dose of around 5–10 ml is appropriate. If the delivery is more complex than a simple lift-out, surgical anaesthesia is required. It is preferable to deliver such patients in the operating theatre where caesarean section may be performed if there is any doubt about the ability to deliver the baby vaginally. Severe fetal distress may occur during attempted instrumental delivery, requiring immediate caesarean section. Therefore the anaesthetist should prepare (and assess) the anaesthetic as if for caesarean section using any of the prescriptions for caesarean delivery (spinal, CSE, epidural) described earlier.

Retained placenta

Regional anaesthesia may be used for manual removal of retained placenta after a careful assessment of blood loss. It is easy to underestimate the blood loss if there has been a continuous trickle of blood for some time. If the woman is not significantly hypovolaemic, the anaesthetic of choice is a spinal, unless there is an epidural *in situ*. Both techniques should provide good surgical anaesthesia with a block extending from at least T10 to the sacral roots.

Repair of trauma to the birth canal

The anaesthetist is often asked to provide anaesthesia for the repair of birth trauma. The full extent of the damage may not be known, as it may not be possible to examine the woman without anaesthesia. The trauma may be extensive and involve disruption of the anal sphincter, which is classified as a third-degree tear. There may be considerable blood loss and it is important to assess this before performing regional anaesthesia. If there is an epidural *in situ*, this can be topped up for the repair. If there is no epidural, then a spinal anaesthetic is the technique of choice; 1.5 ml hyperbaric bupivacaine 0.5% provides good sacral analgesia.

Failed neuroaxial anaesthesia

There are occasions when neuraxial blocks fail. This is most common when topping up a labour epidural for operative delivery, but can also occur in spinal anaesthesia. The key feature is to remember that the greater the accumulated volume of anaesthetic in the epidural or subarachnoid space the greater the likelihood of a high block or a total spinal (see later). Decision making on what to do in this circumstance is dependent on the urgency of the surgery and risk–benefit profile of general anaesthesia compared with further neuraxial block. A CSE with low-dose intrathecal component may be a potential option to avoid general anaesthesia, but decisions need to be made with the involvement of the obstetricians and mother. Calculations also need to be made regarding the total acceptable dose of local anaesthetic according to weight.

Postdelivery analgesia

The anaesthetist is usually involved in the continuing care of the woman after delivery, and this includes the provision of pain relief for:
* normal delivery;
* tears;
* forceps and Ventouse; and
* caesarean section.

Vaginal deliveries

The pain experienced after an uncomplicated vaginal delivery is caused mainly by uterine contractions and also bruising of the perineum. Simple analgesia in the form of paracetamol is usually adequate, although if there is severe bruising of the perineum, episiotomy or tears, NSAIDs are helpful (e.g. diclofenac suppositories). If the woman has had a third-degree tear repaired, she may often have had a regional anaesthetic for the repair, and the use of epidural or intrathecal opioids provides good postoperative analgesia.

Caesarean section

The extensive use of regional anaesthesia for caesarean section has led to intrathecal and epidural opioid analgesia becoming routine practice in most units. Combined with NSAIDs and paracetamol this enables women to mobilise early after caesarean section. Oral opioids are often also needed in the short term. It is prudent to have clear postoperative guidelines for the care of women in the postoperative period, and these should include use of sedation scores. Women who are unable to have NSAIDs do not have such good pain control. Women who have had the caesarean section under general anaesthesia may be managed with PCA using morphine in the same way as other postoperative patients. This is combined with NSAIDs where appropriate.

Transversus abdominis plane (TAP) blocks may be beneficial for women who have had a caesarean section under general anaesthesia but have no benefit in addition to intrathecal/epidural opioids. TAP blocks are performed under ultrasound guidance using approximately 20 ml local anaesthetic (levobupivacaine or ropivacaine) on each side.

Complications of regional anaesthesia and analgesia in obstetrics

Although regional anaesthesia is now very safe and effective, all procedures have potential complications. Repeated attempts at placement of regional blockade increases the risk of complication as well as the chances of disrupting the sterile field. It is important to call for assistance if several attempts of placement have proven unsuccessful. The general complications of regional anaesthesia are described in Chapters 25 and 26.

Shearing of the epidural catheter

An epidural catheter should not be withdrawn through a needle, as this may damage or shear the catheter. Any sheared portion of catheter is inert and sterile and thus unlikely to cause a problem, but a full account should be made in the medical record.

Post–dural puncture headache

The incidence of post–dural puncture headache (PDPH) is 0.5%–1% and is often higher in teaching hospitals. It may occur at the time of insertion of the epidural needle or be caused later by migration of the catheter into the intrathecal space (usually because of a defect in the dura caused during insertion of the needle). The clinical presentation is of an occipital headache that may radiate anteriorly, aggravated by sitting and possibly associated with nausea, distorted hearing, photophobia and, rarely, diplopia resulting from stretching of the sixth cranial nerve as it passes through the dura. The differential diagnoses of meningitis, sub-arachnoid haemorrhage, subdural haematoma, sagittal sinus thrombosis and cerebral space-occupying lesions should be considered and excluded by history, clinical examination and further investigation if needed.

Management of dural puncture and PDPH

Approximately 75% of women who receive a dural puncture with a 16–18G Tuohy needle will suffer from PDPH.

If dural puncture is recognised at the time (clear fluid flowing from the Tuohy needle), there are two options.

- The epidural can be performed in an adjacent interspace. After insertion, all drugs should be given cautiously because some local anaesthetic may migrate intrathecally.
- The epidural catheter can be threaded into the intrathecal space. The catheter must be clearly labelled as a spinal catheter. Analgesia is provided using intermittent intrathecal top-ups (e.g. bupivacaine 2.5 mg). All top-ups must be administered by an anaesthetist. Consideration should be given to leaving the catheter in place for 24 h after delivery because this may reduce the incidence of PDPH. The risks and benefits of this approach must be considered.
- All women who have had a dural puncture must be visited by an anaesthetist after delivery, and evidence of symptoms and signs of dural puncture as listed earlier should be sought. Prophylactic bed rest and an epidural infusion of saline are no longer recommended. Oral fluids should be encouraged to prevent dehydration, and simple analgesics should be prescribed. If conservative management fails to prevent the appearance of PDPH, then a number of other forms of treatment have been suggested.
- Caffeine produces cerebral vasoconstriction, and oral intake may provide symptomatic relief.
- Antidiuretic hormone may relieve symptoms by an unknown mechanism.
- Corticotrophin and sumatriptan have both been used but are probably ineffective.
- Epidural blood patch (EBP) is the definitive treatment of dural puncture. A sample of the patient's own venous blood (approximately 20 ml) is collected under aseptic conditions and injected into the same interspace at which the dural puncture occurred, or an adjacent interspace, to seal the CSF leak. It is about 75% effective (although the quoted range is 70%–98%). The procedure may be repeated with similar rates of success on the second patch. In some centres, a prophylactic blood patch is performed using the resited epidural catheter at the end of labour in an effort to reduce the risk and duration of PDPH, although there is limited evidence to support this. The exclusion of other causes of headache is important.

819

The MBRRACE Report 2014 highlights the death of two women after accidental dural puncture, where cerebral venous sinus thrombosis and subdural haematoma were missed. The report also highlights the importance of follow-up and communications with the general practitioner.

Backache

Backache is common after childbirth and affects 50% of women at some stage in pregnancy. An anaesthetist is often called to assess patients with backache if they have received an epidural. Insertion of an epidural catheter may contribute to short-term acute back pain if it causes:

- an epidural haematoma;
- an epidural infection causing abscess or meningitis; or
- local bruising.

However, long-term backache is not caused by epidural anaesthesia, which has been demonstrated clearly in two prospective studies of more than 1000 obstetric patients who were followed up on the day after delivery and 3 months later. The incidence of new-onset backache was on the order of 40%–50%, but there was no difference in the incidence of backache at 3 months between those who had received an epidural and those who had not. There was a non-significantly slightly higher chance of back pain on day 1, explained by minor local trauma.

Bloody tap

Cannulation of an epidural vessel may occur with either the needle or catheter when performing an epidural. It is important because, if undetected, it can result in intravascular injection and thus local anaesthetic toxicity. If blood flows from the needle, the needle must be withdrawn. If blood is aspirated from the catheter, it should be withdrawn incrementally and flushed with saline until aspiration of blood is no longer possible, ensuring there is still sufficient epidural catheter within the epidural space. If not, it should be reinserted.

An epidural catheter may be positioned with its tip inside a blood vessel in the absence of a bloody tap, and a test dose should always be used.

Hypotension

Hypotension is usually defined as a 25% decrease in systolic or mean arterial pressure or an absolute decrease in systolic pressure of 40 mmHg. Small decreases in pressure are insignificant and may be associated with improved utero-placental blood flow if caused by vasodilatation. Rapidly developing hypotension after spinal anaesthesia may cause unpleasant dizziness and nausea in about 50% of patients if no prophylaxis is given and should be treated with phenylephrine until arterial pressure is restored, while at the same time maintaining normovolaemia and ensuring that there is no aortocaval compression.

Neurological deficit

Neurological deficit may be caused by the drugs used for the procedure or by trauma from the needles or catheter. The incidence of temporary nerve damage is approximately 1 in 1000, permanent nerve damage (more than 6 months' duration) occurs with an incidence of approximately 1 in 13,000, and the incidence of severe injury including paralysis is about 1 in 250,000. When neuropraxia is caused by injury with the epidural needle or catheter, reassurance may be given that these symptoms usually resolve over 3–6 months, but patients should be followed up on an outpatient basis. Several peripheral nerves may be injured during delivery and falsely attributed to the epidural:

- common peroneal nerve by stirrups, causing foot drop;
- lateral cutaneous nerve of the thigh by groin pressure from the lithotomy position, causing anterolateral thigh numbness;
- femoral nerve or sciatic nerve by the lithotomy position, causing weak quadriceps with loss of knee reflex or pain in the back of the leg with loss of ankle reflex, respectively; and
- sacral plexus and obturator nerves – these cross the pelvic rim and rarely may be damaged by occipital presentation or forceps delivery.

Effect on labour and mode of delivery

Epidural analgesia for labour has been shown to prolong the second stage of labour by 15.5 min, but the clinical significance of this is unclear. It also increases the rate of instrumental delivery although this risk may be reduced by low-dose epidural techniques. Epidural analgesia does not increase the incidence of caesarean section or the length of the first stage of labour.

General anaesthesia for the parturient

Since the 1960s, the triennial UK maternal mortality report (currently termed 'Saving Mothers Lives, Improving Mothers' Care') has provided an audit of obstetric and anaesthetic practice. Recent reports have demonstrated decreasing numbers of deaths from anaesthesia. In the 1970s–1980s, the number of deaths directly caused by anaesthesia was 30–50 per 100,000 maternities; from 2009 this number has fallen to 2–4 per 100,000 maternities. The increasing safety of anaesthesia in obstetrics is the result of many factors:

- Increasing use of epidural analgesia in labour
- Increasing use of regional anaesthesia for operative delivery
- Increase in dedicated consultant obstetric anaesthetic sessions
- Improved teaching of obstetric anaesthesia
- Improved assistance for the anaesthetist
- Ongoing learning from triennial enquiries of maternal mortality

Repeated attempts to intubate the trachea whilst losing focus on oxygenation, unrecognised oesophageal intubation and gastric aspiration have been highlighted as direct causes of death in previous reports. General anaesthesia in the parturient is more than 16 times more likely to result in death than a regional anaesthetic; this is also a reflection of the fact that general anaesthesia is usually performed in emergency situations. The reducing use of general anaesthesia in obstetric anaesthesia further exacerbates this problem by decreasing experience and training opportunities.

However, general anaesthesia continues to be required in the following situations:

- In an extreme emergency, e.g. severe fetal distress or maternal haemorrhage
- When there is a contraindication to regional anaesthesia
- When the woman refuses to have a regional anaesthetic; this may be because of a previous bad experience with regional anaesthesia
- If regional anaesthesia has failed or is inadequate

The previous sections on physiology of pregnancy, anatomy and antacid therapy have highlighted many of the problems that should be considered when a pregnant woman presents for a general anaesthetic. It is essential that a thorough preanaesthetic assessment is performed, with airway evaluation and planning in case a difficult airway is encountered. It is mandatory that anaesthetists familiarise themselves with the operating theatre and the anaesthetic equipment, in addition to the guidelines and equipment that are available for difficult and failed intubation. Drugs and equipment should be checked at the beginning of each period of duty on the delivery suite so that an emergency can be dealt with in a calm and ordered manner.

Technique of general anaesthesia in obstetric practice

The method of performing rapid sequence induction is covered elsewhere in the text; however, we highlight some key aspects of importance in obstetrics. The management of failed intubation is covered later.

There is a relatively high incidence of failed intubation in obstetric patients (approximately 1 in 300 compared with 1 in 2220 in non-pregnant patients). The changes associated with pregnancy and labour cause a more rapid rate of oxygen desaturation, which is further compounded by the increasing prevalence of obesity.

Optimum positioning for intubation is of key importance, remembering to compensate for aortocaval compression. Adequate preoxygenation is usually achieved by 3 min of tidal breathing with 100% oxygen at high flow via a tight-fitting face mask. The end-tidal oxygen partial pressure should be more than 80 kPa before RSI. Consideration should be given to nasal oxygenation during induction, as well as gentle face-mask ventilation.

It is standard practice to use thiopental to induce anaesthesia, and a dose of at least 5 mg kg^{-1} is recommended in healthy parturients. Most commonly this is followed rapidly by suxamethonium 1–1.5 mg kg^{-1}. A short-acting opioid is often used at induction to counteract the pressor response of laryngoscopy, particularly in pre-eclampsia, to reduce the risk of hypertensive crisis at induction. Opioids will cause neonatal depression and should be used judiciously. There is also a growing number of obstetric anaesthetists who use propofol and rocuronium (1 mg kg^{-1}) for induction.

The use of suxamethonium originated from the fast action and short duration of action enabling a quick achievement of paralysis sufficient for intubation and early return of spontaneous ventilation in the event of failed intubation. However, life-threatening desaturation may occur before return of neuromuscular function after the administration of suxamethonium. During this period, conditions for intubation and ventilation also become suboptimal, necessitating a further dose of paralysis. Rocuronium 1.2 mg kg^{-1} has a similar speed of onset to suxamethonium in obstetrics, but optimal conditions for intubation and ventilation remain for longer after administration. Rapid reversal of rocuronium necessitates the use of sugammadex, which has additional cost. These drugs are newer agents and there is less experience with them in obstetric practice compared with suxamethonium.

The Fifth National Audit Project (NAP5) has highlighted the issue of awareness in obstetric anaesthesia, with an estimated incidence of 1:670 in general anaesthesia for caesarean section, higher than most other types of surgery. Several factors increase the risk of awareness in obstetrics, including use of lower doses of anaesthetic agents for fear of uterine relaxation or neonatal compromise, the short duration of time between induction and surgical incision, the increased incidence of failed intubation and the omission of opioids. The NAP5 report mentions that thiopental was often underdosed and that there was often a gap in the depth of anaesthesia between induction and maintenance agents. This could have been better covered using higher concentrations of volatile agent, nitrous oxide and higher gas flows to achieve the desired MAC quickly. The debate has also reopened the question of using propofol for induction, which has been linked to fewer cases of awareness. Propofol has lower risks of syringe swap compared with thiopental, which can be confused with other medications. The use of thiopental requires premixing and is more expensive than propofol. Supply problems have meant that thiopental is not readily available in many areas of the world.

Anaesthesia is maintained using nitrous oxide and a volatile anaesthetic agent in oxygen, using positive pressure ventilation. Isoflurane or sevoflurane are commonly used and should be administered to achieve a total end-tidal concentration (volatile and nitrous oxide) of at least 1.0 minimum alveolar concentration (MAC). Higher concentrations cause excessive uterine relaxation, whereas lower concentrations predispose the woman to awareness. If the fetus is compromised, there is evidence that the use of 100% oxygen with a volatile agent may be beneficial by increasing oxygen transfer across the placenta. In this situation a concomitant increase in inspired vapour concentration is needed to maintain the desired MAC without nitrous oxide until after delivery. More conventionally, gas ratios of nitrous oxide and oxygen of 66:33 are used after intubation. After the delivery of the baby, an opioid, such as morphine, may be given with Syntocinon. If suxamethonium is used, an additional non-depolarizing neuromuscular blocking agent (NMBA, e.g. atracurium 25 mg) may be administered after paralysis has worn off, as confirmed by a nerve stimulator. Residual neuromuscular block should be antagonised before tracheal extubation, with the woman in the lateral position and with a slight head-down tilt, or sitting up to reduce the risk of aspiration. Routine postoperative care in an appropriately staffed, fully equipped recovery area is essential. At this time, postoperative pain relief should be optimised and the baby should be given to the mother whenever possible.

Assessment of the pregnant woman presenting for anaesthesia and analgesia

Successive maternal mortality reports highlight the problems of women with intercurrent medical disease and the fact that they are at increased risk in pregnancy and labour. There are many more women with a coincidental significant medical problem becoming pregnant, and it is important that these problems are recognised in the antenatal period. A good history should be taken. The effect of the physiological changes of pregnancy on the disease must be recognised and appropriate investigations instigated.

Women with cardiac or respiratory disease require careful assessment because the physiological changes of pregnancy and delivery may have a profound effect on the disease. Many of these women have good reserves for normal day-to-day activities in pregnancy but are unable to cope with the added stress of labour. The 2016 Confidential Enquiry (MBRRACE) reported that heart disease was the leading cause of maternal death. The report comments on the importance of multidisciplinary work with specialists and being aware that breathlessness and tachycardia can be features of cardiac dysfunction. Aortic dissection is a rare but commonly forgotten differential, with serious consequences. Assessment includes echocardiography, ECG and pulmonary function tests. Assessment of the medical record is particularly relevant if the woman has undergone surgery. Clear plans for labour and delivery need to be written in the record by all the medical team, including the anaesthetist. Many obstetric units now run an anaesthetic obstetric clinic at which high-risk women can be assessed antenatally by a consultant anaesthetist.

The other more common medical conditions occurring in women of childbearing age are neurological disease; significant back problems, including major surgery; drug allergies; previous anaesthetic problems; and difficulties with tracheal intubation.

Obesity, maternal age and smoking are also risk factors that should not be overlooked. Obesity has been highlighted in recent MBRRACE reports as a significant characteristic amongst the women who died. Obesity in pregnancy is associated with an increased risk of a number of serious adverse outcomes, including thromboembolism, gestational diabetes, pre-eclampsia, postpartum haemorrhage, wound infections, miscarriage, stillbirth and neonatal death. There is also a higher caesarean section rate in obese women. The Royal College of Obstetricians and Gynaecologists recommends that all women with a BMI 40 or greater should have an antenatal consultation with an obstetric anaesthetist.

Emergencies in obstetric anaesthesia

The management of acute emergencies has long been a part of anaesthetic practice, and within obstetrics, key emergencies such as haemorrhage and eclampsia should be part of regular multidisciplinary training and updates. It is evident from repeated Confidential Enquiries that the diagnosis and management of critical illness such as sepsis and cardiac disease have now expanded the role of the obstetric anaesthetist into that of the peripartum acute physician. A shift in training and setup of obstetric anaesthesia services should reflect this change.

Haemorrhage

Significant bleeding occurs in 3% of all pregnancies and may happen in either the antepartum or postpartum period.

Antepartum haemorrhage

Seventy percent of all cases of antepartum haemorrhage result from placenta praevia or abruptio placentae. Placenta praevia occurs when the placenta is inserted wholly or in part into the lower segment of the uterus. It is now classified by ultrasound imaging into four grades depending on the relationship and distance to the internal cervical os (Table 43.9). If the placenta lies over the internal cervical os, it is considered a major praevia; if the leading edge of the placenta is in the lower uterine segment but not covering the cervical os, minor or partial praevia exists. Significant bleeding may occur that may necessitate blood transfusion or urgent delivery. There are four factors that increase the potential for significant bleeding.

- Veins on the anterior wall of the uterus are distended.
- If the placenta is anterior, then the surgical incision extends through the placenta, causing significant haemorrhage.
- If the placenta covers the os, then a raw area is left after its delivery. This area of the os does not have the same ability to contract as the normal myometrium and may thus continue to bleed.
- The presence of uterine scarring, such as from a previous caesarean section, predisposes to pathological invasion of the uterine wall to produce a placenta accreta. In placenta accreta the placenta grows through the endometrium to the myometrium. In placenta increta it penetrates into the myometrium. In placenta percreta the placenta penetrates through the myometrium and uterine serosa and into surrounding structures such as the bladder. This may mean that separation of the placenta and uterus is impossible and profuse bleeding occurs, which may require hysterectomy.

Women diagnosed with placenta praevia are delivered by elective caesarean section if it remains within 2 cm of the os on ultrasound. Because the condition may be associated with severe, potentially life-threatening haemorrhage, senior obstetric and anaesthetic staff should be involved with the delivery. Blood should always be cross-matched and equipment should be available to administer a high flow rate of warmed fluids (>1 L min^{-1}). Either general or regional anaesthesia may be used. Regional anaesthesia is associated with a reduced blood loss but may be associated with blood pressure changes that are difficult to manage and a potentially distressed mother. These women should be preoptimised, for example by giving iron supplements antenatally, and cell salvage should be considered. The use of interventional radiology to perform balloon occlusion or embolisation techniques in postpartum haemorrhage has been well reported. Prophylactic arterial catheters can be placed to reduce bleeding in more complex cases, though there is variable evidence for their ultimate value.

Abruptio placentae is defined as the premature separation of the placenta after the 20th week of gestation. It is associated with a perinatal mortality rate of up to 50%. Placental abruption may result in concealed or revealed haemorrhage. Typically the woman presents with abdominal pain, which may be severe, together with signs indicative of acute blood loss in proportion to the amount of blood lost. A trap for the unwary is that placental abruption may be associated with pre-eclampsia; therefore, if the preabruption arterial pressure was markedly elevated, the postabruption blood pressure may still appear normal and so mask hypovolaemia. It is also important to remember that blood loss is often concealed and so may be underestimated; a coagulopathy with low platelets tends to occur early in abruption and should be corrected aggressively.

Postpartum haemorrhage

Postpartum haemorrhage is the most common reason for surgery in the immediate postpartum period. Causes include:
- retained placental tissue, including placenta accreta.
- uterine atony – the failure of the uterus to contract at the site of placental separation. The risk of uterine atony may be increased by:
  - overdistension of the uterus (e.g. polyhydramnios, multiple gestation);
  - prolonged (>8 h) or precipitous (<4 h) labour;
  - multiparity;
  - hypotension; or
  - uterine infection.
- laceration of the birth canal – predisposing factors include instrumental delivery and a large infant.
- hypocoagulable states, such as von Willebrand's disease and HELLP (haemolysis, elevated liver enzymes and low platelets) syndrome.

Anaesthetic management of haemorrhage

Although regional anaesthesia has a role in the management of acute postpartum haemorrhage, the associated sympathetic block interferes with physiological compensatory

Table 43.9 Ultrasound-based grades of placenta praevia	
Grade	**Features**
I	Placenta lies in the lower segment, but its lower edge does not reach the internal cervical os.
II	Placental tissue reaches the margin of the internal cervical os but does not cover it.
III	Placenta partially covers the internal cervical os.
IV	Placenta completely covers the internal cervical os.

mechanisms, potentially aggravating acute hypovolaemia. For this reason, general anaesthesia is the preferred option in this situation unless plasma volume has been fully restored.

Preoperative assessment

Successive triennial maternal mortality reports have highlighted major obstetric haemorrhage as a significant cause of maternal mortality. All units should have a major obstetric haemorrhage protocol, and it is important to be familiar with local guidelines.

Estimation of the degree of blood loss is notoriously unreliable in the obstetric setting, and hence clinical estimation of blood loss and hypovolaemia is necessary. Initial assessment and management of the obstetric patient follows the same principles as any patient with major haemorrhage.

Intraoperative management

Attempts to restore circulating blood volume should precede, but not delay, definitive treatment. Rapid-sequence induction of general anaesthesia is mandatory. Care with induction agents such as thiopental and propofol is required in patients who are hypovolaemic, because profound hypotension may ensue, leading to cardiovascular collapse. Ketamine 1–2 mg kg^{-1} may be useful, as it stimulates the sympathetic nervous system and helps to preserve arterial pressure during induction of anaesthesia.

Anaesthesia may be maintained with N_2O/O_2 mixtures and an opioid such as fentanyl 1–2 µg kg^{-1}, with cautious administration of a volatile anaesthetic agent. Ultimately, hysterectomy may be a life-saving procedure and should be discussed before anaesthesia with a woman at high risk of major haemorrhage. Techniques to conserve the uterus include circumferential uterine suture, intrauterine balloon, internal iliac balloon insertion or embolisation of uterine vessels using interventional radiological techniques. Clotting factors (fresh frozen plasma, cryoprecipitate) and platelets should be administered early without awaiting results. There is a growth in the use of near-patient coagulation tests to guide the administration of blood products in haemorrhage, though the evidence is still limited in obstetrics. A large randomised controlled trial has found that tranexamic acid can reduce death from postpartum haemorrhage with no significant adverse effects. Factor VIIa (Novoseven) has evidence from case series to show a reduction in bleeding if used in postpartum haemorrhage but has associations with thromboembolic events and is not widely used. Cell salvage can be very useful if available.

Failed intubation

Failed intubation of the trachea reflects the relatively high incidence of airway difficulties in obstetric patients (approximately 1 in 300 compared with 1 in 2220 in non-pregnant patients). The increased incidence of difficult intubation in parturients is caused by changes in the soft tissues of the airway resulting in swollen upper airway mucosa, swollen and engorged breasts and full dentition. The decreasing use of general anaesthesia in obstetrics may lead to a relative lack of experience in this technique, with increased anxiety for both junior and senior anaesthetists.

In 2015 the Difficult Airway Society (DAS) and Obstetric Anaesthetists' Association (OAA) developed combined guidelines into the management of failed intubation in obstetric anaesthesia. This is an essential algorithm and should be displayed prominently in all obstetric theatres (Fig. 43.6). It is important to call for help early when unexpected difficulty with laryngoscopy or intubation arises. The algorithm stresses preinduction planning, which includes deciding on the best course of action if airway management is difficult. It also suggests considering the use of gentle face-mask ventilation during induction and nasal oxygen for apnoeic oxygenation. Failed intubation is the inability to intubate after two attempts. Repeated attempts without maintaining oxygenation should be avoided. In the presence of a poor view of the glottis at laryngoscopy, consider reducing or removing the cricoid. The insertion of a supraglottic airway device (SAD, ideally second generation) may facilitate ventilation. In the situation of adequate oxygenation via an SAD, consideration needs to be made about whether to proceed with surgery considering the features pertinent to the individual case (Fig. 43.7).

Pre-eclampsia and eclampsia

Hypertensive disorders are among the leading causes of maternal mortality. Pre-eclampsia is a multisystem disorder and is defined as hypertension after 20 weeks gestation in association with proteinuria, other maternal organ dysfunction e.g. renal insufficiency or fetal growth restriction. Eclampsia is defined as the occurrence of convulsions and/or coma during pregnancy associated with pre-eclampsia with the exclusion of other causes.

Aetiology of eclampsia and pre-eclampsia

The aetiology is unknown, but current knowledge may be summarised as follows:

- *Immunological factors.* In the normal placenta, the vascular bed is of low resistance. In pre-eclampsia there is abnormal migration of the trophoblast into the myometrial tissue, and this leads to constriction of the spiral arteries, which increases the resistance in the vascular bed. Prostacyclin and nitric oxide may be involved in this process.
- *Endothelial factors.* Normotensive pregnant women demonstrate an increase in the activity of the renin-angiotensin-aldosterone system (RAAS) and a reduced response to exogenous angiotensin II. In pre-eclamptic

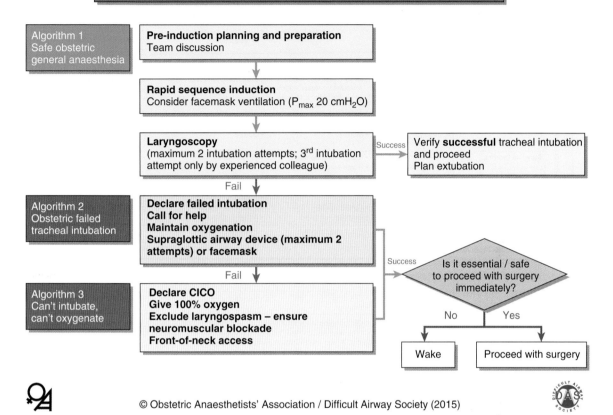

Master algorithm – obstetric general anaesthesia and failed tracheal intubation

Algorithm 1
Safe obstetric
general anaesthesia

Pre-induction planning and preparation
Team discussion

Rapid sequence induction
Consider facemask ventilation (P_{max} 20 cmH$_2$O)

Laryngoscopy
(maximum 2 intubation attempts; 3rd intubation attempt only by experienced colleague)

Success → Verify **successful** tracheal intubation and proceed
Plan extubation

Fail ↓

Algorithm 2
Obstetric failed
tracheal intubation

Declare failed intubation
Call for help
Maintain oxygenation
Supraglottic airway device (maximum 2 attempts) or facemask

Fail ↓

Success → Is it essential / safe to proceed with surgery immediately?

No → Wake
Yes → Proceed with surgery

Algorithm 3
Can't intubate,
can't oxygenate

Declare CICO
Give 100% oxygen
Exclude laryngospasm – ensure neuromuscular blockade
Front-of-neck access

© Obstetric Anaesthetists' Association / Difficult Airway Society (2015)

Fig. 43.6 Obstetric general anaesthesia, failed tracheal intubation and can't intubate, can't oxygenate (CICO) guideline – Difficult Airway Society (DAS) and Obstetric Anaesthetists' Society (OAA) 2015.

women this does not occur, and this has been linked to a lack of nitric oxide production by endothelial cells.

- *Platelet and coagulation factors.* Endothelial dysfunction may lead to a lack of nitric oxide and prostacyclin, altering the balance of platelet function in favour of platelet aggregation.

Clinical presentation of pre-eclampsia

Clinically, pre-eclampsia is a multisystem disorder, and the predominant features in each system are as described next.

Cardiovascular system

- Hypertension in pregnancy is defined as systolic arterial pressure greater than 140 mmHg and/or diastolic arterial pressure greater than 90 mmHg.

- Generalised vasoconstriction leads to an increase in systemic vascular resistance and hypertension.
- Increased capillary permeability leads to a redistribution of plasma into the interstitial space.
- Blood volume is decreased by up to 30% in severe cases
- CVP and pulmonary capillary wedge pressure may be normal.
- Low colloid oncotic pressure combined with increased capillary permeability leads to oedema. Patients with pre-eclampsia may not have a raised arterial pressure, although it is significantly raised above baseline pressure at the beginning of pregnancy.

Central nervous system

- Symptoms and signs include:
  - severe headache;
  - visual disturbances; and
  - hyperreflexia.

Table 1 – proceed with surgery?				
Factors to consider	**WAKE** ←		→	**PROCEED**
Maternal condition	• No compromise	• Mild acute compromise	• Haemorrhage responsive to resuscitation	• Hypovolaemia requiring corrective surgery • Critical cardiac or respiratory compromise, cardiac arrest
Fetal condition	• No compromise	• Compromise corrected with intrauterine resuscitation, pH < 7.2 but > 7.15	• Continuing fetal heart rate abnormality despite intrauterine resuscitation, pH < 7.15	• Sustained bradycardia • Fetal haemorrhage • Suspected uterine rupture
Anaesthetist	• Novice	• Junior trainee	• Senior trainee	• Consultant / specialist
Obesity	• Supermorbid	• Morbid	• Obese	• Normal
Surgical factors	• Complex surgery or major haemorrhage anticipated	• Multiple uterine scars • Some surgical difficulties expected	• Single uterine scar	• No risk factors
Aspiration risk	• Recent food	• No recent food • In labour • Opioids given • Antacids not given	• No recent food • In labour • Opioids not given • Antacids given	• Fasted • Not in labour • Antacids given
Alternative anaesthesia • regional • securing airway awake	• No anticipated difficulty	• Predicted difficulty	• Relatively contraindicated	• Absolutely contraindicated or has failed • Surgery started
Airway device / ventilation	• Difficult facemask ventilation • Front-of-neck	• Adequate facemask ventilation	• First generation supraglottic airway device	• Second generation supraglottic airway device
Airway hazards	• Laryngeal oedema • Stridor	• Bleeding • Trauma	• Secretions	• None evident

Rows "Maternal condition" through "Alternative anaesthesia" are grouped under "Before induction"; rows "Airway device / ventilation" and "Airway hazards" are grouped under "After failed intubation".

 Criteria to be used in the decision to wake or proceed following failed tracheal intubation. In any individual patient, some factors may suggest waking and others proceeding. The final decision will depend on the anaesthetist's clinical judgement.
© Obstetric Anaesthetists' Association / Difficult Airway Society (2015)

Fig. 43.7 Criteria to be used in the decision to wake or proceed after failed tracheal intubation – Difficult Airway Society (DAS) and Obstetric Anaesthetists' Society (OAA) 2015. (From Difficult Airway Society (DAS) and Obstetric Anaesthetists' Society (OAA) 2015.)

• Seizures may occur without warning; 40% of first fits occur in the postpartum period.

Renal system
• Endothelial damage leads to protein loss and further decrease in colloid oncotic pressure.
• Glomerular filtration rate is reduced by 25% compared with normal pregnant women, as a result of glomerular oedema.
• Increases in urea and uric acid concentrations may be used as an indicator of severity.

Haematological system
• A rapidly decreasing platelet count is indicative of a worsening of pre-eclampsia, and low platelets may be associated with HELLP syndrome.
• In general, a platelet count $\geq 80 \times 10^9$ L^{-1} (taken within the last 4 h) is safe for insertion of an epidural catheter. At levels less than this, a clotting screen is advised and the risks and benefits of regional block should be assessed.

Respiratory system
• Pre-eclampsia increases the risk of airway oedema, which may make tracheal intubation hazardous.
• Pulmonary oedema may occur at any time, including up to 24 h after delivery, as a result of increased capillary permeability and decreased colloid oncotic pressure.

Management of pre-eclampsia

Obstetric management is designed to stabilise the mother and deliver the baby. It is essential that the mother is assessed and monitored carefully. This includes full biochemical and haematological screening and monitoring of arterial pressure, heart rate, fluid balance and oxygen saturation. High-dependency care is essential. Treatment of hypertension is essential, and in the acute situation the drugs of choice are oral or i.v. labetalol, oral nifedipine and i.v. hydralazine. Aggressive treatment of severe hypertension (>170 mmHg systolic and/or >110 mmHg diastolic) is important because intracerebral haemorrhage secondary to hypertension (especially systolic) is the main cause of death in pre-eclampsia. Magnesium sulphate should be used in moderate to severe cases as prophylaxis against eclampsia. Magnesium inhibits synaptic transmission at the neuromuscular junction, causes vasodilatation and has a central anticonvulsant effect at the N-methyl-D-aspartate (NMDA) receptor. A loading dose of 4 g (in 100 ml saline) is followed by a maintenance dose of 1 g h^{-1}. Serum concentrations may be monitored along with hourly assessment of peripheral limb reflexes. As serum concentrations increase to more than 10 mmol L^{-1}, there is progressive reduction in reflexes, respiratory arrest and asystole. The therapeutic range is 4–7 mmol L^{-1}.

Pre-eclamptic patients are classically vasoconstricted and hypovolaemic, so careful fluid administration is advisable during treatment of hypertension. There is continued debate about the suitability of crystalloid or colloid in these patients; a detailed discussion of this is outside the remit of this chapter. It is important to remember that the woman may already be receiving antihypertensive therapy, such as methyldopa or nifedipine.

The role of epidural analgesia and anaesthesia in pre-eclampsia

Epidural analgesia is specifically indicated for labour analgesia in pre-eclampsia, provided that the platelet count is adequate, because:

- it provides excellent pain relief;
- it attenuates the hypertensive response to pain;
- it reduces circulating stress-related hormones and hence assists in controlling arterial pressure;
- it improves uteroplacental blood flow; and
- these women have a higher incidence of caesarean section, and the presence of an epidural allows extension of the block.

If hypotension occurs, a crystalloid bolus (500 ml) may be administered, with the patient in a lateral tilt and receiving oxygen. If this is not adequate, a bolus of phenylephrine 50–100 μg may be given; however, because of increased sensitivity of the circulation to exogenous vasopressors, caution is essential. Neuraxial anaesthesia is the anaesthetic of choice if the woman is to be delivered by caesarean section, provided that the coagulation profile and platelet count is suitable. If general anaesthesia is required, maternal stabilisation and blood pressure control is vital before intubation in order to minimise maternal risk of intracranial haemorrhage. One method of doing this is by the administration of short-acting opioids at induction.

Eclampsia

If the woman has an eclamptic fit, the 'ABCs' of basic resuscitation should be started, and it is essential that there is no compression of the aorta or vena cava during resuscitation. The treatment of eclampsia is magnesium sulphate 4 g by slow intravenous bolus as recommended in 1995 by the Eclampsia Trial Collaborative Group.

Thromboembolic disease

Until the 2006–2008 Confidential Enquiry, thromboembolic disease had been the leading cause of maternal mortality for 21 years. The rates have reduced; however, it remains an important cause of morbidity and mortality. The reduction in death rate is probably because guidelines on thromboprophylaxis for high-risk patients have since been introduced and were refined further in 2015.

- All women should be risk-assessed early in pregnancy, and high-risk patients should be given thromboprophylaxis antenatally and for up to 6 weeks postnatally.
- The dose of thromboprophylaxis should be increased appropriately for weight.
- Risk factors include pre-existing conditions such as obesity and smoking, obstetric risk factors such as caesarean section and pre-eclampsia and transient risk factors such as dehydration and systemic infection.
- Local units should have a numerical scoring risk assessment that can be used to guide treatment through pregnancy and the postpartum period.
- Where there is also a risk of bleeding, careful consideration should be made to balance the risk and benefit of thromboprophylaxis.

The presentation of pulmonary embolism ranges from progressive dyspnoea to sudden cardiovascular collapse.

- There should be a high index of suspicion in all parturients with risk factors, with new-onset dyspnoea with consideration of cardiac disease as a key differential.
- Treatment is supportive and anticoagulation.
- Anticoagulation should be started immediately before investigations are completed in highly suggestive cases.
- Usually this will be with low molecular weight heparin (LMWH; e.g. enoxaparin 1 mg kg^{-1} every 12 h antenatally), but unfractionated heparin may be used where regional anaesthetic techniques may be required.

Amniotic fluid embolism

Amniotic fluid embolism (AFE) has been estimated to occur in 2 per 100,000 pregnancies. Mortality rates were previously almost 100% though recent estimates have revised this to 16%–30%. Amniotic fluid embolus is difficult to diagnose definitively, and this may result in both under- and over-reporting of cases. There were 16 deaths caused by AFE in the 2012–2014 Confidential Enquiry. Historically, amniotic fluid embolus was described as a postmortem diagnosis dependent on the pathological finding of fetal squamous cells in the lung tissue. More recently, a clinical diagnosis has been used. Diagnosis is one of exclusion. The classic features are hypoxia, cardiovascular collapse and a coagulopathy. The mechanism of AFE is still unclear, but it is suggested that the entrance into the circulation of amniotic fluid constituents causes the release of various primary or secondary endogenous mediators such as histamine, bradykinins, leukotrienes and endothelin. The haemodynamic response is biphasic, with initial pulmonary vasoconstriction and severe hypoxia followed by left ventricular failure.

Risk factors include advancing age, multiparity and placental abruption.

The woman presents with sudden collapse, usually after a rapid labour, but may present after an obstetric intervention, during labour or even during caesarean section. There may be preceding cyanosis, a confusional state, respiratory distress, left ventricular failure with hypotension and acute pulmonary oedema. This is followed rapidly by development of a consumptive coagulopathy and resultant haemorrhage. Management of this emergency involves resuscitation, with administration of oxygen and maintenance of the airway, including tracheal intubation and cardiopulmonary resuscitation, if necessary. If the fetus is undelivered, immediate caesarean section may be necessary to facilitate maternal resuscitation. Treatment is largely supportive, with early correction of coagulopathy. A protracted period of intensive care treatment may be necessary. All suspected cases of AFE in the UK should be reported to the National Amniotic Fluid Embolism Register at UKOSS.

Sepsis

Sepsis has been prominent in the latest triennial enquiries into maternal mortality. Community-acquired β-haemolytic *Streptococcus* Lancefield Group A *(Streptococcus pyogenes)* has caused an increased number of deaths from genital tract sepsis. It is important that all women are educated about the importance of good personal hygiene, both antenatally and postnatally. The maternity sepsis toolkit has recently been developed alongside NICE guidance into sepsis. This includes the development of red flag features that highlight sick pregnant or postpartum women for early escalation of management:

- Responds only to voice/pain or is unresponsive
- Systolic BP 90 mmHg or lower (or a decrease >40 from normal)
- Heart rate greater than 130 min^{-1}
- Respiratory rate 25 min^{-1} or more
- Needs oxygen to keep SpO$_2$ 92% or greater
- Non-blanching rash, mottled, ashen, or cyanotic
- Has not passed urine for more than 18 h
- Urine output less than 0.5 ml kg^{-1} h^{-1}
- Lactate 2 mmol L^{-1} or more

In hospital, Modified Early Obstetric Warning Scoring system (MEOWS) charts should be used to help in the timely recognition, treatment and referral of women who have, or are developing, a critical illness.

There is a 'golden hour' in the treatment of sepsis, and sepsis care bundles such as the Surviving Sepsis campaign should be followed. These can be summarised as the 'sepsis six': Within 1 h of the recognition of severe sepsis, (1) administer oxygen, (2) take blood culture, (3) give i.v. antibiotics, (4) give i.v. fluids, (5) check serial lactates and (6) measure urine output. Critical care services should also be involved early in the management of these patients, and they should be cared for in an appropriate environment with suitable monitoring.

Maternal and neonatal resuscitation

Severe haemorrhage, amniotic fluid embolism, pulmonary embolism or other even more uncommon causes may result in an acutely collapsed mother. In these circumstances, immediate resuscitation is required following standard resuscitation guidelines, but aortocaval compression should be avoided with tilt, wedging or manual uterine displacement. Unsuccessful resuscitation is often caused by profound hypovolaemia. Perimortem caesarean section should be considered as soon as a pregnant woman has a cardiac arrest. Delivery should be completed within 5 min of cardiac arrest to maximise the chance of both maternal and fetal survival and good outcome.

Neonatal resuscitation

The condition of the infant at birth may be assessed by the following:
- Colour, tone, breathing, heart rate are used for the acute assessment. Although the Apgar score, calculated at 1 and 5 min, is of some use retrospectively, it is not used to guide resuscitation.
- Umbilical cord vein pH is normally 7.25–7.35.

The process of resuscitation of the infant begins with drying the baby and thus gentle physical stimulation. If, at the initial assessment after stimulation, the neonate is blue or white with irregular or inadequate respiration and the heart rate is slow (<60 beat min^{-1}), the airway should be opened and five inflation breaths of air should be given. If the heart rate remains slow despite adequate inflation breaths (chest movement seen), cardiopulmonary resuscitation should be commenced at a ratio of three compressions to one inflation breath. The newborn must be kept warm throughout.

Anaesthesia for interventions other than delivery or extraction of retained products of conception

Cervical cerclage

This is a surgical procedure required occasionally for women with a history or active clinical features of an incompetent

Table 43.10 Anaesthetic drugs in obstetric practice

Drug	Effect
Induction agents	Safe for use in standard clinical doses.
Nitrous oxide	High concentrations for prolonged periods have shown teratogenicity in animals. Short periods of exposure have been used safely in large retrospective surveys.
Volatile agents	Safe in standard doses.
Non-depolarising NMBA	Safe, as ionised drugs do not cross the placenta.
Suxamethonium	Plasma cholinesterase concentration can be reduced, but in practice the recovery from suxamethonium is not usually prolonged.
Neostigmine	Crosses the placenta and can cause fetal bradycardia.
Glycopyrrolate	Quaternary ammonium compound does not cross the placenta.
Atropine	Crosses the placenta and can cause fetal tachycardia.
Opioids	Brief exposure is safe, but recurrent exposure will result in features of withdrawal in the neonate after delivery.
NSAIDs	Use in early pregnancy may be associated with miscarriage, and use in the third trimester may cause premature closure of the ductus arteriosus. Large studies of low-dose aspirin have shown that this is safe.
Local anaesthetics	Generally safe to use. Reduced protein binding can result in a theoretical increased risk of toxicity.
Benzodiazepines	Large studies have shown that single exposure in pregnancy is safe. Exposure immediately before delivery may dispose to neonatal sedation and withdrawal symptoms.

Anaesthetic agents can all be potentially teratogenic in high doses and certain circumstances. Studies of drug safety have mainly involved animals or retrospective reviews of outcome in humans. Most commonly used anaesthetic drugs can be used safely when used in standard clinical concentrations with the maintenance of normal maternal physiology. Large retrospective surveys have shown a small but statistically significant increase in spontaneous abortion after surgery with general anaesthesia in the first or second trimesters. The general principle of avoidance, or using the lowest dose for the shortest time, applies.

cervix, usually presenting as premature, precipitate labour. To reduce the risk of this occurring, a suture (Shirodkar suture) is placed around the cervix, in a procedure lasting 20–30 min. As this is usually performed in the second trimester or later, the anaesthetic considerations for any pregnant woman apply. Regional (spinal) anaesthesia is the technique of choice, with the required block height of T10–S5 being achieved using 1.5 ml hyperbaric bupivacaine 0.5% with or without fentanyl 25 μg. If general anaesthesia must be undertaken, use of an RSI is advised if the patient is at more than 12 weeks' gestation.

The pregnant patient with a surgical (non-obstetric) emergency

The incidence of general surgical emergencies is undiminished in pregnancy, and thus pregnant patients may require anaesthesia for laparotomy or any other procedure. The anaesthetic technique should ensure good delivery of oxygen to the placenta, remembering to use lateral tilt to avoid aortocaval compression from 20 weeks. The use of depressant drugs such as opioids is not contraindicated. Regional techniques are recommended where possible. After the 13th week of gestation, the risk of regurgitation of gastric contents increases, so RSI should always be performed. Good practice is to avoid drugs that may harm the developing fetus. Table 43.10 details drugs generally considered safe. These must always be considered in the clinical context.

References/Further reading

Chaggar, R.S., Campbell, J.P., 2017. The future of general anaesthesia in obstetrics. BJA Education 17 (3), 79–83.

Cook, T.M., Counsell, D., Wildsmith, J.A.W., 2009. Major complications of central neuroaxial block: report on the third National Audit of the Royal College of Anaesthetists. Br. J. Anaesth. 102, 142–151.

Knight, M., Nair, M., Tuffnell, D., Kenyon, S., Shakespeare, J., Brocklehurst, P., et al. (Eds.), 2016. On behalf of MBRRACE-UK. Saving lives, Improving mothers' care - surveillance of maternal deaths in the UK 2012-14 and lessons learned to inform maternity care from the UK and Ireland confidential enquiries into maternal deaths and morbidity 2009-14. National Perinatal Epidemiology Unit, University of Oxford, Oxford.

Mushambi, M.C., Kinsella, S.M., Popat, M., Swales, H., Ramaswamy, K.K., Winton, A.L., et al., 2015. Obstetric Anaesthetists' Association and Difficult Airway Society guidelines for the management of difficult and failed tracheal intubation in obstetrics. Anaesthesia 70, 1286–1306.

Pandit, J.J., Andrade, J., Bogod, D.G., Hitchman, J.M., Jonker, W.R., Lucas, N., et al., 2014. The 5th national audit project (NAP5) on accidental awareness during general anaesthesia: a summary of main findings and risk factors. Anaesthesia 69, 1089–1101.

Chapter 44

Emergency and trauma anaesthesia

Anil Hormis

Patients scheduled for elective surgery are usually in optimal physical and mental condition, with a definitive surgical diagnosis; any coexisting medical disease is defined and well controlled. These patients have often discussed plans for surgery and anaesthesia (including postoperative care) in advance and may be better prepared from a psychological perspective for the challenges of the perioperative period. In contrast, the patient with a surgical emergency may have an uncertain diagnosis and uncontrolled coexisting medical disease, in addition to any physiological derangements resulting from their surgical pathological condition. In the emergency setting, preparation for theatre focusses on identifying, correcting or optimising (where possible) any major physiological abnormalities. In addition, the anaesthetist must be prepared for potential complications arising because of the nature of emergency surgery or anaesthesia. These include vomiting and regurgitation, hypovolaemia, haemorrhage, electrolyte disturbances, acute kidney injury and adverse reactions to drugs in the emergency situation.

Preoperative assessment

Thorough preoperative anaesthetic assessment of the emergency surgical patient is very important. This requires adequate and accurate preoperative evaluation of the patient's general condition, with attention to specific problems that may influence anaesthetic management. The likely surgical diagnosis and the extent and urgency of the proposed surgery must be discussed with surgical and medical colleagues preoperatively. The urgency for surgery is most helpfully conveyed using a recognised classification system, such as the one created by the National Confidential Enquiry into Patient Outcome and Death (NCEPOD) (Table 44.1). The nature and urgency of the planned surgery dictate the extent of preoperative preparation and anaesthetic technique. The classification is useful in prioritising cases on the emergency list.

During the preoperative assessment, the history must be focused and highlight areas that are likely to influence choice of anaesthetic technique, postoperative care and any potential complications. Emergency patients may often be obtunded because of their illness, so a history may have to be elicited from various sources, such as the patient's previous notes and/or relatives or carers.

It is important to ensure that all the history taken from the patient before emergency surgery is just as thorough as for elective surgery (see Chapter 19) including:

*   medical and surgical history;
*   previous anaesthetic history (especially previous airway problems or admissions to ICU);
*   drug history (especially use of anticoagulants and antiplatelet agents);
*   drug allergies;
*   correct identification of fasting times (the same guidelines apply as for elective patients (see Chapter 22), though in extreme surgical emergencies the patient may need to proceed to theatre before these fasting times are achieved);
*   social history; and
*   functional history, including assessment of metabolic equivalents (METs) (see Chapter 19).

Depending upon the urgency of surgery, the physical examination may be targeted to identify significant cardiorespiratory dysfunction or any abnormalities that might lead to technical difficulties during anaesthesia. Valuable information about the patient's condition can also be obtained from the bedside observations chart. In particular, trends in physiological variables such as blood pressure, heart rate, respiratory rate and oxygen saturations may signal a deteriorating condition and even impending decompensation.

Table 44.1 NCEPOD classification of surgical urgency

Code	Category	Description	Target time to theatre	Expected location	Examples	Typical procedures
1	Immediate	Immediate (A) lifesaving or (B) limb- or organ-saving intervention Resuscitation simultaneous with surgical intervention	Within minutes of decision to operate	Next available operating theatre – 'break in' to existing lists, if required	Ruptured aortic aneurysm Major trauma to abdomen or thorax Fracture with major neurovascular deficit	Repair of ruptured aortic aneurysm Laparotomy/ thoracotomy for control of haemorrhage
2	Urgent	Acute onset or deterioration of conditions that threaten life, limb or organ survival; fixation of fractures; relief of distressing symptoms	Within hours of decision to operate and normally once resuscitation complete	Daytime 'emergency list' or Out-of-hours emergency theatre (including at night)	Compound fracture Perforated bowel with peritonitis Critical organ or limb ischaemia Penetrating eye injury	Debridement plus fixation of fracture Laparotomy for perforation
3	Expedited	Stable patient requiring early intervention for a condition that is not an immediate threat to life, limb or organ survival	Within days of decision to operate	Elective list which has 'spare' capacity or Daytime emergency list (not at night)	Tendon and nerve injuries Stable and non-septic patients for wide range of surgical procedures	Repair of tendon and nerve injuries Excision of tumour with potential to bleed or obstruct
4	Elective	Surgical procedure planned or booked in advance of routine admission to hospital	Planned	Elective theatre list booked and planned before admission	Encompasses all conditions not classified as immediate, urgent or expedited	Joint arthroplasty

NCEPOD, National Confidential Enquiry into Patient Outcome and Death.

Cardiovascular system

Basal lung crepitations, pitting oedema and raised jugular venous pressure signify impaired ventricular function and limited cardiac reserve, which significantly increase the risks of emergency surgery and anaesthesia. It is also important to exclude arrhythmias and heart sounds indicative of valvular heart disease, as these influence the patient's response to physiological challenges and thus anaesthetic management. Any significant arrhythmias need to be identified and managed preoperatively.

Respiratory system

Assessment of respiratory function is particularly difficult, as the patient in pain (with or without peritoneal irritation) may be unable to cooperate with pulmonary function testing.

Airway

The standard clinical tests of airway assessment should be used (see Chapter 23) and any previous anaesthetic charts consulted if available. A history of difficult tracheal intubation is of considerable significance; however, a past record of easy tracheal intubation does not guarantee future success. In emergency anaesthesia, airway difficulties may be caused by the patient's usual anatomy but also surgical pathological conditions such as dental abscesses, trauma, bleeding or haematoma. If RSI is contemplated, then contingency plans are required for management of the patient in the event of failure to intubate the trachea. If a high degree of difficulty in tracheal intubation is anticipated, then an awake technique may be necessary (see Chapter 23).

The final stage of the preoperative assessment is to review any relevant laboratory investigations, including ECG, blood tests, radiological imaging and arterial blood gases where appropriate. The guidelines for preoperative investigations in the elective setting (see Chapter 19) should be viewed as the minimum requirements, with most emergency patients routinely requiring additional tests depending on their underlying pathological condition and physiological status. The availability of blood products should be checked if necessary and urgent requests should be made for any additional tests which may influence patient management.

Assessment of circulating volume

Assessment of intravascular volume is essential, as underestimated or unrecognised hypovolaemia may lead to circulatory collapse during induction of anaesthesia, which attenuates the sympathetically mediated increases in arteriolar and venous constriction as well as reducing cardiac output. In any patient in whom fluid is sequestered or lost (e.g. peritonitis, bowel obstruction) or in whom haemorrhage has occurred (e.g. ectopic pregnancy), the anaesthetist should try to quantify the circulating blood and extracellular fluid volumes and correct any deficits.

Intravascular volume deficit

Blood loss may be assessed using the patient's history and any measured losses, but more commonly the anaesthetist must rely on clinical evaluation of the patient's current cardiovascular status. Profound circulatory shock with hypotension, poor peripheral perfusion, oliguria and altered cerebration is easy to recognise. However, a more careful assessment is needed to recognise the early manifestations of haemorrhage, such as tachycardia and cutaneous vasoconstriction. Useful indices include heart rate, blood pressure (especially pulse pressure), the state of the peripheral circulation, pyrexia and urine output. In young, healthy adults, arterial pressure may be an unreliable guide to volume status because compensatory mechanisms can prevent a measurable decrease in arterial pressure until more than 30% of the patient's blood volume has been lost. In such patients, attention should be directed to pulse rate, skin circulation and a narrowing pulse pressure. In elderly patients with widespread arterial disease, limited cardiac reserve and a rigid vascular tree (fixed total peripheral resistance), signs of severe hypovolaemia may become evident when blood volume has been reduced by as little as 15%. However, as baroreceptor sensitivity decreases with age, elderly patients may exhibit less tachycardia for any degree of volume depletion.

Although clinical evaluation remains the most important and most commonly used guide to intravascular volume management, non-invasive and minimally invasive methods of cardiac output measurement can be used (see Chapters 17 and 30). These techniques may be of particular benefit in guiding the immediate resuscitation of frail or critically ill patients in theatre.

Extracellular volume deficit

Assessment of extracellular fluid volume deficit is difficult. Guidance may be obtained from the nature of the surgical condition, duration of impaired fluid intake and presence and severity of symptoms associated with abnormal losses (e.g. vomiting). At the time of the earliest radiological evidence of intestinal obstruction, there may be 1500 ml of fluid sequestered in the bowel lumen (so-called 'third space losses'). If the obstruction is well established and vomiting has occurred, the extracellular fluid deficit may exceed 3000 ml. Table 44.2 describes some of the clinical features seen with varying degrees of severity of extracellular fluid losses. Considerable fluid losses must occur before clinical signs are apparent, and these signs are often subjective in more minor degrees of extracellular fluid deficit. In addition to clinical signs, laboratory investigations may also indicate extracellular fluid volume deficit. Haemoconcentration results in increased haemoglobin concentration and packed cell volume. As dehydration becomes more marked,

Table 44.2 Clinical signs of the extent of extracellular fluid deficit

Body weight lost as water	Fluid lost (ml kg^{-1})	Signs and symptoms
4%–6% (mild)	>35	Thirst Reduced skin elasticity Decreased intraocular pressure Dry tongue Reduced sweating
6%–8% (mild)	>70	As above, plus: Orthostatic hypotension Reduced filling of peripheral veins Oliguria Apathy Haemoconcentration
8%–10% (moderate)	>80	As above, plus: Hypotension Thready pulse with cool peripheries
10%–15% (severe)	100–150	Coma, shock followed by death

renal blood flow diminishes, reducing renal clearance of urea and consequently increasing the blood urea concentration. Patients with moderate volume contraction exhibit a 'prerenal' pattern of uraemia characterised by an increase in blood urea out of proportion to any increase in serum creatinine concentration. Under maximal stimulation from antidiuretic hormone (ADH) and aldosterone, conservation of sodium and water by the kidneys results in excretion of urine of low sodium concentration ($0–15$ mmol L^{-1}) and high osmolality ($800–1400$ mosmol kg^{-1}).

Once the extent of blood volume or extracellular fluid volume loss has been estimated, deficits should be corrected with the appropriate intravenous fluid. The overall priority is to maintain adequate tissue perfusion and oxygenation; therefore correction of intravascular deficit takes precedence. Hypovolaemia as a result of blood loss should be treated with a balanced crystalloid solution (such as Hartmann's solution) until packed red cells (PRCs) are available (see Chapter 12). Resuscitation is usually guided by clinical indices of circulating volume status and organ perfusion. High-risk surgical patients undergoing major surgery may benefit from the use of (non-invasive) cardiac output measuring devices to direct fluid resuscitation towards predetermined goals for cardiac output and systemic oxygen delivery (goal-directed therapy; see Chapter 30). Extracellular fluid deficit is usually corrected after the correction of any intravascular deficit, by adjusting maintenance fluid infusion rates. Losses from vomiting or gastric aspirates are best replaced by crystalloid solutions containing an appropriate potassium supplement. Hartmann's solution is often used, although hypochloraemia is an indication for saline 0.9% (with additional potassium). Lower GI losses, such as those caused by diarrhoea or intestinal obstruction, are normally replaced volume for volume with Hartmann's solution.

The full stomach

Vomiting or regurgitation of gastric contents, followed by aspiration into the tracheobronchial tree whilst protective laryngeal reflexes are obtunded, is one of the most common and most devastating hazards of emergency anaesthesia. Vomiting is an active process that occurs in the lighter planes of anaesthesia. Consequently, it is a potential problem during induction of, or emergence from, anaesthesia but should not occur during maintenance if anaesthesia is sufficiently deep. In light planes of anaesthesia, the presence of vomited material above the vocal cords stimulates spasm of the cords (laryngospasm). In contrast to vomiting, regurgitation is a passive process that may occur at any time, is often 'silent' (i.e. not apparent to the anaesthetist) and, if aspiration occurs, may have clinical consequences ranging from minor pulmonary sequelae to fulminating aspiration pneumonitis

---

Box 44.1 Situations in which vomiting or regurgitation may occur during anaesthesia

Full stomach
With absent or abnormal peristalsis

Peritonitis of any cause
Postoperative ileus
Metabolic ileus (e.g. hypokalaemia, uraemia, diabetic ketoacidosis)
Drug-induced ileus (e.g. anticholinergics or agents with anticholinergic effects)

With obstructed peristalsis

Small or large bowel obstruction
Gastric carcinoma
Pyloric stenosis

With delayed gastric emptying

Diabetic autonomic neuropathy
Fear, pain or anxiety
Late pregnancy
Opioids
Head injury

Other causes

Hiatus hernia
Oesophageal strictures – benign or malignant
Pharyngeal pouch

---

and acute respiratory distress syndrome (ARDS). Regurgitation usually occurs in the presence of deep anaesthesia or at the onset of action of neuromuscular blocking agents (NMBAs), when protective laryngeal reflexes are absent. The most important factors determining the risk and degree of gastric regurgitation are lower oesophageal sphincter function and residual gastric volume, which itself is largely determined by the duration of fasting and rate of gastric emptying. Risk factors for vomiting and/or regurgitation during anaesthesia are shown in Box 44.1.

Lower oesophageal sphincter

The lower oesophageal sphincter (LOS) is a 2–5 cm length of oesophagus with a higher resting intraluminal pressure situated just proximal to the cardia of the stomach. The sphincter relaxes during oesophageal peristalsis to allow food into the stomach but remains contracted at other times. The structure cannot be defined anatomically but may be detected using intraluminal pressure manometry. The LOS is the main barrier preventing reflux of gastric contents into the oesophagus. Many drugs used in anaesthetic practice affect the resting tone of the LOS. Reflux is related not to the

LOS tone *per se,* but to the difference between gastric and LOS pressures; this is termed the *barrier pressure.* Drugs that increase the barrier pressure (e.g. cyclizine, anticholinesterases, α-adrenergic agonists and metoclopramide) decrease the risk of reflux. Anticholinergic drugs, ethanol, tricyclic antidepressants and opioids all reduce LOS pressure, and it is reasonable to assume that these drugs increase the tendency to gastro-oesophageal reflux.

Gastric emptying

Gastric emptying results from peristaltic waves sweeping from the cardia to pylorus at a rate of approximately three per minute. The rate of gastric emptying is significantly delayed if the mixture reaching the duodenum is very acidic or hypertonic (the inhibitory enterogastric reflex), but both the nervous and humoral elements of this regulating mechanism are still poorly understood. Many pathological conditions reduce gastric emptying (see Box 44.1). It is important to understand that the stomach is never 'empty'. In the absence of any of these factors, it is reasonably safe to assume that the risks of regurgitation and aspiration are minimised, provided that solids have not been ingested within the previous 6 h, with only fluids consumed up to 2 h before anaesthesia, and provided that normal peristalsis is occurring. This is the usual case for elective surgical patients. However, in emergency surgery it may be necessary to induce anaesthesia before an adequate period of starvation occurs. In addition, the patient's surgical condition is often accompanied by delayed gastric emptying or abnormalities of peristalsis. In these circumstances, even if the usual period of fasting has been observed it cannot be assumed that the risks of aspiration have been minimised.

In patients who have sustained a significant trauma injury, gastric emptying virtually ceases because of the combined effects of fear, pain, shock and treatment with opioid analgesics. In these patients the interval between ingestion of food and the injury is a more reliable index of residual stomach volume than the period of fasting observed since injury. A patient's sensation of hunger should not be used to indicate an empty stomach; sensations of hunger and satiety are complex and are unreliable indicators of stomach volume. There is currently a considerable interest in bedside ultrasonography as an objective tool in determining the volume of gastric contents, and its use may become more widespread in the coming years.

Injury from the regurgitation/aspiration of gastric contents results from three different mechanisms: chemical pneumonitis (from acid material), mechanical obstruction from particulate material and bacterial contamination. Aspiration of liquid with a pH less than 2.5 is associated with a chemical burn of the bronchial, bronchiolar and alveolar mucosa, leading to atelectasis, pulmonary oedema and reduced pulmonary compliance. Management after aspiration is discussed in Chapter 27.

Anaesthetic techniques

It is important to recognise any patient who may have significant gastric residue and who is in danger of regurgitation (and therefore aspiration). For emergency surgical procedures, if general anaesthesia is necessary, then tracheal intubation is common practice, with an RSI routine if there is significant risk of aspiration.

Preinduction

Although it may be necessary to postpone surgery in the emergency patient to obtain investigations and resuscitate with i.v. fluids, there is usually little benefit in terms of reducing the risk of aspiration of gastric contents; the risk of aspiration must be weighed against the risk of delaying an urgent procedure. Although not completely effective, insertion of a nasogastric tube to decompress the stomach and to provide a low-pressure vent for regurgitation may be helpful. Aspiration through the tube may be useful if gastric contents are liquid, as in bowel obstruction, but is less effective when contents are solid. Cricoid force (see Chapter 23) is still effective at reducing regurgitation even with a nasogastric tube *in situ.* In patients who have any haemodynamic instability preoperatively, consider the use of invasive arterial blood pressure monitoring before induction of anaesthesia. These patients may well go on to need vasopressor infusions (e.g. metaraminol, noradrenaline) intraoperatively and so placing a CVC should be considered either before the patient is anaesthetised or, more commonly, immediately after induction.

Induction

The conduct of RSI is discussed in detail in Chapter 23, and this is the technique used most often for the patient with a full stomach. One of the main disadvantages of the RSI technique is the haemodynamic instability that may result if the dose of induction agent is excessive (hypotension, circulatory collapse) or inadequate (hypertension, tachycardia).

Thiopental has long been regarded as the i.v. induction agent of choice for RSI. It provides a rapid loss of consciousness with a clearly defined endpoint. A dose of 4–5 mg kg^{-1} can reliably be predicted to be sufficient for healthy young patients, but much less (1.5–2 mg kg^{-1}) is required in the older, frail or hypovolaemic patient. In the critically ill patient with a metabolic acidaemia, the unbound fraction of the drug is increased, and this will reduce dose requirements. Ketamine (1–2 mg kg^{-1}) has a slower speed of onset and poorly defined endpoint compared with thiopental. However, it causes the least cardiovascular depression of any induction

835

agent and has now become the agent of choice in severely shocked patients. In comparison, propofol 2–5 mg kg^{-1} causes greater suppression of laryngeal reflexes and may be more familiar to junior anaesthetists because of its everyday use in anaesthesia for elective procedures. However, propofol causes more cardiovascular depression than thiopental and ketamine and should be used with caution in the emergency setting. Intravenous anaesthetic agents are detailed in Chapter 4.

Opioids are often injected along with intravenous anaesthetics at induction of anaesthesia for elective surgery, but 'classical' teaching was that they should be omitted during RSI despite their potential benefits. This was largely because of concerns about delaying the onset of spontaneous respiration in the event of failed tracheal intubation. However, shorter-acting drugs such as alfentanil are now widely used as part of an RSI to reduce induction agent doses and to help obtund the sympathetic response to laryngoscopy, particularly in conditions such as pre-eclampsia (see Chapter 43) or traumatic brain injury (see Chapter 40).

Inhalational induction

If there is reasonable doubt about the ability to perform successful tracheal intubation or to maintain a patent airway in a patient with a full stomach (e.g. the patient with facial trauma, epiglottitis or bleeding tonsil), an inhalational induction may be used with oxygen and sevoflurane. When the patient has reached a deep plane of anaesthesia, laryngoscopy is performed followed by an attempt at tracheal intubation during spontaneous ventilation. Traditionally the patient was placed in the left lateral, head-down position, but current practice favours sitting the patient up and using cricoid force. When anaesthesia is sufficiently deep, a rapid-onset NMBA is injected and the trachea intubated. This technique may be used in any older, frail patients who may not tolerate i.v. induction agents.

Awake fibreoptic intubation

Tracheal intubation with a fibreoptic intubating laryngoscope is often the preferred technique in those patients who are likely to develop refractory airway obstruction when loss of consciousness occurs (e.g. trismus from dental abscess) or who are known or suspected to pose difficulties with tracheal intubation. The procedure is discussed in detail in Chapter 23.

Regional anaesthesia

The use of regional anaesthesia is increasing in the UK, partly because of the growth in the practice of ultrasound-guided regional anaesthetic techniques. Many regional techniques are ideal for emergency procedures on the extremities (e.g.

to reduce fractures or dislocations) and are discussed in detail in Chapter 25. Brachial plexus block by the axillary, supraclavicular or interscalene approach works well for orthopaedic manipulations or surgical procedures involving the upper extremity. It satisfies surgical requirements for analgesia, muscle relaxation and immobility. There are minimal effects on the cardiovascular system, and there is a prolonged period of analgesia postoperatively. For regional anaesthesia of the lower extremity, available techniques include subarachnoid, epidural and sciatic/femoral blocks. Spinal and epidural blocks are contraindicated if there is doubt about the adequacy of extracellular fluid or vascular volumes, as large decreases in arterial pressure may result from the associated pharmacological sympathectomy.

It is a common surgical misconception that subarachnoid or epidural anaesthetic techniques are safer than general anaesthesia for patients in poor physical condition. It must be emphasised that for the *inexperienced* anaesthetist, these techniques are invariably more dangerous than general anaesthesia for the patient with moderate to major trauma or any intra-abdominal emergency condition.

Maintenance of anaesthesia

If RSI has been performed, the patient's lungs are gently ventilated manually whilst heart rate and blood pressure measurements are repeated to assess the cardiovascular effects of the drugs used and of the stimulus of tracheal intubation. Capnography is essential throughout anaesthesia and gives valuable information about perfusion and ventilation of the lungs. When there is evidence of return of neuromuscular transmission (by clinical signs or from a nerve stimulator) as suxamethonium is degraded, a non-depolarising NMBA is administered. The choice depends on the patient's condition and the effect of the induction of anaesthesia on the patient's cardiovascular status. Both rocuronium and atracurium are appropriate drugs for routine use, although the pharmacokinetics of atracurium make it the logical choice for the older patient. Atracurium has virtually no cardiovascular effects in clinical doses and is useful if there is any doubt about renal function.

After induction of anaesthesia, the tracheal tube is connected to a mechanical ventilator and minute volume adjusted to produce normocapnia. Ventilators are now increasingly sophisticated and incorporate a choice of ventilation modes. The choice is usually between pressure- or volume-controlled ventilation. It can be difficult to predict ventilator requirements, but initial settings should aim to produce a tidal volume of 6–8 ml kg^{-1}. The inspiratory flow rate should be adjusted to minimise peak airway pressure (target < 30 cmH$_2$O), and the capnograph waveform and pressure volume loops should be inspected regularly to guide the further adjustment of ventilator settings. Maintenance of core temperature is a very important aspect of intraoperative management; core temperature should be monitored throughout the procedure and hypothermia avoided whenever possible (see Chapter 13).

Before the initial surgical incision is made, analgesia may be supplemented by incremental i.v. doses of opioids. It is important to be familiar with the pharmacokinetics and pharmacodynamics of all agents used and to be aware that these may change during emergency anaesthesia, when acute circulatory changes or impaired organ function often occur.

Fluid management

During emergency intra-abdominal surgery, there may be large blood and fluid losses, which exceed the patient's maintenance fluid replacement. Hartmann's solution (compound sodium lactate) is still the preferred i.v. fluid during emergency surgery. More sophisticated methods of determining intravascular volume status and cardiac output (see Chapter 17) are increasingly used especially in emergency laparotomy, as this form of monitoring is a standard for the UK National Emergency Laparotomy Audit (NELA).

The requirement for blood transfusion varies in different groups of patients. In general, and in the absence of major haemorrhage, the threshold for transfusion of packed red blood cells is a haemoglobin concentration less than 80 g L^{-1}. A higher transfusion trigger is often used for certain patient populations, such as 100 g L^{-1} in patients with ischaemic heart disease, though the evidence for this is not established. Near-patient testing devices and/or sampling from arterial or venous catheters are invaluable aids to guide transfusion during surgery.

At the end of surgery, anaesthesia can be discontinued, if the patient is deemed stable enough for tracheal extubation; the conduct of this is discussed in Chapter 23. It is important to ensure that adequate analgesia has been provided (either by analgesic agents or a regional technique) before awakening. Direct pharyngoscopy may be performed and secretions and debris removed from the pharynx; if a nasogastric tube is *in situ*, it can be aspirated and left on free drainage. If the train-of-four count is more than 3, glycopyrrolate 20 μg kg^{-1} and neostigmine 50 μg kg^{-1} or sugammadex 2 mg kg^{-1} are given as a bolus to antagonise residual neuromuscular block; lung ventilation should be continued to eliminate volatile agents until signs of awakening appear. The end-tidal concentration of volatile anaesthetic is usually less than 0.1 minimum alveolar concentration (MAC) before eye opening occurs. Because the risk of aspiration of gastric contents is as great on recovery as at induction, tracheal extubation should not be performed until protective airway reflexes have returned fully and the patient responds to commands such as 'open your eyes' or 'lift your hand up'. Both the level of consciousness and neuromuscular

Box 44.2 **Indications for postoperative mechanical ventilation**

Prolonged shock/hypoperfusion state of any cause
Severe sepsis (faecal peritonitis, cholangitis, septicaemia) and likely return to theatre in next 24–48 h
Severe ischaemic heart disease
Extreme obesity
Overt aspiration of gastric contents
Severe pulmonary disease
Profound hypothermia

transmission should be assessed to demonstrate the adequacy of reflexes.

Postoperative mechanical ventilation should be considered electively in several circumstances, some of which are listed in Box 44.2. There should be close cooperation between ICU colleagues, surgeons and anaesthetists when the decision is made to continue ventilation.

Emergency laparotomy in the older patient

Older patients undergoing emergency laparotomy are at particularly high risk of complications or death, as highlighted by the UK NCEPOD reports. The decision to perform emergency surgery requires the input of senior surgical, anaesthetic, medicine for the elderly and ICU clinicians. The risks and potential benefits should be carefully assessed, and frail, older patients should not necessarily undergo major surgery followed by prolonged intensive care treatments if it is considered that the burden of surgical treatment and poor prognosis outweigh the likely benefit of surgery. Decision making in this context is complex and should only be made by senior clinicians. It is emphasised that such decisions must be individualised and the views of the patient are paramount. The use of preoperative risk stratification has become a standard of care. There are many scoring systems to use (see Chapter 19), but the P-POSSUM (Portsmouth Physiological and Operative Severity Score for the Enumeration of Mortality and Morbidity) score and the NELA risk tool are commonly used.

Before embarking on emergency, potentially major surgery in frail, older patients with an acute abdomen, some questions must be answered:

- Is it likely that the patient will die *with* or *without surgery*? If the answer is yes, then surgery is *not* indicated unless it is likely that it will contribute to the physical comfort of the patient during the dying process (i.e. contribute to a 'good death').
- Is it likely that the patient would survive a laparotomy if the underlying cause were found to be curable or

treatable (e.g. perforated duodenal ulcer, appendicitis)? If the answer is yes, then surgery is indicated and agreement on the appropriate level and duration of postoperative organ support must be reached.

- If, having embarked on surgery, the underlying cause is found to be treatable but not curable (e.g. perforated carcinoma with metastases, gangrenous bowel), would radical surgery be appropriate, given the patients overall state? If not, aggressive postoperative intensive care is not indicated. If yes, then what would be an appropriate level and duration of postoperative support? These questions need to be answered by experienced clinicians.

National Emergency Laparotomy Audit

The Royal College of Surgeons of England has identified that the delivery of emergency surgical care in England and Wales is currently suboptimal, with higher than expected mortality rates; this has led to the production of a number of recommendations about identifying the patients who are at high risk of mortality. NELA was set up in 2012 and aims to collect data from hospitals regarding compliance to the national standards for patients aged older than 17 years undergoing an expedited, urgent or emergency laparotomy (Table 44.3). NELA also includes information about the structure of the service (e.g. provision of emergency theatres/out-of-hours radiology), process measures (e.g. seniority of clinical staff in theatre, admissions to critical care), and outcome measures (e.g. 30-day mortality, duration of hospital stay).

Major trauma

The management of the patient with major trauma requires a multidisciplinary team effort that is coordinated and systematic. Trauma is the leading cause of death in adults aged younger than 45 years and accounts for around 10% of the world's deaths. Within the UK, deficiencies in expertise and resources at local district general hospitals have resulted in the formation of regional trauma networks, with resources being concentrated at the major trauma centres (MTCs). Trauma patients will often have 'time-critical' injuries and will need specialist interventions or emergency surgery. A successful outcome depends on the quality of the initial resuscitation and correct prioritisation of treatment. Current trauma management is based on major trauma protocols, evolved from Advanced Trauma Life Support teaching and experience from military and civilian trauma management.

Table 44.3 National Emergency Laparotomy Audit (NELA) standards

Risk assessment	Use of the P-POSSUM or NELA score If predicted mortality > 10% care should directly involve a consultant anaesthetist/surgeon
Preoperative	Senior anaesthetic and surgical input if risk of death ≥ 5% Senior intensivist input if risk of death ≥ 10% Sepsis review and antibiotics if needed Appropriate imaging (CT recommended) and report available
Intraoperative	Appropriate antibiotic cover (see Chapter 18) Goal-directed fluid therapy with cardiac output monitoring (see Chapter 17) Maintenance of normothermia Assessment of base excess and lactate Effective analgesia
End of surgery care bundle	Assessment of base excess and lactate Aim for normothermia Nutrition plan ICU admission if: Predicted > 10% mortality Lactate > 4 mmol L^{-1} Hypothermia PaO_2/FIO_2 ratio < 40

P-POSSUM, Portsmouth Physiological and Operative Severity Score for the Enumeration of Mortality and Morbidity.

Major trauma is a dynamic, high-stakes environment with difficult decision making. Excellent teamwork, communication and non-technical skills are fundamental to successful trauma management.

Scoring systems

It is important to understand the common trauma scoring systems, as they underpin many triage decisions and outcome measures.

Abbreviated Injury Scale

The Abbreviated Injury Scale (AIS) grades injuries anatomically according to a detailed 6-point severity scale (1 – minor, 2 – moderate, 3 – serious, 4 – severe, 5 – critical and 6 – maximal (currently untreatable)) in nine body regions (head, face, neck, thorax, abdomen, spine, upper extremity, lower extremity, external/other).

Injury Severity Score

The Injury Severity Score (ISS) is based on the AIS but focusses on six body regions (head/neck, face, chest, abdomen/pelvis, extremities/pelvic girdle, external) and is the sum of the squares of the AIS severity scores of the three most severely injured regions (e.g. ISS = Head 4^2 + Chest 3^2 + Abdomen 2^2 = 29). The score ranges from 1–75 (i.e. a severity of 5 in each group); if any of three scores is a 6 (unsurvivable injury), the score is automatically set to 75. Major trauma is defined as ISS greater than 15 and moderately severe trauma as ISS 9–15.

Revised Trauma Score

The Revised Trauma Score (RTS) is a physiological score based on the initial Glasgow Coma Scale (GCS) score, systolic blood pressure and respiratory rate with a score from 0–4 in each category. The RTS can used to predict survival and as a triage tool.

Trauma management

Effective management of major trauma requires the following:
1. *Rapid primary survey.* Recognition and treatment of any immediately life-threatening injuries, such as airway obstruction, tension/open pneumothorax, massive bleeding (chest, abdomen, pelvis, long bones or external), cardiac tamponade or intracranial injury.
2. *Damage control resuscitation.* Control of haemorrhage, achieving adequate tissue perfusion, hybrid resuscitation (hypotensive and haemostatic) and damage control surgery.
3. *Ongoing, repeated examination* to identify threats to life or limb and all associated injuries.
4. *Definitive care.*

Although these processes are described sequentially, a well-run trauma team will prioritise, communicate, and assess and treat in parallel.

The trauma team

There will normally be a prealert from the ambulance service so that the trauma team is activated before the patient arrives in the emergency department (ED). The composition of the trauma team should be standardised in each hospital (Fig. 44.1). The trauma team leader should brief the team once they are assembled and preparations to receive the patient can begin. The prealert from the ambulance service should consist of the ATMIST handover:
- Age of the patient
- Time of injury

Anaesthetist
- Assess and monitor patient's airway
- Tracheal intubation
- Vascular access
- Invasive monitoring

ED Doctor 1
- Primary survey
- Intercostal drain
- FAST scan

ED Nurse 2

Porter
- Transport of blood samples
- Patient trasfer to CT/theatre
- Collection of blood products

Scribe
- Documentation of findings
- Timing of interventions and decisions
- Patient details

ODP
- Prepare for tracheal intubation, invasive monitoring
- Fluid warmer, forced-air warming
- Pre-RSI checklist

ED Nurse 1
- Apply monitoring
- Assist with i.v. access
- Blood tests

General surgeon
- Abdominal examination

Orthopaedic Surgeon
- Reduction of limb-threatening fractures
- Apply / adjust pelvic binder

Radiographer
- Arranges CT/ radiographic imaging

Trauma Team Leader
- Coordinates team
- Maintains 'hands-off' overview
- Communication with other areas/specialties

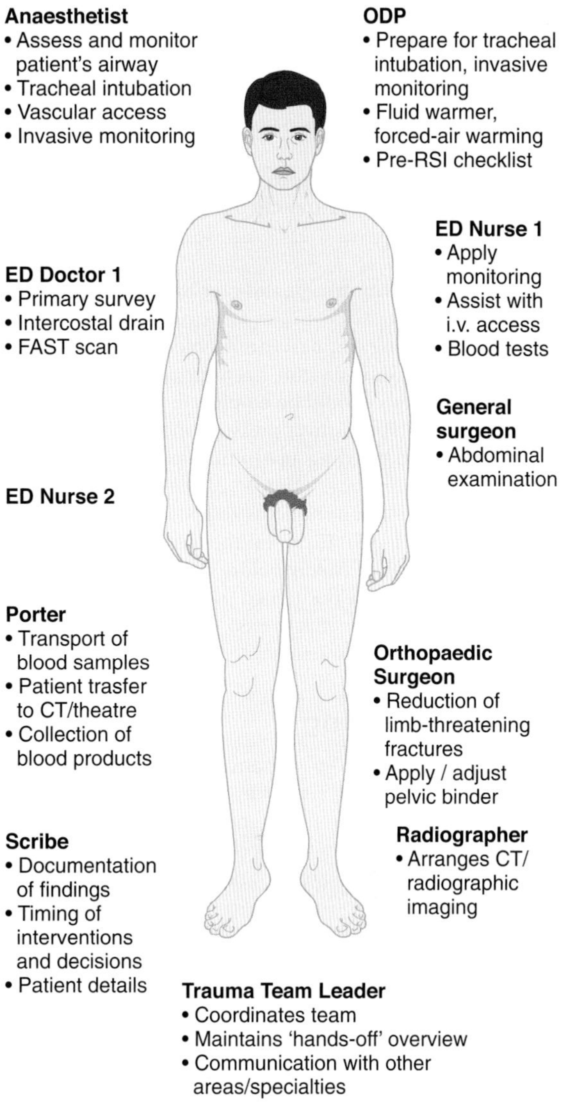

Fig. 44.1 Example of a trauma team, including examples of possible roles and positions. *ED,* Emergency department; *FAST,* focussed assessment with sonography in trauma; *ODP,* operating department practitioner.

- Mechanism of injury
- Injuries identified
- Vital Signs
- Treatments (given), estimated time of arrival, mode of transport (land vs. air), and any specialist resources needed of arrival (e.g. intercostal drain, blood products etc.)

Primary survey/damage control resuscitation

As soon as the patient arrives in the ED, a rapid primary survey is performed at the same time as resuscitation. A cABC approach is taken:

- Catastrophic haemorrhage control; less common in civilian than military trauma but does occur.
- Airway
- Breathing
- Circulation; haemorrhagic and non-haemorrhagic causes may co-exist.

There is a strong emphasis on haemorrhage control. In case control of exsanguinating haemorrhage is needed, the following methods should be employed:

- In the limbs, apply direct pressure and elevate.
- For continued bleeding, use indirect pressure and apply a military tourniquet (Fig. 44.2); ensure the time of application of a tourniquet is recorded in the patient's notes and in indelible ink on the tourniquet.
- A pelvic binder is usually before arrival at the hospital; ensure it is correctly positioned (i.e. sited over the greater trochanters, not the iliac crests), as malpositioning can exacerbate a pelvic fracture.

Airway/breathing

Anaesthetists are usually responsible for managing the patient's airway. As they are at the 'head end', they are also in the best position to assess and monitor the patient's conscious level. Box 44.3 shows some indications for tracheal intubation. In general, airway assessment reveals one of three clinical scenarios:

- *Patient is conscious, alert, talking.* Give high-flow oxygen via face mask. There is no need for immediate airway intervention, and a full clinical evaluation can be done. Persisting signs of shock or the diagnosis of serious underlying injuries might be an indication for planned tracheal intubation and mechanical ventilation.
- *Patient has a reduced conscious level but some degree of airway control and gag reflex still present.* If the patient is

maintaining their airway and breathing adequately, then there is no need for immediate intervention. Give high-flow oxygen via face mask. Tracheal intubation will be necessary, but a clinical evaluation can be done whilst equipment is being readied.

- *Patient has a reduced conscious level, and gag reflex is absent.* If the patient is unable to maintain the airway or respiration is inadequate, tracheal intubation and mechanical ventilation should be carried out at once.

When confronted with an unconscious trauma victim, the anaesthetist must establish the patency of the patient's airway whilst ensuring immobilisation of the cervical spine (cervical collar, sandbags and tape). Unstable cervical spine injuries are relatively uncommon; however, *all* patients should be assumed to be at risk until proven otherwise. If upper airway obstruction is present, the pharynx should be cleared of any debris and a jaw-thrust performed; a chin-lift should be avoided as this causes a greater degree of cervical spine movement. If the patient is apnoeic, face-mask ventilation with 100% oxygen must be started immediately to ensure adequate oxygenation. Tracheal intubation should be performed with care. The cervical collar should be unfastened at the front to allow easier laryngoscopy and the application of cricoid force (if necessary), and the cervical spine should be protected by manual in-line immobilisation; the collar can be reapplied after tracheal intubation is complete. The use of a bougie or videolaryngoscopy may facilitate tracheal intubation and is encouraged. During laryngoscopy it not necessary to obtain the 'best possible' view of the glottic

---

> **Box 44.3 Indications for tracheal intubation in the emergency department**
>
> Inability to maintain and protect own airway regardless of conscious level
> Come with reduced level of consciousness (not obeying commands, not speaking, not eye opening, i.e. GCS ≤ 8)
> Severe agitation preventing lifesaving therapeutic intervention(s)
> Anticipated clinical course (e.g. requirement for urgent intervention in theatre or inter-hospital transfer)
> Refractory hypoxaemia
> Facial/airway/neck burns (often done prophylactically)
> In traumatic brain injury
>   Significantly deteriorating conscious level (≥1 or more points on the motor score), even if not coma
>   Ventilatory insufficiency as judged by blood gases:
> $PaO_2 < 13$ kPa on oxygen and/or $PaCO_2 > 6$ kPa
>   Spontaneous hyperventilation causing $PaCO_2 < 4$ kPa
>   Irregular respirations
>
> *GCS*, Glasgow Coma Scale.

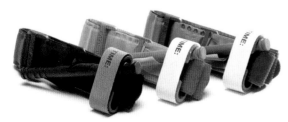

Fig. 44.2 Combat application tourniquet (CAT). (From www.combattourniquet.com.)

Table 44.4 Indications for damage control resuscitation in trauma

Severity of traumatic injuries	Physiological derangement	Laboratory derangement
ISS > 36 Penetrating injuries Open pelvic fracture Truncal haemorrhage/amputation Long bone fracture with lung contusion or head injury	Weak/absent radial pulse Systolic blood pressure < 100 mmHg Heart rate > 100 beats min^{-1} Core temperature < 35°C	Lactate > 2.5 mmol L^{-1} Base deficit > 6 Haemoglobin < 110 g L^{-1} Coagulopathy pH < 7.2

ISS, Injury Severity Score.
Adapted from Giannoudi M., & Harwood, P. (2016) Damage control resuscitation: lessons learned. *European Journal of Trauma & Emergency Surgery.* 42, 273–282.

opening (i.e. Cormack-Lehane grade 1), as this will increase cervical spine movement; a glottic view that allows easy passage of a bougie is adequate (grade 2b/3). There is a higher incidence of failed tracheal intubation in the emergency trauma setting, which is partly attributable to cervical immobilisation. A realistic, feasible airway strategy must be planned and communicated with the trauma team, up to and including a surgical airway. There is rarely a 'wake-up' option in the major trauma situation.

Patients with severe facial trauma who are cooperative and awake despite their injuries may not require immediate tracheal intubation. However, they do need frequent and regular upper airway evaluation to assess the rate of progress of pharyngeal or laryngeal oedema, which may proceed to complete airway obstruction with alarming speed.

If there are clinical signs suggesting a pneumothorax or surgical emphysema and/or a flail segment is apparent, then a thoracostomy (with an intercostal drain subsequently) should be performed simultaneously or before mechanical ventilation is commenced. Persistence of hypoxaemia after institution of mechanical ventilation suggests unrecognised pneumothorax, haemothorax, pulmonary contusion or poor cardiac output (e.g. secondary to hypovolaemia or cardiac tamponade).

Circulation

There has been a significant shift in the resuscitation strategy of the haemodynamically unstable patient, with a move away from 'full' resuscitation and 'definitive' surgery towards a concept of damage control resuscitation (DCR). The term *hybrid resuscitation* is used to describe the combination of *time-limited* permissive hypotension with haemostatic resuscitation. The presence of a central pulse (approximating to systolic blood pressure 70 mmHg) is deemed to be evidence of adequate perfusion, and that is the target until the source of bleeding is controlled. The emphasis is on rapid and effective control of bleeding. Some indications for implementing DCR are shown in Table 44.4.

Haemorrhage is the most common cause of shock in the injured patient, and virtually all patients with multiple injuries have an element of hypovolaemia. In the UK there is a lower incidence of penetrating trauma compared with blunt trauma. Patients with major trauma often require urgent restoration of sufficient circulating blood volume to ensure:

- adequate oxygen delivery to the tissues;
- stabilisation and/or correction of metabolic derangements; and
- correction of acute traumatic coagulopathy (ATC) and prevention of iatrogenic coagulopathy.

Initial response to adequate boluses of warmed isotonic fluids may give some guide as to degree of hypovolemia. However, if a patient has clear signs or a strong history suggestive of significant blood loss, there is little to be gained by administration of crystalloids; blood should be given at the earliest opportunity. All fluids given must be warmed, as the triad of hypothermia, acidosis and clotting derangement can be lethal. Large-bore i.v. access should be inserted into peripheral veins and attached to infusions that are connected to devices capable to effectively warming fluids (ideally blood and blood products) delivered at a high rate (e.g. 'Level 1' transfuser).

Concurrently with i.v. fluid replacement, the team should be instituting damage-control resuscitation measures to try and reduce further blood loss. These include:

- limited crystalloid infusions (tends to dilute coagulation factors and worsen ATC);
- permissive hypotension (if traumatic brain injury (TBI) not suspected) and especially in penetrating trauma (see later);
- treatment of ATC (see later);
- rapid haemorrhage control with early damage control surgery; and

- regaining homeostasis with aggressive temperature management to treat or avoid hypothermia and treatment of hypocalcaemia (common after massive transfusion and worsens ATC).

Permissive hypotension

Permissive hypotension is the strategy of restricting fluid resuscitation and permitting a lower than normal perfusion pressure until the haemorrhage is controlled. This should be strictly time limited (up to 60 min maximum) and ideally will have been started in the prehospital phase. The exact systolic blood pressure targets remain controversial. European guidance suggests systolic blood pressure of 80–100 mmHg with the exception of severe TBI, where the mean arterial pressure should be maintained 80 mmHg or greater. There is still uncertainty about the best way to manage multisystem blunt trauma that occurs in conjunction with TBI, and, in the first instance, management should focus on achieving adequate cerebral perfusion.

Haemostatic resuscitation

Acute traumatic coagulopathy is seen in major trauma patients, with a significant number of patients already coagulopathic by the time they have arrived in the ED. Acute traumatic coagulopathy is induced by a combination of the tissue trauma and shock and is driven by the degree of tissue hypoperfusion (see also Chapter 14 and Box 14.1). The coagulopathy that develops is due to activation of the protein C pathway, which causes hyperfibrinolysis. The administration of tranexamic acid (1 g i.v. bolus and then 1 g infusion over 8 h) within 3 h of injury has been shown to be effective and is now often administered in the prehospital environment.

Massive transfusion is defined arbitrarily as either replacement of more than 50% of a patient's blood volume within 1 h, or replacement of 1–1.5 blood volumes within a 24-h period. Massive haemorrhage protocols are a fundamental component of good clinical care; an example is shown in Fig. 44.3. Transfusion protocols have changed, largely as a result of experience gained in conflict zones. Hospitals will have their own protocols for massive haemorrhage, and these vary in the ratios of PRCs to fresh frozen plasma (FFP) to cryoprecipitate to platelets. Hospital transfusion services now often provide 'shock packs' which contain PRCs and other clotting products in predetermined ratios. Over recent years than has been a move towards the transfusion of PRC/FFP/platelets in 1 : 1 : 1 ratio in cases of major haemorrhage. Packed red cells contain no plasma, platelets, coagulation factors or leucocytes. Therefore the treatment of massive haemorrhage by volume replacement solely with PRCs will not correct ATC and places the patient at high risk of further dilutional coagulopathy. High-dose FFP will correct hypofi-brinogenaemia and most coagulation factor deficiencies. However, if the fibrinogen concentration remains less than 1.5 g L^{-1}, cryoprecipitate or fibrinogen concentrate therapy should be considered. It is necessary to give platelet concentrate for all instances of severe thrombocytopenia (platelet count < 50 × 10^9 L^{-1}). The use of point-of-care coagulation testing (e.g. thromboelastography (TEG) or rotational thromboelastometry (ROTEM)) may be of value and regular liaison with haematology is vital.

The importance of the prevention of hypothermia during massive transfusion cannot be overstated. Hypothermia causes platelet dysfunction, an increased tendency to cardiac arrhythmias and a left shift of the oxygen–haemoglobin dissociation curve, thereby decreasing oxygen delivery to the tissues (see Chapter 10). Hypothermia also decreases the metabolism of citrate and lactate, both of which are usually present in stored PRCs. If the normally rapid metabolism of these substances is slowed, then a profound metabolic acidaemia can develop. Core temperature should be measured continuously during massive transfusion, and every effort must be made to prevent heat loss. Warm air over-blankets are usually helpful. Efficient systems for heating stored blood and allowing rapid infusion are available, but all fluids should be warmed to body temperature if possible. In addition, calcium chelation by citrate can lead to clinically significant hypocalcaemia, which should be treated and monitored.

Cardiac 'pump failure'

Cardiac 'pump failure' in major trauma can lead to persistent hypotension and traumatic cardiac arrest. This can be due to the presence of a tension pneumothorax, but other possibilities include severe myocardial contusion and traumatic pericardial tamponade. Tension pneumothorax causes compression of the mediastinum (heart and great vessels) and presents with extreme respiratory distress, shock, unilateral air entry, a shift of the trachea towards the normal side and distension of the veins in the neck (may not be seen in hypovolemic shock). Tension pneumothorax is a clinical diagnosis and should be treated if suspected; a chest radiograph simply delays treatment. It may be relieved immediately by insertion of a large-gauge cannula through the second intercostal space in the midclavicular line or in the fifth intercostal space in the midaxillary line; however, in around 50% of patients the pleural cavity cannot be reached with a standard cannula. The technique of finger thoracostomy (fifth intercostal space in the mid axillary line) is now recommended for traumatic pneumothoraces and should be performed in patients who have already undergone tracheal intubation and are mechanically ventilated. This should be followed by insertion of an intercostal drain. Patients with blunt chest trauma and fractured ribs may develop a tension pneumothorax rapidly when positive

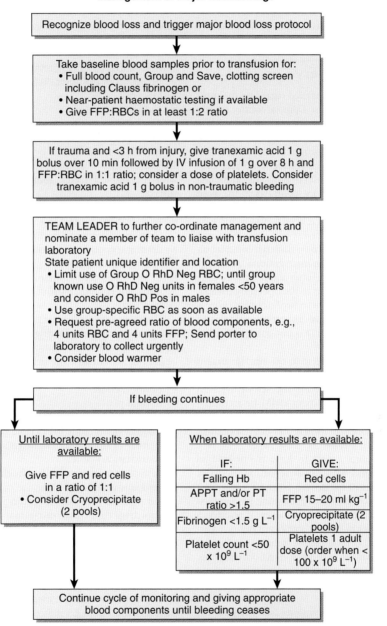

A practical guideline for the haematological management of major haemorrhage

Recognize blood loss and trigger major blood loss protocol

↓

Take baseline blood samples prior to transfusion for:
• Full blood count, Group and Save, clotting screen including Clauss fibrinogen or
• Near-patient haemostatic testing if available
• Give FFP:RBCs in at least 1:2 ratio

↓

If trauma and <3 h from injury, give tranexamic acid 1 g bolus over 10 min followed by IV infusion of 1 g over 8 h and FFP:RBC in 1:1 ratio; consider a dose of platelets. Consider tranexamic acid 1 g bolus in non-traumatic bleeding

↓

TEAM LEADER to further co-ordinate management and nominate a member of team to liaise with transfusion laboratory
State patient unique identifier and location
• Limit use of Group O RhD Neg RBC; until group known use O RhD Neg units in females <50 years and consider O RhD Pos in males
• Use group-specific RBC as soon as available
• Request pre-agreed ratio of blood components, e.g., 4 units RBC and 4 units FFP; Send porter to laboratory to collect urgently
• Consider blood warmer

↓

If bleeding continues

Until laboratory results are available:

Give FFP and red cells in a ratio of 1:1
• Consider Cryoprecipitate (2 pools)

When laboratory results are available:

IF:	GIVE:
Falling Hb	Red cells
APPT and/or PT ratio >1.5	FFP 15–20 ml kg^{-1}
Fibrinogen <1.5 g L^{-1}	Cryoprecipitate (2 pools)
Platelet count <50 x 10^9 L^{-1}	Platelets 1 adult dose (order when < 100 x 10^9 L^{-1})

↓

Continue cycle of monitoring and giving appropriate blood components until bleeding ceases

Fig. 44.3 A practical guideline for the haematological management of major haemorrhage. *APTT,* Activated partial thromboplastin time; *FFP,* fresh frozen plasma; *Hb,* haemoglobin; *Neg,* negative; *PT,* prothrombin time; *RBCs,* red blood cells. (From Hunt, B. J., Allard, S., Keeling, D., et al.; British Committee for Standards in Haematology. (2015) A practical guideline for the haematological management of major haemorrhage. *British Journal of Haematology.* 170, 788–803.)

pressure ventilation is commenced, and the prophylactic insertion of a chest drain should be considered in such patients. Patients who have arrested after a penetrating chest or upper abdominal injury may require a resuscitative thoracotomy if pericardial tamponade is suspected.

Damage control surgery

An early decision by the team is needed regarding the most appropriate pathway for the patient. Damage control surgery has been adopted as a lifesaving and temporary procedure for unstable patients who have sustained major trauma. The concept has arisen from the current understanding that the patient lacks the physiological reserve to survive prolonged definitive surgery at this point in time. Urgent trauma whole-body CT scanning (with i.v. contrast) is the gold standard and provides important anatomical information about injuries. Whole-body CT has been found to increase the probability of survival in patients with major trauma and even unstable patients often now undergo imaging on the way to the operating theatre or interventional radiology suite. Patients with inadequate perfusion and not responding to resuscitation should go straight to the operating theatre. Patients intermediate between these two groups require a more complex decision. The most important action is to make a decision; waiting in the ED is not going to further the patient's care.

- Systolic blood pressure more than 90 mmHg: urgent trauma CT
- Systolic blood pressure 70–90 mmHg: senior decision making; if CT is chosen, the patient MUST be accompanied by the trauma team
- Systolic blood pressure < 70 mmHg and not responding: transfer to operating theatre

Well-run trauma units expect to have major trauma patients through CT and with initial reporting of major findings within 30 min of ED arrival. Focused assessment with sonography for trauma (FAST) scanning by a skilled operator may also provide helpful information if positive; a negative FAST scan does not rule out significant injury. Based on the CT findings and clinical picture, senior members of the trauma team will make a prompt decision regarding intervention: operating theatre for damage control surgery; angiography suite for embolisation; or non-operative continued resuscitation in the ICU.

The use of radiological interventions (see Chapter 46) has increased hugely in the last decade as an alternative to surgery. Most preventable deaths in trauma are due to unrecognised and therefore untreated haemorrhage, particularly in the abdomen or pelvis. Interventional radiology uses minimally invasive endovascular techniques to control haemorrhage by blocking (transcatheter arterial embolisation) or by relining (stent grafting) bleeding vessels. The main objective is to stop the bleeding in parts of the body that are difficult to access by conventional surgical means. It also can prevent the physiological stress that will result if the patient has to undergo major abdominal or pelvic exploratory surgery. Interventional radiology can be used for the treatment of bleeding in the following structures:

- Thoracic aorta
- Abdominal aorta (e.g. retrograde endovascular balloon occlusion of the aorta, REBOA)
- Spleen
- Kidney
- Liver
- Pelvic vessels

At MTCs, there should be 24-h access to this service. The anaesthetist must be involved in ongoing discussions with the surgical teams about the extent and intent of surgery.

The aims of damage control surgery are:

- haemorrhage control (e.g. abdominal packing, clamps, ligation, splinting of fractures);
- decompression of at risk compartments (i.e. head, heart, limbs, abdomen);
- to minimise contamination (e.g. debridement of fractures and wounds, closure or resection of hollow viscus injuries).

The duration of surgery is limited and additional surgical trauma is minimised. During this time, particularly once haemorrhage has been controlled, the anaesthetist should be aiming to normalise physiology by correcting metabolic, fluid and haemostatic derangements. Targets typically include:

- normothermia;
- normal pH;
- fibrinogen greater than 1.5 g L^{-1} normal activated partial thromboplastin time (APTT) and prothrombin time (PT);
- normal or improving lactate (a marker of adequacy of resuscitation); and
- correction of anaemia (haemoglobin $100–110 \text{ g L}^{-1}$ is generally accepted).

For patients who do not require immediate surgery for haemorrhage control, decontamination or decompression, a team decision may need to be made whether to proceed to early total care (definitive treatment of all long-bone fractures) or damage control orthopaedic surgery. These decisions should be based on an overall assessment of patient condition, particularly the trend in blood lactate. If lactate is less than 2.0 mmol L^{-1}, then early total care can be considered; if more than 2.5 mmol L^{-1}, then continued resuscitation or damage control orthopaedic surgery is required.

Trauma anaesthesia

It is sometimes necessary to induce anaesthesia in a patient who is hypovolaemic; this requires meticulous attention to fluid and drug management. A controlled RSI should be performed, but with extreme care regarding dose of induction agent. The depressant effects of i.v. anaesthetic agents are exaggerated in trauma patients because the proportion of the cardiac output going to the heart and brain is increased. In addition, the rate of redistribution and/or metabolism is decreased as a result of reduced blood flow to muscle, liver and kidneys. Ketamine can be used safely in patients with a significant TBI, as the benefits of maintained arterial blood pressure outweigh any concerns about cerebro-metabolic effects. Particular care needs to be taken in the presence of hypovolaemia and TBI, as hypotension is associated with a doubling of mortality. Permissive hypotension should be avoided in patients with TBI, as maintenance of cerebral perfusion pressure is paramount.

After tracheal intubation, the lungs are ventilated at the lowest peak airway pressure consistent with an acceptable tidal volume. Judicious doses of NMBAs and analgesia (usually fentanyl) are given as necessary. As the cardiovascular status normalises and systolic blood pressure exceeds 90 mmHg, anaesthesia should be deepened as tolerated. This should be undertaken cautiously and, in principle, agents that are rapidly reversible or rapidly excreted should be used. In the shock state, there is very rapid uptake of inhalational agents. Reduced cardiac output and pulmonary blood flow decrease the rate of removal of anaesthetic agent from the alveoli, producing a rapid increase in alveolar concentration. Thus the MAC value is approached more rapidly than in normovolaemic patients.

Basic monitoring will have been instituted in the ED. Insertion of arterial lines should not delay time to CT or surgical control of haemorrhage. However, blood may be sampled from an arterial cannula to monitor changes in acid–base state, haemoglobin concentration, coagulation and electrolyte concentrations.

Vascular access

Central venous access is not a high priority in trauma resuscitation but may be essential for i.v. access in the presence of four-limb trauma. Short, large-diameter central access devices (e.g. insertion sheaths for pulmonary artery flotation catheters) are popular in the military. The intraosseous (i.o.) route has been used for many years in children for fluid and drug delivery and is now being used increasingly in adults as it provides rapid access to the circulation in an emergency setting. Insertion devices are now commonplace in both prehospital and in-hospital settings. Sites for i.o. needle placement in adults include the proximal humerus, proximal tibia and distal tibia. The proximal humerus site allows greater flow rates of up to 5 L h^{-1} and is useful for drug and fluid delivery as they enter the central circulation very rapidly, reaching the right atrium in 3 s. It is also the preferred site if there is any lower limb or pelvic injury

> **Box 44.4 Causes of persistent hypotension after trauma**
>
> Surgical or medical (check platelets and clotting screen)
> Continued overt bleeding
> Continued concealed bleeding – chest, abdomen, retroperitoneal space, pelvis, soft tissues of each thigh
> Pump failure – haemothorax, pneumothorax, tamponade, myocardial contusion
> Metabolic problem – acidaemia (only correct pH < 7.1), hypothermia (largely preventable), hypocalcaemia

suspected. Induction agents, NMBAs, fluids and blood products can all be delivered via the i.o. route.

When surgical bleeding has been controlled, the patient's cardiovascular status should improve. However if hypotension persists despite apparently adequate fluid administration, other causes of haemorrhage should be sought (Box 44.4). It is important that the patient is regularly reassessed during prolonged anaesthesia to exclude these latent complications of major trauma.

Analgesic considerations in trauma patients

Traditionally, pain has been managed according to the WHO analgesic ladder (see Chapter 6). It is unlikely to be entirely applicable to acute trauma care, but agents are usually given i.v. or via the intranasal, transmucosal or inhalational route.

Intranasal

The intranasal route is popular in paediatrics and becoming more popular in adults. Highly lipid-soluble drugs such as diamorphine and fentanyl have all been administered by this route, with the ideal delivery tool being a mucosal atomiser device. This route has a fast onset and good bioavailability. Analgesia can be achieved within 3–5 min, with peak concentrations at 10–15 min. For an intranasal fentanyl dose via mucosal atomiser device, initially administer 1.5 µg kg^{-1} divided between nostrils, with a further dose of 0.75–1.5 µg kg^{-1} if required after 10 min.

Oral transmucosal

Highly lipid soluble agents (commonly fentanyl) can be administered in the form of a lollipop or lozenge. Transmucosal absorption provides rapid pain relief and then the ingested drug provides ongoing analgesia. Fentanyl lozenge adult dose is 200 µg initially over 15 min followed by 200 µg if required.

Inhalational

The inhalational route is fast acting and can be patient controlled. Entonox (see Chapter 3) can be used but causes expansion of closed air-containing cavities such as pneumothoraces and thus should be used with caution.

Methoxyflurane is a halogenated volatile anaesthetic agent with analgesic properties that can be inhaled in subanaesthetic doses via an inhaler (Penthrox) to provide PCA in adults. Studies have shown it to be effective analgesic for acute pain, the most common adverse effects being dizziness and headaches. A 3-ml bottle can be used, with a further 3 ml if required. Analgesia is established over 6–10 inhalations, and then intermittent inhalations can be used for maintenance.

Intravenous

Fentanyl ($0.25–1.0\ \mu g\ kg^{-1}$) and ketamine ($0.1–0.5\ mg\ kg^{-1}$) i.v. are commonly used. These agents are discussed in detail in Chapter 6.

Anaesthetic considerations in the prehospital environment

This section examines specifically some of the issues providing trauma care in the prehospital environment and offers some specific guidance on managing patients in this environment. Doctors in emergency medicine, anaesthesia, intensive care or acute medicine are eligible to apply for prehospital emergency medicine (PHEM) subspecialty training in the UK. Hospital staff may find themselves providing prehospital care in several situations:

- as a member of a hospital flying squad or during a major incident;
- as an immediate care practitioner (British Association of Immediate Care (BASICS) doctor);
- on duty (either paid or with the voluntary services) at an event such as a football match or festival;
- good Samaritan acts.

Each of these situations has different clinical and logistical issues, but there are some common themes. For this chapter the main example used is that of hospital staff attending a road traffic collision (RTC). It is unreasonable to expect hospital staff to attend an incident and function effectively without training and preparation. An RTC is also a remote and unsupervised location, and hospitals should deploy only staff with the correct clinical background to work in these situations. Working safely in the prehospital environment demands consideration of hazards at the scene and of the roles of the other emergency services. Doctors and hospital staff are asked to attend if there is a casualty who is physically trapped and who may require analgesics to facilitate extrication.

Team preparation includes having appropriate safety clothing and equipment, such as:

- fire-retardant and waterproof overgarments;
- high-visibility jackets;
- helmets;
- eye and ear protection;
- safety boots; and
- gloves.

Mechanisms of injury

Using the principles of kinematics, it is useful to try and work out the forces involved in collisions and then relate this to the potential injury patterns that might be seen or suspected. Road traffic collisions involving vehicles will broadly fall into the following categories:

- Car against:
  - Pedestrian
  - Cyclist
  - Motorcyclist
- Car against car or other large vehicle (casualty entrapment):
  - Head-on frontal impact
  - Side impact ('T-bone')
  - Rear impact
- Car/cycle/motorcycle against stationary object (e.g. tree):
  - Head-on frontal impact
  - Side impact

Scene safety

On approaching a scene, the rescuer's safety is paramount. If there are already emergency services present, then the medical team need to report to the fire officer in charge (will be wearing a white helmet). He or she will be able to confirm the safety of the scene and also the location and reasons for any cordons. For example, at an RTC, potential hazards include:

- broken glass;
- spilt fuel;
- fire and smoke;
- other traffic moving around the incident; and
- cutting and lifting equipment being used by the fire and rescue service.

Teamwork

Hospital personnel at an incident are there to support the ambulance service, and they need to know whom to report to and how to work with ambulance staff and police. In addition, the fire service may be present to manage hazards and provide cutting equipment if needed for extrication. The police are present to coordinate the incident and the area around it, managing traffic flow and protecting evidence at the scene. Although everyone is concentrating their efforts on saving and treating the casualties, hospital staff need to understand that the other emergency services have their own roles, and the management of the incident continues after they and the casualties have left the scene. Interservice working is addressed by the courses such as the Major Incident Medical Management and Support (MIMMS) course.

Working at the scene

Problems likely to be encountered include the following:

- *Access to the casualty.* The vehicle compartment around the casualty may be deformed and intruded. The vehicle may be on its side, upside down or in a ditch, making access to the casualty difficult.
- *Multiple casualties.* This may complicate the rescue especially if a combination of adults and children are injured at the scene.
- *Lighting.* The emergency services may provide portable lights, but in prehospital care the anaesthetist is often trying to assess and manage a casualty in poor light.
- *Noise.* Noise from generators and vehicles makes auscultation very difficult and interferes with communication with team members and other emergency services.
- *Environment.* Wet weather and cold conditions imply that casualties (and staff not wearing appropriate clothing) become hypothermic quickly.

Logistical considerations

The aim is to move the patient in the best clinical condition possible to the most appropriate hospital in the shortest time possible. In reality, a series of compromises are needed. Before carrying out any procedure, the clinician on the scene needs to ask:

- Is this essential?
- Should it be carried out now, during the move to hospital or at the hospital?
- Am I helping the patient and the situation or causing undue delay?

For example, is it appropriate to struggle for 15 min to set up an i.v. infusion when the hospital is only 5 min travel time away? If the casualty is trapped and needs i.v. analgesia or anaesthesia to facilitate release, then the answer is probably yes, unless there are alternatives. However, if the casualty is ready to leave the scene except for this intervention, then the answer is probably no (unless there is no vehicle available to move the casualty). Decisions such as these depend on many factors, including the overall situation, travel time to hospital, availability of ambulances and the needs of other casualties.

Extrication

Extrication will be supervised and performed primarily by the fire service. The medical team may be asked if they feel the patient is time critical (i.e. has a life-threatening injury and thus needs rapid extrication). If this is not the case, then the fire service will plan a more controlled extrication of the patient. If the patient is able to self-extricate, this should be encouraged.

Clinical considerations

The same principles that were discussed earlier are used in the prehospital setting, with a strong emphasis on haemorrhage control. A cABC approach is taken:

- Catastrophic haemorrhage control
- Airway
- Breathing
- Circulation – haemorrhagic and non-haemorrhagic causes may coexist

Prehospital emergency anaesthesia

In severely injured patients, prehospital tracheal intubation and mechanical ventilation may be desirable in a casualty at risk of aspiration or with a severe head injury. Simple methods should be used first and the situation reassessed because access to the casualty may be improved (e.g. when the roof of the car has been cut off or when the casualty has been released from the vehicle). The NCEPOD Report from 2007 highlighted the deficiencies in airway management in trauma and emphasised the need for prehospital anaesthesia when appropriate. Rapid-sequence induction with oral tracheal intubation is usually the technique of choice, but this should be performed only by appropriately trained individuals with adequate resources. The decision to do it must be based on a risk/benefit assessment. The Association of Anaesthetists have produced guidance on the specific requirements in training, equipment and personnel to undertake this procedure. The same standards of equipment and monitoring are used in this environment. Checklists for all procedures are used extensively in prehospital medicine, with the aim to standardise practice as much as possible.

Cervical spine control

Many road accident casualties are at risk of cervical spine injury. Neck collars and other immobilisation devices limit mouth opening and make airway management difficult. The front of the collar may be removed and paramedics may be asked to substitute manual in-line immobilisation if the anaesthetist is having difficulty establishing a clear airway. There have been publications which question the efficacy

847

and need for cervical spine immobilisation in some patients, but at present it should be instituted in any unconscious trauma patient.

Transfer to hospital

The choice of hospital is decided usually by the medical and ambulance staff on scene and relayed to ambulance control. Ambulance control or the personnel on scene should contact the hospital so that the receiving team is placed on standby and receives as much information about the casualty (or casualties) as possible in advance. The conduct of transfers is discussed in detail in Chapter 48.

In some situations it is necessary to 'load and go' as fast as possible (e.g. some stabbing or gunshot incidents in which the overriding need is surgical intervention). Civilian helicopter ambulances provide a fast method of transporting a patient to hospital, but these have some limitations. The attending staff may be unfamiliar with working in a helicopter, the space around the casualty is restricted compared with a ground ambulance and the environment is noisy. In addition, a second ambulance journey is often required at many UK hospitals to transport the patient from the helicopter landing site to the ED.

Management of major incidents

Major incidents are defined as situations that place an extraordinary burden on healthcare resources as a result of the number or type of casualties involved in an incident, which cannot be met by standard available resources. These can be further classified into natural disaster or manmade, simple or compound (depending on the state of infrastructure such as hospitals, roads and communication systems) and compensated or uncompensated incidents (i.e. is the incident within the scope of existing major incident plans or so large as to overwhelm all plans).

The important principles in managing a major incident are as follows:

- Command and Control
- Safety
- Communication
- Assessment
- Triage
- Treatment
- Transport

Communication and teamwork are essential in a major incident, not only because of the clinical needs of multiple patients but also because a major incident is usually a crime scene for the police. If not a terrorist event or a manmade incident, there will at least be an inquiry into what happened, possibly many depending on the type of incident and if there were multiple deaths. There are three levels of control in a major incident which are mirrored across all the emergency services: bronze (operational); silver (tactical); and gold (strategic). Bronze commanders are the frontline commanders who will have control over a section of the incident, whereas silver commanders have responsibility for multiple sectors and gold has overall incident command at regional level.

Triage is the next crucial step in any major incident. This ensures that the sickest patients are treated first and also that the right patients are sent to the right hospital. Triaging is done using a triage sieve (Fig. 44.4). This is a swift, reliable and reproducible tool that is based on a patient's clinical

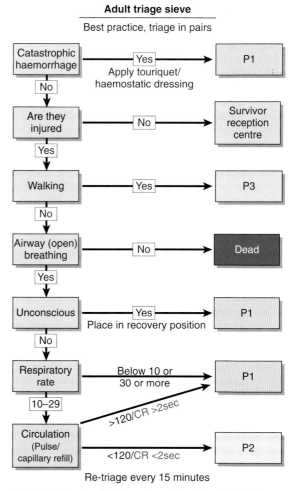

Fig. 44.4 Example of a triage sieve algorithm. *CR,* Capillary Refill. (From http://www.smartmci.com/products/triage/smart_triage_pac.php.)

signs at a particular time. Triage is a dynamic process because patients can change triage category as time progresses, but the key is to make early decisions with ongoing reassessment. Each patient should take no longer than 15 s to assess. It is also important to note that the person triaging must not become involved with delivering care to patients. The three exceptions to this rule are applying a tourniquet, opening an airway to assess for presence of respiratory effort or rapidly repositioning an unconscious patient into the recovery position to maintain a clear airway. Once a triage category has been assigned, patients must be appropriately marked to ensure they are treated with the appropriate expediency.

Treatment at a major incident

As part of its prehospital response plan, every ambulance organisation will set up a casualty clearing centre (CCC) at the site of an incident. This may be in tents or, preferably, a suitable undamaged building with a good supply of energy, water, heat and light. It is at the CCC that the triage sort takes place, and depending on the type and duration of the incident it may be possible to bring some hospital facilities and capabilities forward to the incident. There should be an ambulance pickup point at the CCC to allow for the quick extrication of patients to appropriate hospitals, as well as a nearby command post where fire, ambulance and police commanders should be located.

Every hospital will have a major incident plan. Inside this will be action cards for all the different clinical and administrative personnel. If a major incident is declared, the hospital's major incident plan is activated and several actions take place simultaneously. Hospital switchboard will try and gather as many relevant senior clinicians as possible, a briefing will take place of the current plan and additional beds will be sourced as soon as possible. Practically this means the discharge of any patients who are well enough, emptying the ED, cancellation of elective surgical lists/reallocation of theatre teams, and plans for discharge or transfer of ICU patients. Once this surge capacity has been generated, the hospital can feed back to ambulance control as to how many patients they can accept and of what type. It is important to familiarise yourself with the major incident plan for your hospital and know what is on your action card.

References/Further reading

Association of Anaesthetists, 2017. Safer pre-hospital anaesthesia. http://www.aagbi.org/sites/default/files/Safer%20pre_hospital%20anaesthesia2017.pdf.

CRASH-2 collaborators, Roberts, I., Shakur, H., Afolabi, A., Brohi, K., Coats, T., et al., 2011. The importance of early treatment with tranexamic acid in bleeding trauma patients: an exploratory analysis of the CRASH-2 randomised controlled trial. Lancet 377 (9771), 1096–1101.e2.

Lockey, D.J., Healey, B., Crewdson, K., Chalk, G., Weaver, A.E., Davies, G.E., 2015. Advanced airway management is necessary in prehospital trauma patients. Br. J. Anaesth. 114 (4), 657–662.

National Institute for Health and Care Excellence, 2016. Major trauma guidelines. https://www.nice.org.uk/guidance/ng39.

Sundstrøm, T., Asbjørnsen, H., Habiba, S., Sunde, G.A., Wester, K., 2014. Prehospital use of cervical collars in trauma patients: A critical review. J. Neurotrauma 31 (6), 531–540.

The National Emergency Laparotomy Audit. http://www.nela.org.uk.

Chapter | 45 |

Anaesthesia in resource-poor areas

Mary O'Regan

Background

The variation in resources available to healthcare systems in regional populations of the world is widely acknowledged. The terms *developed* and *developing world* mislead, suggesting binary options and inevitable progress to a complete state. The reality is a skewed spectrum of resource and development dictated by the combined influences of geography, climate, economics, politics, culture and conflict. Development at the weakest end of the spectrum often loses momentum and is easily driven backwards. The poor of the world are exposed to greater personal and environmental health risks; they are less well nourished, have fewer health choices and have less access to health information and high-quality healthcare. The consequence is a burden of illness and disability with devastating consequences for individuals and struggling healthcare systems.

Challenges to the provision of anaesthesia

This chapter focuses on the provision of anaesthesia and critical care in the poorest-resourced communities of the world. The ceiling of what can be achieved may be curbed by an inadequate supply of clean running water, electricity, medicines, equipment, skilled staff, education and transport. Patients may present with low expectations, advanced pathological conditions and complications from the ministrations of traditional healers. While international agencies set goals and contend with the complexity of world health inequity, individuals focus on alleviating pain and suffering at a local level. For the anaesthesia provider, this means attempting to provide safe anaesthesia, analgesia,

critical care and peer education in an unpredictable environment over which they have limited control. A solid foundation of theoretical knowledge and strong practical skills are required. Access to a wider medical community brings valuable support. Consensus standards may encourage significant development even when achieving specific goals proves impossible. An awareness of recent advances and the potential offered by new technologies must be contextualised shrewdly. Cultural awareness and linguistic skills provide valuable insights and facilitate the management of complex medical situations. Highly developed non-technical skills, teamwork, pragmatism and tireless optimism are essential tools against falling standards and professional burnout.

Attention to personal health and safety is particularly important. Workplace dangers include poorly maintained electrical equipment, explosive anaesthetic vapours, contaminated sharps, exposure to lethal pandemics and the risk of violence. Neglect of one's own physical and mental health is hazardous. If the lone anaesthesia provider in a large isolated community is unable to work, the impact for patients can be devastating. Healthcare facilities rarely have enough staff to meet the needs of the community they serve. Staff are obliged to be generalists, and the 24-h emergency management of the most urgent cases dominates the workload.

Population and procedures

The bulk of the surgical work comprises obstetric emergencies and the management of abscesses, wounds and fractures (Box 45.1). The anaesthesia required may be considered basic, but the patient is often in poor condition and requires significant preoperative resuscitation. Preoperative assessment follows universal principles with the emphasis on clinical signs rather than investigations. Special consideration needs to be given

Box 45.1 Common procedures performed in basic or intermediate level healthcare settings

General surgery

Incision and drainage of superficial abscess
Wound toilet and debridement
Suturing and dressing
Hydrocele drainage and reduction
Circumcision
Inguinal hernia repair
Appendicectomy
Prostatectomy
Amputation
Emergency laparotomy
Insertion of intercostal drain

Obstetrics

Uterine evacuation
Caesarean section
Haemorrhage control (uterine & genital tract)
Destructive fetal procedures

Gynaecology

Tubal ligation
Ovarian cystectomy
Salpingo-ophrectomy
Hysterectomy

Orthopaedics and trauma

Cleaning and stabilisation of fractures
Closed and open fixation of fractures

Other

Cataract extraction
Burns surgery
Removal of foreign body (including airway)

to the common conditions affecting the local community. These might include the effects of parasitic disease and severe anaemia (e.g. malaria and schistosomiasis), malnutrition, HIV/AIDS, tuberculosis, massive goitre, pregnancy-induced hypertensive disease, advanced molar pregnancy and the effects of traditional medicines. Populations are usually relatively young, and a large proportion of the patients treated will be infants and children. In some settings, most elective surgical work is performed by visiting specialists. This can be a challenge for the lone anaesthesia provider obliged to meet the requirements of more complex procedures with an unfamiliar team. If a visiting team includes a specialist anaesthesia provider, the resident anaesthetist may be offered a rare opportunity for education and case-based discussion. Visiting teams may depart having overburdened their hosts with challenging patients and their complex postoperative care needs.

Anaesthesia without electricity or pressurised gas supplies

Recommended international standards for the safe provision of anaesthesia were updated and ratified by the World Federation of Societies of Anaesthesiologists (WFSA) in 2010. The WFSA defined three levels of healthcare setting in which general anaesthesia may be delivered (Table 45.1).

The infrastructure standards recommended for even the most basic settings require electricity or pressurised gas supplies to provide oxygen. In reality, many institutions in remote and resource-poor environments are obliged to operate without oxygen for all or some of the time. Anaesthesia providers in these circumstances need to employ simple and safe techniques that offer patients rapid recovery requiring minimal postoperative care. Institutional

Table 45.1 World Federation of Societies of Anaesthesiologists (WFSA) classification of healthcare settings

Setting	Infrastructure	Description
Level 1	Basic	Rural hospitals and health centres Small number of beds Operating room equipped for minor procedures, emergency trauma and obstetrics (excluding caesarean section)
Level 2	Intermediate	District or provincial hospitals 100–300 beds Adequately equipped for major procedures and short-term management of all major life-threatening conditions
Level 3	Optimal	Referral hospitals with at least basic intensive care facilities 300–1000 beds Equipped for specialised surgery and pronged mechanical ventilation

Table 45.2 Basic requirements for anaesthesia in a resource-poor area

Requirements	Notes
Simple and safe techniques	May be provided by less skilled practitioners
Rapid return to street fitness	Minimise postoperative care requirements
Affordable	Maximises the number of patients treatable
Simple and durable equipment	Reusable, local maintenance, portable
Temperature stable, long shelf-life medication	Refrigeration facilities may not be available

self-reliance supports a resilient service. Equipment must be affordable, durable and easy to maintain locally (Table 45.2).

The cost and infrastructure required to deliver liquid oxygen from a vacuum-insulated evaporator (see Chapter 16) makes this an unachievable option for most hospitals in resource-poor environments. Reliance on a cylinder supply alone reduces dependence on electricity but is relatively costly and can be unreliable when delivery depends upon poorly maintained roads and vehicles. Many anaesthetists prefer the low running costs of an oxygen concentrator and reserve a backup oxygen cylinder for emergency use during electricity blackouts. A well-maintained portable oxygen concentrator can provide up to 8 L min^{-1} of 90%–95% oxygen (Fig. 45.1). It draws atmospheric air through a series of dust filters and compresses it before passing it through a zeolite filter column. Nitrogen is reversibly adsorbed onto zeolite, and the residual oxygen-rich gas is passed to a reservoir before delivery to a breathing system. Several zeolite filters operate alternately to avoid filter exhaustion. Modern machines can also provide up to 10 L min^{-1} air, which when mixed with the oxygen output allows titration of inspired oxygen concentration and enough volume to drive basic pneumatic ventilators. Some machines can compress small volumes of oxygen within a reservoir. When combined with an uninterruptible power supply unit (UPS) usefully this prolongs oxygen delivery for up to 20 min after an electricity supply fails.

Conduct of anaesthesia

The mainstays of general anaesthesia in these circumstances are intravenous anaesthesia with ketamine, draw-over inhalational anaesthesia or a combination of both. Spontaneously breathing anaesthesia can be provided with

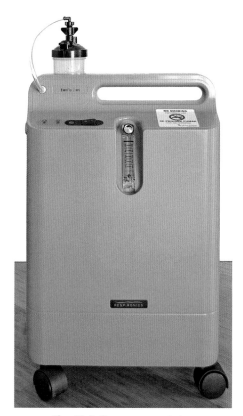

Fig. 45.1 Oxygen concentrator.

a surprisingly small selection of relatively inexpensive and stable pharmacological agents (Table 45.3). Atropine and lidocaine may be administered routinely before ether or halothane anaesthesia to counter hypersalivation and malignant arrhythmias. Spontaneous breathing techniques that require minimal skilled airway intervention are favoured. Regional anaesthesia offers many advantages but is not appropriate for all procedures. Supplies of essential drugs should be maintained, but this often proves impossible.

Monitoring

Monitoring relies upon keen clinical observation rather than technology: a finger on the pulse; observation of skin, mucosal and blood colour; and reference to a modified Guedel classification of depth of anaesthesia may be all that can be provided (see Chapter 22). Battery-powered pulse oximeters are available but may not be affordable. An ECG may be available, but the conducting gel of disposable electrodes quickly desiccates in hot climates, rendering them useless. Cotton wool soaked in saline is a common improvised alternative.

Table 45.3 Suggested minimum drug inventory when resource limitations are extreme

Requirements	Notes
Diazepam	Sedation
Ketamine	Analgesia and anaesthesia
Lidocaine 1%	Locoregional anaesthesia
Lidocaine 5% or bupivacaine 0.5%	Intrathecal anaesthesia
Atropine	
Suxamethonium bromide (powder)	Refrigeration not required
Adrenaline	Diluted for use as a vasoconstrictor
Meperidine or morphine sulphate	
Balanced crystalloid intravenous solution	

Ketamine intravenous anaesthesia

The detailed pharmacology of the versatile drug ketamine is covered elsewhere (see Chapter 4). Ketamine continues to be regarded as a relatively safe drug for induction and maintenance of anaesthesia even in unskilled hands. It has many properties that are particularly desirable in the resource-poor environment:

- it is inexpensive and does not require refrigeration;
- airway reflexes are partially preserved, and patients may maintain their own airway and require minimal airway support;
- it may offer a very limited degree of protection against regurgitation and pulmonary aspiration when tracheal intubation to protect the airway is indicated but impractical;
- at the cost of tachycardia, and within limits, it can preserve blood pressure and cardiac output when there is no time or facilities for preoperative stabilisation of a shocked patient.

Dose

- Induction of anaesthesia in an adult can be achieved by 1–2 mg kg^{-1} slow i.v. injection and in an uncooperative child by 5–10 mg kg^{-1} i.m. The patient's eyes may remain open and nystagmus may be observed. A smaller 2 mg kg^{-1} i.m. dose may sedate a child enough to allow cannulation without distress and resistance within 5–10 min. Anaesthesia can be maintained by intermittent intravenous bolus (0.5 mg kg^{-1}) or a ketamine drip (ketamine 500 mg in 0.9% NaCl or 5% dextrose solution 500 ml started at 2 drops kg^{-1} min^{-1} titrated to effect).

- When i.v. access is impossible (e.g. an extensive burn injury), heavy sedation and analgesia may be achieved in adults approximately 30–60 min after 500 mg administered orally with 5 mg diazepam (ketamine 15 mg kg^{-1} in children). The bitter taste of the drug may need to be disguised in a strong pleasant-flavoured liquid.

- In the absence of opioid analgesia, postoperative pain relief can be provided by ketamine. A loading dose of 0.5–1.0 mg kg^{-1} i.m. is followed by a ketamine infusion. Ketamine 50 mg in 500 ml 0.9% NaCl or 5% dextrose solution is titrated by drip count over 4–12 h (40–120 ml h^{-1}).

Inhalational anaesthesia using draw-over vaporisers

Draw-over anaesthesia is provided using a wide variety of equipment and circuit conformations, some of which have become popular regionally. Ideal draw-over anaesthetic workstations conveniently combine the key components required to deliver general anaesthesia in the absence of an oxygen and electricity supply. These systems use the negative pressure generated by spontaneous breathing or the deployment of a self-inflating bellows to draw environmental air (ideally enriched with oxygen) through a vaporiser for delivery to a patient breathing system. Gas flow through the system is intermittent, dependent on ventilation, low-resistance components and unidirectional valves. A unidirectional patient valve allows expired gas to leave the distal end of the system without environmental air entrainment.

One such basic system combines the highly durable Epstein Macintosh Oxford (EMO) and Oxford Miniature Vaporiser (OMV, Penlon, Abingdon, UK) in series with an Oxford Inflating Bellows (Fig. 45.2). Highly portable units such as the Diamedica Portable Anaesthesia System (DPA 02, Diamedica (UK) Ltd., Devon, UK) have been developed for in-the-field use (Fig. 45.3). More sophisticated workstations such as the Glostavent systems (Diamedica (UK) Ltd.) (Fig. 45.4) can include an oxygen concentrator and basic pneumatic ventilator for use when electricity is available. These can also support prolonged ventilation in an intensive care setting. An uninterruptable power supply unit acts as a voltage stabiliser protecting the oxygen concentrator from power surges and sudden power failures, which can be frequent and prolonged.

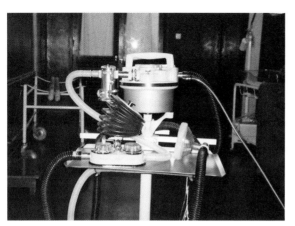

Fig. 45.2 A basic draw-over anaesthesia system in use from 1956 until the present day. An Epstein Macintosh Oxford Vaporiser (EMO) is in series with an Oxford Miniature Vaporiser (OMV) and Oxford Inflating Bellows (OIB). Air drawn into the EMO inlet may be supplemented with the small volume of oxygen filling the low-volume reservoir during expiration. An Ambu-E1 patient valve connects the circuit to the face mask or endotracheal tube. (Reproduced with permission of Dr Mary O'Regan.)

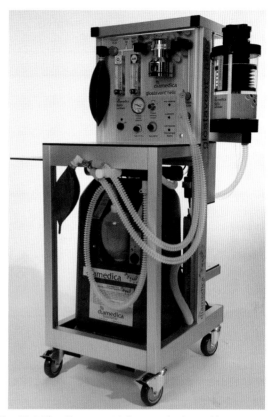

Fig. 45.4 The Glostavent Helix anaesthetic machine incorporating an oxygen concentrator and ventilator (Diamedica (UK) Ltd.). (Reproduced with permission from Mr Robert Neighbour.)

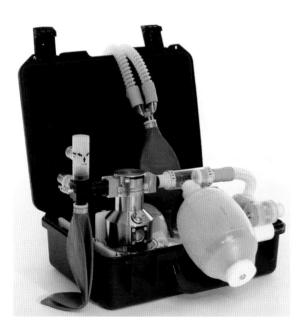

Fig. 45.3 A modern portable draw-over anaesthesia system (DPA 02, Diamedica (UK) Ltd., Devon, UK). (Reproduced with permission from Mr Robert Neighbour.)

As with plenum (continuous flow) vaporisers, the output of a draw-over vaporiser is determined by a dial that alters the proportion of fresh gas bypassing or entering the vaporising chamber. The performance of a very basic system such as the Goldman vaporiser (no longer in production) may be greatly influenced by the volume of volatile agent it contains, fresh gas flow rate and operating temperature (which declines sharply over time as volatile agent is vaporised). More sophisticated draw-over vaporisers such as the OMV (Fig. 45.5) or the Diamedica vaporiser (DDV, Diamedica (UK) Ltd.) buffer temperature change and compensate for the effects of variable gas flow within normal working limits. Wick design balances the conflicting requirements for efficient vaporisation and ease of dismantling for cleaning and maintenance. These vaporisers are small, light and very portable. The same vaporiser may be used interchangeably with several volatile agents, including halothane, isoflurane and sevoflurane. They perform well

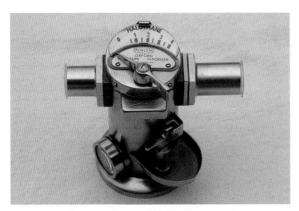

Fig. 45.5 Oxford Miniature Vaporiser (OMV) (Penlon, Abingdon, UK). (Reproduced with permission from frankshospitalworkshop.com.)

even during low-pressure continuous flow anaesthesia (useful with a Mapleson F circuit in paediatric practice). A degree of calibration may be achieved using interchangeable setting dial plates. Anaesthesia providers more familiar with precision plenum vaporisers need to adjust their practice and compensate for conditions that result in a less predictable vaporiser output.

Draw-over equipment pitfalls

The most durable draw-over systems are only as safe as their weakest link. Failure of one component can put many patients at risk or paralyse an anaesthetic service vital to the community of a huge geographical area. Anaesthesia providers need to understand how their equipment functions and know its limitations and nuances. Breathing system valves may appear similar superficially but behave very differently in breathing systems. Equipment must be stored in a protective environment and be subject to a programme of local maintenance activity. Patient valves will resist gas flow or allow upstream atmospheric air entrainment unless they are regularly disassembled, cleaned and carefully dried. Care is needed during reassembly to avoid valve leaflet pinching, which may trap the mechanism in an open or closed position. Vaporisers may seize so that the settings dial can no longer be turned. This usually is due to atmospheric dust and the build-up of sticky residues derived from preservatives such as thymol in volatile agents. Similar residues may gradually clog a wick system, reducing effective surface area and efficiency, with the risk of awareness during anaesthesia. A vaporiser should be drained between infrequent uses. It should be regularly disassembled for cleaning with a soft cloth and a detergent recommended by the manufacturer. Ether can be used to dissolve the thymol residues left behind by halothane.

Failure to recognise modifications of apparently familiar equipment can cause confusion and untoward incidents. Unlike plenum vaporisers, most draw-over units are designed for gas flowing from right to left through the device. There are left-to-right versions of some draw-over vaporisers (e.g. the OMV-50 used in the Tri-Service anaesthetic apparatus). Vaporiser orientation errors may lead to delivery of unpredictable vapour concentrations. When reliant on aged and donated apparatus, an anaesthesia provider is often obliged to work with equipment of differing international specifications. One must improvise and accept reuse of equipment designed for single use. Although delivery of hypoxic gas mixtures to a patient using standard draw-over systems is almost impossible, misguided modification of standard anaesthetic circuits has led to deaths from hypoxia, hypercarbia and barotrauma. There are a variety of tubing and connector diameters and vaporiser inlet and outlet taper sizes. Leakage from joints with incompatible tapers can lead to loss of vapour from a system or upstream entrainment of air and dilution of vapour delivered to the patient. Donated pieces of equipment may be connectible but be tragically incompatible.

Ether (diethyl ether)

The safety profile, availability, and affordability of industrial-grade ether has ensured its continued use in some resource-poor environments.

Physical properties

Ether is a colourless, highly volatile liquid with a characteristic smell. This sole inhalational agent can provide deep anaesthesia, profound analgesia even at subanaesthetic doses, and excellent muscle relaxation.

Systemic effects

RS
- Respiratory stimulant and bronchodilator; offers a significant margin of safety when supplemental oxygen is not available.
- Pungent: stimulates tracheobronchial secretion and irritates the airways resulting in breath-holding, coughing and laryngospasm.

CVS
- Preserves baroreceptor reflexes, does not depress the myocardium and stimulates the sympathetic nervous system. It can provide a level of cardiovascular stability during anaesthesia of a shocked patient that is difficult to achieve with modern volatile agents.

GI
- Postoperative nausea and vomiting is very common.

855

Other

- Ether is highly flammable and under the influence of light and air can form explosive peroxides. As the vapour is heavier than air, escaping ether fumes will accumulate at floor level and present a significant fire and explosion risk. Precautions need to be taken to avoid static electricity or other ignition sources. If an oxygen concentrator is used, it should be housed securely at head height to separate it from ether fumes at floor level. A simple wide-bore tube from the expired limb of the patient expiratory valve to the outside environment provides a crude but effective passive scavenging system.
- Industrial-grade ether is supplied in large-volume containers or drums. This requires that it is decanted on site and by hand into more practical containers that may be taken into the operating theatre. This poses an obvious risk if efficient fume cupboard facilities are not available.

Pharmacology

Ether is moderately potent (Minimum alveolar concentration 1.92) and usually administered in concentrations ranging from 5%–15%. It has a very high blood/gas partition coefficient (12) and consequently inhalational induction of anaesthesia is slow, technically challenging for the anaesthesia provider and unpleasant for the patient. Whenever possible, anaesthesia providers prefer to reserve its use for maintenance of anaesthesia after a smoother induction using ketamine or halothane. This explains why draw-over systems often have several vaporisers in series (see Fig. 45.2).

Halothane

The pharmacology of halothane and comparison with more modern volatile agents is covered in Chapter 3. It is disappearing from contemporary practice where superior drugs are affordable. Reduced global demand and a decline in profitability has prompted suppliers to increase its price or cease to import it altogether. Poorly resourced anaesthesia services reliant on halothane as an inexpensive mainstay for inhalational anaesthesia are increasingly vulnerable. Isoflurane does not offer the smooth induction experienced with halothane, and sevoflurane remains relatively expensive and unaffordable.

Regional anaesthesia

Regional blockade meets many of the desired basic requirements of adult anaesthesia in a resource-poor area. Mastery of intrathecal anaesthesia, axillary approach to the brachial plexus block, inguinal field block and penile block gives an anaesthesia provider a useful basic set of low-risk alternatives to general anaesthesia. Suboptimal sensory blocks may be accepted with pragmatism by clinicians and patients. Augmentation with small doses of ketamine and local infiltration by the surgeon may be required. Many of the commonly performed surgical procedures can be managed with regional techniques (see Box 45.1), yet spinal anaesthesia, plexus blocks and peripheral nerve blockade remain underused techniques in some settings. There are several reasons for this:

- The opportunity to learn plexus and peripheral nerve block techniques may only present itself during rare visits from expert practitioners. The practice of these tutors is increasingly reliant on ultrasound location of neural structures, and the number of experts confident teaching landmark techniques is dwindling.
- Local anaesthesia is cheap, but the reliability afforded by use of nerve stimulators and ultrasound equipment may be an unachievable capital outlay.
- When supplies of needles and local anaesthetic agents fail for prolonged periods, clinician experience, confidence and ambition can become eroded.
- If vasopressors are not available, a deliberately conservative spinal block may be performed (e.g. T10 sensory block for caesarean section). The patient may experience considerable discomfort, and anaesthesia is inevitably augmented with near-anaesthetic doses of i.v. ketamine.
- Surgeons may perceive general anaesthesia to be quicker and safer and can dictate the choice of technique. In this setting, surgeons are often required to work without the assistance of a trained anaesthesia provider. If they perform an intrathecal injection themselves, they may be reliant on the skills of a theatre domestic worker to monitor the patient during and after surgery. With experience, this kind of assistant can become a very skilled patient attendant. Good communication and familiarity within this team mitigates risk to some degree. Unfortunately, the consequences of a single mismanaged complication such as high spinal or severe hypotension during surgical haemorrhage can shake the surgeon-anaesthetist's confidence and permanently change practice in favour of i.v. ketamine anaesthesia. One peripatetic surgeon or anaesthesia provider may influence the anaesthetic practice of an entire region for decades.

Common complications resulting from inappropriate equipment and drugs may also deter regular use of regional techniques:

- Use of 5% lidocaine for intrathecal anaesthesia risks neuraxial toxicity but is relatively affordable compared with safer alternatives.
- Sharing a single unrefrigerated vial of local anaesthetic between many patients over a period of days may be a necessity but introduces the risk of bacterial meningitis.
- Fine-gauge and pencil-point needles, even when available, are unpopular as they cannot be cleaned and sterilised effectively for reuse. Use of sharply bevelled 20G spinal

needles, 20G spinal introducer needles and 18G peripheral cannulae to perform intrathecal anaesthesia is widespread, and mild to moderate post–dural puncture headache is relatively common.

Perioperative blood loss

Significant blood loss, severe anaemia and coagulopathy are difficult situations to manage without access to refrigerated stores of viral-screened donated blood products. Anaesthesia providers may be working without the facility to quantify a clinically detected anaemia. Efforts should be made to treat preoperative anaemia, but these are often logistically impossible. A crude point-of-care assessment of anaemia can be provided during surgery by observing the consistency of blood sampled and the behaviour and appearance of several drops placed on absorbent paper.

Techniques employed to manage or minimise perioperative blood loss include the following:

- Severely restrictive transfusion triggers.
- Maintainance of normothermia and avoidance of hypertension.
- Positioning of the patient to avoid increased venous pressure at the operative site; the use of a tourniquet should be considered.
- Meticulous devascularisation should be achieved by surgical methods or infiltration with dilute adrenaline solutions.
- Tranexamic acid is relatively inexpensive and may be the only affordable pharmacological intervention.
- Same-day predonation of whole blood by the patient or close relatives. Suitable hardware for several hours' blood storage and bedside basic cross-matching are required. Transmission of bloodborne infection is a significant risk.
- Autologous transfusion of salvaged blood is an option if the surgical field is uncontaminated; blood free in the peritoneum can be scooped up, filtered through gauze into a bowl and gravity syphoned into a suitably treated donation bag.
- When blood transfusion is not available and a severely anaemic patient is bleeding, one may be obliged to accept hypovolaemia. Acute crystalloid dilution of haemoglobin concentration less than 30 g L^{-1} usually results in hypoxia secondary to gross pulmonary oedema.

Intensive care

Intensive and high-dependency care services remain a distant aspiration for most healthcare settings in resource-poor areas. The mismatch between service provision and demand is stark, particularly for the neonate, infant, young child and parturient. In most sub-Saharan hospitals the burden of puerperal sepsis, obstetric haemorrhage, eclampsia and severe pre-eclampsia would easily justify a large obstetric critical care unit. Even in small rural hospitals, neonatal sepsis, severe malaria and meningitis in childhood are common enough to justify paediatric high-dependency and intensive care facilities.

Many factors impede the development of critical care services. These include lack of technology (e.g. monitors and ventilators), laboratory support, suitable accommodation and skilled nursing. Attempts to replicate the technology-based critical care unit model used by well-resourced facilities can be misguided. The sickest patients may end up attached to monitors but isolated from the main ward activity and the staff that might respond to their needs. The reality of many so-called critical care units in the poorest hospitals is a spotlessly clean room, furnished with redundant equipment and reserved for local VIPs. Where genuine critical care is provided, resource is commonly concentrated on patients who require respiratory support immediately after surgery or trauma; other patient groups are poorly provided for. Effective units develop a model of care appropriate to their own institution. They have generous nurse-to-patient ratios and provide basic monitoring and organ support very well. If an appropriate cannula is available, central venous pressure can be measured using a manometer constructed from a loop of giving set infusion tubing. Prolonged mechanical respiratory support can be challenging without pressurised gas or electricity. Some units have successfully trained domestic staff and relatives to provide prolonged manual ventilation. It is often necessary to allow patients who have their tracheas intubated to breathe spontaneously through a tracheal tube until they are well and awake enough to protect their own airways.

Even basic critical care can have a significant impact on the survival of carefully selected individuals. It can legitimise the performance of more complex surgical procedures and provide a valuable training resource that promotes better care for all inpatients. Skilled staff providing critical care within, or close to, general wards can provide a degree of outreach care. Unfortunately, poor patient outcomes constantly threaten the sustainability of these units. Triage to such a limited resource is problematic. Without adherence to clear and sensible admission criteria, clinicians are often tempted to prioritise their sickest patients, for whom recovery is unlikely with or without critical care. A district health commissioner struggling to provide basic primary healthcare for large communities may not be able to justify the concentration of great resource on a few patients with relatively poor prognoses. Relatives too have difficult choices to make. They may be astute enough to interpret the application of an oxygen face mask or insertion of a nasogastric tube as sign that chance of recovery is declining sharply. In this context the costs of accompanying a patient away from home and mounting medical bills may become unsustainable. In many low-resource hospitals, clinicians are reluctant to start high-dependency interventions for fear that it will precipitate a family abandoning hope and taking their relative home to die.

Education and training

Non-physician anaesthetists provide most of the anaesthetic care delivered in resource-poor environments. Some have no formal training or qualifications but may have gained considerable skill by apprenticeship. Where formal training does occur, courses tend to be relatively short and place strong emphasis on received wisdom and practical skills. Selection of candidates for training may be determined by influences other than an individual's aptitude or educational achievements. Trainees often accept considerable personal, financial and domestic hardship to study far away from home. Teaching may be delivered in an unfamiliar language and assume a level of mathematical and scientific understanding that their basic education did not provide. These students of anaesthesia are generally highly motivated and acutely aware that this brief period as a trainee may be their sole opportunity for professional development. Even if they fail to reach an ascribed standard, they may return to their communities to be the only anaesthesia provider for a large population over many decades. They may face many challenging clinical cases without advice or anaesthesia colleagues to confer with. In this context, trainers need to be mindful that every learning opportunity is precious and must be exploited to the full. Basic educational deficits that hinder progress need to be addressed early. Non-physician anaesthetists must be equipped to justify, communicate and assert their clinical opinions if these are to be accepted by surgical colleagues. Course content must be relevant to the environment to which the trainee will return. The sensitive and perceptive visiting expert can play a key role supplementing limited local educational resource. Their broader perspective and attitudes may inspire and empower trainees and trainers. Friendships formed and social media communities can support professional and personal development over a lifetime of anaesthetic practice even if contact is relatively infrequent.

Chapter | 46 |

Anaesthesia outside the operating theatre

Sally Hancock

General anaesthesia outside the operating theatre suite is often challenging for the anaesthetist. Although the principles of remote site anaesthesia are common to many situations, each specialised environment poses its own unique problems. In hospital the anaesthetist must provide a service for patients with standards of safety which are equal to those in the main operating theatre department. Outside the hospital, this level of service may be more dependent on location and available resources.

Anaesthesia in remote locations within the hospital

In-hospital remote locations include radiology, radiotherapy and emergency departments, and wards with areas designated for procedures such as electroconvulsive therapy (ECT), assisted conception, cardioversion and intrathecal chemotherapy administration.

General considerations and principles

Anaesthetists are often required to use their skills (e.g. administer anaesthesia, analgesia, sedation, resuscitate, cannulate, etc.) outside the familiar operating theatre environment. When requests are made for anaesthetic intervention in remote locations, there are multiple considerations for the anaesthetist. These include the following:

1. *Appropriate personnel.* Only senior experienced anaesthetists, who are also familiar with the particular environment and its challenges, should normally administer anaesthesia in remote locations. Patients are often challenging, and additional skilled anaesthetic help may not be readily available compared with an operating theatre suite.

2. *Equipment.* The remote clinical area may not have been designed with anaesthetic requirements in mind. Anaesthetic apparatus often competes for space with bulky equipment such as scanners, and in general, conditions are less than optimal, including poor lighting. Monitoring capabilities and anaesthetic equipment should be of the same standard as those used in the operating department and should meet the minimum standards set by the Association of Anaesthetists. The updated 2015 guidelines include guidance on monitoring neuromuscular blockade, depth of anaesthesia and cardiac output. The anaesthetist who is unfamiliar with the environment should spend time becoming accustomed to the layout and equipment. Compromised access to the patient requires careful consideration, and advanced planning helps to prepare for unanticipated scenarios. Basic requirements such as i.v. fluids should be located, as these may be stored in an area away from the procedure room, and the presence of general and specific emergency drugs and equipment should be verified before starting the procedure.

3. *Patient preparation.* Preparation of the patient may be inadequate because the patient is from a ward where staff are unfamiliar with preoperative protocols, or patients may be unreliable, such as those presenting for ECT.

4. *Assistance.* An anaesthetic assistant (e.g. operating department practitioner) should be present, although this person may be unfamiliar with the environment, and maintenance and stocking of anaesthetic equipment may be less than ideal. Consequently the anaesthetist must be particularly vigilant in checking the anaesthetic machine, particularly because it may be disconnected and moved when not in use.

5. *Communication.* Communication between staff from other specialties and the anaesthetist may be poor. This may lead to failure in recognising each other's requirements.

The use of the WHO checklist is particularly important in these areas and often highlights issues that may have been overlooked.

6. *Recovery.* Recovery facilities are often non-existent, and anaesthetists may have to recover their own patients in the suite. Consequently, they must be familiar with the location of recovery equipment, including suction, supplementary oxygen and resuscitation equipment. Alternatively, patients may be transferred to the main hospital recovery area. This requires the use of routine transfer equipment, which should ideally be available as a grab-bag kept alongside monitoring equipment, and a portable oxygen supply. This ensures that nothing is forgotten and avoids delays in searching for various pieces of equipment. The bag should be regularly checked and maintained.

There should be a nominated lead anaesthetist responsible for remote locations in which anaesthesia is administered in a hospital. This individual should liaise with the relevant specialties (e.g. radiologists, psychiatrists) to ensure that the environment, equipment and guidelines are suitable for safe, appropriate and efficient patient care.

Anaesthesia in the radiology department

In most hospitals, members of the anaesthetic department are called upon to anaesthetise or sedate patients for diagnostic and therapeutic radiological procedures. These procedures include angiography and subsequent intervention, CT scanning and MRI. The major requirement of all these imaging techniques is that the patient remains almost motionless. Thus general anaesthesia may be necessary when these investigations and interventions are performed in children, the critically ill or uncooperative patient and/or if the procedure is likely to be painful or prolonged.

Radiological studies may require administration of conscious sedation; chloral hydrate may be used in young children and benzodiazepines, opioids or propofol in adults. This is discussed in more detail in Chapter 4, but essential practice elements include the following:

- Personnel responsible for the sedation should be familiar with the effects of the medication and skilled in resuscitation (including airway management).
- All the equipment and drugs required for resuscitation should be readily available and checked regularly.
- It is undesirable for a single operator to be responsible for both the radiological procedure and administration of sedation because there is the potential to be distracted from one responsibility and to allow adverse events to go untreated.
- Guidelines for prescribing, evaluating and monitoring sedation should be readily available.

- Particular care should be taken with high-risk groups such as frail and older patients and those with cardiovascular or respiratory disease.
- Patients should be starved before sedation, vital signs monitored and documented, and appropriate recovery and discharge criteria used.

Iodine-containing intravascular contrast agents are used routinely during angiographic and other radiological investigations. The anaesthetist must always be aware of the risk of an anaphylactoid contrast reaction. In recent years, low-osmolar contrast media have been introduced; these cause less pain on injection and have fewer adverse effects than the older contrast agents (3% vs. 15%).

Factors contributing to the development of adverse reactions include:

- speed of injection;
- type and dose of contrast used;
- intra-arterial contrast injection (coronary and cerebral angiography are associated with a greater risk of anaphylactoid contrast reaction); and
- patient susceptibility (e.g. allergy, asthma, extremes of age (younger than 1 and older than 60 years), cardiovascular disease and a history of previous reaction to contrast medium)

Nausea and vomiting are common and reactions may progress to urticaria, hypotension, arrhythmias, bronchospasm and cardiac arrest. Fatal reactions are rare, occurring in about 1 in 100,000 procedures. Treatment depends on the severity of the reaction but usually consists of i.v. fluids, supplemental oxygen and careful monitoring (see Chapter 27). An anaphylaxis protocol and kit should be readily available containing appropriate drugs and fluids.

Adequate hydration is important because high-osmolarity contrast dye can potentially cause dose-dependent contrast-induced nephropathy (CIN) (see Chapter 11). Risk factors include: dehydration; pre-existing acute kidney injury; and repeated administration of contrast. The circulating volume should be maintained or expanded using oral fluids and i.v. saline 0.9% or bicarbonate. There is little evidence to support therapies such as *N*-acetylcysteine or diuretics, but they are sometimes used. The incidence and severity of CIN has decreased with the use of lower-osmolar contrast media, and severe CIN requiring renal replacement therapy is rare. A urinary catheter may be useful for patients undergoing long procedures.

Healthcare workers are exposed to X-rays in the radiology and imaging suites. The greatest source is usually from fluoroscopy and digital subtraction angiography. Exposure to ionising radiation from a CT scanner is relatively low, although the patient dose is high because the X-rays are highly focused. Radiation intensity and exposure decrease with the square of the distance from the emitting source. The recommended distance is 2–3 m. This precaution, together with lead aprons, thyroid shields and movable lead-lined glass screens, keeps exposure at a safe level. A personal-dose monitor should be worn by personnel who work frequently in an X-ray environment. All female patients between the ages of 12 and 55, along with those who have experienced earlier menarche or later menopause, should be offered pregnancy testing before exposure to ionising radiation. In the emergency situation this may be deferred in the interests of time and the risk/benefit ratio to the patient.

Computed tomography

General principles
A CT scan provides a series of tomographic axial 'slices' of the body. Each image is produced by computer integration of the differences in radiation absorption coefficients between different normal tissues and between normal and abnormal tissues. The image of the structure under investigation is generated by a cathode ray tube and the brightness of each area is proportional to the absorption value. One rotation of the gantry produces an axial slice, or 'cut'. A series of cuts is made, usually at intervals of 7 mm, but this may be larger or smaller depending on the diagnostic information sought. The circular scanning tunnel contains the X-ray tube and detectors, with the patient lying in the centre of the doughnut during the study.

Anaesthetic management
Computed tomography is non-invasive and painless, requiring neither sedation nor anaesthesia for most adult patients; however, it is noisy and claustrophobic, and a few patients may require conscious sedation to alleviate fears or anxieties. Patients who cannot co-operate (most often paediatric and head trauma patients or those who are under the influence of alcohol or drugs) or those whose airway is at risk may need general anaesthesia to prevent movement, which degrades the image. Anaesthetists may also be asked to assist in the transfer from the ICU and in the care of critically ill patients who require CT scans.

General anaesthesia is preferable to sedation when there are potential airway problems or when control of ICP is critical. Because the patient's head is inaccessible during the CT scan, the airway needs to be secured. The scan itself requires only that the patient remains motionless. If ICP is high, controlled ventilation is necessary to ensure tight control of $PaCO_2$. Because these patients are often in transit to or from critical care areas or the emergency department (ED), a total intravenous technique with neuromuscular blockade is usually the technique of choice, with tracheal intubation and controlled ventilation. Use of volatile anaesthetic agents during the scan is acceptable but may involve changing from one technique to another for transfer. In addition, the anaesthetic machine may be left unplugged when not in use in the scanner, and reconnecting and checking it may be distracting and time consuming. A portable ventilator

with end-tidal CO_2 monitoring removes the need to change breathing systems. If the scan is likely to take a long time, it may be advisable to change from cylinder to piped oxygen supply to conserve supplies for transfer. If during the scan the anaesthetist is observing the patient from inside the control room, it is imperative that alarms/monitors have visual signals which may be seen easily.

Anaesthetic complications while in the CT scanner include:
- kinking of the tracheal tube or disconnection of the breathing system, particularly during positioning and movement of the gantry;
- hypothermia in paediatric patients;
- disconnection of drips and lines during transfer; and
- haemodynamic instability during movement on to the scanning table (e.g. in the trauma setting).

Magnetic resonance imaging

General principles
Magnetic resonance imaging (MRI) is an imaging modality that depends on magnetic fields and radiofrequency pulses to produce its images. The imaging capabilities of MRI are superior to those of CT for examining intracranial, spinal and soft tissue lesions. It may display images in the sagittal, coronal, transverse or oblique planes and has the advantage that no ionising radiation is produced.

An MRI imaging system traditionally requires a large magnet in the form of a tube, which is capable of accepting the entire length of the human body. Wider bore and open scanners have more recently been developed, which allow the patient to stand up to reduce the feeling of claustrophobia. This also means that more obese patients or those with significant deformities (e.g. severe kyphosis) can now be scanned. A radiofrequency transmitter coil is incorporated in the tube which surrounds the patient; the coil also acts as a receiver to detect the energy waves from which the image is constructed. In the presence of the magnetic field, protons in the body align with the magnetic field in the longitudinal axis of the patient. Additional perpendicular magnetic pulses are applied by the radiofrequency coil; this causes the protons to rotate into the transverse plane. When the pulse is discontinued, the nuclei relax back to their original orientation and emit energy waves which are detected by the coil. The magnet is more than 2 m in length and weighs approximately 500 kg. The magnetic field is applied constantly even in the absence of a patient. It may take several days and great expense to re-establish the magnetic field if it is removed, and so the magnet is only quenched in an emergency.

The magnetic field strength is measured in tesla units (T). One tesla is the field intensity generating 1 newton of force per 1 ampere of current per 1 metre of conductor. One tesla equals 10,000 gauss; the Earth's surface strength is 0.5–1.0 gauss. MRI strengths usually vary from 1 to 3 T, although some research facilities have scanners which may produce fields up to 9.4 T. The force of the magnetic field decreases exponentially with distance from the magnet, and a safety line at a level of 5 gauss is usually specified. Higher exposure may result in pacemaker malfunction, and unscreened personnel should not cross this safety line. At 50 gauss, ferromagnetic objects become dangerous projectiles. The magnetic fields present are strong static fields, which are present all around the magnet area, and fast-switching and pulsed radiofrequency fields in the immediate vicinity of the magnet.

The final magnetic resonance (MR) image is made from very weak electromagnetic signals, which are subject to interference from other modulated radio signals. Therefore, the scanner is contained in a radiofrequency shield (Faraday cage). A hollow tube of brass is built into this cage to allow monitoring cables and infusion lines to pass into the control room. This is termed the waveguide.

Anaesthetic management

Staff safety. Staff safety precautions are essential. The supervising magnetic resonance (MR) radiographer is operationally responsible for safety in the scanner, and anaesthetic staff should defer to him or her in matters of safety. Screening questionnaires identify those at risk, and training should be given in MR safety, emergency procedures arising from equipment failure and evacuation of the patient. Anaesthetists should also understand the consequences of quenching the magnet and be aware of recommendations on exposure and the need for ear protection. Long-term effects of repeated exposure to MRI fields are unknown, and pregnant staff should be offered the option not to work in the scanner. All potentially hazardous articles should be removed (e.g. watches, mobile telephones bleeps, pens and stethoscopes). Bank cards, credit cards and other belongings containing electromagnetic strips become demagnetised in the vicinity of the scanner, and personal computers, pagers, mobile telephones and calculators may also be damaged.

Patient safety. Ferromagnetic objects within or attached to the patient pose a risk.

- Jewellery, hearing aids or drug patches should be removed.
- Absolute contraindications to MRI include implanted surgical devices such as cochlear implants, intraocular metallic objects and metal vascular clips.
- Pacemakers remain an absolute contraindication in most settings, although MRI-conditional pacemakers have now been developed.
- Programmable shunts for hydrocephalus may malfunction because the pressure setting may be changed by the magnetic field, leading to over- or underdrainage.
- The use of neurostimulators such as spinal cord stimulators for chronic pain is increasing. These devices may potentially fail or cause thermal injury on exposure to

the magnetic field. Each must be considered individually; some may be safe if strict guidelines are adhered to.
- Joint prostheses, artificial heart valves and sternal wires are generally safe because of fibrous tissue fixation. Patients with large metal implants should be monitored for implant heating. A description of the safety of various devices is available on dedicated websites.
- All patients should wear ear protection because noise levels may exceed 85 dB.

In most scanners the body cylinder of the scanner surrounds the patient totally; manual control of the airway is impossible, and tracheal intubation or use of a supraglottic airway device (SAD) is essential when general anaesthesia is necessary. The patient may be observed from both ends of the tunnel and may be extracted quickly if necessary. Because there is no hazard from ionising radiation, the anaesthetist may approach the patient in safety.

Technological advances mean that intraoperative MRI is now possible, and MRI scanners are becoming integrated into operating theatres to allow real-time imaging during complex neurosurgery. There are additional risks associated with its use including contamination of the surgical field, the need for patient repositioning and the requirement for non-ferromagnetic surgical instruments (see Chapter 40).

Equipment. The magnetic effects of MRI impose restrictions on the selection of anaesthetic equipment. Any ferromagnetic object distorts the magnetic field sufficiently to degrade the image. It is also likely to be propelled towards the scanner and may cause a significant accident if it makes contact with the patient or with staff. Equipment used in the MRI scanner is designated 'MR-conditional', 'MR-safe' or 'MR-unsafe'.

- *MR-conditional* equipment pose no hazards in a specified MR environment with specified conditions of use. The conditions in which it may be used must accompany the device, and it may not be safe to use it outside these conditions. Consideration needs to be given to replacing equipment if a scanner is replaced by one of higher field strength.
- *MR-safe* equipment pose no safety hazard in the MR room, but may not function normally or may degrade the image quality.

The layout of the MRI room or suite determines whether the majority of equipment needs to be inside the room (and therefore MR-conditional or MR-safe), or outside the room with suitable long circuits, leads and tubing to the patient. Suitable anaesthetic machines and ventilators are manufactured and may be positioned next to the magnetic bore to minimise the length of the breathing system. They require piped gases or special aluminium cylinders for oxygen and nitrous oxide. Consideration also needs to be given to i.v. fluid stands, infusion pumps and monitoring equipment, including stethoscopes and nerve stimulators. Laryngoscopes may be non-magnetic, but standard batteries should be replaced with non-magnetic lithium batteries. Supraglottic airway devices without a metal spring in the pilot tube valve should be available.

Monitoring. All monitoring equipment must be appropriate for the environment. Technical problems with non-compatible monitors include interference with imaging signals and radiofrequency signals from the scanner inducing currents in the monitor which may give unreliable monitor readings. Special monitors are available or unshielded ferromagnetic monitors may be installed just outside the MRI room and used with long shielded or non-ferromagnetic cables (e.g. fibre-optic or carbon fibre). Ambient noise levels are such that visual alarms are essential. The 2010 Association of Anaesthetists guidelines on services for MRI suggest that monitoring equipment should be placed in the control room outside the magnetic area. A non-invasive automated arterial pressure monitor, in which metallic tubing connectors are replaced by nylon connectors, should be used. Distortion of the ECG may occur. Interference may be reduced by using short braided leads connected to compatible electrodes placed in a narrow triangle on the chest. There should be no loops in cables because these may induce heat generation and lead to burns. Side-stream capnography and anaesthetic gas concentration monitoring require a long sampling tube, which leads to a time delay of the monitored variables. The use of 100% oxygen during the scan should be indicated to the radiologist reporting the images because this may produce artefactually abnormal high signal in CSF spaces in some scanning sequences.

Conduct of anaesthesia. The indications for general anaesthesia during MRI are similar to those for CT. A complex scan may take up to 20 min, and an entire examination more than 1 h. Most MRI scans are performed within normal working hours; exceptions may be neuraxial MRI scanning for acute evaluation of the brain or spinal cord.

Anaesthesia is usually induced outside the MRI room in an adjacent dedicated anaesthetic area where it is safe to use ferromagnetic equipment (outside the 5 gauss line). Short-acting drugs should be used to allow rapid recovery with minimal adverse effects. Sedation of children by organised, dedicated and multidisciplinary teams for MRI has been shown to be safe and successful. However, general anaesthesia allows more rapid and controlled onset, with immobility guaranteed. All patients must be transported into the magnet area on MRI-appropriate trolleys. During the scan, the anaesthetist should ideally be in the control room but may remain in the scanning room in exceptional circumstances if wearing suitable ear protection. If an emergency arises, the anaesthetist needs to be aware of the procedure for rapid removal of the patient to a safe area.

Increasingly, ICU patients require MRI scanning. Careful planning is required and screening checklists should be used. Non-essential infusions should be discontinued and essential infusions may need to be transferred to MRI-safe pumps. This may induce a period of instability in the patient while the infusions are being moved, and high requirements for drugs such as vasopressors may be a relative contraindication to scanning. The tracheal tube pilot balloon valve spring should be secured away from the scan area. Pulmonary artery catheters with conductive wires and epicardial pacing catheters should be removed to prevent microshocks. Simple CVCs appear safe if disconnected from electrical connections.

Gadolinium-based contrast agents are used in MRI and are generally safe, with a high therapeutic ratio. However, the use of these contrast agents in patients with renal failure may precipitate a life-threatening condition called nephrogenic systemic fibrosis. In patients with a glomerular filtration rate (GFR) less than 30 ml min^{-1} 1.73 m^{-2}, only minimal amounts of contrast should be given (if deemed absolutely necessary) and not repeated for at least 7 days.

Diagnostic and interventional angiography

General principles

Direct arteriography using percutaneous arterial catheters is used widely for the diagnosis of vascular lesions. Catheters are usually inserted by the Seldinger technique via the femoral artery in the groin or the radial artery in the wrist, and injection of contrast medium provides images which are viewed by conventional or digital subtraction angiography. In addition, it is becoming increasingly common to consider vessel embolisation both in the elective preoperative setting (e.g. vascular tumours or malformations) and in the emergency management of major haemorrhage (e.g. major trauma or massive obstetric or gastrointestinal haemorrhage). The procedure involves the injection of an embolic material to stimulate intravascular thrombosis, resulting in occlusion of the vessel. There is a risk of distal organ damage if the blood supply is completely occluded. Non-invasive angiographic techniques used with CT or MRI have reduced the need for direct arteriography for diagnosis of some vascular lesions. The advent of spiral and double helical CT scanners allows whole vascular territories to be mapped within 30 s and produces superior images, including three-dimensional pictures. Magnetic resonance imaging is sensitive to the detection of flow and, together with more sophisticated scanning and data collection techniques, is used increasingly for assessment of vascular structures.

Anaesthetic management

Most angiographic procedures may be carried out under local anaesthesia, with sedation if necessary during more complex investigation. If the procedure is likely to be prolonged, general anaesthesia may be more appropriate. The same applies to nervous patients, those unable to co-operate and children. Complete immobility is required during the investigation and particularly if any interventional procedures are to be performed. Major trauma patients and those with life-threatening haemorrhage are nearly always sedated, with ventilation controlled, before arrival in the angiography suite.

Complications of angiography

Local
- Haematoma and haemorrhage
- Vessel wall dissection
- Thrombosis
- Perivascular contrast injection
- Adjacent nerve damage
- Loss and knotting of guide wires and catheters

General
- Contrast reactions of varying severity
- Emboli from catheter clots, intimal damage and air
- Sepsis

Interventional neuroradiology
Cerebral angiography may be used to demonstrate tumours, arteriovenous malformations, aneurysms, subarachnoid haemorrhage (SAH) and cerebrovascular disease. Since the ISAT (International Subarachnoid Aneurysm Trial) in 2002 (which compared coiling in patients with a ruptured aneurysm of good clinical grade with surgical clipping) showed a favourable initial outcome, endovascular treatment has become the technique of choice for most patients with aneurysmal SAH. Subsequent follow-up has found a need for retreatment in a significant proportion of patients because of reaccumulation of the aneurysm; however, the morbidity and mortality are still less than that of open clipping.

Coiling is ideally performed as soon as possible after ictus to reduce the risk of rebleeding (5%–10% in the first 72 h). Early intervention also allows the aneurysm to be protected before the onset of vasospasm, which increases the procedural risk and makes vascular navigation more difficult. Detachable coils are used to pack the aneurysm to prevent rebleeding.

Anaesthetic considerations
- These patients are often systemically unwell as a result of SAH and may be profoundly cardiovascularly unstable during induction of anaesthesia.
- Many of these patients have intracranial hypertension and cerebral vasospasm; consequently, control of arterial pressure and carbon dioxide tension are essential.
- Obtunding the pressor response to tracheal intubation and careful positioning to avoid increasing CVP are necessary to prevent elevation of ICP.
- Neuromuscular blockade is usually used with positive pressure ventilation to maintain $PaCO_2$ 4.5–5.0 kPa. A moderate reduction in $PaCO_2$ causes vasoconstriction of

normal vessels, slows cerebral circulation and contrast medium transit times and improves delineation of small vascular lesions.
- Transient hypotension and bradycardia or asystole may occur during cerebral angiography with contrast dye injection. This usually responds to volume replacement and atropine.
- Complications during interventional neuroradiology include haemorrhage from rupture of the vessel (which may necessitate reversal of anticoagulation with protamine) or ischaemia as a result of thromboembolism (e.g. clot forming around the catheter tip), vasospasm, embolic material or hypoperfusion. All complications may occur rapidly and with devastating results. Occasionally, urgent craniotomy or external ventricular drainage of CSF may be required.
- Heparin and glycoprotein IIb/IIIa inhibitors (e.g. abciximab) may be required if an occlusive clot forms along with oral (n.g.) or i.v. aspirin.

Mechanical thrombectomy
Hyperacute stroke therapy is evolving to include vessel recanalisation by mechanical thrombectomy. Standard treatment of i.v. thrombolysis is less effective for proximal large arterial occlusion (e.g. middle cerebral artery), and so endovascular approaches are increasingly being used. Endovascular thrombectomy has been shown to be associated with improved functional outcomes at 90 days. However, there are considerable logistical issues in terms of time constraints (at present <12 h from onset of symptoms) and the provision of peri-procedural care.

Patients present as time-critical emergencies. The anaesthetic technique used will depend on the individual patient, but the overriding issue is that treatment should not be delayed. Co-operative patients may undergo thrombectomy under local anaesthesia with or without sedation, whereas those who are uncooperative or at risk of aspiration may need a general anaesthetic. Full monitoring should be instituted, but procedures such as arterial line insertion and bladder catheterisation should not delay the start of the procedure. Blood pressure should be maintained between 140–220 mmHg (180 mmHg in those who have received i.v. thrombolysis). Postoperatively patients should be returned to a high-dependency or stroke unit to continue neurological monitoring.

Cardiac catheterisation
General anaesthesia is required mainly for children, whereas sedation is usually adequate in adults. In children (premature neonates to teenagers), congenital heart disease may cause abnormal circulations and intracardiac shunts, often presenting with cyanosis, dyspnoea, failure to thrive and congestive heart failure. Patients may also have coexisting non-cardiac congenital abnormalities. Neonatal patients may be deeply

cyanotic and critically ill. Initial echocardiography often gives a diagnosis, but cardiac catheterisation is required for treatment or determining the possibility of surgery. These procedures include pressure and oxygen saturation measurements, balloon dilatation of stenotic lesions (e.g. pulmonary valve), balloon septostomy for transposition of the great arteries and ductal closure.

The ideal anaesthetic technique would avoid myocardial depression, hypertension and tachycardia; preserve normocapnia; and maintain spontaneous respiration of air. All techniques have their limitations. Positive pressure ventilation causes changes in pulmonary haemodynamics and therefore influences measurements of flow and pressure. Spontaneous respiration with volatile agents may be unsuitable for patients with significant cardiac disease. The onset of action of anaesthetic drugs is affected by cardiac shunts and congestive failure. Contrast medium in the coronary circulation may cause profound transient changes in the ECG. Therefore ECG and invasive arterial pressure monitoring should be used to allow rapid assessment of arrhythmias and hypotension. Children with cyanotic heart disease may be polycythaemic, thereby predisposing to thrombosis.

Transcatheter aortic valve implantation

Transcatheter aortic valve implantation (TAVI) involves placing a prosthetic valve inside the old valve using a balloon catheter and is generally performed in patients who are considered unfit for conventional valve replacement surgery. It may be performed by a femoral or transapical approach or, more rarely, via transaortic or subclavian routes. Procedures carried out by the femoral route are increasingly being done under local anaesthesia with sedation, whereas the other approaches require general anaesthesia. Facilities for cardiopulmonary bypass may need to be on standby, meaning that the catheter lab becomes relatively crowded. The anaesthetist needs to be aware of potential complications including cardiac tamponade, coronary occlusion and arrhythmias. When the valve is being deployed, the ventricle is fast paced to decrease stroke volume and prevent the valve being expelled; however, this may result in ventricular fibrillation.

Pacemaker and implantable cardioverter defibrillator insertion

Pacemaker and implantable cardioverter defibrillator (ICD) devices may be inserted in the cardiac catheter laboratory under local or general anaesthesia depending on the circumstances. Implantation requires placing transvenous leads in the cardiac chambers and subcutaneous tunnelling to the device pocket. Testing of cardioverter defibrillator units should be performed under general anaesthesia and the benefit of using direct arterial monitoring considered. Radiofrequency ablation (RFA) may also be performed for patients with aberrant conduction pathways. This may be a prolonged procedure requiring general anaesthesia with the obvious potential for arrhythmias. Radiofrequency ablation may also be used for tumour ablation as an alternative to surgery.

Endovascular aortic aneurysm repair

Endovascular aortic aneurysm repair (EVAR) may be performed either in theatre or in the radiology suite (see Chapter 39) under general or regional anaesthesia, with or without sedation. These patients are at high risk for general anaesthesia, especially for emergency EVAR. If performed in the radiology suite the team must be prepared for the management of acute haemorrhage, cardiovascular instability and transfer of the patient to the operating department if the procedure is unsuccessful.

Vertebroplasty

Percutaneous vertebroplasty and kyphoplasty are commonly carried out by spinal surgeons or radiologists for the management of pain and deformity after vertebral collapse as a result of osteoporosis, metastatic cancer spread or trauma. The procedure may be carried out under local anaesthesia with sedation or general anaesthesia. The patient lies prone, and under fluoroscopic guidance, cement is injected into the vertebral body via transpedicular wide-bore needles. If kyphoplasty is being performed, a balloon is inflated first to correct loss of vertebral body height. Injection is sometimes painful, and if done under local anaesthesia, potent analgesia will be necessary (e.g. remifentanil or ketamine). The main complications are cement embolisation, which may result in cardiovascular collapse, or extrusion of cement into the vertebral canal, which may lead to temporary or permanent neurological deficit.

Transjugular intrahepatic portosystemic shunt procedures

Transjugular intrahepatic portosystemic shunt (TIPSS) procedures are increasingly being carried out in the management of refractory portal hypertension to decrease the risk of developing complications such as variceal bleeding or ascites. A shunt is created between the portal and hepatic veins to decrease vascular resistance. Complications include: bleeding and liver injury; hepatic encephalopathy (as a result of increased nitrogen load from the gut); hepatic ischaemia; and acute deterioration in cardiac function as a result of increased preload after shunting. Patients are often acutely unwell, with ascites, poor cardiovascular reserve and disordered fluid balance.

Anaesthesia for radiotherapy

Radiotherapy is used in the management of a variety of malignant diseases, some of which occur in childhood. These include the acute leukaemias, Wilms' tumour, retinoblastoma and central nervous system tumours. High-dose X-rays are administered by a linear accelerator, and all staff must remain outside the room to be protected from radiation.

Anaesthesia in paediatric radiotherapy presents several problems:

- treatment is administered daily over a 4- to 6-week period and necessitates repeated doses of sedation or general anaesthesia;
- the patient must remain alone and motionless for short periods during treatment, but immediate access to the patient is required in an emergency;
- monitoring is difficult because the child may be observed only on a closed-circuit television screen during treatment; and
- recovery from anaesthesia must be rapid, because treatment is organised usually on an outpatient basis, and disruption of normal activities should be minimised.

Before treatment begins, the fields to be irradiated are plotted and marked so that the X-rays may be focused on the tumour to avoid damaging the surrounding structures. This procedure requires the child to remain still for 20–40 min and takes place in semidarkness. Radiotherapy treatment is of much shorter duration; two or three fields are irradiated for 30–90 s each. Anaesthesia or sedation may be required for both the focusing and the administration of radiation.

Anaesthetic considerations

- Often these children have a Hickman line *in situ* to ensure reliable i.v. access for a range of medications and blood sampling.
- Intravenous induction is the most common. The dead space volume of Hickman lines must always be remembered, and they should be kept sterile. Failure to flush these lines immediately after administering drugs may lead to disastrous consequences when the anaesthetic drugs are flushed into the bloodstream at a later time. Agents such as ketamine are unsatisfactory because sudden movements may occur, and excessive salivation may risk airway compromise.
- When anaesthesia has been induced, the child is placed on a trolley and anaesthesia maintained with volatile anaesthesia delivered via an SAD.
- No analgesia is required, and tracheal intubation is generally not necessary. There is virtually no surgical stimulation, and patients may be maintained at relatively light anaesthetic levels, allowing for rapid emergence and recovery.

The same principles apply when providing anaesthesia for children undergoing other oncology procedures such as bone marrow aspiration, lumbar puncture and administration of intrathecal chemotherapy.

Anaesthesia for electroconvulsive therapy

Electroconvulsive therapy is controlled electrical stimulation of the central nervous system to cause seizures. It is often administered in a dedicated ward area within a psychiatric hospital.

Indications

- Severe depression (including postnatal and psychotic depression)

Contraindications

- Increased intracranial pressure
- Recent cerebrovascular accident
- Phaeochromocytoma
- Cardiac conduction defects
- Cerebral or aortic aneurysms

The mechanism of the therapy remains unknown. The electrical stimulus applied transcutaneously to the brain results in generalised tonic activity for about 10 s followed by a generalised clonic episode lasting up to 1 min or more. The handheld electrodes are placed in the bifrontotemporal region for bilateral ECT, or with both electrodes over the non-dominant hemisphere for unilateral therapy. The duration of the seizure may be important for outcome and depends on age, stimulus site, stimulus energy and drugs, including anaesthetics. Seizure activity lasting 25–50 s is optimal for the antidepressant effect. Treatment may initially be 2 or 3 times per week for 3 weeks.

Anaesthetic considerations

- Potential drug interactions with tricyclic antidepressants, monoamine oxidase inhibitors and lithium should be considered.
- Pretreatment with glycopyrrolate may be useful to reduce bradycardia and oral secretions.
- After preoxygenation, an i.v. induction agent and a neuromuscular blocker are administered:
  - Propofol is the most commonly used i.v. anaesthetic agent, replacing methohexital in this role. If seizure activity is deemed inadequate, etomidate is sometimes used, although consideration must be given to the potential effect of adrenal suppression with repeated administration. Thiopental is used occasionally but may shorten the duration of the seizure.
  - Partial neuromuscular blockade is required to allow monitoring of the duration of the peripheral seizure and to reduce physical symptoms in an attempt to help avoid trauma and minimise postseizure muscle pain. Suxamethonium is often used in a dose of 0.5 mg kg^{-1} because it has a short duration. Subsequent doses for ECT may be modified as appropriate. Use of other neuromuscular blockers (e.g. mivacurium) may necessitate short postprocedural artificial ventilation

and may not be as effective in preventing muscle contractions.

- A bite block is inserted when face-mask ventilation with oxygen is achieved, and then the stimulus is applied to produce a seizure. Ventilation should continue until the patient is breathing because hypoxia and hypercapnia may shorten the seizure.
- Seizures cause parasympathetic followed by sympathetic discharge, producing bradycardia followed by tachycardia and hypertension.
- Myocardial and cerebral oxygen demands increase and cardiac arrhythmias, with changes in blood pressure of variable magnitude and significance, depending on any underlying medical conditions (e.g. hypertension, coronary artery disease, peripheral vascular disease), may occur. Cardiovascular drugs such as esmolol or labetalol may be required to minimise the acute haemodynamic changes of ECT in high-risk patients.
- Emergence agitation, nausea, headache and fracture dislocations are other described complications.
- Anaesthetic drug administration and the patient's response should be accurately recorded, as in other anaesthetic situations. This is particularly important with ECT because the therapy is repeated frequently over several weeks, and consistent conditions are required to obtain the best ECT stimulus response.

Anaesthesia in the Emergency Department

Anaesthetists' involvement in the ED varies among hospitals, depending on the skills of the resident ED medical staff. The following clinical conditions usually require an anaesthetist to attend the ED:

- preoperative assessment and resuscitation before emergency surgery (e.g. major trauma or ruptured aortic aneurysm);
- specialist airway management for a patient with respiratory failure or acute airway compromise;
- intensive care admission for a patient needing ventilatory and/or other organ support;
- resuscitation as part of the cardiac arrest or trauma team;
- patients requiring specialist cannulation skills;
- anaesthesia for patients requiring procedures such as cardioversion or gastric lavage; and
- anaesthesia for patients requiring CT scan (e.g. suspected intracranial haemorrhage);

Detailed management of these situations is discussed elsewhere (see Chapters 44 and 48).

The anaesthetist attending ED should be trained and experienced enough to manage these seriously ill patients, and trained anaesthetic assistance is mandatory. Ideally there should be dedicated trolleys containing specific anaesthetic equipment that should be regularly checked and restocked. Drug boxes are often available containing drugs for emergency tracheal intubation and transfer. These do not usually contain opioids, and so these should be requested separately. Governance of drugs in the ED is important, and everything should be documented meticulously. Accurate clinical records should be kept throughout the period spent in ED and during any transfers (e.g. to CT scan). This is often difficult as many things are happening at once but is just as important as in theatre, particularly where blood products have been given. Patients are often aggressive because of the effects of drugs or pathological conditions and may also pose infection risks to staff. This should be clearly communicated to all staff in any receiving areas.

Chapter | **47** |

Anaesthesia and organ transplantation

Chris Snowden, Emily Bonner

Improvements in surgical and perioperative technique, immunosuppression regimens and organ preservation over the last century have meant that organ transplantation is now considered the primary treatment for organ failure. Solid organ transplants (kidney, liver, heart, lung and pancreas) make up the majority of procedures (Fig. 47.1), although the range of organs and tissues available for transplantation is continually expanding.

The improvement in long-term outcomes of transplantation means that most recipients are now able to lead a normal life after transplant. However, recipients are more likely than the general population to require elective surgery for malignancy or emergency procedures (especially for acute gastrointestinal pathological conditions). All anaesthetists require knowledge of both general and organ-specific problems relating to non-transplantation surgery in transplant recipients.

General considerations in organ transplantation

Epidemiology

The types of organs transplanted is similar in the UK, Europe and the USA (see Fig. 47.1). In contrast, the aetiologies of the indications for transplantation differ between healthcare systems. For example, liver transplantation in the UK is performed predominantly for alcohol-related liver disease, whereas hepatitis dominates in the USA. The success of transplantation surgery is reflected in high survival rates for all transplantation procedures (Table 47.1).

Transplant recipient listing/organ allocation

Defined protocols for listing potential recipients are set nationally and are important for equitable and appropriate transplantation. In general, patients who are likely to have better than 50% survival at 5 years are potential organ recipients. However, because transplantation outcome is much better than this, there remains a mismatch between the number of patients listed for transplant and those eventually receiving an organ (Fig. 47.2). Many patients, even when they have been listed as potential organ recipients, will ultimately die on the waiting list.

Organ allocation is prioritised differently across the world, with differences between healthcare systems and prognostic criteria. The majority of systems have developed organ allocation based around severity of the patient's illness, risk of death without transplantation and duration spent on a waiting list, with the overall aim being to prevent waiting list death. In the UK, 'case of need' also takes preference in specific cases where there is a rapidly deteriorating organ function (e.g. acute liver failure, heart failure).

Organ procurement

As the number of patients with end-stage disease increases, the organ supply/demand gap remains and the limiting factor to successful transplantation is the availability of acceptable donor organs. The mainstay of organ procurement has been from donation after brain death (DBD), often resulting from trauma. Initiatives to both increase the numbers of organs available and to increase the quality of the available organs have been applied, and include:

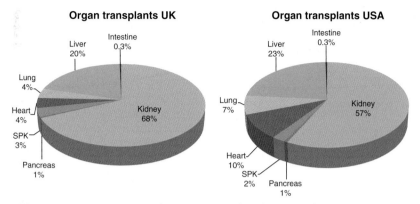

Fig. 47.1 Organ transplantation activity comparison between USA and UK (2015–2016). SPK, Simultaneous Pancreas Kidney Transplant. (Data from United Network for Organ Sharing (USA) and UK Blood Transfusion Service).

Table 47.1 Patient survival after first organ transplantation

	1-year survival (%)	2-year survival (%)	5-year survival (%)
Kidney (live related)	99	98	94
Kidney (DBD)	96	95	90
Kidney (DCD)	95	93	84
Liver (DBD)	93	91	82
Liver (DCD)	81	80	71
Heart	82	79	71
Lung (DBD)	82	74	59
Lung (DCD)	86	78	64
Pancreas (DBD)	96	94	81
Pancreas (DCD)	100	100	95
Simultaneous pancreas kidney (DBD)	96	93	87
Simultaneous pancreas kidney (DCD)	99	94	94

DBD, Donation after brain death; *DCD,* donation after circulatory death.
Data from UK Blood Transfusion Service, Year of Transplant 2009–2011.

1. Different sources of donation:
   a. Donors after circulatory death (DCD)
   b. Live-related donors—kidney and liver transplantation
   c. Split-organ donation—liver
2. Acceptance of 'marginal' organs through the following:
   a. Better methods of organ preservation—including *ex vivo* perfusion techniques
   b. Increasing donation from older persons where outcomes are acceptable
   c. Improved ICU management and end-of-life care

Anaesthetic management: general principles

Organ donation procedure

Deceased donor donation

Management of the DBD donor commences in the ICU after donor death has been confirmed by neurological criteria (see

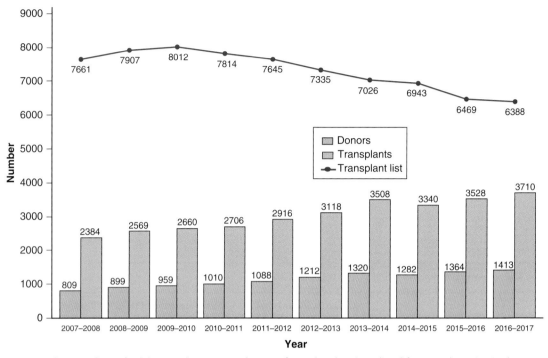

Fig. 47.2 Trends in numbers of solid organ donors, transplants performed and patients listed for transplantation in the UK. (Data from UK Blood Transfusion Service.)

Chapter 48). Donor management by the anaesthetist follows on directly from these donor management and end-of-life care pathways in the ICU. Management of the DCD donor commences as soon as death is pronounced and requires early intervention in terms of *in vivo* organ perfusion.

Acquisition of donated organs occurs in the operating theatre and requires careful haemodynamic management to ensure appropriate organ quality for subsequent transplantation. The procedure involves a midline laparotomy and sternotomy and has the potential for:

- blood loss;
- hypothermia;
- cardiovascular instability; and
- spinal reflex movements.

Appropriately experienced individuals provide donor support during the procedure. Vasoactive infusions are likely to have been commenced during ICU care and are continued during the procedure. Hypertension may also occur and requires volatile anaesthetic agents, opioids or vasodilators. Volatile anaesthetic agents may also provide some degree of ischaemic preconditioning and are often used during hepatic and cardiac donation procedures. There are inadequate data to suggest that spinal reflex responses require anaesthetic suppression. However, many anaesthetists would administer a neuromuscular blocking agent to prevent the

appearance of spinal reflexes, as these may be disturbing to staff who are unfamiliar with their cause.

Live-related organ donation

Whole organ donation from a close relative has revolutionised renal transplantation; donation of part of an organ (a liver lobe) has also being introduced for liver transplant recipients. Organ donation from a previously fit individual to a patient with end-stage disease requires careful consideration of the ethical issues. Careful management of sequential procedural timing to allow immediate donor organ implantation will avoid storage injury. If these issues are fully addressed, the outcome after living-related donation is amongst the best of all transplantation procedures.

Organ transplantation procedure

Preoperative assessment of transplant recipients

Any organ allocation system that offers transplantation to patients based on end-organ disease severity requires thorough multisystem preoperative anaesthetic assessment to ensure that extended outcome benefit is not curtailed by disease of other organ systems. All transplant procedures are classified as high risk. Because the majority of postoperative deaths occur in the early perioperative period and recipients are increasing in age and comorbidities, preanaesthetic assessment is vital.

Preoperative assessment usually occurs some time before the actual operative procedure and can usefully be divided into:

(a) specific disease—related to end-organ disease, such as hepatopulmonary syndrome, portopulmonary hypertension (liver), autonomic neuropathy (pancreas); or

(b) non-specific disease—such as ischaemic heart disease, chronic obstructive pulmonary disease (COPD).

Assessment of eligible recipients is particularly focussed on the cardiorespiratory system. The use of functional reserve assessment by subjective (e.g. metabolic equivalents (METS) estimation) or objective (e.g. cardiopulmonary exercise testing) has been advocated in many forms of major surgery, as a decision point for more invasive forms of cardiovascular assessment (see Chapters 19 and 30). Renal dysfunction is a key determinant in the early recovery of many transplantation procedures, and assessment of the likely requirement for early postoperative renal support is essential. End-stage disease is associated with nutritional deficiencies that may worsen during the catabolic phase after major surgery. Preoperative information and psychological support are very important; patients may need assistance in maintaining acceptable compliance with postoperative medication regimens, which are essential for good recovery after transplantation.

Intraoperative management

Most transplantation procedures can be usefully separated into four specific phases:

1. *Dissection phase.* This phase entails the removal of the diseased organ from the recipient. Blood loss is common. Preparation for acceptance of the new organ is paramount to ensure that the next phase is as short as possible.

2. *Implantation.* Implantation of the donor organ occurs immediately on removal of the diseased organ. Once an organ is removed, any benefit from residual organ function is eliminated. In cardiothoracic transplantation, removal usually relies on cardiopulmonary bypass, whereas in liver/pancreas/kidney procedures, a period of no organ function is tolerated. When the donor organ is removed from the relative protective effects of the *ex vivo* preservation environment (cold ischaemia), the period of implantation provides a period of 'warm ischaemia', which is potentially damaging to subsequent organ function and must be minimised.

3. *Reperfusion.* Once the organ has been surgically implanted, the blood supply has to be reconnected thus providing reperfusion of the new organ. This phase can be complicated by haemodynamic compromise caused by myocardial depression and vasodilatation; pharmacological support is often needed.

4. *Postreperfusion.* Once reperfusion has been completed, the postreperfusion phase allows checking of surgical anastomosis, restoration of haemodynamic stability and optimisation of the environment for appropriate organ function.

Postoperative management

Most transplantation patients are managed in a high-dependency area after solid organ transplantation. Ensuring adequate haemodynamic support through appropriate monitoring and rapid response to changes in patient status ensures adequate organ perfusion and reduces early complications that may lead to early transplant failure.

Transplant recipients undergoing non-transplant procedures

Transplant recipients presenting for non-transplant surgery may have residual evidence of chronic disease, be immuno-compromised and/or have reduced organ functional reserve. In an emergency situation the effect of acute illness may also complicate further anaesthetic management. Appropriate anaesthetic management aims for transition through the perioperative period without risk of further transplanted organ impairment or postoperative rejection.

Preoperative considerations

Transplanted organ status
The interval between organ transplantation and subsequent elective surgery determines the likelihood, nature and complexity of anaesthetic problems. Within the first 6 months after transplantation, the major considerations for the anaesthetist are those of graft rejection and acute changes in physiology. One year after successful transplantation, the risk of chronic rejection remains. Although many standard biochemical tests of renal, liver and cardiac function are normal in transplant recipients, the functional reserve of most transplanted organs is reduced.

Function of other organ systems
Although some systemic manifestations of the original organ failure are reduced by successful transplantation, residual disease in remote organs associated with pretransplant disease may remain. Cardiovascular issues are common to many multisystem diseases requiring transplantation, especially renal, pancreatic, and liver disease and are a common cause of ongoing mortality after transplantation. Paradoxically, the presence of coronary artery disease in heart transplant recipients is less likely unless rejection is present. Although most patients will have been fully investigated before

transplantation, more recent investigations are usually warranted for subsequent surgical procedures.

Immunosuppression

Immunosuppressive regimens enable long-term transplantation benefit and prevent graft rejection, which usually occurs within the first year after transplantation. Older steroid-based regimens are being substituted with newer agents with fewer generalised adverse effects. As a general rule, all current immunosuppressive therapy should be continued throughout the perioperative period. However, if gastrointestinal absorption is likely to be compromised after surgery, oral immunosuppressive drugs should be converted to i.v. preparations. Complete omission of immunosuppressive regimens must be limited to the most extreme cases, where sepsis is potentially life threatening and where the risk of graft rejection becomes a secondary issue.

Presence of infection

In addition to the presence of infection causing the initial requirement for transplantation (e.g. hepatitis or cytomegalovirus infection), the development of *de novo* infection must be investigated. However, the diagnosis may be difficult in transplant recipients because typical presenting features may be absent. Fever may not be present, and given that some drug regimens cause leucopoenia, an increased white cell count for a particular patient may lie within the 'normal' range. In elective situations a recent culture screen for infection should have been performed before surgery and will guide further management. There is no evidence to support an increase in the use or duration of prophylactic perioperative antibiotics in the transplant recipient.

Intraoperative considerations

The overriding principles for anaesthetic management of transplant recipients are to reduce the degree of surgical stress, avoid injury to the transplanted organ and protect against infection.

Avoidance of surgical stress

Laparoscopic surgical techniques have the advantage of reducing surgical stress. However, especially in the case of abdominal solid organ transplants, this must be balanced with the increased intra-abdominal pressures during laparoscopy and the potential to reduce organ perfusion. Regional analgesic techniques also reduce surgical stress but may have relative contraindications if coagulation (liver), haemodynamic (cardiac) or autonomic (e.g. renal, pancreatic) dysfunction is present.

Reducing injury to transplanted organ

The use of anaesthetic agents that are non-toxic to the transplanted organ is important, given reduced organ reserve. Large volumes of radiological contrast agents, aminoglycosides and NSAIDs are best avoided in renal transplant recipients.

Anaesthetic drugs rarely affect liver transplant function and, importantly, paracetamol in analgesic doses is not contraindicated. It is vital to maintain adequate perfusion of the transplanted organ, and hypovolaemia must be avoided. Minimally invasive techniques to optimise fluid balance and cardiac output are recommended in major surgery (see Chapter 30). Perfusion pressures must be maintained for renal transplant recipients, and direct arterial monitoring is indicated for all but the most minor procedures. Other measures to maintain organ perfusion, in addition to maintaining circulating volume, include avoidance of:

- high CVPs;
- high concentrations of PEEP;
- excessive doses of volatile anaesthetic agents (liver);
- high airway pressures (lung); and
- excessive airway manipulation (lung).

Direct injury to cardiac function in heart transplant recipients is less likely during non-cardiac surgery.

Infection

Strict asepsis must be adhered to at all times, especially when inserting central venous access lines or performing regional anaesthetic techniques or during airway manipulation. Dedicated *in situ* total parenteral nutrition (TPN) lines should not be used for the administration of anaesthetic drugs.

Postoperative considerations

Postoperative management of transplant recipients usually requires enhanced postoperative care facilities. Analgesia is provided with regional techniques, thereby preventing the administration of i.v. or oral agents that have the potential for transplanted organ toxicity. Reduced metabolism and excretion of analgesic agents, especially opioids, may require alteration in drug dose, and more rapid-acting agents are commonly used in liver and renal transplant recipients. The administration of additional steroid doses to prevent the possibility of adrenal unresponsiveness is controversial. Some authors suggest that supplementation is not required unless the maintenance dose of steroid is more than 20 mg prednisolone per day. In the absence of clear evidence, the use of prolonged doses of steroids is best avoided.

Anaesthesia for organ transplantation and transplant recipients: organ-specific considerations

Renal transplantation

Renal transplantation is the most common type of solid organ transplantation and has high success in that most recipients are rendered dialysis free. The success of the live-related kidney program has allowed patients with more severe comorbidities to undergo transplantation. Common indications for renal transplantation include diabetic nephropathy (often combined as simultaneous kidney–pancreas transplant), hypertensive nephrosclerosis and polycystic kidney disease.

Preoperative assessment

Ischaemic heart disease is often present because of the association between chronic kidney disease and cardiac risk factors, including hypercholesterolemia, diabetes and hypertension. Preoperative anaemia is managed with varying strategies including erythropoietin. Most patients will be dialysed before transplant to avoid perioperative hyperkalaemia, volume overload, acidosis and uraemia. Preoperative dialysis will often negate the need for posttransplant dialysis even if postoperative graft function is delayed. However, the removal of large volumes of fluid with intravascular depletion should be avoided to prevent aggressive intraoperative fluid therapy being needed to maintain graft flow.

Intraoperative

Arteriovenous fistulae are common, and care should be taken to position both peripheral and central cannulae away from pre-existing fistulae. The fistula arm should be padded and positioned appropriately to prevent traction or compression injuries during surgery. Both central venous cannulae and pre-emptive haemodialysis catheter insertion may be challenging from multiple previous cannulation attempts. Ultrasonic assessment of the vasculature to rule out pre-existing venous stenosis is advised.

Induction of anaesthesia can be achieved with standard intravenous anaesthetic agents and rapid-acting opioids. Metabolites of morphine are excreted in the urine, and although this should not affect intraoperative analgesic dosing, postoperative dosing may need to be reduced. Rapid-sequence induction should be considered in patients with potential autonomic dysfunction and risk of aspiration, but acute hyperkalaemia with suxamethonium is possible. Neuromuscular blocking agents undergoing Hofmann degradation and ester hydrolysis (e.g. atracurium, cisatracurium) are required. Maintenance of anaesthesia may be either inhalational or with TIVA combinations that are independent of renal clearance (e.g. propofol/remifentanil). Analgesia can be provided with paracetamol and incremental doses of opioid. NSAIDs are relatively contraindicated because of reduction of blood flow in the renal vasa recta compromising graft function. Regional blockade (e.g. transverse abdominus plane) has been used as a useful opioid-sparing analgesic adjunct. Careful consideration needs to be given to the risks and benefits of central neuraxial blockade when postoperative anticoagulation for dialysis is required.

Adequate graft perfusion requires careful maintenance of MAP and fluid management, often adjusted according to preoperative blood pressure levels. A recently dialysed patient may require fluid loading to maintain cardiac output, optimise graft perfusion and reduce viscosity. However, fluid overload should be avoided, especially where anuria is present. Cardiac output monitoring is useful; the oesophageal Doppler does not require arterial cannulation, and this may be relevant for patients who may need future fistula formation.

Postoperative

Preserving adequate flow through the transplanted kidney continues into the postoperative period. Early graft failure occurs in approximately 5% of procedures. Primary non-function is the most common cause; acute rejection also occurs but is less prevalent. Potential complications in the early postoperative period include bleeding, acute vascular thrombus and urinary leak. Ureteric stents are usually placed at the end of the operation to bridge the ureteric anastomosis and are removed approximately 6 weeks after transplant under local anaesthesia.

Anaesthesia for renal transplant recipients
Surgical presentation

Common indications for non–transplant-related surgery are urological complications or the need for further fistula formation where transplantation has been unsuccessful. Systemic complications of renal disease, including osteoporosis, may require orthopaedic intervention. Gastrointestinal and cardiac diseases are also more common in these patients and may require surgical intervention.

Anaesthetic considerations

Renal transplant recipients presenting for elective surgery retain pre-existing diabetes-related illnesses, ischaemic heart disease, hypertension and pulmonary disease. They are also maintained on relatively severe immunosuppressive regimens, with associated risk of adverse effects.

Preoperatively, serum creatinine concentrations are often normal, but glomerular filtration rate and renal plasma flow are usually reduced on direct measurement (see Chapter 11). This may have a covert effect on drug metabolism and excretion. Nephrotoxic drugs (e.g. contrast agents) should be administered in reduced doses, whereas NSAIDs are relatively contraindicated. Residual hypertension is a common finding after transplantation, with 50% of renal recipients requiring therapy at 1 year after transplant.

Because the transplanted kidney has no autoregulatory mechanisms, it is particularly susceptible to damage if perfusion pressure is reduced. Therefore an appropriate arterial pressure must be maintained by both the judicious use of vasopressor therapy and the avoidance of hypovolaemia, especially where preoperative dialysis has been performed. In this regard, a non-invasive monitor of circulating volume, with or without invasive arterial pressure monitoring, is appropriate.

Regional anaesthesia is safe in renal transplant recipients and should be considered. Drugs used for general anaesthesia should be rapid acting and independent of renal excretion. All inhalational agents may be used safely. Early experimental reports of high doses of fluoride ions after prolonged sevoflurane maintenance have not being substantiated in humans (see Chapter 3).

Liver transplantation

Liver transplantation is the second most common transplant surgery worldwide. The requirement for liver transplantation is likely to increase given an increased incidence of fatty liver and alcohol-related illnesses in younger individuals. The paucity of donor organs has dictated that live-related transplantation is now being performed in some centres. Survival rates for liver transplantation are high: 85%–95% at 1 year and 75% at 5 years. Common indications for transplantation include alcoholic liver disease, viral hepatitis (e.g. hepatitis B and C), biliary cirrhosis, and drug-induced liver failure.

Preoperative assessment

Assessment includes an initial screening for multisystem abnormalities in the cardiorespiratory system, abdominal anatomy, nutritional requirements and psychological assessment. Given the severe physiological stress of surgery, assessment of physiological reserve is imperative through a combination of routine echocardiography (including indirect measurement of pulmonary artery pressure) and tests aimed at recreating the physiological demands experienced during liver transplantation. Cardiopulmonary exercise testing is increasingly the dynamic test of choice, although dobutamine stress echocardiography is also used. Specific sequelae of end-stage chronic liver disease, including portopulmonary hypertension, hepatopulmonary syndrome and hepatorenal syndrome, should be actively diagnosed, as preoperative therapy may be instituted early to allow successful transplantation. Previously these conditions were seen as absolute surgical contraindications to liver transplant.

Intraoperative

Each operative phase poses significant anaesthetic challenges. The dissection phase includes mobilisation of the structures around the liver with subsequent division of the hepatic portal vein, hepatic artery and bile duct. Cardiovascular instability may ensue from decompression of abdominal ascites and subsequent fluid shifts. Severe haemorrhage may occur from disruption of distended abdominal varices (secondary to portal hypertension) and pre-existing coagulopathy. Coagulopathy often worsens during donor organ implantation (anhepatic phase), as there is no hepatic synthesis of clotting factors. Worsening lactic acidosis is also observed because lactate metabolism is absent. Liver reperfusion remains one of the most physiologically challenging periods in any abdominal operation, with potential for sudden and significant rise in potassium leading to cardiac arrhythmias and cardiac arrest. New techniques in donor retrieval, including continuous normothermic perfusion of grafts, are promising in addressing postreperfusion syndrome. Successful reperfusion will promote early resolution of lactic acidosis and provide haemodynamic stability within hours. Hyperfibrinolysis may develop as a result of accelerated graft release of tissue plasminogen activator; antifibrinolytics (e.g. tranexamic acid) may be required.

Intraoperative monitoring

Appropriate recipient selection excludes patients with severe pulmonary hypertension from listing with a diminishing intraoperative requirement for a pulmonary artery catheter. Non-invasive cardiac output monitoring (e.g. pulse contour devices) is often employed, with intraoperative transoesophageal echocardiography (TOE) becoming increasingly popular to monitor cardiac filling during reperfusion. However, resources required for service implementation and concern over the presence of oesophageal varices may limit TOE use. Routine use of arterial blood gases gives guidance for transfusion, along with vital information regarding acid–base balance, ventilation and electrolyte levels.

Blood conservation

Perioperative bleeding can be either surgical or related to coagulation deficiencies. Use of cell salvage is advocated. Targeted treatment of coagulopathy is guided by point-of-care viscoelastic testing with either thromboelastography (TEG) or rotational thromboelastometry (ROTEM) (see Chapter 14).

Postoperative

Postoperatively patients are transferred to the ICU for a period of artificial ventilation. Liver transplantation has a high incidence (15%–20%) of early reoperation for surgical bleeding from the gallbladder bed, from any vascular anastomosis or from portal varices. Surgical bleeding may be difficult to differentiate from coagulopathy and may lead to a 'negative' laparotomy. Where there has been delayed normalisation of coagulation, haematoma formation may lead to abdominal tamponade, which must be released to avoid compromise of renal and liver function.

Hepatic artery or portal vein thrombosis may lead to graft failure, and these are surgical emergencies. Most centres use ultrasound investigation of the graft postoperatively to ensure vessel patency. Worsening metabolic acidosis and coagulopathy are signs of impending thrombosis, and early diagnosis will allow return to the operating theatre to attempt rescue of a threatened graft. Complete thrombosis of vessels is difficult to rectify and may require urgent retransplantation.

Anaesthesia for liver transplant recipients

Surgical presentation

Liver transplant recipients often present surgically for biliary tract drainage procedures and incisional hernia repair. Further abdominal surgery may be complex, and haemorrhage is a real possibility.

Preoperative status

Early graft function leads to rapid return to normal hepatic function, including coagulation and drug metabolism. Many of the systemic manifestations of liver disease, including pulmonary abnormalities, also return to normal. Resolution of pleural effusions, ascites and pulmonary shunting occurs within the first few weeks. The haemodynamic stigmata of chronic liver disease (systemic vasodilatation and high cardiac output) usually return to a normal level within months of transplantation. Clinical evidence of sepsis may suggest active cholangitis, and this should be treated before biliary drainage procedures are performed. Preoperative investigations should include clotting studies, liver function tests and electrolytes. The presence of ongoing viral illness is important for both theatre safety and blood transfusion.

Intraoperative management

Similar to the renal allograft, lack of autoregulation makes the organ susceptible to ischaemia-reperfusion injury. Hypovolaemia, high concentrations of PEEP, and increased central venous pressures may lead to worsening of liver function. Regional anaesthesia is not contraindicated unless clotting dysfunction remains an issue. Unpredictable drug metabolism is important within the first few months after liver transplantation. However, if liver function tests have returned to baseline, it can be assumed that the response to anaesthetic drugs will be normal. Vecuronium is not contraindicated in this population, although it is probably prudent to use atracurium wherever coexisting renal disease is present. Paracetamol in standard analgesic doses is not contraindicated.

Cardiac transplantation

The primary indication for cardiac transplantation is end-stage heart failure refractory to medical or surgical therapy. All patients are New York Heart Association (NYHA) class III–IV, with a predicted 1-year survival of less than 75%. The commonest cause is ischaemic cardiomyopathy. Severe irreversible pulmonary hypertension is an absolute contraindication to cardiac transplantation because of the increased afterload placed on the donor heart. For these patients, heart–lung (*en bloc*) transplant may be an option.

Preoperative

Presentation of patients for cardiac transplant can vary widely, with some being ambulatory outpatients whereas others are critically ill in ICUs. Patients on the transplant waiting list are maintained with complex combination of first-line therapies (e.g. diuretics, beta-blockade, calcium channel blockers, angiotensin-converting enzyme (ACE) inhibitors) and second-line treatments (e.g. ventricular assist devices).

Intraoperative

Induction of anaesthesia can cause severe cardiovascular instability because all patients are highly dependent on endogenous sympathetic drive. A technique using high-dose opioid, supplemented with a benzodiazepine and small concentrations of a volatile anaesthetic agent, is appropriate. Arterial and central venous cannulae are inserted, with or without requirement for pulmonary artery catheterisation. Transoesophageal echocardiography is a standard monitoring technique to assess cardiac status, volume changes and the presence of intracardiac thrombi.

Cardiopulmonary bypass (CPB) with variable levels of hypothermia is used during surgery (see Chapter 42). Explantation of the native heart is immediately followed by implantation that involves four major anastomoses: left and right atrial; aortic; and pulmonary artery anastomoses. Once completed, the aortic cross-clamp is removed and electromechanical activity will usually commence. The patient is then rewarmed, and weaning from CPB is commenced. Inotropic support and cardiac pacing are employed at an early stage. Because of loss of sinus node function in the graft, pacing may be required longer term. Failure to wean from CPB is most commonly due to right ventricular failure with increased pulmonary artery pressures. Reduction of pulmonary vascular resistance (PVR) is often necessary using strategies including adequate oxygenation and ventilation, avoidance of acidosis, hypercapnia or hypothermia, inotropic support for the right ventricle and pulmonary vasodilator therapy (e.g. inhaled nitric oxide and prostaglandins). The new graft is preload dependent, and it is vital to maintain adequate circulating volume whilst avoiding large increases in CVP and overdistension of the right ventricle. Coagulopathy is common postimplantation and after discontinuation of CPB. Aprotinin was widely used to reduce the quantity of blood products transfused. However, after recent concerns about its safety, alternative antifibrinolytics (e.g. tranexamic acid) are now used.

Postoperative

Tracheal extubation occurs once haemodynamic stability is achieved and the risk of bleeding is minimised. Inotropic drugs are only required for 36–72 h, intercostal drains removed 24–48 h after transplant, and patients usually discharged from critical care at 72 h. Early reoperation may be required because of surgical bleeding, with an inherent risk of cardiac tamponade.

Anaesthesia for cardiac transplant recipients

Surgical presentation

Cardiac recipients often present to the non-transplant anaesthetist for abdominal surgery. Cardiopulmonary bypass in conjunction with a debilitated immune system and high-dose immunosuppressant drugs make these patients more susceptible to intra-abdominal complications and mucosal perforation. Furthermore, sternal wound breakdown may require multiple surgeries with complex tissue grafting procedures.

Preoperative status

The transplanted organ must not be considered normal in terms of its innervation and haemodynamic responses. Autonomic denervation leads to a loss in vagal control of the sinoatrial node and a persistent tachycardia. The ECG may show two P waves because of remnants of the explanted organ conduction system. There may also be arrhythmias, bundle branch blocks and requirement for pacemaker insertion. Cardiac function is usually normal, with early preload dependency improving steadily as an appropriate cardiac response to increased catecholamine concentrations occurs. Most successfully transplanted patients eventually return to having a normal cardiac output, stroke volume and ejection fraction. The highest risk of rejection occurs within the first 6 months after transplantation and is diagnosed by myocardial biopsy and increased troponin concentrations. Chronic rejection is angiographically present in 20% of patients at 5 years after transplantation. It often presents as progression of coronary artery disease without angina, because sympathetic innervation is reduced.

Anaesthetic considerations

Preoperatively, hypertension (often induced by ciclosporin A) is present in two-thirds of patients and may require

adjustment of drug therapy or treatment. Permanent pacemakers must be checked before the procedure and appropriate measures taken for intraoperative management. Persistent atrial arrhythmias may suggest rejection and require further investigation.

Intraoperatively the use of regional anaesthesia is somewhat controversial but is unlikely to cause major complications if cardiac function is normal. Right internal jugular vein cannulation is best avoided because it provides venous access for frequent myocardial biopsies. Drugs affecting the autonomic system are of minimal use in these patients because the heart is denervated after transplantation. Direct-acting drugs, including dobutamine, ephedrine and noradrenaline, are used if chronotropic or inotropic drugs are required. Cardiac output is commonly preload-dependent, and fluid therapy should be optimised, guided by appropriate monitoring techniques (e.g. TOE, non-invasive cardiac output devices) and avoiding reductions in afterload.

Pulmonary transplantation

Transplantation may be either single-lung (SLT) or double-lung (DLT) or may occur in combination with a heart transplant (*en bloc*). Common indications for pulmonary transplantation include COPD (45%), cystic fibrosis, pulmonary fibrosis, pulmonary hypertension and other conditions (e.g. Eisenmenger's complex).

Preoperative

Scoring systems for transplant suitability differ according to the indication for transplantation; full lung function assessment predominates in all the criteria. Pulmonary function testing, arterial blood gases and functional testing (6-minute walk test or cardiopulmonary exercise testing) are important. Chest radiograph and CT imaging are necessary to measure the size of the chest cavity and exclude any underlying malignancy or invasive pulmonary disease. Cardiac investigation with echocardiogram and right-sided heart catheterisation are used to assess cardiac contractility and underlying pulmonary hypertension. The presence and severity of gastroesophageal reflux (and hence aspiration risk) must be assessed. Sputum culture is required to assess for fungal or bacterial colonisation of the tracheobronchial tree and indolent invasive pulmonary disease.

Intraoperative

Aims of general anaesthesia are to maintain systemic vascular resistance, preserve myocardial contractility and avoid any increase in pulmonary vascular resistance. Induction using high-dose opioid and a benzodiazepine is usual, although ketamine is a useful alternative in the presence of significant pulmonary hypertension. A double-lumen endobronchial tube is inserted and exchanged to a single-lumen tracheal tube at transplant completion. Patients with obstructive pulmonary pathological conditions may benefit from the bronchodilatory effects of inhalational anaesthetic agents, but high incidences of awareness have been reported during lung transplantation. Therefore propofol infusion alongside inhalational agents or TIVA-based techniques are often used; TIVA also provides some preservation of hypoxic pulmonary vasoconstriction. Cardiopulmonary bypass use is dictated by pathological condition (e.g. primary pulmonary hypertension), haemodynamic instability, refractory hypoxia or hypercarbia. Intrathoracic cooling is used to reduce warm-perfusion graft injury, but global intraoperative hypothermia can worsen pulmonary hypertension, increase the risk of arrhythmias and lead to coagulopathy. Circulating volume must be optimised to maintain perfusion whilst avoiding pulmonary oedema in the transplanted lung.

Postoperative

Effective postoperative analgesia is imperative. Thoracic epidural analgesia is often the mode of choice, performed before waking the patient and when heparin has been fully reversed. Paravertebral blockade may be used as an alternative in SLT. Primary graft dysfunction presents in a similar way to acute lung injury/acute respiratory distress syndrome (ARDS) and can occur on reperfusion to varying degrees of severity. If severe enough to compromise oxygenation, treatment with inhaled nitric oxide or inhaled prostaglandins is administered. Early re-exploration is required for surgical bleeding and repair of anastomotic leaks.

Anaesthesia for pulmonary transplant recipients
Preoperative status

Lung volumes and function after both SLT and DLT are reduced in the first month after transplantation but improve over the next 6 months. Successful DLT results in return of full lung function, and gas exchange and exercise tolerance are likely to be normal at 3 months; SLT has a more variable return of function depending on the underlying disease process. Persistent hypercapnia suggests graft dysfunction. The commonest complications of both forms of lung transplantation are infection and rejection. Rejection often presents as an obliterative bronchiolitis at around 8–12 months after transplant and is present in up to 70% of patients who survive for 5 years.

Surgical presentation

Lung transplant patients may present for investigation of airway stenosis, drainage of infection or diagnostic bronchoscopy. There is also an increased risk of intra-abdominal lymphoproliferative disease requiring incidental surgery.

Anaesthetic considerations

Many patients will have recent pulmonary function tests available, but a worsening of functional symptoms since previous testing requires investigation. A recent echocardiogram may be appropriate to exclude developing cardiac disease. Baseline blood gases are useful where supplemental oxygen is required, especially in SLT recipients. Recent chest infection should trigger preoperative sputum culture with appropriate therapy. Upper airway anatomy and airway responses are often abnormal. Double-lung (or combined heart–lung) recipients have no airway reflexes, whereas SLT patients retain airway and carinal responses. However, the presence of an allograft with normal structure in combination with a lung retaining the original disease process may cause specific ventilatory problems. Pulmonary blood flow diverts preferentially to the allograft, and during lateral positioning, especially where the diseased lung is dependent, difficult oxygenation and hypoxia may occur. Different lung compliances may lead to barotrauma; differential lung ventilation must be considered in this situation. However, given altered airway anatomy, the siting of a double-lumen tube may be very difficult, and other methods of lung isolation may be required.

Pancreas transplantation

The indication for pancreatic transplantation is almost exclusively long-standing, poorly controlled diabetes mellitus, mainly in patients with type 1 diabetes or selected patients with type 2. Isolated pancreas transplant alone is less common than simultaneous kidney–pancreas transplantation where renal impairment is present, as combined transplantation has a better outcome for both grafts. Although patients have the ability to be free from insulin administration and dialysis, there is a trade-off in terms of long-term immunosuppressive therapy with associated risks.

Preoperative

The complications associated with long-standing diabetes dominate preoperative assessment. Significant degrees of autonomic neuropathy, postural hypotension, uncontrolled hypoglycaemic episodes and complex insulin regimens are common. Cardiovascular disease is usual, and both non-invasive and invasive cardiological investigations with subsequent intervention are an important component of assessment (see Chapter 19).

Intraoperative

A combined general and regional anaesthetic technique is used. The choice of regional technique is often dependent on the severity of diabetic neuropathy. Although cautious epidural anaesthesia has been used, intrathecal opioids may be the best option with a lower risk of prolonged hypotension. A maintenance glucose/insulin regimen is used during implantation of the donor pancreas. After successful reperfusion and early graft function, the requirement for exogenous insulin rapidly decreases and it is usual for the recipient to return to a high-dependency unit (HDU) with no insulin requirement. A monoclonal antibody (e.g. alemtuzumab) is administered at the time of reperfusion with the aim of preventing early rejection; these drugs may cause hypotension.

Postoperative

Management in the HDU is focused on adequate glucose control and early assessment of postoperative bleeding. Restored renal function is not always immediate, and haemodialysis may be required. Postoperative anticoagulation is important to prevent devastating early graft thrombosis; this occurs in 10%–15% of transplants with ensuing graft loss. Enteric or urinary drainage of exocrine pancreatic secretions is an integral component of the surgical procedure because the secretions may cause injury to internal organs. Direct urinary drainage may lead to large bicarbonate losses, which may require intravenous replacement.

Anaesthesia for pancreas transplant recipients

Although early graft function allows rapid discontinuation of exogenous insulin therapy, postoperative stabilisation of the patient on an appropriate immunosuppressive regimen may delay full recovery for some weeks. Residual requirement for insulin must be noted, and a similar insulin regimen to those for other patients with diabetes presenting for surgery should be used. The systemic effects of long-term, uncontrolled diabetes may remain even after successful pancreas transplantation. Patients may have persistent ischaemic heart disease, often silent, that must be investigated where there has been recent functional deterioration. Discontinuation of antithrombotic agents prescribed after previous coronary intervention must be considered. Persistent autonomic neuropathy is common and leads to a delay in gastric emptying, hypotension and a vagolytic response to surgery. Wherever there is a combination of antithrombotic medication and autonomic dysfunction, the use of regional anaesthesia must be carefully considered.

References/Further reading

NHSBT—UK Transplantation Resource at https://nhsbtdbe.blob.core.windows.net/umbraco-assets-corp/4657/activity_report_2016_17.pdf

US Transplantation Report. https://unos.org/data/transplant-trends/#transplants_by_organ_type+year+2017

Chapter | 48 |

The intensive care unit

Daniel Harvey, Jonathan Thompson

This chapter provides an overview of general adult intensive care, the key components of which are resuscitation and stabilisation; physiological optimisation to prevent deterioration and organ failure; support of failing organ systems; and management and communication with patients and family of likely treatment outcomes, including potential failure. Levels of care have been described from level 0 (ward-based care) to level 3 (patients requiring advanced respiratory support alone or a minimum of two organs being supported) (Box 48.1). However, the ideal is a comprehensive system where the needs of all critically ill hospital patients are met with consistency rather than just those who are admitted to designated intensive care (ICU) or high-dependency (HDU) units.

In the UK the ICU generally accounts for 1%–2% of the total number of acute hospital beds. The design of ICUs varies from hospital to hospital, but they are designated areas with high nurse-to-patient ratios (1:1, 1:2), continuous medical staff availability, provision for invasive monitoring and the ability to deliver organ support technologies. Minimum standards for the provision of intensive care services are published by the Faculty of Intensive Care Medicine (see further reading).

Staffing an intensive care unit

The ICU team is multidisciplinary and involves contributions from a variety of medical and nursing staff, including physiotherapists, rehabilitation teams, dieticians, psychologists and pharmacists. Each has complementary experience and skills and good teamwork ensures high standards of quality patient care. Models of ICU decision making differ, broadly defined as 'closed' (ICU team takes primary responsibility for admission, management and discharge decisions) 'semi-open' (shared decision-making with referral multidisciplinary team, or MDT) and 'open' (decisions led by referring teams). However, such categories fail to appreciate the shared models in which patient decision-making is individualised; all decisions should also involve the patient and appropriate family members according to professional guidance and relevant legislation (see Chapter 21). Excellence in communication is paramount, both within the ICU and with other teams.

ICU consultants

Twenty-four-hour cover by a named consultant with appropriate expertise increases the quality of ICU care and decreases mortality. Difficult therapeutic and ethical decisions are often required; it is essential that these are taken by an individual with sufficient experience to allow a reasonable assessment of the likely outcome. Because of the nature of critical illness, the ICU consultants should be informed immediately of any significant change in their condition. Similarly, they should be informed of any potential admissions and see all patients within 12 h of admission and twice daily thereafter. The consultant's base specialty is less important than his or her appropriate training and experience.

ICU residents

The ICU junior medical staff have a pivotal role in the monitoring and co-ordination of all aspects of care. Each patients' clinical state should be reassessed frequently because it may change quickly. There are many training opportunities available in the unit, and training should be focused on a competency-based programme.

Box 48.1 Levels of ICU care

Level 0
- Requires hospitalisation
- Patient's needs can be met through normal ward care

Level 1
- Patients recently discharged from a higher level of care
- Patients in need of additional monitoring/clinical interventions
- Patients requiring critical care outreach service support, clinical input or advice

Level 2
- Patients needing preoperative optimisation
- Patients needing extended postoperative care
- Patients stepping down to from level 3 care
- Patients receiving single organ support including basic cardiovascular, renal or respiratory support

Level 3
- Patients receiving advanced respiratory support alone.
- Patients requiring a minimum of two organs supported

ICU nursing staff

Nurses provide most of the direct patient care in the ICU; they have greatly extended roles, experience and responsibility. They undergo specific training to enable them to perform titration of fluid replacement, analgesia, vasoactive drug therapy and weaning from mechanical ventilation. It is essential that the bedside nurse is present and takes part during discussions with patients or their representatives in order to provide consistency in communication and decision making. These discussions must be recorded accurately in the patient's notes. The majority of ICU nurses have enormous experience with critically ill patients and are an invaluable resource in ensuring therapies are appropriate and patient centred.

Physiotherapists

Physiotherapists provide therapy for maintenance of respiratory function, including pulmonary secretion clearance, neuromuscular rehabilitation, and expertise on suitability for weaning from mechanical ventilation. Physiotherapy is used to help preserve joint and muscle function in the bedbound patient and promote independent mobilisation where possible. Early mobilisation and rehabilitation is considered important in recovery from critically illness, and advice from physiotherapists on a patient's changing physical status is invaluable.

Pharmacists

Polypharmacy is inevitable in the critically ill and there is great potential for drug interactions and incompatibility of infusions. Drug doses should be modified in critical illness because of altered pharmacodynamics or pharmacokinetics, especially in patients with hepatic or renal failure (see Chapters 1 and 20). Pharmacists have a vital role in providing detailed advice on drug therapies.

Dieticians

Maintenance of gut integrity and nutrition are important priorities in critical illness. The dietician will assess the patient's nutritional status and requirements and provide individually tailored support.

Microbiologist

Critically ill patients are at high risk of nosocomial infections. Contributing factors include:
- the underlying pathological process itself and its consequences;
- impaired organ function and disturbed homeostasis;
- treatments such as immunosuppressant drugs, including steroids;
- the presence of surgical/traumatic wounds, multiple invasive vascular catheters and other devices;
- loss of protective airway reflexes and the potential for pulmonary aspiration;
- alterations in gut mucosal integrity and normal microbial flora;
- the environmental presence of multiresistant micro-organisms.

To treat sepsis effectively and prevent the spread of resistant pathogens, there should be a nominated microbiologist, familiar with the flora and resistance patterns of the unit, to advise daily on microbiology results and antibiotic therapy.

Outreach teams

The critical care outreach team collaborates between the unit and other areas of the hospital. Its main aims are:
- to identify the deteriorating patient early with the aim of averting admission to ICU or facilitating appropriate ward-based treatments;
- to alert the ICU admission team and assist timely admission to the unit if required;
- to aid in appropriate discharge and follow-up from critical care.

A number of scoring systems based on abnormal physiological variables, such as the National Early Warning Score (NEWS) (Table 48.1), can be recorded by ward staff;

NEWS Score	3	2	1	0	1	2	3
Respiratory rate; breaths min⁻¹		≤8	9–11	12–20		21–24	≥25
SpO₂ Scale 1 (%)	≤91	92–93	94–95	≥96			
SpO₂ Scale 2ᵃ (%)	≤83	84–85	86–87	88–93; 93–94 on air	93–94 on O₂	95–96 on O₂	≥97 on O₂
Breathing air or supplemental oxygen		Oxygen		Air			
Systolic BP; mmHg	≤90	71–100	101–110	111–219			≥220
Pulse; beats min⁻¹	≤40		41–50	51–90	91–110	111–130	≥131
ACVPU	U, P, V, C			A			
Temperature; °C	≤35		35.1–36	36.1–38	38.1–39	≥39.1	

Table 48.1 National Early Warning Score (NEWS) 2

ᵃUse scale 2 if target range is 88%–92% as determined by clinician (e.g. in hypercapnic respiratory failure).
AVPU is a simple assessment where A, alert; C, new-onset confusion disorientation or agitation; V, responds to verbal commands only; P, responds to pain; U, completely unresponsive.
Aid to clinical assessment to be used as part of initial evaluation of acute illness in all adult patients (aged 16 or more) and monitored throughout their hospital stay.
The NEWS-2 system uses 6 variables that are already monitored. Scores recommend frequency of monitoring, urgency of clinical review and competencies of the clinical team needed.
NEW score of ≥5 should trigger urgent clinical review and action.
NEW score of ≥7 should trigger urgent clinical review and action by a tea, with critical care competencies and usually transfer to a higher dependency area.
Potentially unreliable in patients with high spinal cord injury because of associated autonomic dysfunction.
Adapted from https://www.rcplondon.ac.uk/projects/outputs/national-early-warning-score-news-2.

the outreach team can be contacted once a trigger score has been reached. Care should be taken with younger, fitter patients, who have good physiological reserve and whose NEWS score may not deteriorate until physiological decompensation occurs (e.g. in presence of bleeding or severe sepsis). Children and obstetric, neurological, renal and other specialty groups have adapted scores to allow for altered background physiological status.

ICU admission and ethical decision-making

Early referral by the specialty medical team for an opinion regarding admission to ICU is preferable, before acute life-threatening deterioration occurs. The use of early warning scores based on vital signs can be helpful in this regard.

Most interventions in ICU are painful and potentially distressing. Mortality, morbidity and functional outcomes are often uncertain, resources are finite and costs are high.

Even if financial resources were unlimited, the time that professionals have is finite. If the capacity of an individual patient to benefit or survive critical illness is limited, complex ethical issues can arise surrounding admission, provision and discontinuation of intensive care therapy. Hence it is important to identify those patients who will not benefit from further resuscitation or critical care support because of their acute illness or underlying diseases, so that harmful or futile interventions are not undertaken. Examples include very frail patients and those receiving palliative care. In these cases, appropriate ward-based care can be agreed and instituted. However, generic admission policies are usually unhelpful; decisions should be individualised to each patient, accounting for their wishes, values and outcomes most relevant to them.

The harms and benefits of all proposed interventions should be explained and understood by patients, families and the wider MDT, but this is often difficult to achieve within the time frames available for emergent decisions. Often patients do not have capacity to understand the complexity of the situation, and a shared decision in the 'best interests' of the patient should be taken by ICU teams, referring specialties and patient family or friends. Importantly, best interests should include all outcomes important to the patient, including social and emotional factors in addition to medical outcomes. Best interests decisions can be difficult and distressing for both staff and the patient's family. If a patient has made an advance directive, its contents must be respected, although application is often ethically and legally challenging and such documents remain rare in UK practice.

In essence the aim of intensive care is to support patients while they recover from the acute process that has generated the need for admission to ICU. It is not to prolong death when there is very little or no hope of meaningful recovery. In many cases, unless the outlook is obviously hopeless, patients may be admitted for a trial of treatment to assess the degree of reversibility and capacity for improvement over time. Conversely, admission of patients with little or no prospect of survival may occasionally be justified and appropriate. For example, admission to ICU of patients with perceived devastating brain injuries will ensure safety in prognostication, allow time for relatives to comprehend the situation and potentially reduce the impact of their bereavement, and facilitate appropriate palliative care.

Decisions about admission to ICU, institution or limitation/withholding of therapy, and withdrawal of life-sustaining treatment should be made using the fundamental principles of medical ethics:
1. Respect for autonomy
2. Beneficence
3. Non-maleficence
4. Distributive justice

Although many doctors can recount these four principles, application of them in practice is often partial. Instead many clinicians rely on heuristic default behaviours when faced with difficult decisions. This is problematic as it is rarely responsive to an individual patient's circumstances or preferences. Where possible the patient's previously expressed, autonomously held wishes and views should be respected, but patients and families do not have the automatic right to treatment regardless of the impacts elsewhere. Despite the potential for conflict inherent in such decision making, a shared decision can nearly always be made. Where disagreements occur they are often a result of misunderstanding and the breakdown of communication and relationships. Many legal systems will have a mechanism for the courts to take ultimate decisions in situations of conflict, but recourse to these 'solutions' is very rarely needed, and decisions taken in this way have very high emotional, financial and social costs.

Assessment of patients

When dealing with a newly admitted patient with acute disease, assessment and resuscitation often take place simultaneously and follow the standard pattern of recognising and dealing with problems in the order of airway, breathing and circulation. It is essential to approach the assessment of the patient in a systematic manner.

History

Often the patient is unable to give a full and accurate history. All possible details should be obtained from the patient's notes, a thorough handover from referring or transferring staff, old notes (which may need to be retrieved from the referring hospital), and information from the patient's primary care doctor. Speaking to the patient's relatives gives invaluable insight into the patient's premorbid condition. It is important that details in the history are not overlooked as it is relatively easy for misinformation to be perpetuated from one handover to the next.

Examination

It is imperative to adhere to unit policy regarding infection control. Scrupulous hand hygiene and the use of gloves and aprons are necessary before examination of the patient. A systematic approach is vital. Remember that although the patient may appear to be unconscious, hearing and other senses may still be intact, and dignity and respect should be maintained at all times.

Airway

Note how the airway has been secured, how long any tube (tracheal/tracheostomy) has been in place, relevant cuff pressures and type and volume of respiratory secretions. In a patient with traumatic injuries, ensure that the cervical spine has been stabilised appropriately.

Breathing

Auscultate the lungs to check for bilateral and equal air entry and added sounds. Check the type and adequacy of ventilation, as well as latest arterial blood gas results, and review the most recent and relevant past imaging data. If intercostal drains are present, ascertain their duration and drainage.

Circulation

Note the heart rate, rhythm, arterial pressure, jugular venous pressure (JVP), heart sounds, CVP, peripheral perfusion using clinical evaluation and monitored variables. Look for the presence of dependent or peripheral oedema. Venous and arterial catheter sites may reveal evidence of infection. Note the type and dose of positive inotropic or other vasoactive drugs required.

Disability (central nervous system)

Ascertain the patient's level of consciousness as well as the dose and duration of sedative/analgesic drugs. Scoring systems for sedation are widely used (see later). It is increasingly standard practice to perform daily sedation holds unless contraindicated (e.g. raised ICP after traumatic brain injury). Make a note of evidence of focal neurological deficits, seizures, or weakness and whether there are purposeful symmetrical movements to verbal command or painful stimulus. Specialist monitoring may be used to measure ICP and cerebral perfusion pressure (CPP).

Gastrointestinal tract

Examination of the abdomen will reveal whether it is soft, tender or distended. The absence of bowel sounds may be misleading in a patient who is sedated and undergoing artificial ventilation; bowel activity is better ascertained from the observation chart. It should be noted whether the patient is being fed enterally or parenterally. If enteral feeding is being provided, note whether the patient is absorbing the feed and whether any prokinetic drugs are required; stress ulcer prophylaxis is routine. Other information gained from examination may include recent surgical activity, the function of stomas, appearance of wounds and contents of abdominal drains.

Renal system

The important features are urine output, current and cumulative fluid balance and abnormalities of serum electrolytes or acid–base balance. The patient may be receiving renal replacement therapy, so make sure catheters and anticoagulation are adequate.

Limbs/skin and wounds

Look for evidence of adequate perfusion (ensure documentation of primary and secondary surveys after trauma), presence of peripheral pulses, adequate capillary refill and evidence of swelling, tenderness, DVT or compartment syndrome. Surgical wounds and trauma sites should be inspected for adequate healing or infection.

Catheters and infection

All invasive catheters and tubing should be inspected for signs of local exit site infection; their duration should be noted as well as review of their ongoing requirement. Evidence suggesting catheter-related sepsis should prompt removal of lines and culture, but they should not be routinely replaced as a method of preventing infection. Note the patient's temperature with changes over time and check against markers of infection such as pulse, white cell count (WCC), C-reactive protein (CRP) and procalcitonin.

Investigations/interventions

Many units use a standard *pro forma* for admission documentation and other algorithms or protocols to encourage consistent high standards of clinical care. Prescription charts, laboratory results (haematology, biochemistry and microbiology), radiological images, and other investigations should be reviewed daily, making particular note of antibiotic requirements and appropriateness of stress ulcer and venous thromboembolism (VTE) prophylaxis.

Management plans

Finally a management action plan needs to be formulated, with special regard to pre-existing, active and ongoing problems. A plan for each organ system requiring support should be put into place as well as for ventilation and/or weaning. A review of nutrition, 24-h fluid balance and changes to drug therapy should also be undertaken and any planned procedures or interventions should be discussed. Communicate back any change in plans to the relevant nursing staff and bear in mind that relatives appreciate honest, up-to-date progress reports. It is important to note that patient confidentiality should never be compromised via discussion or documentation. Full assessment and examination should be repeated at least daily even in stable patients, because the physiological state of critically ill patients can change rapidly.

Transfers

Patients require intra- or interhospital transfers for a variety of reasons, including investigations (e.g. radiological imaging), treatment, provision of specialised services (e.g. transfer to major trauma centre), lack of ICU bed capacity or repatriation. Though usually accomplished safely, any transfer involves risks; the decision should be made by a senior clinician, planned carefully, and the patient's condition stabilised as far as possible beforehand (Box 48.2). Local protocols should be instituted and followed. At least two experienced, competent attendants should accompany the patient; for level 2 and 3 critically ill patients this should involve an anaesthetist or intensivist competent in airway management and resuscitation. Meticulous preparation is needed, including communication with the receiving unit. Vital drugs, monitoring and equipment should be available. An oxygen supply, venous access, monitoring with power backup, emergency drugs, tracheal intubation equipment and the necessary infusions/pumps should be available.

Airway

- Airway safe or secured by tracheal intubation
- Tracheal tube position confirmed on chest radiograph

Ventilation

- Adequate spontaneous respiration or ventilation established on transport ventilator
- Adequate gas exchange confirmed by arterial blood gases
- Sedated and paralysed as appropriate

Circulation

- Heart rate and blood pressure optimised
- Tissue and organ perfusion adequate
- Any obvious blood loss controlled
- Circulating blood volume restored
- Haemoglobin adequate
- Minimum of two routes of venous access
- Arterial catheter and central venous access if appropriate

Neurological

- Seizures controlled, metabolic causes excluded
- Raised intracranial pressure appropriately managed

Trauma

- Cervical spine protected
- Pneumothoraces drained
- Intrathoracic and intra-abdominal bleeding controlled
- Intra-abdominal injuries adequately investigated and appropriately managed
- Long bone/pelvic fractures stabilised

Metabolic

- Blood glucose > 4 mmol L^{-1}
- Potassium < 6 mmol L^{-1}
- Ionised calcium > 1 mmol L^{-1}
- Acid–base balance acceptable
- Temperature maintained

Monitoring

- ECG
- Blood pressure
- Oxygen saturation
- End-tidal carbon dioxide
- Temperature

Adapted from the Intensive Care Society. (2011) *Guidelines for the transport of the critically ill adult*, 3rd ed. London, Intensive Care Society.

Monitoring in ICU

Patients in ICU are monitored continuously using a variety of invasive and non-invasive techniques (Table 48.2). It is important to know that all equipment is working, accurate and calibrated correctly, and device monitoring is used for this purpose (see Chapter 17). The following sections describe the monitors that are used predominantly in the ICU; other monitors used during anaesthesia are discussed in Chapter 17.

Arterial pressure

Arterial cannulation allows continuous measurement of arterial blood pressure, serial blood gas and other sampling. Significant respiratory variation in the amplitude of the arterial pressure wave ('respiratory swing') is characteristic of hypovolaemia. This pulse pressure variability (which relates to stroke volume variability caused by changes in venous return) can be formally measured by modern monitoring systems and is described as a percentage. Abnormal arterial waveforms can be seen in hyperdynamic circulations and conditions such as aortic stenosis, aortic regurgitation and left ventricular failure. Normal waveforms give an indication of cardiac output, myocardial contractility and outflow resistance.

Echocardiography

Echocardiography is emerging as a very useful tool in the critically ill, especially in the assessment of haemodynamics and response to therapeutic interventions; however, this often can prove challenging. Focused echocardiography is used to answer specific clinical questions as an extension to the clinical examination (e.g. to assess myocardial activity, filling or the presence of a pericardial collection). There are a number of systematic approaches to echocardiography that can be employed, depending on the skill and experience of the operator. It is likely that the use of echocardiography in critical care will increase in the future.

Ultrasound

Ultrasound has an established role in venous and arterial access (see Chapter 17) and is also being used increasingly by intensivists for much wider assessment, including the respiratory system (pleural fluid, consolidation, oedema, pneumothorax), abdominal organs and vascular system. As the technology continues to improve, evidence of utility improves and additional training in this modality is essential for safe and appropriate use.

Table 48.2 Minimum and additional monitoring in critically ill patients

Monitor	Comments
Minimum	Basic monitoring for all patients
ECG, pulse rate, SpO_2, arterial pressure, urine output, temperature	
Fluid input/output	• All inputs and outputs including calculation of overall fluid balance (minimum 24-hourly)
Drug infusions	• Drug type, concentrations, infusion rates, volumes
Conscious level	• Sedation score routine; other assessment of conscious level (e.g. GCS, CAM-ICU) where indicated
Additional (level 2/3)	

Cardiovascular	• Invasive arterial monitoring
	  • Arterial pressure, adequacy of oxygenation (PaO_2, SaO_2), ventilation ($PaCO_2$) pH, acid–base abnormalities, lactate, cardiac output using pulse-contour analysis
	• CVC
	  • CVP, infusion of vasoactive or irritant drugs; $ScvO_2$, arteriovenous PCO_2 difference, cardiac output (e.g. lithium dilution techniques)
	• Cardiac output
	• Pulmonary artery catheter

Neurological	• GCS, CAM-ICU or other • CSF drainage • Processed EEG/CFAM • ICP • JVS

Respiratory and ventilator function	• Airway pressures, lung volumes (often via the ventilator)
	  • Lung compliance, resistance, gas trapping, intrinsic PEEP
	• Capnography
	  • Confirmation of tracheal tube position, ventilation, gas flow patterns
	• Arterial plethysmography
	• Tracheal tube cuff pressure
	• Oesophageal pressure

Gastrointestinal	• Input/output for enteral feed and aspirates, bowel output and stool chart • Intra-abdominal pressure
Additional fluid input/output	• All outputs from external stomas or drains • Inputs and outputs
Haematological	• FBC, laboratory or near-patient coagulation tests (e.g. TEG or ROTEM)

CAM-ICU, Confusion assessment method for ICU; *CFAM*, cerebral function analysis monitor; *GCS*, Glasgow Coma Scale score; *JVS*, jugular venous saturation; *TEG*, thromboelastograph; *ROTEM*, rotational thromboelastometry.

Neurological monitoring

Indications for ICP monitoring vary between units but most commonly is undertaken in patients with a traumatic brain injury (TBI) and an abnormal CT scan of the brain. The transducer may be extradural, subdural, intraventricular or intraparenchymal. The ICP monitoring also allows calculation of CPP (see Chapter 40); both variables can then be used to guide management. Jugular venous bulb oxygen saturation is an indirect indicator of cerebral oxygen utilisation and provides a measure of global cerebral oxygenation. It involves a catheter being placed retrogradely up the internal jugular vein. Electroencephalogram or evoked potentials may be used to diagnose and monitor seizures or underlying brain electrical activity in patients with refractory epilepsy or severe brain injury.

Institution of intensive care

It is impossible to provide a comprehensive review of all the conditions requiring intensive care and their full treatment regimens in one chapter. The following includes an overview of the management of some common problems in patients presenting to the ICU.

Respiratory system

Respiratory failure is one of the commonest reasons for admission to the ICU (Table 48.3). It may be the primary reason for admission or a feature of a non-respiratory pathological process, such as acute respiratory distress syndrome (ARDS) in sepsis. There are basic two types of respiratory failure.

Type 1 respiratory failure – $PaO_2 < 8$ kPa with normal/low $PaCO_2$

Lung alveolar function is impaired in a number of pathological processes, such as pneumonia, pulmonary oedema and ARDS. The combination of blood flowing through unven-

tilated areas of lung results in ventilation-perfusion mismatch or 'shunt'. The resultant hypoxaemia is initially accompanied by hyperventilation, in a physiological bid to reduce carbon dioxide tension and increase arterial oxygen saturation. However, this can only usually be sustained for a limited time and progressive exhaustion ensues, with a concomitant increase in $PaCO_2$ and decrease in PaO_2. Respiratory arrest will occur without intervention.

Type 2 respiratory failure – $PaO_2 < 8$ kPa and $PaCO_2 > 8$ kPa

This occurs when there is hypoxaemia and hypoventilation from a variety of causes, such as chronic obstructive pulmonary disease (COPD), reduced central respiratory drive, neuromuscular conditions and chest wall deformity. Although the primary problem is hypercapnia, which may eventually result in progressive carbon dioxide narcosis and respiratory arrest, there is typically accompanying hypoxia. The patient with COPD may have a chronically raised $PaCO_2$, which is well tolerated. The associated reduction in respiratory centre sensitivity is not well understood and probably overstated. Such patients may rely on hypoxia to drive ventilation and will deteriorate when given enough additional oxygen to correct their hypoxaemia.

Assessment of the patient with respiratory failure

Clinical assessment is often the most rapid way to evaluate the patient with respiratory failure (Box 48.3):
- Can the patient talk in full sentences?
- Is the patient awake and orientated?
- What is the pulse, BP and respiratory rate?
- Is the patient using accessory muscles of respiration?
- Can the patient cough effectively to clear secretions?
- Is the patient clammy and sweating?
- Does the patient appear exhausted? Exhaustion and impending respiratory failure that is likely to require ventilatory support is an end-of-bed diagnosis.

Table 48.3 Causes of respiratory failure	
Reduced central drive	Brainstem injury
	Stroke
	Drug effects (e.g. opioids)
	Metabolic encephalopathy
Airway obstruction	Tumour
	Infection
	Sleep apnoea
	Foreign body
Lung pathological conditions	Asthma
	COPD
	Pneumonia
	Fibrosis
	ALI/ARDS
	Lung contusion
Neuromuscular defects	Spinal cord lesion
	Phrenic nerve disruption
	Myasthenia gravis
	Guillain–Barré syndrome
	Critical illness polyneuropathy
Musculoskeletal	Trauma
	Severe scoliosis

ALI, Acute lung injury; *ARDS*, acute respiratory distress syndrome; *COPD*, chronic obstructive pulmonary disease.

Box 48.3 Signs of impending respiratory arrest

Marked tachypnoea, or hypoventilation, patient exhausted
Use of accessory muscles
Cyanosis and desaturation, especially if on supplemental oxygen
Tachycardia or bradycardia if periarrest
Sweaty, cool/clammy peripheries
Mental changes, confusion and leading to coma in extreme conditions

A full history, including previous functional status, and physical examination are mandatory. Serial arterial blood gases are required to determine the extent of the respiratory failure and response to any therapy. The chest radiograph and other available investigations such as peak expiratory flow rate (PEFR) will aid evaluation of the patient's condition.

Management of respiratory failure

Management is directed at correcting hypoxia/hypercarbia and reversing the underlying condition if possible. Simple manoeuvres such as supplying supplemental oxygen should be instituted initially. Give oxygen via face mask, preferably humidified. Higher concentrations of oxygen can be achieved with a reservoir system, and a fixed performance device (e.g. Venturi mask; see Chapters 15 and 29) may be preferable in titrating oxygen concentrations in those COPD patients who rely on hypoxia to drive their ventilation. The effect of oxygen therapy should be assessed by pulse oximetry and arterial blood gas analysis after around 30 min.

Other therapies may be useful, such as bronchodilators, steroids, diuretics and physiotherapy, in the first instance depending on the mechanism of respiratory failure. Many patients may be dehydrated because of poor fluid intake and increased losses and will require i.v. fluids. If there is no improvement over time, additional respiratory support may be necessary. Options include the following:

Continuous positive airway pressure
Continuous positive airway pressure is provided via a tightly fitting mask or hood. A high gas flow (greater than the patient's peak inspiratory flow rate) is required to keep the positive pressure set by the expiratory valve (5–10 cmH$_2$O) almost constant throughout the respiratory cycle. CPAP increases functional residual capacity (FRC), reduces alveolar collapse and improves oxygenation, but it requires a co-operative patient with no facial injuries. It does not generally help the patient with type 2 respiratory failure. There is a small risk of aspiration as a result of stomach distension, and it should not be used in patients after recent gastro-oesophageal resection surgery. High-flow nasal cannulae can provide titrated oxygen therapy and is a well-tolerated alternative to CPAP therapy for some patients.

Non-invasive ventilation
Non-invasive ventilation (NIV) techniques have been successfully used to treat acute exacerbations in patients with COPD, pulmonary oedema and as a weaning aid. Biphasic or bilevel positive airway pressure (BiPAP or BPAP) is a common form where a set inspiratory pressure enhances the patient's own respiratory effort to increase achievable tidal volume and the set expiratory pressure is analogous to CPAP. Many institutions are able to provide NIV in an emergency department or hospital ward, either as a temporary emergency measure or for patients who are deemed unlikely to benefit from invasive mechanical ventilation. Non-invasive ventilation is also used for patients with intractable respiratory failure (e.g. high spinal cord lesions) in the community. If the clinical condition continues to deteriorate in conjunction with worsening arterial blood gases in a patient with potentially reversible pulmonary disease, then invasive mechanical ventilation will be necessary.

Invasive mechanical ventilation

The usual indication for invasive mechanical ventilation is in patients with potentially reversible pathological conditions who are unable to maintain adequate oxygenation or who develop hypercapnia (Box 48.4). In some cases, blood gases may be normal but are predicted to deteriorate because the patient is becoming exhausted.

Tracheal intubation
To enable mechanical ventilation to be carried out effectively, a cuffed tube must be placed in the trachea either via the mouth or nose or directly through a tracheostomy stoma. In the emergency situation an orotracheal tube is usually inserted. Despite the use of tracheal or tracheostomy tubes that have a high-volume, low-pressure tracheal cuff, two additional complications may occur during prolonged artificial ventilation:

- Microaspiration of oral secretions or feed. Frequent tracheal suction by nurses and physiotherapists is needed. In addition, newer tracheal tubes with a specific subglottic suction port are available. Use of these has been shown to decrease the incidence of ventilator-associated pneumonia and they are routinely used in many ICUs.
- Pressure from the tracheal cuff can cause ischaemic damage to the underlying tracheal mucosa. Tracheal cuff pressures should be monitored regularly and maintained at less than 25 cmH$_2$O.

If the patient is conscious, anaesthesia should be induced judiciously with a titrated dose of an i.v. anaesthetic agent using a coinduction technique and neuromuscular blocking agent (NMBA). The Fourth National Audit Project of the

---

Box 48.4 Indications for ventilatory support

- Reduced conscious level
- Exhaustion
- Tachypnoea
- Reduced PaO_2 despite increasing oxygen therapy
- Increased $PaCO_2$
- Acidaemia
- Cardiovascular instability (e.g. cardia/bradycardia, hypotension)

RCoA and Difficult Airway Society (NAP4) reported a higher rate of adverse outcomes and significant deficiencies of airway management in ICUs. This has led to the development of an algorithm for tracheal intubation in the critically ill patient (Fig. 48.1).

The critically ill patient is often exquisitely sensitive to i.v. anaesthetic drugs and reductions in preload as a result of institution of positive pressure ventilation, and cardio-vascular collapse may occur; consequently, full resuscitation equipment must be immediately available; resuscitation with i.v. fluids and vasoactive drug infusions are often required. If the patient is unconscious, an NMBA alone may be necessary (but not obligatory) to facilitate the passage of the tracheal tube; however, an i.v. anaesthetic induction technique and NMBA should always be used in patients with head injury to prevent an increase ICP during laryngoscopy and tracheal intubation (see Chapter 40). The usual precautions relating to cervical spine protection and risk of aspiration if not fasted (see Chapter 44) should be employed if applicable. When the upper airway or larynx is obstructed and conventional tracheal intubation is not possible (e.g. epiglottitis or laryngeal trauma), the emergency airway of choice is a scalpel cricothyroidotomy (Fig. 48.2).

Many patients are hypoxaemic, and it is essential that 100% oxygen is administered before tracheal intubation. CPAP, NIV and high-flow nasal oxygenation are of particular value in preoxygenation of critically ill patients, as standard methods (see Chapter 23) are only partially effective.

Sedation and analgesia. Once tracheal intubation has been performed, sedative drugs will be required to tolerate the tube and facilitate effective mechanical ventilation. The balance between providing adequate sedation to permit patient co-operation with organ system support and oversedation, which leads to a number of detrimental effects (Table 48.4), is often challenging. The aims of sedation include patient comfort and analgesia and minimisation of anxiety, to allow a calm, co-operative patient who is able to sleep when undisturbed and able to tolerate appropriate organ support. Requirements for sedation change according to the clinical condition and need for therapies and so should be reviewed constantly. A validated sedation score (e.g. the Richmond Agitation and Sedation Score; RASS) can help nurses deliver titrated and appropriate amounts of sedatives. Patients must never be paralysed and awake; however, agitation and distress may interfere with ventilation and other care, increase oxygen demands and increase the risk of psychological problems later. Sedative drugs should be reduced or interrupted daily ('sedation hold'); this reduces length of mechanical ventilation, incidence of delirium, mortality and possibly long-term psychological dysfunction.

Tracheostomy

In addition to being performed as part of major head and neck surgery (e.g. laryngectomy; see Chapter 37), tracheos-

Table 48.4 Problems and potential consequences of excessive sedation in ICU patients

Problem	Potential consequence
Accumulation with prolonged infusion	Delayed weaning from supportive care
Detrimental effect on cardiovascular system	Increased requirement for vasoactive drugs
Detrimental effect on pulmonary function	Increased ventilation/perfusion mismatch
Tolerance	Withdrawal on stopping sedation
No rapid eye movement (REM) sleep	Sleep deprivation, delirium and psychosis
Reduced intestinal motility	Impairment of enteral feeding
Potential effects on immune/endocrine function	Drugs such as opioids may have a role in immunomodulation and risk of infection
Adverse effects of specific drugs	For example, propofol infusion syndrome

tomy in the ICU is usually performed as an elective procedure.

The main indication is to aid weaning from mechanical ventilation; tracheostomy allows more gradual weaning and withdrawal of sedative drugs and increases patient comfort. It is most useful in patients:

- with prolonged and ongoing requirements for ventilatory support;
- unable to protect their airway e.g. reduced level of consciousness or neurological injury; and
- with longer-term need for bronchial toilet (e.g. excessive secretions and/or inadequate cough).

The timing of tracheostomy remains controversial and should be individualised to the clinical situation. Percutaneous dilatational tracheostomy is increasingly performed by intensivists and is associated with fewer complications, lower infection rate, and shorter procedural time compared to formal surgical tracheostomy. When performed in the ICU, percutaneous tracheostomy also avoids the logistical problems and risks associated with interhospital transfer to the operating theatre. Percutaneous dilatational tracheostomy is performed using a Seldinger technique and dilatation of the trachea and tract from the skin, using simultaneous bronchoscopy to allow direct visualisation of tracheostomy placement and final position. Ultrasound of the neck before

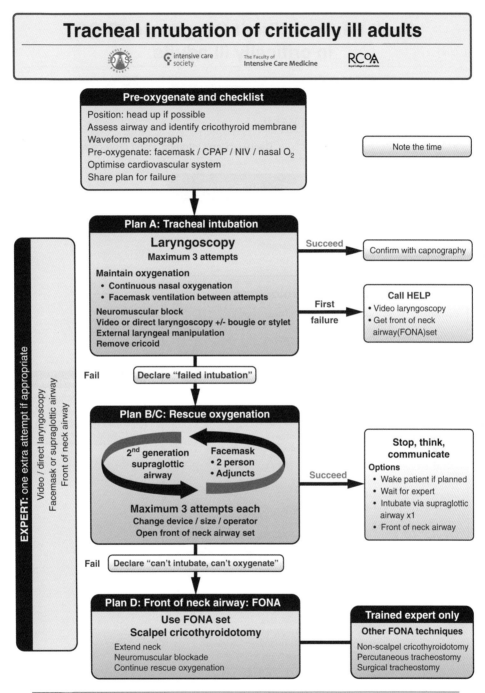

Fig. 48.1 Guidelines for tracheal intubation of the critically unwell patient. (From Higgs, A., McGrath, B. A., & Goddard, C., et al. (2017) Guidelines for the management of tracheal intubation in critically ill adults. *British Journal of Anaesthesia.* 120, 323–352.)

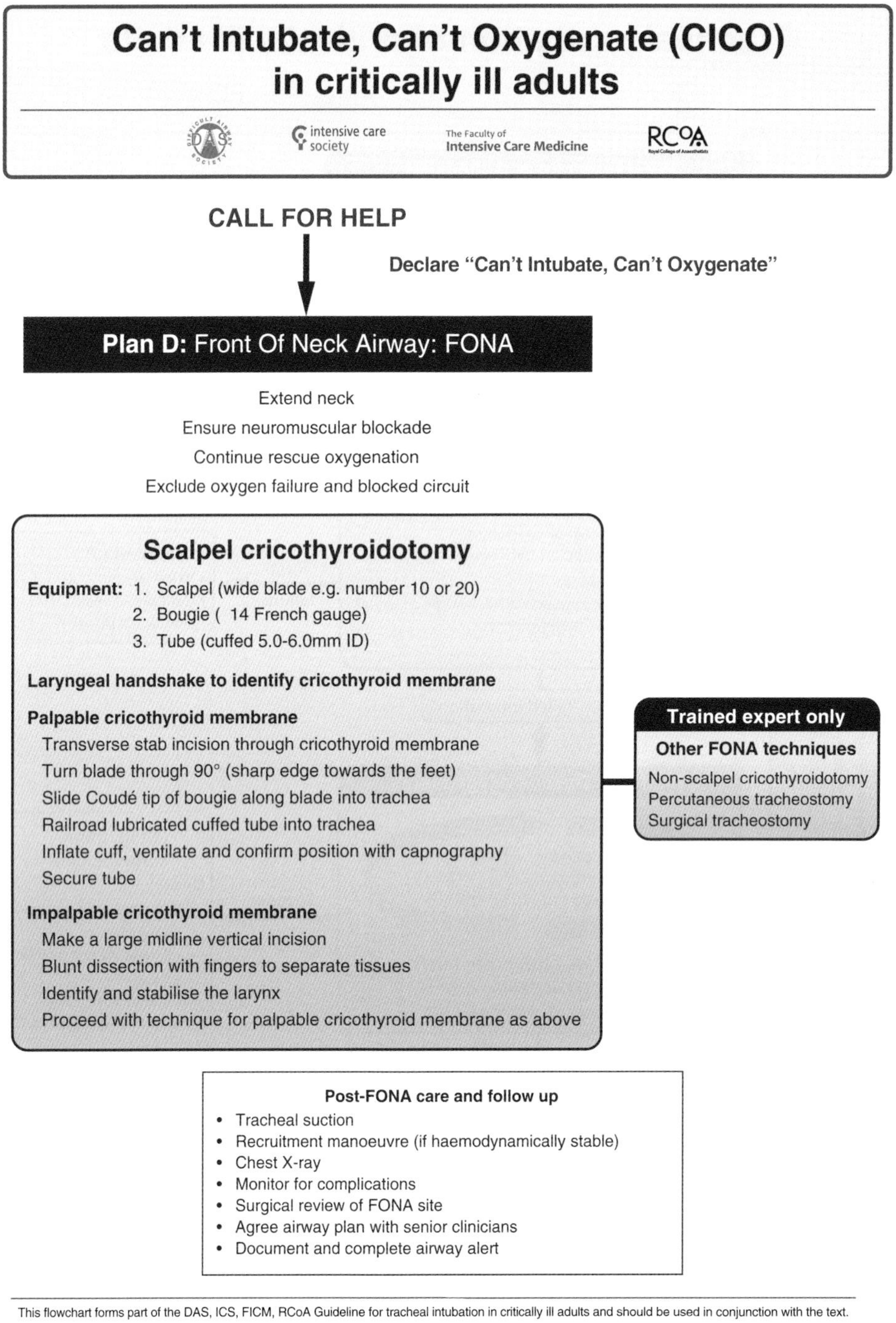

Can't Intubate, Can't Oxygenate (CICO) in critically ill adults

  intensive care society   The Faculty of **Intensive Care Medicine**   RCoA Royal College of Anaesthetists

CALL FOR HELP

Declare "Can't Intubate, Can't Oxygenate"

Plan D: Front Of Neck Airway: FONA

Extend neck
Ensure neuromuscular blockade
Continue rescue oxygenation
Exclude oxygen failure and blocked circuit

Scalpel cricothyroidotomy

Equipment: 1. Scalpel (wide blade e.g. number 10 or 20)
2. Bougie (14 French gauge)
3. Tube (cuffed 5.0-6.0mm ID)

Laryngeal handshake to identify cricothyroid membrane

Palpable cricothyroid membrane

Transverse stab incision through cricothyroid membrane
Turn blade through 90° (sharp edge towards the feet)
Slide Coudé tip of bougie along blade into trachea
Railroad lubricated cuffed tube into trachea
Inflate cuff, ventilate and confirm position with capnography
Secure tube

Impalpable cricothyroid membrane

Make a large midline vertical incision
Blunt dissection with fingers to separate tissues
Identify and stabilise the larynx
Proceed with technique for palpable cricothyroid membrane as above

Trained expert only

Other FONA techniques

Non-scalpel cricothyroidotomy
Percutaneous tracheostomy
Surgical tracheostomy

Post-FONA care and follow up
- Tracheal suction
- Recruitment manoeuvre (if haemodynamically stable)
- Chest X-ray
- Monitor for complications
- Surgical review of FONA site
- Agree airway plan with senior clinicians
- Document and complete airway alert

This flowchart forms part of the DAS, ICS, FICM, RCoA Guideline for tracheal intubation in critically ill adults and should be used in conjunction with the text.

Fig. 48.2 Guidelines for 'cannot intubate, cannot oxygenate' in the critically unwell patient. (Reproduced from Royal College of Physicians. (2017) *National Early Warning Score (NEWS) 2: Standardising the assessment of acute-illness severity in the NHS. Updated report of a working party.* London, RCP.)

the procedure is useful to identify underlying blood vessels. Relative contraindications include high oxygen or PEEP requirements ($FiO_2 > 0.6$, PEEP ≥ 8), morbid obesity, cervical spine injury, neck immobility, and coagulopathy.

Overview of modes of ventilation

Different manufacturers have used different terms for similar modes of ventilation. This can cause confusion for the inexperienced.

Volume-controlled ventilation
The simplest form of volume-controlled ventilation is controlled mandatory ventilation (CMV). The patient's lungs are ventilated at a preset tidal volume and rate (e.g. tidal volume 500 ml, rate 12 breaths min^{-1}). The tidal volume delivered is predetermined and the peak pressure required to deliver this volume varies depending upon other ventilator settings and the patient's pulmonary compliance. A major disadvantage of CMV is that high peak airway pressures may result and this can lead to lung damage or barotrauma. Therefore it is only really suitable for patients who are heavily sedated or paralysed and who are making no respiratory effort. It is used occasionally where measured airway pressure may not reflect alveolar or intrathoracic pressure (e.g. profound bronchospasm).

Pressure-controlled ventilation
Pressure-controlled modes of ventilation are used commonly and are preferred in patients with poor pulmonary compliance. A peak inspiratory pressure is set and so tidal volume delivered is a function of the peak pressure, inspiratory time and pulmonary compliance. By using lower peak pressures and slightly longer inspiratory times, the risks of barotrauma can be reduced. As the patient's condition improves and lung compliance increases, the tidal volume achieved for the same settings will increase and the inspiratory pressure can therefore be reduced. Biphasic or bilevel positive airway pressure (BiPAP) is a variation of pressure-controlled ventilation which permits spontaneous breaths by the patient at all times during the ventilator cycle.

Synchronised intermittent mandatory ventilation
Modes of ventilation have been developed that allow preservation of the patient's own respiratory efforts by detecting an attempt by the patient to breathe in and synchronising the mechanical breath with spontaneous inspiration; this technique is termed synchronised intermittent mandatory ventilation (SIMV). If no attempt at inspiration is detected over a period of some seconds, then a mandatory breath is delivered to ensure that a safe total minute volume is provided. Most modern ventilator modes are synchronised even if not specifically described by their names.

Pressure support ventilation/assisted spontaneous breathing
Breathing through a ventilator can be difficult because respiratory muscles may be weak and ventilator circuits and tracheal tubes provide significant resistance to breathing. During pressure support ventilation (PSV), the ventilator senses a spontaneous breath and augments it by addition of positive pressure. This reduces the patient's work of breathing and increases tidal volume. Automatic calibration to offset the resistance of the airway is often included. Both SIMV and PSV require a method of detecting the patient's own respiratory effort, in order to trigger the appropriate ventilator response. This is commonly achieved by flow sensors detecting small changes in gas flow within the circuit.

Inverse ratio ventilation
Inverse ratio ventilation is not a separate mode of ventilation but describes the use of an inspiratory phase that is of longer duration than the expiratory phase (typical ratios between 1.5:1 and 3:1), using pressure- or volume-controlled modes. This maintains alveolar recruitment and improves oxygenation allowing lower concentrations of both peak and end-expiratory pressures. It is usually used in patients with acute lung injury. Adverse effects include increased gas-trapping and decreased cardiac output/venous return.

Airway pressure release ventilation
Airway pressure release ventilation (APRV) is essentially an exaggerated form of inverse ratio ventilation using a pressure-controlled mode (BiPAP). Airway pressure release ventilation was initially described as providing continuous moderate pressure (typically 20 cmH_2O) for a prolonged part of the respiratory cycle (typically 4–5 s), with brief interruptions (0.5–1 s) to zero or low pressure; the patient can breathe spontaneously throughout. In this way, CPAP is maintained and the short duration of release reduces the potential for alveolar decruitment

Positive end-expiratory pressure
Positive end-expiratory pressure has the advantage of alveolar recruitment and maintenance of functional residual capacity, which improves lung compliance. Some patients, such as those with expiratory airflow limitation, can develop air trapping and a degree of so-called intrinsic PEEP; modern ventilators can calculate this. If intrinsic PEEP is high, the concentration of additional extrinsic PEEP can become crucial as there is a potential risk of sustained lung hyperinflation if external PEEP is greater than the concentration of intrinsic PEEP. Although PEEP is beneficial for the vast majority of mechanically ventilated patients, it can reduce venous return and cardiac output at higher concentrations (see later). This has led to the concept of 'best PEEP' where the effects of PEEP on oxygenation and cardiac output are titrated to maximise oxygen delivery.

'Open-lung' ventilation techniques

Airway pressure release ventilation, inverse ratio ventilation and the use of high PEEP are termed 'open-lung' ventilator techniques that seek to maintain relatively high airway pressures for a large proportion of the respiratory cycle. Other modes based on a similar physiological premise include high-frequency oscillatory ventilation (HFOV; see later). Though open-lung ventilation techniques improve gas exchange, there is limited evidence for effects on clinical outcomes.

Problems associated with mechanical ventilation

Patients undergoing mechanical ventilation are crucially dependent on technology and the expertise of staff to minimise the risk of complications. Important aspects of care include humidification of gases; regular physiotherapy; tracheal toilet; and continuous monitoring of SpO_2, end-tidal CO_2, inspired O_2 concentration, minute volume, and airway pressures (see Chapter 17). Constant risks associated with mechanical ventilation include tracheal tube dislodgement and difficult reintubation, laryngeal/tracheal damage, ventilator-associated pneumonia (see later), need for sedation, and adverse cardiovascular effects. Positive pressure ventilation decreases venous return; this causes a reduction in cardiac output and oxygen delivery, particularly in the presence of hypovolaemia or impaired cardiovascular function. The effects are often more marked with high PEEP values and open-lung ventilation techniques.

Ventilator-induced lung injury (VILI) encompasses several components, including barotrauma, where high pressures are applied to the airway, especially if lung compliance is reduced. This may cause clinically obvious pneumothorax, pneumomediastinum, pneumoperitoneum and subcutaneous emphysema. Volutrauma may occur if excessive tidal volumes are applied; the clinical manifestations are similar to barotrauma. In addition, repeated opening and closure of alveolar units stimulates 'shear stress' with release of cytokines and other inflammatory mediators, even with lower tidal volumes; this is termed atelectrauma. Trauma to the lungs by any of these mechanisms may cause lung damage, systemic inflammation and extrapulmonary organ failure.

Problem solving in ventilated patients

The first priorities are to exclude and, if necessary, correct hypoxaemia or hypercapnia and to detect any adverse effects or complications of ventilation. When a problem arises, consider whether the underlying issue is related to the ventilator (by manually ventilating the patient's lungs), an equipment issue (e.g. function/position/blockage of the tracheal tube; see later) or the patient's pathophysiology (e.g. progression of the lung problem, such as ARDS, or development of a new problem, such as pneumothorax or bronchospasm)? When the problem has been identified, correct management will rectify the situation and is often directed at changes in ventilatory settings and sedation.

Endobronchial intubation is a common complication during mechanical ventilation as the tracheal tube may migrate down the trachea when the patient is moved during normal nursing procedures. Intubation of the right main bronchus cannot be detected reliably by observation of chest movements or by auscultation of the chest because of the exaggerated transmission of breath sounds during mechanical ventilation, although absent or asynchronous chest movement may occur when pulmonary collapse has taken place. Endobronchial intubation is one of the causes of a sudden decrease in compliance, and restlessness and coughing often occur if the end of the tube irritates the carina. If this is suspected, the tube should be withdrawn gradually by up to 5 cm while lung compliance and chest expansion are observed carefully. The position of the tracheal tube should always be confirmed by a chest radiograph; occasionally direct visualisation with bronchoscopy is required to ensure correct tracheal tube/tracheostomy position.

Ventilation strategies

The concept of VILI by overdistension, shear stress injury and oxygen toxicity has been increasingly recognised over the past few years. Several strategies are used to reduce VILI:

- Limiting peak pressure to 30 cmH$_2$O
- Limiting tidal volume to 4–6 ml kg^{-1}
- Acceptance of higher than normal $PaCO_2$ (with pH > 7.2), so-called permissive hypercapnia
- Acceptance of PaO_2 7–8 kPa, SaO_2 > 90%
- Use of higher PEEP to improve alveolar recruitment
- Use of longer inspiratory times as with inverse ratio ventilation or APRV
- Use of ventilation modes that allow and support spontaneous respiratory effort

The acceptable threshold for the values listed here is not known and has to be considered on an individual patient basis.

High-frequency oscillation ventilation

High-frequency oscillatory ventilation is a means of reducing transpulmonary pressure while providing adequate gas exchange in patients with poor lung compliance. Small tidal volumes (lower than dead space) are generated by an oscillating a diaphragm across the open airway resulting in a sinusoidal or square gas flow pattern. Peak airway pressure is reduced but mean airway pressure is increased, allowing for alveolar recruitment and improved oxygenation. Oxygenation improves, but recent large randomised trials have shown no improvement in mortality.

Prone positioning

When prone, the volume of lung compressed by the mediastinal structures decreases, pleural pressure becomes more uniform and ventilation-perfusion mismatch is reduced. The technique is very labour intensive; at least four people are needed to turn the patient and great care is required to ensure that the airway and vascular catheters and cannulae are not dislodged. The evidence base is mixed; it appears to depend on the specific cohort of patients, timing and duration of prone therapy.

Extracorporeal membrane oxygenation

Extracorporeal membrane oxygenation (ECMO) is an option if other conventional techniques of providing ventilatory support have failed. Research continues into the most appropriate timing and duration of ECMO therapy. Partial cardiopulmonary venovenous bypass is initiated using heparin-bonded vascular catheters, and extracorporeal oxygenation and carbon dioxide removal are achieved using a membrane oxygenator. An ultra-low-volume, low-pressure regimen of ventilation is continued to allow the lungs to recover. Results of ECMO appear favourable in selected patients, but in the UK the availability of ECMO in adults is limited to a few centres, so the additional risks, benefits and timing of transfer of the severely hypoxaemic patient must be considered. Smaller, more portable lung assist devices, primarily for carbon dioxide removal, are under investigation.

Weaning from mechanical ventilation

Weaning is the process by which the patient's dependence on mechanical ventilation is gradually reduced to the point where spontaneous breathing sufficient to meet metabolic needs is sustained. Because of the adverse effects of mechanical ventilation, weaning should be undertaken at the earliest opportunity, and the decision to commence weaning is based largely on clinical judgement.

Ideally, before weaning, the condition requiring mechanical ventilation should have resolved and a patient should:
- be awake and co-operative with intact neuromuscular and bulbar function; and have:
  - stable cardiovascular function with minimal requirements for inotropic or vasopressor drugs;
  - no ongoing respiratory metabolic acidosis;
  - inspired oxygen requirements < 50%;
  - low sputum production; and
  - adequate nutritional status.

In addition, ventilatory support should be not be withdrawn completely until these criteria have been confirmed by sustained evaluation and the patient can protect the airway and generate a good cough.

Weaning is a dynamic process and will involve reduction in level of ventilatory support. Pressure support ventilation and assisted support breathing (ASB) are forms of partial ventilatory support that are used in combination with other modes (e.g. BiPAP, SIMV, APRV, CPAP) during weaning. The degree of support should be gradually weaned so that the patient contributes increasingly to the work of breathing. Introduction of ventilator independence can be rapid, such as in a spontaneous breathing trial. This involves allowing the patient to breathe spontaneously with the application of PEEP only, ideally for 30 min and up to a maximum of 2 h. A successful spontaneous breathing trial usually indicates that tracheal extubation will be successful, and if not, a repeat trial can be performed daily. A gradual form of weaning is to allow a short period of spontaneous breathing without ventilatory assistance (e.g. initially 1–5 min) with close observation and monitoring of the patient. The duration and frequency of these trials is increased as the patient's condition improves.

It may take from a few hours to several weeks before total independence from ventilatory support is achieved. Weaning may also be facilitated by the use of a tracheostomy tube, which has the advantage of reducing dead space and allowing sedation to be discontinued, as they are much better tolerated than a translaryngeal tube. Extended periods of spontaneous breathing are possible with easy re-establishment of support if required, such as to aid sleep.

Cardiovascular system
Shock

Most critically ill patients require support of the cardiovascular system at some time. Failure of the cardiovascular system to deliver an adequate supply of oxygenated blood to organs and tissues results in shock, which if unchecked will result in organ failure and death. Common mechanisms of tissue hypoperfusion include:
- hypovolaemia (e.g. haemorrhage and burns);
- septic shock (e.g. pneumonia);
- cardiogenic shock (e.g. myocardial infarction);
- neurogenic shock (e.g. high cervical spinal cord injury); and
- adrenocortical insufficiency.

There may be many elements contributing to shock in an individual patient, and common features include hypotension, tachycardia, oliguria, increased serum lactate and metabolic acidaemia. As initial compensatory mechanisms fail, multiple organ dysfunction ensues; hepatic, gastrointestinal, and pancreatic impairment and disseminated intravascular coagulation may all occur.

Management should be directed at:
- treatment of the underlying pathological condition;
- optimisation of circulating blood volume;
- optimisation of cardiac output;
- optimisation of blood pressure;
- restoration of vascular tone;

- optimisation of oxygen delivery; and
- support of any organ failure.

Applied cardiovascular physiology

A fundamental principle of management for any critically ill patient is the maintenance of adequate oxygen delivery to the tissues. It is important to understand the factors affecting oxygen delivery and consumption and how these may be monitored and manipulated (see Chapters 9 and 10). Oxygen delivery (DO_2) is calculated as the product of cardiac output and arterial oxygen content. Arterial oxygen content is determined by arterial oxygen saturation (SaO_2) and haemoglobin concentration.

$$DO_2 = \text{cardiac output} \times \text{arterial } O_2 \text{ content}$$
$$= \text{cardiac output} \times [(SaO_2 \times \text{haemoglobin} \times 1.34) + PaO_2]$$
$$= 850 - 1200 \text{ ml min}^{-1}$$

Therefore sufficient oxygen delivery can be achieved with good oxygen saturation, haemoglobin concentration 80–100 g L^{-1} and adequate cardiac output.

Oxygen consumption ($\dot{V}O_2$) is the total amount of oxygen consumed by the tissues. The difference between the amount of oxygen carried to the tissues (arterial oxygen delivery) and the amount of oxygen returned to the heart (venous oxygen delivery) indicates the total amount of oxygen consumed by the tissues:

$$\dot{V}O_2 = \text{cardiac output} \times (\text{arterial } O_2 \text{ content} - \text{mixed venous oxygen content})$$
$$= 240 - 270 \text{ ml min}^{-1}$$

Mixed venous oxygen saturation reflects the amount of oxygen returning to the pulmonary capillaries, because it was not used by the tissues to support metabolic function. The pulmonary artery is the site where SvO_2 values should be measured. It is important to sample only at this site to allow for adequate mixing of blood from the superior and inferior vena cavae and coronary sinus. Oxygen saturation sampled from a catheter in the superior vena cava ($ScvO_2$), can be used as a surrogate for SvO_2, though it mainly reflects oxygen supply and demand from the head and neck and upper extremities. If SvO_2 is in the normal range (60%–80%), the clinician may assume that tissue perfusion is adequate. If SvO_2 decreases to less than 60%, a decrease in oxygen delivery and/or an increase in oxygen consumption has occurred. Increased plasma lactate concentrations suggest anaerobic metabolism, which supports this diagnosis, although the cellular metabolism of lactate in shock states is complex and is best considered a marker of shock rather than a direct contributor to pathophysiology. If SvO_2 is more than 80%, an increase in oxygen supply and/or a decrease in demand has occurred. An increase in oxygen delivery can

be caused by an increased FIO_2, haemoglobin concentration or cardiac output. A decrease in oxygen consumption can be seen in hypothermic states or in patients who are anaesthetised, mechanically ventilated and receiving NMBAs. In sepsis or poisoning, oxygen uptake into the tissues may also be decreased.

In health there is little fluctuation of cardiac output within the normal range of heart rate (60–160 beats min^{-1}). However, the critically ill, especially those with pre-existing heart disease and older patients, tolerate extremes of heart rate much less well. At low heart rates, cardiac output falls as a function of reduced heart rate, despite maintenance of stroke volume. Tachycardia results in reduced available time for the ventricles to fill and a subsequent fall in stroke volume. With an increase in heart rate, myocardial consumption also increases and this, coupled with reduced diastolic coronary artery perfusion, can lead to significant myocardial ischaemia. Factors affecting cardiac output are discussed in detail in Chapter 9.

Optimisation of the cardiovascular system

The specific management of particular shock states is beyond the scope of this chapter but a rational approach is to first ensure optimal preload with the administration of i.v. fluid and/or packed red cells. This is often best achieved using a dynamic measure, such as stroke volume responsiveness via a cardiac output monitor or pulse pressure variation. If blood pressure, urine output, tissue perfusion and other measures of cardiac output still remain low, positive inotropic or vasopressor drugs may be required. These should be started at low doses and titrated to effect. There is little evidence base to recommend one drug regimen over another, and all should be used with caution as adverse effects can arise. The pharmacology of vasoactive drugs is detailed in Chapter 9. If the predominant problem is thought to be loss of systemic vascular resistance as a result of sepsis or other causes, then it is logical to start with a vasoconstrictor to increase arterial pressure. Agents used commonly include noradrenaline and phenylephrine, which both act on α_1 receptors. Vasopressin is often given as a second-line agent to help restore vascular reactivity and tone. If cardiac contractility is considered to be a problem, then a positive inotrope may be helpful. The vasodilatation produced by some positive inotropes may be beneficial in the presence of a high systemic vascular resistance, which is seen in cardiogenic shock.

Cardiac rhythm disturbances are common in critical illness. Ensure that general resuscitation measures are adequate and treat any electrolyte disturbances (especially potassium and magnesium). Specific treatment may be required, such as amiodarone or digoxin for supraventricular tachycardia (see Chapter 9). Other cardiovascular conditions to consider include myocardial ischaemia, cardiac failure and cardiogenic shock.

Gastrointestinal system

The gastrointestinal tract is important in the pathophysiology of critical illness. Not only is it a common site for surgical intervention and a common source of intra-abdominal sepsis, but the gut is a large 'third space' for fluid loss within the lumen of the gut and may also act as a bed for altered blood flow (arteriovenous shunting) during shock states. It can become a reservoir for bacteria and endotoxins which may translocate into the portal, lymphatic and systemic circulations, producing systemic inflammatory response syndrome (SIRS), sepsis and multiorgan failure, particularly during periods of altered blood flow.

Micro-organisms from the gut can also colonise and infect the respiratory tract, and the gastrointestinal tract itself can be a site for secondary nosocomial infections, such as *Clostridium difficile* colitis. The maintenance of gastrointestinal integrity and function is therefore of major importance during critical illness, and adequate splanchnic blood flow is thought to be crucial. Early resuscitation in shock states is essential and both volume resuscitation and vasopressors should be used early to aid perfusion pressure. In those patients who are adequately resuscitated, early enteral nutrition may also be of value in helping to preserve mucosal integrity and gastrointestinal function.

Manifestations of gastrointestinal tract failure

Gastrointestinal tract failure may present in a number of ways: delayed gastric emptying, failure to absorb feed, ileus, pseudo-obstruction, diarrhoea, stress ulceration, gastrointestinal haemorrhage, acalculous cholecystitis, liver dysfunction, and gastrointestinal ischaemia. Investigation of such dysfunction should, in the first instance, exclude potential remediable abdominal pathological conditions, which often requires the need for imaging, radiological drainage or surgical exploration (e.g. abscesses, ischaemic bowel, peritonitis).

Nutrition

It is important to provide adequate nutrition during critical illness, especially as many patients are likely to be already nutritionally deficient from pre-existing illness. When providing nutritional support, estimation of energy and nitrogen requirements are made to attenuate the negative effects of the catabolic phase. However, it is generally accepted that underfeeding is better than overfeeding in terms of mortality, but failure to provide at least 25% of calculated requirements results in greater risk of infection and death. Nutrition is discussed further in Chapter 13.

Water- and fat-soluble vitamins are provided in commercially available enteral feed preparations, whereas folic acid and vitamin B12 need to be prescribed independently.

Trace elements and minerals such as calcium, magnesium and iron can also be added according to need. Glutamine, arginine, fish oils, selenium and a variety of antioxidants have been the focus of research into immunonutrition. Currently there is no clear evidence for an improved outcome (many of the studies involved administration of a cocktail of combined substrates) and some substances may only be of benefit in specific critical illness subgroups, with higher mortality associated in alternative groups of patients.

Enteral feeding

It is usually accepted practice to initiate enteral feeding early, although in the resuscitative phase of critical illness, nutrients may not be utilised efficiently. Enteral feeding should be considered before the parenteral route but can be associated with significant complications, such as undernutrition and high gastric aspirates. Prokinetic drugs (metoclopramide, erythromycin) and the use of a head-up tilt may promote gastric emptying. Diarrhoea can be a problem, and the use of pre- and probiotics may help normalise gut flora. There is a risk of aspiration with enteral feeding, and recently there has been increased use of postpyloric feeding; there is no strong evidence that this reduces aspiration.

Parenteral feeding

If enteral feeding is contraindicated, such as for surgical reasons, or cannot be established successfully, then parenteral (i.v.) feeding is initiated. It requires dedicated central venous access and advice from the nutrition team, so that complications relating to overfeeding, hyperglycaemia, hypertriglyceridaemia, uraemia, metabolic acidaemia and electrolyte imbalance can be avoided. Hepatobiliary dysfunction (including derangement of liver enzymes and fatty infiltration of the liver) may also occur and is usually caused by the patient's underlying condition and overfeeding. Parenteral nutrition is discussed in Chapter 13.

Refeeding syndrome

Refeeding syndrome results from shifts in fluid and electrolytes that may occur when a chronically malnourished patient receives artificial feeding, either parenterally or enterally. It results in hypophosphataemia but may also feature abnormal sodium and fluid balance as well as changes in glucose, protein and fat metabolism and is potentially fatal. Thiamine deficiency, hypokalaemia and hypomagnesaemia may also be present. Patients at high risk include those chronically undernourished and those who have had little or no energy intake for more than 10 days. Ideally these patients require refeeding at an initially low level of energy replacement alongside vitamin supplementation.

Stress ulcer prophylaxis

Early enteral feeding promotes and maintains gastric mucosal blood flow, provides essential nutrients to the mucosa and reduces the incidence of stress ulcers. If enteral feeding cannot be established, alternative prophylactic measures need to be prescribed, commonly H_2-antagonists (e.g. ranitidine) or a proton pump inhibitor, although there is some evidence that these agents increase the risk of ventilator-associated pneumonia by facilitating bacterial overgrowth in the stomach and subsequent microaspiration.

Blood glucose

Targets for blood glucose control remain controversial: The potential benefits of 'tight' control (plasma glucose 4–6 mmol L^{-1}) have not been confirmed in all critically ill patients and increases the risk of episodic hypoglycaemia. Control is usually achieved by an infusion of insulin running alongside a dextrose-based infusion, to allow titration of blood glucose concentrations; a target of 6–8 mmol L^{-1} is common. High blood glucose (>11 mmol L^{-1}) worsens outcomes in brain injury and cardiac ischaemia. Greater emphasis should probably be placed on avoiding glucose variability and easier continuous bedside blood glucose monitoring.

Fluid balance

Ensuring adequate fluid balance is a fundamental requirement in treating the critically ill patient. Normal approximate intake in a 70-kg man is 1500 ml from liquid, 750 ml in food and 250 ml from metabolism. In health, output matches input, with insensible losses accounting for approximately 500 ml (see Chapter 12). In addition to providing adequate water, electrolytes should be replaced; normal daily sodium and potassium requirements are 50–100 mmol day^{-1} and 40–80 mmol day^{-1}, respectively. A typical maintenance regimen should be based on a balanced salt solution (e.g. Hartmann's solution), as excessive administration of 0.9% saline may result in hyperchloraemic acidosis.

Fluid balance is almost invariably disturbed in the critically ill patient. Common causes include widespread capillary leak associated with sepsis and inflammatory conditions leading to peripheral and pulmonary oedema, gastrointestinal dysfunction, fluid sequestration and diarrhoea. Fluid losses occur from burns, fistulae and wounds, whereas increased insensible losses are associated with pyrexia and poor humidification of inspired ventilator gases. High urinary output states such as diabetes insipidus will also result in water loss. Therefore fluid and electrolyte replacement should be dictated by the underlying clinical condition, the overall fluid balance and the serum biochemistry.

A traditional reliance on artificial colloid solutions has decreased recently, largely because of concerns over the short- and long-term complications of starch solutions. Consequently many units use crystalloids exclusively, including for rapid resuscitation. Albumin solutions have some theoretical advantages in sepsis states, but there is no good evidence base for widespread use. Blood and blood products should be used in cases of haemorrhage and coagulopathy (see Chapter 14), guided by local policy and senior advice.

Renal dysfunction

Renal dysfunction is common in critical illness and the cause is often multifactorial. Pre-existing renal disease may be worsened by the patient's new pathological condition or the use of nephrotoxic drugs.

Acute kidney injury (AKI) is defined as an abrupt (within 48 h) reduction in kidney function. The commonly used Kidney Disease: Improving Global Outcomes (KDIGO) diagnostic criteria for AKI are based on the specific changes from baseline in patients who have achieved an optimal state of hydration (see Chapter 11, Table 11.4). This classification includes relatively small increases in serum creatinine, as these are associated with adverse outcomes. When managing a patient with AKI, focus the history and examination to distinguish potential causes (Table 48.5). These are classically distinguished as prerenal, renal and postrenal, although several factors contribute in most patients. A sudden cessation of urine output should be assumed to be caused by obstruction until proved otherwise.

In most cases of AKI in the critically ill the primary cause is prerenal, but up to 20% of cases will have other significant pathological conditions. Serial blood biochemistry results

Table 48.5 Causes[a] of renal dysfunction or acute kidney injury in critical illness

Prerenal (>70%)	Renal (>20%)	Postrenal (5%–10%)
Sepsis	Nephrotoxic drugs	Kidney outflow obstruction
Hypovolaemia	Autoimmune disease	Ureteric obstruction
Hypotension	Hepatorenal syndrome	Bladder outlet obstruction
Dehydration	Trauma (rhabdomyolysis)	Blocked urinary catheter
Major surgery	Renovascular disease	
Burns		
Abdominal compartment syndrome		

[a]Several potential causes often coexist, and some conditions contribute in different ways.

Table 48.6 Distinguishing features of prerenal and renal causes of acute kidney injury		
	Prerenal	**Renal**
Urinary sodium; mmol L^{-1}	<10	>30
Urinary osmolality	High	Low
Urine: plasma urea ratio	>10:1	<8:1
Urine microscopy	Normal	Tubular casts

Box 48.5 **Indications for renal replacement therapy (RRT)**[a]

Oliguria/anuria (urine output < 200 ml/12 h)
Hyperkalaemia (K$^+$ > 6.5 mmol L^{-1} or increasing rapidly)
Serum urea > 35 mmol L^{-1}
Serum creatinine > 400 μmol L^{-1}
Serum sodium < 110 or > 160 mmol L^{-1b}
Pulmonary oedema unresponsive to diuretics
Metabolic acidaemia (pH < 7.1)
Symptomatic uraemia (encephalopathy, pericarditis, bleeding)
Dialysable toxins (e.g. lithium, aspirin, methanol, ethylene glycol, theophylline)

[a]If one criterion is present, RRT should be considered. If two criteria are simultaneously present, RRT is strongly recommended
[b]Use with caution to avoid over-rapid correction of serum sodium
From Bellomo, R. (2013) Renal replacement therapy. In: Bersten, A. D., & Soni, N. (eds.) *Oh's intensive care unit manual*, 7th ed. Oxford, UK, Elsevier.

are essential, and urine tests can be helpful (unless the patient has received diuretics) in distinguishing prerenal from intrinsic renal failure (Table 48.6). Other investigations may be needed as determined by the clinical scenario: creatinine kinase/urinary myoglobin; vasculitic screen; and imaging, such as renal tract ultrasound.

Oliguria is a normal part of the postoperative stress response (see Chapters 11 and 13), but the lack of an appropriate biomarker makes it difficult to differentiate pathophysiological oliguria from relative hypovolemia. Therefore, in the case of oliguria (urine output < 0.5 ml kg^{-1} h^{-1} for at least 2 consecutive hours), consider a fluid challenge of 250–500 ml. As renal filtration is pressure dependent, renal perfusion pressure should be maintained. If circulating volume is adequate, consider the early use of vasopressors or inotropes to maintain MAP greater than 65 mmHg, or greater than 80% of the patient's usual MAP. If the cause of oliguria remains unclear and there is no response, look for and treat sepsis and consider stopping any nephrotoxic drugs. The use of loop diuretics if the patient remains oliguric is controversial but may aid fluid balance with benefits in other organ systems. Intrinsic AKI is a recognised component of SIRS, and so if cardiac output, MAP and renal perfusion pressure have been restored with fluids and drugs and there remains no response to diuretics, renal replacement therapy is likely to be required (see below).

Acute kidney injury has three potential outcomes: return to baseline function, the development of chronic kidney disease, or persistent renal failure. Most cases of AKI occurring in ICU resolve over time (acute tubular necrosis pattern, may take up to 6 weeks).

Renal replacement therapy

Continuous renal replacement therapy (RRT) is used in the ICU because the gradual correction of biochemical abnormalities and removal of fluid results in greater haemodynamic stability compared with intermittent haemodialysis. The indications for RRT are shown in Box 48.5. Two main processes are utilised. *Dialysis* refers to the passage of solutes across a membrane by diffusion down a concentration

gradient. The degree of diffusive transfer depends on the characteristics of the solute and the membrane, the concentration gradient between blood and dialysate, and the rat of delivery of the solute. Solutes can also be removed from blood by convection, whereby a pressure gradient is created across the membrane and solutes are swept across the membrane with the ultrafiltrate. Convective transport is determined by the flow rates (and hence the pressure gradients and membrane porosity) but is independent of the concentration gradient between blood and filtrate.

Continuous venovenous haemofiltration

Continuous venovenous haemofiltration (CVVH) is the simplest form of continuous RRT. As the patient's blood passes through a filter, plasma water, electrolytes and small molecular weight molecules pass through down a pressure gradient (Fig. 48.3A). This filtrate is discarded and replaced by a balanced electrolyte solution. Typically 200–500 ml h^{-1} of filtrate are removed and replaced. Overall negative fluid balance can be achieved by replacing less fluid than is removed. As no dialysate is used, solute movement is entirely dependent on convective transport, which is a slower removal process, so clearance of small molecules and solutes is inefficient. This can require large volumes of filtrate to be removed and replaced in order to achieve acceptable clearance of solutes.

Continuous venovenous haemodialysis

Continuous venovenous haemodialysis (CVVHD) depends on diffusive solute transfer because of the countercurrent flow of dialysate fluid through the haemofilter (Fig. 48.3B). Fluids, electrolytes and small molecules can move in both directions across the filter, depending on hydrostatic pressure, ionic charge, protein binding and concentration gradients. Overall creatinine clearance is greatly improved compared with haemofiltration alone. In CVVHD, provided the volume of dialysis fluid passing out from the system matches the volume of dialysis fluid passing in, there is no net gain or loss of fluid to the patient. By allowing more dialysate fluid to pass out of the filter than passes in, fluid can be effectively

removed from the patient, with removal rates of up to 200 ml h^{-1} possible.

Continuous venovenous haemodiafiltration

The term continuous venovenous haemodiafiltration (CVVHDF) is used for systems that intentionally combine both the processes of diffusion and convection employed by haemodialysis and haemofiltration, respectively. Dialysis

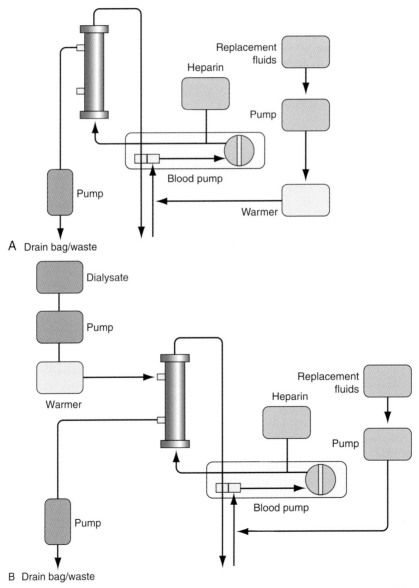

Fig. 48.3 (A) Continuous venovenous haemofiltration (CVVH) circuit. (B) Continuous venovenous haemodialysis (CVVHD) circuit.
Continued

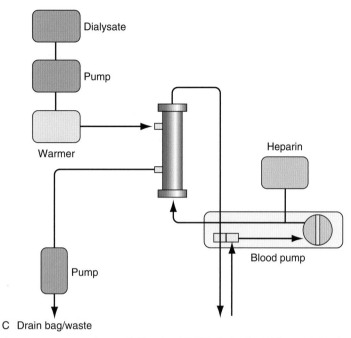

Fig. 48.3, cont'd (C) Continuous venovenous haemodiafiltration (CVVHDF) circuit. (With permission from Bellomo, R. (2013) Renal replacement therapy. In: Bersten, A. D., & Soni, N. (eds.) *Oh's intensive care unit manual,* 7th edn. Oxford, UK, Elsevier.)

fluid is passed across the filter to remove solutes by osmosis, but at the same time ultrafiltrate is removed and replaced (Fig. 48.3C).

Vascular access for RRT

Renal replacement therapies require dedicated vascular access (using a 10–14F catheter). Arteriovenous RRT is rarely used in the ICU. For venovenous access, a single large vein is cannulated percutaneously with a double-lumen catheter using the Seldinger technique. All catheters have a lumen that functions as the 'arterial' outflow limb of the circuit and a second lumen which functions as the 'venous' inflow limb of the circuit. The 'arterial' port removes blood from holes in the side of the catheter and blood is returned down the 'venous' lumen through a single hole at the catheter tip to minimise recirculation of filtered blood. As blood is passing through an extracorporeal circuit, anticoagulation is required to prevent clotting and obstruction of the filter, unless the patient has severe coagulopathy. This is infused directly into the dialysis circuit. Citrate is now the preferred anticoagulant as it reduces the risk of filter clotting, bleeding and heparin-induced thrombocytopaenia compared with heparin. Replacement of calcium and magnesium are required, and caution is need in patients with liver failure who are unable to metabolise citrate. Prostacyclin infusions are occasionally used but can cause vasodilatation and

hypotension. The complications associated with RRT are shown in Box 48.6.

Neurological system

Despite the wide range of pathological conditions that require admission to ICU for specialised neurological support, some specific treatment regimens are common to them all. The most important principle underlying neurocritical care, irrespective of the primary cause of neurological damage, is the prevention of secondary injury caused by hypoxaemia, hypotension, hypercapnia, seizures, hyperglycaemia and other metabolic disturbance.

As cerebral blood volume is influenced by carbon dioxide tensions, ventilation should be targeted to achieve a $PaCO_2$ of 4.5–5 kPa to minimise increases in ICP. Aggressive hyperventilation needs to be avoided as hypocapnia induces cerebral vasoconstriction and may promote cerebral ischaemia in the context of brain injury (see Chapter 40). The inspired oxygen concentration needs to be adjusted to sustain SaO_2 more than 94%. The use of deep sedation will usually require vasopressors to maintain blood pressure within the normal range. Ideally MAP should be maintained at more than 80 mmHg and systolic pressure more than 120 mmHg; even isolated periods of systolic pressures less than 90 mmHg have been found to be associated with worse outcome in

Box 48.6 **Complications of continuous renal replacement therapy**

- Associated with anticoagulation:
  - Bleeding (gastrointestinal tract, catheter site)
  - Heparin-induced thrombocytopenia (HIT)
  - Citrate toxicity/hypocalcaemia
- Catheter related:
  - Sepsis
  - Thrombosis
  - Arteriovenous fistulae
  - Arrhythmia
  - Pneumothorax
  - Pain
  - Disconnection
- Hypothermia
- Anaemia, thrombocytopenia
- Hypovolaemia
- Hypotension, worsening gas exchange in lungs
- Membrane reactions (bradykinin release, nausea, anaphylaxis)
- Electrolyte abnormalities (hypophosphataemia, hypokalaemia; hypocalcaemia or hypomagnesaemia with citrate)
- Metabolic: acidaemia (bicarbonate loss), alkalaemia (overbuffering)
- Air embolism
- Drug related (altered pharmacokinetics)

TBI. Intravenous administration of glucose should be avoided, as hyperglycaemia increases cerebral metabolic rate, and i.v. insulin should be infused if the blood glucose concentration exceeds 11 mmol L^{-1}.

The plasma osmolality and serum sodium concentration should be monitored carefully because hypo-osmolality of the plasma creates an osmotic gradient across the blood–brain barrier which can provoke cerebral oedema. Hyperthermia (even mild) should be avoided, as this increases cerebral metabolism and worsens outcomes. However, the benefits of induced hypothermia are unclear, as it affects other systems. For example, hypothermia worsens coagulopathy, predisposes to infection and could be detrimental in the case of cerebral haemorrhage. Instead of therapeutic hypothermia, the term *targeted temperature management* summarises the balance between avoidance of hyperthermia and maintenance of mild hypothermia/normothermia. There is good evidence to support its use after cardiac arrest to reduce the impact of hypoxic brain injury, and there are theoretical benefits in other similar situations.

Patients with severe TBI (Glasgow Coma Scale score (GCS) < 8) and/or focal signs should be referred to a regional neurosurgical centre, as they may require ICP monitoring or neurosurgical intervention. Discussion and review of CT scans should be undertaken with the neurosurgeons before transfer. Transfer should be in accordance with national guidelines and will include the following:

- Exclude and treat other life-threatening injuries elsewhere (e.g. chest and abdominal bleeding).
- Secure the airway definitively.
- Staff should be trained in airway and head injury management.
- Place a urinary catheter (especially if mannitol has been administered).
- SpO_2, end-tidal CO_2 ECG and blood pressure should be monitored continuously.
- End-tidal CO_2 should be maintained at 4–4.5 kPa. It is important to remember that end-tidal CO_2 may correlate poorly with $PaCO_2$ in early phases of resuscitation; $PaCO_2$ should be checked before departure.
- If the patient has had a seizure, load with anticonvulsants (e.g. phenytoin 15–18 mg kg^{-1} or levetiracetam 1 g).
- Brain CT imaging should be completed and hard/electronic copies available.
- Transfer should be complete within 4 h, without delays for non-urgent intervention (e.g. central venous access).

In patients with severe head injury and an abnormal admission CT scan, it may be appropriate to target CPP by direct measurement of ICP and MAP. It is recommended that the arterial catheter transducer is placed at the level of the patient's tragus when calculating CPP. Intracranial pressure should be maintained within the normal range if possible; sudden increases may occur in patients who are restless or hypertensive; adequate sedation and analgesia are important components of therapy. Deep sedation with neuromuscular blockade may be necessary to minimise cerebral metabolism, and therapy can be guided using the EEG to attain burst suppression. Cerebral perfusion pressure can be manipulated with fluid loading and the use of vasopressor agents and many protocols aim to maintain CPP greater than 65 mmHg. However, in the patient with loss of cerebral autoregulation, a high CPP may result in increased cerebral oedema. Identification of the presence of intact autoregulation may be possible using multimodality monitoring in the neuro-ICU and is the focus of research efforts. The loss of autoregulation may be suggested by correlation between MAP and ICP instead of the inverse correlation (within physiological limits).

Other useful measures to consider when managing the patient with acute neurological injury include nursing in a head-up position to improve venous drainage, increasing serum osmolality to 300–310 mOsm L^{-1} using mannitol or hypertonic saline, and the control clinical and subclinical seizures, as these have a detrimental effect on cerebral metabolism. At all times therapy should be adjusted to maximise oxygen delivery, minimise oxygen consumption, preserve cerebral blood flow and normalise ICP.

Other aspects of intensive care

Venous thromboembolism prophylaxis

The critical care population is at higher risk of thrombo-embolism (VTE) than general medical patients for a number of reasons, including disordered coagulation; maximal inflammatory response; presence of intravascular catheter devices; injuries specifically implicated in VTE, such as pelvic and long bone injuries; and long periods of immobility. Similarly, these patients are also at increased risk from anticoagulation therapy because of disease process/concurrent interventions and treatment, so pharmacological prophylaxis with low molecular weight heparins (LMWH) can potentially be problematic.

Low molecular weight heparins are associated with a lower incidence of haemorrhage and heparin-induced thrombocytopaenia than unfractionated heparin. Unless contraindicated, mechanical means of VTE prophylaxis (e.g. intermittent pneumatic compression and antiembolic stockings) should also be given to all patients. Early mobilisation and physiotherapy, where possible, and avoiding dehydration can also help reduce the risk of VTE.

ICU-acquired muscle weakness

Neuromuscular abnormalities resulting in skeletal muscle weakness are a common occurrence in the critically ill. Some degree of loss of muscle mass is likely in all cases of immobility and critical illness. However, more severe problems are common, and they can be described as two distinct conditions, namely polyneuropathy and myopathy. However, it is likely that these two entities often coexist, and although the exact incidence remains variable amongst studies, their presence is associated with multiple adverse outcomes, including higher mortality, prolonged duration of mechanical ventilation, and increased duration of stay.

The pathogenesis of such nerve and muscle damage is not well defined but probably involves inflammatory injury of nerve and/or muscle that is potentiated by functional denervation and corticosteroids. The latter is a well-identified risk factor for developing acquired muscle weakness. Other risk factors include sepsis, hyperglycaemia, neuromuscular blockade and increasing severity of illness. The clinical diagnosis of ICU-acquired neuromuscular disorders is suspected in the presence of unexplained weakness in patients recovering from critical illness. Weakness can be so severe as to be confused with coma. Other metabolic, pharmacologic, and central nervous system causes of weakness must be ruled out before establishing the diagnosis. Electrophysiological testing is useful primarily to exclude other (possibly treatable) causes of severe weakness, such as Guillain–Barré

syndrome or cervical spine problems. Physical rehabilitation may accelerate recovery, and the National Institute for Health and Care Excellence has published guidelines recognising the value of rehabilitation during and after critical care.

Healthcare-associated infection

Unfortunately, healthcare-association infection (HAI) is common amongst patients in ICU, in whom risk factors such as immunocompromise, tracheal intubation, the presence of intravascular and urinary catheters, antimicrobial therapy, stress ulcer prophylaxis and protracted durations of stay are common. Catheter-related bloodstream infections, ventilator-associated pneumonia, *C. difficile* diarrhoea, and emergence of antibiotic-resistant bacteria such as methicillin-resistant *Staphylococcus aureus* (MRSA) and vancomycin-resistant *Enterococcus* (VRE) remain important causes of mortality, morbidity and increased financial burden. Routine surveillance of HAI rates is essential to identify problematic pathogens and to develop initiatives to reduce their incidence.

Preventative measures are multifactorial and start with good standards of hospital environmental cleanliness. Protective garments should be worn for all patient contact; however, gloves are not a substitute for hand washing, and poor hand hygiene is a major factor in nosocomial infection.

Catheter-related bloodstream infection

Catheter-related bloodstream infections (CRBSIs) are common in the ICU and result from venous and arterial catheters becoming coated in plasma proteins after insertion. Bacteria are then able to migrate from the skin and catheter hubs to become embedded in this protein sheath, with both external and endoluminal colonisation occurring. There is a direct relationship between the number of organisms colonising the catheter and the risk of CRBSI. Mortality from CRBSI may be as high as 25%, and diagnosis is made from a positive blood culture with the same organism grown from the access device.

To reduce rates, the ongoing need for invasive catheters should always be considered in the first instance. Consider the site of insertion; the subclavian vein has the least risk of CRBSI compared with the internal jugular and femoral veins, respectively. Strict aseptic technique should be adhered to during insertion and during all handling of catheters. If the device is to be used for parenteral nutrition, ensure that there is a dedicated catheter or lumen for this. If there is a suspicion of CRBSI, the catheter should be removed and antibiotic therapy tailored to the culture result.

Antibiotic therapy

Appropriate antibiotic use is imperative, and local policies as well as advice from the microbiologist are important sources of information. If appropriate empirical therapy is started within 1 h of the onset of sepsis/septic shock, in-hospital mortality is reduced. De-escalation when a causative pathogen is identified reduces inappropriate use and minimises superinfection. Selective decontamination of the digestive tract (SDD) is a technique designed to eradicate aerobic, potentially pathogenic bacteria colonising the oropharynx and upper gastrointestinal tract, thus eliminating an important risk factor for nosocomial pneumonia. It has not been widely adopted in the UK because of its inconsistent effects on mortality and concerns about the potential for selecting antibiotic-resistant pathogens.

Ventilator-associated pneumonia

Ventilator-associated pneumonia (VAP) is a common nosocomial infection occurring in patients receiving mechanical ventilation for more than 48 h. There is no gold standard for diagnosis, so the exact incidence remains difficult to estimate, but mortality is in the order of 30%. Aerobic gram-negative bacilli colonise the oropharynx and upper gastrointestinal tract (augmented by the use of H_2-receptor antagonists), and these pathogens gain access to the lungs with movement aided by the positive pressure of mechanical ventilation. Clinical scores use focal infiltrates on chest radiographic image, increased FIO_2 requirements, sputum production, temperature, and inflammatory markers to suggest the presence of VAP. Quantitative culture of bronchoalveolar lavage (BAL) specimens can aid diagnosis. Treatment is the timely administration of appropriate antibiotics, and preventative measures include scrupulous hand hygiene, good oral hygiene, nursing the patient semirecumbent, ensuring adequate tracheal cuff inflation, improved tracheal cuff design, supraglottic suction, rational use of H_2-receptor antagonists, avoiding the need for tracheal reintubation where possible, and potentially SDD. Care bundles to standardise simple aspects of care have been shown capable of reducing hospital acquired infections successfully (see later).

Psychological problems

Longer-stay patients in intensive care can suffer significant psychological morbidity. A combination of the underlying pathological condition, sedative and analgesic drugs, an environment of loud noise and bright lights, and frequent nursing input can all lead to sensory overload, which may result in anxiety, depression, delirium and hallucinations during treatment. Research into the longer-term consequences of surviving critical illness has suggested that for a significant number of patients there may not only be continuing physical debilitation, but they are also at risk of subsequent depression, post-traumatic stress disorder and moderate to severe loss of cognitive function. Family dynamics may become altered, as can financial security, so it is important to identify patients at risk of physical and non-physical morbidity and work towards short- and medium-term agreed rehabilitation goals in an attempt to optimise recovery.

Delirium

Delirium is often underdiagnosed but is associated with increased duration of hospital stay and is an independent predictor of increased mortality at 6 months. It is often described as hyperactive, hypoactive or a mixture of both. A validated tool such as the Confusion Assessment Method for the Intensive Care Unit (CAM-ICU) can be used to detect delirium (Fig. 48.4). Preventative measures include avoidance of pharmacological precipitants where possible (although this may be impossible in practice) and employing non-pharmacological interventions such as clear communication, provision of clocks, calendars, diaries and the patient's own familiar objects. In addition, consistent nursing care, controlling excess noise and creating a day/night cycle are also helpful. Allowing self-care where possible and ensuring that the patient has his or her own glasses, dentures or personal items can often be as important as treating any organic cause. If preventative measures fail and no organic cause can be found, treatment with haloperidol and other drugs may be helpful.

Care bundles

There is an increasing evidence for the utility of care bundles for specific conditions. They consist of a number of evidence-based practices each of which has been found to improve outcome and are easily achievable. When performed collectively, reliably and continuously these bundles confer a greater probability of survival. The most familiar bundles are the Surviving Sepsis campaign resuscitation (6 h) and management (24 h) bundles and ventilator care bundles. The ventilator care bundle comprises the following components to reduce ALI and ARDS:

- Low tidal volumes (4–6 ml kg^{-1} ideal body weight)
- Plateau airway pressure less than 30 cmH$_2$O
- Sedation holds and use of sedation scores
- Permissive hypercapnia
- Semirecumbent positioning (head up by 45 degrees unless contraindicated) during ventilation to reduce the incidence of VAP
- Lung recruitment by PEEP to prevent alveolar collapse
- Avoidance of NMBAs
- Protocol-driven weaning

Ventilator-associated pneumonia rates have been shown to be reduced by combining sedation holds, semirecumbent nursing, stress ulcer prophylaxis, VTE prophylaxis and daily oral hygiene with chlorhexidine. Good nursing care should

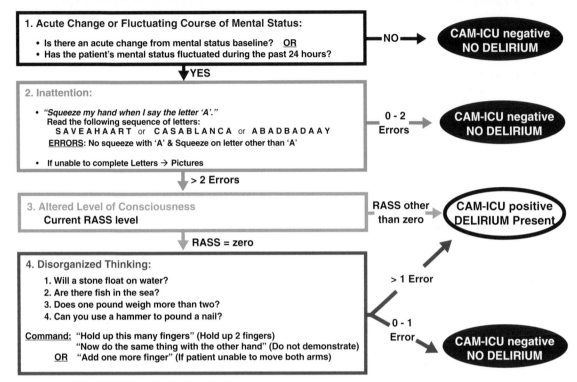

Confusion Assessment Method for the ICU (CAM-ICU) Flowsheet

1. Acute Change or Fluctuating Course of Mental Status:
- Is there an acute change from mental status baseline? **OR**
- Has the patient's mental status fluctuated during the past 24 hours?

NO → CAM-ICU negative / NO DELIRIUM

↓ **YES**

2. Inattention:
- *"Squeeze my hand when I say the letter 'A'."*
  Read the following sequence of letters:
  S A V E A H A A R T or **C A S A B L A N C A** or **A B A D B A D A A Y**
  ERRORS: No squeeze with 'A' & Squeeze on letter other than 'A'
- If unable to complete Letters → Pictures

0 - 2 Errors → CAM-ICU negative / NO DELIRIUM

↓ **> 2 Errors**

3. Altered Level of Consciousness
Current RASS level

RASS other than zero → CAM-ICU positive / DELIRIUM Present

↓ **RASS = zero**

4. Disorganized Thinking:
1. Will a stone float on water?
2. Are there fish in the sea?
3. Does one pound weigh more than two?
4. Can you use a hammer to pound a nail?

Command: "Hold up this many fingers" (Hold up 2 fingers)
"Now do the same thing with the other hand" (Do not demonstrate)
OR "Add one more finger" (If patient unable to move both arms)

> 1 Error → CAM-ICU positive / DELIRIUM Present

0 - 1 Error → CAM-ICU negative / NO DELIRIUM

Fig. 48.4 Flowchart for the Confusion Assessment Method for the Intensive Care Unit (CAM-ICU). (From http://www.icudelirium .org/docs/CAM_ICU_flowsheet.pdf.)

not be underestimated and is an important contributor to good overall outcome.

Outcome after intensive care

Attempts to predict outcome after discharge from critical care has led to the development of a number of scoring systems, which generally involve collection of large quantities of data, stratifying these data to produce a risk score in order to predict survival for a patient population. However, there are flaws with this approach, including problems of diagnostic categorisation; the initial hospital diagnosis may bear little relation to the subsequent, often multiple pathological conditions in the individual patient. Although scoring systems are helpful in predicting population outcomes, their potential for application to individual cases is limited. Patients may survive discharge from the ICU, but mortality

remains high on the wards and at home, so that 6-month or 1-year outcomes of mortality and morbidity may prove better endpoints than the traditional 28-day mortality.

Assessments of functional disability, quality of life and return to work among patients who have survived an admission to intensive care are more difficult to quantify than death, but the small numbers of studies which have been undertaken suggest that mortality and morbidtiy are significantly higher than would be expected in matched individuals for several years. In addition, a significant proportion of patients report impaired quality of life and many remain unable to work for prolonged periods after discharge. However, the majority of patients who survive can return to a reasonable quality of life.

Several scoring systems are used:
- *APACHE II*. The Acute Physiology and Chronic Health Evaluation score takes into account pre-existing comorbidities as well as acute physiological disturbance and correlates well with the risk of death in an intensive care

population, but not on an individual basis. However, it remains one of the more widely used tools. A score is calculated on the worst physiological derangement occurring within the first 24 h after admission, age and chronic health status.

- *APACHE III.* This has superseded the APACHE II score, with variations in the physiological measures.
- *Simplified Acute Physiology Score (SAPS).* This scoring system uses 12 physiological variables assigned a score according to the degree of derangement.
- *Therapeutic Intervention Score System (TISS).* A score is given for each procedure performed on the ICU, so that sicker patients require more procedures. However, procedures undertaken are both clinician and unit specific and so TISS is less useful for comparing outcomes between different units.
- *Sequential Organ Failure Assessment (SOFA).* This tracks changes in the patient's condition regarding their respiratory, cardiovascular, hepatic, neurological, renal and coagulation status.

The importance of national collaborative audit and research in improving the practice of critical care is well recognised, and the Intensive Care National Audit and Research Centre for England and Wales (ICNARC) collects demographic data, diagnostic criteria, physiological scoring and outcome for the majority of patients admitted to ICU.

Death in intensive care

Death is common, and good palliative care for patients and their families is a fundamental component of ICU care. Unfortunately, despite maximal support and care, some patients succumb to the overwhelming nature of the underlying disease process. Few deaths are directly attributable to an unexpected primary cardiorespiratory arrest once the patient is fully supported in ICU; hence 'do not attempt cardiorespiratory resuscitation' (DNACPR) orders are less relevant to critical care than care on the general ward.

Futility and withdrawal

Approximately 70% of deaths in the ICU occur after withdrawal of support, where continued treatment would not achieve patient-centred goals and carries significant burdens; however, the cause of death remains the underlying pathological process. This typically follows a period of continued deterioration or a failure to improve, despite appropriate supportive therapy. There is no legal distinction between the withdrawal of life-sustaining treatment or limiting or withholding treatment. It is important to note that withdrawal of *treatment* does not equate with

withdrawal of *care* given by nurses and doctors including symptom relief.

The process of withdrawal entails a reduction/removal of interventions, with the understanding that the patient is very likely to deteriorate and die without such support. Consideration should always be given as to whether patients would have wished to donate their organs after their death before a decision to withdraw life-sustaining therapies; teams should be prepared to discuss the patient's wishes with the support of a specialist nurse for organ donation.

Once the decision is made and agreement with the family and admitting team obtained, all treatments and therapies should be reviewed and only those contributing to symptom control continued. These may include treatments which could be considered to prolong the dying process and hence potential suffering. Additional analgesia and anxiolysis (sedatives) are often required to prevent or alleviate pain and distress. Feeding and hydration may be continued if these will not prolong or worsen the dying process. Death may occur quickly or be prolonged over hours or days depending on the clinical situation.

Depending on the speed of decline, patients may die in ICU or be discharged to ward-based care. Occasionally patients may improve despite all odds, and clinicians should be prepared to revisit such clinical decisions over time. Such an outcome does not mean that the harm/benefit analysis leading to the decision to limit or withdraw advanced organ support was incorrect.

Neurological death

Suspicion of brainstem death is raised by the loss of all cranial reflexes and unconsciousness in the setting of severe brain injury and the absence of sedative agents. Destruction of the brainstem may occur from compression from above or from direct injury. As the brainstem is compressed, systemic features may include hypertension and bradycardia (Cushing's reflex), followed by hypotension and vasodilatation. Hypothalamic and pituitary function is lost (diabetes insipidus) and reduced thyroid hormone synthesis occurs. Hypothermia is common because of a loss of thermoregulation.

Professional guidance should be rigorously followed in the diagnosis of death by neurological criteria. Preconditions for brainstem death testing include:

- the presence of identifiable pathological condition causing irreversible damage; and
- exclusion of potential confounders for reduced conscious level such as hypothermia, depressant drugs and potentially reversible circulatory, metabolic, and endocrine disturbances.

The tests are a series of clinical examinations undertaken by two medical practitioners, one of whom is a consultant and both of whom have been registered with the General Medical Council for more than 5 years. Two sets of tests are performed, and time of death is recorded when the first test indicates brainstem death.

- Pupils must be fixed and unresponsive to light (cranial nerves II, III).
- Corneal reflex is absent (cranial nerves V, VII).
- Vestibulo-ocular reflexes are absent; that is, no eye movement occur after injection of ice-cold saline into the auditory meatus (cranial nerves, III, IV, VI, VIII).
- No facial movement occurs in response to supraorbital pressure (cranial nerves V, VII).
- No gag reflex is present to posterior pharyngeal wall stimulation (cranial nerve IX).
- No cough or other reflex is present in response to carinal stimulation with a suction catheter passed down the tracheal tube (cranial nerve X).
- No respiratory movements occur on disconnection from the ventilator; hypoxia is prevented by preoxygenation and oxygen insufflation via a tracheal catheter. $PaCO_2$ should increase to more than 6.65 kPa with pH reducing to less than 7.25.
- Spinal reflexes may be present or exaggerated and do not preclude the diagnosis of brainstem death.

Organ donation

All patients in whom death might reasonably be predicted after withdrawal of life-sustaining therapy, including those in whom death has already been diagnosed by neurological criteria, should be considered for organ donation. Such consideration should include early discussion with a specialist nurse for organ donation before an approach to the patient's family, which should only be done by those trained to do so. Solid organ donation can occur after declaration of death by neurological (donation after brain death, DBD) or circulatory (donation after circulatory death, DCD) criteria.

In DCD a complex process of matching organs to suitable recipient patients and organ is undertaken before withdrawal of life-sustaining therapy, followed by confirmation of death after a period of 5 min has elapsed since the cessation of cardiac output to that ensure autoresuscitation cannot occur. The patient is then transferred to the operating theatre, where organ retrieval takes place.

In DBD maximum viability of organs can be ensured by the use of a donor management protocol after the determination of death. Such protocols include maintenance of adequate circulating volume, tissue oxygenation and MAP to prevent further end-organ damage and impairment. The specific loss of anterior pituitary hormone function in the context of neurological death requires supplementation with vasopressin and corticosteroids. Although there is also a loss of thyroid function, specific replacement of free thyroxine has not shown an improvement in organ outcomes. Organs can be retrieved when the surgical teams are in place before stopping artificial ventilation.

Discharge from intensive care

For those patients who survive, discharge from ICU is appropriate when their condition has improved so that they no longer warrant intensive care support. Careful discussion with the relatives and admitting teams should be undertaken with clear documentation of decisions made in relation to re-escalation of treatment, readmission to ICU, whether or not to attempt resuscitation and other ongoing management.

Those patients whose levels of care are to be reduced need to be sufficiently fit for discharge so that their underlying disease process is stable and/or improving. Consideration needs to be made regarding where such patients are to be discharged to. Often discharge is to a high-dependency unit or, if the patient is fit enough, back to a general ward, with outreach review. If the patient has been transferred from another hospital, ideally he or she should be returned to the referring hospital as soon as treatment can be safely undertaken there. Discharges should be made during daytime hours, as discharges made outside these times are more likely to experience deterioration and readmission.

Follow-up clinics

Follow-up clinics are an important aspect of continued treatment of a patient's physical and emotional well-being, as well as a means of service evaluation and an opportunity for patients to reflect and give feedback on their experience. After periods of critical illness, patients typically experience impaired physical and mental functioning as a result of the underlying disease processes or complications occurring on the ICU. In the UK, follow-up clinics are increasingly provided in an attempt to address some of these issues.

References/Further reading

Bersten, A.D., Soni, N. (Eds.), 2013. Oh's intensive care unit manual, seventh ed. Elsevier.

Confusion Assessment Method for the ICU (CAM-ICU). Available from: http://www.icudelirium.org/delirium/monitoring.html.

Guidelines for the transport of the critically ill adult patient (3rd edition 2011). Intensive Care Society 2011. Available from: http://www.ics.ac.uk/ICS/guidelines-and-standards.aspx.

Guidance for the provision of Intensive Care Services. Faculty of Intensive Care Medicine 2015. Available from: https://www.ficm.ac.uk/standards-and-guidelines/gpics.

A code of practice for the diagnosis and confirmation of death. Academy of Medical Royal Colleges 2008. Available from: http://www.aomrc.org.uk/publications/reports-guidance/ukdec-reports-and-guidance/code-practice-diagnosis-confirmation-death/.

Index

Page numbers followed by 'f' indicate figures, 't' indicate tables, 'b' indicate boxes, and 'e' indicate online content.

Cannabinoids
for non-cancer pain management, 522
for PONV treatment, 126t–127t, 129
Cannot intubate, cannot oxygenate (CICO), 890f
Cannulas
arterial, 332b
narrow-bore, 493–494, 493f
with high pressure source ventilation, 492–493
wide-bore, 493–494
Cannulation, 794
Capacitance, 284
Capacity, consent, 434
Capsaicin, for non-cancer pain management, 522
Carbamino carriage, CO_2 in blood, 193
Carbetocin, pregnancy and, 808
Carbohydrate metabolism, 236
anaerobic glycolysis, 235
cellular respiration pathway, 234–235
gluconeogenesis, 236
glucose, 235f
glycolytic pathway, 235f
Krebs citric acid cycle, 235f
pentose phosphate pathway, 236
Carbohydrate mobilisation, stress response, 241
Carbon dioxide, 175–176, 176f
cerebral blood flow and, 759–760
cylinders, 293
colour of, 293t
sizes of, 293t
end-tidal
fall in, 576f–577f
rise in, 577f–579f
in gas and vapour analysis, 344–346
inspired, rise in, 577f–579f
transport, 190–193, 191f
CO_2 carried in blood, 193, 194f
diffusion, 190
O_2 carried in blood, 190–192
oxygen therapy, 192–193
Carbon dioxide absorbers, 56
equipment checks, 444
Carbon dioxide electrode, in blood gas analysis, 347
Carbonic anhydrase, 7t–9t
inhibitors, 208
ophthalmic anaesthesia, 725t–726t
Carboprost, pregnancy and, 809
Carcinoid tumour, 749–750
5-HT antagonists, 750
Cardiac arrest
diagnosis, 603
in-hospital. see In-hospital cardiac arrest
local anaesthesia, 608
periarrest arrhythmias, 609–612, 610f–611f
potentially reversible causes, 607
prone position, 608
see also Cardiopulmonary resuscitation
Cardiac catheterisation, 864–865
for cardiopulmonary bypass, 788–789, 789t
Cardiac cycle, 155–157, 156f
Cardiac disease, obstetric anaesthesia assessment and, 822
Cardiac events, preoperative prediction, 394–395, 395t–396t
Cardiac failure, treatment of, 410
Cardiac impulse, 151–152
Cardiac muscle contraction, 153–155, 154f–155f
Cardiac myocyte action potential, 152–153, 152f
Cardiac output (CO), 157–158, 335–338
cardiac surgery monitoring and, 790–792
chemical indicator dilution in, 336
Doppler ultrasonography in, 337, 338f
early recovery period, 626
Fick principle in, 335
high-risk patient perioperative management, 641
indicator dilution in, 335–336, 336f
in inhaled anaesthetic agents, 51
obesity, and 660
pregnancy and, 800
pulse contour analysis in, 337
thermal indicator dilution in, 336–337
thoracic electrical bioimpedance in, 338
transoesophageal echocardiography in, 338
Cardiac 'pump failure', 842–844
Cardiac rhythm, 798
Cardiac surgery
anaesthesia for, 785–799
induction of, 794
technique in, 793–797
analgesia in, 799
bleeding in, 798–799
investigations for, 790
monitoring for, 790–792
number of older patients undergoing, 785
pathophysiology of, 792–793, 793f
postoperative care for, 798–799
premedication for, 793–794
preoperative assessment for, 788–790
cardiac catheterisation, 788–789, 789t
CT/MRI in, 789
echocardiography, 789
exercise electrocardiography, 788
preoperative drug therapy in, 789–790
radionuclide imaging for, 789
risk assessment in, 790, 791t
Cardiac tamponade, 607
Cardioactive drugs, intravenous anaesthetic agent in, 70t
Cardiopulmonary bypass (CBP), 787–788, 787f, 795–796
acid-base balance in, 795–796
anaesthesia before, 794–795
anticoagulation in, 787
bleeding in, 797
cell salvage in, 795
coagulation control in, 795
connecting tubes in, 788
filters in, 788
fluid prime in, 788
haemodynamics after, 797–798
low cardiac output state, 796–797
manometer in, 788
myocardial preservation in, 795
organ transplantation, 875–876
oxygen delivery in, 795
oxygenator in, 788
perfusion on, 795
pumps in, 788
serum potassium concentration in, 796
suction in, 788
venous reservoir for, 788
weaning from, 796–797
Cardiopulmonary exercise testing (CPET), 389–390, 390f
high-risk patient identification, 639, 640f
Cardiopulmonary resuscitation (CPR), 602–603
during, 606–607, 606t
airway management, 608
circulation, 608–609
do-not-attempt-resuscitation decisions, 615
extracorporeal, 609
high-quality, 603
in hospital, 603, 604f
mechanical, 609
operating room, 607–608
postresuscitation care, 612–614
airway, 612
breathing, 612
circulation, 612
disability, 612–613
organ donation, 614
prognostication, 613–614, 614f
ventilation, 608
Cardiorespiratory investigations, preoperative assessment of, 386–388
Cardiovascular collapse, 576f–577f

Index

Index

Haemorrhage *(Continued)*
  antepartum, 823
  aortic clamping, 741
  in cardiac surgery, 798–799
  in cardiopulmonary bypass, 797
  massive, 842, 843*f*
  in obstetric anaesthesia, 822–824
  postpartum, 823
Haemostasis, 251–258, 387*t*–388*t*
Haemostatic resuscitation, major
    trauma anaesthesia and, 842
HAFOE devices. *see* High air flow
    oxygen enrichment (HAFOE)
    devices
Hagen-Poiseuille formula, 274, 276
HAI. *see* Healthcare-associated infection
Hair hygrometer, 280
Haldane effect, 64
Half-life, 16
Haloperidol, 89
Halothane, 49, 50*t*, 56–57, 856
  in cardiovascular system, 57
  in central nervous system, 57
  in gastrointestinal system, 57
  hepatic dysfunction associated with, 57
  hepatitis, 57
  hepatotoxicity and, incidence, 57–61,
      58*f*–60*f*
  pharmacology of, 57
  physical properties of, 56
  in respiratory system, 56–57
  structural formulae of, 54*f*
  systemic effects of, 56–57
  uses of, 56
  in vaporiser, 298
Handover, early recovery period,
    618–619, 619*b*
Handwashing, 371
Harmonic mean (HM), 26
Head and neck
  cancer surgery, anaesthesia for,
      719–720
  plastic surgery, 753–754
Headache, postoperative care, 634
Head-down position, 689
Head-injured patients, intensive care
    management of, 770–771
Healthcare-associated infection (HAI),
    901
  see also specific infections
Heart block, cardiopulmonary bypass
    and, 798
Heart failure, preoperative therapy, 404
Heart rate, 155
  control of, 153, 153*f*
  neonates, 669, 669*t*
Heat, 277–278
Heat and moisture exchanging (HME),
    280
Heat balance, 244–246

Heat loss
  greater than heat production
      (phase 2), 246–247
  gynaecological/genitourinary surgery,
      695
  neonates, 670
  neurosurgical anaesthesia, 762
  thermoregulation, 244
Heidbrink valve, 271
Helium, 65
  cylinders, 293
    colour of, 293*t*
    sizes of, 293*t*
Henderson-Hasselbalch equation, 4
  buffer systems, 228–229
Henry's law, 280
Heparin-induced thrombocytopaenia
    (HIT), 256
Hepatic disease
  intravenous anaesthetic agent in, 70*t*
  opioid pharmacokinetics, 111
Hepatic dysfunction, day surgery and,
    684
Hepatic failure, 416
Hepatic function
  in propofol, 72
  thiopental in, 77
Hepatorenal syndrome, 416
Hepatotoxicity, of halothane, 57–61,
    58*f*–60*f*
Herbal remedies, anaesthesia
    interactions, 384
Hernia
  diaphragmatic, 680–681
  surgery, 698
High air flow oxygen enrichment
    (HAFOE) devices, 629–630, 630*f*
High altitude, respiratory physiology at,
    197–199, 198*t*
High spinal block, 594*f*–595*f*
High-density lipoproteins (HDLs), 237
High-dependency units (HDUs)
  definition of, 879
  high-risk patient identification, 641
  see also Intensive care unit
High-frequency jet ventilation (HFJV),
    315
High-frequency oscillation ventilation,
    892
High-frequency ventilation, 315–316,
    316*t*
High-quality cardiopulmonary
    resuscitation, 603
High-risk patients
  identification, 638–639
    for postoperative care, 640–641
  inotropic support, 644–645
  perioperative management, 641–643
    anaesthetic choice, 641
    fluid restriction regimens, 643

fluid therapy, 641–643
  oxygen delivery, 641
  stroke volume, 641–642, 642*f*–643*f*
postoperative management, 643–645
prediction scoring systems, 639
preoperative interventions, 639–640
recovery, 645
risk reduction, 639–640
surgical alternatives, 639
High-risk surgery, 638–645
  definition of, 638
Hip fracture, 706–707, 706*t*
Hip resurfacing arthroplasty, 705–706
Histamine, intravenous induction
    complications, 448
Histamine H_1 receptor antagonists, for
    PONV treatment, 126*t*–127*t*,
    127–128
History-taking
  ICU admission, 882
  of obstructed airway management,
      500
HM. *see* Harmonic mean
Hoarseness, 635
HOCM. *see* Hypertrophic
    cardiomyopathy
Honesty, 362
Hormone production, placenta and, 806
Hosmer-Lemeshow test, 36–37
Hot-wire flowmeters, in measuring gas
    flow, 342–343
Hüfner's constant, 163
Human albumin solution (HAS), 260*t*
Human chorionic gonadotrophin
    (hCG), 806
Human error, complications of
    anaesthesia, 558
Human factors, in difficult airway
    management, 495
Human fallibility, quality and safety, 367
Human immunodeficiency virus (HIV),
    431
Human placental lactogen (hPL), 806
Humidification, 279–280
  of respiratory tract, 280
  in ventilators, 314, 315*f*
Humidity, 279–280
Humility, 362
Hyaluronidase, 732–733
Hydralazine, 171
Hydrocortisone, 7*t*–9*t*
Hydromorphone, 113
  metabolism and excretion of, 110*t*–111*t*
  structure, 108*f*
Hydrothorax, 626
Hydroxychloroquine, anaesthesia
    interactions, 382*t*–384*t*
Hyoscine, for PONV treatment,
    126*t*–127*t*, 128
Hyperacute stroke therapy, 864

Index

Ketamine (*Continued*)
  emergency anaesthesia and, 835–836
  in eye, 75
  in gastrointestinal system, 75
  high-risk patient in, 75
  indications for, 71*t*, 75
  major trauma anaesthesia and, 844–845
  mechanism of action of, 68
  neonates, 672, 678
  for non-cancer pain management, 522
  paediatric anaesthesia and, 75
  pharmacokinetics of, 75
  pharmacology of, 74–75
  physical characteristics and presentation of, 74
  precautions for, 75
  properties of, 73*t*
  in respiratory system, 74–75
  sedation and, 75
  in skeletal muscle, 75
  in uterus and placenta, 75
Ketamine intravenous anaesthesia, 853
  dose for, 853
Ketoacidosis, diabetic, 423
Ketones, 238, 238*f*
Ketorolac trometamol, pharmacokinetics, 118
Kidney
  anatomy of, 200, 201*f*
  function of, 200–215
    assessment of, 210–212, 211*t*
    measurement of, 211*t*
  microcirculation of, 202*f*
  pharmacology of drugs acting on, 207–210
    distal convoluted tubule, 209–210
    diuretics, 207–208
    loop of Henle, 208–209
    proximal convoluted tubule, 208
    whole nephron, 208
  roles of, 200
Kidney Disease: Improving Global Outcomes (KDIGO) diagnostic criteria, for acute kidney injury, 212, 213*t*
Krebs citric acid cycle, 235*f*
Kruskal-Wallis test, 33
Kyphoplasty, 865

L

Labetalol, 169
Laboratory tests, blood coagulation, 252
Labour, 809–810
  analgesia during, 812–815
    inhalational, 813
    non-pharmacological, 812–813
    parenteral (systemic), 813
    regional, 813
  failed neuroaxial anaesthesia in, 818
  feeding and antacid prophylaxis in, 811
  first stage of, 810
  foetal monitoring and, 810
  forceps and ventouse delivery, 818
  general anaesthesia for, 820–822
  pain and pain relief in, 811–816, 812*f*
    effect of, on mother and foetus, 811–812
  pain pathways in, 805–806, 806*f*
  postdelivery analgesia for, 818–819
  regional anaesthesia for, 816–820
    complications of, 819–820
  repair of trauma to birth canal, 818
  retained placenta in, 818
  second stage of, 810
  third stage of, 810
Labyrinthine disturbances, as postoperative epidural block complications, 546
Lack system, 303, 303*f*
Lactate dehydrogenase, 235
Lactation, drugs in obstetric anaesthesia, 808
Lactic acidosis, 230
Lamina cribrosa, 724*f*
Laminar flow, of fluids, 273–274, 274*f*
Laparoscopic surgery, 691–692
Laparotomy, emergency, in the older patient, 837–838
Laryngeal granulomata, 635
Laryngeal mask airway (LMA), 458, 458*t*
  neonates, 674
Laryngeal oedema, 623
Laryngeal spasm (laryngospasm), 584*f*–585*f*
  as complications of tracheal extubation, 482
  hypoventilation, 623
  inhalational anaesthesia complications, 447–448
  in thiopental, 78
Laryngectomy, 719
Laryngoscopes/laryngoscopy, 459–464, 460*f*
  bronchoscope, 463–464
  difficult, 475–476, 476*f*
    risk of, specific tests to predict, 477–479
  flexible intubating, 463–464
  Macintosh, 460, 460*f*
  neonates, 673–674, 673*t*
  obesity, 658
  specialised blades, 461
  upper airway obstruction, 501
  videolaryngoscopes, 461–463, 462*f*–463*f*
Lasers, 288*f*
Lasting Power of Attorney (LPA), 437
Latent heat of vaporisation, 278
Lateral position, 452*f*
  spinal blockade in, 538–541, 539*f*–540*f*
Lateral positioning, 690–691
Lateral rectus muscle, 728*f*
Latex, anaphylactic reaction of, 569
Laudanosine, 139
Leakage, in flowmeter, 294
Lean production system, 370
Least squares correlation, 33
Leflunomide, anaesthesia interactions, 382*t*–384*t*
Left anterior descending artery, 786*f*
Left ventricle, ejection in, weaning from cardiopulmonary bypass and, 796
Left ventricular failure, 408
Legs. *see* Lower limbs
Length, 266, 267*t*
Lens, 729*f*
Leukocytes, 250
Levator, 728*f*
Levator palpebrae superioris muscle, 729*f*
Levobupivacaine, 96
  doses of, 95*t*
  for epidural block, 545
    in Caesarean section, 817
  features of, 91*t*
  pharmacology of, 97
  for spinal anaesthesia, 541
Levosimendan, 167
Liberty
  restraint and deprivation of, 438
  safeguards and intensive care, 438
Licox PMO, in brain oxygenation, 353
Lidocaine
  doses of, 95*t*
  for epidural block, 545
    in Caesarean section, 817
  features of, 91*t*
  lactation and, 808
  for pain, 512–513
  pharmacology of, 96
  for spinal anaesthesia, 686
Ligands, 11, 12*f*
Light guide, of lasers, 288
Lignocaine, 7*t*–9*t*
Limbs
  ICU admission, 883
  plastic surgery for, 754
Limits of agreement, 33–34
Linear regression, 34*f*
Linearity, in clinical measurement, 324
Lines, ICU admission, 883
Lingual drug administration, 19
Lipid metabolism, 237–239
Lipid solubility
  in local anaesthetics, 94
  materno-foetal concentration gradient, 807

Index

Index